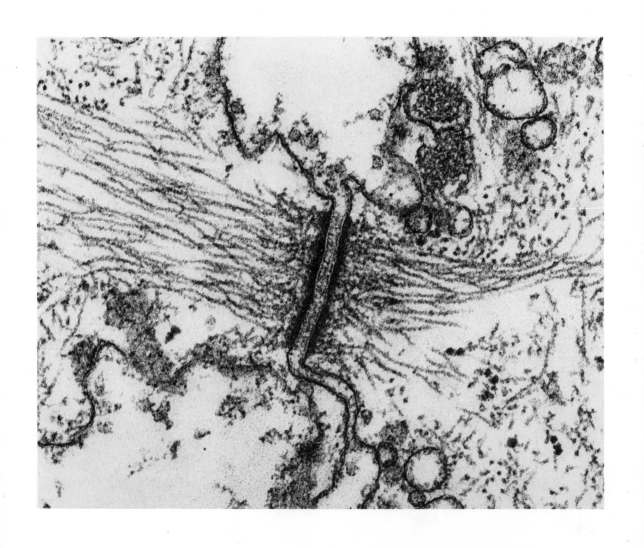

# PERIODONTICS

in the tradition of Gottlieb and Orban

# PERIODONTICS

## in the tradition of Gottlieb and Orban

Edited by

## DANIEL A. GRANT, D.D.S.

Clinical Professor, Surgical Sciences (Periodontics), University of
Southern California School of Dentistry
Los Angeles, California;
Clinical Professor, Periodontology
Loyola University School of Dentistry
Chicago, Illinois;
Private Practice
San Diego, California

## IRVING B. STERN, D.D.S.

Affiliate Professor of Oral Biology,
University of Washington School of Dentistry
Seattle, Washington;
Formerly, Professor and Chairman, Department of Periodontology
Tufts University School of Dental Medicine
Boston, Massachusetts;
and Professor of Periodontics,
University of Washington School of Dentistry
Seattle, Washington;
Private Practice
Seattle, Washington

## MAX A. LISTGARTEN, D.D.S.

Professor and Chairman
Department of Periodontology
University of Pennsylvania
School of Dental Medicine
Philadelphia, Pennsylvania;
Private Practice
Philadelphia, Pennsylvania

SIXTH EDITION

With 1617 illustrations and 8 full-color plates

## The C. V. Mosby Company

ST. LOUIS • WASHINGTON, D.C. • TORONTO    1988

**MOSBY**

A TRADITION OF PUBLISHING EXCELLENCE

Editor: Donna Saya Sokolowski
Assistant editor: Melba Steube
Production editor: Helen C. Hudlin
Designer: Rey Umali

Sixth edition

Copyright © 1988 by The C. V. Mosby Company

Previous editions copyrighted 1958, 1963, 1968, 1972, 1979

Printed in the United States of America

The C. V. Mosby Company
11830 Westline Industrial Drive, St. Louis, Missouri 63146

Library of Congress Cataloging-in-Publication Data
Periodontics in the tradition of Gottlieb and Orban.

　　　Rev. ed. of: Periodontics in the tradition of Orban and Gottlieb / Daniel A. Grant, Irving B. Stern, Frank G. Everett. 5th ed. 1979.
　　　Includes bibliographies and index.
　　　1. Periodontics.　I. Grant, Daniel A.,
II. Stern, Irving B.　III. Listgarten, Max A.　IV. Orban,
Balint J. (Balint Joseph), 1899-1960.　V. Gottlieb,
Bernhard, 1885-　　.　[DNLM: 1.　Periodontal Diseases.
WU 240 D44756]
RK361.P465　1987　　　617.6′32　　　87-5815
ISBN 0-8016-2017-1

GW/MV/MV　9　8　7　6　5　　　　　　　02/D/295

*To our families*
*whose assistance and understanding*
*have made this work possible*

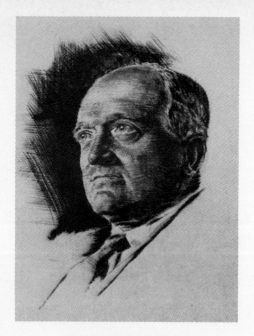

**BERNHARD GOTTLIEB**
1885-1951

Father of the biologic concept
of periodontics

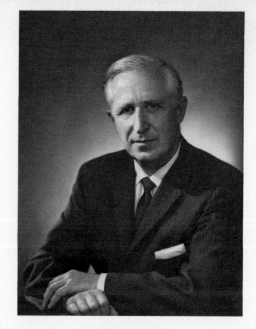

**BALINT ORBAN**
1899-1960

A clinician of consummate skill;
a researcher of an incomparable power
of observation and an unprejudiced
intellect in interpretation; a teacher of
inspiring genius and unstinting generosity;
a human being of empathy and humility

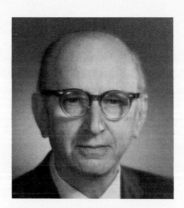

**FRANK G. EVERETT**
1907-1976

Clinician, researcher, educator;
a man of intellect,
an indefatigable worker,
a trusted colleague

# PREFACE

When this book was conceived in the mid 1950s, the goals of simplicity in organization and writing and the inclusion of pertinent data were established. These goals remain. With time, additional goals were added.

*Periodontics* is a learning textbook. It is written for the undergraduate dental student, the general practitioner, and the dental hygienist. Its content and style direct it to the graduate student and the practicing specialist.

Credibility and readability are the design of this book. Clarity and simplicity in language has been our objective, and the organization of chapters is intended to provide cohesiveness of material. The marginal notes serve as a programmed guide for the reader.

The goal of *Periodontics* is to supply the reader with the knowledge necessary to treat periodontal diseases as an integral part of the practice of dentistry.

The effective treatment of periodontal ailments requires that the dentist be well grounded in basic biologic principles and that the prevention and treatment of periodontal diseases be practiced as a part of all dentistry. The dental treatment of the general patient has periodontal considerations, even when extractions and prosthetics are involved. Periodontal treatment can succeed only when needed associated restorative treatment is performed. The converse is also true: successful restorative treatment requires associated periodontal treatment. Dentitions can be preserved and the well-being of the patient promoted only when complete treatment is given. The ability to integrate all phases of dental treatment must be mastered by the general dentist, even in cases in which the cooperation of the specialist is enlisted.

Periodontics, interrelated as it is with all parts of dental practice and with obvious relationships to basic science, is the part of dentistry that can best be used to promote a unified approach to dental treatment. This concept embraces an integration of periodontics, general practice, and biologic principles in a clinical approach called *complete therapy*.

Daniel A. Grant
Irving B. Stern
Max A. Listgarten

# ACKNOWLEDGMENTS

When this book was conceived about 35 years ago, we realized that with the continuing explosion of knowledge, a persisting challenge would be present: how to weigh what is currently popular with its validity. Demonstrably, what is modish is not necessarily enduring. The recent literature is filled with therapies once popular and since discarded or shelved as unimportant, with biologic interpretations once accepted and now rejected, and with experiments once cited and since refuted. Because prominent objectives of *Periodontics* were readability, clarity, and credibility, their fulfillment has exacted a demanding discipline. The vast scope of periodontics has required help of other workers in periodontology. This text is the result of our efforts with the assistance of other workers in the areas indicated, whose contributions are gratefully acknowledged.

The orientation of this text to the dental student was pursued throughout the writing. Undergraduate students and teachers were asked to review material in an effort to make the text simple and understandable. Despite inevitable change, evidence of their efforts may be found in this sixth edition. Our gratitude is hereby expressed to Michael Alfano, D.D.S., Ph.D.; Charles R. Amen, D.D.S.; Paul Baer, D.D.S.; George Bernard, D.D.S., Ph.D.; Richard E. Bradley, D.D.S., M.S.; Richard Chace, D.D.S.; C. Kenneth Collings, D.D.S., M.A.; Mario Droppelmann, D.D.S.; Cyril Enwonwu, Sc.D., M.D.S., B.D.S.; R.D. Emslie, B.D.S., M.S., F.D.S.; Harold E. Grupe, Sr., D.D.S.; Stanley P. Hazen, D.D.S., M.S.; William Hiatt, D.D.S.; Alvin C. Hileman, D.M.D., M.S.; Leonard Hirschfeld, D.D.S.; Bennett Klavan, D.D.S.; Herbert B. Laffitte, D.D.S.; Jan Lindhe, L.D.S., Odont.D.; Bruce Mackler, Ph.D.; Irwin Mandel, D.D.S.; Nicholas R. Marfino, D.D.S., M.S.; Melvin Morris, D.D.S.; Claude L. Nabers, D.D.S., M.S.D.; John Nabers, D.D.S.; Michael G. Newman, D.D.S.; Timothy O'Leary, D.D.S.; Richard C. Oliver, D.D.S., M.S.D.; R.J. Rizzo, D.D.S.; Robert G. Schallhorn, D.D.S., M.S.D.; Hubert E. Schroeder, D.M.D.; Harry Sicher, M.D.; Richard Stallard, D.D.S., Ph.D.; Roger V. Stambaugh, D.D.S., M.S.; Stanley R. Suit, D.D.S., M.S.; Else Theilade, D.D.S.; Patrick Toto, D.D.S., M.S.; D.E. Van Scotter, D.D.S.; Frank M. Wentz, D.D.S., Ph.D., M.S.; and Helmut A. Zander, D.D.S., M.S.

# CONTRIBUTORS

Manuscripts for chapters or parts of chapters were submitted by the distinguished contributors listed below:

Microbiology (plaque)

Sigmund Socransky, D.D.S.
A.D. Haffajee, D.D.S.
Forsyth Dental Center
Boston, Massachusetts

The epidemiology, etiology, and public health aspects of periodontal disease

Aubrey Sheiham, B.D.S.
University College
The Dental School
London, England

Vesicular and bullous diseases (desquamative gingivitis)

Jose Luis Castellanos, D.D.S.
Universidad de Bajio
Guanajuato, Mexico

Scaling and root planing

Susan B. Wilson, R.D.H., D.Ed.
University of Southern California
School of Dentistry
Los Angeles, California

Bone grafts and transplants

James Mellonig, D.D.S.
Naval Graduate School of Dentistry
Bethesda, Maryland

Interrelated endodontics-periodontics
The periodontally diseased furcation

Marlin Gher, D.D.S.
United States Navy
San Diego, California

Implants

Daniel van Steenberghe, M.D., L.D.S., Ph.D.
Catholic University of Leuven
Leuven, Belgium

Charles Berman, D.D.S.
Hackensack, New Jersey

Other revised sections of chapters from the 5th edition:

Calculus

Jorgen Theilade, D.D.S., B.Sc.D., M.S.
Forsyth Dental Center
Boston, Massachusetts

Immunology and host response

Jon Suzuki, D.D.S., Ph.D.
University of Maryland
College of Dentistry
Baltimore, Maryland

Howard R. Creamer, Ph.D.
The Oregon Health Sciences University
School of Dentistry
Portland, Oregon

Steven C. Schonfeld, D.D.S., Ph.D.
University of Southern California
School of Dentistry
Los Angeles, California

Edward H. Montgomery, Ph.D.
The University of Texas
Health Science Center at Houston
Dental Branch
Houston, Texas

Pharmacology

Max Goodson, D.D.S., Ph.D.
Forsyth Dental Center
Boston, Massachusetts

Classification

Thomas W. Weatherford III, D.V.M., D.M.D., M.S.
University of Alabama
School of Dentistry
Birmingham, Alabama

Plaque control, root sensitivity

Joyce Litch, D.D.S., R.D.H., M.S.
University of the Pacific
School of Dentistry
San Francisco, California

Periodontal osseous resection

Robert E. Lamb, D.D.S., M.S.D.
James O. Bartlett, D.D.S.
University of the Pacific
School of Dentistry
San Francisco, California

Mucogingival surgery

Walter B. Hall, D.D.S., M.S.
University of the Pacific
School of Dentistry
San Francisco, California

In addition, we wish to recognize the contributions of the following who reviewed and revised chapters and provided material for this edition:

Donald Adams, D.D.S., M.S.
The Oregon Health Sciences University
School of Dentistry
Portland, Oregon

Oded Bahat, D.D.S., M.S.D.
University of Southern California
School of Dentistry
Los Angeles, California

Sol Bernick, Ph.D.
University of Southern California
School of Medicine
Los Angeles, California

Israel Speckman Borg, D.D.S.
Mexico City, Mexico

Anthony Gargiulo, D.D.S., M.S.
Loyola University
School of Dentistry
Maywood, Illinois

O.M. Gupta, B.D.S., D.M.D., M.S., M.S.D., D.P.H.
Howard University
College of Dentistry
Washington, D.C.

Phillip Hoag, D.D.S.
University of Illinois
College of Dentistry
Chicago, Illinois

Mansoor H. Jabro, B.D.S., M.S.D.
Creighton University
Boyne School of Dental Science
Omaha, Nebraska

Charles Joseph, D.D.S., Ph.D.
University of Southern California
School of Dentistry
Los Angeles, California

Katsuei Mori, D.D.S.
Tokyo, Japan

Jon E. Peterson, D.D.S.
San Diego, California

Gerald J. Tussing, D.D.S., M.S.D.
University of Nebraska
College of Dentistry
Lincoln, Nebraska

Material on saliva was provided originally by Dr. Irwin Mandel. Dr. Michael J. Levine added material on salivary glycoproteins in plaque, and Dr. Murray Robinovitch reviewed the chapter on saliva. The chapter on nutrition was originally written by Dr. Cyril Enwonwu and revised by Dr. Michael Alfano. Dr. Stanley Hazen contributed to the chapter on calculus. The chapter on immune mechanisms contains the work of Dr. Bruce Mackler. Dr. Anthony Gargiulo contributed material on dimensions of the dentogingival junction. Marmoset specimens, microscopic slides of which appear in the text, were provided by Dr. Barnett Levy; the histologic preparation was by Dr. Sol Bernick.

Dr. William S. Lavine provided material on neutrophil function in periodontosis. Dr. Oded Bahat updated the important chapter on the periodontal flap. Dr. Phillip Hoag reviewed and modified the chapter on maintenance. Dr. Charles Joseph collaborated in the revision of the chapter on scaling and root planing.

Dr. Leonard Hirschfeld provided information for the chapters on prognosis and the treated patient. Mrs. Valerie Haynes Schwartz and Miss Danielle Grant assisted in plaque control. Material on bone grafts was contributed by Drs. Gerald Bowers, William Hiatt, Robert Schallhorn, John Nabers, Harold Meader, and Edward F. Sugarman. Histologic material on wound healing was provided by Drs. Malbern Wilderman, Mick Dragoo, Jan Egelberg, and Max Crigger. Other histologic material was contributed by Drs. Hubert Schroeder, Roy Page, and George Bernard.

Dr. Bennett Klavan and Dr. Patrick Pierre contributed to furcation involvements. Dr. Clifford Ochsenbein contributed to osseous resection. Dr. Richard Chace wrote material for the treated patient. Dr. Herman Corn and Dr. Edwin Rosenberg contributed to preprosthetic surgery. Manuel H. Marks contributed material on orthodontic therapy. Dr. Terry Tanaka reviewed the chapter on treatment of periodontal trauma. Virginia Grant struggled to keep us organized.

Assistance in illustrative material and text were provided by distinguished contributors:

Daniel Etienne, D.C.D., M.S.
Paris, France

Alain Fontanelle, D.C.D., M.S.
Paris, France

Hilton Israelson, D.D.S.
Richardson, Texas

Robert Jaffin, D.D.S.
Hackensack, New Jersey

Clifford D. Kopp, D.D.S.
New York, New York

Michelle Lavier, D.C.D., M.S.
Paris, France

Dan M. Loughlin, D.D.S.
Arlington, Texas

Andre Saadoun, D.D.S.
Los Angeles, California

We express our appreciation for the contributions that have so enhanced and added to our own work. *In all areas, we either wrote or revised contributed material, and the final wording and the concepts expressed herein are our responsibility.*

# CONTENTS

## PART FOUR:  Elements of Therapeutic Judgment

## PART FIVE:  Initial Nonsurgical Therapy

## PART SIX:  Surgery

## PART SEVEN:  Occlusal and Reconstructive Aspects of Therapy

# PART EIGHT:   Maintenance

## COLOR PLATES

# PART ONE

## Introduction

# CHAPTER 1

# Periodontal health and disease

**Problem of prevention and treatment**

**Periodontal structure: the gingiva**
Surface characteristics

**Papillae and vasculature as early indicators of disease**

---

The purpose of this text is to teach students and practitioners of dentistry to recognize, prevent, treat and, where possible, cure periodontal diseases. Throughout, the principles underlying clinical practice will be related to the scientific, philosophic, or conceptual reasons for them. Naturally, these interrelationships may be perceived differently as our scientific knowledge progresses. Understanding the biology of supporting tissues of the teeth and the environment in which they exist promotes a more meaningful application of therapeutic practices and leads to greater success in the treatment of periodontal diseases.

The teeth are supported by the alveolar processes of the maxilla and mandible. Bundles of collagen fibers course between and insert into the cementum and the alveolar bone to hold the teeth in place. The teeth are surrounded by the periodontal tissues (Greek *peri,* "around"; *odont-,* "tooth"), which provide the support that is essential to function. The gingiva covers the alveolar bone and surrounds the neck of each tooth. The ability to chew normally with one's own teeth depends in part on the health of the periodontium.

Periodontal diseases affect the health of the periodontium and may lead to a loss **Pocket** of alveolar bone and loosening of the teeth. As a result of pathologic changes, the gingival attachment to the tooth may become displaced apically, while the gingiva seemingly remains in place, resulting in a loose sleeve of diseased gingiva lying against the tooth. The space between this detached gingiva and the tooth is called a *pocket.* The ultimate result of progressive pocket formation, bone loss, and tooth mobility is the loss of a tooth or teeth.

Periodontal diseases are found in all people, in all nations. In the United States more than half the people over 40 years of age have lost at least one tooth because of periodontal disease. In fact, 23 million adults have lost all their teeth, many to periodontal disease, which accounts for 50% of the missing teeth in adults in the United States, with two out of three middle-aged individuals affected.[1-4] Of 127 million adults with some or all their teeth, 94 million have periodontal disease with 32 million considered to have advanced disease. The disease process may well have been present in these people in their youth, but the signs were not evident to them or to their dentists.

## Problem of prevention and treatment

Periodontal diseases are preventable and controllable to a large degree. These diseases are most effectively treated in the early stages. Since the dentist's professional obligation is to keep teeth healthy and to prevent their loss, knowledge of periodontal disease and its prevention and treatment are of paramount concern to the dentist and to the patient. In fact, without such knowledge, a dentist cannot be considered fully competent. Undiagnosed periodontal disease continues to be a problem for the profession and the patient. This problem is compounded by patients' lack of awareness of the disease and disbelief in their own susceptibility.[5] The relatively infrequent use of all facets of the periodontal examination by the practitioner adds to the problem.[5]

**Periodontal diseases**
The various diseases of the periodontium are collectively termed *periodontal diseases*. Their treatment is referred to as *periodontal therapy*. The clinical science that deals with the periodontium in health and disease is called *periodontology*, the practice of which is *periodontics*.

Before any further consideration of periodontal diseases and their treatment, recognition of the healthy periodontium is essential as is also the ability to discern the minute and gross changes that accompany periodontal disease. The dentist who cannot recognize periodontal diseases cannot proceed to treat them. Such a shortcoming is detrimental to the patient, who may ultimately suffer pain, discomfort, and tooth loss. The patient's need for complete mouth care will not be realized, and the function of dentistry will not be fulfilled.

## Periodontal structure: the gingiva

Fundamentally the oral mucosa may be classified into three different types: the gingiva and the covering of the hard palate (*masticatory* mucosa), the dorsum of the tongue (*specialized* mucosa), and the remainder of the oral mucous membrane (*lining* mucosa).

### SURFACE CHARACTERISTICS

**Normal gingiva**
The gingiva (masticatory mucosa) is the part of the oral mucous membrane attached to the teeth and the alveolar processes of the jaws (Fig. 1-1). Normal clinical features of the gingiva include the following:[6]

1. *Color.* The color of normal gingiva is pale pink but may vary according to degree of vascularity, epithelial keratinization, pigmentation, and thickness of the epithelium.
2. *Papillary contour.* Papillae should fill the interproximal spaces. With increasing age the papillae and other parts of the gingiva may recede slightly, together with the underlying alveolar crest. A blunt rather than pointed papillary contour may therefore be considered to be normal for older persons.
3. *Marginal contour.* The gingiva should slope coronally to end in a thin edge. Mesiodistally the gingival margins should be scalloped in form.
4. *Texture.* Stippling is generally present to varying degrees on vestibular surfaces of the gingiva. This type of surface has been described as "orange peel" in appearance.
5. *Consistency.* The gingiva should be firm and tightly anchored to the teeth and underlying alveolar bone.
6. *Sulcus.* The sulcus is the groove or shallow space between the gingiva and the tooth. A healthy sulcus is minimal in depth (less than 1 mm). However, a sulcus up to 3 mm in depth may be compatible with health.
7. *Gingival groove.* The gingival groove is a shallow indentation on the vestibular surface of the gingiva. It may parallel the gingival margin at the level of the apical extent of the junctional epithelium. When present, its location does not correspond to the sulcus bottom.

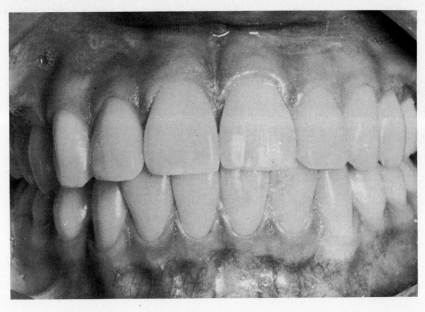

**Fig. 1-1.** Surface characteristics of the clinically normal gingiva. (Courtesy A.L. Ogilvie, Vancouver, British Columbia.)

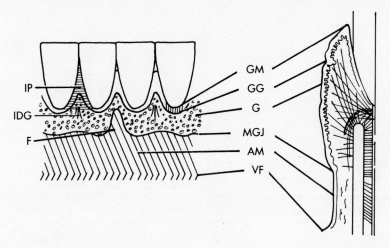

**Fig. 1-2.** Diagrammatic illustration of surface characteristics of the clinically normal gingiva showing: *IP,* interdental papilla; *IDG,* interdental grooves; *F,* frenum; *GM,* gingival margin; *GG,* gingival groove; *G,* gingiva; *MGJ,* mucogingival junction; *AM,* alveolar mucosa; *VF,* vestibular fornix.

Although the gingiva is subject to mechanical stresses during mastication, its structure is adapted to resist these stresses.

The gingiva is demarcated from the loosely anchored and movable alveolar mucosa by a recognizable line, the *mucogingival junction* (Figs. 1-2 and 1-3, *A-D*). This line of demarcation between the gingiva and the alveolar mucosa occurs on the outer (vestibular) surfaces of both jaws. A similar line may occur on the inner (oral) surface of the mandible between the mucosa and the floor of the mouth. There is no clear dividing line on the palate because the mucosa of the hard palate is keratinized, firmly attached to bone, and continuous with the gingiva. The mucogingival junction, although clinically and anatomically evident, is subject to considerable variation in shape and position. It is clinically recognizable by the color change distinguishing it from

**Gingiva and mucogingival junction**

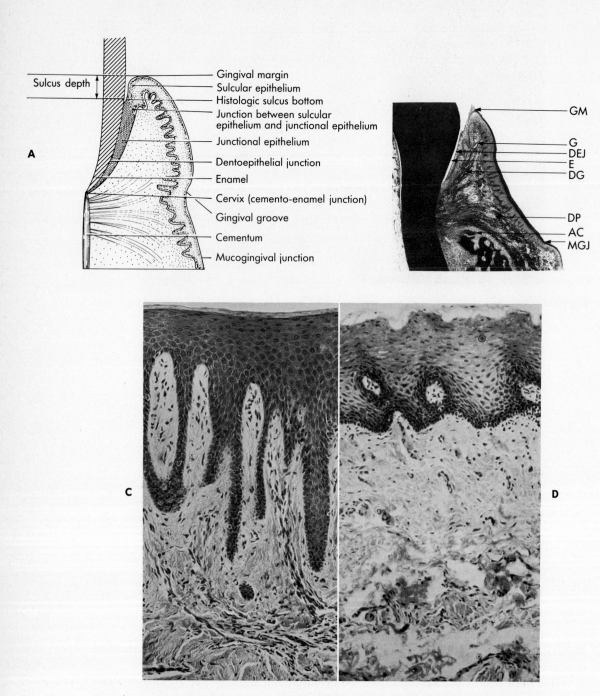

**Fig. 1-3. A,** Diagrammatic illustration of a cross section of tooth and gingiva. **B,** Buccolingual section of dog premolar showing: *GM,* gingival margin; *G,* gingiva; *DEJ,* dentoepithelial junction; *E,* enamel space; *DG,* dentogingival fibers; *DP,* dentoperiosteal fibers; *AC,* alveolar crest; *MGJ,* mucogingival junction. Difference between gingiva, **C,** and alveolar mucosa, **D,** is that the surface of the gingival epithelium is keratinized, whereas that of the alveolar mucosa is not. Epithelial ridges and connective tissue papillae of the gingiva are long as compared with those of the alveolar mucosa. (**C** and **D** courtesy G.P. Ivancie, Denver, Colorado.)

Labels in diagram A:

Sulcus depth

Gingival margin
Sulcular epithelium
Histologic sulcus bottom
Junction between sulcular epithelium and junctional epithelium
Junctional epithelium
Dentoepithelial junction
Enamel
Cervix (cemento-enamel junction)
Gingival groove
Cementum
Mucogingival junction

Labels in image B:

GM
G
DEJ
E
DG
DP
AC
MGJ

the gingiva and by the elasticity and mobility of the alveolar mucosa apical to it.

The term *vestibular* is used to describe surfaces that face the vestibule, thus eliminating the need or differentiating between buccal and labial. This tends to simplify descriptions and coincides with proper anatomic usage. The vestibular cavity is bounded anterolaterally by the mucous membranes of the lips and cheeks and internally by the teeth and gingiva. *Vestibular* would therefore apply to any tooth surface facing the vestibular cavity. Similarly the term *oral* describes the palatal and lingual surfaces. The oral cavity proper is bounded anterolaterally by the teeth and gingiva, superiorly by the soft and hard palate, inferiorly by the tongue and mucous membranes of the floor of the mouth, and posteriorly by the pillars of the fauces, the opening into the oral pharynx.

The *interdental gingiva* occupies the interdental space. It is more or less pyramidal in form in the incisor region. Between the posterior teeth it forms an interdental "col."[7] The interdental gingiva of posterior teeth has been compared to a "sagging pup tent" (Fig. 1-4). The interdental gingiva and the oral and vestibular portions of the gingiva are attached to the tooth surfaces by junctional epithelium and by gingival connective tissue fibers.

With recession, the pointed interdental papillae become progressively more blunt (Fig. 1-5). Where a diastema is present, the interdental tissue assumes the form of a blunt ridge or sometimes a concave saddle (Fig. 1-6).

The term *"free" gingiva* has been used in the past to describe that portion of the clinically healthy marginal gingiva not attached to the tooth.[8] However, where there is no disease, there is little, if any, "free" gingiva. The term *"attached" gingiva*, has been used to describe the gingiva apical to the "free" gingiva.[8-15] It is attached to the tooth and alveolar process by means of connective tissue fibers.

The World Workshop* has recommended dropping the terms "free" and "attached" gingiva, since in the normal, healthy state, there is little or no sulcus depth (see Fig. 1-2). Both divisions of the gingiva should be referred to as "gingiva." When the sulcus is deepened, prosthodontists speak of "attached" and "free" gingiva.

Vertical growth of the alveolar process and a slow rate of tooth eruption gradually

---

*International Conference on Research in the Biology of Periodontal Diseases, Chicago, June 12-15, 1977.

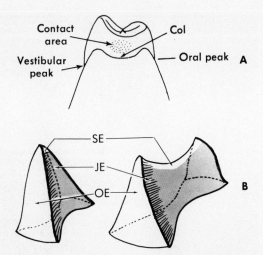

**Fig. 1-4. A,** Diagrammatic representation of the interdental papilla showing the col and peaks. **B,** Interdental papillae showing pyramidal form between anterior teeth and "sagging pup tent" form between posterior teeth. *SE,* sulcular epithelium; *JE,* junctional epithelium; *OE,* oral epithelium.

**Fig. 1-5.**  Diagram of marginal gingiva before and after recession. **A,** Mandibular anterior section, labial view. **B,** Mandibular anterior segment, labiolingual section. **C,** Mandibular posterior segment, buccal view. **D,** Mandibular molar, buccolingual section. (From Carranza, F.A.: Glickman's clinical periodontology, ed. 6, Philadelphia, 1984, W.B. Saunders Co.)

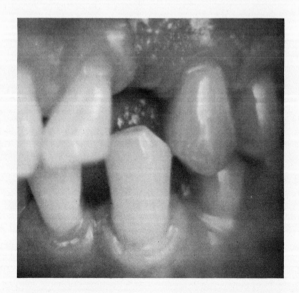

**Fig. 1-6.**  Saddlelike appearance of the interdental tissue in a diastema. Gingiva surrounds the tooth like a collar.

increase the width of the gingiva[15] while the location of the mucogingival junction tends to remain relatively stable.[13]

In youngsters, the gingival margin is located on enamel. The margin gradually recedes so that in the adult it is at or below the cementoenamel junction. Exposure of the anatomic crown because of gingival recession is referred to as *passive eruption* or *passive exposure*.[16]

Variations in gingival contour, thickness, and height depend on the following positional factors: presence of diastemata (see Figs. 1-6 to 1-8), degree of eruption (see Figs. 1-7 to 1-9), missing teeth, and positioning of the teeth in the arch. In instances of rotation, overlapping, and labial or lingual (vestibular or oral) placement of teeth (see Figs. 1-11 and 1-16), the gingival margin is altered in height. Viewed from the vestibule, the gingiva are receded when the teeth are in vestibular version. If the tooth is in oral version, the gingival margin tends to be displaced coronally, and has a thickened, rolled edge (see Fig. 1-16).[17] The reverse relationships exist when teeth are viewed from the oral aspect. The position of the tooth in the arch may influence the form of the alveolar bone over the root. The thickness of the alveolar bone also plays a role in determining gingival form.

The degree of scalloping of the gingival margin will be affected primarily by the degree of convexity or concavity of the tooth surface. Highly convex root surfaces will be associated with a markedly scalloped gingival margin. Teeth with relatively flat contours will have flat, even, nonscalloped gingival margins. On the other hand, the margin will tend to creep coronally over concave surfaces—for example, root surfaces directly coronal to a furcation.

**Width of gingiva**

The normal gingiva is bounded by the mucogingival junction[18] and by the gingival margin. This zone varies in width among individuals and in different areas of the same mouth. It is usually widest about the maxillary incisors and molars and on the lingual surface of the mandibular first molars. It is narrower in the mandibular premolar region.[10] In the mandibular second and third molar region it is sometimes 1 mm in width or may even be nonexistent. The gingiva is generally wider in the maxilla than in the mandible. The gingiva may increase in width with age.[11-14] Figs. 1-7 to 1-14 demonstrate the range of normal gingival width at various ages.

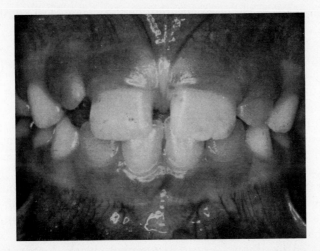

**Fig. 1-7.** Mixed dentition in an 8-year-old boy. Gingival color is pale pink. During eruption the gingival margins (see maxillary central incisors) are thicker and flat over a flat tooth surface. Crowns of the central and lateral incisors are not fully exposed. Where teeth are in proximal contact, the papillae fill the interdental spaces. (Courtesy M. Droppelmann, Valparaiso, Chile.)

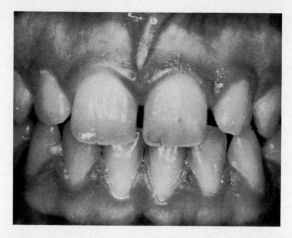

**Fig. 1-8.** At 14 years, the gingiva begins to become more adultlike in appearance and scalloped over a convex tooth surface. The maxillary gingival margins are rolled as passive exposure of the crown proceeds. Gingival color is pale pink.

Fig. 1-9 is of a 20-year-old woman whose gingival form is ideal. The gingiva is knife edged, and festooning is regular. The gingiva is delicate in texture, and the mucogingival line is not strongly delineated.

The gingival form of a 44-year-old man in Fig. 1-10 is similar to that of the patient in Fig. 1-9. However, the degree of keratinization and the amount of stippling are more pronounced.

The photograph of a 46-year-old woman in Fig. 1-11, *A*, is more than 14 years old, but the appearance of the gingiva cannot be distinguished from that in a more recent photograph taken at age 60 (Fig. 1-11, *B*).

The degree of difference between the tissues of the 75-year-old patient in Fig. 1-12 and younger patients is not great.

Fig. 1-13 is of a 47-year-old patient. Note the slight festooning about the teeth. There is a faint pigmentation in the attached gingiva of the anterior teeth.

Fig. 1-14 shows all characteristics of ideal gingival form in a 21-year-old black woman. The gingiva is made more apparent by the generalized pigmentation of this zone.

**Stippling**  The surface of the gingiva is characterized by an orange peel–like appearance called *stippling* (Fig. 1-15). The stippling may be fine or coarse and may vary in different individuals; it may also vary according to age and sex.[19,20] The stippling is finer in girls than it is in boys. It is normally absent in some locations (e.g., the molar area). In addition to stippling, the epithelial surface may contain scattered minute protuberances that contribute to its texture.[20] Stippling reflects the contours of the epithelial connective tissue boundary in health. In health, the interdental "col"[21,22] is tightly attached to the adjacent teeth surfaces through a junctional epithelium and through collagen fibers.

**Alveolar mucosa**  The alveolar mucosa differs from the gingiva in structure, function, and color. The gingiva is firmly adherent to the underlying bone and is immovable, whereas the alveolar mucosa is loosely connected and movable. The alveolar mucosa is sharply demarcated clinically from the gingiva by the mucogingival line.[18]

**Color**  Pigmentation of the gingiva occurs frequently in blacks,[23] Orientals, and Indians and is also seen in whites of Mediterranean, Turkish, and Arab ancestry. It may be general or localized and regularly or irregularly distributed.[23] The pigment may vary from faint to intense, but it is normal and should not be confused with the changes

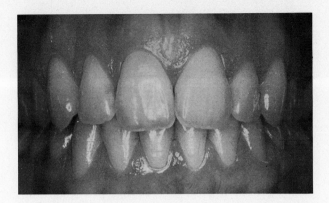

**Fig. 1-9.**   Gingival tissues of a 20-year-old woman.

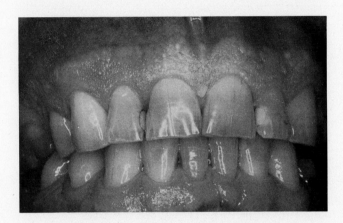

**Fig. 1-10.**   Gingival tissues of a 44-year-old man.

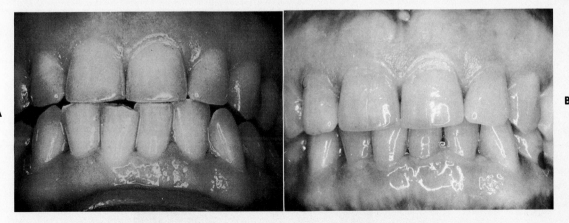

**Fig. 1-11.   A,** Gingival tissues of a 46-year-old woman. **B,** Same patient at age 60.

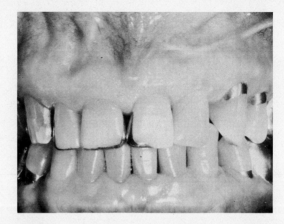

**Fig. 1-12.** Gingival tissues of a 75-year-old woman.

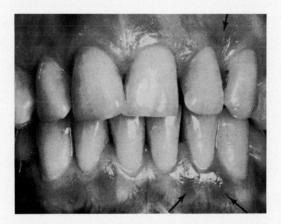

**Fig. 1-13.** Gingiva of a 47-year-old woman. Arrows point to pigmented areas.

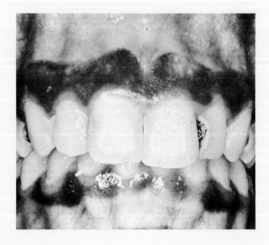

**Fig. 1-14.** Gingiva of a 21-year-old woman. Note the pigmentation.

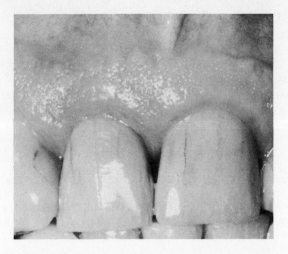

**Fig. 1-15.**  Stippling (depressed points) of the attached gingiva.

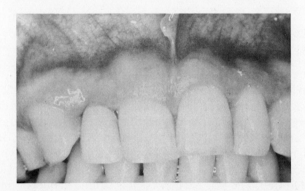

**Fig. 1-16.**  Maxillary right central incisor is extruded. Left incisor is vestibular (labial) to it. When viewed from the oral aspect, the gingival margin of the right incisor is attached further coronally. This difference in height of attachment is a result of the difference in position of teeth in the arch.

that accompany periodontal disease. Pigmentation ranges from light brown to black. The exact hue is subject to individual variation. Since epithelium is translucent, the color depends on the vascularity and thickness of the subjacent connective tissue, which may be altered by the degree of keratinization of the epithelium.

In health, there is no change in coloration between the different areas of the gingiva. The lining mucosa of the cheek and lips, the vestibular fornix, and the alveolar mucosa differ from the gingiva in pinkness because the epithelium at these sites is thin, nonkeratinized, and essentially translucent so that the underlying tissue produces a reddish or faintly bluish hue.

**Contour and demarcation**

In addition to variations in color, there are variations in papillary and marginal contour, texture, and consistency of normal gingival tissues, as is apparent in Figs. 1-7 to 1-16. Furthermore, differences exist in the width of the gingiva. The position and prominence of the frenum and muscle attachments are also subject to individual variation.

**Papillary gingiva**

One must be able to look at a patient's gingiva and dentition and understand how these various factors influence normal gingival form. Furthermore, and perhaps more importantly, one must also be able to detect the earliest changes produced by periodontal disease. The gingival papillae, formed from gingival tissue that extends interdentally, are important clinically and diagnostically since they show early signs of periodontal disease.[24]

Treatment of periodontal disease is always more successful and accomplished with more ease when it is instituted early. In such instances treatment tends to be interceptive and the tissue changes reversible. In the later stages of disease, treatment arrests the disease but usually cannot restore lost tooth support. Interceptive and preventive treatment is preferred to curative treatment. An old tenet in medicine states that the best treatment is the least treatment that will restore health.

## Papillae and vasculature as early indicators of disease

**Clinical signs**

To be able to detect the early stages of gingival inflammation or gingivitis, one must recognize the following symptoms in the interdental papillae and marginal gingivae:

1. Redness
2. Tendency to bleed easily
3. Tenderness
4. Sponginess
5. Slight swelling
6. Development of probing depth

These symptoms are all present in the patient with gingivitis shown in Plate 1, *A*. One papilla is red and bleeding (*lower arrow*). The upper arrow indicates an enlarged papilla. If these signs are ignored, the condition may deteriorate. Edema and inflammation may extend from the interdental papilla to the gingival margin. In Plate 1, *B*, changes in color are evident in the papillae and marginal gingivae, and inflammatory enlargement (edema) obliterates the stippling. In Plate 1, *C*, a hyperplastic inflammatory enlargement is evident. The papilla has spread laterally over the tooth surface and has become blunted. The disease process has extended deeper into the interdental tissues involving the bone and is now termed *periodontitis*. Were the disease to continue, the interdental papillae might be destroyed, and the vessels of the inflamed area would become more prominent because they dilate in the areas of inflammation (*arrows*) (Plate 1, *D*).

In some instances in which the gingiva is thick, fibrotic, and well stippled, inflammatory changes tend to be concealed; yet in Plate 1, *E*, edema has caused a loss of stippling over the mandibular incisor and canine. In addition, frank pus is exuding from the pocket over the canine and the lateral incisor (*arrows*). Such cases are rather insidious since they are not as evident to the untrained eye as is the disease seen in the patient in Plate 1, *F,* where the disease process is very obvious.

Inflammatory changes are accompanied by an increased blood supply to the gingiva.[25] Why are these inflammatory changes so clinically evident? First, the epithelium is translucent. Second, the gingiva has a rich and extensive blood supply that increases in inflammation. The capillaries form a plexus extending throughout the gingiva and into the marginal gingiva (Figs. 1-17 and 1-18), where capillary loops are subjacent to the epithelium.[25] In inflammatory conditions the permeability of these vessels is increased. There is vascular proliferation and vascular leakage (Figs. 1-19 to 1-21). Furthermore, blood vessels are found closer to the pocket surface.[26] The combination of a translucent epithelium, collagen fiber destruction, and increased vascularity contributes to increased redness. Vascular leakage promotes edematous changes in surface texture and contour. Swollen, enlarged gingiva may give rise to increased probing depth (pseudopockets).

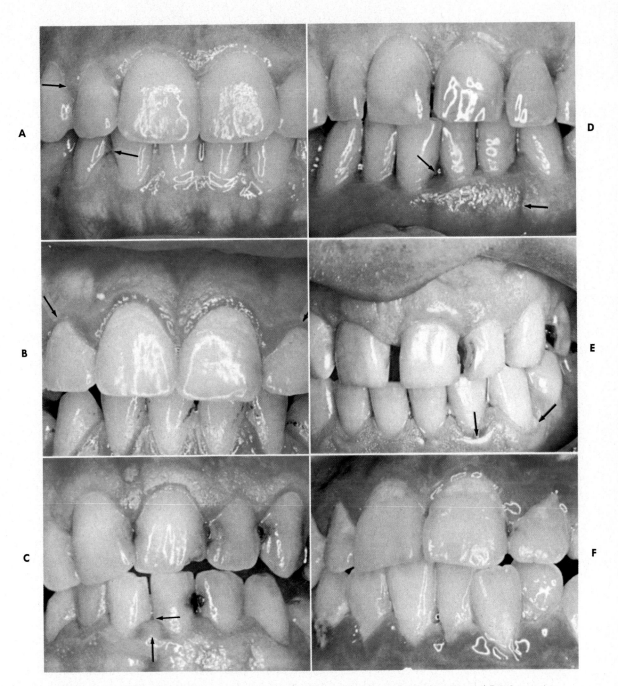

**Plate 1.** **A,** Slight swelling of the interdental papilla *(upper arrow)*; bleeding papilla *(lower arrow)*. **B,** Inflammation of papillary and marginal gingivae *(arrows)*. Papillae are hyperplastic, edematous, and stippling is obliterated. **C,** Enlargement of papilla *(arrows)*. The papilla has become blunted. **D,** Continued inflammation has led to a loss of papillary tissue *(arrow)*. **E,** In the presence of denser tissue, the inflammatory changes tend to be concealed. Some stippling persists, although loss of stippling may occur where pockets exist *(arrows)* and exudation can be seen *(arrows)*. **F,** Generalized inflammation exhibiting change in color, loss of stippling, edema, and gingival enlargement.

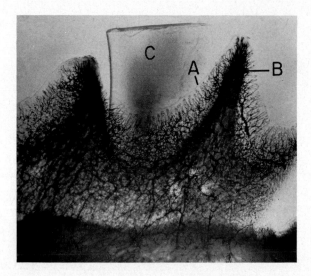

**Fig. 1-17.** Dog gingiva perfused with India ink showing distribution of blood vessels. *A,* Marginal gingiva; *B,* interdental papilla; *C,* tooth. (Courtesy D.A. Rolfs, Wenatchee, Washington.)

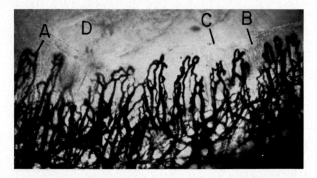

**Fig. 1-18.** Same animal as in Fig. 1-17; higher magnification. *A,* Capillary loops pass toward the epithelium; *B,* epithelium extends between connective tissue papillae; *C,* marginal gingiva; *D,* tooth surface. (Courtesy D.A. Rolfs, Wenatchee, Washington.)

With time inflammation may extend into the underlying tissues of the periodontium. This is accompanied by loss of bone, which becomes evident in roentgenograms. Untreated, the disease process may result in the loosening, migration, and ultimate loss of the tooth (Fig. 1-22, *A* and *B*).

The bacterially induced diseases of the periodontium include gingivitis (inflammation of the gingiva without bone destruction) and periodontitis (inflammation and destruction of the deeper structures of the periodontium, including alveolar bone). These diseases were at one time believed to progress slowly and continuously.[27-29] Currently, it is thought that gingivitis and periodontitis have intermittent periods of quiescence or nondestructive activity and periods of destruction, which are sometimes very rapid. A model of destructive periodontal disease in which bursts of activity occur for short periods of time in individual sites with intervening periods of remission is now preferred to the "continuous disease" hypothesis. The possibility exists that exacerbations of the disease are coupled with the activity of specific bacterial infections or with periods of impaired host resistance.[30-32]

Periodontal disease is best considered as the outcome of an ongoing host-parasite interaction between pathogenic microorganisms that have colonized the periodontal

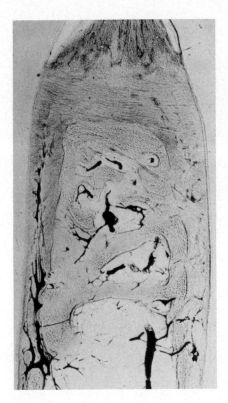

**Fig. 1-19.** The gingival vasculature in this periodontally healthy, perfused spider monkey is regular with even, nonenlarged vascular loops entering the papillae between rete ridges. (From Grant, D.A., and Bernick, S.: J. Dent. Res. **52:**Abstract no. 770, 1973.)

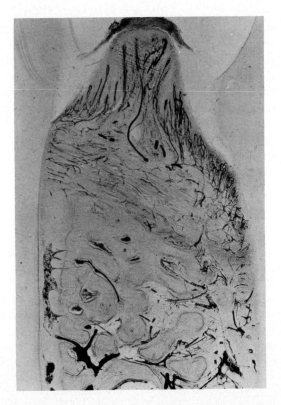

**Fig. 1-20.** In mild gingival inflammation, the vessels of the subepithelial vascular plexus become enlarged (perfused spider monkey). (From Grant, D.A., and Bernick, S.: J. Dent. Res. **52:**Abstract no. 770, 1973.)

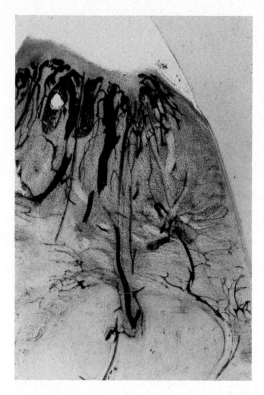

**Fig. 1-21.** *In severe inflammation, the regularity of the subepithelial vascular channels is altered. Vessels are greatly enlarged, gingival collagen is destroyed, and the spaces created are then occupied by proliferating capillaries and inflammatory cells. The gingiva appears deep or bright red clinically (perfused spider monkey). (From Grant, D.A., and Bernick, S.: J. Dent. Res. **52:**Abstract no. 770, 1973.)*

pocket and host tissues that resist such bacteria or their products. Inadequate antimicrobial defense strategies of the host frequently result in the loss of normal structural components such as the collagen fibers of the gingiva and periodontal ligament and the replacement of these fibers by dense infiltrates of inflammatory cells. These lesions are the result of imbalances in the host-parasite equilibrium, which may lead to periodic, short-lived episodes of tissue destruction. The cumulative effect of these episodic events gives rise to an increased loss of dental support that may lead to the eventual loss of one or more teeth.

There are, in addition to nonspecific forms of gingivitis and periodontitis, other diseases of the periodontal tissues. Among those are a group of acute conditions such as periodontal abscess (Plate 2, *A*), pericoronitis (Plate 2, *B*), necrotizing ulcerative gingivitis (Plate 2, *C*), acute primary herpetic gingivostomatitis (Plate 2, *D* and *E*), and benign mucous membrane pemphigoid (Plate 2, *F*). These conditions require rapid diagnosis and immediate treatment to alleviate the discomfort the patient is experiencing. These and other conditions such as cysts, pregnancy gingivitis (Plate 3, *A*), juvenile periodontitis, recession (Plate 3, *B*), overgrowth, periodontal traumatism, gingival enlargement (Plate 3, *C*), plaque and calculus (Plate 3, *D*), frenum pull (Plate 3, *E*), diabetes (Plate 3, *F*), and many other topics will be discussed in the chapters that follow.

It should be noted that treatment strategies may vary depending on the patient's needs, economic status, priorities concerning health care and the presence of discomfort, loss of function, and esthetic considerations. Private practitioners treating indi-

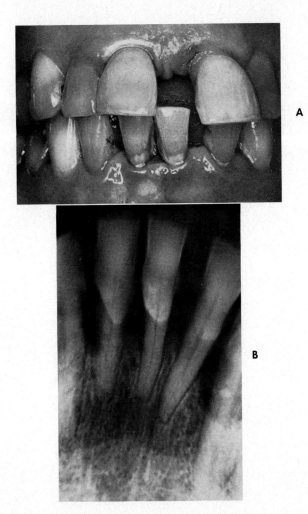

**Fig. 1-22.** **A,** Progressive inflammation of periodontal tissues. Deposits are evident on the tooth surface. The teeth have migrated and produced diastemata. **B,** Roentgenogram of the mandibular teeth shown in **A.** Note the loss of bone and the deposits of calculus.

vidual patients may have different standards of successful therapy than public health dentists who are trying to accommodate the periodontal health needs of a large population in a system trying to contain upwardly spiralling health care costs. Societal considerations may dictate the acceptance of a chronic, "slow-moving" disease and some tooth loss with its attendant disadvantages. Thus periodontics represents a complex and variable approach to the treatment of a wide range of individuals and populations that calls for flexibility and a depth of understanding on the part of the practitioner. It is the aim of this textbook to give the knowledge and background necessary to provide such a depth of understanding.

To begin with we shall discuss the histology of the periodontal tissues since an understanding of tissue structure and function is an important prerequisite to the diagnosis and treatment of periodontal diseases.

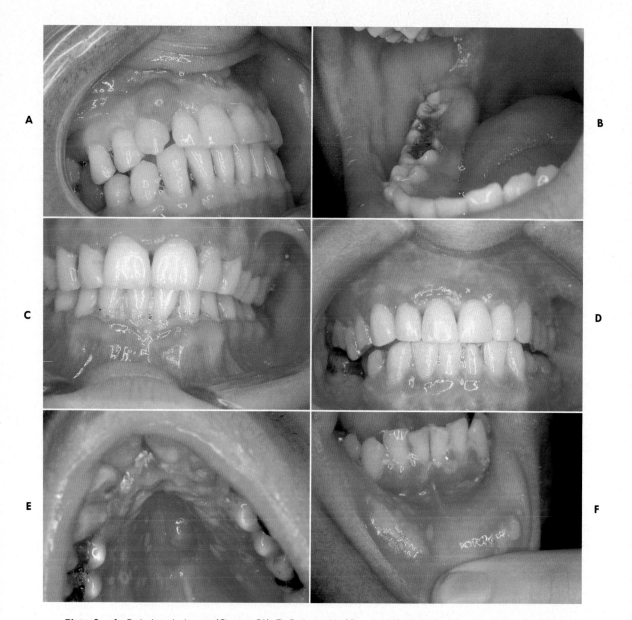

**Plate 2.** **A,** Periodontal abscess (Chapter 21). **B,** Pericoronitis (Chapter 20). **C,** Necrotizing ulcerative gingivitis (Chapter 18). **D** and **E,** Acute primary herpetic gingivostomatitis (Chapter 19). **F,** Benign mucous membrane pemphigoid (Chapter 22).

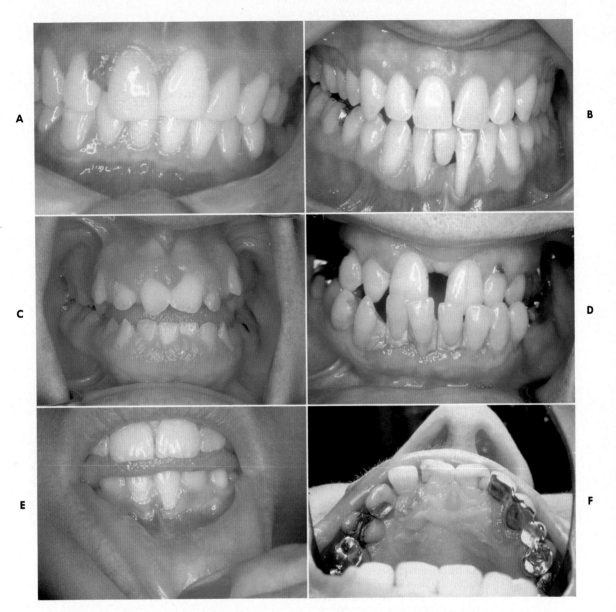

**Plate 3.   A,** Pregnancy gingivitis (Chapter 15). **B,** Recession (Chapters 23 and 40). **C,** Gingival enlargement (hereditary fibromatosis) (Chapter 24). **D,** Plaque and calculus (Chapters 3, 9, 15, 16, 31 and 32). **E,** High frenum and frenum pull (Chapters 23 and 40). **F,** Granulation tissue in a diabetic patient (Chapters 1 and 15).

## REFERENCES

1. Allen, E.F.: Statistical study of the primary causes of extraction, J. Dent. Res. **23**:453, 1944.
2. McHugh, W.D., et al.: Evaluation of the NIDR periodontal disease research activity. Report of the ad hoc scientific evaluation panel, 1976, National Institute of Dental Research, p. 1.
3. Challenges for the Eighties, National Institute of Dental Research. Long-range research plan, 1983, U.S. Department of Health and Human Services, Public Health Services, Nat. Inst. Health, p. 37.
4. Harden, J.F.: Periodontal disease in America: a personal and national tragedy, J. Public Health Dent. **43**:106, 1983.
5. Brady, W.: Periodontal disease awareness, J. Am. Dent. Assoc. **109**:706, 1984.
6. Orban, B.: Clinical and histologic study of the surface characteristics of the gingiva, Oral Surg. **1**:827, 1948.
7. Cohen, B.: Morphologic factors in the pathogenesis of periodontal disease, Br. Dent. J. **107**:31, 1959.
8. Ainamo, J., and Löe, H.: Anatomical characteristics of gingiva: a clinical and microscopic study of the free and attached gingiva, J. Periodontol. **37**:5, 1966.
9. Bowers, G.M.: A study of the width of attached gingiva, J. Periodont. Res. **1**:163, 1966.
10. Lang, N.P., and Löe, H.: The relationship between the width of keratinized gingiva and gingival health, J. Periodontol. **43**:623, 1972.
11. Ainamo, J., and Talari, A.: The increase with age of the width of attached gingiva, J. Periodont. Res. **11**:182, 1976.
12. Rose, S.T., and App, G.R.: A clinical study of the development of the attached gingiva along the facial aspect of the maxillary and mandibular anterior teeth in the deciduous, transitional and permanent dentitions, J. Periodontol. **44**:131, 1973.
13. Ainamo, A.: Influence of age on the location of the maxillary mucogingival junction, J. Periodont. Res. **13**:189, 1978.
14. Ainamo, A., Ainamo, J., and Poikkeus, R.: Continuous widening of the band of attached gingiva from 23 to 65 years of age, J. Periodont. Res. **16**:595, 1981.
15. Ainamo, A., and Ainamo, J.: The width of attached gingiva on supraerupted teeth, J. Periodont. Res. **13**:194, 1978.
16. Gottlieb, B., and Orban, B.: Active and passive eruption of the teeth, J. Dent. Res. **13**:214, 1933.
17. Morris, M.: The position of the margin of the gingiva, Oral Surg. **11**:969, 1958.
18. Fleisch, L., Cleaton-Jones, P., and Austin, J.C.: A histological and scanning electron microscopy study of the mucogingival junction in the vervet monkey, J. Periodont. Res. **11**:189, 1976.
19. Wentz, F.M., Maier, A.W., and Orban, B.: Age changes and sex differences in the clinically "normal" gingiva, J. Periodontol. **23**:13, 1952.
20. Rosenberg, H.M., and Massler, M.: Gingival stippling in young adult males, J. Periodontol. **38**:473, 1967.
21. Kohl, J.T., and Zander, H.A.: Morphology of interdental gingival tissues, Oral Surg. **14**:287, 1961.
22. Cohen, B.: Comparative studies in periodontal disease, Proc. R. Soc. Med. **53**:275, 1960.
23. Dummett, C.O., and Barens, G.: Oromucosal pigmentation: updated review, J. Periodontol. **42**:726, 1971.
24. Massler, M., Schour, I., and Chopra, B.: Occurrence of gingivitis in suburban Chicago school children, J. Periodontol. **21**:146, 1950.
25. Hock, J., and Nuki, K.: A vital microscopy study of the morphology of normal and inflamed gingiva, J. Periodont. Res. **6**:81, 1971.
26. Dragoo, M., et al.: Root planing with and without chlorhexidine rinses, Int. J. Periodont. Rest. Dent. **4**(3):9, 1984.
27. Löe, H., et al.: The natural history of periodontal disease in man: the rate of periodontal disease destruction before 40 years of age, J. Periodontol. **49**:67, 1978.
28. Löe, H., et al.: The natural history of periodontal disease in man: study design and baseline data, J. Periodont. Res. **13**:550, 1978.
29. Löe, H., et al.: The natural history of periodontal disease in man: tooth mortality before 40 years of age, J. Periodont. Res. **13**:563, 1978.
30. Socransky, S.S., et al.: An approach to the definition of periodontal disease syndromes by cluster analysis, J. Clin. Periodontol. **9**:460, 1982.
31. Goodson, J.M., et al.: Patterns of progression and regression of advanced destructive periodontal disease, J. Clin. Periodontol. **9**:472, 1982.
32. Socransky, S.S., et al.: New concepts of destructive periodontal disease, J. Clin. Periodontol. **11**:21, 1984.

## ADDITIONAL SUGGESTED READING

Becker, W., Becker, B.E., and Berg, L.: Periodontal treatment without maintenance: a retrospective study in 44 patients, J. Periodontol. **55**:505, 1984.

Listgarten, M.A.: A re-evaluation of selected diagnostic techniques: potential influence on the clinical practice of periodontics, J. Can. Dent. Assn. **50**:549, 1984.

Listgarten, M.A., et al.: Three-year longitudinal study of the periodontal status of an adult population with gingivitis, J. Clin. Periodontol. **12**:225, 1985.

Listgarten, M.A.: Pathogenesis of periodontitis, J. Clin. Periodontol. **13**:418, 1986.

McFall, W.T., Jr.: Tooth loss in 100 patients with periodontal disease: a long-term study, J. Periodontol. **53**:539, 1982.

# PART TWO

## Structure, Physiology, and Pathophysiology of the Periodontium

# CHAPTER 2

# Gingiva and dentogingival junction

## Periodontal structure (the periodontium)

*Periodontium*[1] is the functional unit of tissues supporting the tooth. The tooth and periodontium together are called the *dentoperiodontal unit.* The tissues of the periodontium include the gingiva, the junctional epithelium, the periodontal ligament, the cementum, and the alveolar process. They are biologically interdependent. The harmonious relationship between the different parts of the periodontium is maintained under normal conditions despite the constant changes that take place in periodontal tissues throughout life.

The maintenance of these tissues in health depends upon normal cellular activity that permits normal tissue responses to environmental conditions or insult. These adaptations may be seen on gross anatomic, microscopic, ultramicroscopic, and biochemical levels. Pathologic changes in cellular and tissue metabolism or in cellular environment also alter the morphology and function of the cells. These changes appear as the clinical and microscopic signs of periodontal disease.

The main support of the tooth is provided by the periodontal ligament, which connects the cementum layer covering the root surface of the tooth to the alveolar bone lining the *alveolus,* or tooth socket, into which the root fits. The gingiva provides relatively little physical support. Its main function is to protect the supporting tissues from the oral environment.

## Histologic features

The bulk of the gingiva is composed of connective tissue. Scattered within the fibrous network are a variety of cells including neural and vascular elements that are immersed in a markedly hydrated ground substance through which soluble substances can diffuse. The connective tissue elements are protected by an epithelial covering that not only serves as a barrier to mechanical and bacterial injury and immunologic insult but also attaches the coronal portion of the gingiva to the tooth surface. Let us consider the epithelium.

## GINGIVAL EPITHELIUM

The gingival epithelium is comprised of the oral epithelium, the sulcular epithelium, and the junctional epithelium (Fig. 2-1), all of which are stratified squamous epithelia.[2-7]

**Oral epithelium**

The *oral epithelium* may have a keratinized (Fig. 2-2) or parakeratinized surface.[8,9] The basal surface of the epithelium contains prominent ridges that interdigitate with connective tissue papillae in the marginal gingiva.[10,11] Ridge intersections correspond to surface depressions, which give the gingiva its "stippled" appearance[12-16] (Fig. 2-3). These ridges are much less pronounced in the alveolar mucosa.[11]

**Sulcular epithelium**

The *sulcular epithelium* is a stratified squamous epithelium that generally is nonkeratinized (Figs. 2-4 to 2-7) but may undergo partial keratinization.[2,4,7] It is continuous with the oral epithelium at the gingival margin and lines the lateral wall of the sulcus. The base of the sulcus is formed by junctional epithelium, which is continuous with the sulcular epithelium (see Fig. 2-1). The sulcular and oral epithelia are relatively impermeable to the passage of cells and fluid when compared with the junctional epithelium.[17-20]

**Junctional epithelium**

The *junctional epithelium* is a stratified squamous nonkeratinizing epithelium (Fig. 2-5) originally described by Gottlieb as the *epithelial attachment*[21] and then by Waerhaug as the *epithelial cuff*.[22] The term *epithelial attachment* describes the connecting interface attaching the tissue to the tooth. The junctional epithelium produces the attachment material. The junctional epithelium extends apically from the sulcus bottom to form a collar of epithelium around each tooth (see Fig. 2-1). This epithelial collar may be located entirely over enamel, on enamel and cementum, or entirely on cementum, depending on the stage of dental eruption and degree of gingival recession.[23] The junctional epithelium is attached to the gingival connective tissue on one side and to the tooth on the other. The junctional epithelium is widest near the sulcus bottom, where it may be 10 to 30 cells thick, gradually narrowing apically to a few

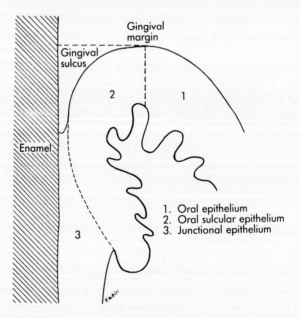

1. Oral epithelium
2. Oral sulcular epithelium
3. Junctional epithelium

**Fig. 2-1.** Diagrammatic view of gingival sulcus region. (From Listgarten, M.A.: Oral Sci. Rev. **1:**3, 1972.)

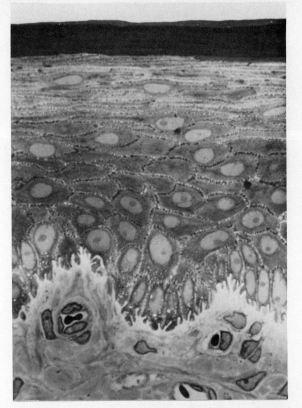

**Fig. 2-2.** Histologic section of orthokeratinized gingival surface. (Epon section—toluidine and methylene blue stain.)

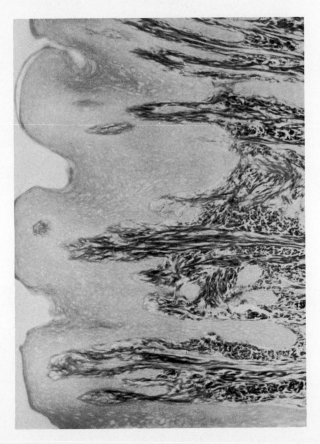

**Fig. 2-3.** Gingival specimen showing stippling. Note the relation of the connective tissue fiber bundles to the stippled surface. (Mallory stain.)

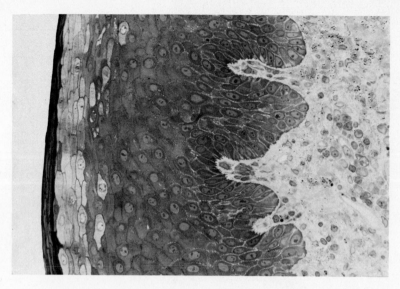

**Fig. 2-4.**   Histologic section of parakeratinized sulcular epithelium. (Epon section—toluidine and methylene blue stain.)

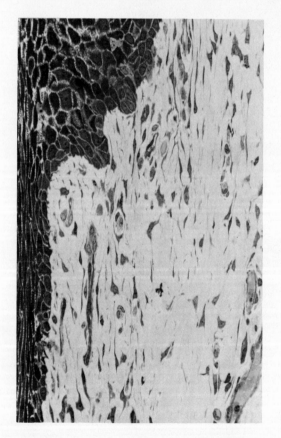

**Fig. 2-5.**   Histologic section of nonkeratinized junctional epithelium. (Epon section—toluidine and methylene blue stain.)

cells in thickness[24,25]; desquamation occurs at its coronal surface. Unlike the oral and sulcular epithelia, the junctional epithelial surface abutting on the connective tissue is generally devoid of ridges. The junctional epithelium is the most permeable of the gingival epithelia. Intercellular spaces of the junctional epithelium are the preferred route for tissue fluid and inflammatory cells migrating from the connective tissue to the sulcus.[17-20,26-32]

The oral epithelium consists of a *stratum basale, stratum spinosum, stratum granulosum,* and *stratum corneum* (Fig. 2-6), also referred to as basal, prickle-cell (or

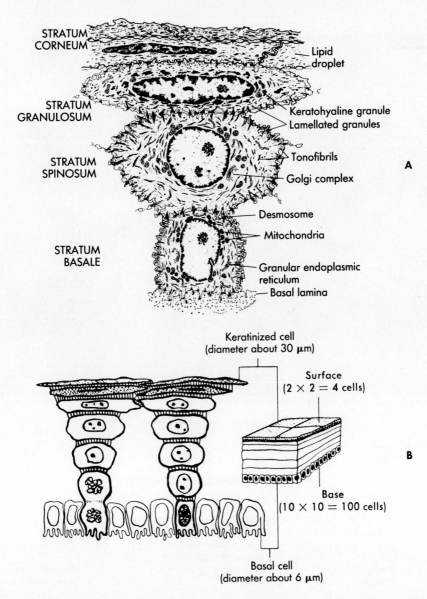

**Fig. 2-6.  A,** Schema of the various layers of stratified squamous epithelium as seen by electron microscopy. **B,** Diagram of epithelial cell size in the stratum basale and stratum corneum. About four cornified cells may cover a hundred basal cells in area. Since one cell should desquamate for each cell formed, there are no fewer cells in the stratum corneum. They have simply become flattened and compacted, one cell above the other. (**A** courtesy Dr. A. Weinstock, in Ham, A.W., and Cormack, D.H.: Histology, ed. 8, Philadelphia, 1979, J.B. Lippincott Co.; **B** from Mehregan, A.H., and Pincus, H.: Cancer **17:**609, 1964.)

spinous), granular, and cornified layers, respectively.[2-6,33] The sulcular epithelium is usually not cornified in humans.

The basal cell layer consists of relatively small cuboidal or polyhedral cells in contact with a *basal lamina* (Fig. 2-7) that connects them to the underlying connective tissue. *Hemidesmosomes* are localized specializations of the cell periphery that attach the cell to the basal lamina. The basal lamina, in turn, is attached to the connective tissue surface.[2-4,24,33-37]

The cells of the gingival epithelia are replaced every 1 to 2 weeks. Junctional epithelium has the fastest turnover rate, estimated at 1 week or less; oral epithelium

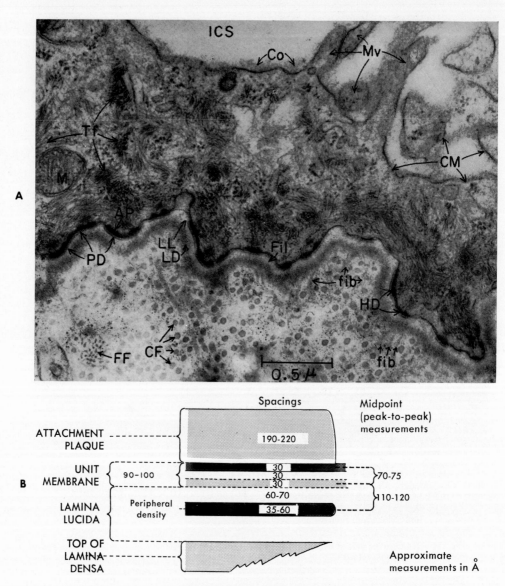

**Fig. 2-7. A,** Electron micrograph of human gingiva. Portion of a basal cell with basal lamina and hemidesmosomes. *AP,* attachment plaque of hemidesmosome; *CF,* collagen fibrils in cross section; *CM,* cell membrane; *Co,* cell membrane coating; *Fib,* anchoring fibrils; *FF,* fine fibrils resembling oxytalan fibrils; *HD,* hemidesmosome; *ICS,* intercellular space; *LD,* lamina densa; *LL,* lamina lucida; *M,* mitochondrion; *Mv,* microvilli; *Tf,* tonofilaments. Specks in the connective tissue are staining artifacts. **B,** Approximate dimensions of a hemidesmosome. (**A** from Stern, I.B.: Periodontics, **3:**224, 1965.)

has the longest, approximately 2 weeks.[38-42] New cells are produced by cell division in the basal layer, while superficial cells are lost by desquamation into the oral cavity. There is a proliferative compartment of cells that divide rapidly and thereby maintain the integrity of the epithelium. Another population of basal cells is serrated and heavily packed with *tonofilaments*. These are adaptations (serrations and filaments) for attachment to connective tissue.

The basal lamina is a product of the epithelial cells.[43-45] It consists of a nonfibrillar form of collagen classified as *type IV collagen*[46,47] and a unique glycoprotein, *laminin*.[48]

Ultrastructurally the basal lamina of gingival epithelium is approximately 100 na-

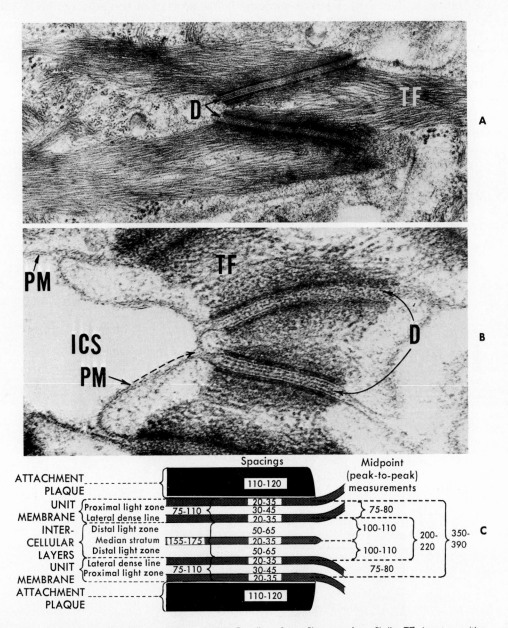

**Fig. 2-8. A,** Desmosomes *(D)* from human gingiva. Bundles of tonofilaments, (tonofibrils, *TF*), insert on either side of the junction. **B,** Higher magnification of two desmosomes *(D)* showing internal structure and relationship to plasma membrane *(PM)*. *ICS*, intercellular space; *TF*, tonofilaments. **C,** Diagrammatic representation of a desmosome and dimensions of various components in **A** expressed in Å. (From Stern, I.B.: Periodontics **3:**224, 1965.)

nometers (1000 Å) wide. It is composed of an electron-lucent *zona (lamina) lucida* adjacent to the cells and an electron-dense *densa* in contact with the connective tissue.[49-51] *Anchoring fibrils* are short, curved, banded fibrils of connective tissue origin that insert into the underside of the basal lamina.[52-54] They attach the basal lamina to the connective tissue (Fig. 2-7) and are composed of a recently described type VII collagen.

The cytoplasm of the basal cells contain widely dispersed *tonofilaments*, also referred to as *cytokeratins*. They are one of the precursors of *keratin*.[55-57] The cells are attached to one another by a few types of intercellular junctions, the major type being *desmosomes* (Fig. 2-8). Each desmosome is the product of two adjacent cells, each contributing approximately one half of its structure. They are the main intercellular junction throughout the epithelium. *Tight junctions (macula occludens, fascia occludens)* and *gap junctions* (Fig. 2-9) are found infrequently.[2,5,49,51] There are fewer desmosomes between basal cells. Their numbers increase rapidly in the supra basal layers.[2,49-51]

The *stratum spinosum* is the major epithelial layer. It is composed of large cells (Figs. 2-10 and 2-11), with well-developed arrays of desmosomes.[49,51] The concentration of tonofilaments increases from the basal layer toward the surface.[58,59] In the spinous layer the tonofilaments aggregate into dense bundles, the *tonofibrils*, which converge toward the attachment plaques of desmosomes.[49,51]

The *stratum granulosum* (Fig. 2-12) is generally less well defined than its counterpart in skin.[2] Lamellar (membrane-coating) granules[60-62] may be released from the

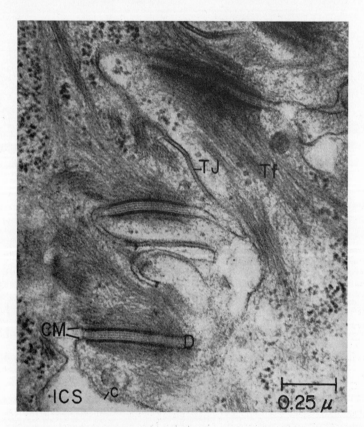

**Fig. 2-9.** Electron micrograph of rat cheek. Note at least two types of cell junctions, namely desmosomes *(D)* and tight (gap?) junctions *(TJ)*. In this preparation the tight junctions and gap junctions cannot be readily distinguished. *C,* cell coat; *CM,* cell membrane; *ICS,* intracellular junction; *Tf,* tonofilaments. (From Stern, I.B.: Periodontics **3:**224, 1965.)

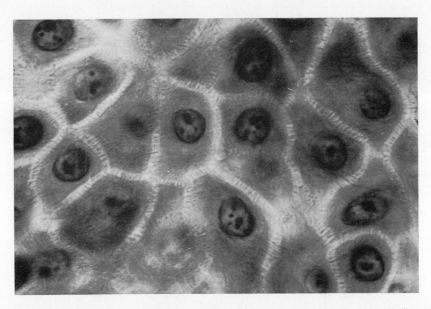

**Fig. 2-10.** Histologic section of stratum spinosum (prickle-cell layer) of human gingival epithelium showing intercellular junctions and tonofibrils.

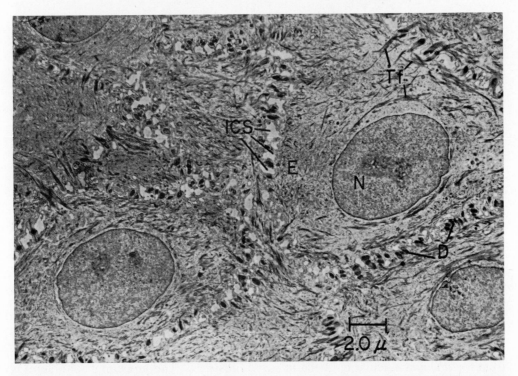

**Fig. 2-11.** Electron micrograph of stratum spinosum of human gingiva. Epithelium cells *(E)* containing round nuclei *(N)* are connected to one another by desmosomes *(D)*. *ICS,* intercellular space (×6000). (From Stern, I.B.: Periodontics **3:**224, 1965.)

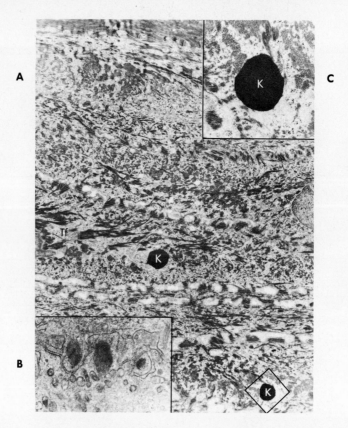

**Fig. 2-12.** **A,** Stratum granulosum (granular layer) of human gingival epithelium. This layer is characterized by flattened cells containing spherical keratohyalin granules *(K)* and coarse bundles of tonofilaments *(Tf)*. The transition from this layer to the stratum corneum is sudden (× 7000). **B,** Membrane-coating granules near the superficial surface of a stratum granulosum cell (× 22,000). **C,** Higher magnification of **A**. (× 23,000). (From Listgarten, M.A.: Oral Sci. Rev. **1**:3, 1972.)

superficial cell surfaces into the intercellular spaces where they contribute to glyco-lipids that function in the permeability barrier of epithelium.[63-65] The stratum granulosum is characterized by the presence of *keratohyalin granules*, which are round, electron-dense cytoplasmic inclusions, approximately 0.1 μm in diameter.[2,5,49,51] They contain a histidine-rich protein, *filaggrin*,[66-70] which is the matrix protein that aggregates the tonofilaments (cytokeratins or intermediate filaments) to form keratin.

The *stratum corneum* consists of very flat cells that have lost their nuclei and cytoplasmic organelles (Fig. 2-13). The cells have thickened cell membranes. They are filled with compacted tonofilaments and isolated lipid droplets.[2,6,49,51] The intercellular junctions gradually disintegrate as the cells approach the surface. Nuclei and isolated organelles may be retained in the most superficial cells when keratinization is incomplete (parakeratinization).

## JUNCTIONAL (ATTACHMENT) EPITHELIUM

**Dentogingival junction**

The microscopic structure of the junctional epithelium (Figs. 2-14 and 2-15) differs from the oral and sulcular epithelia in several respects.[4] The junctional epithelium is the only gingival epithelium with two distinct basal laminas. It has a basal lamina on each surface. One basal lamina is continuous with that of sulcular epithelium. This basal lamina mediates the attachment of the junctional epithelium to the connective

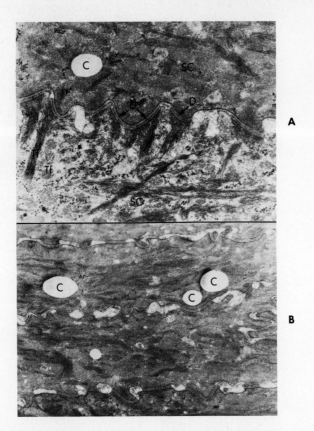

**Fig. 2-13. A,** Junction of stratum granulosum *(SG)* and stratum corneum *(SC).* The cornified cell membrane is markedly thickened. *C,* clear lipid droplet; *D,* desmosome; *Tf,* tonofibril (× 25,000). **B,** Stratum corneum layer. Note absence of cell organelles and dense content of tonofilaments. *C,* lipid droplet (× 18,000). (From Listgarten, M.A.: Oral Sci. Rev. **1:**3, 1972.)

tissue and is known as the *external basal lamina* of the junctional epithelium (Fig. 2-16). The other, the *internal basal lamina,* attaches the junctional epithelium to the tooth surface.[4]

Unlike the oral and sulcular epithelium, the junctional epithelium does not keratinize.[24,25,34,35] The concentration of tonofilaments does not increase between the basal layer and the desquamating surface.[25] The cells produced in the basal layer migrate coronally and desquamate into the sulcus so that the coronal surface of the junctional epithelium is its desquamating surface.[2]

The desquamating surface area is relatively small when compared to the proliferative basal cell area (Fig. 2-16). It appears that the rate of cellular desquamation in relation to surface area for junctional epithelium is greater than that for sulcular or oral epithelium. This increased flow of cells toward the sulcus bottom may enhance repair and maintenance of junctional epithelium and the integrity of the gingival sulcus.[2,71]

The junctional epithelial cells are adapted for adherence to the tooth surface unlike keratinized cells, which cannot adhere.[71,72] This may be important following injury to the junctional epithelium and its epithelial attachment. There are fewer intercellular junctions in the junctional epithelium than in the oral or sulcular epithelium.[73] This may explain both its susceptibility to tearing during probing[74-80] and its greater permeability to migrating cells and fluids.[17-20,26,28,31,80-82]

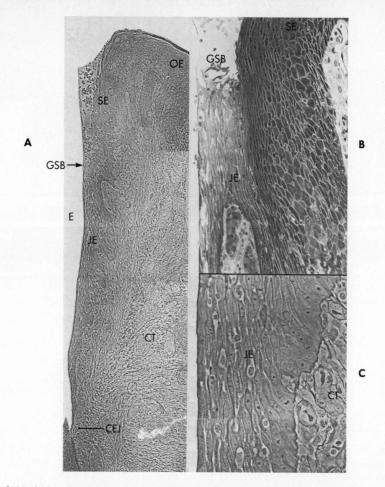

**Fig. 2-14.** **A,** Vertical section through the dentogingival region. The junctional epithelium *(JE)* is attached to the gingival connective tissue *(CT)* and the enamel *(E,* enamel space). *CEJ,* cementoenamel junction; *GSB,* gingival sulcus bottom; *OE,* oral epithelium; *SE,* sulcular epithelium (×100). **B,** Higher magnification of sulcus region. The gingival sulcus bottom *(GSB)* is the coronal end of the junctional epithelium *(JE)*. Sulcular epithelium *(SE)* forms the lateral wall of the sulcus and overlaps the junctional epithelium (×250). **C,** Inflammatory cells migrate through the junctional epithelium *(JE)* toward sulcus. *CT,* gingival connective tissue (×480). (From Schroeder, H.E.: Differentiation of human oral stratified epithelia, Basel, 1981, S. Karger.)

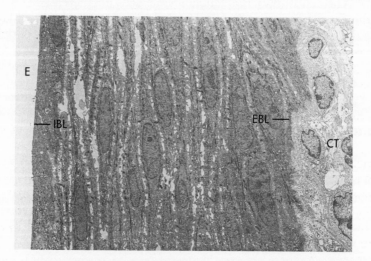

**Fig. 2-15.** Electron micrograph of midportion of junctional epithelium. An internal basal lamina *(IBL)* and an external basal lamina *(EBL)* attach the epithelium to the tooth and gingival connective tissue *(CT)*, respectively. *E,* enamel space (×9000). (From Schroeder, H.E.: Differentiation of human oral stratified epithelia, Basel, 1981, S. Karger.)

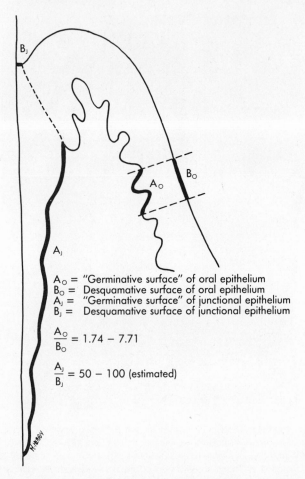

$A_O$ = "Germinative surface" of oral epithelium
$B_O$ = Desquamative surface of oral epithelium
$A_J$ = "Germinative surface" of junctional epithelium
$B_J$ = Desquamative surface of junctional epithelium

$$\frac{A_O}{B_O} = 1.74 - 7.71$$

$$\frac{A_J}{B_J} = 50 - 100 \text{ (estimated)}$$

**Fig. 2-16.** Diagram illustrating the ratio between the "germinative surface" and the corresponding desquamative surface for oral epithelium $A_O$:$B_O$ and junctional epithelium $A_J$:$B_J$. Since the proliferative rates are similar, the desquamation rate in the sulcus region must be much greater than on the vestibular surface. (From Listgarten, M.A.: Oral Sci. Rev. **1**:3, 1972.)

## DEVELOPMENT OF THE EPITHELIAL ATTACHMENT AND GINGIVAL SULCUS

**Formation of the epithelial attachment and gingival sulcus**

The unerupted crown is covered with a layer of *reduced enamel epithelium* (Fig. 2-17), consisting of *reduced ameloblasts* and the external cells of the reduced enamel epithelium.[5] These cells are derived from the stratum intermedium, with some contributions from the stellate reticulum and outer enamel epithelium. The reduced ameloblasts cannot divide, while the outer cells of the reduced enamel epithelium retain mitotic ability[83] (Fig. 2-18). After amelogenesis, the ameloblasts form a basal lamina and hemidesmosomes, which contribute to the primary epithelial attachment.

As the erupting tooth approaches the oral cavity, the reduced enamel epithelium covering the erupting crown nears the epithelium covering the alveolar ridge. The basal cell layers of these epithelia begin to proliferate. As the cusps emerge into the oral cavity, the proliferating cells on the outer surface of the reduced enamel epithelium start to migrate toward the newly formed sulcus and desquamate into the sulcus itself. In the process they displace the reduced ameloblasts still adherent to the cusp tips. The area of the cusp tip is the region where junctional epithelium first replaces reduced enamel epithelium.

The junctional epithelium is the product of the proliferative activity of the outer

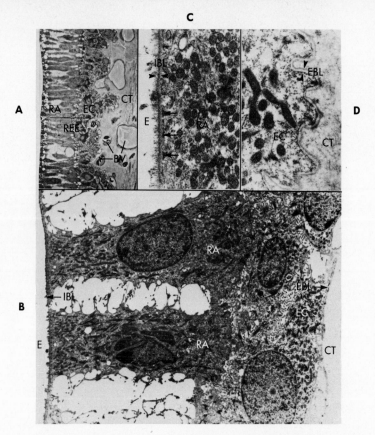

**Fig. 2-17.** **A,** Reduced enamel epithelium of monkey incisor. *BV,* blood vessels; *CT,* follicular connective tissue; *EC,* external cells of reduced enamel epithelium; *RA,* reduced ameloblasts; *REE,* reduced enamel epithelium (×440). **B,** Electron micrograph of junction between reduced ameloblasts *(RA)* and enamel space *(E). CT,* follicular connective tissue; *EBL,* external basal lamina; *EC,* external cell of reduced enamel epithelium; *IBL,* internal basal lamina (×3900). **C,** Reduced ameloblast *(RA)* lining enamel space *(E). IBL,* internal basal lamina; arrows point at hemidesmosomes along cell membrane of *RA* (×18,000). **D,** Junction between reduced enamel epithelium and follicular connective tissue *(CT). EBL,* external basal lamina; *EC,* external cell of reduced enamel epithelium (×18,000). (From Listgarten, M.A.: Oral Sci. Rev. **1:**3, 1972.)

cells of the reduced enamel epithelium. As these cells proliferate, they migrate toward the enamel surface as well as coronally. In the process they displace the reduced ameloblasts from the enamel surface, becoming attached to the tooth via a similar interface.[83]

**Primary and secondary epithelial attachment**

The junction of reduced ameloblasts to the enamel forms the *primary epithelial attachment.* The interface between the junctional epithelium and the tooth surface forms the *secondary epithelial attachment* (Fig. 2-18).

The proliferative activity of the outer cells of the reduced enamel epithelium, which begins near the cusp tip, proceeds by degrees in an apical direction. In the process, the reduced ameloblasts are gradually displaced by the newly formed junctional epithelial cells. This process continues until the entire relatively static reduced enamel epithelium is replaced by junctional epithelium with a relatively rapid rate of turnover estimated to be from 1 week to 10 days.[4]

The low density of intercellular junctions in the junctional epithelium accounts for the readily distensible intercellular spaces. The parallel orientation of the cells to the tooth surface and the lack of a keratinized layer at the desquamative surface of the junctional epithelium also contribute to the relatively high permeability of the junctional epithelium to bacterial and other products from the oral cavity.[84] Inflammatory cells and fluid originating from local blood vessels pass through the junctional epi-

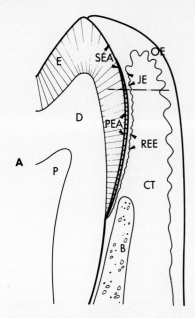
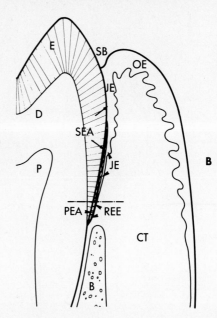

**Fig. 2-18.**    Diagrammatic view of the dentogingival region shortly after eruption. **A,** At the time of eruption most of the enamel *(E)* surface is covered with reduced enamel epithelium *(REE)*, which is connected to the enamel by a primary epithelial attachment *(PEA)*. Near the cusp tip, some ameloblasts have become transformed into junctional epithelial cells that are attached to the enamel by a secondary epithelial attachment *(SEA)*. **B,** After further eruption, proliferation of the outer cells of the reduced enamel epithelium contributes to the gradual replacement of the reduced enamel epithelium *(REE)* by a junctional epithelium *(JE)*. B, bone; *CT,* gingival connective tissue; *D,* dentin; *OE,* oral epithelium; *P,* pulp; *SB,* sulcus bottom. (From Schroeder, H.E., and Listgarten, M.A.: Fine structure of the developing epithelial attachment of human teeth. In Wolsky, A., editor: Monographs in developmental biology, vol. 2, Basel, 1971, S. Karger.)

thelium into the sulcus. Inflammatory cell infiltration of the epithelium tends to undermine its structural integrity.[85] The low cohesive forces between the junctional epithelial cells, together with repeated traumatic injury of the coronal portion of this epithelium, lead to frequent tears that are rapidly repaired because of the rapid migration rate of the epithelium (see Fig. 2-16).

The gradual gingival recession that uncovers the anatomic crown[85a] and possibly some of the root surface is known as *passive eruption* or *exposure.* Passive eruption has been classified into *four* stages, depending on the position of the dentoepithelial junction on the tooth[33]:

*Stage 1.*    The dentoepithelial junction is located on enamel.

*Stage 2.*    The dentoepithelial junction is located on enamel as well as cementum.

*Stage 3.*    The dentoepithelial junction is located entirely on cementum, extending coronally to the cementoenamel junction.

*Stage 4.*    The dentoepithelial junction is on cementum, and the root surface is exposed as a result of further migration of the dentoepithelial junction on the cementum.

## CUTICULAR STRUCTURES AT THE DENTOEPITHELIAL JUNCTION

Although the junctional epithelium may be directly attached to enamel, cementum, or both, a number of organic layers may be interposed between the tooth surface *per se* and the junctional epithelium.[4] These have been called *pellicles* and *cuticles* and their origin, composition, and importance have been the subject of debate.[86-96] There are a number of hypotheses as to their origin.

It has been suggested that these surface coatings be classified as either *endogenous,* that is of developmental origin, or *acquired* coatings, which are salivary or bacterial

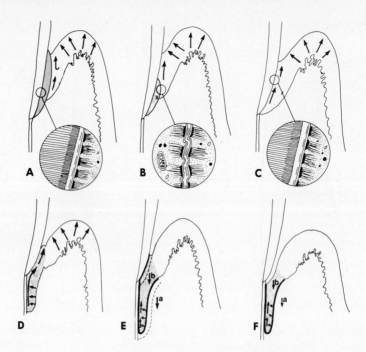

**Fig. 2-19.** *Dynamics of migration of the tissues of the dentoepithelial junction.* **A,** *The dentoepithelial junction first consists of reduced ameloblasts attached by hemidesmosomes to the lamina lucida. The oral epithelial cells migrate to the gingival surface and keratinize (arrows). Some cells join the reduced enamel epithelium, to which they attach.* **B,** *The reduced ameloblasts are gradually displaced by the junctional epithelium, cells of which are joined by desmosomes and by tight and gap junctions. When the reduced enamel epithelium gives rise to the junctional epithelium (x), mitotic activity is increased. Here the cells of the outer enamel epithelium, and possibly the stratum intermedium, form a locus of proliferation.* **C,** *With the complete replacement of the reduced enamel epithelium by the junctional epithelium, the attachment occurs by the same mechanism as shown in* **A.** **D,** *In time the junctional epithelium may be found attaching to both the enamel and the cementum. How does this apical migration occur?* **E,** *The junctional epithelium renews itself in a matter of days, as does the gingival epithelium. Cells migrate in the pathways denoted by the arrows in* **D.** *The cells of the junctional epithelium travel from basal lamina to the epithelial attachment. In inflammation, the basal cells at* a *migrate apically and laterally into areas of collagenolysis. They form a new basal lamina. Arrow at* b *represents a deepening of the sulcus.* **F,** *Even when the junctional epithelium has completely migrated onto cementum, the attachment is still mediated by the basal lamina and by hemidesmosomes.*

products.[95] The endogenous coatings are the ones most likely to be found between the tooth and the junctional epithelium. They include incompletely mineralized enamel matrix that forms a *subsurface pellicle* on enamel, reduced enamel epithelial remnants, *afibrillar coronal cementum,* and the *dental cuticle.* These may occur singly or in combination—for example, dental cuticle over coronal cementum (Fig. 2-20).[97]

*Afibrillar coronal cementum* is described in Chapter 3. It forms before tooth eruption in areas where reduced enamel epithelium has degenerated. The exposed enamel may become covered with a thin layer of coronal cementum that may eventually be covered, in turn, by junctional epithelium.

*Dental cuticle* probably is a product of the junctional epithelium.[4,95] Continued production of basal lamina by the junctional epithelium may produce a thickened layer of basal lamina, which is then seen as dental cuticle.

The dental cuticle may be an acquired coating, possibly a product of inflammation. Acquired coatings include acquired surface pellicles, which are produced by adsorption of salivary, dietary, microbial, and hematogenous materials to tooth surfaces and possibly to calculus.[98]

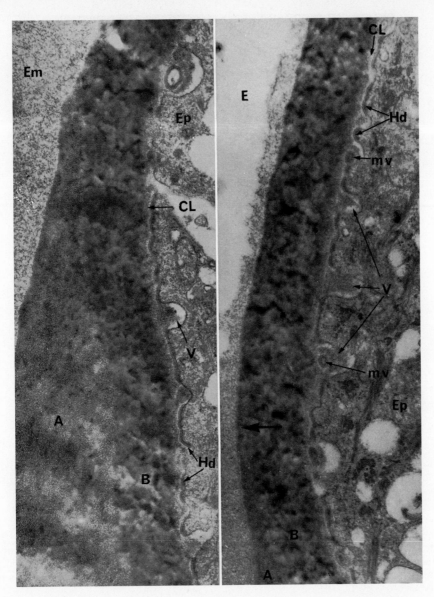

**Fig. 2-20.**   Mandibular deciduous molar of 5-year-old boy. Junctional epithelial cell *(EP)* is attached to the dental cuticle *(B)* via a basal lamina *(CL)* and hemidesmosomes *(Hd)*. The dental cuticle in turn is attached directly to enamel *(E,* enamel space; *Em,* enamel matrix) or to a layer of afibrillar coronal cementum *(A)*, which covers the enamel. *Mv,* microvilli; *V,* structure resembling discharging vacuole (×39,000). (From Listgarten, M.A.: Am. J. Anat. **119:**147, 1966.)

## GINGIVAL CONNECTIVE TISSUE

Gingival connective tissue is composed of a *lamina propria,* which consists primarily of densely packed *collagen* and reticular fibers with occasional *elastic* and *oxytalan* fibers embedded in a ground substance that also contains a variety of cells, vascular elements, and nerves.

Gingival connective tissue has fingerlike projections, *papillae* (Fig. 2-21), extending into depressions on the undersurface of the oral and sulcular epithelia.[10,11] The connective tissue papillae are the *papillary layer* of the lamina propria, while the zone of reticular fibers forms the *reticular layer.* A submucosa is lacking.

**Lamina propria**

**Papillary and reticular layer**

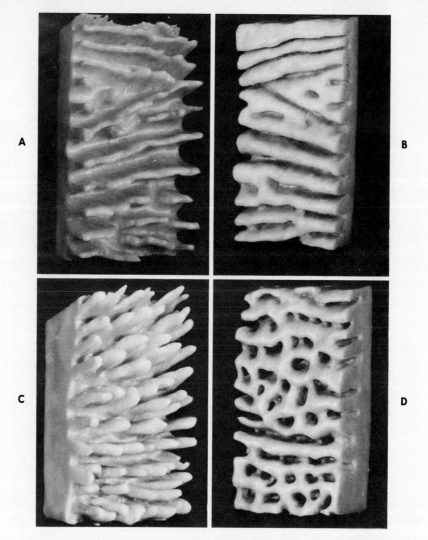

**Fig. 2-21.** Wax reconstruction of gingival epithelium/connective tissue interface. **A** and **C,** Connective tissue. **B** and **D,** Epithelium. (Reprinted from The three-dimensional concept of the epithelium connective tissue boundary of gingiva by T. Karring and H. Löe from Acta Odontol. Scand. **28:**917, 1970, by permission of Norwegian University Press [Universitetsforlaget AS], Oslo.)

## Gingival fibers

Collagen fibers from the reticular layer insert into the periosteum of the alveolar process and into the cementum. The fibers of the gingiva are classified into groups depending on their location, origin, and insertion.[99-104] These fiber groups are intimately blended and are sometimes difficult to differentiate. The various gingival fibers are shown in Fig. 2-22.

1. *Dentogingival group.* These fibers extend from the cementum apical to the junctional epithelium and course laterally and coronally into the lamina propria of the gingiva.
2. *Alveologingival group.* The fibers of this small group arise from the alveolar crest and insert coronally into the lamina propria.
3. *Circular group.* This small group of fibers encircles the teeth.
4. *Transseptal group.* A group of prominent horizontal fibers that extend interproximally between adjacent teeth are called *transseptal* fibers.

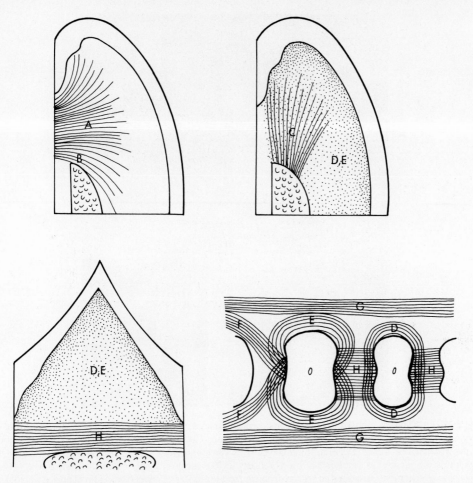

**Fig. 2-22.** Diagrammatic representation of the main gingival fiber groups. *A,* Dentogingival. *B,* Dentoperiosteal. *C,* Alveologingival. *D,* Circumferential. *E,* Semicircular. *F,* Transgingival. *G,* Intergingival. *H,* Transseptal.

5. *Dentoperiosteal group.* On the oral and vestibular surfaces of the jaws, a prominent fiber group called *dentoperiosteal* extends from the tooth, passing over the alveolar crest to blend with fibers of the periosteum of the alveolar bone.
6. *Semicircular group.* These fibers from the mesial or distal root surface of a tooth extend around the vestibular or oral surface to insert on the opposite side of the same tooth.
7. *Transgingival group.* Fibers from proximal root surfaces radiate through the embrasures to blend with fibers on the vestibular and oral surfaces.
8. *Intergingival group.* These fibers run parallel to dentition on vestibular and oral surfaces.

Fibers that connect the cementum to the alveolar bone are the principal fibers of the periodontal ligament and will be described in Chapter 3.

## FIBRILLAR ELEMENTS

Connective tissue fibers are made up of collagen (Fig. 2-23). Collagen accounts for approximately 60% of the total protein of gingiva. Its molecule is rodlike, 300 nm long and 1.5 nm in diameter, and consists of three helically packed polypeptide chains, the $\alpha$-chains. The $\alpha$-chains are classified as $\alpha1$-, $\alpha2$-, $\alpha A$- and $\alpha B$-chains.[46,105] In addition, several $\alpha1$-chains with different chemical compositions have been identified. Five types of collagen have been described in detail.[105-107] As many as 10 types have been reported.

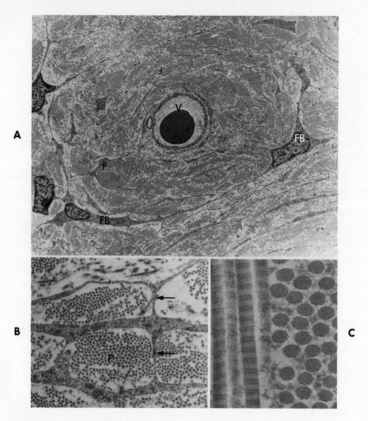

**Fig. 2-23. A,** Gingival connective tissue is composed primarily of collagen fibers *(F)*, which in turn consist of up to hundreds of fibrils; in this electron micrograph they are sectioned transversely. Fibroblasts *(FB)* are responsible for the maintenance and remodelling of the collagenous framework. Their cytoplasmic processes, which extend throughout the connective tissue, allow the fibroblasts to form an interconnected cellular network. *V,* Venule containing an erythrocyte. **B,** Magnified section of above. Note the junction between processes of adjacent fibroblasts *(arrows).* F, collagen fiber. **C,** Collagen fibrils cut longitudinally and transversely. Note typical cross-striations.

**Collagen structure**

    The most common form, type I collagen, is composed of two α-chains and an α2-chain. This is abbreviated as an $[\alpha 1(I)]_2 \alpha 2$ molecular structure. Type I collagen accounts for most of the collagen in skin, mucosa, bone, dentin, and cementum. Type I collagen molecules are aggregated into striated *fibrils* (Fig. 2-23, C) with an axial periodicity of about 70 nm. The fibrils in turn are grouped into bundles of various sizes—the collagen *fibers* (Fig. 2-23, A, B). These are the smallest structural units detectable with light microscopy.

    Small, loosely packed collagen fibers in perivascular and perineural locations and beneath epithelial linings have been described as reticular fibers.[108,109] They take up silver stains preferentially and are called *argyrophilic fibers.* Such fibers may be composed of type III collagen, i.e., $[\alpha 1(III)]_3$ rather than type I collagen.[45,46,105-108] Basement membranes may contain both type IV[46-48,107,108] and type V collagen[107] as well as glycoprotein constituents.

    There are few elastic fibers in gingival connective tissue. They are detectable in perivascular locations (Fig. 2-24) where they appear as small aggregations of fibers consisting of an amorphous elastin component surrounded by microfibrillar elements.[110-114]

    *Oxytalan fibers,*[115-125] which may be interspersed among the collagen fibers, appear ultrastructurally similar to the microfibrillar component of elastic fibers (Fig. 2-25).

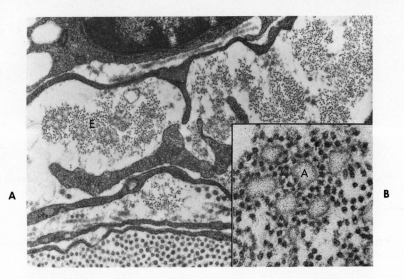

**Fig. 2-24.** **A,** Elastin fibers *(E)* in a perivascular location. **B,** Fibers are typically composed of an amorphous *(A)* and a microfibrillar *(F)* component.

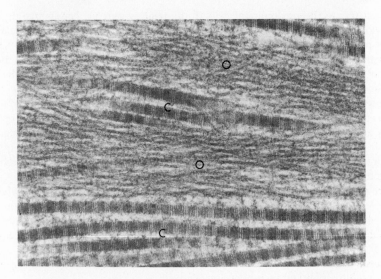

**Fig. 2-25.** Oxytalan fibers *(O)* adjacent to collagenous fibers *(C)*.

They may represent an immature form of elastic fiber, rather than an unravelling of collagen fibrils.[124-127] Oxytalan fibers resist acid oxidation.[115] They can be distinguished from elastic fibers ultrastructurally by the absence of the amorphous elastin component.[116,120,121,124]

*Anchoring fibrils* may be found in intimate contact with the basal lamina of epidermal and mucosal epithelium.[52,54] They are short, curved fibrils with a different banding pattern than type I collagen.[2] They are composed of recently described type VII collagen. They help to anchor the basal lamina to the adjacent connective tissue (Figs. 2-7 and 2-26).

## Ground substance

Fibers are surrounded by a highly hydrated ground substance composed of proteoglycans and glycoproteins.[128] The ground substance facilitates cell movement and

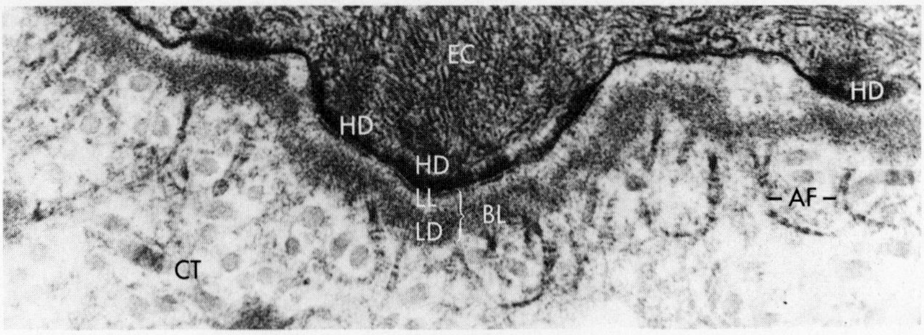

**Fig. 2-26.** Curving, striated anchoring fibrils *(AF)* appear to anchor the lamina densa *(LD)* of the basal lamina *(BL)* to the underlying connective tissue *(CT)*. *EC,* epithelial cell; *HD,* hemidesmosomes; *LL,* Lamina lucida (×44,000). (From Listgarten, M.A.: Oral Sci. Rev. **1:**3, 1972.)

the diffusion of various biologically active substances, including gases, minerals, nutrients, waste products, hormones, enzymes, and so on.

### Connective tissue cells

Several types of cells can be identified in the lamina propria.

1. *Fibroblasts* are the predominant cells in the healthy gingival connective tissue.[129] They are widely distributed between the gingival fibers and are found in perivascular locations. They play a major role in the maintenance of gingival connective tissue. They are responsible for the synthesis of different collagen types[130-134] and possibly other types of fibers[135] as well as the glycoproteins and proteoglycans of the ground substance.[136] In addition, they play an active role in the resorption and remodeling of the collagenous framework.[137-143]

2. *Mast cells* are generally located perivascularly and are seen rarely within the epithelium.[144] They are identified by their unique cytoplasmic granules.[145,146] They produce histamine, which mediates the early stages of inflammation. They decrease in mild inflammation and increase in chronic inflammation.[147-149] They also produce heparin, which may modulate the rate of bone resorption.[150]

3. There are few *macrophages, monocytes, lymphocytes, plasma cells* and *polymorphonuclear leukocytes* in healthy tissues. They tend to be more numerous near the junctional epithelium. Their role is defensive. The macrophages are mononuclear cells that act primarily as scavengers while monocytes, lymphocytes, and plasma cells[151] act as mediators of immune responses.

4. *Osteoblasts and osteoclasts* are found close to the alveolar process. They are responsible for bone formation and resorption, respectively.

5. *Cementoblasts and cementoclasts* are responsible for cementum formation and resorption, respectively.

### VASCULAR SUPPLY

The major arterial supply to the maxillary gingiva includes the posterosuperior alveolar, the infraorbital, the greater palatine, and the sphenopalatine arteries. The mandibular gingiva is supplied by branches of the inferior alveolar artery, including the mental, the sublingual, and the buccal arteries. The gingival blood supply originates from periosteal arterioles that course over the alveolar processes and form anastomoses with vessels from the periodontal ligament and marrow spaces.[152,153] The arterioles supply a capillary plexus that courses below the various gingival epithelia.[154] Fine capillary loops extend into the papillary layer of the oral epithelium. Beneath the junctional epithelium, the plexus lacks distinct capillary loops.[155-157] However, the vessels are readily affected by injurious stimuli.[26,155-160] In the presence of chronic irritation, they will enlarge and acquire varicosities.[161,162]

Leakage of fluid and diapedesis of leukocytes into the lamina propria subjacent to

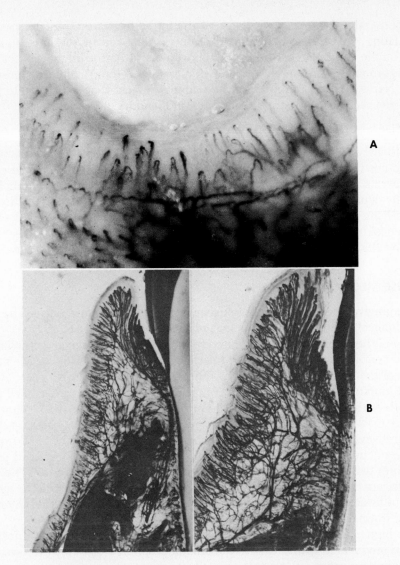

**Fig. 2-27. A,** Vital micrograph of capillary loops near the surface of a healthy human marginal gingiva. **B,** Micrographs of India ink–injected vessels in the gingiva of a perfused monkey. (**B** courtesy of D.W. Cohen, Philadelphia, Pennsylvania.)

the junctional epithelium is the major source of *sulcular fluid* and of inflammatory cells found within the intercellular spaces of the junctional epithelium.[163,164]

The venous and lymphatic vessels[165] follow a course closely paralleling that of the arteriolar supply (Fig. 2-27). The lymphatics from the maxillary gingiva drain into the deep cervical lymph nodes. Those from the mandibular gingiva drain into the submental, submandibular, and cervical lymph nodes. Their main function is to return fluids and filterable plasma components to the blood via the thoracic duct. Lymphatic capillaries differ from blood capillaries by the presence of intraluminal valves, the lack of red blood cells in the vessels, and the absence of a continuous basal lamina around the vessels at the ultrastructural level. In addition, gaps frequently occur between cells of the endothelial lining.

## NERVE SUPPLY

The nerve supply follows a course resembling that of the vascular supply. The maxillary gingiva is supplied by terminal branches of the posterior, middle, and anterosuperior alveolar nerves, branches of the infraorbital nerve, greater palatine, and nasopalatine nerves. The mandibular gingiva is supplied by the buccal and mental nerves on the vestibular side and the sublingual nerve on the lingual aspect. Terminal branches from the inferior alveolar nerve may provide some additional sensory innervation. Nerve endings terminate as free nonmyelinated fibers sensitive to pain or in specialized receptors for temperature, pressure, and tactile sensations.[166-170]

## EPITHELIAL-MESENCHYMAL INTERACTIONS

Epithelial and connective tissues are each essential to the maintenance and function of the other through a phenomenon called *inductive interaction*.[171] The connective tissue exerts a major effect on the differentiation of the overlying epithelium.[172-174] Thus the dense lamina propria under gingival and palatal mucosa tends to influence the overlying epithelium to keratinize. By contrast, the loose and elastic submucosa of the cheek will direct the overlying epithelium to remain nonkeratinized. Epithelial cells have the genetic potential to differentiate into either keratinized or nonkeratinized forms.

## DEFENSE MECHANISMS OF THE GINGIVA

The gingival tissues are continuously coated by bacteria and saliva. They are subjected to mechanical stresses from mastication and brushing.

Among the mechanisms of defense are gingival and junctional epithelial cell desquamation and a rapid transit time. Superficial injuries are resisted by the keratinized surface of the gingiva and repaired by the rapidity of cell turnover.

The junctional epithelium lacks keratinization and its cells are oriented parallel to the tooth surface. Thus vertical tears are likely to occur even with minor stresses (such as mastication or oral hygiene). Rapid repair, in a week or less, is due to the high turnover rate of this epithelium, coupled with the high rate of cell desquamation into the sulcus. The injured epithelium is shed coronally and is replaced with intact epithelium arising from the progenitor cell pool in the basal layer.[2] The excellent vascularization and comparatively high turnover rate of the connective tissue compartment favor the rapid repair of more extensive gingival injuries and the healing of surgical wounds.

The high permeability of junctional epithelium to diffusible substances permits bacterial products to gain access to the lamina propria.[17-20,26-31] However systemic and local immune reactions against these products counteract their penetration. Immune reactions may also neutralize their noxious properties.[19]

One of the most important defenses against bacterial infection is the ability of the host to mobilize large numbers of polymorphonuclear leukocytes, especially neutrophils.[175-177] These cells, which migrate from the vascular plexus adjacent to the junctional epithelium, are able to penetrate the junctional epithelium and migrate toward the gingival sulcus. They are capable of phagocytizing and killing a variety of microorganisms.

## GINGIVAL SULCULAR FLUID

Sulcular fluid is an inflammatory exudate from the leaky venules adjacent to the sulcus and junctional epithelium. It is one of the first detectable signs of gingival inflammation.[163,164,178] Increased sulcular fluid flow begins before the onset of some of the cardinal signs of gingival inflammation.[179,180] Sulcular fluid is believed to contribute to gingival defense. Fluid flow is capable of flushing particulate materials such as carbon particles and bacteria from the sulcus.[180,181] However soluble substances from the oral cavity may diffuse against the current of sulcular fluid and reach the underlying connective tissue. A number of substances, some with high molecular weights are capable of penetrating the gingival tissues in this fashion through the intercellular spaces of the junctional epithelium. Among these are histamine,[26] albumin,[81,182] endotoxins,[29,183,184] and horseradish peroxidase.[18,20,31]

Leukocytes may enter the sulcus where they have an antibacterial function.[4,164,175,185-189] Additional protection is provided by antibodies to plaque bacteria and complement.[190-196] Assorted enzymes, primarily of lysosomal origin, may also provide some protection.[164,197-207] Sulcular fluid may also serve as a vehicle for antibacterial drugs. The sulcular fluid levels of some drugs (e.g., tetracyclines) may exceed their blood level by two- to ten-fold.[208-213]

## REFERENCES

1. Orban, R., and Sicher, H.: The oral mucosa, J. Dent. Educ. **10:**94, 1946.

2. Listgarten, M.A.: Normal development, structure, physiology and repair of gingival epithelium. In Melcher, A.H., and Zarb, G.A., editors: Gingival epithelium, Oral Sci. Rev. **1:**3, 1972.

3. Listgarten, M.A.: Changing concepts about the dento-epithelial junction, J. Can. Dent. Assn. **36:**70, 1970.

4. Schroeder, H.E., and Listgarten, M.A.: Fine structure of the developing epithelial attachment of human teeth. In Wolsky, A., editor: Monographs in developmental biology, vol. 2, Basel, 1971, S. Karger.

5. Schroeder, H.E.: Gingival tissue. In Cohen, B., and Kramer, I.R.H., editors: Scientific foundations of dentistry, London, 1976, William Heinemann Medical Books Ltd., p. 426.

6. Selvig, K.A.: Structure and metabolism of the normal periodontium. In Klavan, B., et al., editors: International conference on research in the biology of periodontal disease, Chicago, 1977, University of Illinois College of Dentistry, p. 2.

7. Caffesse, R.G., et al.: The effect of mechanical stimulation on the keratinization of sulcular epithelium, J. Periodontol. **53:**89, 1982.

8. Weinmann, J.P., and Meyer, J.: Types of keratinization in the human gingiva, J. Invest. Dermatol. **32:**87, 1959.

9. Weiss, M.D., Weinmann, J.P., and Meyer, J.: Degree of keratinization and glycogen content in the uninflamed and inflamed gingiva and alveolar mucosa, J. Periodontol. **30:**208, 1959.

10. Karring, T., and Löe, H.: The three-dimensional concept of the epithelium connective tissue boundary of gingiva, Acta Odontol. Scand. **28:**917, 1970.

11. Klein-Szanto, A.J.P., and Schroeder, H.E.: Architecture and density of the connective tissue papillae of the human oral mucosa, J. Anat. **123:**93, 1977.

12. Orban, B.: Clinical and histologic study of the surface characteristics of the gingiva, Oral Surg. **1:**827, 1948.

13. Fehr, C., and Mühlemann, H.R.: The surface of the free and attached gingiva studied with the replica method, Oral Surg. **8:**649, 1955.

14. Soni, N.N., Silberkweit, M., and Hayes, R.L.: Histological characteristics of stippling in children, J. Periodontol. **34:**427, 1965.

15. Rosenberg, H.M., and Massler, M.: Gingival stippling in young adult males, J. Periodontol. **38:**473, 1967.

16. Owings, J.R.: A clinical investigation of the relationship between stippling and surface keratinization of the attached gingiva, J. Periodontol. **40:**588, 1969.

17. McDougall, W.A.: Pathways of penetration and effects of horseradish peroxidase in rat molar gingiva, Arch. Oral Biol. **15:**621, 1970.

18. McDougall, W.A.: Penetration pathways of a topically applied foreign protein into rat gingiva, J. Periodont. Res. **6:**89, 1971.

19. McDougall, W.A.: The effect of topical antigen on the gingiva of sensitized rabbits, J. Periodont. Res. **9:**153, 1974.

20. Tanaka, T.: Transport pathway and uptake of microperoxidase in the junctional epithelium of healthy rat gingiva, J. Periodont. Res. **19:**26, 1984.

21. Gottlieb, B.: Der Epithelansatz am Zahne, Dtsch. Mschr. Zahnheilk. **39:**142, 1921.

22. Waerhaug, J.: Gingival pocket: anatomy, pathology, deepening and elimination, Odont. Tidskr. **60:**Suppl. No. 1, 1952.

23. Gottlieb, B., and Orban, B.: Active and passive eruption of the teeth, J. Dent. Res. **13:**214, 1933.

24. Schroeder, H.E.: Ultrastructure of the junctional epithelium of the human gingiva, Helv. Odont. Acta **13:**65, 1969.

25. Schroeder, H.E., and Münzel-Pedrazzoli, S.: Morphometric analysis comparing junctional and oral epithelium of normal gingiva, Helv. Odont. Acta **14:**53, 1970.

26. Egelberg, J.: Diffusion of histamine into the gingival crevice and through the crevicular epithelium, Acta Odontol. Scand. **21:**271, 1963.

27. Fine, D.H., Pechersky, J.L., and McKibben, D.H.: Penetration of human gingival sulcular tissue by carbon particles, Arch. Oral Biol. **14:**1117, 1969.

28. Gavin, J.B.: The effect of histamine on the permeability of gingiva, New Zealand Dent. J. **68:**291, 1972.

29. Schwartz, J., Stinson, F.L., and Parker, R.B.: The passage of tritiated bacterial endotoxin

across intact gingival crevicular epithelium, J. Periodontol. **43**:270, 1972.

30. Jensen, R.L., and Folke, L.E.A.: The passage of exogenous tritiated thymidine into gingival tissues, J. Periodontol. **45**:786, 1974.

31. Kahnberg, K.-E., Morgan, P., and Lindhe, J.: The cellular response to topically applied horseradish peroxidase in the gingiva of normal and immunized dogs. I. A histometric and ultrastructural study, J. Periodont. Res. **13**:46, 1978.

32. Yamasaki, A., et al.: Ultrastructure of the junctional epithelium of germfree rat gingiva, J. Periodontol. **50**:641, 1979.

33. Stern, I.B.: Oral mucous membrane. In Bhaskar, S.N., editor: Orban's oral histology and embryology, ed. 10, St. Louis, 1986, The C.V. Mosby Co.

34. Listgarten, M.A.: Electron microscopic study of the dento-gingival junction of man, Am. J. Anat. **119**:147, 1966.

35. Rebstein, F.: La jonction entre l'épithélium et l'email chez l'homme: étude histologique et histochimique, Parodont. Acad. Rev. **1**:207, 1967.

36. Yamasaki, A., et al.: Dento-epithelial junction in erupted rat molars, J. Electron Microsc. (Tokyo) **24**:45, 1975.

37. Kobayashi, K., Rose, G.G., and Mahan, C.J.: Ultrastructure of the dentoepithelial junction, J. Periodont. Res. **11**:313, 1976.

38. Skougaard, M.R., and Beagrie, G.S.: The renewal of gingival epithelium in marmosets (*Callithrix jacchus*) as determined through autoradiography with thymidine-H, Acta Odontol. Scand. **20**:467, 1962.

39. Skougaard, M.: Turnover of the gingival epithelium in marmosets, Acta Odontol. Scand. **23**:623, 1965.

40. Skougaard, M.: Cell population kinetics of the gingival epithelium, Copenhagen, 1965, International Science Publication.

41. Skougaard, M.R.: Cell renewal with special reference to the gingival epithelium. In Staple, P.H., editor: Advances in oral biology, vol. 4, New York, 1970, Academic Press, Inc., p. 261.

42. Anderson, G.S., and Stern, I.B.: The proliferation and migration of the attachment epithelium on the cemental surface of the rat incisor, Periodontics **4**:115, 1966.

43. Dodson, J.W., and Hay, E.D.: Secretion of collagenous stroma by isolated epithelium grown *in vitro*, Exp. Cell Res. **65**:215, 1971.

44. Kefalides, N.A.: Basement membranes: structural and biochemical considerations, J. Invest. Dermatol. **65**:85, 1975.

45. Birkedal-Hansen, H., et al.: Multiple collagen gene expression with type III predominence in rat mucosal keratinocytes, Collagen Rel. Res. **2**:287, 1982.

46. Trelstad, R.L.: The developmental biology of vertebrate collagens, J. Histochem. Cytochem. **21**:521, 1973.

47. Yaoita, H., Foidart, J.-M., and Katz, S.I.: Localization of the collagenous component in skin basement membrane, J. Invest. Dermatol. **70**:191, 1978.

48. Stanley, J.R., et al.: Structure and function of basement membrane, J. Invest. Dermatol. **79**:69s, 1982.

49. Listgarten, M.A.: The ultrastructure of human gingival epithelium, Am. J. Anat. **114**:49, 1964.

50. Stern, I.B.: Electron microscopic observations of oral epithelium. I. Basal cells and the basement membrane, Periodontics **3**:224, 1965.

51. Schroeder, H.E., and Theilade, J.: Electron microscopy of normal human gingival epithelium, J. Periodont. Res. **1**:95, 1966.

52. Susi, F.R., Belt, W.D., and Kelly, J.W.: Fine structure of fibrillar complexes associated with the basement membrane in human oral mucosa, J. Cell Biol. **34**:686, 1967.

53. Briggaman, R.A., Dalldorf, F.G., and Wheeler, C.E., Jr.: Formation and origin of basal lamina and anchoring fibrils in adult human skin, J. Cell Biol. **51**:384, 1971.

54. Briggaman, R.A., and Wheeler, C.E.: The epidermal-dermal junction, J. Invest. Dermatol. **65**:71, 1975.

55. Dale, B.A., Stern, I.B., and Huang, L-Y.: Identification of fibrous proteins in fetal rat epidermis by electrophoretic and immunologic techniques, J. Invest. Dermatol. **66**:230, 1976.

56. Osborn, M.: Components of the cellular cytoskeleton: a new generation of markers of histogenetic origin, J. Invest. Dermatol. **82**:443, 1984.

57. Sun, T-T., et al.: Keratin classes: molecular markers for different types of epithelial differentiation, J. Invest. Dermatol. **81**:109s, 1983.

58. Schroeder, H.E., and Münzel-Pedrazzoli, S.: Application of stereologic methods to stratified gingival epithelia, J. Microsc. **92**:179, 1970.

59. Schroeder, H.E., and Amstad-Jossi, M.: Epithelial differentiation at the mucogingival junction: a stereological comparison of the epithelia of the vestibular gingiva and alveolar mucosa, Cell Tissue Res. **202**:75, 1979.

60. Matoltsy, A.G., and Parakkal, P.F.: Membrane coating granules of keratinizing epithelia, J. Cell Biol. **24**:297, 1965.

61. Frithiof, L., and Wersall, J.: A highly ordered structure in keratinizing human oral epithelium, J. Ultrastr. Res. **12**:371, 1965.

62. Martinez, I.R., and Peters, A.: Membrane-coating granules and membrane modifications in keratinizing epithelia, Am. J. Anat. **130**:93, 1971.

63. Squier, C.A.: The permeability of keratinized and non-keratinized oral epithelium to horseradish peroxidase, J. Ultrastr. Res. **43:**160, 1973.

64. Hayward, A.F., and Hackermann, M.: Electron microscopy of membrane-coating granules and cell surface coat in keratinized human oral epithelium, J. Ultrastr. Res. **43:**205, 1973.

65. Wertz, P.W., and Downing, D.T.: Glycolipids in mammalian epidermis: structure and function in the water barrier, Science **217:**1261, 1982.

66. Dale, B.A., Lonsdale-Eccles, J.D., and Holbrook, K.A.: Stratum corneum basic protein: an interfilamentous matrix protein of epidermal keratin. In Bernstein, I.A., and Seiji, M., editors: Biochemistry of normal and abnormal epidermal differentiation, Tokyo, 1980, University of Tokyo Press, p. 311.

67. Lonsdale-Eccles, J.D., Haugen, J.A., and Dale, B.A.: A phosphorylated keratohyalin-derived precursor of epidermal stratum corneum basic protein, J. Biol. Chem. **255:**2235, 1980.

68. Steinert, P.M., et al.: Characterization of a class of cationic proteins that specifically interact with intermediate filaments, Proc. Nat. Acad. Sci. (USA) **78:**4097, 1981.

69. Dale, B.A., Lonsdale-Eccles, J.D., and Lynley, A.M.: Two-dimensional analysis of proteins of rat oral epithelia and epidermis, Arch. Oral Biol. **27:**529, 1982.

70. Dale, B.A., Thompson, W.B., and Stern, I.B.: Distribution of histidine-rich basic protein, a possible keratin matrix protein, in rat oral epithelium, Arch. Oral Biol. **27:**535, 1982.

71. Schroeder, H.: Differentiation of human oral stratified epithelia, Basel, 1981, S. Karger, p. 147.

72. Squier, C.A.: Keratinization of the sulcular epithelium: a pointless pursuit? J. Periodontol. **52:**426, 1981.

73. Geisenheimer, J., and Han, S.S.: A quantitative electron microscopic study of desmosomes and hemidesmosomes in human crevicular epithelium, J. Periodontol. **42:**396, 1971.

74. Weinreb, M.M.: The epithelial attachment, J. Periodontol. **31:**186, 1960.

75. Armitage, G.C., Svanberg, G.K., and Löe, H.: Microscopic evaluation of clinical measurements of connective tissue attachment levels, J. Clin. Periodontol. **4:**173, 1977.

76. Spray, J.R., et al.: Microscopic demonstration of the position of periodontal probes, J. Periodontol. **49:**148, 1978.

77. Listgarten, M.A.: Periodontol probing: what does it mean? J. Clin. Periodontol. **7:**165, 1980.

78. Van der Velden, U.: Periodontal probing: clinical and histological investigations, Thesis, University of Amsterdam, 1981.

79. Jansen, J., Pilot, T., and Corba, N.: Histologic evaluation of probe penetration during clinical assessment of periodontol attachment levels: an investigation of experimentally induced periodontal lesions in beagle dogs, J. Clin. Periodontol. **8:**98, 1981.

80. Fowler, C., et al.: Histologic probe position in treated and untreated human periodontal tissues, J. Clin. Periodontol. **9:**373, 1982.

81. Tolo, K.: Transport across stratified non-keratinized epithelium, J. Periodont. Res. **6;**237, 1971.

82. Nasjleti, C.E., and Caffesse, R.G.: Dextran penetration through nonkeratinized and keratinized epithelia in monkeys, J. Periodontol. **55:**424, 1984.

83. Glavind, L., and Zander, H.A.: Dynamics of dental epithelium during tooth eruption, J. Dent. Res. **49:**549, 1970.

84. Listgarten, M.A.: Pathogenesis of periodontitis, J. Clin. Periodontol. **13:**418, 1986.

85. Stern, I.B.: Current concepts of the dentogingival junction: the epithelial and connective tissue attachments to the tooth, J. Periodontol. **52:**465, 1981.

85a. Smith, R.G.: A longitudinal study into the depth of the clinical gingival sulcus of human canine teeth during and after eruption, J. Periodont. Res. **17:**427, 1982.

86. Gottlieb, B.: Ätiologie und Prophylaxe der Zahnkaries, Z. Stomatol. **19:**129, 1921.

87. Kronfeld, R.: The epithelial attachment and so-called Nasmyth's membrane, J. Am. Den. Assn. **17:**1889, 1930.

88. Dawes, C., Jenkins, G.N., and Tonge, C.H.: The nomenclature of the integuments of the enamel surface of teeth, Brit. Dent. J. **115:**65, 1963.

89. Hodson, J.J.: A critical review of the dental cuticle with special reference to recent investigations, Int. Dent. J. **16:**350, 1966.

90. Dawes, C.: The nature of dental plaque, films, and calcareous deposits, N.Y. Acad. Sci. **153:**102, 1967.

91. Meckel, A.H.: The nature and importance of organic deposits on dental enamel, Caries Res. **2:**104, 1968.

92. Schwartz, R., and Massler, M.: Tooth accumulated materials: a review and classification, J. Periodontol. **40:**407, 1969.

93. Newman, H.N.: The organic films on enamel surfaces. I. The vestigial enamel organ, Brit. Dent. J. **135:**64, 1973.

94. Newman, H.N.: The organic films on enamel surfaces. II. The dental plaque, Brit. Dent. J. **135:**106, 1973.

95. Listgarten, M.A.: Structure of surface coatings of teeth: a review, J. Periodontol. **47:**139, 1976.

96. Newman, H.N.: Ultrastructural observations on the human pre-eruptive enamel cuticle, Arch. Oral Biol. **25:**49, 1980.

97. Listgarten, M.A.: Phase-contrast and electron microscopic study of the junction between reduced enamel epithelium and enamel in unerupted human teeth, Arch. Oral Biol. **11:**999, 1966.

98. Listgarten, M.A., and Ellegaard, B.: Electron microscopic evidence of a cellular attachment between junctional epithelium and dental calculus, J. Periodont. Res. **8:**143, 1973.

99. Goldman, H.: The topography and role of the gingival fibers, J. Dent. Res. **30:**331, 1951.

100. Arnim, S.S., and Hagerman, D.A.: The connective tissue fibers of the marginal gingiva, J. Am. Dent. Assn. **47:**271, 1953.

101. Melcher, A.H.: The interpapillary ligament, Dent. Pract. **12:**461, 1962.

102. Smukler, H., and Dreyer, C.J.: Principal fibres of the periodontium, J. Periodont. Res. **4:**19, 1969.

103. Glenwright, H.D.: Observations on circular and longitudinal gingival collagen fibres in the rhesus monkey, Dent. Pract. **20:**337, 1970.

104. Page, R.C., et al.: Collagen fibre bundles of the normal marginal gingiva in the marmoset, Arch. Oral Biol. **19:**1039, 1974.

105. Melcher, A.H., and Eastoe, J.E.E.: The connective tissues of the periodontium. In Melcher, A.H., and Bowen, W.H., editors: Biology of the periodontium, New York, 1969, Academic Press, Inc., p. 167.

106. Nimni, M.E.: Metabolic pathways and control mechanisms involved in the biosynthesis and turnover of collagen in normal and pathological connective tissues, J. Oral Path. **2:**175, 1973.

107. Eyre, D.R.: Collagen: molecular diversity in the body's protein scaffold, Science **207:**1315, 1980.

108. Chavrier, C., et al.: Connective tissue organization of healthy human gingiva: ultrastructural localization of collagen types I-III-IV, J. Periodont. Res. **19:**221, 1984.

109. Melcher, A.H.: Gingival reticulin: identification and role in histogensis of collagen fibers, J. Dent. Res. **45:**426, 1966.

110. Greenlee, T.K., Jr., Ross, R., and Hartman, J.L.: The fine structure of elastic fibers, J. Cell Biol. **30:**59, 1966.

111. Ross, R., and Bornstein, P.: Elastic fibers in the body, Sci. Am. **224:**44, 1971.

112. Bodley, H.D., and Wood, R.L.: Ultrastructural studies on elastic fibers using enzymatic digestion of thin sections, Anat. Rec. **172:**71, 1972.

113. Brissie, R.M., Spicer, S.S., and Thompson, N.T.: The variable fine structure of elastin visualized with Verhoeff's iron hematoxylin, Anat. Rec. **181:**83, 1974.

114. Sandberg, L.B., Soskel, N.T., and Leslie, J.G.: Elastin structure, biosynthesis, and relation to disease states, New Engl. J. Med. **304:**566, 1981.

115. Fullmer, H.M., and Lillie, R.D.: The oxytalan fiber: a previously undescribed connective tissue fiber, J. Histochem. Cytochem. **6:**425, 1958.

116. Carmichael, G.C., and Fullmer, H.M.: The fine structure of the oxytalan fiber, J. Cell Biol. **28:**33, 1966.

117. Griffin, C.J., and Harris, R.: The fine structure of the developing periodontium, Arch. Oral Biol. **12:**971, 1967.

118. Harris, R., and Griffin, C.J.: The protein polysaccharide complex of the developing human periodontium, Arch. Oral Biol. **12:**1107, 1967.

119. Carmichael, G.C.: Observations with the light microscope on the distribution and connections of the oxytalan fibre of the lower jaw of the mouse, Arch. Oral Biol. **13:**765, 1968.

120. Sheetz, J.H., Fullmer, H.M., and Narkates, A.J.: Oxytalan fibers: identification of the same fiber by light and electron microscopy, J. Oral Pathol. **2:**254, 1973.

121. Soames, J.V., and Davies, R.M.: Elastic and oxytalan fibres in normal and inflamed dog gingivae, J. Periodont. Res. **10:**309, 1975.

122. Fullmer, H.M., Sheetz, J.H., and Narkates, A.J.: Oxytalan connective tissue fibers: a review, J. Oral Pathol. **3:**291, 1975.

123. Sims, M.R.: The oxytalan fiber system in the mandibular periodontal ligament of the lathyritic mouse, J. Oral Pathol. **6:**233, 1977.

124. Soames, J.V., and Davies, R.M.: Ultrastructure of elastic and oxytalan fibres in dog gingivae, J. Periodont. Res. **13:**173, 1978.

125. Sampson, W.J.: A comparative light microscopic evaluation of oxytalan fiber staining with a variety of dye substances, Stain Tech. **54:**181, 1979.

126. Selvig, K.A.: Nonbanded fibrils of collagenous nature in human periodontal connective tissue, J. Periodont. Res. **3:**169, 1968.

127. Edmunds, R.S., et al.: Light and ultrastructural relationship between oxytalan fibers in the periodontal ligament of the guinea pig, J. Oral Pathol. **8:**109, 1979.

128. Balazs, E.A., editor: Chemistry and molecular biology of the intercellular matrix: vol. I, Collagen, basal laminae, elastin; vol. II, Glycosaminoglycans, proteoglycans; vol. III, Structural organization and function of the matrix, New York, 1970, Academic Press Inc.

129. Johnson, N.W., and Hopps, R.M.: Cell dynamics of experimental gingivitis in macaques: the nature of the cellular infiltrate with varying degrees of gingivitis, J. Periodont. Res. **10:**177, 1975.

130. Ko, S.D., Narayanan, A.S., and Page, R.C.: Influence of cell cycle on collagen synthesis by human gingival fibroblasts, J. Periodont Res. **16:**302, 1981.

131. Narayanan, A.S., and Page, R.C.: Connective tissues of the periodontium: a summary of current work, Collagen Rel. Res. **3:**33, 1983.

132. Limeback, H., Sodek, J., and Aubin, J.E.: Variation in collagen expression by cloned periodontal ligament cells, J. Periodont. Res. **18:**242, 1983.

133. Hassell, T.M., and Stanek, E.J. III: Evidence that healthy human gingiva contains functionally heterogeneous fibroblast subpopulations, Arch. Oral Biol. **28:**617, 1983.

134. Bordin, S., Page, R.C., and Narayanan, A.S.: Heterogeneity of normal human diploid fibroblasts: isolation and characterization of one phenotype, Science **223:**171, 1984.

135. Yajima, R., Rose, G.G., and Mahan, C.J.: Human gingival fibroblast cell lines *in vitro*. II. Electron microscopic studies of fibrogenesis, J. Periodont. Res. **15:**267, 1980.

136. Baumhammers, A., and Stallard, R.: [35]S-sulfate utilization and turnover by the connective tissues of the periodontium, J. Periodont. Res. **3:**187, 1968.

137. Ten Cate, A.R.: Morphological studies of fibrocytes in connective tissue undergoing rapid remodelling, J. Anat. **112:**401, 1972.

137a. Listgarten, M.A.: Intracellular collagen fibrils in the periodontal ligament of the mouse, rat, hamster, guinea pig, and rabbit, J. Periodont. Res. **8:**335, 1973.

138. Frank, R.M., et al.: Collagen resorption by fibroblasts in human gingiva, J. Biol. Bucc. **5:**343, 1977.

139. Rose, G.G., Yajima, T., and Mahan, C.J.: Human gingival fibroblast cell lines in vitro. I. Electron microscopic studies of collagenolysis, J. Periodont. Res. **15:**53, 1980.

140. Svoboda, E.L.A., and Deporter, D.A.: Regional variation in collagen phagocytosis in rat gingiva: an electron microscope stereologic investigation, J. Periodont. Res. **16:**298, 1981.

141. Yamasaki, A., Rose, G.G., and Mahan, C.J.: Collagen degradation by human gingival fibroblasts. I. In vivo phagocytosis, J. Periodont. Res. **16:**309, 1981.

142. Golub, L.M., et al.: Minocycline reduces gingival collagenolytic activity during diabetes: preliminary observations and a proposed new mechanism of action, J. Periodont. Res. **18:**516, 1983.

143. Schneir, M.L., Ramamurthy, N.S., and Golub, L.M.: Extensive degradation of recently synthesized collagen in gingiva of normal and streptozotocin-induced diabetic rats, J. Dent. Res. **63:**23, 1984.

144. Barnett, M.L.: Mast cell in the epithelial layer of human gingiva, J. Ultrastruct. Res. **43:**247, 1973.

145. Weinstock, A., and Albright, J.T.: The fine structure of mast cells in normal human gingiva, J. Ultrastruct. Res. **17:**245, 1967.

146. Barnett, M.L.: The fine structure of human connective tissue mast cells in periodontal disease, J. Periodont. Res. **9:**84, 1974.

147. Zachrisson, B.U.: Mast cells of the human gingiva. II. Metachromatic cells at low pH in healthy and inflamed tissue, J. Periodont. Res. **2:**87, 1967.

148. Zachrisson, B.U.: Mast cells of the human gingiva. III. Histochemical demonstration of immature mast cells in chronically inflamed tissue, J. Periodont. Res. **3:**136, 1968.

149. Zachrisson, B.U.: Mast cells of the human gingiva. IV. Experimental gingivitis, J. Periodont. Res. **4:**46, 1969.

150. Goldhaber, P.: Heparin enhancement of factors stimulating bone resorption in tissue culture, Science **147:**407, 1965.

151. Weinstock, A.: Plasma cells in human gingiva: an electron microscope study, Anat. Rec. **162:**289, 1968.

152. Lindhe, J.: Textbook of clinical periodontology, Copenhagen, 1963, Munksgaard, p. 57.

153. Mormann, W., Meier, C., and Firestone, A.: Gingival blood circulation after experimental wounds in man, J. Clin. Periodontol **6:**417, 1979.

154. Keller, G.J., and Cohen, D.W.: India ink perfusions of the vascular plexus of oral tissues, Oral Surg. **8:**539, 1955.

155. Egelberg, J.: The blood vessels of the dentogingival junction, J. Periodont. Res. **1:**163, 1966.

156. Kindlova, M.: Changes in the vascular bed of the marginal periodontium in periodontitis, J. Dent. Res. **44:**456, 1965.

157. Gavin, J.R.: Ultrastructural features of chronic marginal gingivitis, J. Periodont. Res. **5:**19, 1970.

158. Nuki, K., and Hock, J.: The organization of the gingival vasculature, J. Periodont. Res. **9:**305, 1974.

159. Hansson, B.O., Lindhe, J., and Brånemark, P-I.: Microvascular topography and function in clinically healthy and chronically inflamed dento-gingival tissues: a vital microscopic study in dogs, Periodontics **6:**264, 1968.

160. Hock, J., and Nuki, K.: A vital microscopy study of the morphology of normal and inflamed gingiva, J. Periodont. Res. **6:**81, 1971.

161. Lindhe, J., et al.: Clinical and structural alterations characterizing healing gingiva, J. Periodont. Res. **13:**410, 1978.

162. Hock, J.: Vascular morphology in noninflamed healed gingiva of dogs, J. Clin. Periodontol. **6:**37, 1979.

163. Alfano, M.: The origin of gingival fluid, J. Theoret. Biol. **47:**127, 1974.

164. Cimasoni, G.: Crevicular fluid updated. In Myers, H.M., editor: Monographs in oral science, vol. 12, Basel, 1983, S. Karger.

165. Bernick, S., and Grant, D.A.: Lymphatics in the gingiva, J. Dent. Res. **57:**810, 1978.

166. Gairns, F.W., and Aitchison, J.A.: A preliminary study of the multiplicity of nerve endings in the human gum, Dent. Rec. **70:**180, 1958.

167. Bernick, S.: Innervation of teeth and periodontium after enzymatic removal of collageous elements, Oral Surg. **10**:323, 1957.

168. Luzardo-Baptista, M.: Intraepithelial nerve fibers in the human oral mucosa, Oral Surg. **35**:372, 1973.

169. Martinez, I.R., Jr., and Pekarthy, J.M.: Ultrastructure of encapsulated nerve endings in rat gingiva, Am. J. Anat. **140**:135, 1974.

170. Fortman, G.J., and Winkelmann, R.K.: The Merkel cell in oral human mucosa, J. Dent. Res. **56**:1303, 1978.

171. Slavkin, H.C., et al.: Dermal-epidermal interactions: cultivation of embryonic rabbit gingiva and studies of heterotypic tissue recombinants on the chick chorio-allantoic membrane, Arch. Oral Biol. **17**:585, 1972.

172. Karring, T., Ostergaard, E., and Löe, H.: Conservation of tissue specificity after heterotopic transplantation of gingiva and alveolar mucosa, J. Periodont. Res. **6**:282, 1971.

173. Karring, T., Lang, N.P., and Löe, H.: The role of gingival connective tissue in determining epithelial differentiation, J. Periodont. Res. **10**:1, 1975.

174. Mackenzie, I.C., and Hill, M.W.: Maintenance of regionally specific patterns of cell proliferation and differentiation in transplanted skin and oral mucosa, Cell Tiss. Res. **219**:597, 1981.

175. Page, R.C., and Schroeder, H.E.: Pathogenesis of inflammatory periodontal disease: a summary of current work, Lab. Invest. **33**:235, 1976.

176. Ranney, R.R.: Pathogenesis of periodontal disease. In Klavan, B., et al., editors: International conference on research in the biology of periodontal disease, Chicago, 1977, University of Illinois College of Dentistry, p. 222.

177. Page, R.C., and Schroeder, H.E.: Periodontitis in man and animals: a comparative review, Basel, 1982, S. Karger.

178. Brill, N., and Krasse, B.: The passage of tissue fluid into the clinically healthy gingival pocket, Acta Odontol. Scand. **16**:233, 1958.

179. Brill, N., and Bjorn, H.: Passage of tissue fluid into human gingival pockets, Acta Odontol. Scand. **17**:11, 1959.

180. Brill, N.: Removal of particles and bacteria from gingival pockets by tissue fluids, Acta Odontol. Scand. **17**:431, 1959.

181. Green, L.H., and Kass, E.H.: Quantitative determination of antibacterial activity in the rabbit gingival sulcus, Arch. Oral Biol. **15**:491, 1970.

182. Ranney, R.R., and Zander, H.A.: Allergic periodontal disease in sensitized squirrel monkeys, J. Periodontol. **41**:12, 1970.

183. Tolo, K.: Transport across stratified nonkeratinized epithelium, J. Periodont. Res. **6**:237, 1971.

184. Rizzo, A.A.: Absorption of bacterial endotoxin into rabbit gingival pocket tissue, Periodontics **6**:65, 1968.

185. Ranney, R.R., and Montgomery, E.H.: Vascular leakage resulting from topical application of endotoxin to the gingiva of the beagle dog, Arch. Oral Biol. **18**:963, 1973.

186. Egelberg, J.: The topography and permeability of vessels at the dento-gingival junction in dogs, J. Periodont. Res. **2**:Suppl. No. 1, 1967.

187. Freedman, H.L., Listgarten, M.A., and Taichman, N.S.: Electron microscopic features of chronically inflamed human gingiva, J. Periodont. Res. **3**:313, 1968.

188. Frank, R.M., and Cimasoni, G.: Ultrastructure de l'epithelium cliniquement normal du sillon et de la jonction gingivo-dentaires, Z. Zellforsch. **109**:356, 1970.

189. Attström, R.: Studies on neutrophil polymorphonuclear leukocytes at the dento-gingival junction in gingival health and disease, J. Periodont. Res. **6**:Suppl. No. 8, 1971.

190. Schroeder, H.E.: Transmigration and infiltration of leucocytes in human junctional epithelium, Helv. Odont. Acta **17**:6, 1973.

191. Brill, N., and Bronnestam, R.: Immunoelectrophoretic study of tissue fluid from gingival pockets, Acta Odontol. Scand. **18**:95, 1960.

192. Brandtzaeg, P.: Immunochemical comparison of proteins in human gingival pocket fluid, serum and saliva, Arch. Oral Biol. **10**:795, 1965.

193. Holmberg, K., and Killander, J.: Quantitative determination of immunoglobuline (IgG, IgA, and IgM) and identification of IgA-type in the gingival fluid, J. Periodont. Res. **6**:1, 1971.

194. Shillitoe, E.J., and Lehner, T.: Immunoglobulins and complement in crevicular fluid, serum and saliva in man, Arch. Oral Biol. **17**:241, 1972.

195. Attström, R., et al.: Complement factors in gingival crevice material from healthy and inflamed gingiva in humans, J. Periodont. Res. **10**:19, 1975.

196. Schenkein, H.A., and Genco, R.J.: Gingival fluid and serum in periodontal diseases. I. Quantitative study of immunoglobulins, complement components, and other plasma proteins, J. Periodontol. **48**:772, 1977.

197. Schenkein, H.A., and Genco, R.J.: Gingival fluid and serum in periodontal diseases. II. Evidence for cleavage of complement components C3, C3 proactivator (factor B) and C4 in gingival fluid, J. Periodontol. **48**:778, 1977.

198. Bang, J., Cimasoni, G., and Held, A.J.: High levels of β-glucuronidase in human gingival fluid, J. Dent. Res. **48**:1142, 1969.

199. Sueda, T., Cimasoni, G., and Held, A.-J.: High levels of acid phosphatase in human gingival fluid, Arch. Oral Biol. **12:**1205, 1967.
200. Ishikawa, I., and Cimasoni, G.: Alkaline phosphatase in human gingival fluid and its relation to periodontitis, Arch. Oral Biol. **15:**1401, 1970.
201. Frank, R.M., and Cimasoni, G.: Electron microscopy of acid phosphatase in the exudate from inflamed gingivae, J. Periodont. Res. **7:**213, 1972.
202. Tynelius-Bratthall, G., and Attström, R.: Acid phosphatase, hyaluronidase, and protease in crevices of healthy and clinically inflamed gingiva in dogs, J. Dent. Res. **51:**279, 1972.
203. Valazza, A., et al.: Acid phosphatase, beta-glucuronidase, and cathepsin D in microamounts of gingival fluid, J. Dent. Res. **51:**862, 1972.
204. Golub, L.S., Stakiw, J.E., and Singer, D.L.: Collagenolytic activity of human gingival crevice fluid, J. Dent. Res. **53:**1501, 1974.
205. Friedman, S.A., Mandel, I.D., and Herrera, M.S.: Lysozyme and lactoferrin quantitation in the crevicular fluid, J. Periodontol. **54:**347, 1983.
206. Kitawaki, M., et al.: Neuraminidase activity in human crevicular fluid, J. Periodont. Res. **18:**318, 1983.
207. Collins, A.A., and Gavin, J.B.: An evaluation of the antimicrobial effect on the fluid exudate from the clinically healthy gingival crevice, J. Periodontol. **32:**99, 1961.
208. Bader, H.I., and Goldhaber, P.: The passage of intravenously administered tetracycline in the gingival sulcus of dogs, J. Oral Therap. Pharm. **2:**324, 1966.
209. Ciancio, S.G., Mather, M.L., and McMullen, J.A.: An evaluation of minocycline in patients with periodontal disease, J. Periodontol. **51:**530, 1980.
210. Gordon, J.M., et al.: Concentration of tetracycline in human gingival fluid after single doses, J. Clin. Periodontol. **8:**117, 1981.
211. Walker, C.B., et al.: Gingival crevicular fluid levels of clindamycin compared with its minimal inhibitory concentrations for periodontal bacteria, Antimicrob. Agents Chemother. **19:**867, 1981.
212. Gordon, J.M., et al.: Tetracycline: levels achievable in gingival crevice fluid and *in vitro* effect on subgingival organisms. I. Concentrations in crevicular fluid after repeated doses, J. Periodontol. **52:**609, 1981.
213. Walker, C.B., et al.: Tetracycline: levels achievable in gingival crevice fluid and *in vitro* effect on subgingival organisms. II. Susceptibilities of periodontal bacteria, J. Periodontol. **52:**613, 1981.

### ADDITIONAL SUGGESTED READING

Osborn, M.: Intermediate filaments as histologic markers: an overview, J. Invest. Dermatol. **81:** 1048s, 1983.

# CHAPTER 3

# Periodontal ligament

Periodontal ligment
Macroscopic features
Microscopic features
Physiologic and functional considerations

## Periodontal ligament

The periodontal ligament is a dense, fibrous connective tissue attaching the tooth to the alveolar bone. Its primary function is to support the tooth in the alveolus and to maintain the physiologic relation between the cementum and the bone. Its collagen fibers are inserted in the alveolar bone and the cementum layer covering the root. The ligament is quite cellular, well innervated and vascularized, and contains epithelial cell aggregates.

### MACROSCOPIC FEATURES

If a sound tooth is extracted from its socket, the periodontal ligament is torn and the periodontal fibers inserted into the cementum are retained on the root surface. If the tooth is dipped into a diluted dye solution (e.g., 0.5% methylene blue), the fibers are stained dark blue. In healthy teeth they cover the entire root up to the cementoenamel junction. In teeth with advanced periodontal disease, where the supporting structures have been partially destroyed, the fibers may be evident only in the apical portion of the root. The areas of destruction are unstained (Fig. 3-1).

The periodontal ligament occupies the narrow interval between the calcified surfaces of the cementum and the alveolus (Fig. 3-2). It is detectable in radiographs as a radiolucent line paralleling the root surface. The periodontal ligament varies in thickness between 0.1 to 0.25 mm depending on age, stage of eruption of the tooth, and its functional characteristics.[1] It tends to be somewhat thicker in adolescents than in older subjects (Table 3-1). It reaches maximal dimensions when teeth are in heavy function. In teeth without antagonists the ligament is considerably thinner and is thinner still in impacted teeth (Table 3-2).

The lamina dura in radiographs is a radiodense line that represents the alveolar bone proper (Fig. 3-2). Under normal function the periodontal ligament tends to be narrowest near the middle of the root and wider near the crest and apex. Widening of the periodontal ligament may be caused by occlusal hyperfunction or, rarely, by systemic disease (e.g., scleroderma).[2]

It is estimated that 53% to 74% of the ligament volume consists of collagen or oxytalan fibers and 1% to 2% of vascular elements.[3] The remainder consists of cells

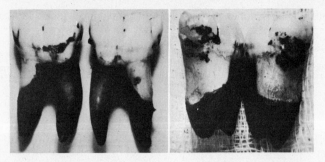

**Fig. 3-1.** Partially destroyed periodontal ligament adherent to the root surface of extracted teeth from patients with juvenile periodontitis is stained with 0.5% aqueous methylene blue dye. (From Kaslick, R.S., and Chasens, A.I.: Oral Surg. **25:**327, 1968.)

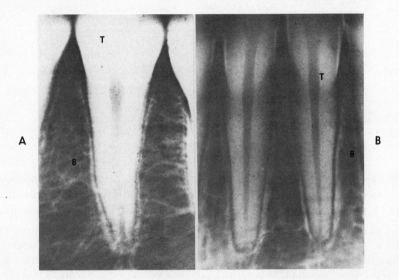

**Fig. 3-2.** Radiographically the periodontal ligament appears as a radiolucent *(black)* line between the relatively radiodense tooth *(T)* and the radiodense alveolar bone *(B)* adjacent to the ligament. This white line in bone (radiodensity) is called the *lamina dura* in x rays. **A,** Normal periodontal ligament. **B,** Widened periodontal ligament caused by hyperfunction (occlusal trauma).

and neural elements. The surface area of alveoli varies from 150 to 275 mm$^2$ for single-rooted teeth to upward of 450 mm$^2$ for multirooted molars.[4] The *root trunk* of maxillary molars accounts for 32% of the total root surface.[5]

In recently erupted teeth as many as 50,000 fiber bundles may insert into each mm$^2$ of root surface. The mean fiber bundle density in fully functional teeth averages around 28,000/mm$^2$, while in nonfunctional teeth (e.g., impacted teeth) the fiber bundle density may drop to around 2000/mm$^2$ (Fig. 3-3).[6] The mean diameter of collagen fiber bundles tends to be smallest at eruption, around 2 to 3 μm. In the fully functional tooth, the diameter may almost double.[6] Since the diameter is double, there is a reduced number of fiber bundle insertions in the fully functional tooth.

## MICROSCOPIC FEATURES
### Histogenesis

The organization and function of the periodontal ligament can be better understood by following its histologic development.[7-14] The periodontal ligament develops from connective tissue elements during embryonic life. A recognizable ligament is formed before

**Table 3-1** Variations in periodontal ligament width according to age and location on the tooth

| Age range | No. of teeth / No. of jaws | Average near alveolar crest (mm) | Average near midroot (mm) | Average near apex (mm) | Overall mean (mm) |
|---|---|---|---|---|---|
| 11-16 | 83/4 | 0.23 | 0.17 | 0.24 | 0.21 |
| 32-50 | 36/5 | 0.20 | 0.14 | 0.19 | 0.18 |
| 51-67 | 35/5 | 0.17 | 0.12 | 0.16 | 0.15 |

From Coolidge, E.D.: The thickness of the human periodontal membrane, J. Am. Dent. Assoc. **24**:1260, 1937.

**Table 3-2** Variations in periodontal ligament width according to functional state and location on the tooth

| Functional state | No. of teeth / No. of jaws | Average near alveolar crest (mm) | Average near midroot (mm) | Average near apex (mm) | Overall mean (mm) |
|---|---|---|---|---|---|
| Teeth in heavy function | 44/8 | 0.20 | 0.14 | 0.19 | 0.18 |
| Teeth without antagonists | 20/12 | 0.14 | 0.11 | 0.15 | 0.13 |
| Embedded teeth | 5/12 | 0.09 | 0.17 | 0.18 | 0.08 |

From Coolidge, E.D.: The thickness of the human periodontal membrane, J. Am. Dent. Assoc. **24**:1260, 1937. Modified by Schroeder, H.E.: Orale Strukturbiologie, Stuttgart, 1976, Georg Thieme Verlag, p. 212.

eruption of the primary teeth and the permanent molars (teeth without predecessors). Secondary succedaneous teeth develop a ligament after they erupt into the oral cavity (Fig. 3-4). The formation of the ligament is illustrated in four sequential steps.

1. Short, brushlike, closely spaced cemental fibers extend from the cementum (Figs. 3-5 and 3-6). A few isolated alveolar fibers extend from the alveolar wall. Between these two groups of fibers are loose collagenous fibers that are aligned parallel to the long axis of the tooth. About seven eighths of the ligament's width (Figs. 3-5 and 3-6, A) is made up of the loosely aligned longitudinal fibers.
2. The alveolar fibers increase in size and number. They become longer and splay out (arborize) at their ends. The alveolar fibers are more widely separated than the cemental fibers (Fig. 3-6, B).
3. The alveolar and cemental fibers continue to lengthen and appear to join (Fig. 3-6, C).
4. When the tooth becomes functional, the fiber bundles increase in width and are apparently continuous between bone and cementum (Figs. 3-4 and 3-6, D).

The organization of the ligament occurs first in the cervical region of the tooth and proceeds apically (Figs. 3-4[13,14] and 3-5).

**Intermediate plexus**

An intermediate plexus is demonstrable in the continuously erupting guinea pig molar.[15] The concept of an intermediate plexus in humans arose from studying erupting teeth and from the observation of an apparent mingling of the alveolar and cemental fibers near the center of the ligament in fully erupted teeth. Sicher[16,17] and Orban[18] believed that a splicing and unsplicing in the region of the intermediate plexus permitted the rearrangement of fibers during eruptive and migratory tooth movements. This concept is of historical interest only and is no longer held.

Once the tooth has erupted into clinical occlusion, such an intermediate plexus is no longer demonstrable.[13,14,19-22] The principal fiber bundles become thickened and apparently continuous.[13]

Growth changes and tooth movement are possible because of the constant remodelling and turnover of the structural elements of the ligament and bone. These

| FUNCTIONAL STAGE | TANGENTIAL SECTION | DENSITY/1000 μm² MEAN ± SD | DIAMETER, μm MEAN ± SD |
|---|---|---|---|
| Preeruptive and eruptive | 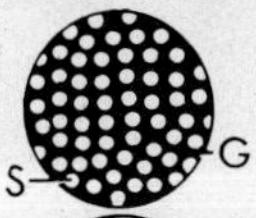 | 53.4 ± 13.5 | 3.0 ± 0.02 |
| Normal functioning | 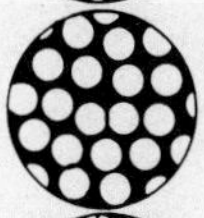 | 28.0 ± 3.2 | 4.0 ± 0.3 |
| Completely embedded | 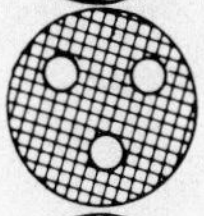 | 2.1 ± 5.3 | 4.1 ± 0.3 |
| Excessive destruction of crown | 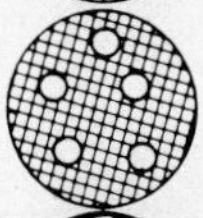 | 5.5 ± 0.4 | 3.8 ± 0.4 |
| Fixed bridge abutment | 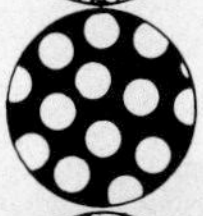 | 21.3 ± 5.2 | 4.6 ± 0.6 |
| Removable partial denture abutment | 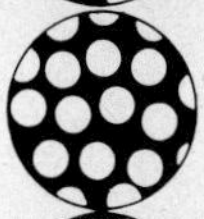 | 17.0 ± 0.6 | 4.6 ± 0.6 |
| Excessive bone loss | 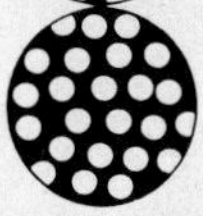 | 20.0 ± 8.1 | 3.8 ± 0.03 |

**Fig. 3-3.** Density and diameter of Sharpey's fibers in the superficial layers of cementum. (Modified from Akiyoshi, M., and Inoue, M.: Bull. Tokyo Med. Dent. Univ. **10:**41, 1963.)

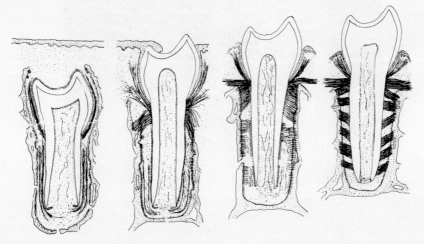

**Fig. 3-4.** Diagrammatic representation of the periodontal ligament of a premolar (a secondary tooth) before and during eruption. These stages differ in a permanent molar (which is not a succedaneous tooth) in that the permanent molar has well-defined fibers in the preeruptive stages. (From Grant, D.A., and Bernick, S.: J. Periodontol. **43:**17, 1972.)

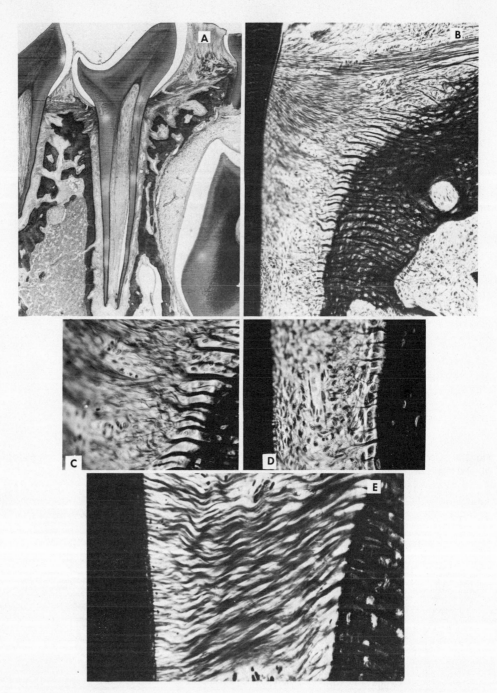

**Fig. 3-5. A,** Squirrel monkey premolars during eruption. At the stage of first occlusal contact, these secondary teeth show only dentogingival, alveolar crest, and horizontal fibers as organized groups. The remainder of the ligament is in a formative stage. **B,** Higher magnification of the alveolar crest shows that fiber formation is evident at the cementoenamel junction. Further, apically, the cemental and alveolar fibers have yet to join. **C,** Higher magnification shows the thick alveolar fibers at the osseous crest that have become arborized and extended toward the cemental fibers. **D,** Midroot, thick, widely spaced alveolar fibers are separated from the fine closely spaced cemental fibers by loosely organized collagen fibers. **E,** With function the principal fibers become thickened and appear to extend without interruption between cementum and bone. (From Grant, D.A., and Bernick, S.: J. Periodontol. **42:**17, 1972.)

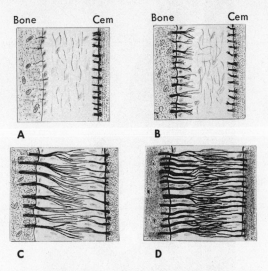

**Fig. 3-6.** Diagrammatic representation of the formation of periodontal ligament fibers during eruption. Although the chronology differs, the sequence of principal periodontal fiber formation is the same for teeth with and without predecessors. In each the developmental pattern occurs as follows: **A,** Fibers first emanate from cementum *(Cem)*. These are short and closely spaced. The osteoblast-lined alveolar bone shows no fiber extrusions or only a rare isolated fiber. The greatest part of the periodontal ligament space is occupied by collagenous elements similar in appearance to those of the dental sac. **B,** Fibers, thicker and more widely spaced than those from cementum, emerge from bone to extend briefly toward the tooth and then splay out (arborize) at their ends. The central three fourths of the periodontal ligament space is occupied by loosely structured collagenous elements. **C,** Alveolar fibers extend into the central zone to join lengthening cemental fibers, eliminating the intermediate loosely organized fibers. **D,** With occlusal function the principal fibers become more closely packed, thicker, and apparently continuous between bone and cementum. (From Grant, D.A., and Bernick, S.: J. Periodontol. **43:**17, 1972.)

processes have been studied by radioautographic[23-29] and biochemical analytic techniques.[29-33] It should be noted that while the extracellular elements of the ligament (fibers, ground substance) have a relatively high turnover rate, the cellular turnover is relatively slow.[34-36] Even with continuous labelling procedures, the ligament cells become labelled slowly and a large pool of cells remains unlabelled, either because they are not able to divide or because they are slow cycling. The number of labelled cells can be increased by the extraction of antagonist teeth in experimental animals. This triggers more rapid eruption, thereby affecting the rate of remodelling and cellular turnover.[29,37] Labelling studies[38] with ³H-thymidine have shown that labelling is greatest in the central zone of the ligament around blood vessels, while cell density is greatest toward bone and cementum. This suggests that undifferentiated progenitor cells in the vicinity of blood vessels produce osteoblasts and cementoblasts that later migrate toward bone and tooth, respectively.

### Fiber organization and function

Traditionally, periodontal ligament fibers have been organized into principal fiber groups,[39,40] which are identified by their location and direction (Figs. 3-7 to 3-9):

**Principal fibers**

1. *Alveolar crest group.* The fiber bundles of this group radiate from the crest of the alveolar process and are attached to the cervical cementum.
2. *Horizontal group.* The bundles of this group run at right angles to the long axis of the tooth, from cementum to bone near the crest.
3. *Oblique group.* The bundles course obliquely and are attached in cementum somewhat apically from their attachment to bone. These fiber bundles are most numerous and constitute the main support of the tooth.
4. *Apical group.* The bundles radiate from the apical region of the root to the surrounding bone (Fig. 3-10).

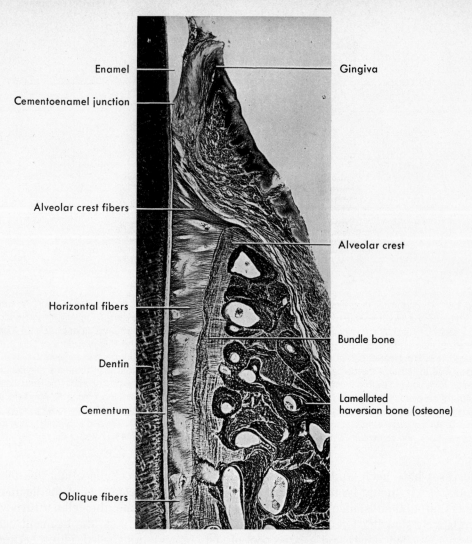

Enamel

Cementoenamel junction

Alveolar crest fibers

Horizontal fibers

Dentin

Cementum

Oblique fibers

Gingiva

Alveolar crest

Bundle bone

Lamellated
haversian bone (osteone)

**Fig. 3-7.** Principal fibers of the periodontal ligament. Note the attachment of the fibers to the bone on one side and to the cementum on the other. Bundle bone containing Sharpey's fibers is evident.

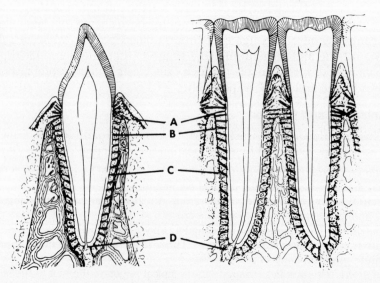

**Fig. 3-8.** Diagram of the principal fiber groups of the periodontal ligament: *A*, Alveolar crest fibers; *B*, horizontal fibers; *C*, oblique fibers; *D*, apical fibers. The oblique fibers are the largest group, followed in order by the apical, horizontal, and alveolar crest groups. Interradicular fibers are not shown. (Modified from Schour, I.: Noyes' oral histology and embryology, ed. 8, Philadelphia, 1960, Lea & Febiger.)

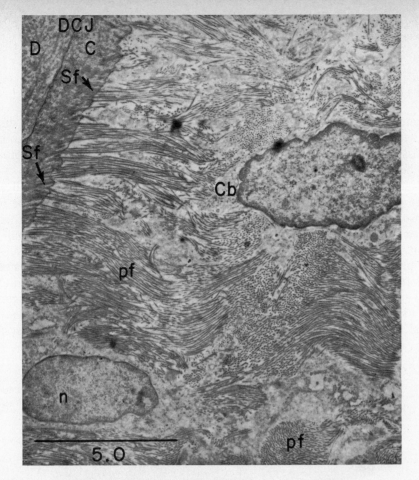

**Fig. 3-9.** Electron micrograph of periodontal fibrils *(pf)* of a rat inserted in cementum, *(C)*. Note the wavy course of the fibrils. Two cementoblasts are evident *(Cb)*, as are their nuclei, *(n)*. *D* indicates the dentin; *DCJ,* the dentin-ocemental junction; *Sf,* Sharpey's fibrils (so called because they are submicroscopic fibrils embedded in cementum). (From Stern, I.B.: Am. J. Anat. **115:**377, 1964.)

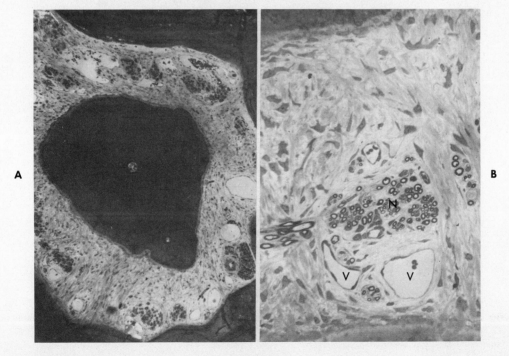

**Fig. 3-10.** **A,** Cross section of a monkey root, near apex. The radial arrangement of the principal fibers near the apex is not as well defined as in more coronal cross sections. Numerous blood vessels and nerve fibers are present. **B,** Magnified serial section of **A.** Note the thin-walled blood vessels *(V)* and the numerous myelinated axons in the nerve bundle *(N).*

5. *Interradicular group.* This group courses over the crest of the interradicular septum in the furcations of multirooted teeth.

Although the principal fiber bundles run from cementum to bone, their direction is not just radial. The paths of the various groups can be somewhat tangential and may cross one another. In this manner the fibers seem to reinforce one another and may be better suited for support.

Collagen fibers account for the major bulk of the fibers in the periodontal ligament. Most are principal fibers (Fig. 3-11). However, some fibers appear to course parallel to the root surface, forming a loose intersecting network (Fig. 3-12). This has been described as an *indifferent fiber plexus.*[41,42] It is most evident in the apical half of the ligament.

The principal fiber bundles emanating from bone are more widely separated than those from cementum. The alveolar fibers are thick, relatively short, and tend to splay out into smaller fibers that blend and mesh with the closely approximated cemental fibers[13] (Figs. 3-5 and 3-13, *A*). Thus, while they tend to run in parallel arrays, the principal fibers actually form an interconnected meshwork rather than a system of parallel cables.[20]

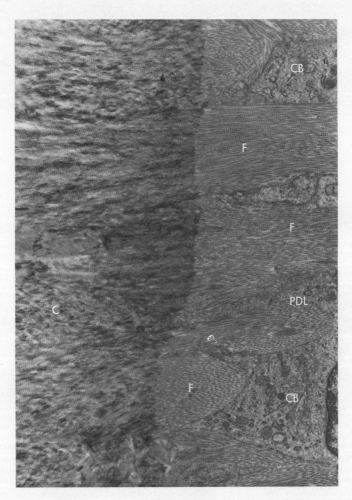

**Fig. 3-11.** Electron micrograph of junction between periodontal ligament *(PDL)* and acellular fibrillar cementum *(C)*. Most of the collagen fibrils in the ligament form principal fibers *(F)* that enter and become part of the cemental organic matrix. *CB,* cementoblasts.

The ends of the principal fibers embedded in cementum and bone are called *Sharpey's fibers*.[43] They are the mineralized portions of the principal fibers (Fig. 3-13, *B*). Indifferent fibers may also become incorporated into the mineralized matrices. While the principal fibers are formed primarily by periodontal fibroblasts, osteoblasts and cementoblasts contribute mostly to the synthesis of indifferent fibers and matrix. The matrix envelops the fibers and mineralizes to form either bone or cementum. Thus periodontal fibroblasts collaborate with either osteoblasts or cementoblasts in the synthesis of the alveolar bone proper and cementum.[3] The Sharpey's fibers entering alveolar bone (Fig. 3-13, *A*) are fewer and wider than those entering cementum.[13,20,44,45]

**Sharpey's fibers**

The dynamic state of the periodontal tissues (bone, cementum, and ligament) permits the tooth to move in relation to its bony housing and to adapt to altered functional states. Teeth migrate mesially throughout life. This mesial migration is reflected histologically by the presence of long, distinct Sharpey's fibers in the alveolus, distal of the tooth with distinct appositional lines in bone and a relatively smooth osteoblast-lined surface (Fig. 3-13).

By contrast, the bone bordering the mesial surface of the tooth shows evidence of resorption, alternating with short cycles of bone formation. The change from bone resorption to bone formation is identified histologically by a scalloped *reversal line* in

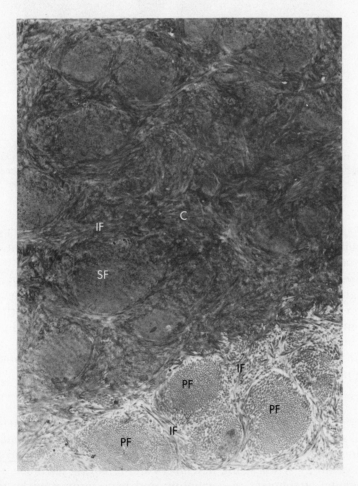

**Fig. 3-12.**  Tangential section through cementum and periodontal ligament in apical half of the root. The circular cross sections through the principal fibers *(PF)* are surrounded by an "indifferent" fiber plexus *(IF)*. This arrangement persists in the adjacent cementum *(C)*. *SF,* Sharpey's fiber.

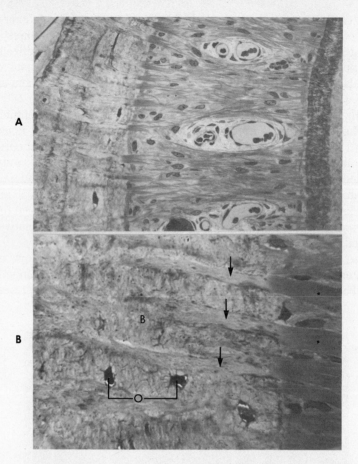

**Fig. 3-13. A,** Cross section of periodontal ligament in coronal half of root. The principal fibers form a branching, interconnected network of fibrillar collagen throughout the ligament. The principal fibers enter bone and cementum as mineralized Sharpey's fibers. **B,** Sharpey's fibers *(arrows)* within alveolar bone *(B)*. O, osteocytes; *, principal fibers of the ligament.

the alveolar bone. The short cycle of bone formation produces a thin layer of new bone containing relatively short Sharpey's fibers that reanchor the ligament to the bone following resorption (Fig. 3-14).

Interspersed among the collagen fibers are *oxytalan fibers* morphologically similar to those in gingiva. They run in an occluso-apical direction, associated with blood vessels and nerve fibers.[46,47] They may also follow the direction of the principal fibers, on occasion inserting into cementum. More oxytalan fibers are seen on the cemental than on the bony side of the ligament.

*Elastic fibers* are infrequent. They are confined to the loose connective tissue surrounding neurovascular channels.

### Cells

A number of different cell types are present in the periodontal ligament, including epithelial cell aggregates and those which are part of the neural and vascular channels. The main function of periodontal ligament cells is to maintain the normal organization of the fiber system by synthesizing new fibers and removing old ones. The integrity of the periodontal attachment to cementum and bone is ensured by the constant remodelling of these surfaces.

*Undifferentiated mesenchymal cells* predominate in the central portion of the lig-

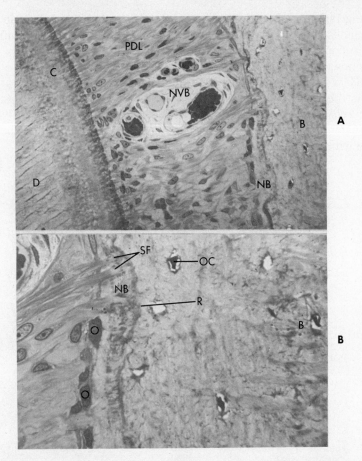

**Fig. 3-14.  A,** Periodontal ligament adjacent to the mesial surface of the alveolus. *B,* alveolar bone; *C,* acellular fibrillar cementum; *D,* dentin; *NB,* new bone; *NVB,* neurovascular bundle; *PDL,* periodontal ligament. **B,** Higher magnification of **A.** *B,* alveolar bone; *NB,* new bone; *O,* osteoblasts; *OC,* osteocyte in lacuna; *R,* reversal line; *SF,* short Sharpey's fibers.

ament, in close proximity to blood vessels.[10] These cells are considered to be progenitor cells for more differentiated cell types—fibroblasts, cementoblasts, and osteoblasts.[7-10]

*Fibroblasts* make up the major cellular population of the ligament. They are spindle-shaped and polarized, with their long axis parallel to the principal fibers.[48-50] They function to synthesize collagen, which aggregates into fibrils and fibers extracellularly.[23-25, 27-51] They also synthesize the proteoglycan matrix surrounding the fibers.[26] Fibroblasts also participate in the resorption of collagen fibrils, segments of which can be found in phagocytic vacuoles in cells.[52-62] The degradation of collagen is facilitated by a collagenase, the activity of which increases in periodontitis[63] and decreases with administration of tetracycline-like drugs.[64] Finally, fibroblasts are believed to play a role in eruption because of their contractile properties.[65-68]

There are at least five distinct types of collagen.[69] Type I comprises most of the collagen of skin, bones, dentin, cementum, and the mucosal lamina propria. Type II is found in cartilage. Type III is found in fetal skin but is also a minor component in tissues in which type I collagen is dominant. Types IV and V are not fibrillar proteins. They are typically recovered from basal laminae. As many as 10 types of collagen have been described.

The production of different collagens is apparently caused by the heterogeneity of the fibroblast population.[70-73] Cloned periodontal ligament fibroblasts are capable of synthesizing types I, III, and V collagens. However the ratios of these types vary in different clones, one clone producing almost pure type I collagen.[71] Differences have also been reported among cultured gingival fibroblasts in their ability to synthesize noncollagenous proteins and glycosaminoglycans.[70-73]

*Osteoblasts* originate from undifferentiated fibroblast-like cells located perivascularly.[74,75] As the cells migrate toward the alveolar bone they differentiate into *osteoprogenitor cells, preosteoblasts,* and eventually *osteoblasts.* Osteoblasts are best observed in regions of active osteogenesis or bone remodelling. They may become trapped in lacunae within bone as *osteocytes* (see Fig. 3-13).

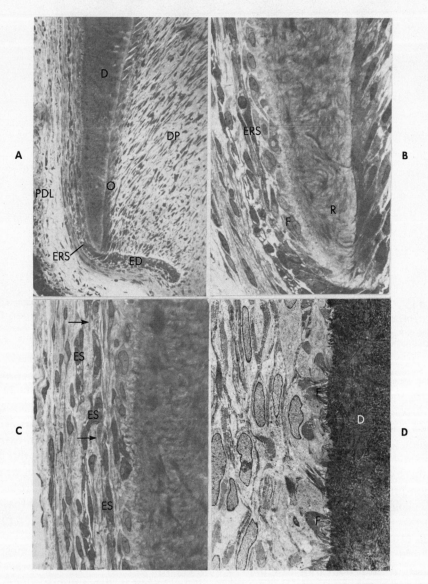

**Fig. 3-15.** **A,** Developing periodontal ligament *(PDL)* near apical foramen of developing premolar root. *D,* dentin; *DP,* dental pulp; *ED,* epithelial diaphragm; *ERS,* epithelial root sheath; *O,* odontoblast layer. **B,** Higher magnification of **A.** As the epithelial diaphragm rounds the growing root tip *(R),* it becomes displaced away from the dentin surface by collagen secreting cells *(F)* to form Hertwig's epithelial root sheath *(ERS).* **C,** Section just coronal to **B.** The epithelial root sheath loses its integrity as shown by the appearance of gaps between portions of the sheath *(arrows)* and isolated epithelial strands *(ES).* **D,** Electron micrograph of **C** showing early formation of periodontal ligament fibers *(F)* perpendicular to the surface of the root dentin *(D).* Most of the adjacent cells and fibers are still orientated parallel to the root surface.

*Cementoblasts* originate from undifferentiated cells in a manner similar to osteoblasts. They line the cemental surface where cementogenesis is occurring. In areas of rapid cementogenesis they may become trapped within lacunae as *cementocytes*.

*Osteoclasts and odontoclasts* are multinucleated cells that are morphologically and functionally indistinguishable. Osteoclasts function in an integrated manner with osteoblasts to remodel existing alveolar bone. Odontoclasts can resorb mineralized dental tissue, including cementum. They do not appear to be coupled to cementoblastic activity. Cemental remodelling is rare and localized.

*Epithelial cells* are routinely noted in the ligament close to cementum.[76-85] Their distribution depends on the stage of tooth eruption and age of the subject. They originate from Hertwig's epithelial root sheath, which becomes displaced from the dentin surface[86] and perforated just coronal to the epithelial diaphragm during cementogenesis (Fig. 3-15). The perforations slowly enlarge so that the perforated sheath gradually turns into a delicate network of epithelial cords that may undergo further loss of continuity.[77,78,83] The epithelial remnants are known as *cell rests of Malassez* (Fig. 3-16). While they retain the ability to proliferate,[80-82] their function is unknown. In some instances the cells rests of Malassez may be continuous with the junctional epithelium.[83,85]

*Defense cells* are comparatively few in the disease-free periodontal ligament. They include *macrophages, polymorphonuclear* and *mononuclear leukocytes,* and *mast cells.* They play important roles in the response to injury and in wound healing and repair.

Generally the cellular density in periodontal ligament is greatest in young individuals and decreases with age.[87,88] This has been demonstrated both in animals[87] and in humans.[88] Labelling with tritiated thymidine, an indicator of mitotic activity, decreases with age.[87] Cellular density also increases with heavy function and decreases with lack of function.

## Blood vessels and lymphatics

The periodontal ligament is well vascularized. The blood supply originates from three main sources: (1) branches of the alveolar artery that enter the periodontal ligament from the apical region and course in a coronal direction, (2) branches of the

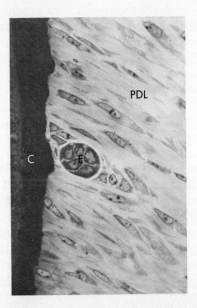

**Fig. 3-16.** Epithelial cell rest of Malassez *(E)* in the periodontal ligament of a mouse molar in a typical location, close to the cementum *(C)* surface. *PDL,* periodontal ligament.

interradicular arteries that penetrate the periodontal ligament through alveolar foramina and arborize in a coronal and apical direction, and (3) gingival vessels that enter
the periodontal ligament in the crestal region and anastomose with the vascular network of the ligament. The density of the foramina in the alveolar wall increases from
the canine region posteriorly.[89]

The anastomosing network of arterioles and venules in the periodontal ligament
tends to run predominantly in an occluso-apical direction, approximately midway between tooth and bone. In addition to their nutrient function and the removal of cellular
waste, the blood vessels of the ligament act as a hydraulic shock-absorbing system,
cushioning the tooth against light occlusal forces.[90-93]

Lymphatic vessels form a network that is located alongside the blood vessels and
drain to the same nodes as adjacent gingival lymphatics.[94-96]

### Nerves

The periodontal ligament contains both sensory and autonomic nerve endings.[97,98]
The sensory nerves penetrate the ligament through the apical foramen, as myelinated
fibers that pass occlusally, gradually losing their myelin sheath. Other nerve endings
reach the ligament through foramina in the alveolar wall and branch occluso-apically.
Nerves may terminate as free endings without a myelin sheath or in a number of
specialized receptors with a variety of ultrastructural features.[98-101]

The sensory nerve endings are able to identify pain and pressure. The mechanoreceptors for pressure are extremely sensitive and are able to detect minute particles
between occluding tooth surfaces. While proprioceptive functions have been attributed
to the ligament nerves, there is little loss in proprioception in edentulous patients.[102]

The autonomic innervation that originates from the superior cervical ganglion is
primarily responsible for the control of smooth muscles associated with the periodontal
vasculature.[98]

### PHYSIOLOGIC AND FUNCTIONAL CONSIDERATIONS

The periodontal ligament performs the following functions:

### Formative functions

The periodontal ligament develops from the mesenchymal tissues of the dental
follicle—the innermost layer of mesenchyme in contact with the enamel organ. Transplantation experiments to extraoral sites[7,8] have indicated that the cells in the follicle
are able to give rise to alveolar bone, periodontal ligament, and cementum. This potential to synthesize three distinct tissues is retained in the mature ligament and
contributes to the maintenance and repair of the supporting tissues of the teeth.

Autoradiography of tritiated proline uptake and dissipation[24,28] combined with biochemical microassay investigations[29-34] indicate a high turnover rate for periodontal
collagen. The turnover is approximately two- to six-fold greater than gingiva, skin, or
alveolar bone.[31] At this point this technique suffers from the errors of uptake and
recycling of proline by proteins other than collagen. The pool expansion technique
assigns a half-life of 8.8 plus or minus 1 day to rat molar periodontal ligament collagen.
This technique, however, suffers from sampling errors.[32] Most of the collagen synthesized is type I with 20% or less type III.[32a] These observations coupled with the finding
that the half-life of labelled proteins in periodontal ligament (6 to 8 days) is considerably
shorter than that of dentogingival fibers (25 days)[34] indicate that the ligament is capable
of rapid regeneration. Consequently, quick remodelling can be expected when orthodontic or other forces are applied to teeth as well as rapid repair following injury or
surgical intervention.

Continuous long-term labelling of mouse periodontal ligament indicates that maximum labelling is reached after 25 days.[36] At that time only 30% of the cells are labelled.

This suggests that 70% of the unlabelled cells do not cycle or cycle very slowly. Stimulation of the ligament cells through wounding or orthodontic tooth movement may raise the percentage of labelled cells to 60%.[36] Most of the labelling occurs in cells around blood vessels in the central portion of the ligament with the subsequent migration of cells toward the bone and cementum.[38]

## Supportive functions

The periodontal ligament anchors the teeth to their alveoli and provides a multistage shock-absorbing system to protect the ligament from injury during mastication.[91-93] Light forces are cushioned by the fluid content of the vasculature. As pressure forces the fluid content of the vasculature. As pressure forces the fluid out of ligament vessels, the interfibrillar matrix may become squeezed into adjacent narrow spaces.[103-106] The principal fibers provide the final stage of cushioning occlusal forces, transmitting them to the walls of the alveolus and possibly causing alveolar bone to flex.[107]

Normal functional stresses maintain the normal width and cellularity of the ligament. Single-rooted teeth tend to rotate about a point located near the junction of the lower and middle thirds of their roots.[108] This results in a wider ligament coronally and near the root apex.[1,109] In multirooted teeth the axis of rotation is probably located between the roots, near the apical third.

If a tooth loses its antagonist, the absence of occlusal forces no longer counteracts the tendency of the tooth to erupt. Despite the lack of convincing evidence,[110] the most likely source of eruptive forces are the fibroblasts in the periodontal ligament.[65-68,111-113] The loss of normal function results not only in gradual supereruption but also in a narrowing of the ligament and a loss of cellularity.[1,109,114] Similar but more extreme changes can be observed around impacted teeth. Supereruption may be accompanied by thickening of the apical cementum as well as a widening of the gingiva.

## Nutritive and sensory functions

The nutritive functions are provided by the blood vessels that bring nutrients and oxygen to the ligament. These diffuse to the cellular elements, while waste products and assorted metabolites diffuse into the vasculature.

The sensory functions of the ligament are primarily confined to pain and tactile sensation. Proprioceptive functions have also been postulated, but proprioception does not appear to be significantly affected by the absence of teeth.

## REFERENCES

1. Coolidge, E.D.: The thickness of the human periodontal membrane, J. Am. Dent. Assoc. **24:**1260, 1937.
2. Alexandridis, C., and White, S.C.: Periodontal ligament changes in patients with progressive systemic sclerosis, Oral Surg. **58:**113, 1984.
3. Schroeder, H.E.: Orale Strukturbiologie, Stuttgart, 1976, Georg Thieme Verlag, p. 212.
4. Jepsen, A.: Root surface measurements and a method for x-ray determination of root surface area, Acta Odontol. Scand. **21:**35, 1963.
5. Hermann, D.W., et al.: The potential attachment area of the maxillary first molar, J. Periodontol. **54:**431, 1983.
6. Akiyoshi, M., and Inoue, M.: On the functional structure of cementum, Bull. Tokyo Med. Dent. Univ. **10:**41, 1963.
7. Ten Cate, A.R., and Mills, C.: The development of the periodontium: the origin of alveolar bone, Anat. Rec. **173:**69, 1971.
8. Ten Cate, A.R., Mills, C., and Solomon, G.: The development of the periodontium: a transplantation and autoradiographic study, Anat. Rec. **170:**365, 1971.
9. Freeman, E., and Ten Cate, A.R.: Development of the periodontium: an electron microscopic study, J. Periodontol. **42:**387, 1971.
10. Ten Cate, A.R.: Cell division and periodontal ligament formation in the mouse, Arch. Oral Biol. **17:**1781, 1972.
11. Ten Cate, A.R.: Formation of supporting bone in association with periodontal ligament organization in the mouse, Arch. Oral Biol. **20:**137, 1975.
12. Levy, B., and Bernick, S.: Studies on the biology of the periodontium of marmosets. II. Development and organization of the periodontal ligament of deciduous teeth in marmosets (*Callithrix jacchus*), J. Dent. Res. **47:**27, 1968.

13. Grant, D., and Bernick, S.: The formation of the periodontal ligament, J. Periodontol. **43:**17, 1972.

14. Grant, D.A., et al.: A comparative study of periodontal ligament development in teeth with and without predecessors in marmosets, J. Periodontol. **43:**162, 1972.

15. Sicher, H.: Bau und Funktion des Fixationapparates der Meerschweinchenmolaren, Z. Stomatol. **21:**580, 1923.

16. Sicher, H.: The principal fibers of the periodontal membrane, Bur. **55:**2, 1954.

17. Sicher, H.: The axial movement of continuously growing teeth, J. Dent. Res. **21:**201, 1942.

18. Orban, B.: Beziehungen zwischen Zahn und Knochen Bewegung der Zahnkeime. Z. Anat. u. Entwicklungs. **83:**804, 1927.

19. Bernick, S.: The organization of the periodontal membrane fibres of the developing molars of rats, Arch. Oral Biol. **2:**57, 1960.

20. Zwarych, P.D., and Quigley, M.B.: The intermediate plexus of the periodontal ligament: history and further observations, J. Dent. Res. **44:**383, 1965.

21. Miura, F., et al.: Development and organization of periodontal membrane and physiologic tooth movement, Bull. Tokyo Med. Dent. Univ. **17:**123, 1970.

22. Melcher, A.H., and Correia, M.A.: Remodelling of periodontal ligament in erupting molars of mature rats, J. Periodont. Res. **6:**118, 1971.

23. Crumley, P.J.: Collagen formation in the normal and stressed periodontium, Periodontics **2:**53, 1964.

24. Carneiro, J.: Synthesis and turnover of collagen in periodontal tissues. In Leblond, C.P., and Warren, K.B., editors: Use of radioautography in investigating protein synthesis, New York, 1965, Academic Press, Inc., pp. 247-257.

25. Carneiro, J., and de Moraes, F.F.: Radioautographic visualization of collagen metabolism in the periodontal tissues of the mouse, Arch. Oral Biol. **10:**833, 1965.

26. Baumhammers, A., and Stallard, R.E.: S$^{35}$-sulfate utilization and turnover by the connective tissues of the periodontium, J. Periodont. Res. **3:**187, 1968.

27. Skougaard, M.R., Levy, B.M., and Simpson, J.: Collagen metabolism in skin and periodontal membrane of the marmoset, Scand. J. Dent. Res. **78:**256, 1970.

28. Kameyama, Y.: Autoradiographic study of $^3$H-proline incorporation by rat periodontal ligament, gingival connective tissue and dental pulp, J. Periodont. Res. **10:**98, 1975.

29. Kanoza, R.J.J., et al.: A biochemical analysis of the effect of hypofunction on collagen metabolism in the rat molar periodontal ligament, Arch. Oral Biol. **25:**663, 1980.

30. Sodek, J.: A new approach to assessing collagen turnover by using a microassay: a highly efficient and rapid tunrover of collagen in rat periodontal tissues, Biochem. J. **160:**243, 1976.

31. Sodek, J.: A comparison of the rates of synthesis and turnover of collagen and non-collagen protein in adult rat periodontal tissues and skin using a microassay, Arch. Oral Biol. **22:**655, 1977.

32. Imberman, M., et al.: A reassessment of collagen half-life in rat periodontal tissues: application of the pool expansion approach, J. Periodont. Res. **21:**396, 1986.

32a. Sodek, J.: A comparison of collagen and non-collagenous protein metabolism in rat molar and incisor periodontal ligaments, Arch. Oral Biol. **23:**977, 1978.

33. Sodek, J., et al.: Collagen synthesis is a major component of protein synthesis in the periodontal ligament in various species, Arch. Oral Biol. **22:**647, 1977.

34. Minkoff, R., and Engstrom, T.G.: A long-term comparison of protein turnover in subcrestal vs. supracrestal fibre tracts in the mouse periodontium, Arch. Oral Biol. **24:**817, 1979.

35. Gould, T.R.L., Brunette, D.M., and Dorey, J.: Cell turnover in the periodontal ligament determined by continuous infusion of H$^3$-thymidine using osmotic minipumps, J. Periodont. Res. **17:**662, 1982.

36. McCullouch, C.A.G., and Melcher, A.H.: Continuous labelling of the periodontal ligament of mice, J. Periodont. Res. **18:**231, 1983.

37. Rippin, J.W.: Collagen turnover in the periodontal ligament under normal and altered functional forces. II. Adult rat molars, J. Periodont. Res. **13:**149, 1978.

38. McCullouch, C.A.G., and Melcher, A.H.: Cell density and cell generation in the periodontal ligament of mice, Am. J. Anat. **167:**43, 1983.

39. Black, G.V.: Special dental pathology, Chicago, 1915, Medico-Dental Publishing Co.

40. Schour, I.: Noyes' oral histology and embryology, ed. 8, Philadelphia, 1960, Lea & Febiger.

41. Shackleford, J.M.: The indifferent fiber plexus and its relationship to principal fibers of the periodontium, Am. J. Anat. **131:**427, 1971.

42. Shackleford, J.M.: Scanning electron microscopy of the dog periodontium, J. Periodont. Res. **6:**45, 1971.

43. Quigley, M.B.: Perforating (Sharpey's) fibers of the periodontal ligament and bone, Alabama J. Med. Sci. **7:**336, 1970.

44. Eccles, J.D.: Studies on the development of the periodontal membrane: the principal fibres of the molar teeth, Dent. Pract. Dent. Rec. **10:**31, 1959.

45. Eccles, J.D.: The development of the periodontal membrane in the rat incisor, Arch. Oral Biol. **9:**127, 1964.

46. Sims, M.R.: Oxytalan-vascular relationships

observed in histologic examination of the periodontal ligaments of man and mouse, Arch. Oral Biol. **20:**713, 1975.

47. Sims, M.R.: Electron-microscopic affiliations in oxytalan fibres, nerves and the microvascular bed in the mouse periodontal ligament, Arch. Oral Biol. **28:**1017, 1983.

48. Garant, P.R., and Cho, M.-I.: Cytoplasmic polarization of periodontal ligament fibroblasts: implications for cell migration and collagen secretion, J. Periodont. Res. **14:**95, 1979.

49. Beertsen, W., Everts, V., and Brekelmans, M.: Unipolarity of fibroblasts in rodent periodontal ligament, Anat. Rec. **195:**535, 1979.

50. Pitaru, S., and Melcher, A.H.: Orientation of gingival fibroblasts and newly synthesized collagen fibers in vitro: resemblance to transseptal and dento-gingival fibers, J. Periodont. Res. **18:**483, 1983.

51. Nimni, M.E.,: Metabolic pathways and central mechanisms involved in the biosynthesis and turnover of collagen in normal and pathological connective tissues, J. Oral Pathol. **2:**175, 1973.

52. Listgarten, M.A.: Intracellular collagen fibers in the periodontal ligament of the mouse, rat, hamster, guinea pig and rabbit, J. Periodont. Res. **8:**335, 1973.

53. Ten Cate, A.R., and Syrbu, S.: A relationship between alkaline phosphatase activity and the phagocytosis and degradation of collagen by the fibroblast, J. Anat. **117:**351, 1974.

54. Eley, B.M., and Harrison, J.D.: Intracellular collagen fibrils in the periodontal ligament of man, J. Periodont. Res. **10:**168, 1975.

55. Ten Cate, A.R., and Deporter, D.A.: The degradative role of the fibroblast in the remodeling and turnover of collagen in soft connective tissue, Anat. Rec. **182:**1, 1975.

56. Garant, P.R.: Collagen resorption by fibroblasts: a theory of fibroblastic maintenance of the periodontal ligament, J. Periodontol. **47:**380, 1976.

57. Shore, R.C., and Berkovitz, B.K.B.: An ultrastructural study of periodontal ligament fibroblasts in relation to their possible role in tooth eruption and intracellular collagen degradation in the rat, Arch. Oral Biol. **24:**155, 1979.

58. Svoboda, E.L.A., Brunette, D.M., and Melcher, A.H.: *In vitro* phagocytosis of exogenous collagen by fibroblasts from the periodontal ligament: an electron microscopic study, J. Anat. **128:**301, 1979.

59. Yajima, T., Rose, G.G., and Mahan, C.J.: Human gingival fibroblast cell lines *in vitro*. II. Electron microscopic studies of fibrogenesis, J. Periodont. Res. **15:**267, 1980.

60. Birek, P., et al.: Epithelial rests of Malassez *in vitro:* phagocytosis of collagen and the possible role of their lysosomal enzymes in collagen degradation, Lab. Invest. **43:**61, 1980.

61. Deporter, D.A., and Ten Cate, A.R.: Collagen resorption by periodontal ligament fibroblasts at the hard tissue-ligament interfaces of the mouse periodontium, J. Periodontol. **51:**429, 1980.

62. Yamasaki, A., Rose, G.G., and Mahan, C.J.: Collagen degradation by human gingival fibroblasts. I. In vivo phagocytosis, J. Periodont. Res. **16:**309, 1981.

63. Christner, P.: Collagenase in the human periodontal ligament, J. Periodontol. **51:**455, 1980.

64. Golub, L.M., et al.: Minocycline reduces gingival collagenolytic activity during diabetes: preliminary observations and a proposed new mechanism of action, J. Periodont. Res. **18:**516, 1983.

65. Beertsen, W., Everts, V., and van den Hoof, A.: Fine structure of fibroblasts in the periodontal ligament of the rat incisor and their possible role in tooth eruption, Arch. Oral Biol. **19:**1087, 1974.

66. Beertsen, W.: Migration of fibroblasts in the periodontal ligament of the mouse incisor as revealed by autoradiography, Arch. Oral Biol. **20:**659, 1975.

67. Harris, A.K., Stopak, D., and Wild, P.: Fibroblast traction as a mechanism for collagen morphogenesis, Nature **290:**249, 1981.

68. Bellows, C.G., Melcher, A.H., and Aubin, J.E.: An *in vitro* model for tooth eruption utilizing periodontal ligament fibroblasts and collagen lattices, Arch. Oral Biol. **28:**715, 1983.

69. Eyre, D.R.: Collagen: molecular diversity in the body's protein scaffold, Science **207:**1315, 1980.

70. Hassell, T.M., and Stanek, E.J. III: Evidence that healthy human gingiva contains functionally heterogeneous fibroblast subpopulations, Arch. Oral Biol. **28:**617, 1983.

71. Limeback, H., Sodek, J., and Aubin, J.E.: Variation in collagen expression by cloned periodontal ligament cells, J. Periodont. Res. **18:**242, 1983.

72. Bordin, S., Page, R.C., and Narayanan, A.S.: Heterogeneity of normal human diploid fibroblasts: isolation and characterization of one phenotype, Science **223:**171, 1984.

73. Narayanan, A.S., and Page, R.C.: Connective tissues of the periodontium: a summary of current work, Collagen Rel. Res. **3:**33, 1983.

74. Roberts, W.E., Goodwin, W.C., Jr., and Heiner, S.R.: Cellular response to orthodontic force, Dent. Clin. North Am. **25:**3, 1981.

75. Roberts, W.E., Mozsary, P.G., and Klingler, E.: Nuclear size as a cell-kinetic marker for osteoblast differentiation, Am. J. Anat. **165:**373, 1982.

76. Reeve, C.M., and Wentz, F.J.: The prevalence, morphology, and distribution of the epithelial cell rests in the human periodontal ligament, Oral. Surg. **15:**785, 1962.

77. Simpson, H.E.: The degenerations of the

rests of Malassez with age as observed by the apoxestic technique, J. Periodontol. **36:**288, 1965.

78. Simpson, H.E.: A three-dimensional approach to the microscopy of the periodontal membrane, Proc. Roy. Soc. Med. **60:**537, 1967.

79. Nylen, M., and Grupe, H., Jr.: Ultrastructures of epithelial cells in human periodontal ligament explants, J. Periodont. Res. **4:**248, 1969.

80. Trowbridge, H.O., and Shibata, F.: Mitotic activity in epithelial rests of Malassez, Periodontics **5:**109, 1967.

81. Johansen, J.R.: Incorporation of tritiated thymidine by the epithelial rests of Malassez after attempted extraction of rat molars, Acta Odontol. Scand. **28:**463, 1970.

82. Gilhuus-Moe, O., and Kvam, E.: Behaviour of the epithelial remnants of Malassez following experimental movement of rat molars, Acta Odontol. Scand. **30:**139, 1972.

83. Grant, D.A., and Bernick, S.: A possible continuity between epithelial attachment and epithelial rests in miniature swine, J. Periodontol. **40:**87, 1969.

84. Spouge, J.D.: A new look at the rests of Malassez: a review of their embryological origin, anatomy, and possible role in periodontal health and disease, J. Periodontol. **51:**437, 1980.

85. Spouge, J.D.: The rests of Malassez and chronic marginal periodontitis, J. Clin. Periodontol. **11:**340, 1984.

86. Grant, D., and Bernick, S.: Morphodifferentiation and structure of Hertwig's root sheath in the cat, J. Dent. Res. **50:**1580, 1971.

87. Tonna, E.A.: Histological age change associated with mouse paradontal tissues, J. Gerontol. **28:**1, 1973.

88. Severson, J.A., et al.: A histological study of age changes in the adult human periodontal joint (ligament), J. Periodontol. **49:**189, 1978.

89. Birn, H.: The vascular supply of the periodontal membrane, J. Periodont. Res. **1:**51, 1966.

90. Picton, D.C.A.: The effect of external forces on the periodontium. In Melcher, A.H., and Bowen, W.H., editors: Biology of the periodontium, London, 1969, Academic Press, Inc., p. 363.

91. Wills, D.J., Picton, D.C.A., and Davies, W.I.R.: A study of the fluid systems of the periodontium in macaque monkeys, Arch. Oral Biol. **21:**175, 1976.

92. Moxham, B.J., and Berkowitz, B.K.B.: The effects of external forces on the periodontal ligament: the response to axial loads. In Berkowitz, B.K.B., Moxham, B.T., and Newman, H.N., editors: The periodontal ligament in health and disease, New York, 1982, Pergamon Press, p. 249.

93. Walker, T.W., Ng, G.C., and Burke, P.S.: Fluid pressures in the periodontal ligament of the mandibular canine tooth in dogs, Arch. Oral. Biol. **23:**753, 1978.

94. Edwall, L.G.A.: Vasculature of the periodontal ligament. In Berkowitz, B.K.B., Moxham, B.T., and Newman, H.N., editors: The periodontal ligament in health and disease, Oxford, 1982, Pergamon Press, p. 151.

95. Levy, B., and Bernick, S.: Studies on the biology of the periodontium of marmosets. V. Lymphatic vessels of the periodontal ligaments, J. Dent. Res. **47:**1166, 1968.

96. Bernick, S., and Grant, D.A.: Lymphatic vessels of healthy and inflamed gingiva, J. Dent. Res. **57:**810, 1978.

97. van Steenberghe, D.: The structure and function of periodontal innervation: a review of the literature, J. Periodont. Res. **14:**185, 1979.

98. Hannam, A.G.: The innervation of the periodontal ligament. In Berkowitz, B.K.B., Moxham, B.T., and Newman, H.N., editors: The periodontal ligament in health and disease, New York, 1982, Pergamon Press Inc., p. 173.

99. Griffin, C.J.: The fine structure of end-rings in human periodontal ligament, Arch. Oral Biol. **17:**785, 1972.

100. Griffin, C.J., and Spain, H.: Organization and vasculature of human periodontal ligament mechanoreceptors, Arch. Oral Biol. **17:**913, 1972.

101. Berkowitz, B.K.B., Shore, R.C., and Moxham, B.J.: The occurrence of a lamellated nerve terminal in the periodontal ligament of the rat incisor, Arch. Oral Biol. **28:**99, 1983.

102. Willis, R.D., and DiCosimo, C.J.: The absence of proprioceptive nerve endings in the human periodontal ligament: the role of periodontal mechanoreceptors in the reflex control of mastication, Oral Surg. **48:**108, 1979.

103. Bien, S.M.: Hydrodynamic damping of tooth movement, J. Dent. Res. **45:**907, 1966.

104. Atkinson, H.F., and Ralph, W.J.: An experimental model for the investigation of the tooth support mechanism, Arch. Oral Biol. **20:**261, 1975.

105. Kardos, T.B., and Simpson, L.D.: A theoretical consideration of the periodontal membrane as a collagenous thixotropic system and its relationship to tooth eruption, J. Periodont. Res. **14:**444, 1979.

106. Ferrier, J.M., and Dillon, E.M.: The water binding capacity of the periodontal ligament and its role in mechanical function, J. Periodont. Res. **18:**469, 1983.

107. Davies, R., and Picton, D.C.A.: Dimensional changes in the periodontal membrane of monkey's teeth with horizontal thrusts, J. Dent. Res. **46:**114, 1967.

108. Muhlemann, H.R.: The determination of tooth rotation centers, Oral Surg. **7:**392, 1954.

109. Kronfeld, R.: Histologic study of the influence of function on the human periodontal membrane, Am. J. Dent. Assoc. **18:**1242, 1931.
110. Moxham, B.J., and Berkowitz, B.K.B.: The periodontal ligament and physiological tooth movements. In Berkowitz, B.K.B., Moxham, B.T., and Newman, H.N., editors: The periodontal ligament in health and disease, New York, 1982, Pergamon Press Inc., p. 215.
111. Parfitt, G.H.: The physical analysis of tooth supporting structures. In Anderson, D.J., et al., editors: The mechanisms of tooth support, Bristol, 1967, J. Wright & Sons, p. 154.
112. Ness, A.R.: Eruption: a review. In Anderson, D.J., et al., editors: The mechanisms of tooth support, Bristol, 1967, J. Wright & Sons, p. 84.
113. Zajicek, G.: Fibroblast cell kinetics in the periodontal ligament of the mouse, Cell Tiss. Kinet. **7:**479, 1974.
114. Anneroth, G., and Ericsson, S.G.: An experimental histological study of monkey teeth without antagonist, Odont. Rev. **18:**345, 1967.

**ADDITIONAL SUGGESTED READING**

Anderson, D.J., Hannam, A.G., and Matthews, B.: Sensory mechanisms in mammalian teeth and their supporting structures, Physiol. Rev. **50:**171, 1970.

# CHAPTER 4

# Cementum

Classification

Cementum-associated cells

Structural characteristics of radicular cementum
Acellular fibrillar cementum
Cellular fibrillar cementum

Development of radicular cementum

Development and structure of coronal cementum

Developmental and acquired anomalies associated with cementogenesis

---

Cementum is a mineralized connective tissue that covers the roots of teeth. Its main function is to attach the periodontal ligament fibers to the teeth. Occasionally cementum may extend over enamel. Cementum is similar in structure and composition to bone. Yet it differs from bone in several important respects including its microscopic organization, its lack of vascularity, and the absence of continuous remodelling.

## Classification

Cementum can be classified by its *location* on the tooth, its *cellularity,* and by the *presence or absence of collagen fibrils* in its organic matrix.

Radicular and coronal cementum

Acellular and cellular cementum

Fibrillar and afibrillar cementum

*Radicular cementum* refers to the cementum that covers the root. In humans, radicular cementum accounts for the bulk of cementum.[1,2] *Coronal cementum* refers to cementum found over enamel.[1,2] In human teeth it is thin and poorly developed.[3-5] Coronal cementum is most developed on teeth of herbivores[6-13] where it helps in anchoring teeth with long crowns and relatively short or absent roots. *Acellular cementum*[1,2] refers to cementum lacking embedded cells, while *cellular cementum*[1,2] contains cells in lacunae located within the mineralized matrix (Fig. 4-1). *Fibrillar cementum,*[4,11,14-22] the most common form, contains well-defined, densely packed collagen fibrils in its matrix. By contrast, the organic matrix of *afibrillar cementum*[4,5,11,23-25] lacks this dense array of collagen fibrils, although isolated fibrils may be encountered. It is comparatively rare.

Little cementum is formed before eruption and prior to teeth reaching functional occlusion. This cementum is generally acellular and contains comparatively few col-

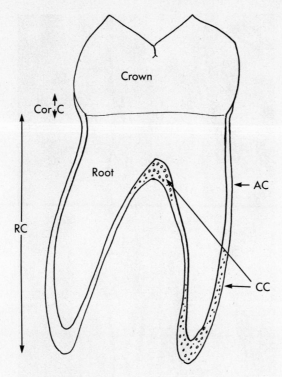

**Fig. 4-1.** Diagram illustrating the distribution of cementum on the tooth surface. The cementum covering the anatomic crown of the tooth is coronal cementum *(Cor C)*. The roots are covered with radicular cementum *(RC)*. Cellular cementum *(CC)* can be found on the apical third of the roots and within furcations. Acellular cementum *(AC)* covers the coronal two thirds of the root and extends over the cervical portion of the crown.

lagen fibrils, which are loosely packed and more or less perpendicular to the dentin-ocemental junction. This constitutes the *primary cementum* layer. Subsequent to occlusal contact, additional layers of cementum are deposited over the primary cementum to form *secondary cementum* (Fig. 4-2). Its matrix contains a much denser array of collagen fibrils. It may be acellular or cellular.[14]

**Primary and secondary cementum**

## Cementum-associated cells

The cells associated with cementum are comparatively few and generally reside within the periodontal ligament.

### Cementoblasts

The earliest cementoblasts originate from ectomesenchymal cells in the dental follicle surrounding developing teeth.[26-28] Cementoblasts may also develop later from undifferentiated mesenchymal cells persisting in the center of the periodontal ligament. Cementoblasts are responsible for producing a loose network of collagen fibrils and a proteoglycan ground substance that surrounds the principal fibers of the periodontal ligament. They probably also participate in the mineralization of the cementum. They are morphologically similar to periodontal fibroblasts,[20-22] and are differentiated primarily by their location within the periodontal ligament, along the forming cemental surface (Fig. 4-3). Their cytoplasmic volume and basophilia may increase during periods of active cementogenesis.

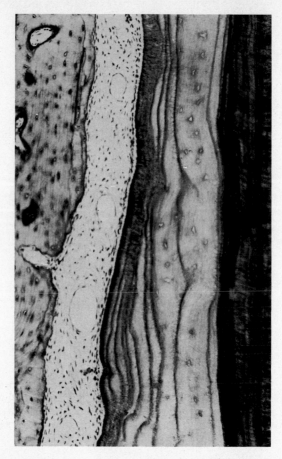

**Fig. 4-2.** Secondary cellular cementum is sandwiched between a base and an outer coat of acellular cementum. The lamellar (layered) arrangement reflects the appositional growth pattern of cementum.

## Cementocytes

Cementocytes are found only in cellular cementum (Fig. 4-4). They are located within *lacunae* and have numerous cytoplasmic processes coursing in *canaliculi* that are preferentially directed toward the ligament. Their cytoplasmic volume and the density of cytoplasmic organelles is markedly reduced when compared to cemento-blasts.[19,21] While these cells remain vital, their metabolic activity is low. Labelling experiments in rodents suggest that these cells retain the capability of synthesizing as well as resorbing the cementum lining the lacunae,[22,29] but their lytic potential has been questioned.[30]

## Periodontal fibroblasts

Technically these cells belong to the periodontal ligament where they are respon-sible, in part, for the synthesis of the principal fibers. Since the latter become embedded in and form an important component of cementum, periodontal fibroblasts indirectly participate in the formation of cementum.

## Cementoclasts (odontoclasts)

These multinucleated giant cells are indistinguishable from osteoclasts. They are responsible for the extensive root resorption that leads to primary tooth exfoliation and for the localized cemental resorption that is commonly encountered in adult dentitions.

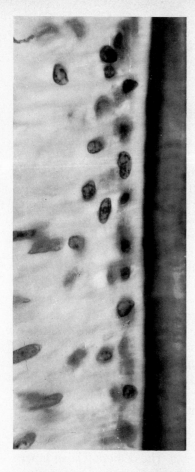

**Fig. 4-3.** Cementoblasts on the surface of a recently formed layer of uncalcified cementum (or cementoid).

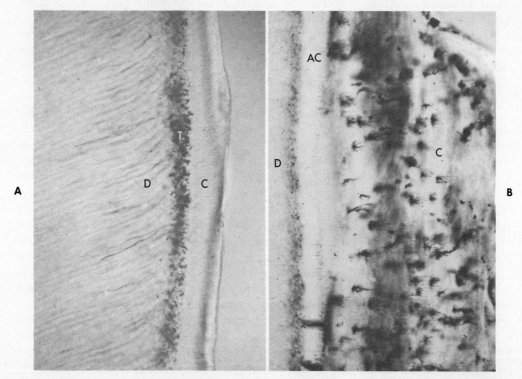

**Fig. 4-4.** **A,** Ground section of acellular fibrillar cementum in the coronal half of the root. Tomes' granular layer *(T)*, which is part of the peripheral dentin *(D)*, is in contact with the relatively thin cementum layer *(C)*. **B,** Ground section of cellular fibrillar cementum in the apical third of the root. A thin layer of acellular cementum *(AC)* separates the dentin *(D)* from the cellular cementum *(C)*. Note lacunar canaliculi preferentially oriented toward periodontal ligament side *(to the right)*.

Such resorption occurs on mesial surfaces in association with mesial migration and may occur with occlusal trauma and during orthodontic or periodontal therapy.

## Structural characteristics of radicular cementum

Radicular cementum is the most prominent form of cementum in human teeth both quantitatively and in terms of its functional importance. It is almost entirely made up of fibrillar cementum and it helps to anchor the root to the alveolar wall via the periodontal ligament. The coronal two thirds of cementum is generally acellular. The apical third and the furcations of multirooted teeth are lined with cellular cementum, which frequently lies over a thin layer of acellular cementum (Fig. 4-4, B).

### ACELLULAR FIBRILLAR CEMENTUM

Acellular, fibrillar cementum covers the coronal half of the root. It is a thin, transparent, mineralized tissue, which in ground sections of teeth appears clear and devoid of cells (Fig. 4-4, A). In demineralized, stained microscopic sections the cementum forms as a distinct layer external to and clearly differentiated from dentin. It does not contain the characteristic tubules of dentin and does not include the zone of irregularly mineralized dentin known as Tomes' granular layer. In stained sections the acellular, fibrillar cementum is characterized by well-defined *appositional lines (resting lines)* more or less parallel to one another and the root surface. The lines reflect the slow, cyclical, appositional growth pattern of cementum that continues throughout life (see Fig. 4-2). Consequently, the rather thin layer of cementum noted on recently erupted teeth will tend to increase in thickness with age.[31,32]

The thickness of the acellular, fibrillar cemental layer varies from a few micrometers at the time of eruption to 60 μm or more in elderly subjects. The cemental layer tapers off in a coronal direction to end in the vicinity of the cervical region. On the other hand, apically the thickness of cellular cementum may exceed 500 μm.[31]

In most instances cementum overlaps the cervical enamel (60% to 65%), thereby giving rise to poorly developed patches of coronal cementum. Sometimes cementum touches, but does not overlap, the enamel (30%) and infrequently (5% to 10%) there is a gap of exposed dentin between the enamel and cementum. All of these relationships may occur on a single tooth (Fig. 4-5).[7]

Despite its mineralized nature and the absence of included cells, acellular, fibrillar cementum is readily penetrated by various aqueous solutions[33-35] and presumably, following gingival recession, by bacterial toxins.[36-38] Attempts to clarify the depth to which bacterial toxins can penetrate cementum have produced controversial results.

Of the mineralized dental tissues, cementum is the least mineralized. However it is somewhat more mineralized than bone.[39-41] Electron micrographs of demineralized cementum reveal an organic matrix principally composed of an array of densely packed collagen fibrils[14-16,18-21] with the typical type I collagen bands in register with one another (Fig. 4-6, A). A fine granular matrix surrounds the collagen fibrils. The bulk of the fibrils are oriented more or less perpendicularly to the root surface (Fig. 4-6, B).[42,43] These fibrils are mainly derived from principal fibers of the periodontal ligament, which become incorporated into the first formed cementum. In time, more of the periodontal fibers gradually become embedded into the cementum matrix by the action of the cementoblasts. The cementoblasts produce loosely packed collagen fibrils that form a meshwork surrounding the principal fibers of the ligament (Fig. 4-7) in a plane parallel to the cementum surface.[16,18] These *indifferent cementum fibrils,*[44] as well as the principal fibers, are surrounded by a proteoglycan ground substance also synthesized by cementoblasts. This organic layer becomes mineralized shortly after its deposition on the root surface (Fig. 4-8).

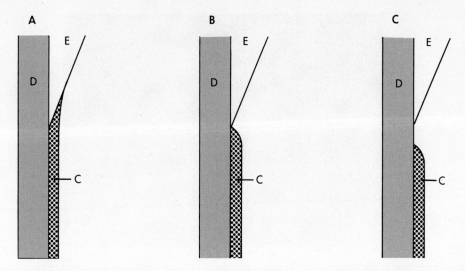

**Fig. 4-5.** Relationships of cementum to the apical enamel border. **A,** Cementum *(C)* overlaps enamel *(E)*. **B,** Cementum abuts enamel. **C,** Cementum is separated from enamel, exposing a gap of dentin *(D)*.

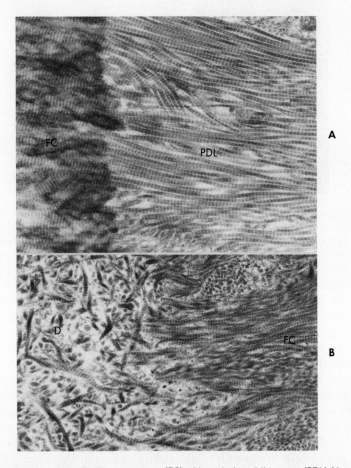

**Fig. 4-6.** **A,** Junction of acellular fibrillar cementum *(FC)* with periodontal ligament *(PDL)*. Note that individual fibrils within cementum tend to blend with adjacent fibrils. Collagen fibrils in *FC* are continuous with those in *PDL*. In cementum, the striations of the collagen fibrils are frequently in register with neighboring fibrils. **B,** Junction of acellular fibrillar cementum *(FC)* with dentin *(D)*. The dentinocemental junction can be readily identified by the different orientation of the collagen fibrils in dentin and cementum.

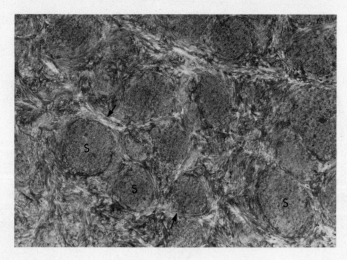

**Fig. 4-7.** Section of cementum parallel to the surface. Sharpey's fibers *(S)* have a circular cross section. Note that they are surrounded by collagen fibrils that lie in a plane perpendicular to Sharpey's fibers *(arrows)*.

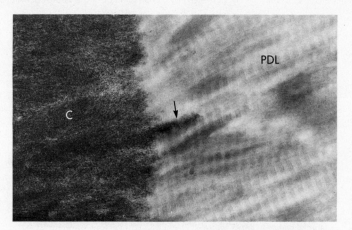

**Fig. 4-8.** Section through the junction of undemineralized cementum *(C)* and periodontal ligament *(PDL)*. The electron-dense needle-shaped hydroxyapatite crystallites obliterate the collagen fibrils and their typical striations. Note mineralization of a single fibril ahead of the mineralizing front *(arrow)*.

The cementoblasts control the rate of cementum matrix deposition as well as its mineralization. During active cementogenesis, the cementoblasts form a distinct layer of cuboidal cells lining the cemental surface. They may be separated from the mineralized front by a layer several micrometers wide of nonmineralized cementum matrix, the *cementoid* or *precementum* (see Fig. 4-3). The cementoid layer tends to increase in thickness with increasing cementogenetic activity. Its continuity is interrupted by principal fibers that pass from the ligament into the cementum. During periods of inactivity the cementoid layer as well as the cementoblasts may temporarily disappear. A cementoid layer may be rare in old age.[44a] During active cementogenesis, the cementoblasts exhibit a prominent cytoplasm, which features a well-developed Golgi region and rough-surfaced endoplasmic reticulum.[22] Cytoplasmic projections extend toward the cementum, frequently surrounding collagen fibers anchored in the cementum.

The mineralized portion of the principal fibers embedded in the cementum are referred to as *Sharpey's fibers*,[43] a descriptive term that is applicable to all mineralized fiber insertions. The mineralized component consists of thin, needle-shaped crystals of hydroxyapatite that permeate the entire organic framework and account for approximately 61% by weight (33% by volume) of radicular cementum. The remaining fractions consist of organic matrix 27% by weight (31% by volume) and water 12% by weight (36% by volume). The degree of mineralization varies in different layers of cementum. Generally, the mineral content tends to be highest at the surface, close to the dentinocemental junction and within resting lines.[16,19,45,46] The cemental mineralization of teeth in teenagers tends to be less than in older subjects.[47] In periodontally diseased teeth, the cervical cementum exposed to the oral environment may develop a hypermineralized surface layer,[48-52] presumably from the calcium- and phosphate-rich saliva.

Loosely packed collagen fibrils and large interfibrillar spaces containing an amorphous organic matrix are seen near the dentinocemental junction. In addition, the junction between dentin and cementum can be localized ultrastructurally by the difference in orientation of collagen fibrils (see Fig. 4-6, *B*). In dentin, collagen fibrils tend to curve, are not aggregated into distinct bundles, and exhibit little, if any, preferential orientation. Cemental collagen fibrils, on the other hand, tend to be straight and form bundles that are more or less perpendicular to the dentinocemental junction. Peripheral to its junction with dentin, the bundles of fibrils (fibers) within acellular, fibrillar cementum may not be readily apparent since the dense packing of the collagen fibrils masks individual fibers in the matrix (see Fig. 4-6, *A*).[53]

## CELLULAR FIBRILLAR CEMENTUM

Cellular fibrillar cementum is found primarily over the apical half of the root and in the furcation of multirooted teeth. Although similar to acellular fibrillar cementum, it differs in several respects: namely, the presence of cementocytes in cemental lacunae; the irregularity of formation, as reflected by the pattern of resting lines; its greater rate of formation, reflected in greater thickness and the spacing of the resting lines;[54] the degree of mineralization that may vary significantly from one layer to another; and the more prominent Sharpey's fibers in cellular cementum. At midroot, cellular cementum is frequently formed over a previously deposited layer of acellular cementum (see Fig. 4-2).

The cellularity of this type of cementum is best observed in ground sections. While the actual cells may be lost in processing, the lacunae and the numerous canaliculi that radiate from them can be identified. In contrast to osseous lacunae, which do not exhibit any preferential canalicular orientation, cemental lacunae tend to have a majority of canaliculi directed toward nutritive sources in the periodontal ligament (see Fig. 4-4, *B*).

In stained sections of demineralized teeth, the resting lines are not as parallel to one another and as regularly spaced as in acellular, fibrillar cementum. Instead, the lines frequently follow an irregular outline, sometimes running into adjacent lines. This appositional pattern suggests that cellular cementum is deposited at different rates in different areas of the root surface.[42,43,54] Despite the irregularity of cellular cementogenesis, the average rate of formation exceeds that of acellular cementum. This increased rate of formation may result in trapping cementoblasts within the newly formed cementoid layer and the consequent formation of cementocytes.

Like that of acellular fibrillar cementum, the organic matrix of cellular cementum is composed predominantly of collagen fibrils within a proteoglycan ground substance. Most of the collagen fibrils are oriented perpendicularly to the cementum surface and appear as distinct fiber bundles continuous with the principal fibers entering the periodontal ligament. Indifferent collagen fibrils arranged parallel to the cementum surface course between the other collagen fibers. Indifferent collagen fibrils tend to be more prominent in cellular than in acellular cementum, thus preventing the fiber bundles from becoming closely packed (Figs. 4-9 and 4-10). In acellular cementum, collagen fibers derived from the principal fibers of the ligament frequently lose their identity as a result of close packing. By contrast, the fibers in cellular cementum remain as distinct bundles, mineralized to varying degrees.[16,18,19]

Sharpey's fibers in cellular cementum tend to be well mineralized on the periphery, while the central core remains unmineralized.[55,56] By scanning electron microscopy of deproteinized root surfaces, this pattern of mineralization exhibits a surface with dome-like prominences (the individual Sharpey's fibers) many of which contain a central pit (Fig. 4-10) caused by the loss of the nonmineralized fibrils from the core of the fiber.[55] In addition to the irregular mineralization of Sharpey's fibers, the degree of mineralization may vary between adjacent *lamellae* of cementum, i.e., the cementum layers between the resting lines.

Cellular, fibrillar cementum gradually increases in thickness with age. In the apical region the average thickness of cementum may vary from approximately 0.2 mm in teenagers to 0.6 mm or more in the elderly.[31] In overerupted teeth, the thickness of the apical cementum may be considerably greater.

## Development of radicular cementum

Root formation is initiated and controlled by *Hertwig's epithelial root sheath*, a double-layered apical extension of the odontogenic epithelium that ends as the epithelial diaphragm.[57,58] This structure induces the differentiation of odontoblasts from the mesenchymal cells of the dental papilla. The odontoblasts proceed to form a layer of predentin in contact with the basal lamina of the epithelial root sheath. The predentin mineralizes almost immediately to form dentin. As root formation proceeds apically, the dentin wall gradually thickens by continuous apposition on its pulpal surface. The epithelial diaphragm also guides the number and shape of the roots being formed.

Just coronal to the root end (see Fig. 3-15, *B*), Hertwig's epithelial root sheath is displaced away from dentin. This displacement appears to occur as the result of collagen-producing cells invading the epithelial root sheath from the dental follicle. These cells produce collagen within the intercellular spaces of the sheath as well as between the sheath and the dentin wall.[18,58-62]

The collagen-producing cells that perforate the epithelial sheath produce a dense collagenous matrix in contact with the dentin surface, with fibers oriented parallel to the root surface. The cells are ultrastructurally similar to fibroblasts with their long axis oriented parallel to the root surface. Little if any cementum is detectable at this stage of root development in human teeth (see Fig. 3-15, *D*).

In rodent teeth, cementum formation occurs earlier than in human teeth and at a comparatively more rapid rate. Cementogenesis in rodents may give rise to an atypical cementum layer with trapped remnants of Hertwig's epithelial root sheath.[22,30,60] This layer has been described as *intermediate cementum*.[58] It is not routinely found in human teeth, nor should it be confused with Tomes' granular layer of dentin (see Fig. 4-4, *A*).[63] In rodent teeth the collagen fibrils in the first formed cementum tend to be parallel to the dentin surface,[14,15] a finding that is not typical of human or monkey cementum (see Fig. 4-6, *B*).

Just before eruption in primary teeth and permanent molars, or shortly after eruption in secondary teeth, the dental follicle becomes reorganized into a periodontal ligament (see Chapter 3, pp. 59-61). In the earliest stage of this remodelling process collagen fibers appear that are oriented perpendicularly to and in contact with the dentin surface. The ultrastructural organization of the root substance at this time confirms that most

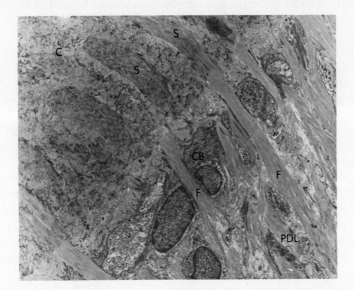

**Fig. 4-9.**    Cementum in apical third of root. Principal fibers *(F)* in the periodontal ligament *(PDL)* insert into cementum *(C)* at a more or less perpendicular angle, as mineralized Sharpey's fibers *(S). CB,* cementoblast.

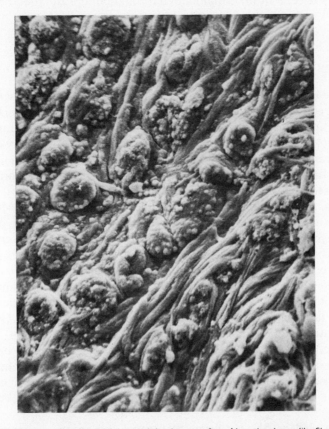

**Fig. 4-10.**    Scanning electron micrograph of deproteinized root surface. Note the dome-like Sharpey's fibers, which project from the cementum surface. This preparation does not exhibit well-defined hollow cores.

of the root surface lacks cementum. Cementogenesis can be said to begin when newly formed fibers, perpendicular to the root surface, are surrounded by a mineralizing ground substance that anchors them to the dentin surface.

As the teeth erupt and become functional, the cementoblasts contribute to the appositional growth of cementum (secondary cementum) by progressively embedding periodontal ligament fibers (principal fibers) and indifferent fibers into a mineralizing proteoglycan ground substance. Cementogenesis continues throughout life but at a comparatively slow rate and in cycles of deposition followed by periods of rest. Occlusal function is not required for cementogenesis. Loss of occlusal function is associated with thick layers of cementum. Teeth that have never been in function or have lost their antagonists following eruption have thick cementum as well.[1,64]

In the coronal half of the root, the cementoblasts on the surface retreat as new cementum is formed. The functional width of the periodontal ligament is maintained primarily by remodelling at the surface of the alveolar bone. In the apical half of the root and in furcations where the growth of cementum is more rapid, cementoblasts may become trapped within the precementum (cementoid) lacunae and become cementocytes. In the case of nonfunction, the width of the periodontal ligament is narrowed, primarily by the apposition of cementum.

Although evidence of localized resorption of acellular and cellular cementum is common,[65] this mineralized tissue does not turn over as does alveolar bone by an integrated process of alternating bone resorption and formation. Instead, deposition of cementum is far more prevalent than resorption.[30] This ensures that the anchorage of ligament fibers to cementum is maintained throughout life and that transient episodes of trauma are repaired.

## Development and structure of coronal cementum

Following completion of amelogenesis, the enamel surface of human teeth remains lined with an epithelial covering—the reduced enamel epithelium. During the subsequent preeruptive period, portions of the reduced enamel epithelium covering the cervical enamel may disappear, thereby exposing sections of the cervical enamel and isolated patches on the cervical half of the crown to adjacent follicular connective tissue. This is frequently followed by the deposition of thin layers of coronal cementum over the exposed enamel surface.[3-5]

In humans, this cementum is afibrillar and acellular (Fig. 4-11). It consists of an organic matrix devoid of collagen fibrils, although isolated fibrils are occasionally detectable. In demineralized specimens examined by transmission electron microscopy, the matrix appears to be finely granular with distinct appositional lines.[4,5] The mineral component is composed of fine crystals of hydroxyapatite.[5,66]

Cross sections through the cervical region indicate that coronal cementum is often continuous with the radicular cementum layer.[4,5,24] The demarcation between the two is readily identified by the difference in their fibrillar content. Occasionally the fibrillar cementum will overlap the afibrillar cementum over enamel. In longitudinal sections of teeth the coronal cementum may appear as a spurlike extension of the radicular cementum. The structural difference between the two may not be detectable by light microscopy. Patchy depositions of coronal cementum over cervical enamel may appear as isolated, flat islands of cementum without connection to radicular cementum.[5]

Cellular as well as fibrillar forms of coronal cementum are common in herbivores,[6,8-13] rabbits,[23] and guinea pigs.[67] A cellular, afibrillar form of coronal cementum has been reported in the bottom of the developmental fissures of human teeth.[25]

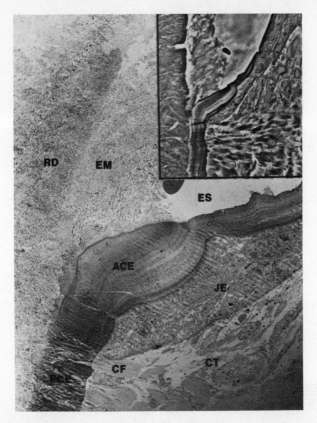

**Fig. 4-11.** Electron micrograph of afibrillar cementum "spur" *(ACE)* overlapping apical border of enamel space *(ES)* created by demineralization during tissue processing for microscopy. *CF*, collagen fiber; *CT*, connective tissue of gingiva; *FCE*, fibrillar root cementum; *EM*, enamel matrix; *RD*, dentin. *Inset*, phase-contrast micrograph of serial section.

## Developmental and acquired anomalies associated with cementogenesis

There are certain anomalies in cementogenesis that may have an impact on the susceptibility of teeth to periodontal disease and the treatment of affected teeth. Some of these will be described briefly:

### Enamel projections

If amelogenesis is not turned off before the start of root formation, enamel may continue to form over portions of the root normally covered by cementum from odontogenic epithelium destined to form Hertwig's root sheath. This may occur in localized areas, particularly in furcations of mandibular molars.[68] It is hypothesized that enamel projections may predispose teeth to periodontal defects involving the furcations.

### Enamel pearls

This anomaly consists of globules of enamel on the root surface in the cervical region (Fig. 4-12). They resemble small pearls, up to several millimeters in diameter.[68,69] They appear to form as a result of the localized failure of Hertwig's root sheath to separate from the dentin surface, thereby allowing cementogenesis to proceed. The adhering epithelium becomes amelogenetic and deposits circumscribed globules of enamel, which in turn may become covered with a layer of afibrillar cementum. The

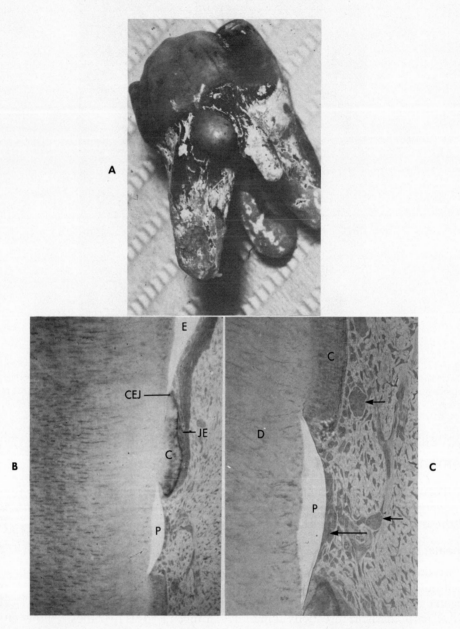

**Fig. 4-12.** **A,** Large enamel pearl near cervical region of maxillary molar. **B,** Small enamel pearl *(P)* just apical to the cementoenamel junction *(CEJ)*. The junctional epithelium *(JE)* has migrated from the crown *(E)* over the cementum *(C)* separating the enamel of the crown *(C)* from the enamel of the pearl *(P)*. **C,** Magnified portion of **B.** Note cell rests *(arrows)* and reduced enamel epithelium *(large arrow)* covering the enamel pearl *(P)*. *C,* cementum; *D,* dentin.

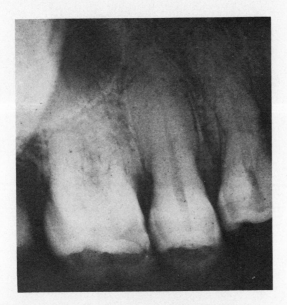

**Fig. 4-13.** Radiograph of hyperplastic cementum (hypercementosis) on maxillary premolar.

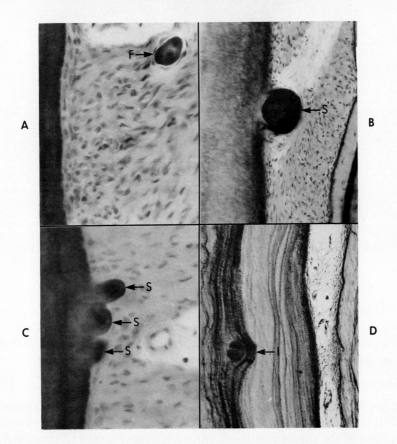

**Fig. 4-14.** **A-C,** Sessile *(S)* and free *(F)* cementicles in periodontal ligament. **D,** Interstitial cementicle *(I)* within cementum layer.

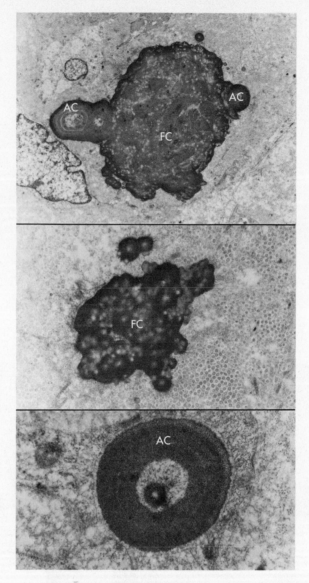

**Fig. 4-15.** Electron micrograph of free cementicles composed of afibrillar cementum *(AC)* and/or fibrillar cementum *(FC)*.

clinical relevance of enamel pearls is their ability to promote periodontal lesions by acting as plaque-retentive structures. While they may mimic calculus clinically and radiographically, they cannot be scaled off and elimination can only be accomplished by grinding. Large pearls may contain pulpal extensions.

### Hypercementosis (hyperplastic cementum)

This is an anomaly consisting in the formation of abnormally thick radicular cementum.[70] It may affect individual teeth or many teeth. Hypercementosis may occur as a thickening of the cementum layer, generally more marked in the apical third of the root (Fig. 4-13). It may also take the form of multiple, localized, knoblike or spike-shaped projections, which give the root an irregular contour. It may fill concavities or root surfaces as selective depositions.

Generalized hypercementosis[71,72] may be hereditary. It has been described in conjunction with Paget's disease.[73] Localized hypercementosis may be observed in impacted teeth as well as teeth without antagonists.[1,66] Spike-shaped projections tend to form on the tension side of teeth along principal fiber insertions. Knoblike projections may form by fusion of free cementicles with the root surface.[69] Hypercementotic anomalies may favor the anchorage of teeth but may also present problems with scaling of the root surface or in extraction of the affected teeth.

## Cementicles

These are globular masses of acellular cementum, generally less than 0.5 mm in diameter, which form within the periodontal ligament.[70] They generally exhibit concentric appositional layers of afibrillar and/or fibrillar cementum (Figs. 4-14 and 4-15) and may lie free within the periodontal ligament (*free* cementicles) or become fused to the radicular cemental surface (*sessile* or *attached* cementicles). Eventually, attached cementicles may become totally incorporated in cementum (*interstitial* cementicles). It has been postulated that cementicles originate from foci of degenerating cells or epithelial cell rests in the periodontal ligament. Generally, cementicles are not of clinical significance unless they become exposed to the oral environment where they may act as sites for plaque retention.

### REFERENCES

1. Kronfeld, R.: The biology of cementum, J. Am. Dent. Assn. **25:**1451, 1938.
2. Gottlieb, B.: Biology of the cementum, J. Periodontol. **13:**13, 1942.
3. Meyer, W.: Normal histology and histogenesis of the human teeth and associated parts, Philadelphia, 1935, J.B. Lippincott Co., p. 151.
4. Listgarten, M.A.: Phase-contrast and electron microscopic study of the junction between reduced enamel epithelium and enamel in unerupted human teeth, Arch. Oral Biol. **11:**999, 1966.
5. Schroeder, H.E., and Listgarten, M.A.: Fine structure of the developing epithelial attachment of human teeth. In Wolsky, A., editor: Monographs in developmental biology, vol. 2, Basel, 1971, S. Karger.
6. Kronfeld, R.: Einige histologische Befunde an Schafzähnen, Schweiz. Mschr. Zahnheilk. **37:**392, 1927.
7. Hopewell-Smith, A.: The normal and pathological histology of the mouth, ed. 2, vol. 1, Philadelphia, 1918, P. Blackiston & Son Co.
8. Weinreb, M.M., and Sharav, Y.: Tooth development in sheep, Am. J. Vet. Res. **25:**891, 1964.
9. Mills, P.B., and Irving, J.T.: Coronal cementogenesis in cattle, Arch. Oral Biol. **12:**929, 1967.
10. Cuttress, T.W., and Healy, W.B.: Calcified deposits on sheep incisor teeth, J. Dent. Res. **46:**1363, 1967.
11. Listgarten, M.A.: A light and electron microscopic study of coronal cementogenesis, Arch. Oral Biol. **13:**93, 1968.
12. Mills, P.B., and Irving, J.T.: Deciduous central incisor tooth development and coronal cementogenesis in cattle, Arch. Oral Biol. **14:**803, 1969.
13. Ainamo, J.: Morphogenetic and functional characteristics of coronal cementum in bovine molars, Scand. J. Dent. Res. **78:**378, 1970.
14. Stern, I.: An electron microscopic study of the cementum, Sharpey's fibers and periodontal ligament in the rat incisor, Am. J. Anat. **115:**377, 1964.
15. Selvig, K.A.: An ultrastructural study of cementum formation, Acta Odontol. Scand. **22:**105, 1964.
16. Selvig, K.A.: The fine structure of human cementum, Acta Odontol. Scand. **23:**423, 1965.
17. Selvig, K.A.: Ultrastructural changes in cementum and adjacent connective tissue in periodontal disease, Acta Odontol. Scand. **24:**459, 1966.
18. Selvig, K.A.: Studies on the genesis, composition and fine structure of cementum, University of Bergen, Thesis, 1967, Universitatsforlaget, Bergen.
19. Furseth, R.: A microradiographic and electron microscopic study of the cementum of human deciduous teeth, Acta Odontol. Scand. **25:**613, 1967.
20. Bevelander, G., and Nakahara, H.: The fine structure of the human periodontal ligament, Anat. Rec. **162:**313, 1968.
21. Furseth, R.: The fine structure of the cellular cementum of young human teeth, Arch. Oral Biol. **14:**1147, 1969.
22. Jande, S.S., and Belanger, L.F.: Fine structural study of rat molar cementum, Anat. Rec. **167:**439, 1970.
23. Listgarten, M.A., and Kamin, A.: The development of a cementum layer over the enamel surface of rabbit molars: a light and electron

microscopic study, Arch. Oral Biol. **14:**961, 1969.

24. Listgarten, M.A.: Afibrillar dental cementum in the rat and hamster, J. Periodont. Res. **10:**158, 1975.

25. Silness, J., et al.: Cellular afibrillar coronal cementum in human teeth, J. Periodont. Res. **11:**331, 1976.

26. Trott, J.R.: The development of the periodontal attachment in the rat, Acta Anat. **51:**313, 1962.

27. Kenney, E.B., and Ramfjord, S.P.: Cellular dynamics of root formation in rhesus monkeys, J. Dent. Res. **48:**114, 1969.

28. Ten Cate, A.R., Mills, C., and Solomon, G.: The development of the periodontium: a transplantation and autoradiographic study, Anat. Rec. **170:**365, 1971.

29. Belanger, L.F.: Resorption of cementum by cementocyte activity ("cementolysis"), Calc. Tiss. Res. **2:**229, 1968.

30. Frank, R.M., and Steuer, P.: Etude ultrastructurale du cément cellulaire chez le rat, J. Biol. Bucc. **5:**121, 1977.

31. Zander, H.A., and Hurzeler, B.: Continuous cementum apposition, J. Dent. Res. **37:**1035, 1958.

32. Hurzeler, B., and Zander, H.A.: Cementum apposition in periodontally diseased teeth, Helv. Odont. Acta **3:**1, 1959.

33. Stones, H.H.: The permeability of cementum, Brit. Dent. J. **56:**273, 1934.

34. Wainwright, W.W.: The permeability of human dental root structures to radioactive iodine, J. Periodontol. **23:**95, 1952.

35. Linden, L.A.: Microscopic observations on fluid flow through cementum and dentine; an in vitro study on human teeth, Odont. Rev. **19:**4, 1968.

36. Aleo, J.J., et al.: The presence and biologic activity of cementum-bound endotoxin, J. Periodontol. **45:**672, 1974.

37. Nakib, N.M., et al.: Endotoxin penetration into root cementum of periodontally healthy and diseased human teeth, J. Periodontol. **53:**368, 1982.

38. Daly, C.G., et al.: Histological assessment of periodontally involved cementum, J. Clin. Periodontol. **9:**266, 1982.

39. Selvig, K.A.: Differences between cementum and bone tissue, Norske Tannlaegeforenings Tidskr. **78:**71, 1968.

40. Ishikawa, J., et al.: Microradiographic study of cementum and alveolar bone, J. Dent. Res. **43:**936, 1964.

41. Schroeder, H.E.: Orale Strukturbiologie, Stuttgart, 1976, Georg Thieme Verlag, p. 145.

42. Egli, A.R.: Über die Struktur des Faserzementes, Schweiz. Monatschr. Zahnheilk. **56:**23, 1946.

43. Gustafson, A.G., and Persson, P.A.: The relationship between the direction of Sharpey's fibers and the deposition of cementum, Odont. Tidskr. **65:**457, 1957.

44. Shackleford, J.M.: The indifferent fiber plexus and its relationship to principal fibers of the periodontium, Am. J. Anat. **131:**427, 1971.

44a. Grant, D.A., and Bernick, S.: The periodontium of aging humans, J. Periodontal. **43:**660, 1972.

45. Soni, N.N., van Huysen, G., and Swenson, H.M.: A microradiographic and x-ray densitometric study of cementum, J. Periodontol. **33:**372, 1962.

46. Furseth, R., and Johansen, E.: The mineral phase of sound and carious human dental cementum studied by electron microscopy, Acta Odontol. Scand. **28:**305, 1970.

47. Nakata, T.M., Stepnick, R.J., and Zipkin, I.: Chemistry of human dental cementum: the effect of age and fluoride exposure on the concentration of ash, fluoride, calcium, phosphorus and magnesium, J. Periodontol. **43:**115, 1972.

48. Selvig, K.A., and Zander, H.A.: Chemical analysis and microradiography of cementum and dentin from periodontally diseased human teeth, J. Periodontol. **33:**303, 1962.

49. Yamada, N.: Fine structure of exposed cementum in periodontal disease, Bull. Tokyo Med. Dent. Univ. **15:**409, 1968.

50. Selvig, K.: Biological changes at the tooth-saliva interface in periodontal disease, J. Dent. Res. **48:**846, 1969.

51. Selvig, K.A., and Hals, E.: Periodontally diseased cementum studied by correlated microradiography, electron probe analysis and electron microscopy, J. Periodont. Res. **12:**419, 1977.

52. Wirthlin, M.R., et al.: The hypermineralization of diseased root surfaces, J. Periodontol. **50:**125, 1979.

53. Listgarten, M.A.: Electron microscopic study of the dento-gingival junction of man, Am. J. Anat. **119:**147, 1966.

54. Formicola, A.J., Krampf, J.I., and Witte, E.T.: Cementogenesis in developing rat molars, J. Periodontol. **42:**766, 1971.

55. Kvam, E.: Topography of principal fibers, Scand. J. Dent. Res. **81:**533, 1973.

56. Selvig, K.A.: Structure and metabolism of the normal periodontium. In Klavan, B., et al., editors: International conference on research in the biology of periodontal disease, Chicago, 1977, University of Illinois College of Dentistry, p. 2.

57. Bhussry, B.R.: Development and growth of teeth. In Bhaskar, S.N., editor: Orban's oral histology and embryology, ed. 10, St. Louis, 1985, The C.V. Mosby Co.

58. Armitage, G.C.: Cementum. In Bhaskar, S.N., editor: Orban's oral histology and embryology, ed. 10, St. Louis, 1985, The C.V. Mosby Co.

59. Selvig, K.A.: Electron microscopy of Hertwig's epithelial sheath and of early dentine and cementum formation in the mouse incisor, Acta Odontol. Scand. **32:**105, 1963.

60. Lester, K.S.: The incorporation of epithelial cells by cementum, J. Ultrastr. Res. **27:**63, 1969.

61. Simpson, H.E.: The degeneration of the rests of Malassez with age as observed by the apoxestic technique, J. Periodontol. **36:**288, 1965.

62. Simpson, H.E.: A three-dimensional approach to the microscopy of the periodontal membrane, Proc. Roy. Soc. Med. **60:**537, 1967.

63. Shackleford, J.M.: The structure of Tomes' granular layer in dog premolar teeth, Anat. Rec. **170:**357, 1971.

64. Kronfeld, R.: Die Zementhyperplasien an nicht-funktionierenden Zähnen, Z. Stomatol. **25:**1218, 1927.

65. Henry, J.L., and Weinmann, J.P.: The pattern of resorption and repair of human cementum, J. Am. Dent. Assn. **42:**271, 1951.

66. Listgarten, M.A.: A mineralized cuticular structure with connective tissue characteristics on the crown of human unerupted teeth in amelogenesis imperfecta: a light and electron microscopic study. Arch. Oral Biol. **12:**877, 1967.

67. Listgarten, M.A., and Shapiro, I.M.: Fine structure and composition of coronal cementum in guinea pig molars, Arch. Oral Biol. **19:**679, 1974.

68. Gorlin, R.J., and Goldman, H.M.: Thoma's oral pathology, ed. 6, St. Louis, 1970, The C.V. Mosby Co.

69. Gottlieb, B.: Zementexostosen, Schmelztropfen und Epithelnester. Österr. Z. Stomatol. **19:**515, 1921.

70. Shafer, W.G., Hine, M.K., and Levy, B.M.: A textbook of oral pathology, ed. 2, Philadelphia, 1963, W.B. Saunders Co., p. 237.

71. Zemsky, J.L.: Hypercementosis and heredity: an introduction and plan of investigation, Dent. Items Int. **53:**355, 1931.

72. Frank, R.M., and Nicolas, P.: Contributions à l'étude de la pathologie du cément, Bull. Group. Int. Rech. Sci. Stomatol. **5:**30, 1962.

73. Morgan, G.A., and Morgan, R.R.: Oral and skull manifestations of Paget's disease, J. Can. Dent. Assn. **35:**208, 1969.

## ADDITIONAL SUGGESTED READING

Schroeder, H.E.: The periodontium, Berlin, 1986, Springer-Verlag, p. 23.

Moor, J., et al.: The distribution of bacterial lipopolysaccharide (endotoxin) in relation to periodontally involved root surface, J. Clin. Periodontol. **13:**748, 1986.

# CHAPTER 5

# Alveolar process

**Alveolar process**
Function
Anatomy

**Microscopic features**

**Bone cells**

**Remodelling and repair of alveolar bone**

---

## Alveolar process

**Alveolar bone proper and supporting bone**

The alveolar process is the part of the maxilla or mandible that forms and supports the teeth. As a result of functional adaptation, two parts of the alveolar process may be distinguished: the *alveolar bone proper* and the *supporting bone*.[1] The alveolar bone proper consists of a thin lamella of bone (cortical bone) surrounding the root. Fibers of the periodontal ligament are embedded in this bone (Fig. 5-1). The supporting bone surrounds the alveolar bone proper and provides additional functional support. Supporting bone consists of (1) the compact cortical plates of the vestibular and oral surfaces of the alveolar processes (outer cortical plates) and (2) the cancellous, trabecular, or spongy bone sandwiched between these cortical plates and the alveolar bone proper (inner cortical plate).

**Lamina dura and cribriform plate**

In roentgenograms the alveolar bone proper (inner wall of the socket or inner cortical plate) appears as an opaque line called the *lamina dura* (Fig. 5-2). The alveolar bone proper is perforated by many openings through which the blood vessels, lymphatics, and nerves of the periodontal ligament pass[1,2] (Fig. 5-3). It is also called the *cribriform plate* because of these perforations. The outer cortical plate is covered by a fibrous and cellular *periosteum*. The inner cortical plate (alveolar bone proper) contains the Sharpey's fibers of the periodontal ligament fibers.

The inner and outer cortical plates meet at the *alveolar crest* where they may fuse. The inner cortical plates of adjacent alveoli are also frequently fused interdentally. The alveolar crest more or less parallels the outline of the cervical margin of the enamel 1 to 3 mm apical to it, with a greater distance seen in older individuals.[3]

**Interdental septa**

The *interdental septa* (singular, septum) are the bony partitions that separate adjacent alveoli. Coronally, at the cervical region, the septa are thinner and here the inner cortical plates are fused and cancellous bone is frequently missing (Fig. 5-4, *A*). Apically the septa are thicker and generally contain intervening cancellous bone and sometimes haversian bone.

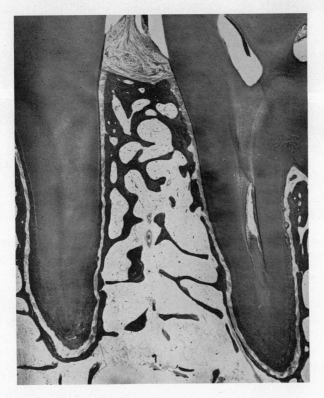

**Fig. 5-1.** Alveolar bone proper and the supporting cancellous bone form the alveolar process.

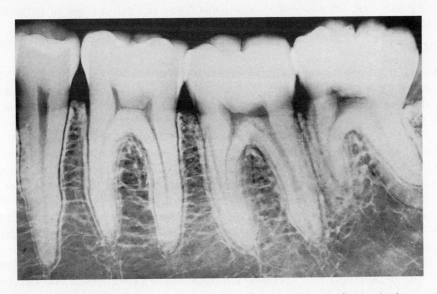

**Fig. 5-2.** Alveolar bone proper appears in the roentgenogram as a dense white line (lamina dura) separated from the root surface by a radiolucent periodontal ligament. The surrounding supporting bone is cancellous.

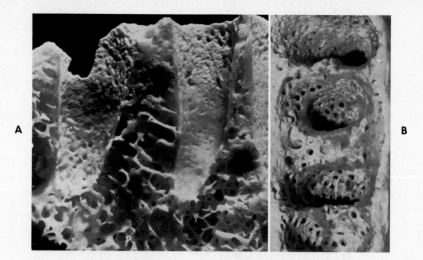

**Fig. 5-3.** **A,** Section of the alveolar bone of a human jaw. **B,** Occlusal view into two molar sockets. The wall of the tooth socket (alveolar bone proper) is perforated, forming a cribriform plate. (**A** from the collection of J.B. Weinmann.)

The shape of the alveolar crest, under normal conditions, depends on the contour of the enamel of adjacent teeth (Fig. 5-4, *B*), the relative positions of the adjacent cementoenamel junctions (*C*), the degree of eruption of the teeth (*C*), the vertical positioning of the teeth (*D*), and the orovestibular width of the teeth[3,4] (*E*). In general, the bone about each tooth follows the contour of the cervical line.

## FUNCTION

The alveolar bone proper adapts itself to the functional demands of the teeth in a dynamic manner. It is formed for the express purpose of supporting and attaching the teeth. The alveolar process depends on the presence of teeth for its existence.[5] If teeth fail to develop (e.g., in anodontia), it will not form. If teeth are lost or extracted,[6] it will tend to involute (resorb).

## ANATOMY

**Roentgeno-grams**

Roentgenograms of cross sections of the alveolar process (Fig. 5-5) show its cortical and cancellous portions. The cortical plates are generally thicker in the mandible. The cortical plates and the cancellous bone are also generally thicker on the oral aspects of the mandible and the maxilla, but there is individual variation.[7]

Anteriorly, along the vestibular aspect of the alveolar arch, is the depression of the incisive fossa, bordered distally by the cuspid eminences. Here the bone is thin, and there may be little or no cancellous bone. Posteriorly, in the premolar and molar regions, the bone is thicker, and, generally, cancellous bone separates the cortical plate from the alveolar bone proper.

**Thickness of alveolar process**

Since the teeth are responsible for the alveolar process, its general form and shape follow the arrangement of the dentition. In addition, the thickness of the alveolar process has a direct bearing on the external contour.[8] When the alveolar process is thin, there are prominences over the roots and interdental depressions between the roots (Fig. 5-6). When the processes are thick, these prominences and depressions may be lacking.

**Alveolar crest**

The margin of the alveolar process (*alveolar crest*) is normally rounded or beaded (Fig. 5-7, *arrows*). However, occasionally the bone margin ends in a fine sharp edge.

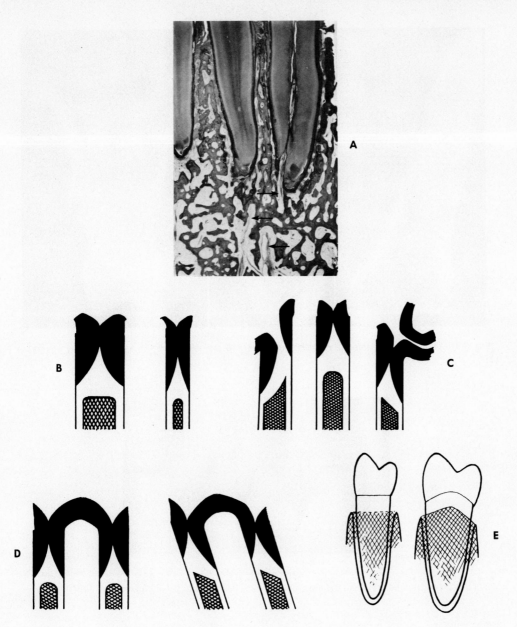

**Fig. 5-4.** **A,** Low magnification of a mesiodistal histologic section of mandibular anterior teeth. Note the cancellous supporting bone, which contains nutrient canals *(arrows)*. The coronal portion of the interdental septa consists of the fused cortical plates of the alveolar bone proper (**B** to **E**). Diagrammatic illustration of the variations in shape of the interdental alveolar crest, depending on the following anatomic features: **B,** Contour of the enamel and width of the interdental space. **C,** State of eruption. **D,** Position of the teeth. **E,** Shape of the cementoenamel junction and orovestibular width of the tooth.

This occurs only when the bone is extremely thin, for example, on the vestibular surface of the incisors and canines *(arrow)* (Fig. 5-7).

Dehiscences and fenestrations are common defects in the alveolar process.[9-11] An alveolar dehiscence is a dipping of the crestal bone margin exposing the root surface.[7,12-15] The defect may be wide and irregular and extend to the middle of the root or farther (Fig. 5-8).

**Dehiscences and fenestrations**

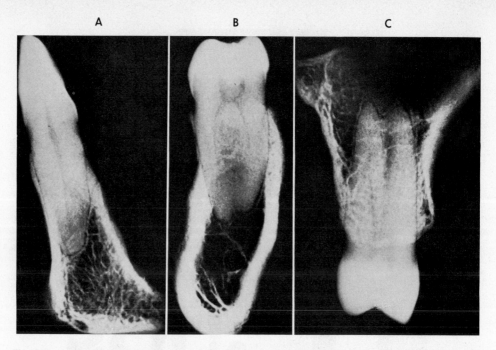

**Fig. 5-5.** Vertical sections through **A,** mandibular incisor; **B,** mandibular molar; and **C,** maxillary premolar.

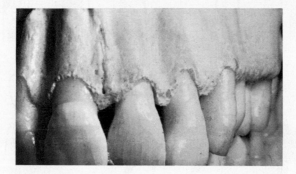

**Fig. 5-6.** Dried skull showing prominences over the roots and depressions between the roots. These are not as evident in the posterior region where the alveolar process is thick. (Courtesy J. Easley, Seattle, Washington.)

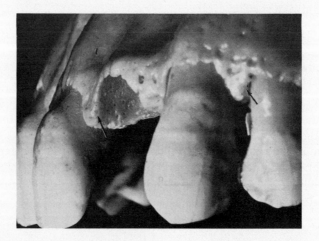

**Fig. 5-7.** Rounded margin of alveolar process *(arrows)*. Note the fine edge on the vestibular surface of the canine. (Courtesy J. Easley, Seattle, Washington.)

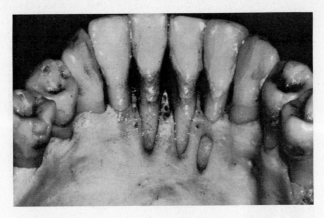

**Fig. 5-8.** *Dihiscences and fenestration on the vestibular surface of the mandibular incisors. (Courtesy D. Keene, Daytona Beach, Florida.)*

The alveolar fenestration is a circumscribed hole in the cortical plate over the root and does not communicate with the crestal margin (Fig. 5-8). It varies in size and can be located anywhere along the root surface. These irregularities are sometimes found in the alveolus before tooth eruption and may represent variations in bone form or may occur following pathologic resorption.

The variations of alveolar bone form about malpositioned teeth are so specific that one can predict the shape of the bone by noting the position of the tooth. When a tooth is prominent, the bone will be thin on the side of prominence and thick on the opposite side. **Tooth position and osseous form**

A variation of this condition arises when a tooth (e.g., a premolar) has rotated 90 degrees. In such a case the oral and vestibular aspects of the alveolar process will be relatively thick, since the tooth is narrow mesiodistally.

Another form change that accompanies tooth malposition is the level of the alveolar crest. Where a tooth is prominent, the crest will be located apical to its otherwise normal position. On the opposite side of the tooth, the margin will be in a more coronal position. When a tooth is in supraversion (extruded), the alveolar crest may be more coronal than on adjacent teeth.

The contour of the crestal margin of the process is often described as scalloped, yet this is not always the case. The marginal contour varies with the shape of the root.[13] When a root surface is flat, the alveolar contour is straight or flat. When the root surface is convex, the contour is scalloped. If the root surface is concave, the bone margin may arch coronally. When the bone is thin, the scalloping is accentuated, and, when the bone is thick, the scalloping is reduced. **Contour of crestal bone margin**

The form of the interdental septum follows the alignment of adjacent cemento-enamel junctions. In the posterior part of the mouth, the septa are relatively flat when viewed from the vestibule. The septa form peaks primarily in the anterior portion of the mouth. In general the interdental embrasures of posterior teeth are relatively wide and the septa are wider and possess more cancellous bone than the septa of the anterior teeth. **Form of interdental septum**

When teeth are in close approximation, the intervening interdental septum is extremely narrow and in some cases is absent (Fig. 5-9). This anatomic feature is commonly observed between the distobuccal root of the maxillary first molar and the mesiobuccal root of the neighboring second molar. If periodontal disease attacks such a region the destruction of the supporting tissues may be rapid and may lead to the loss of the septum between the roots and eventually to the loss of teeth.

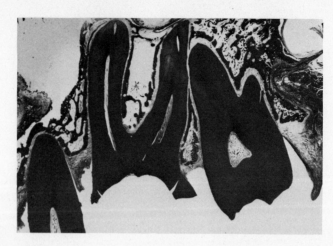

**Fig. 5-9.**   Histologic section of closely approximated roots and absence of intervening septum.

**Maxillary sinuses**

Another important anatomic consideration is that of the relationship of maxillary posterior teeth to the maxillary sinuses. The *maxillary sinuses,* which are barely detectable in the newborn, gradually enlarge through childhood and adolescence. In the young adult the root apices of the maxillary posterior teeth are separated from the sinus floor by a thin, but substantial osseous partition. With expansion of the sinuses, the thickness of this partition tends to decrease with age. The level of the sinus floor may then become located coronal to the root apices. (Fig. 5-10). Expansion of the sinuses may occur more rapidly following extraction. The cortical plate between teeth next to extraction sockets and the sinus may become paper thin.[16] As a result, oroantral perforations can occur during surgical procedures or extractions.

**Embryo-genesis of alveolar bone**

**Woven bone**

The alveolar bone of the maxilla develops in mesenchyme. In the mandible, the alveolar process develops from the mesenchyme of the first branchial arch, initially adjacent to Meckel's cartilage. As the first deciduous tooth buds appear in both maxilla and mandible, *woven bone* spicules loosely surround each developing tooth. Growth of each deciduous—and later permanent—tooth is accompanied by growth of the trabeculae of alveolar bone. As the permanent tooth develops, the root of its deciduous predecessor is progressively resorbed. Ultimately the deciduous tooth is shed, and the permanent tooth occupies the alveolar socket. Growth of each permanent molar takes place within its own separately forming socket. The genesis of alveolar bone is similar to intramembranous ossification elsewhere in the body. Trabeculae of woven bone grow and anastomose, extending from the developing maxillary and mandible proper to form the alveolar processes.

Woven bone first forms in areas predestined to become bone when mesenchymal cells form aggregations that differentiate into osteoblasts. These cells have a well-developed cytoplasm, a slightly eccentric nucleus, and, as in most specialized cells, a large ratio of cytoplasm-to-nuclear volume (Fig. 5-11, *A*). The process of forming a calcifying extracellular matrix begins in the center of the spherule of aggregated osteoblasts, collagen, proteoglycans, and matrix vesicles secreted by the osteoblasts. The first sign of hydroxyapatite calcification is seen within the matrix vesicle[17-19] (Fig. 5-11, *B*). Later the hydroxyapatite crystals growing by epitaxy form spheroids 1500 to 3000 Å in diameter. These are the bone nodules that coalesce into seams of woven bone and extend in, on, and between collagen fibrils.[17] Ultrastructurally, seams of woven bone have a nodular appearance (Fig. 5-12), which is seen in the light microscope as purple-stained irregularities in hematoxylin-eosin sections of woven bone. As the woven bone grows into trabeculae, osteoblasts are trapped in the growing calcified

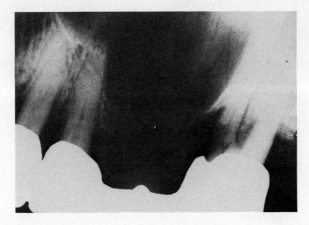

**Fig. 5-10.**    Radiograph of maxillary posterior region. Note that the expanded sinus has encroached on the alveolar process, thinning the osseous partition between the sinus floor and the root surfaces in the alveolar ridge.

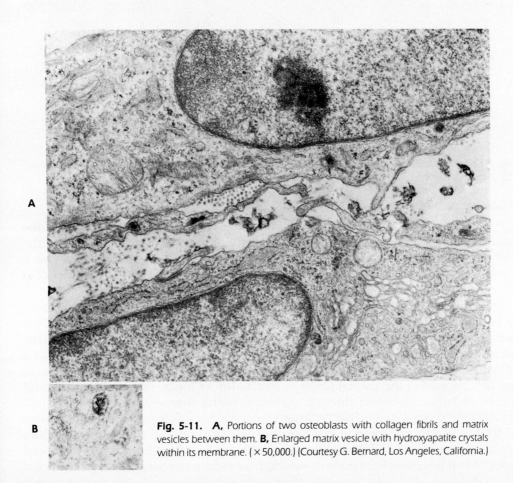

**Fig. 5-11.    A,** Portions of two osteoblasts with collagen fibrils and matrix vesicles between them. **B,** Enlarged matrix vesicle with hydroxyapatite crystals within its membrane. ( × 50,000.) (Courtesy G. Bernard, Los Angeles, California.)

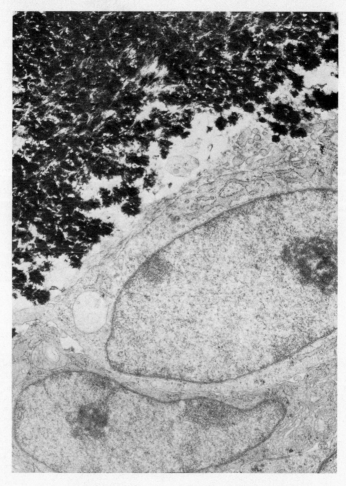

**Fig. 5-12.** Portions of two osteoblasts adjoining an area of woven bone. Note the coalesced bone nodules. (Courtesy G. Bernard, Los Angeles, California.)

matrix and are now termed *osteocytes* (Fig. 5-13). On the trabecular surfaces of the woven bone, collagen is secreted in oriented sheets that calcify by epitaxy from the hydroxyapatite crystals in the woven bone.[20] The successive layers of collagen, each sheet oriented in a different plane, give the bone the leaflet-on-leaflet appearance called

**Lamellar bone**  *lamellar bone*.

  Shortly after the first woven bone has formed, osteoclasts are found on the surfaces of both the woven and lamellar bone of the trabeculae (Fig. 5-14). They begin the process of resorbing and, with osteoblasts, remodelling the bone into its proper shape at each stage of development. Secretion of calcifying extracellular matrix and resorption of ossified tissue constitute the process of bone remodelling, which continues throughout life. Because of the natural forces of mesial drift of the teeth and the normal and abnormal forces generated through the teeth during function, there is a constant

**Bone turnover**  remodelling process and active turnover of alveolar bone.[21] Woven bone is only seen in fetal or developing bones and is normally only found in the adult during fracture repair, that is, in areas of rapidly growing bone or as embryonic remnants in sutural lines. When bone is being rapidly remodeled, osteoclasts are activated to resorb bone. Multinucleated osteoclasts are said to originate from osteoprogenitor cell coalescences[22] or from circulating monocytes.[23,24] In fact, both may be the sources of multinucleated

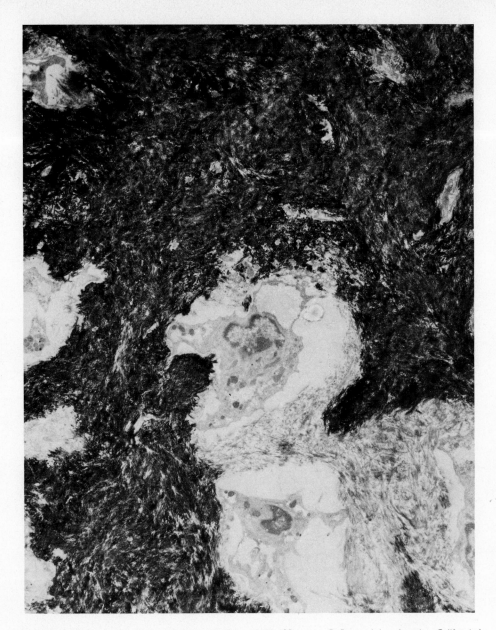

**Fig. 5-13.** *Osteocytes forming within the calcifying matrix. (Courtesy G. Bernard, Los Angeles, California.)*

resorptive cells in bone. Monocytes[25,26] and osteoblasts[27] may also resorb bone directly.

## Microscopic features

To summarize and restate, *osteoblasts*, or bone-forming cells, secrete *osteoid*. Osteoid is the organic matrix that gradually mineralizes into bone. As osteoid production proceeds, osteoblasts as well as capillaries become surrounded by the growing bone. The trapped osteoblasts become *osteocytes*, each located in a *lacuna*.

Early bone is described as *woven bone* and is characterized by a high cellularity. In woven bone osteocytes are plump, star-shaped cells, within irregularly shaped,

**Cells**

**Woven bone**

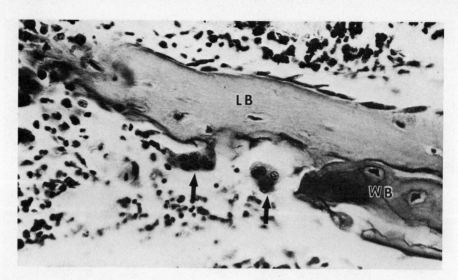

**Fig. 5-14.** Woven bone *(WB)* on the surface of lamellar bone *(LB)*. Osteoblasts are aligned on the surface of the bone, as are two osteoclasts *(arrows)*. (Courtesy G. Bernard, Los Angeles, California.)

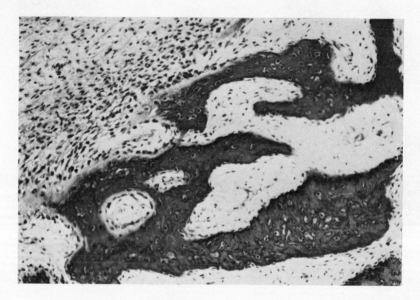

**Fig. 5-15.** Histologic section of embryonic woven bone in the jaw region. Note the high cellular content.

**Bone matrix**

closely packed lacunae. They are connected to adjacent osteocytes by cytoplasmic processes that course through a network of *canaliculi* that radiate from each lacuna (Fig. 5-15). The bone matrix is composed of loosely arranged bundles of collagen fibers of irregular sizes ranging up to 13 μm in diameter. Its degree of mineralization is highly variable. The demineralized matrix stains intensely with basophilic as well as eosinophilic stains. It is a highly labile type of bone that is rapidly formed and resorbed. *Osteocytic osteolysis*—that is, bone resorption by osteocytes within lacunae—is a common occurrence.

**Lamellar (bundle) bone**

As the child grows to adolescence, *lamellar bone* gradually replaces woven bone (Fig. 5-16, *A*). Lamellar bone is a highly organized form of bone. The matrix consists of collagen bundles of uniform size, 2 to 4 μm in diameter. The collagen bundles are

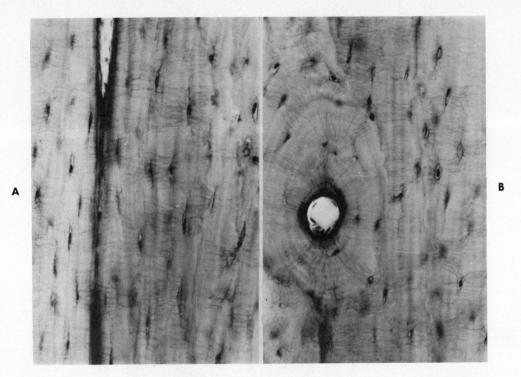

**Fig. 5-16.** Histologic sections of lamellar bone with rows of lacunae parallel to the resting lines between adjacent lamellae. **A,** Outer circumferential lamellae. **B,** Haversian system (osteone) and outer circumferential lamellae.

**Table 5-1.** Composition of bone and cementum by weight and volume

|  | Composition | Water | Organic matrix | Mineral |
|---|---|---|---|---|
| Bone | By weight | 25 | 30 | 45 |
|  | By volume | 40 | 37 | 23 |
| Cementum | By weight | 12 | 27 | 61 |
|  | By volume | 36 | 31 | 33 |

From Schroeder, H.E.: Orale Strukturbiologie, Stuttgart, 1976, Georg Thieme Verlag.

embedded in a proteoglycan ground substance and are generally arranged in parallel arrays. The bone is less mineralized than cementum. The proportions of water, minerals, and organic matrix are shown in Table 5-1.

The osteocytes in lamellar bone are more uniform in size and smaller than in woven bone. They are often spindle shaped and lie in rows of lacunae oriented with their long axis parallel to collagen fibers. The demineralized matrix of lamellar bone is preferentially stained by eosinophilic stains. Resting lines tend to be more basophilic (Figs. 5-16 and 5-17).

Bone formation is primarily by *apposition* by osteoblasts that line the bone surface. As they become embedded in osteoid to form osteocytes, new osteoblasts differentiate from adjacent cells, or *preosteoblasts*. These in turn are derived from undifferentiated mesenchymal cells or *osteoprogenitor* cells. The cyclical deposition of new bone results in formation of *circumferential lamellae* of bone separated by *resting* or *appositional lines*. This type of bone is seen on bone-forming surfaces, such as the alveolar wall during tooth movement or the outer cortical plates during jaw growth.

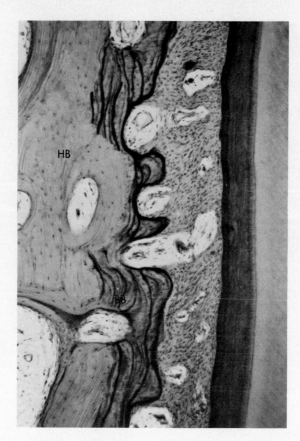

**Fig. 5-17.** Remodelling of bundle bone *(BB)* from the endosteal surface and its replacement by haversian bone *(HB)*.

On the bone side of the periodontal ligament, principal fibers of the ligament are embedded in bone via *Sharpey's fibers,* a mineralized portion of the fiber that actually becomes part of the bone matrix. Where bone apposition is dominant, Sharpey's fibers are relatively long, extending deep into the alveolar bone (see Figs. 3-13 and 5-23). Bone containing bundles of Sharpey's fibers (see Figs. 5-17 and 5-23, *B*) is sometimes

**Bundle bone** referred to as *bundle bone.*[28] It can also be found in regions of tendon insertions. Where bone resorption is dominant, Sharpey's fibers are short and abut directly on a *reversal line* (see Fig. 3-14). A reversal line is similar to a resting line between cycles of bone deposition. However it tends to have a scalloped outline because it delineates the surface outline that existed at the end of the last resorption cycle, just before its reversal to a relatively brief cycle of bone deposition. The scalloped outline is caused by the outline of resorption bays created by resorbing cells.

**Haversian system** Bone may be laid down in concentric lamellae about a central blood vessel. Such an arrangement is termed an *haversian system.* In a three-dimensional reconstruction, the lamellae arranged circumferentially about the course of a vessel form a cylindric *osteone.* Haversian systems result from remodelling of previously formed bone, including woven or lamellar bone (Figs. 5-16 and 5-17). The residual bone between adjacent haversian systems is described as *interstitial bone.* Recently formed osteones that have not become remodelled are called *primary osteones.* If these become partly resorbed and replaced by adjacent osteones, they become *secondary osteones.* The presence of secondary and even tertiary osteones is indicative of old bone (Figs. 5-17 and 5-18).

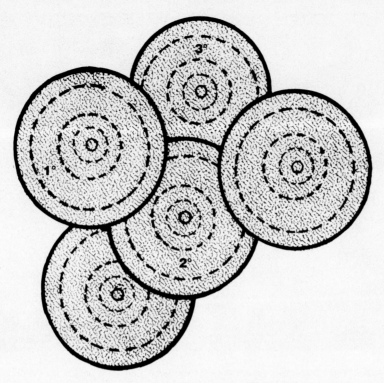

**Fig. 5-18.** Diagrammatic representation of primary (1°), secondary (2°), and tertiary (3°) osteones.

Bone resorption is mediated primarily through large, multinucleated *osteoclasts*, although mononuclear cells, including macrophages and osteocytes may also resorb bone. *Osteoclasts* generally lie within scalloped depressions on the bone surface, called *Howship's lacunae* (Figs. 5-19 to 5-21). During bone remodelling, bone resorption and bone apposition at a given site may alternate in a highly regulated manner. Both processes may occur at the same time and in close proximity (Figs. 5-20 and 5-21).

In mature bone, the lamellar structure is best observed in compact bone (see Figs. 5-16 and 5-17). Cancellous bone, which remodels more rapidly, is less likely to exhibit well-defined lamellae. The spongelike network of spaces in cancellous bone (see Fig. 5-1) is occupied by *marrow*. The hematopoietic marrow seen in infants is progressively replaced by fatty or fibrous marrow in adults in which sparsely distributed hematopoetic cell remnants may be found.

The outer surface of the alveolar process is lined with a layer of *periosteum*. This **Periosteum** fibrous layer is cellular where it contacts the bone surface. The cells include osteoblasts, osteoclasts, and their precursor cells. The periosteum contains the neural, vascular, as well as the cellular elements necessary for the maintenance of normal bone function and repair. On the alveolar surfaces, the periodontal ligament serves in the same capacity as the periosteum. The *endosteum* is the corresponding cellular layer found within marrow spaces.

## Bone cells

Bone cells include *osteocytes, osteoblasts, preosteoblasts,* and *osteoprogenitor cells* (see Fig. 5-20).

Osteoblasts are primarily engaged in bone formation. Actively secreting osteoblasts **Osteoblasts**

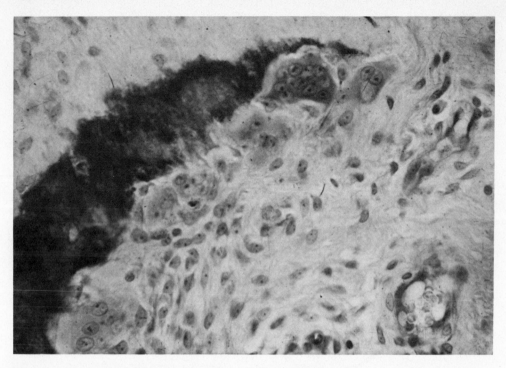

**Fig. 5-19.** Multinucleated osteoclasts are actively resorbing bone. Osteoid is present on the opposing surface. (From Grant, D.A.: J. Periodontol. **38:**409, 1967.)

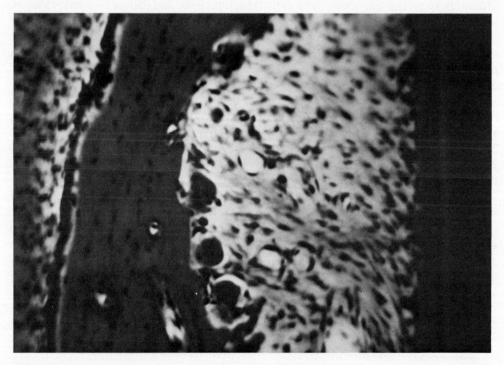

**Fig. 5-20.** Osteoclasts are actively resorbing bone on one surface of alveolar bone proper. Cells like preosteoblasts or osteoblasts are aligned on the endosseous surface of the same bone. (Courtesy W. Paule, Los Angeles, California.)

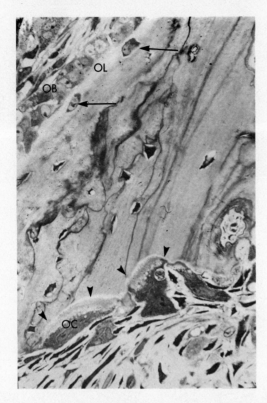

**Fig. 5-21.** Bone trabeculum undergoing bone apposition by osteoblasts *(OB)* on one side and resorption by osteoclasts *(OC)* on the other. Note the scalloped outline of the Howship's lacunae *(arrowheads)*. Two osteocytes *(arrows)* can be seen within the osteoid layer *(OL)*.

are lined up along the osseous surface as a sheet of plump, basophilic cells with large nuclei (Figs. 5-20, 5-21, and 5-22). They have well-developed golgi regions with a dense network of rough-surfaced endoplasmic reticulum. Cytoplasmic extensions may traverse the osteoid layer to make contact with those of adjacent osteocytes. Where active osteogenesis is absent, the bone surface may be lined with flattened cells lacking a rough endoplasmic reticulum. They are considered to be *osteoprogenitor cells.* They are capable of dividing and differentiate into *preosteoblasts,* which are no longer able to divide and may evolve further into osteoblasts.[29]

Osteocytes are derived from osteoblasts and are capable of resorbing and forming bone (see Fig. 5-20). Osteocytes have a reduced volume of cytoplasm and cellular organelles when compared to osteoblasts.[30] Their cytoplasmic processes radiate from the cell body through numerous canaliculi to connect with cells in adjacent lacunae (Fig. 5-22, *B*). Osteocytes respond to changing hormonal levels.[31] They are able to resorb the bone of the lacunar walls (osteocytic osteolysis)[32,33] and to deposit new bone. When *osteoblasts* become embedded in bone to form *osteocytes,* new osteoblasts differentiate from adjacent *preosteoblasts.* The preosteoblasts are derived from undifferentiated mesenchymal *(osteoprogenitor)* cells. **Osteocytes**

Osteoclasts are large multinucleated cells found in depressions of the bone surface (see Figs. 5-19 to 5-22). They are the main cell type capable of bone resorption (others are osteocytes and macrophages). The surface facing bone is highly convoluted forming a "ruffled border."[33] The cytoplasm of the osteoclast contains numerous vesicles, lysosomes, and mitochondria, but little endoplasmic reticulum. The size and concentration of vesicles increases in proximity to the ruffled border, which is the zone where **Osteoclasts**

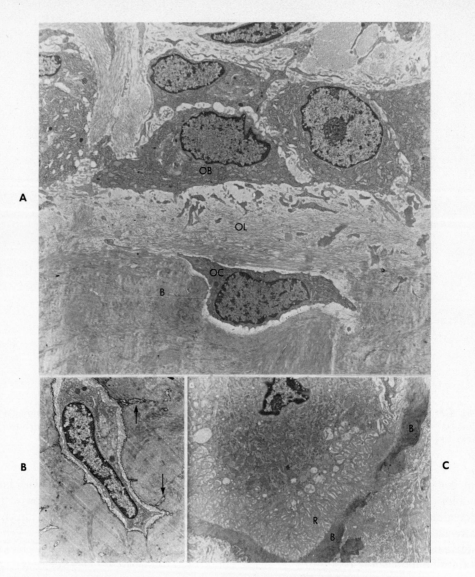

**Fig. 5-22.  A,** Electron micrograph of osteoblasts *(OB)* lining an osteoid layer *(OL)*. Note the bone cell *(OC)* partially enclosed in bone *(B)* about to become an osteocyte. **B,** Osteocyte within a lacuna. The cytoplasmic volume is considerably reduced from that seen in osteoblasts. Cytoplasmic processes extend from the cell through canaliculi in the bone *(arrows)*. **C,** Ruffled border of an osteoclast *(R)* in the process of resorbing a bony spicule *(B)*.

active bone resorption takes place. Free apatite crystallites and frayed collagen fibrils are found between the cytoplasmic processes of the ruffled border. The periphery of the ruffled border, by contrast, closely contacts the bone surface and seals the resorptive, ruffled border zone. This region is referred to as the *clear zone* because the adjacent cytoplasm lacks organelles and particulate elements.[34]

Osteoclasts originate from macrophages of hematopoietic origin.[28,35-37] These cells fuse to form typical multinucleated cells or they may participate in bone resorption as single nuclear cells. Fibroblast-derived collagenase may also contribute to bone resorption.[38]

The number and activity of osteoclasts may be increased by *parathyroid hormone* (PTH) (although they do not possess PTH receptors), and is decreased by *calcitonin*.[29] *1,25-Dihydroxycholecalciferol*, a vitamin D–related hormone, stimulates the enlargement of the ruffled border and resorptive activity without affecting cell numbers.[28] Its effect appears to be mediated via osteoblasts and osteocytes.[39] In addition to the above hormones, locally produced agents such as *osteoclast-activating factor* (OAF)[40] and possibly other *lymphokines* and *prostaglandins* also influence bone resorption.[28]

## Remodelling and repair of alveolar bone

The structure of alveolar bone proper varies, on different sides of the tooth, with different functional demands. Under physiologic conditions teeth migrate continuously in a mesial direction toward the midline. This is called *physiologic mesial drift*.[27,41] The migration leads to a resorption of the inner wall of the alveolus on the mesial side of the tooth and the formation of new bone on the distal surface. The resorption may be the result of mild compression of the periodontal ligament by the migrating tooth. New bone formation is caused by tension on the periodontal fibers on the distal surface (Figs. 5-23 and 5-24). The unique bone that is formed here is known traditionally as bundle bone because of the presence of Sharpey's fibers, which are fibers of the periodontal ligament embedded in the newly formed bone lamellae on the side of tension. In areas of rapid bone deposition without equal resorption, bone lamellae containing residual Sharpey's fibers give alveolar bone its unique bundle bone appearance even after the Sharpey's fibers are no longer continuous with periodontal ligament fibers. The physiologic migration of teeth occurs both mesially and occlusally. This latter eruptive movement influences the structure of the alveolus, causing bone formation at both the alveolar fundus and the alveolar crest.[42]

Physiologic tooth migration continues throughout life but slows or halts in old age. The alveolar bone adapts and reconstructs itself continuously. Pathologic changes occur when this process of adaptation is disturbed. Changes in function must result in a tissue response (Figs. 5-23 and 5-24). The question may be asked, "How is the connective tissue attachment of the tooth maintained during bone resorption?"

Some portions of the bone surface may be covered by a thin layer of new bone that anchors short Sharpey's fibers. This new bone is formed during relatively brief periods of bone deposition, which allows the root to remain anchored to bone despite a predominance of bone resorption over deposition. The new bone is separated from the old bone by a *reversal line*. Reversal lines tend to have to have a scalloped outline that delineates the surface of the last resorptive activity. The outline is the result of resorptive bays created by osteoclasts. Bone apposition is periodic and periods of quiescence followed by bone apposition produces resting lines between appositional lamellae of bone.

Supporting bone also adapts to functional requirements. Bone is resorbed if functional requirements are reduced, and additional bone is formed if functional influences demand it. The loss of occlusal function will lead to a disuse atrophy of the supporting bone. Increased functional demands will produce denser bone (more bone per unit volume). On the other hand, demands beyond the physiologic tolerance of bone tissue will result in a decreased bone density (less bone per unit volume). The bone of the alveolar process is in a constant state of flux. It is influenced primarily by functional stimuli and also by systemic factors.

Alveolar bone constantly renews its structure. This turnover results from the delicate coupling of bone resorption and bone deposition. It has been estimated that 3.5% of the entire skeleton undergoes active remodelling at any given time.[43] The rate of remodelling of alveolar bone is particularly rapid and thus permits functional adaptation to changing conditions.[44] For example, eruption of the tooth into the oral cavity requires resorption of the overlying bone and the remodelling of the alveolar bone with bone apposition at the crest. Where bone remodelling is inhibited—for example, in certain

*Margin notes:*

**Structure, function, and physiologic tooth migration**

**Reversal lines**

**Turnover of bone**

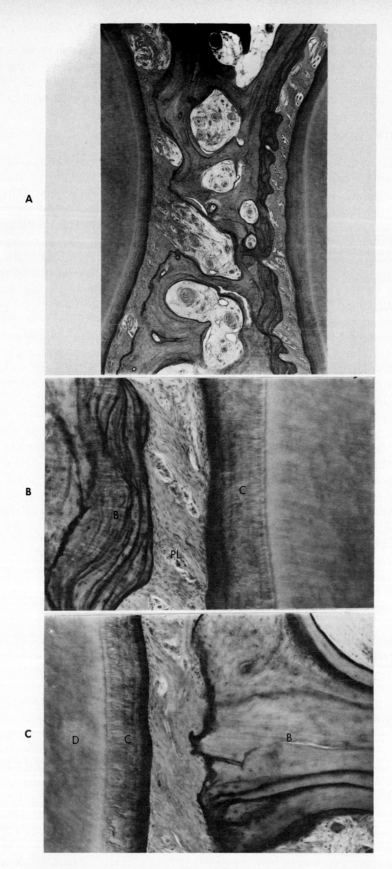

**Fig. 5-23. A,** Histologic section in the occlusal plane of the interdental septum. **B,** Higher magnification of **A** showing bundle bone *(B)* next to the periodontal ligament *(PL)* on the bone-forming side of the alveolus. **C,** Higher magnification of a serial section of **A** on the bone-resorbing side of the alveolus. Note the lack of bundle bone. *C,* cementum; *D,* dentin.

d ← m        d

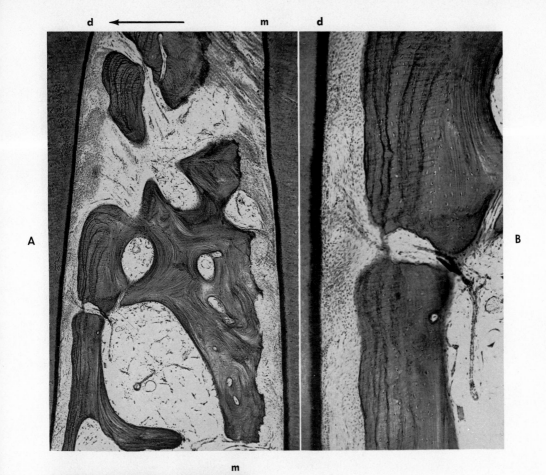

A                                                          B

m

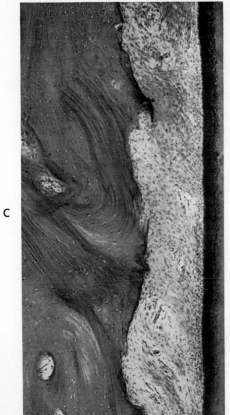

C

**Fig. 5-24.** Interdental septum. **A,** Incremental lines and formation of bundle bone occur alongside the distal *(d)* tooth surface. Resorption of lamellated bone has taken place alongside the mesial *(m)* surface of the adjacent tooth. This indicates the mesial direction of tooth drift *(in the direction of the arrow).* **B,** Higher magnification of the distal surface of the alveolar septum. **C,** Higher magnification of the mesial surface.

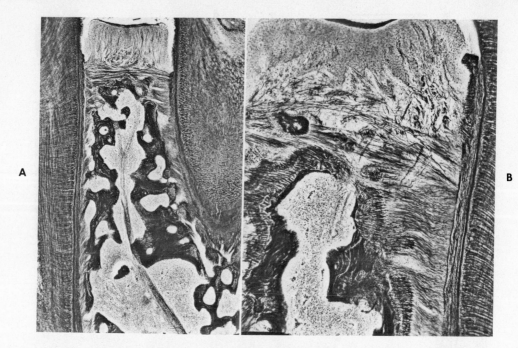

**Fig. 5-25.** **A,** A vascular channel in the alveolar septum (which consists of cancellous bone) arborizes to supply the periodontal ligament and, **B,** leaves the alveolar bone at the coronal corners of the crest to enter the gingiva. (From Grant, D.A., and Bernick, S.: J. Dent. Res. **52,** Abstract no. 770, 1973.)

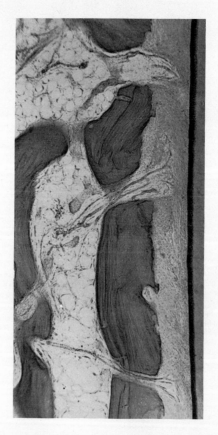

**Fig. 5-26.** Blood vessels enter the periodontal ligament through openings in the alveolar bone.

rat strains with genetically defective bone resorption[45]—tooth eruption is retarded or prevented.

The blood supply to the alveolar bone comes from branches of the alveolar artery. **Vitality of** The periosteal vessels run over the oral and vestibular plates of bone and contribute **bone** to the circulatory supply of the gingiva and the periodontal ligament. The major supply comes from the alveolar vessels that pass up the center of the alveolar septum (Fig. **Blood supply** 5-25), sending branches laterally from the marrow spaces, and by way of canals through the cribriform plate to the periodontal ligament[46,47,48] (Fig. 5-26). The interdental vessel passes upward to supply the septum and the interdental papilla. In the periodontal ligament the vessels generally take a longitudinal course with ascending and descending branches and parallel longitudinal vessels with interconnecting loops[46] (Fig. 5-27). The physiologic and pathologic features of the vascular supply to the periodontium are of major importance to the understanding and therapy of periodontal diseases.

Studies in rodent molars suggest that periodontal fibers may pass completely through the alveolar septal bone to insert into the cementum of the adjacent teeth.[49-52] This was not demonstrable in marmosets.[52]

The tooth and its investing tissues (periodontal ligament, bone, cementum) con- **Ankylosis** stitute a developmental and functional entity.[53] The organization into cementum, periodontal ligament, and alveolar bone appears to be a matter of inductive organizational

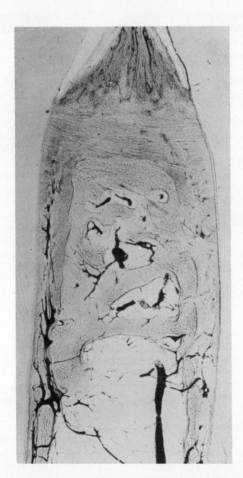

**Fig. 5-27.** Vessels enter the pulp, periodontal ligament, and interdental alveolar septum. The septal vessels arborize to enter the periodontal ligament, forming two or more parallel ascending and descending channels with interconnecting loops. (From Grant, D.A., and Bernick, S.: J. Dent. Res. **52,** Abstract no. 770, 1973.)

influences.[54-56] Since ankylosis rarely occurs, the suggestion has been made that the periodontal ligament possesses some inhibitory quality in this regard. Generalized injury or removal of the periodontal ligament may lead to *ankylosis*—that is, the fusion of the mineralized root surface with alveolar bone. Such injuries have been provoked experimentally or may occur as a result of accidents or clinical procedures. If a tooth is accidentally exfoliated or extracted, it may be possible to replace it in its socket. If the periodontal ligament remains viable, repair of the attachment apparatus may occur.[57-62] The ligament not only contains precursor cells for the entire line of cementum and bone cells but is able to protect the cementum surface from resorption and to prevent ankylosis of the root and bone. Any procedure that will damage the ligament cells—such as dehydration, sterilization procedures, root planing or excessive extraoral handling—may cause enough damage to lead to root and bone resorption and in some cases ankylosis. The periodontal ligament, cementum, and alveolar bone comprise a structure with a function and biology unique among the ligaments and joints of the body.

## REFERENCES

1. Bhaskar, S.N.: Maxilla and mandible (alveolar process). In Bhaskar, S.N., editor: Orban's oral histology and embryology, ed. 9, St. Louis, 1980, The C.V. Mosby Co.
2. Birn, H.: The vascular supply of the periodontal membrane, J. Periodont. Res. **1:**51, 1966.
3. Ritchey, B., and Orban, B.: The crests of the interdental alveolar septa, J. Periodontol. **24:**75, 1953.
4. MacMillan, H.W.: The structure and function of the alveolar process, J. Nat. Dent. Assn. **11:**1059, 1924.
5. MacMillan, H.W.: A consideration of the structure of the alveolar process, with special reference to the principle underlying its surgery and regeneration, J. Dent. Res. **6:**251, 1924-1926.
6. Landberger, R.: Histologische Untersuchungen über das alveolare Wachstum in seiner Beziehung zu der Entwicklung des Zahnkeimes, Dtsch. Mschr. Zahnheilk. **41:**417, 1923.
7. Parfitt, G.J.: An investigation of the normal variations in alveolar bone trabeculation, Oral Surg. **15:**1453, 1962.
8. Easley, J.R.: Methods of determining alveolar osseous form, J. Periodontol. **38:**112, 1967.
9. Stahl, S.S., Cantor, M., and Zwig, E.: Fenestrations of the labial alveolar plate in human skulls, Periodontics **1:**99, 1963.
10. Elliott, J.R., and Bowers, G.M.: Alveolar dehiscence and fenestrations, Periodontics **1:**245, 1963.
11. Caffesse, R.G., Barletta, B.O., and Carranza, F.A.: Defectos oseos en la tabla vestibular superior de maxilares humanos, Res. Assoc. Odontol. Argent. **52:**238, 1963.
12. Hirschfeld, I.: A study of skulls in the American Museum of Natural History in relation to periodontal disease, J. Dent. Res. **5:**241, 1923.
13. Nabers, C.L., Spear, G.R., and Beckham, L.C.: Alveolar dehiscence, Tex. Dent. J. **78:**4, 1959.

14. Larato, D.C.: Alveolar plate fenestrations and dehiscences of the human skull, Oral Surg. **29:**816, 1970.
15. Larato, D.C.: Periodontal defects in the juvenile skull, J. Periodontol. **41:**473, 1970.
16. Vidíc, B.: Maxillary sinus. In Bhaskar, S.N., editor: Orban's oral histology and embryology, ed. 10, St. Louis, 1985, The C.V. Mosby Co.
17. Bernard, G.W., and Pease, D.C.: An electron microscopic study of initial intramembranous osteogenesis, J. Anat. **125:**271, 1969.
18. Bonucci, E.: Fine structure of early cartilage calcification, J. Ultrastruc. Res. **20:**33, 1967.
19. Anderson, H.C.: Vesicles associated with calcification in the matrix of epiphyseal cartilage, J. Cell. Biol. **41:**59, 1969.
20. Bernard, G.W.: The ultrastructural interface of bone crystals and organic matrix in woven and lamellar endochondral bone, J. Dent. Res. **48:**781, 1969.
21. Stein, G., and Weinmann, J.: Die physiologische Wanderung der Zähne, Z. Stomatol. **23:**733, 1925.
22. Young, R.: Specialization of bone cells. In Frost, H.M., editor: Bone biodynamics, Boston, 1964, Little, Brown & Co.
23. Fishman, A., and Hay, E.D.: Origin of osteoclasts from mononuclear leucocytes in regenerating new limbs, Anat. Rec. **143:**329, 1962.
24. Minken, C., et al.: The affects of PTH and adenylcyclase in murine mononuclear phagocytes, Biochem. Biophys. Res. Commun. **76:**875, 1977.
25. Mundy, G.R., et al.: Direct resorption of bone by human monocytes, Science **196:**1109, 1977.
26. Kahn, A.J., Stewart, C.C., and Teitelbaum, S.L.: Contact mediated bone resorption by human monocytes in vitro, Science **199:**988, 1978.
27. Puzas, J.E., and Brand, J.S.: Collagenolytic activity from isolated bone cells, Biochim. Biophys. Acta **429:**964, 1976.

28. Vaughan, J.: The physiology of bone, ed. 3, Oxford, 1981, Clarendon Press.
29. Rasmussen, H., and Bordier, P.: The physiological and cellular basis of metabolic bone disease, Baltimore, 1974, Williams & Wilkins.
30. Baud, C.A.: Submicroscopic structure and functional aspects of the osteocyte, Clin. Orthop. **56:**227, 1968.
31. Baud, C.A., and Boivin, G.: Effect of hormones on osteocyte function and perilacunar wall structure, Clin. Orthop. **136:**270, 1978.
32. Belanger, L.F.: Osteolytic osteolysis, Calc. Tiss. Res. **4:**1, 1969.
33. Hancox, N.M., and Boothroyd, B.: Motion picture and electron microscope studies on the embryonic avian osteoclast, J. Biophys. Biochem. Cytol. **11:**651, 1961.
34. Holtrop, M.E., and King, G.J.: The ultrastructure of the osteoclast, Clin. Orthop. **123:**177, 1977.
35. Chambers, T.J.: Multinucleate giant cells, J. Pathol. **126:**125, 1978.
36. Owen, M.: Histogenesis of bone cells, Calc. Tiss. Res. **25:**205, 1978.
37. Marks, S.C., Jr., and Walker, D.G.: The hematogenous origin of osteoclasts: experimental evidence from osteopetrotic (microphthalmic) mice treated with spleen cells from beige mouse donors, Am. J. Anat. **161:**1, 1981.
38. Deporter, D.A.: The possible role of the fibroblast in granuloma-induced bone resorption in the rat, J. Pathol. **127:**61, 1979.
39. Rodan, G.A., and Martin, T.J.: Role of osteoblasts in hormonal control of bone resorption: a hypothesis, Calc. Tiss. Internat. **33:**349, 1981.
40. Horton, J.E., et al.: Bone resorbing activity in supernatant fluid from cultured human peripheral blood leukocytes, Science **177:**793, 1972.
41. Picton, D.C.A.: The effect of external forces on the periodontium. In Melcher, A.H., and Bowen, W.H., editors: Biology of the periodontium, New York, 1969, Academic Press, Inc., p. 363.
42. Weinmann, J.P., and Sicher, H.: Bone and bones, fundamentals of bone biology, ed. 2, St. Louis, 1955, The C.V. Mosby Co.
43. Rasmussen, H.: The parathyroids. In Williams, R.H., editor: Textbook of endocrinology, ed. 4, Philadelphia, 1968, W.B. Saunders Co., p. 847.
44. Baumhammers, A., Stallard, R.E., and Zander, H.A.: Remodelling of alveolar bone, J. Periodontol. **36:**439, 1965.
45. Handelman, C.S., Morse, A., and Irving, J.T.: The enzyme histochemistry of the osteoclasts of normal and "ia" rats. Amer. J. Anat. **115:**363, 1964.
46. Grant, D.A., and Bernick, S.: Development of the periodontal ligament. In Berkowitz, B.K.B., Moxham, B.T., and Newman, H.N., editors: The periodontal ligament in health and disease, Oxford, 1982, Pergamon Press, p. 211.
47. Fröhlich, E.: Die Bedeutung der peripheren Durchblutung des Parodontiums für die Entstehung und Therapie der Zahnbetterkrankungen, Forum Parodontologicum, Dtsch. Zahnärztl. Z. **19:**154, 1964.
48. Grant, D., and Bernick, S.: Formation of the periodontal ligament, J. Periodontol. **43:**17, 1972.
49. Quigley, M.B.: Perforating (Sharpey's) fibers of the periodontal ligament and bone, Alabama J. Med. Sci. **7:**336, 1970.
50. Cohn, S.A.: A new look at the orientation of cementoalveolar fibers of the mouse periodontium, Anat. Rec. **166:**292, 1970.
51. Bernick, S., et al.: The intraosseous orientation of the alveolar component of marmoset aveolodental fibers, J. Dent. Res. **56:**1409, 1977.
52. Cohn, S.A.: A re-examination of Sharpey's fibers in alveolar bone of the marmoset (*Sanguinis fuscicollis*), Arch. Oral Biol. **17:**261, 1972.
53. Baume, L.J.: Tooth and investing bone: a developmental entity, Oral Surg. **9:**736, 1956.
54. Melcher, A.H.: Repair of wounds in the periodontium of the rat: influence of periodontal ligament on osteogenesis, Arch. Oral Biol. **15:**1183, 1970.
55. Harndt, E.: Paradentitis und Paradentose, Munich, 1950, Carl Hanser Verlag.
56. Melcher, A.H.: Biological processes in resorption, deposition and regeneration of bone. In Stahl, S.S.: Periodontal surgery: biologic basis and technique, Springfield, Ill., 1976, Charles C Thomas, Publisher.
57. Andreasen, J.O., and Hjorting-Hansen, E.: Replantation of teeth. I. Radiographic clinical study, Acta Odontol. Scand. **24:**263, 1966.
58. Andreasen, J.O., and Hjorting-Hansen, E.: Replantation of teeth. II. Histological study of 22 replanted anterior teeth in humans, Acta Odontol. Scand. **24:**287, 1966.
59. Emmertsen, E., and Andreasen, J.O.: Replantation of extracted molars: a radiographic and histologic study, Acta Odontol. Scand. **24:**327, 1966.
60. Sherman, P.: Intentional replantation of teeth in dogs and monkeys, J. Dent. Res. **47:**1066, 1968.
61. Hammer, J.E., Reed, O.M., and Stanley, H.R.: Reimplantation of teeth in the baboon, J. Am. Dent. Assn. **81:**662, 1970.
62. Andreasen, J.O.: Periodontal healing after replantation and autotransplantation of permanent incisors, Internat. J. Oral Surg. **60:**54, 1981.

**ADDITIONAL SUGGESTED READING**

Andreasen, J.O., and Kristerson, L.: The effect of limited drying or removal of the periodontal ligament: periodontal healing after replantation of mature permanent incisors in monkeys, Acta Odontol. Scand. **39:**1, 1981.

Atrizadeh, F., Kennedy, J., and Zander, H.: Ankylosis of teeth following thermal injury, J. Periodont. Res. **6:**157, 1971.

Baron, R., and Saffar, J.-L.: A quantitative study of bone remodeling during experimental disease in the golden hamster, J. Periodont. Res. **13:**309, 1978.

Farley, J.R., Wergedal, J.E., and Baylink, D.J.: Fluoride directly stimulates proliferation and alkaline phosphatase activity of bone-forming cells, Science **222:**330, 1983.

Giovannolli, J.-L.: Que faut-il penser des proximités radiculaires, Rev. Orthop. Dent Fac. **15:**387, 1981.

Jeansonne, B.G., et al.: Cell to cell communication of osteoblasts, J. Dent. R. **58:**1415, 1979.

Line, S.E., Polson, A.M., and Zander, H.A.: Relationship between periodontal injury, selective cell repopulation and ankylosis. J. Periodontol. **45:**725, 1974.

Maugh, T.H. II: Human skeletal growth factor isolated, Science **217:**819, 1982.

Rygh, P.: Ultrastructural changes of the periodontal fibers and their attachment in rat molar periodontium incident to orthodontic tooth movement, Scand. J. Dent. Res. **81:**467, 1973.

Schroeder, H.E.: Orale Strukturbiologie, Stuttgart, 1976, Georg Thieme Verlag, p. 162.

Schroeder, H.E.: The periodontium, Berlin, 1986, Springer-Verlag, p. 129.

Tonna, E.A.: Factors (aging) affecting bone and cementum, J. Periodontol. **47:**267, 1976.

Urist, M.R., DeLange, R.J., and Finerman, G.A.M.: Bone cell differentiation and growth factors, Science **220:**680, 1983.

Williams, R.C., et al.: Flurbiprofen: a potent inhibitor of alveolar bone resorption in beagles, Science **227:**640, 1985.

# Periodontal structure in ageing humans

**Structural changes**
Vasculature
Periodontal ligament
Cementum
Alveolar bone
Gingiva and alveolar mucosa
Gingival epithelium
Collagen

**Summary of structural changes**

---

A progression of clinical changes in the periodontium from young to old was shown in Chapters 1 and 2. The periodontal tissues in health were discussed in Chapters 2 to 5. Chapter 6 is concerned with what may occur in the periodontal tissues in old age.

Senescence includes changes in the adult organism that occur with time. Such changes may be intrinsic and chronologically related, or they may be extrinsic and attributable to the environment. Unfortunately the distinction between the physiologic time-related changes and the environmental pathologic changes is often unclear.[1]

**Definition**

## Structural changes

It is important to recognize age changes in the periodontium since these may affect function. While the opinion has been stated that age changes may prepare the way for a pathologic state,[2] this latter hypothesis cannot be correlated with epidemiologic data and the evidence is equivocal.[3-5]

Age changes affect the following periodontal tissues:[6,7]

1. Vasculature
2. Periodontal ligament
3. Cementum
4. Alveolar bone
5. Gingiva and alveolar mucosa

### VASCULATURE

Arteriosclerosis is a frequent finding in ageing humans.[6] It may be seen in large vessels with muscular elements in the vessel wall (Fig. 6-1), vessels in the alveolar

**Arterio-sclerosis**

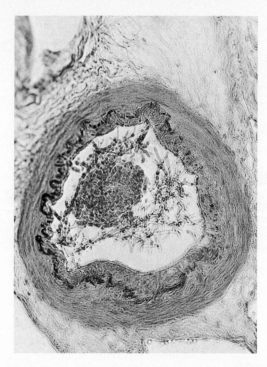

**Fig. 6-1.** Alveolar artery from a 76-year-old man showing changes characteristic of arteriosclerosis, including intimal thickening with cellular and fibrous proliferation. (From Grant, D.A., and Bernick, S.: J. Periodontol. **41:**170, 1970.)

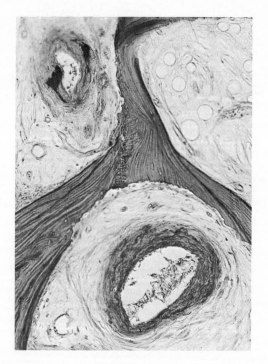

**Fig. 6-2.** Subdivision of the alveolar artery in the spongiosa around the mandibular first molar, showing a thickening of the vessel wall and a narrowed and plaque-lined lumen. Superiorly a smaller vessel shows extensive calcification of its lateral and superior portions. Note the resorptive bays lining endosteal marrow spaces (72-year-old man). (From Grant, D.A., and Bernick, S.: J. Periodontol. **41:**170, 1970.)

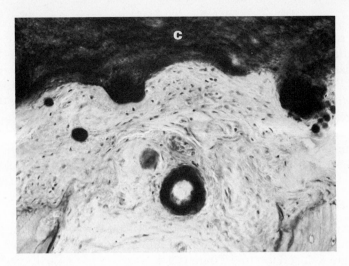

**Fig. 6-3.** In a periodontal ligament arteriole from a 76-year-old-man, calcification has involved all three layers of the vessel producing a pipestem arteriole. *c,* Cementum. (From Grant, D.A., and Bernick, S.: J. Periodontol. **41:**170, 1970.)

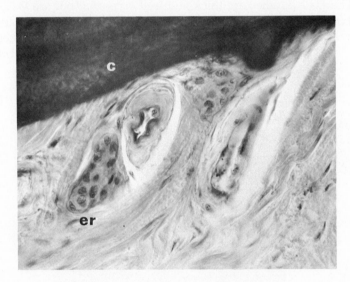

**Fig. 6-4.** Arteriole in the periodontal ligament of a mandibular premolar in a 76-year-old man. The vessel exhibits a narrowed lumen and concentric lamination, giving it an onionskin appearance. The vessel borders an enlarged epithelial rest aggregate. *c,* Cementum; *er,* epithelial rest. (From Grant, D.A., and Bernick, S.: J. Periodontol. **41:**170, 1970.)

bone (Fig. 6-2), and vessels in the periodontal ligament (Figs. 6-3 and 6-4). The relationship of this vascular pathologic condition to other changes in the periodontium is inconclusive. The relative ischemia that arteriosclerosis may produce in periodontal tissues because of a reduction in blood flow has been hypothesized as predisposing these tissues to disease[8] or provoking other changes such as fibrosis, loss of cellularity, and focal calcification.[9] It may also relate to reduced bone metabolism and may be correlated with slower or altered wound healing.[10]

The reduced arterial flow may be related to changes that have been observed elsewhere in the body and in experimental animals. For instance, the loss of ground substance may be a result of a reduced supply of oxygen associated with diminished

**Loss of ground substance**

arterial flow.[11] Also, basement membranes have been reported to be thicker in old persons and markedly distinct from the surrounding ground substance.[12]

**Connective tissue changes**

Several other changes are noted in the periodontal tissues. There is a decrease in connective tissue cellularity and an increase in the number and coarseness of collagenous fibers.[13,14] Studies have shown a decrease in protein-bound hexose and mucoproteins.[15] Other studies describe a steadily decreasing number of DNA-synthesizing cells with age.[16] The number of synthesizing cells is significantly greater in younger animals, and a greater number of cells are capable of regeneration.[17] The rate of collagen synthesis decreases with age in rats when measured by in vitro labeling technique.[18] Also, it has been shown that the cells of the periodontal ligament of old mice do not renew as rapidly as those of young animals.[16]

## PERIODONTAL LIGAMENT

**Changes in old age**

The principal fibers of the periodontal ligament are thicker in ageing humans than in younger individuals. The well-organized bundles are broad and wavy. The interfibrillar areas are reduced in size.[1] There is a decrease in the ratio of ground substance to collagen (Fig. 6-5). Fewer fibroblasts, osteoblasts, and cementoblasts can be seen[1] (Fig. 6-6). A decrease occurs in the labeling index and the cell density in the periodontal ligament of ageing rats.[19] The staining characteristics of periodontal fibers are altered[9,20] (Fig. 6-7). The fiber bundles are thick and well organized but are less distinct since they contain fewer reticular or argyrophilic fibers (Fig. 6-8). Young collagen takes up silver nitrate readily (argyrophilia). Old collagen, on the other hand, takes up the stain only slightly. The contrast between the principal fibers of the young and old is apparent (Fig. 6-9).

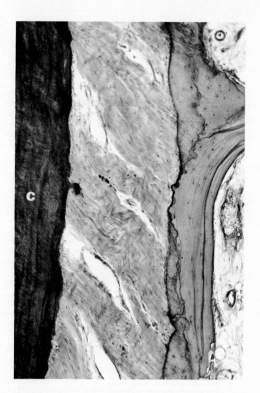

**Fig. 6-5.** Principal fibers are thick and show reduced cellularity. They are strongly PAS positive. The spaces between the fiber bundles are reduced in size. The cementum (c) is also thick. (From Grant, D.A., and Bernick, S.: J. Periodontol. **43:**660, 1972.)

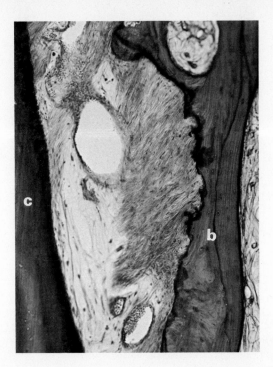

**Fig. 6-6.**   Few osteoblasts and cementoblasts are seen bordering bone and tooth. A lessened cellularity of the principal fibers is also evident. The bone margin is irregular and deeply stained. No recent cellular activity is evident. *c,* Cementum; *b,* alveolar bone. (From Grant, D.A., and Bernick, S.: J. Periodontol. **43:**660, 1972.)

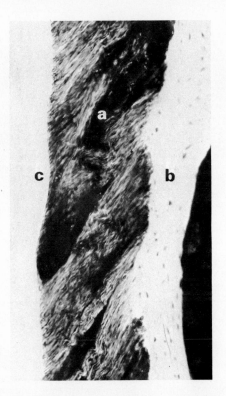

**Fig. 6-7.**   An increase in neutral carbohydrates *(a)* is observed when the periodontal ligament of a 72-year-old man is exposed to Alcian blue-PAS stain. Fibers of younger individuals show little neutral carbohydrates. *c,* Cementum; *b,* alveolar bone. (From Grant, D.A., and Bernick, S.: J. Periodontol. **43:**660, 1972.)

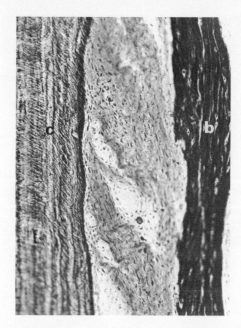

**Fig. 6-8.** Silver nitrate impregnation emphasizes the thickened character of the fiber bundles. *c,* Cementum; *b,* bone. (From Grant, D.A., and Bernick, S.: J. Periodontol. **43:**660, 1972.)

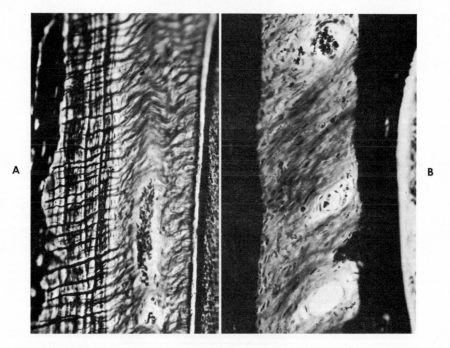

**Fig. 6-9.** When the periodontal ligament of a young marmoset, **A,** is compared to that of an old animal, **B,** several differences are noteworthy: more intense argyrophilia of the fibers in younger animal, greater thickness of the fibers in the older animal, and the less intensive staining of the fibers in the older animal. Sharpey's fibers are easily demonstrable in the younger marmoset, whereas in the older animal they cannot be seen in bone.

The periodontal ligament shows degenerative hyaline changes[1] (Fig. 6-10). At times, cells within lacunae are demonstrable.[1,9] These are characteristic of fibrocartilage and indicate a chondroid degeneration, probably a sequel to injury. Both the hyalinization and the chondroid degeneration may be (1) causally related to or an accompaniment of a reduced vascular supply, (2) a response to injury, or (3) an undetermined effect of ageing.

**Hyalinization and chondroid degeneration**

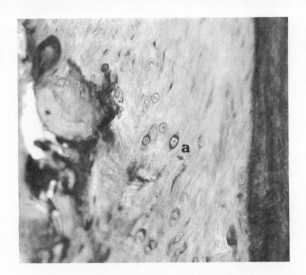

**Fig. 6-10.** Hyaline and chondroid degeneration in the periodontal ligament of an ageing human. *a*, Cartilage-like cells. (From Grant, D.A., and Bernick, S.: J. Periodontol. **43:**660, 1972.)

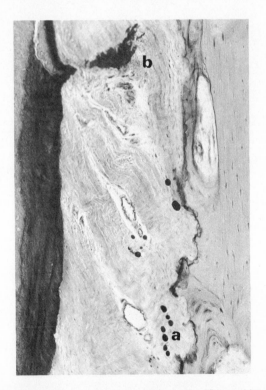

**Fig. 6-11.** Two types of calcified bodies are seen in the ligament of a 72-year-old man: small calcospherites *(a)* and larger irregularly shaped calcified bodies *(b)*. (From Grant, D.A., and Bernick, S.: J. Periodontol. **43:**660, 1972.)

**Calcification**

Calcified bodies are common in the periodontal ligament of elderly humans.[1] Two types of rounded calcospheroid-like bodies are demonstrable: small rounded calcospherites and larger, irregularly shaped calcifications. The calcospherites appear to be formed in relation to fiber bundles. They coalesce to form the larger rounded or irregularly shaped bodies (Fig. 6-11). Occasionally they increase in number and appear to calcify a complete fiber bundle, producing an ankylosis[1,21] (Fig. 6-12).

**Epithelial rests**

Epithelial rests in the periodontal ligament show altered forms of aggregation.[1] Rest aggregates tend to contain more cells with both proliferative and degenerative morphology.[22] The aggregates are frequently encircled by a thickened basement membrane (Fig. 6-13). Rather than being situated near the root surface (as in young persons), these epithelial rests are found irregularly located in the periodontal ligament, near the tooth, midway between the tooth and bone, and near bone.[1,9] Whereas some rests may degenerate (Fig. 6-14), others may become calcified[1] (Fig. 6-15).

## CEMENTUM

**Hypertrophy**

Cementum deposition appears to be continuous through life; a direct relationship has been shown between age and cementum thickness.[14,23,24] Cemental deposition is less near the cementoenamel junction and greater in the apical area. The laminar deposition results in a broad zone of cementum clothing the root (Fig. 6-16).

Indications exist that cemental deposition slows in old age.[1] In addition, the attachment of cementum to dentin may be weakened. The frequent cemental tears seen in specimens of ageing humans (Fig. 6-17) may be related to age changes in the ground substance of cementum, to reduced vascular supply, or to thickened and less extensible ligament fibers embedded in the cementum.[1]

Spurring of cementum is sometimes the result of the fusion of calcospheroid bodies near cementum or of the calcification of epithelial rest aggregates[1] (see Fig. 6-15).

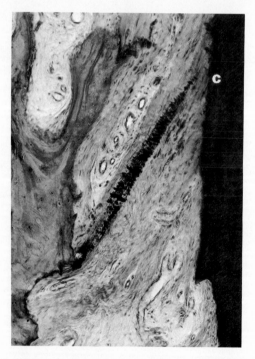

**Fig. 6-12.** *Sometimes the calcospheroid bodies are so numerous that an entire fiber bundle becomes calcified, linking the tooth to bone. c, Cementum. (From Grant, D.A., and Bernick, S.: J. Periodontol.* **43:**660, 1972.)

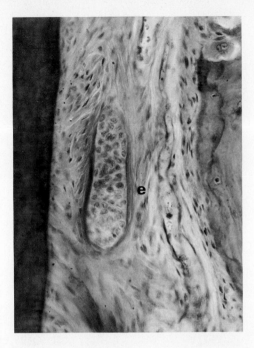

**Fig. 6-13.**  Enlarged epithelial rest (e) situated midway in the periodontal ligament with a thick PAS-positive basement membrane. (From Grant, D.A., and Bernick, S.: J. Periodontol. **43:**660, 1972).

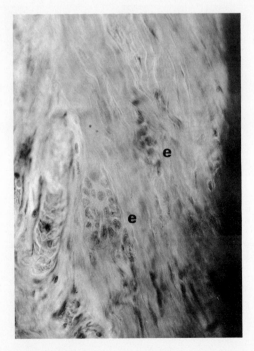

**Fig. 6-14.**  Degeneration of epithelial rests (e) and hyalinization of principal fibers in an ageing human. (From Grant, D.A., and Bernick, S.: J. Periodontol. **43:**660, 1972.)

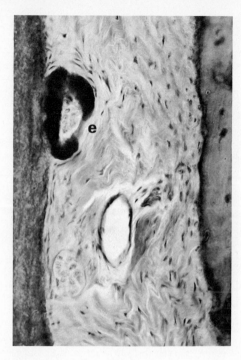

**Fig. 6-15.** Calcification of an epithelial rest *(e)* in a 55-year-old man. (From Grant, D.A., and Bernick, S.: J. Periodontol. **43:**660, 1972.)

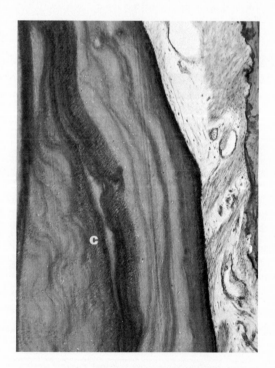

**Fig. 6-16.** Midroot area of a premolar showing the thick layers of cementum *(c)* as a result of continuous apposition in a 92-year-old woman. (From Grant, D.A., and Bernick, S.: J. Periodontol. **43:**660, 1972.)

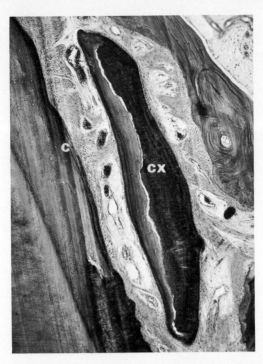

**Fig. 6-17.** A large fragment of cementum *(cx)* has been torn from the tooth and has become a part of the alveolar bone proper. Bone has been deposited on the fragment. A periodontal ligament remains between the detached fragment of cementum and the bone. A second periodontal ligament has formed between the secondary cementum on the tooth surface and the bundle bone deposited on the detached cementum fragment. *c,* Cementum, *cx,* detached cemental fragment. (From Grant, D.A., and Bernick, S.: J. Periodontol. **43:**660, 1972.)

## ALVEOLAR BONE

In observation of postmortem specimens, alveolar bone shows age changes ( Figs. 6-6, 6-11, 6-15, and 6-18).[1] The alveolar bone proper has a darkly stained margin, which may be interpreted as an ageing characteristic of bone.

Little evidence of continued bone apposition is present in senescence. In view of this, physiologic tooth migration may be slowed or even halted in old age.[1] (See discussion on physiologic tooth migration in Chapters 5 and 22.) Topographic labeling, with [3]H-proline autoradiography, is reduced in the periodontal bone of ageing mice.[25] **Physiologic migration**

Attrition of tooth substance on occlusal and incisal surfaces and at the contact points is a well-recognized characteristic of ageing. **Attrition of tooth substance**

Wear on occluding tooth surfaces can be related to use (as occurs in chewing), occupational wear (as in primitive Eskimos who soften leather with their teeth), or parafunctional habits (as in bruxism). The attrition may be slow or rapid. The loss of tooth substance is of extrinsic origin and is related to the environment; since time is a factor, it is also chronologically related to senescence.

Attrition of contact points and contact planes occurs with ageing and is the result of the friction imparted by the slight vertical movement of teeth during function. This movement is permitted by the periodontal ligament.

Vertical (interocclusal) dimension and arch continuity are usually maintained into old age, since wear is compensated for by bone apposition on distal surfaces and at the fundus of the sockets. Continuous apposition of cementum at the apex also helps to compensate for such wear.[24] If continuous apposition of bone is slowed or even halted (as in senescence), such compensation for attrition does not occur. Together with atrophy of musculature, a decreased vertical facial height may result (closed bite).[1]

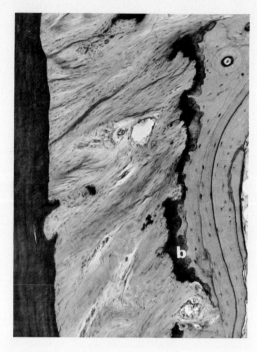

**Fig. 6-18.**   The margin of the alveolar bone proper (b) of an ageing human is darkly stained, possibly a concomitant of ageing. Physiologic tooth migration appears to be slowed or even halted. (From Grant, D.A., and Bernick, S.: J. Periodontol. **43:**660, 1972.)

The vascularity of bone appears to be diminished.[1] Moreover, the continuous remodeling of the alveolar bone that occurred throughout earlier life may alter the blood supply by changing vascular pathways.[1]

**Osteoporosis**   Osteoporosis has been reported in ageing,[26,27] particularly in the alveolar bone of postmenopausal women, but the decrease in the trabeculation of alveolar bone sometimes seen roentgenographically is more often related to loss of function (extraction of an opposing tooth).

## GINGIVA AND ALVEOLAR MUCOSA

The gingiva is reported to be increasingly fibrotic in old age, and the amount of surface keratinization is said to be decreased.[13] Elastoid degeneration is reported in the collagen fibers of the alveolar mucosa. Arteriosclerotic vessels have been described.[6,7]

## GINGIVAL EPITHELIUM

The mitotic index of human gingival epithelium is not significantly different in older humans; however, there is a significant increase in cell density, which may indicate a slower rate of maturation.[28]

## COLLAGEN

As might be anticipated, the age changes that can be seen in cellular, fibrillar, calcified, and ground substance components of the periodontium are similar to those which have been described in connective tissues elsewhere in the body.

The changes in periodontal tissues correlate well with age changes in collagen. Clausen,[29] Verzar,[30] Gross,[31] and Milch[32] have summarized these; all agree that there is an increase in the thickness of collagen fibrils and that the chemical and physical

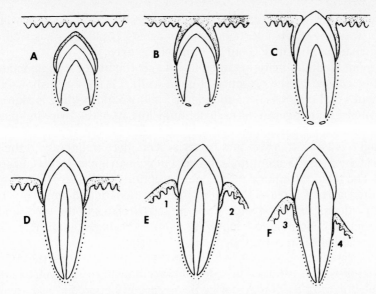

**Fig. 6-19.** Diagram of the development and changing position of the gingival attachment to the surface of the tooth. **A,** Erupting tooth is below the epithelium of the oral mucous membrane. The enamel is covered by reduced enamel epithelium. **B,** Reduced enamel epithelium and epithelium of the oral mucous membrane come into contact. **C,** Tip of the enamel erupts through the epithelium. No connective tissue is exposed. The epithelium is attached to the enamel, and there is no break in continuity. **D,** Tooth erupts into occlusion. The epithelium is still attached to the enamel. Apical end of the junctional epithelium is at the cementoenamel junction. **E** and **F,** Changing position of the dentogingival junction is demonstrated: *1,* Bottom of the gingival sulcus is on the enamel, and the apical end of the junctional epithelium is at the cementoenamel junction; *2,* bottom of the sulcus is still on the enamel, but the apical end of the attachment has shifted to the cementum; *3,* bottom of the sulcus is at the cementoenamel junction, and the apical end of the attachment has moved onto the cementum; *4,* entire junctional epithelium has shifted apically, exposing cementum. (From Orban, B., and Köhler, J.: Z. Stomatol. **22:**353, 1924.)

properties of collagen are altered. There is (1) an increase in the tensile strength of collagen fibers, (2) an increase in thermal contraction, (3) a decrease in in vitro extensibility, (4) a reduction in the amount of soluble collagen, (5) a decrease in water content, and (6) an increased resistance to proteolytic enzymes. Some of these changes may be related to the loss of acid mucopolysaccharide and water as well as to increased cross-linkages.

The progressive exposure of the root surface with age has been called *passive eruption*[33] or *passive exposure*. It is related to the slow, gradual migration of junctional epithelium onto cementum in the absence of overt, clinical periodontal disease. Four stages of passive eruption have been described (Fig. 6-19). Recession of the gingival margin may occur because of inflammatory periodontal disease or trauma to the gingiva (e.g., toothbrush trauma). The occurrence of recession as a characteristic of ageing is unproved.

**Passive eruption**

## Summary of structural changes

The longevity of individuals in the United States has increased from 45 years in 1900 to 75 years in the 1980s.[34] According to one estimate, about 18% of the population will be 65 or older by the year 2000[34] and 75% of dental patients may be in this age group.[35] Older people are retaining more of their natural dentition.[36] Caries rates are declining.[37] There are, however, problems in some of the elderly related to decreased masticatory efficiency, speech problems, and decreased salivation[36] with some medications. Yet the problems often ascribed to ageing, are not normally part of the ageing physiology. They are the result of pathologic processes. Thus dentists will have to be conversant with the normal sequences in an ageing population[38] as well as with the pathologic changes that may occur in some of the aged.[1,5,39]

Since more teeth are being retained in old age, the increase in periodontitis in the aged may be caused by the presence of more teeth.[40] It has been shown that inflammation ensues and progresses more quickly[41] and wound healing is slower.[38,39] Some of the morphologic changes in the periodontium are part of the "winding-down process" in ageing.[1,6] Periodontal fibers are thicker and their staining characteristics are different.[1] Collagen is less extensible and injury is seen more frequently in the periodontal ligaments of the aged.[1] Cementum is thicker but with an apparent greater susceptibility to injury.[1] The repair of injured periodontal structures is not always by the restoration of the injured part.[1] Cartilage may form in the periodontal ligament.[1,21] This is associated with a decreased blood supply and probably relates to the ubiquitous presence of arteriosclerosis.[6] Sometimes, following injury, the periodontal ligament becomes calcified and ankylosis results.[1]

There is slowing and even a halt in bone remodeling.[1] Thus the replacement of extracted teeth with prostheses in order to prevent overeruption, malpositioning, and tilting of neighboring teeth may not be necessary. Function and esthetics will be the principal reasons for tooth replacement. Osteoporosis is common.[26,27]

Periodontal disease increases in prevalence and severity with increasing age.[5,42] The increase may be caused by the cumulative effect of the number of "bursts" of periodontal destruction, a deterioration in plaque removal efficiency, or to the increased number of teeth retained into old age and therefore affected by plaque-induced disease.[40,43-45]

Attention should be directed toward the decline in immunofunction with age.[2,46-48] While direct relationships with periodontal diseases have yet to be demonstrated, the purported association of increased age with altered salivary function might be significant.[49] Salivary mucins and antibacterial proteins (lactoferrin, lactoperoxidase, secretory IgA, lysozyme) regulate bacterial colonization patterns, thereby modulating and possibly permitting dental disease. The increase in root caries with age may be a case in point.[37] Dry mouth, a common complaint in the aged, may be related.

While ageing and a decline in immunocompetence may be related vis-a-vis the progression of periodontal disease, no evidence of such a causal relationship has been made.[50]

The periodontally diseased, but otherwise healthy, patient can be treated.[51] A consideration is that the reduced longevity of the aged may alter the prognosis and treatment plan prescriptions.

## REFERENCES

1. Grant, D.A., and Bernick, S.: The periodontium of ageing humans, J. Periodontol. **43:**660, 1972.
2. Makinodan, T.: Immunobiology of aging, J. Am. Geriatr. Soc. **24:**249, 1976.
3. Hugoson, A. and Jordan, T.: Frequency distribution of individuals aged 20-70 years according to severity of periodontal disease, Com. Dent. Oral Epidemiol. **10:**187, 1982.
4. Bossert, W.A., and Marks, H.H.: Prevalence and characteristics of periodontal disease in 12,800 persons under periodic dental treatment, J. Am. Dent. Assoc. **52:**129, 1956.
5. Douglass, C., et al.: The potential for increase in the periodontal diseases of the aged population, J. Periodontol. **54:**721, 1983.
6. Grant, D.A., and Bernick, S.: Arteriosclerosis in periodontal vessels of ageing humans, J. Periodontol. **41:**170, 1970.
7. Severson, I., et al.: A histologic study of age changes in the adult human periodontal joint (ligament), J. Periodontol. **49:**189, 1978.
8. Doyle, J.L., et al.: Experimental arteriosclerosis and the periodontium, J. Periodontol. **40:**350, 1969.
9. Hill, M.W.: The influence of aging on skin and oral mucosa, Gerondont. **3:**35, 1984.
10. Holm-Pedersen, P., Fenstad, A.M., and Folke, A.M.: DNA, RNA and protein synthesis in

healing wounds in young and old mice, Mech. Ageing Den. **3:**173, 1974.

11. Oliver, J.: Anatomic changes of normal senescence. In Stieglitz, F.J., editor: Geriatric medicine, Philadelphia, 1954, J.B. Lippincott Co.

12. Chvapil, M.: Connective tissues. In Shock, E.D., editor: Perspectives in experimental gerontology, Springfield, Ill., 1966, Charles C Thomas, Publisher.

13. Wentz, F.M., Maier, A.W., and Orban, B.: Age changes and sex differences in the clinically normal gingiva, J. Periodontol. **23:**13, 1952.

14. Klingsberg, J., and Butcher, E.O.: Comparative histology of age changes in oral tissues of rat, hamster and monkey, J. Dent. Res. **39:**158, 1960.

15. Flieder, D.E.: Cytochemistry of human oral mucosa, J. Dent. Res. **41:**112, 1962.

16. Jensen, J.L., and Toto, P.D.: Radioactive labeling of the periodontal ligament in ageing rats, J. Dent. Res. **47:**149, 1968.

17. Toto, P.D., and Borg, M.: Effect of age changes on the premitotic index in the periodontium of mice, J. Dent. Res. **47:**40, 1968.

18. Schneir, M., Furute, D., and Berger, K.: Collagens of oral soft tissues, J. Periodont. Res. **11:**235, 1976.

19. Toto, P.D., Rubenstein, A.S., and Garguilo, A.: Labeling index and cell density of ageing rat oral tissues, J. Dent. Res. **54:**6, 1975.

20. Götze, W.: Über Altersveränderungen des Parodontiums, Dtsch. Zahnaerztl. Z. **20:**465, 1965.

21. Everett, F.G., and Bruckner, R.J.: Cartilage in the periodontal ligament space, J. Periodontol. **41:**165, 1970.

22. Reeve, C.M., and Wentz, F.M.: The prevalence, morphology and distribution of epithelial rests in the human periodontal ligament, Oral Surg. **15:**785, 1962.

23. Zander, H.A., and Hürzeler, B.: Continuous cementum apposition, J. Dent. Res. **37:**1035, 1958.

24. Ive, J.C., Shapiro, P.A., and Ivey, J.L.: Age-related changes in the periodontium of pigtail monkeys, J. Periodont. Res. **15:**420, 1980.

25. Tonna, E.A.: Topographic labeling method used ³H-proline autoradiography in assessment of ageing parodontal bone in the mouse, Arch. Oral Biol. **21:**729, 1976.

26. Somerman, M.J.: Mineralized tissue in aging, Gerondont. **3:**93, 1984.

27. Kribbs, P.J., and Chesnut, C.H. III: Osteoporosis and dental ostopenia in the elderly, Gerondont. **3:**101, 1984.

28. Ryan, E.J., Toto, P.D., and Garguilo, A.W.: Ageing in human attached gingival epithelium, J. Dent. Res. **53:**74, 1974.

29. Clausen, B.: Ageing of connective tissues. In Asboe-Hansen, G., editor: Hormones and connective tissue, Baltimore, 1966, Williams & Wilkins.

30. Verzar, F.: Ageing of the collagen fibers. In Hall, D.A., editor: International review of connective tissue research, vol. 2, New York, 1961, Academic Press, Inc.

31. Gross, J.: Ageing of connective tissue, the extracellular components. In Bourne, G.H., editor: Structural aspects of ageing, New York, 1961, Hafner Publishing Co., Inc.

32. Milch, R.A.: Aging of connective tissues. In Shock, E.D., editor: Perspectives in experimental gerontology, Springfield, Ill., 1966, Charles C Thomas, Publisher.

33. Orban, B., and Köhler, J.: Die physiologische Zahnfleischtasche, Epithelansatz und Epitheltiefenwucherung, Z. Stomatol. **22:**353, 1924.

34. Slavkin, H.C.: Developmental and immunogenetic features of biologic aging, J. Am. Dent. Assoc. **109:**451, 1984.

35. Levy, B.M., and Konigsberg, I.: Gerontology and the practice of general dentistry, Gerondontol. **3:**255, 1984.

36. Baum, B.J.: The dentistry-gerontology connection, J. Am. Dent. Assoc. **108:**899, 1984.

37. Banting, D.W.: Dental caries in the elderly, Gerondontol. **3:**55, 1984.

38. Church, H., and Dolby, A.E.: The effect of age on the cellular immune response to dento-gingival plaque extract, J. Periodont. Res. **13:**120, 1978.

39. Van der Velden, U.: The effect of age on the periodontium, J. Clin. Periodontol. **11:**281, 1984.

40. Baum, B.J.: Characteristics of participants in the oral physiology component of the Baltimore longitudinal study of aging, Community Dent. Oral Epidemiol. **9:**128, 1981.

41. Holm-Pedersen, P., Auerback, N., and Theilade, E.: Experimental gingivitis in young and elderly individuals, J. Clin. Periodontol. **2:**14, 1975.

42. Löe, H., et al.: The natural history of periodontal disease in man, J. Periodontol. **49:**607, 1978.

43. Kelly, J.E., and Harvey, C.R.: Basic data on dental examination findings of persons 1-74 years, United States, 1971-74, D.H.E.W. Pub. No. 79-1662, Sec. 11, #214, Washington, D.C., 1979, U.S. Printing Office.

44. Mandell, I.D.: Preventive dentistry for the elderly, Spec. Care Dent. **3:**157, 1983.

45. Hanson, G.C.: An epidemiologic investigation on the effect of biologic aging on the breakdown of periodontal tissue, J. Periodontol. **44:**269, 1973.

46. Peterson, W.J.: Immunity, age and loss of immunohomeostasis, Gerondont. **3:**259, 1981.

47. Roper, R.E., et al.: Periodontal disease in aged individuals, J. Periodontol. **43:**304, 1972.

48. Beck, J.D.: The epidemiology of dental diseases in the elderly, Gerondont. **3:**5, 1984.

49. Mandel, I.D.: Oral defenses and disease: salivary gland function, Gerondont. **3:**47, 1984.
50. Page, R.C.: Periodontal diseases in the elderly: a critical evaluation of current information, Gerondont. **3:**63, 1984.
51. Ettinger, R.L.: Clinical decision-making in the dental treatment of the elderly, Gerondont. **3:**157, 1984.

**ADDITIONAL SELECTED READING**

Baum, B.J. and Bodner, L.: Aging and oral motor function: evidence for altered performance among older persons, J. Dent. Res. **62:**2, 1983.
Niessen, L.C. and Jones, J.A.: Oral health changes in the elderly: their relationship to nutrition, Postgrad. Med. **75:**231, 1984.
Stahl, S.S., and Fox, L.M.: Histological changes of the oral mucosa associated with certain chronic diseases, Oral Surg. **6:**339, 1953.

# Saliva

Saliva bathes the oral tissues and is basic to the health status of the oral cavity. It plays a major role in the maintenance of health and in the production of disease by permitting or inhibiting the formation of plaque, calculus, and the proliferation of selected microorganisms. Saliva also contains immunoglobulins, white blood cells, lipids, electrolytes, and proteins and is important to the host's resistance to periodontal diseases.

The traditional view of saliva is that it is primarily a digestive fluid, initiating the digestion of starch through the secretion of amylase. Breakdown of starch to maltose indeed occurs in the mouth, but food is rapidly cleared through the oral cavity; most of the digestion of starch results from the action of pancreatic, not salivary, amylase. The salivary contribution to the digestive process is primarily preparative and gastronomic: the formation of the food bolus allows for more efficient mastication and swallowing, and the maintenance of a proper fluid environment provides for optimal functioning of the taste buds.

The most important attributes of the salivary secretions are protective in nature, helping to maintain the integrity of the teeth, tongue, and mucous membranes of oral and oropharyngeal areas. When the protective action of saliva is lost, its critical importance becomes apparent.

Malfunction of the salivary glands (because of obstruction, drug effects, irradiation, nerve damage, or disease) results in dry mouth, or *xerostomia*. The mucosa becomes dry, rough, and sticky; it bleeds readily and is subject to infection. The tongue becomes red, smooth, slimy, and hypersensitive to irritation and loses taste acuity. In the edentulous patient, dentures become extremely difficult to manage. When teeth are present, there is a heavy accumulation of plaque, materia alba, and debris; caries progress rapidly and extensively; and periodontal disease can become exacerbated. **Xerostomia**

In *mouth breathing,* which may be the result of malocclusion, anterior open bite, habit, adenoids, deviated nasal septum, sinusitis, allergies, or incomplete lip closure, **Mouth breathing**

135

a drying of the gingiva also occurs, which may produce a gingivitis characterized by a shiny erythematous surface with rolled gingival margins. In adolescents this condition may result in a hyperplastic gingival response.

For these and other reasons, the secretion and composition of saliva are of direct concern to the dentist.

## Characteristics

Whole saliva—the fluid collected by expectoration—is really a mixture of variable composition containing contributions from the major salivary glands (parotid, submaxillary, sublingual) and the minor salivary glands (minor sublingual, labial, buccal, glossopalatine, palatine, lingual), as well as bacteria, cells, food debris, and, in some instances, gingival fluid.

Total salivary fluid produced during a 24-hour period is about 1000 ml. About 90% of this fluid is derived from the parotid and submaxillary glands (in roughly equal amounts), about 5% from the sublingual glands, and up to 5% from the minor salivary glands. Since the unstimulated flow rate of the major salivary glands is less than 0.05 ml/min/gland at rest (with no external stimulation) and 0.5 (or greater) ml/min/gland with stimulation, it is apparent that 80% to 90% of the daily production of saliva is the result of stimulation. This stimulation is mainly gustatory and masticatory and is associated with eating. During most of the day and all night, salivary flow is minimal.

### COLLECTION

**Whole saliva**

The most commonly used procedure for collection of saliva is to have the subject spit stimulated whole saliva into a plastic or glass receptacle after chewing paraffin or rubber bands. Citric acid–impregnated filter paper placed on the tongue at intervals may also be used. The ease of collection of whole saliva should be weighed against the complexity of the mix secured and the contamination by nonsalivary components. More definitive starting materials for studies of salivary proteins can be secured with the use of special collecting devices.

**Parotid saliva**

The collection device in use today is patterned after the simple collector developed by Lashley in 1916.[1] The collector is composed of two concentric circles fabricated from plastic or metal. The inner circle fits over the opening of Stensen's duct, on the inner aspect on the cheek opposite the upper first molar tooth. The exit portal from this circle is connected by way of plastic tubing to a collecting receptacle. The outer circle is connected with tubing to a small rubber bulb, which, when squeezed, exhausts air from the outer ring, draws into it the cheek surrounding the opening of Stensen's duct, and holds the collector in place. Parotid saliva can be collected at rest or unstimulated or with gustatory stimulation provided by application of citric acid (usually 2%) to the tongue or sucking sour lemon candy.

**Submandibular sublingual saliva**

Secretion from the paired submandibular-sublingual glands exits from Wharton's ducts, located in the floor of the mouth, under the tongue directly behind the lower anterior teeth. The nature of the tissues in this area makes it difficult to use a universal collecting device. A reasonably usable device can be made with a basic preformed plastic collector that is modified with dental impression materials to fit the individual subject.[1]

### SECRETION

**Mechanism**

Salivary secretion is controlled by a salivary center in the medulla. This center is composed of the superior and the inferior salivary nuclei. Stimulation of flow is generated mainly by unconditioned reflex stimulation and is primarily gustatory (by way of taste buds) and masticatory (through proprioceptors in the periodontal ligament and the muscles of mastication). Olfactory stimuli, oral pain and irritation, and pharyngeal irritation are also stimulatory. Conditioned reflexes as well as emotional and psychic factors have also been shown to affect salivary flow rate.[2]

Neural control of salivary secretion is largely parasympathetic, but there is also a sympathetic component to neural regulation in human salivary glands. The parasympathetic pathway to the parotid glands includes (1) the glossopharyngeal (ninth) nerve from the inferior salivatory nucleus to the tympanic nerve, (2) the tympanic nerve to the otic ganglion, and (3) the auriculotemporal nerve from ganglion to gland. The parasympathetic pathway to the submaxillary and sublingual glands is by way of (1) the chorda tympani branch of the seventh nerve from the superior salivatory nucleus to the submandibular ganglion, and (2) postganglionic branches of the lingual nerve to the respective glands.

Sympathetic control of all salivary glands is maintained through postganglionic fibers from the superior cervical ganglion.

**Pharmaco-logic agents**

A major factor affecting salivary secretion, especially in older persons, is the large number of pharmacologic agents that can reduce salivary flow. Many drugs produce dry mouth (xerostomia) as a side effect. Such sequelae as dry mouth, taste aberrations, and rampant cervical and root caries are often results of the effect of pharmacologic agents on salivary flow. Common examples of these drugs are barbiturates, antihistamines, atropin-like agents (for digestive disorders, ulcers, and Parkinson disease), psychoactive agents such as chlorpromazine (Thorazine) and amytriptyline (Elavil), and antihypertensive drugs.

**Flow rate factors**

Other factors that can affect flow rate are (1) psychic factors, such as pain or threat of pain; (2) interference with taste perception; (3) size of gland; (4) age changes in the gland such as atrophy and fatty and inflammatory infiltrates; (5) light deprivation; (6) systemic disease such as hypothyroidism; (7) diseases of the salivary gland; and (8) irradiation of the glands in tumor therapy of the face and neck area.

## COMPOSITION

**Electrolytes**

Table 7-1 lists the concentration of parotid and submaxillary components for which there are quantitative data. Plasma values are included for comparison.

In general, it can be seen that the parotid concentrations are somewhat higher than the submaxillary-sublingual. The principal exception is calcium. Submaxillary-sublingual calcium is twice that of the parotid concentration. Thus electrolytes are actively transported. Saliva is not an ultrafiltrate of plasma.

On stimulation of 2% citric acid applied to the tongue, the flow rate is increased. The concentrations of sodium, chloride, bicarbonate, and calcium increase; magnesium, phosphate, urea, ammonia, and uric acid decrease. Potassium concentration is independent of flow rate. Protein increases in the submandibular-sublingual secretion but is variable in the parotid. The pH increases with flow rate.

**Nonelectro-lytes**

Glucose is present in very low concentration in saliva. It becomes elevated in diabetes but still appears at about 1% of blood concentration. Lipids and amino acids are also present in low concentrations in saliva.

**pH**

Saliva is slightly acidic before secretion into the oral cavity. It becomes slightly alkaline on excretion from the gland because of a loss of $CO_2$ (carbonic acid in solution). Since bicarbonate concentration increases with increasing flow rate, salivary pH becomes elevated at high flow rates.

**Proteins**

Compared to that in blood, the concentration of proteins in saliva is extremely low.[3] Table 7-2 presents a summary of the proteins of parotid and submaxillary-sublingual saliva that have been identified.[3-7]

The major component of parotid saliva is amylase, which is present in a number of molecular forms known as *isoenzymes*.[4-7] Amylase activity in the submaxillary gland

**Table 7-1.** Salivary composition in normal adults

| | Mean values | | |
|---|---|---|---|
| Flow rate (ml/min/gland) | Parotid 0.7 | Submaxillary 0.6 | Plasma |
| mEq/L | | | |
| Potassium ($K^+$) | 20 | 17 | 4 |
| Sodium ($Na^+$) | 23 | 21 | 140 |
| Chloride ($Cl^-$) | 23 | 20 | 105 |
| Bicarbonate ($HCO_3^-$) | 20 | 18 | 27 |
| Calcium ($Ca^{++}$) | 2 | 3.6 | 5 |
| Magnesium ($Mg^{+++}$) | 0.2 | 0.2 | 2 |
| Phosphorous ($HPO_4^-$) | 6 | 4.5 | 2 |
| mg/100 ml | | | |
| Urea | 15 | 7 | 25 |
| Ammonia | 0.3 | 0.2 | |
| Uric acid | 3 | 2 | 4 |
| Glucose | <1 | <1 | 80 |
| Total lipid | 2.8 | 2 | 500 |
| Cholesterol | <1 | — | 160 |
| Fatty acids | 1 | — | 300 |
| Amino acids | 1.5 | — | 50 |
| Total proteins | 250 | 150 | 7% |
| pH | | 6.8-7.2 | 7.35 |

**Table 7-2.** Proteins of parotid and submaxillary saliva

| Parotid | Submaxillary |
|---|---|
| PRODUCED IN ACINAR CELLS | |
| Amylase (high) | Amylase (low) |
| Cationic glycoproteins (high) | Cationic glycoproteins (low) |
| Anionic glycoproteins (low) | Anionic glycoproteins (high) |
| Secretory component | Secretory component |
| Kallikrein | Kallikrein |
| Lactoperoxidase | Lactoperoxidase |
| Lactoferrin | Lactoferrin |
| Proline rich | High-molecular weight glycoproteins (blood group substance) |
| Basic polypeptides | Phosphoproteins |
| Histidine-rich | |
| PRODUCED IN NONACINAR REGIONS OF THE SALIVARY GLANDS, OR ORIGIN UNKNOWN | |
| Secretory IgA | Secretory IgA |
| Lysozyme (low to moderate) | Lysozyme (high) |
| Phosphatases, esterases, β-glucuronidase | Phosphatases, esterases, β-glucuronidase |
| Ribonucleases (moderate) | Ribonucleases (low) |
| Lactic acid dehydrogenases | |
| LEAKAGE FROM BLOOD | |
| Albumin, IgG and IgM, lipoprotein, and traces of other serum proteins (orosomucoid, ceruloplasmin, etc.) | |

is only about 20% that in the parotid. There is virtually no amylase in sublingual or minor salivary gland secretions since these glands are almost exclusively mucous (with no serous cells).

The viscous quality of whole saliva is attributed to salivary "mucin." It would appear that salivary "mucin" is a mixture of many glycoproteins, some common to all the salivary glands and some produced exclusively by the submaxillary-sublingual or minor salivary glands. The glycoproteins produced by the mucous cells of the submaxillary-sublingual and minor glands are probably responsible for the viscoelastic properties of saliva. The glycoproteins are mainly anionic (negatively charged) and appear to be heterogeneous, some with molecular weights that may approach several million. These larger species are currently under active investigation, and considerable information is becoming available.[3] There is also a basic proline-rich glycoprotein.

**Glycoproteins**

In the parotid gland, serous cells produce a major glycoprotein quite different from the mucous cell product.[3,7,8] It is cationic (positively charged), nonviscous, of relatively low molecular weight, and has an amino acid profile unlike mucous glycoproteins.

Acinar cells of both the parotid and the submaxillary gland produce a glycoprotein (about 50,000 molecular weight) known as secretory component. This, together with immunoglobulin A (one of the gamma globulins), forms a specific structural entity, the *secretory IgA* (produced in exocrine glands), which is active on mucosal surfaces.[9] The cells also produce small amounts of lactoferrin, an iron-binding glycoprotein.

**Secretory IgA**

The secretory immunoglobulin (IgA) found in saliva is produced by plasma cells in the connective tissue of the glands, particularly around the intralobular ducts. It leaves the plasma cell as a dimeric molecule. The two halves of the dimer are held together by a polypeptide known as the "J" piece. The dimer then enters the epithelial cells of the striated duct[10] or possibly the acinar cells.[9] There it joins with the secretory component (or piece), which acts to stabilize the molecule and aids in its release into the lumen of the duct. Over 90% of the IgA in saliva is of the secretory variety. Secretory IgA neutralizes viruses and can act as an antibody to bacterial antigens and probably food antigens as well. It is relatively resistant to proteolytic enzymes and hence can survive in the oral cavity and the gastrointestinal tract.[9]

The mucous cells of the submaxillary-sublingual and minor salivary glands produce "blood group-substance" high-molecular weight glycoproteins that have blood group activity. Portions of the glycoprotein molecule are characteristic for the blood type of the individual. About 80% of the population are secretors; they secrete the specific blood type of glycoproteins in their saliva. The nonsecretors synthesize a precursor blood group substance (the Lewis substance) in their glands. Salivary "mucin" and "blood group substance" may prove to be the same entity.

The antibacterial enzyme, lysozyme, is found in both parotid and submaxillary secretions. It is formed (or concentrated) in basal cells of the striated ducts.[10] Lysozyme is a muramidase; that is, it splits bacterial cell walls in the glycopeptide region that contains muramic acid. Lysozyme may act together with other antibacterial systems in saliva (IgA) as a general scavenger of susceptible bacterial cell walls.

**Lysozyme**

Another important component of the salivary antibacterial system is the enzyme sialoperoxidase. Together with hydrogen peroxide and thiocyanate, sialoperoxidase can affect lactobacilli and cariogenic streptococci.[11] A similar system exists in mother's milk and is considered to be part of the early defense mechanism of the newborn. Comparable peroxidase activity (myeloperoxidase) is part of the antibacterial weaponry of the leukocyte. A system has been introduced for oral use that is purported to generate an ideal level of hydrogen peroxide for endogenous sialoperoxidase activity against *Streptococcus mutans* and other plaque organisms.[12]

**Sialoperoxidase**

Originally described in bovine milk, lactoferrin is widely distributed in body fluids and in granules of polymorphonuclear leukocytes. Theoretically, this red, iron-binding

**Lactoferrin**

glycoprotein should be an effective antibacterial agent in saliva by withholding iron from facultative and aerobic organisms and by producing a "nutritional" immunity.[13]

**Other proteins**

A considerable number of other enzymes have been identified in both parotid and submaxillary-sublingual saliva. These include acid and alkaline phosphatases, nonspecific esterases, ribonucleases, and kallikrein. The enzyme, lactic acid dehydrogenase (LDH), has been found in parotid saliva but not in submaxillary-sublingual saliva.

Both basic (positively charged) and acidic (negatively charged) proteins with rather unusual amino acid compositions have been found to exist in human parotid saliva. The basic proteins include a group that possesses very high levels of proline, glycine, and glutamic acid–glutamine (74% to 88% of the total residues in the proteins)[14] and some basic histidine-rich polypeptides.[15] Four major acidic proline-rich proteins have been isolated and shown to possess levels of dicarboxylic acids, proline, and glycine, as well as a marked affinity for hydroxyapatite and tooth powder.[16,17] These proteins, as well as some minor acidic proline-rich proteins,[18] a tyrosine-rich acidic peptide,[19] and a histidine-rich acidic peptide,[20] have been suggested as likely candidates in the formation of tooth pellicle because of their tendency to adsorb hydroxyapatite or tooth powders. The tyrosine-rich protein has also been shown to possess a marked ability to inhibit calcium phosphate precipitation in supersaturated solutions.[21] Some of the acidic proline-rich proteins exhibit this property to a lesser degree.

Serum proteins can be identified in saliva by immunologic techniques. They are present in low concentration and appear to enter the secretion by "leakage." Only albumin is present at any appreciable level (about 1 mg/100 ml). In salivary gland disease in which ductal integrity is altered (e.g., parotitis or Sjögren disease), albumin levels are markedly elevated.[22] The finding that IgG is present in saliva in much lower amounts than IgA supports the observation that the salivary IgA is produced in the gland. In blood, the IgG-to-IgA ratio is about 10:1; in saliva it is the reverse.

**Bacterial adherence and aggregating factors**

Bacterial adherence and aggregating factors are really glycoproteins from all three major salivary glands. There are two factors with separate activities. One factor becomes part of the salivary pellicle that coats the teeth (immediately after cleaning) and enhances bacterial adherence to the tooth surface. The other factor is an agglutinating factor that agglutinates bacterial units in the mouth, reducing the number of units and facilitating their reduction by swallowing. Caries-resistant individuals have a lesser amount of adherence factor (usually for *Streptococcus sanguis*) and more agglutinating factor. The reverse is true of caries-prone individuals.

**Formed elements**

Saliva contains epithelial cells from the oral mucosa as well as leukocytes (salivary corpuscles) from the gingival sulcus.[23,24]

## Role in oral health

The inorganic and organic components of saliva endow the secretions with considerable protective potential:

1. *Lubrication and protection.* The glycoproteins and mucoids produced by the major and minor salivary glands form a protective coating for the mucous membrane. This coating is a barrier against irritants acting directly on the membrane. It is also a barrier against (a) proteolytic and hydrolytic enzymes produced in plaque, (b) potential carcinogens (smoking, chemicals, etc.), and (c) desiccation (mouth breathing). The mucoid layer may be considered comparable in some respects to gastric mucin, which protects the stomach from the hydrochloric acid produced therein.
2. *Buffering action.* Primarily because of its bicarbonate content and secondarily because of phosphate and amphoteric proteins, saliva has considerable buffer capacity. This protective function occurs in the plaque, directed against acidogenic microorganisms, and

occasionally on the mucous membrane surface, where acids from foods or regurgitation may occur.

3. *Maintenance of tooth integrity.* Saliva functions to maintain the integrity of the tooth in a number of ways: (a) it provides minerals for posteruptive maturation; (b) it provides ions such as calcium and phosphate in sufficient amounts to counteract tooth dissolution by saliva (solubility product principle); and (c) it forms a film of glycoprotein on the teeth (the pellicle) that may act as a diffusion barrier, thus preventing loss of tooth mineral. Saliva contains at least one special peptide or protein that apparently allows saliva to contain supersaturated amounts of calcium and phosphate ions by counteracting nucleation of calcium phosphate salts.[21] Thus spontaneous precipitation of calcium phosphate within the saliva and on the tooth surfaces is prevented.

4. *Antibacterial activity.* Saliva contains a number of components that can, by themselves or together, marshal an impressive defense against bacterial and viral invasion.[22,25] Great interest is now focused on secretory IgA, which has been demonstrated to be effective against a number of viruses and bacteria.[9] The manner in which IgA operates in the mouth against plaque organisms is the subject of considerable research. Coating of oral streptococci by IgA has been demonstrated.[26,27] Since IgA does not activate complement (which in turn sets a complex defense mechanism in motion), the manner by which it exerts an antibacterial effect remains to be established. The most reasonable explanation is that bacterial cells coated with secretory IgA have a reduced tendency to adhere to teeth and mucous membrane surfaces. Hence they may clump and be swallowed. The exact relationship between the production of secretory IgA and dental disease is still unclear. There may be a negative correlation between the accumulated dental caries experience in permanent teeth (DMF score) and IgA production. Conversely, the periodontal index (PI) appears to be positively correlated; that is, the higher the PI, the *greater* the amount of IgA produced by the parotid salivary gland.[28] Obviously, much more work is required to clarify the role of secretory IgA in the oral cavity as it relates to periodontal disease.

　　Lysozyme (as mentioned) breaks up cell walls of susceptible bacteria. Evidence exists that it has more of a general scavenger function than has heretofore been considered.[13,25]

Several antilactobacilli systems in saliva have been studied.[29] The sialoperoxidase–thiocyanate–hydrogen peroxide system has received greatest attention. Evidence also exists that the antibacterial activity can involve potentially cariogenic streptococci[11] as well as reducing plaque accumulation.[12]

Lactoferrin also exhibits a bactericidal effect on cariogenic streptococci[30] at levels comparable to that usually found in salivary secretions.

## Role in oral disease

The role of saliva in oral disease is most apparent when salivary flow is markedly reduced; this has been discussed earlier. Where salivary flow is relatively normal, saliva is still of interest to the dentist in the following areas: (1) pellicle and plaque deposition, (2) plaque mineralization to form calculus, and (3) dental caries.

### PELLICLE AND PLAQUE DEPOSITION

Saliva influences supragingival plaque deposition and activity in a variety of ways. An organic coating forms when the crown of the tooth emerges and is exposed to saliva. This coating is called *dental pellicle*. The deposition of pellicle occurs in stages: (1) bathing of the tooth surfaces by salivary fluids, which contain numerous protein constituents; (2) selective adsorption of certain negatively and positively charged glycoproteins,[31] (electrostatic attraction of charged molecules is a factor); (3) loss of solubility of the adsorbed proteins by surface denaturation and acid precipitation; and (4) alteration of the glycoproteins by enzymes from bacteria and the oral secretions. The pellicle is involved in the first step of plaque formation.

The pellicle is actively involved in the initiation of bacterial colonization. Adherence factors in proteins in the pellicle[31] can increase the binding of specific bacteria (*Streptococcus sanguis*) to the tooth. The initial step in dental plaque formation involves the adherence of bacteria to the salivary coated tooth surface. This salivary coat (pellicle) is primarily composed of high–molecular weight glycoproteins derived from salivary glands. The bacteria that adhere to and colonize the pellicle are initially *S. sanguis,* followed by *Actinomyces viscosus.* Recently, mucins purified from human and monkey submandibular-sublingual salivas have been used to determine the specificity of interaction with streptococci[32] (Table 7-3). Studies reveal that sialic acid residues on the mucins were necessary for the binding of *S. sanguis* but not *S. mutans.* These findings indicate that such microorganisms possess different receptors for the salivary molecules. These receptors are lectin-ligand interactions. In addition to their role in dental plaque formation, salivary mucins free in the fluid environment may provide nonimmune protection by agglutinating bacteria and making them more susceptible to swallowing.

Once an initial layer of bacteria attaches to the pellicle surface, plaque buildup can progress at a rapid pace, depending on the influence of self-cleansing mechanisms and effectiveness of personal oral hygiene. The second colonizer of the tooth surface is *Actinomyces viscosus.* These organisms have two types of fibrils on their surfaces. Type I fibrils are for tooth surface adherence. Type II fibrils are for cell-to-cell interactions. In the maturation stage, saliva continues to provide adherence substances and other proteins to the intercellular matrix, and bacterial intercellular adhesion results. Salivary proteins and carbohydrates serve as a substrate for metabolic activity of the bacteria. Salivary calcium, phosphorus, magnesium, sodium, and potassium become part of the gel-like interstices of the plaque and influence mineralization and demineralization, cell adhesion, and diffusion of bacterial products. Buffer components from saliva affect plaque pH. Salivary urea and ammonia have a profound effect on bacterial activity and final plaque pH.

## PLAQUE MINERALIZATION AND CALCULUS FORMATION

The most apparent effect of saliva on plaque is that of mineralization to form calculus.

The mineral components of supragingival calculus are derived almost exclusively from the salivary fluids. Deposition is most rapid and heaviest opposite the orifices of the salivary glands. Parotid and submaxillary saliva is usually saturated with respect to brushite and hydroxyapatite (the major minerals of calculus), and hence saliva is

**Table 7-3.**   Salivary-bacterial agglutination effect of sialic acid removal

| Microorganism | Human salivary mucin (molecular weight: 1.6 to 1.8 × 10⁵) | | Monkey salivary mucin (molecular weight: 1 × 10⁶) | |
|---|---|---|---|---|
| | + Sialic acid | − Sialic acid | + Sialic acid | − Sialic acid |
| *S. sanguis* strain 10556 | + | − | + | − |
| *S. sanguis* strain 10558 | + | − | + | − |
| *S. mutans* strain BHT | + | + | + | + |
| *S. mutans* strain B13 | + | + | + | + |

Modified from Levine, M.J., et al.: Specificity of salivary-bacterial interactions: role of terminal sialic glycoproteins with *Strepetococcus sanguis* and *Streptococcus mutans*, Infect. Immun. **19:**107, 1978.

considered a metastable solution. When extremely heavy calculus formers were compared to light formers, submaxillary calcium concentration was usually elevated in the rapid formers to levels above 10 mg/100 ml.[33] No differences were found in parotid calcium or in phosphorus concentration in any of the secretions.[33] Where salivary calcium concentration is elevated (i.e., in such clinical conditions as cystic fibrosis, asthma, and, to a lesser extent, diabetes mellitus), increased calculus formation is apparent.[34,35] Elevations in salivary proteins and urea are also characteristic of heavy calculus formers.[36]

Examination of the salivary proteins that may play a role in plaque mineralization indicates that esterase, pyrophosphatase, and possibly acid phosphatase and lysozyme may be involved.[31,33] Persons who are heavy calculus formers have higher levels of salivary glycoproteins than noncalculus formers. It is possible that they may have glycoproteins not found in noncalculus formers.[37] On the basis of immunochemical examination, however, the proteins in heavy calculus formers do not appear to be antigenically unique.[33] Most probably, heavy calculus formers have more than one protein associated with mineralization.

**Light vs. heavy calculus formers**

### DENTAL CARIES

A voluminous literature attests to the interest in the relationship between saliva and caries.[3] Theoretically, saliva can affect caries in five general ways by acting (1) to mechanically cleanse and thus lessen plaque accumulation; (2) to reduce enamel solubility by plaque modification through calcium, phosphate, and fluoride; (3) buffer and neutralize the acids either produced by cariogenic organisms or introduced directly through diet; (4) by direct antibacterial activity; and (5) by aggregation or clumping bacteria and reducing adherence to tooth surfaces.

## Role in salivary gland disease

Investigation of the flow rate and composition of saliva (sialochemistry) is proving to be of great value in the differential diagnosis of diseases of the salivary glands.[1,38] Salivary changes have been noted in inflammatory disease, Sjögren disease, sarcoidosis, salivary gland calculi, and enlargement of salivary glands because of alcoholic cirrhosis.

### CARIES IN THE ADULT

The epidemiology of caries in the adult population is being studied.[39] Periodontal disease and root caries are statistically strongly associated, with 39% to 58% of the population having one or more root lesions. The peak age group of 50-59 has 22% Root Caries Index (RCI) (22% of surfaces at risk are carious) and three teeth per subject involved. Mandibular posterior teeth have the highest incidence, followed by maxillary anterior, maxillary posterior, and finally mandibular anterior teeth. In periodontal patients, past root caries experience, lactobacillus counts, and age are all helpful in predicting new lesions. Impaired salivary flow leads to more root caries.[40,41]

Root caries are of concern in the management of periodontal disease, particularly their prevention during treatment. *Actinomyces viscosus* is the most common isolate from root caries' lesions. Other isolates include *A. naeslundii, A. odontolyticus, A. eriksonii, Rothia dentocariosa, Nocardia,* and *S. mutans.* In the pathogenesis of root caries, new surfaces are at risk because of recession, and new ecologic niches are created by prostheses under or adjacent to retainers and on exposed over-denture tooth surfaces. The prevention of root caries includes caries' risk assessment as an aid to patient management, home care, nutritional counseling, and fluoride therapy (topical).

**Root caries**

In assessment, four separate evaluations form the basis of the caries risk:

1. Rate of salivary flow
2. Buffering capacity of saliva
3. Bacteriologic quantification of *Streptococcus mutans* and lactobacilli
4. Dietary history

The benefits resulting from evaluation of data from these procedures are two-fold— they include identification of patients "at risk" for dental caries, and they provide a mechanism to monitor progress of home care and nutritional programs to decrease or eliminate caries' risk. Caries' risk assessment requires the participation of the clinician, bacteriologist and a salivary biochemist.[42-47]

## Role in systemic disease

There is a rapidly expanding body of data on the value of salivary examination in the diagnosis of systemic disease and the monitoring of abnormal substances through saliva. In such diseases as cystic fibrosis, asthma,[48] several forms of hypertension, and diseases of the adrenal cortex, saliva has been shown to be abnormal. In toxicity resulting from overdose of digitalis, salivary examination can be diagnostic. Excess of mercury in the body can be monitored through saliva. Many other substances are now being studied.[1,38] The dentist may render valuable help to total health care by examining salivary flow rate and composition.

## Summary

Saliva is a complex secretion that plays a major role in general and oral health and disease. It lubricates and protects the structures of the mouth and influences the nature of the oral microbial flora and even the chemical composition of the teeth. Saliva plays a role in the formation of plaque and calculus and is therefore intimately related to caries and periodontal disease.

Agglutination-, adherence-, and coaggregation-promoting factors of saliva play a key role in the accumulation of dental plaque as well as in bacterial succession within the plaque. It is also extremely important in the resistance of the body to these periodontal diseases and caries.[49-57]

**REFERENCES**

1. Wotman, S., and Mandel, I.D.: The salivary secretions in health and disease. In Rankow, R.W., and Polayes, I.M., editors: Diseases of the salivary glands, Philadelphia, 1976, W.B. Saunders Co.
2. Burgen, A.S.V., and Emmelin, N.G.: Physiology of the salivary glands, Baltimore, 1961, Williams & Wilkins.
3. Mandel, I.D.: Relation of saliva and plaque to caries, J. Dent. Res. **53:**246, 1974.
4. Caldwell, R.C., and Pigman, W.: Disc electrophoresis of human saliva in polyacrylamide gel, Arch. Biochem. Biophys. **110:**91, 1965.
5. Meyer, T.S., and Lamberts, B.L.: Zone electrophoresis of human parotid saliva in acrylamide gel, Nature **205:**1215, 1965.
6. Steiner, J.C., and Keller, P.: An electrophoretic analysis of the protein components of human parotid saliva, Arch. Oral Biol. **13:**1213, 1968.
7. Levine, M.J., and Ellison, S.A.: Immunoelectrophoretic and chemical analyses of human parotid saliva, Arch. Oral Biol. **18:**838, 1973.
8. Mandel, I.D., Thompson, R.H., Jr., and Ellison, S.A.: Studies on the mucoproteins of human parotid saliva, Arch. Oral Biol. **10:**499, 1965.
9. Tomasi, T.B., Jr., and Bienenstock, J.: Secretory immunoglobulins, Adv. Immunol. **9:**1, 1968.
10. Kraus, F.W., and Mestecky, J.: Immunohistochemical localization of amylase, lysozyme and immunoglobulins in the human parotid gland, Arch. Oral Biol. **16:**781, 1971.
11. Morrison, M., and Steele, W.F.: Lactoperoxidase, the peroxidase in the salivary gland. In Person, P., editor: Biology of the mouth, Washington, D.C., 1968, American Association for the Advancement of Science.
12. Koch, G., Edlund, K., and Hoogendoorn, H.:

Lactoperoxidase in the prevention of plaque accumulation, gingivitis and dental caries. II. Effect of mouthrinses with amyloglucosidase and glucoseoxidase on plaque accumulation on teeth in individuals on a sucrose diet, Odontol. Rev. **24:**367, 1973.

13. Mandel, I.D.: Nonimmunologic aspects of caries resistance, J. Dent. Res. **55:**C22, 1976.

14. Levine, M., and Keller, P.J.: The isolation of some basic proline-rich proteins from human parotid saliva. Arch. Oral Biol. **22:**37, 1977.

15. Baum, B.J., Bird, J.L., and Longton, R.W.: Polyacrylamide gel electrophoresis of human salivary histidine-rich polypeptides, J. Dent. Res. **56:**1115, 1977,

16. Bennick, A., and Connell, G.E.: Purification and partial characterization of four proteins from human parotid saliva, Biochem. J. **123:**455, 1971.

17. Oppenheim, F.G., Hay, D.I., and Franzblau, C.: Proline-rich proteins from human parotid saliva. I. Isolation and partial characterization, Biochemistry **10:**4233, 1971.

18. Hay, D.I.: The interaction of human parotid salivary proteins with hydroxyapatite, Arch. Oral Biol. **18:**1517, 1973.

19. Hay, D.I.: The isolation from human parotid saliva of a tyrosine-rich acidic peptide which exhibits high affinity for hydroxyapatite surfaces, Arch. Oral Biol. **18:**1531, 1973.

20. Hay, D.I.: Fractionation of human parotid salivary proteins and the isolation of an histidine-rich acidic peptide which shows high affinity for hydroxyapatite surfaces, Arch. Oral Biol. **20:**553, 1975.

21. Schlesinger, D.H., and Hay, D.I.: Complete covalent structure of statherin, a tyrosinerich acidic peptide which inhibits calcium phosphate precipitation from human parotid saliva, J. Biol. Chem. **252:**1689, 1977.

22. Mandel, I.D., Mandel, L., and Baurmash, H.: Salivary studies in parotitis, IADR Abstract No. 492, 1969.

23. Orban, B., and Weinman, J.P.: The cellular elements of saliva, J. Am. Dent. Assoc. **26:**2008, 1939.

24. Klinkhamer, J.M.: Quantitative evaluation of gingivitis and periodontal disease. II. The mobile mucous phase of oral secretions, Periodontics **6:**253, 1968.

25. Genco, R.J., Evans, R.I., and Ellison, S.A.: Dental research in microbiology with emphasis on periodontal disease, J. Am. Dent. Assoc. **78:**1016, 1969.

26. Brandtzaeg, P., and Fjellanger, I.: Adsorption of gamma A immunoglobulin onto oral bacteria, J. Bacteriol. **96:**242, 1968.

27. Williams, R.C. and Gibbons, R.J.: Inhibition of bacterial adherence by secretory IgA: a mechanism of antigen disposal, Science **177:**697, 1972.

28. Ørstavik, D. and Brandtzaeg, P.: Secretion of parotid IgA in relation to gingival inflammation and dental caries experience in man, Arch. Oral Biol. **20:**701, 1975.

29. Dogon, I.I., and Amdur, B. II.: Further characterization of an antibacterial factor in human parotid secretions active against *Lactobacillus casei,* Arch. Oral Biol. **10:**605, 1965.

30. Cole, M.F., et al.: Studies with human lactoferrin and *Streptococcus mutans.* In Stiles, H.M., Loesche, W.J., and O'Brien, T.C., editors: Proceedings: microbial aspects of dental caries, Sp. Supp. Microbiol. Abstr. **2:**353, 1976.

31. Hay, R.J., Gibbons, R.M., and Spinell, D.M.: Characteristics of some high molecular weight constituents with bacterial aggregating activity from whole saliva and dental plaque, Caries Res. **5:**111, 1971.

32. Levine, M.J., et al.: Specificity of salivary-bacterial interactions: role of terminal sialic glycoproteins with *Streptococcus sanguis* and *Streptococcus mutans,* Infect. Immun. **19:**107, 1978.

33. Mandel, I.D.: Biochemical aspects of calculus formation. II. Comparative studies of saliva in heavy and light calculus formers, J. Periodont. Res. **9:**211, 1974.

34. Wotman, S., et al.: The occurrence of calculus in normal children, children with cystic fibrosis and children with asthma, J. Periodontol. **44:**278, 1973.

35. Marder, M.Z., Abelson, D.C., and Mandel, I.D.: Salivary alterations in diabetes mellitus, J. Periodontol. **46:**567, 1975.

36. Draus, F.J., Tarbet, W.J., and Miklos, F.L.: Salivary enzymes and calculus formation, J. Periodont. Res. **3:**232, 1968.

37. Ericson, T.: Salivary glycoproteins, Acta Odontol. Scand. **26:**3, 1968.

38. Mandel, I.D., and Wotman, S.: The salivary secretions in health and disease, Oral Sci. Rev. **8:**25, 1976.

39. Nyvad, B., and Fejerskov, O.: Root surface caries: clinical, histopathological and morphological features and clinical implications, Int. Dent. J. **32:**312-326, 1982.

40. Katz, R.V., et al.: Prevalence and intraoral distribution of root caries in an adult population, Caries Res. **16:**265-271, 1982.

41. Rewald, N., and Hamp, S.E.: Prediction of root surface caries in patients treated for advanced periodontal disease, J. Clin. Periodontol. **8:**400-414, 1981.

42. Ericsson, G. Clinical investigation on the salivary buffering action, Acta. Odontol. Scand. **17:**131, 1959.

43. Frostall, G. A Colormetric screening test for evaluation of the buffer capacity of saliva, Swed. Dent. J. **4:**81, 1980.

44. Gold, O.G., Jordan, H.V., and Van Houte, J.: A selective medium for *Streptococcus mutans,* Arch. Oral Biol. **18:**1375, 1973.

45. Westergren, G., and Krasse, B.: Evaluation of

a micromethod for determination of *Streptococcus mutans* and lactobacillus infection, J. Clin. Microbiol. **1:**82, 1978.

46. Krasse, B.: Approaches to prevention. In Stiles, H.M., Loesche, W.J., and O'Brien, T.C., editors: Proceedings: microbial aspects of dental caries, Sp. Suppl. Microbiol. Abstr. **3:**867, 1976.

47. Syed, S.W., and Loesche, W.J.: Survival of human dental plaque flora in various transport media, Appl. Microbiol. **24:**638, 1972.

48. Hyyppa, T.: Studies in immunologic and inflammatory factors in saliva in patients with asthma and in patients with periodontitis, J. Clin. Periodontol. **8:**500, 1981.

49. Thomas, E.L., Bates, K.P., and Jefferson, M.M.: Peroxidase antimicrobial system of human saliva: requirements for accumulation of hypothiocyanate, J. Dent. Res. **60:**785, 1981.

50. Smith, D.J., et al.: Salivary IgA antibody to *Actinobacillus actinomycetemcomitans* in a young adult population, J. Periodont. Res. **20:**8, 1985.

51. Sandholm, L., and Gronblad, E.: Salivary immunoglobulins in patients with juvenile periodontitis and their healthy siblings, J. Periodontol. **55:**9, 1984.

52. Güven, O., and DeVisscher, J.: Salivary IgA in periodontal disease, J. Periodontol. **53:**334, 1982.

53. Suber, J.F., et al.: Parotid saliva agglutinins for sheep erythrocytes as a measure of ongoing inflammation in periodontal disease, J. Periodontol. **55:**512, 1984.

54. Hardman, P.K., and Hardman, J.T.: Salivary ABO antibodies and periodontal disease, J. Periodontol. **54:**351, 1983.

55. Smith, A.J., et al.: Changes in salivary periodontal activity observed during experimentally-induced gingivitis, J. Clin. Periodontol. **11:**373, 1984.

56. Tenovvo, J., Pruitt, K.M., and Thomas, E.L.: Peroxidase antimicrobial system of human saliva: hypothiocyanite levels in resting and stimulated saliva, J. Dent. Res. **61:**982, 1982.

57. Sakamoto, W., Fukudo, H., and Nishikaze, O.: Kininogen and kallikrein in saliva of periodontally diseased subjects, J. Dent. Res. **60:**6, 1981.

## ADDITIONAL SELECTED READING

Boackle, R.J., et al.: The effects of human saliva on the hemolytic activity of complement, J. Dent. Res. **57:**103, 1978.

Demetriou, N., Krikos, G., and Bambionitakis, A.: Relation between gingival fluid and mixed and parotid IgA, J. Periodontol. **49:**64, 1978.

Falkler, W.A., Jr., Hawley, C.E., and Mongiello, J.R.: *Leptotrichia buccalis* hemagglutination in cell binding and salivary inhibition studies, J. Periodont. Res. **13:**425, 1978.

Hay, D.I., et al.: Relationship between concentration of human salivary statherin and inhibition of calcium phosphate precipitation in stimulated parotid saliva, J. Dent. Res. **63:**857, 1984.

Iijama, K., et al.: Collagenase activity in human saliva, J. Dent. Res. **62:**709, 1983.

Nakamura, M., and Slots, J.: Salivary enzymes: origin and relationship to periodontal disease, J. Periodont. Res. **18:**559, 1983.

Navazesh, M., and Christensen, C.M.: A comparison of whole mouth resting and stimulated salivary measurement procedures, J. Dent. Res. **61:**1158, 1982.

Shomers, J.P., et al.: The isolation of a family of cysteine-containing phosphoproteins from human submandibular-sublingual saliva, J. Dent. Res. **61:**973, 1982.

Shomers, J.P., et al.: Properties of cysteine-containing phosphoproteins from human submandibular-sublingual saliva, J. Dent. Res. **61:**397, 1982.

Zahradnik, R.T., Propas, D., and Moreno, E.C.: Effect of salivary pellicle formation time on *in vitro* attachment and demineralization by *Streptococcus mutans*, J. Dent. Res. **57:**1036, 1978.

# CHAPTER 8

# Microbiology (plaque)

## Oral microbiota

Infection is defined as a disease that occurs in the presence of bacteria. Thus caries and bacterially induced periodontal disease are infections.

The mouth has an indigenous microbiota. Various organisms are normally present on the tongue. Others may be found on the teeth or in juxtaposition to the sulcus and within periodontal pockets. Still others are found on other oral mucous membranes. Each location has a characteristic flora. The indigenous microbiota constitutes a normal part of the oral environment and may have no adverse effect as long as the host-parasite relationship is in balance. Consequently bacteria may exist in the mouth without producing disease.

Withdrawal of toothbrushing in healthy human experimental subjects results in a growing accumulation of microbial plaque and the development of gingivitis.[1,2] If this bacterial plaque is removed by oral hygiene, the gingivitis is reversible. From these and other studies, it has become obvious that bacteria cause gingivitis[3] (Fig. 8-1).

When periodontally healthy individuals are compared to those with inflammatory periodontal disease, more and different bacteria, both marginal and subgingival, can be recovered from the diseased patient,[4,5] From this relationship, one may draw the conclusion that some of these bacteria act as pathogens. However, one must remember that microbial activity and host response are interrelated; certain microorganisms may cause disease, but the host may interfere with their pathogenic potential and in some cases completely neutralize it. Host immune responses may also promote differential colonization and growth of the species resident in the periodontal microbiota.

### ACQUISITION

Acquisition of the oral microbiota starts at birth.[6,7] Among the great variety of microorganisms entering the mouth of the edentulous infant, only certain species become established (i.e., those that are suited for growth in the oral environment). These microorganisms are to a large extent derived from the oral flora of persons in

**Location**

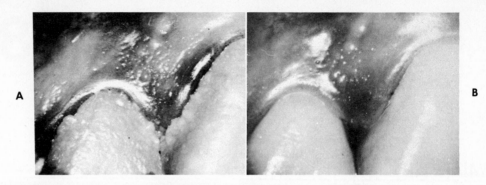

**Fig. 8-1.** **A,** Dental plaque and gingivitis developed during 21 days without any oral hygiene. Before that, the teeth were clean and the gingiva healthy. **B,** Same area 8 days after resumption of efficient oral hygiene. The teeth are again clean and the gingiva healthy. (Courtesy H. Löe and E. Theilade, Aarhus, Denmark.)

contact with the infant. Organisms from the vagina, skin, food, air, and clothing appear only as transients.

During the first few months after birth, the oral microbiota are dominated by streptococci and contain small and variable numbers of staphylococci, lactobacilli, and *Neisseria*, *Veillonella*, and *Candida* species.[6,7] These early colonizers of the edentulous mouth are mainly facultative (aerotolerant—grow with or without oxygen); however, the presence of the anaerobic *Veillonella* species suggests that the facultative organisms create a favorable environment on the tongue for selected anaerobic species. The streptococci on the tongue produce lactic acid, which *Veillonella* species must have to grow.

As the teeth erupt, microorganisms also colonize the teeth, mainly in the fissures and the gingival sulcus region.[8] The sulcular ecosystem provides unique growth conditions; additional bacterial groups including *Actinomyces*, *Rothia*, *Bacterionema*, *Bacteroides*, *Fusobacterium*, *Leptotrichia*, and *Selenomonas* species as well as spirochetes are found.[6]

**Salivary microbiota**

Saliva within the salivary glands is free of bacteria. Saliva flowing from the ducts passes over tooth and mucosal surfaces coated by bacteria and becomes contaminated with microorganisms and their products. Since the microflora of saliva depends on the shedding of organisms from different oral surfaces, it shows great variation in bacterial content and composition. This variation is apparent between individuals and even within individuals at different times. The salivary microbiota is to a large extent derived from the dorsum of the tongue; however, it is not representative of any single oral site.

## SURFACE COATINGS ON TEETH

Deposits acquired after eruption of the teeth may be classified as exogenous structures, consisting chiefly of (1) pellicle, (2) dental plaque, and (3) dental calculus.[9-12]

**Acquired pellicle**

The acquired salivary pellicle is thin (0.05 to 1 μm thick), acellular, and essentially bacteria free.[11,12] It consists of various high molecular–weight glycoproteins derived from the mucous salivary glands selectively adsorbed to enamel or cementum. The pellicle is reformed in minutes if removed from the teeth. It may cover the entire tooth surface. Its formation is not a prerequisite to plaque formation. However, because of its rapid rate of formation, it precedes the first stage in plaque formation. In some areas pellicle becomes colonized by bacteria.[11] Pellicle is also formed on appliances in the mouth and on plastic strips inserted around the teeth for study purposes.[12,13]

**Dental plaque**

Dental plaque consists of soft bacterial deposits firmly adhering to the organic films that cover teeth and intraoral appliances[13-18] (Fig. 8-2). It can be removed by tooth-

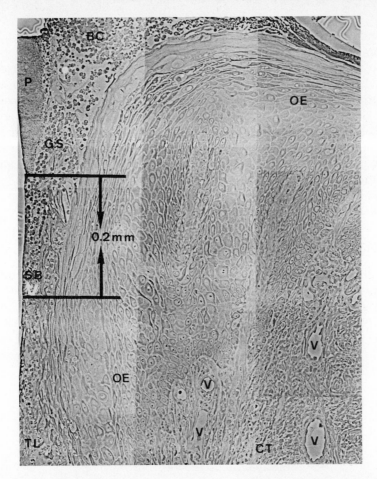

**Fig. 8-2.** The intimate relationship of plaque microbiota to the tissues of the gingival sulcus is evident in this phase-contrast photomicrograph. *P,* Plaque; *GS,* gingival sulcus; *SB,* bottom of the sulcus; *TL,* transmigrating leukocytes accumulating in the junctional epithelium and in the sulcus. *BC,* blood clot from taking biopsy; *OE,* oral epithelium; *CT,* connective tissue; *V,* blood vessels. (Courtesy H.E. Schroeder, Zurich, Switzerland.)

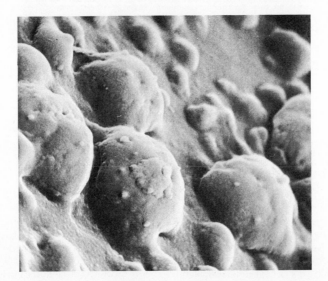

**Fig. 8-3.** Scanning electron micrograph of the surface of an upper central incisor near the sulcus 1 hour after prophylaxis. The formation of these globules is the earliest indication of plaque formation. ( × 12,800.) (From Critchley, P., and Saxton, C.A.: Int. Dent. J. **20:**408, 1970.)

brushing and by scaling. It reforms *rapidly* after removal (Fig. 8-3), although the rate of formation varies among individuals.

Dental plaque is a complex, metabolically interconnected, highly organized bacterial ecosystem. It consists of dense masses of microorganisms embedded in an intermicrobial matrix. There are different plaque ecosystems, with varying compositions and physiology. Some plaque populations may be innocuous, whereas others, in sufficient concentration, may disturb the balance of the host-parasite relationship and cause either dental caries, various periodontal diseases, or both. Thus an understanding of dental plaque, its formation, composition, biochemical characteristics, and biologic effects on the host is important.

**Dental calculus**

Dental calculus (Chapter 9) is plaque that has undergone mineralization. Its surface is generally covered with a layer of nonmineralized plaque.

## Dental plaque

**Formation**

Dental plaque occurs as adherent supragingival and subgingival microbial layers. Plaque formation begins with the microbial colonization of a tooth surface (Figs. 8-3 and 8-4) by selected bacterial species.[12-17] Further increase in the size of plaque occurs

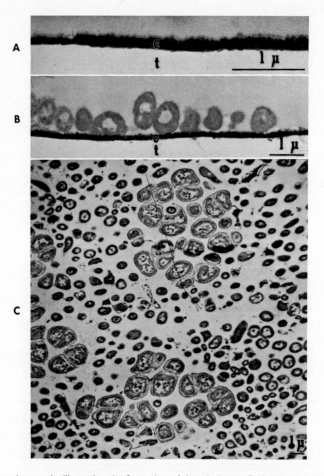

**Fig. 8-4.**  Electron micrographs illustrating the formation of dental plaque. **A,** Acquired pellicle, *(c)* deposited from salivary proteins. *t,* Space representing tooth surface. (×29,000.) **B,** First microorganisms attached to the salivary pellicle *(c). t,* Space representing tooth surface. (×14,500.) **C,** Dental plaque consisting primarily of microorganisms, which seem to proliferate in separate microcolonies. The intermicrobial substance is electron lucent and therefore appears clear. (×5400.) (Courtesy J. Theilade, Aarhus, Denmark.)

by proliferation of the microorganisms within plaque and the contribution of salivary glycoproteins to the intermicrobial matrix. Aggregation of more organisms from saliva and adjacent tooth and gingival regions to those already adhering also occurs (Fig. 8-5). If toothbrushing is suspended, small isolated plaque colonies (Fig. 8-6) form in 1 to 4 days.[16] They are scattered over the tooth surface but are mainly found along the gingival margin. In 2 to 5 days the colonies fuse to form a continuous deposit (Fig. 8-7). After about 10 days without oral hygiene, the plaque may reach maximum extension and thickness; further growth is counterbalanced by the amounts worn off by the friction of masticating food, etc. Various streptococci and gram-positive rods form a prominent part of the microbiota in the early supramarginal (supragingival) plaque colonies.[16] Later in the process of plaque development, the ecology becomes more complex[17] since the various microbial species may proliferate as the environment becomes most suitable for them.[18] Thus facultative microorganisms proliferate first, supragingivally and at the gingival margin, and create a low oxygen tension in which anaerobic microorganisms can grow (Fig. 8-8).

**Location**

Whereas the acquired pellicle covers all tooth surfaces, plaque is prominent in areas protected against friction from food, tongue, lips, and cheeks. In the gingival sulcus, plaque formation may occur undisturbed. How far plaque can extend coronally depends on which frictional forces may act on the individual exposed tooth surfaces. Even vigorous chewing of hard foods (apples, raw carrots) inhibits the occlusal extension of supramarginal plaque only to a limited extent, if at all.[18a,19] It has no inhibitory effect on plaque formation on proximal surfaces or in the gingival sulcus.[20] The direct maxillary palatal surfaces are regularly subjected to friction from the tongue and food particles and are to a degree self-cleansing; however, other areas of the gingiva are not.

Plaque may be supragingival—that is, located on the clinical crowns—or subgingival, located in the gingival sulcus and periodontal pockets. Supragingival plaque receives nutrients from saliva and ingested food, whereas the subgingival plaque is in

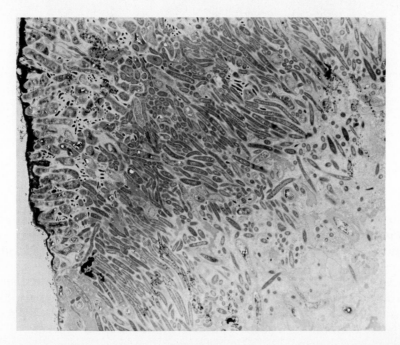

**Fig. 8-5.** *Established microbial plaque near the vestibular gingival margin of the maxillary premolar. A deep layer of coccoid and rodlike microorganisms is covered by a superficial layer of filamentous organisms, which are in turn covered by disintegrating polymorphonuclear leukocytes. (× 9000.) (Courtesy H.E. Schroeder, Zurich, Switzerland.)*

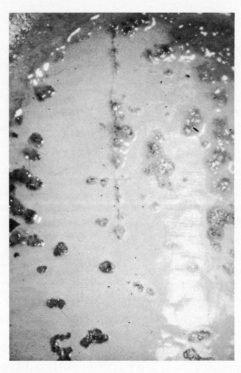

**Fig. 8-6.** Plaque stained with basic fuchsin on a vestibular tooth surface 1 day after cleansing (×30). Note the discrete, small, hemispheric accumulations (plaque colonies). (Courtesy J. Carlsson, Umeå, Sweden.)

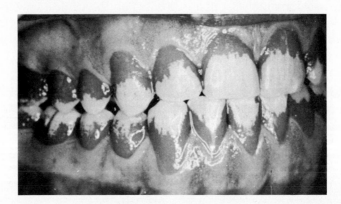

**Fig. 8-7.** Dental plaque formed during 5 days without any oral hygiene. Basic fuchsin is used to demonstrate plaque extending occlusally from the gingival margin.

close contact with gingival exudate, leukocytes, and epithelium (see Fig. 8-2) and is supplied primarily from tissue fluids.

**Structure**     Ultrastructurally (see Fig. 8-5) the inner layer of the plaque consists of densely packed, predominantly coccoid and rod-shaped bacteria; the body of the plaque in addition has many filamentous bacteria oriented perpendicularly to the surface. In subgingival plaque the surface layer in contact with the gingival tissues contains many motile, gram-negative rods and spirochetes.[21] Remnants of the salivary pellicle are usually, but not always, seen at the tooth-plaque interface.

Recent studies of dental plaque have employed improved anaerobic techniques as well as more selective sampling of single pocket sites that distinguish location (su-

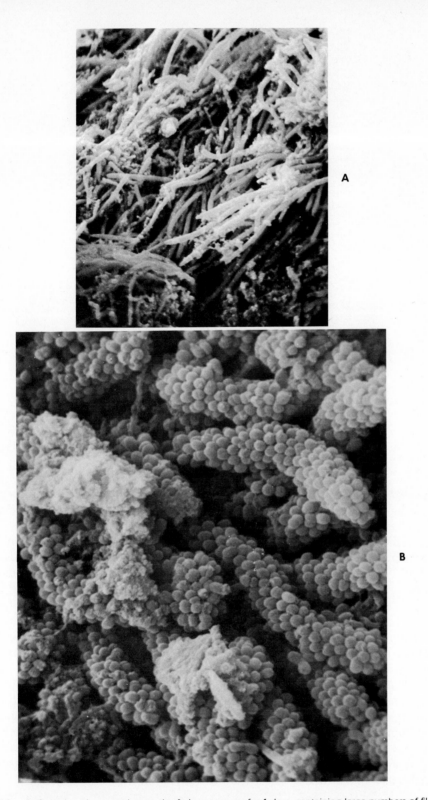

**Fig. 8-8.** **A,** Scanning electron micrograph of plaque grown for 4 days, containing large numbers of filamentous organisms at the surface. (×6000.) **B,** Scanning electron micrograph of plaque illustrating the "corncob" formation of microorganisms on plaque surface. The corncob consists of coccoid bacteria, about 1 μm in diameter, adhering to and completely surrounding the central core composed of one or more filamentous microorganisms. (×4500.)

*Continued.*

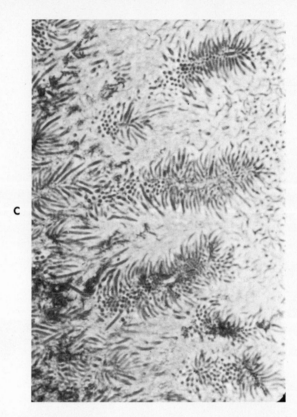

**Fig. 8-8, cont'd.   C,** Longitudinal section of the external surface of 2-month-old subgingival plaque. Note "test-tube–brush" formation. Spirochetes abound in the outermost layer of the plaque facing the soft tissue. (× 1500.)

pragingival or subgingival,) strata (depth of sample toward the base of the pocket), and lateral positioning of the plaque population (adherent and nonadherent popula-tions).[5,12,22-25]

**Matrix**  The microorganisms of plaque are surrounded by an extracellular organic matrix, the intermicrobial substance, which is a granular and fibrillar material in electron micrographs.[15] A portion of the intermicrobial substance consists of proteins derived from saliva and gingival exudate.[26] Some salivary proteins have been shown to cause aggregation of bacteria.[27]

**Polysac-charides**  Polysaccharides produced extracellularly by several bacterial species in plaque are another major component of the intermicrobial substance. Prominent among these extracellular polysaccharides are various glucans (polymers of glucose) and fructans or levans (fructose polymers) produced from dietary sucrose.[28,29] Although the role of plaque polysaccharides as "universal glue" for the bacteria may have been exaggerated, at least the insoluble, $\alpha 1$, $\beta$-linked glucans of *Streptococcus mutans* appear to function in binding this organism to the tooth. In addition, levans and some $\alpha 1$, $\beta$-linked glucans constitute important storage carbohydrates for the plaque bacteria. In the absence of dietary sucrose, plaque may be less abundant. However, plaque is formed even in the absence of any food intake through the mouth, as has been demonstrated in patients fed through a stomach tube.[30]

## PATHOGENIC POTENTIAL

**Total micro-scopic count**  Total counts of microorganisms in dental plaque from the gingival sulcus area are about $10^8$ microorganisms/mg of plaque. This concentration is similar to that of mi-

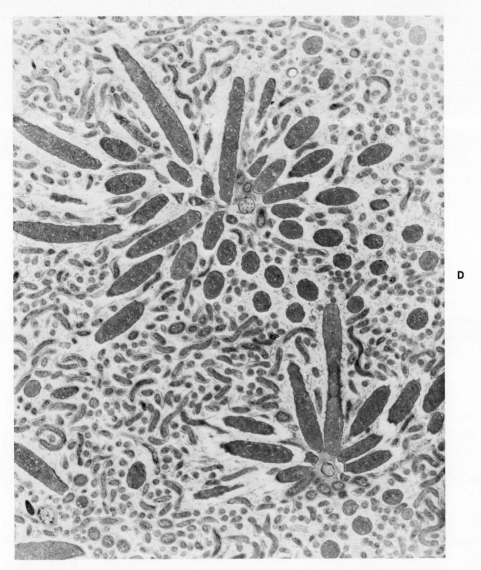

**D**

**Fig. 8-8, cont'd. D,** *Periodontitis. Coarse "test-tube–brush" formations consisting of a large central filament surrounded by large, peritrichously flagellated filamentous bacteria. Background consists of a spirochete-rich flora. (×4300.) (**A** courtesy C.A. Saxton, Isleworth, Middlesex, England; **B** courtesy Z. Skobe, Forsyth Dental Center, Boston, Massachusetts.)*

croorganisms packed by centrifugation of a liquid culture, which means that there is little intermicrobial matrix present between the microorganisms.[31] The gingival region of a person with periodontal disease may harbor 200 mg of plaque, which is an astronomic number of microorganisms in contact with the gingival tissues.

Viable counts of gingival sulcus plaque by aerobic and anaerobic culture techniques average about $1.6 \times 10^7$ to $4.1 \times 10^7$ organisms/mg. The major part of the gingival plaque microbiota is composed of obligate anaerobes. Improvements of anaerobic harvesting and culturing techniques are steadily increasing the recovery of plaque microorganisms.

**Total viable count**

The complexity of the plaque microbiota can be seen in gram-stained smears, in which gram-positive and gram-negative organisms can be distinguished as well as several morphologic types (cocci, rods, fusiforms, filaments, spirilla, and spirochetes).

**Gram-stained smears**

Spirochetes, however, do not stain, so that quantification is difficult in gram-stained smears.

**Enzymes**

A possible mechanism of the destruction of periodontal tissues is through the action of enzymes. Enzymes are produced by the gingival microbiota and act on the intercellular substance of sulcular epithelium, the collagen fibers, and ground substance of connective tissue. Mucopolysaccharidases, notably hyaluronidase, and proteases have been demonstrated in gingival plaque by several investigators.[31-33]

These enzymes may cause a breakdown of proteins and mucopolysaccharides of the intercellular spaces of the junctional epithelium. This may facilitate penetration of various microbial products into the gingival connective tissue. As microbial mucopolysaccharidases, proteases, and collagenases enter the connective tissue, they may disrupt or destroy tissue directly or destroy it indirectly by inducing inflammation. The role of bacterial enzymes in the pathogenesis of periodontitis is not clear at this time and is largely circumstantial and hypothetical.

**Metabolites**

Plaque microorganisms metabolize carbohydrates, amino acids, and proteins, and the various metabolites accumulate in plaque.[31,33] Organic acids produced by fermentation of carbohydrates are essential to caries development. It is unknown whether these acids have any effect on the gingiva. Hydrogen sulfide is produced by several plaque microorganisms and is present in plaque and gingival exudate. Even small concentrations of hydrogen sulfide in air are known to cause irritations of mucous membranes and skin. Ammonia as well as other cytotoxic products are also formed by microbial degradation of amino acids.

**Cell wall components**

Two microbial cell wall components are known to be toxic for mammalian tissue and may be involved in periodontal disease; the first and most completely studied is endotoxin, which is a lipopolysaccharide constituent of gram-negative microorganisms; the second is the mucopeptide complex of gram-positive bacteria.

**Endotoxin**

Endotoxin is a lipopolysaccharide complex with a molecular weight of over 1 million. It is a constituent of the cell wall of all gram-negative bacteria and may be extracted by enzymes, phenol, ether, and other reagents. Injection of endotoxin into experimental animals results in fever, necrotic reactions, diarrhea, or even death. Even in small amounts, endotoxin injected into the oral mucosa may cause inflammation and resorption of adjacent bone. Endotoxin in minute concentrations has a chemotactic effect on neutrophilic granulocytes and induces phagocytosis by these cells.

Free endotoxin is present in dental plaque[34] and in inflamed gingiva.[35] The penetration of clinically healthy gingival epithelium of the dog by radioactive endotoxin has been demonstrated.[36] It can easily be absorbed from gingival pockets and could thereby contribute to the inflammatory process either by a direct toxic effect or through its action as an immunogen.

**Chemotactic factors**

Chemotactic substances are elaborated by plaque bacteria[37] and may attract neutrophilic granulocytes migrating from the connective tissue into the gingival sulcus. In addition, endotoxin may interact with serum and release a chemotactic factor from complement.[38] The white blood cells that accumulate in the gingival tissues and the sulcus are important in host defense. However, they may also release lysosomal enzymes and other products that have the capacity to destroy tissue (see Chapter 12).[39]

**Bacterial antigens**

In addition to the direct initiation of the inflammatory response by microbial products, periodontal inflammation may be produced indirectly by immunopathologic processes set in action by the penetration of microbial antigens into the tissues.

**Other agents**

Although bacteria are numerically and clinically the most significant microbial forms found in the oral cavity, other infective agents may be present from time to time,

**Viruses**

for example, herpes virus, or the etiologic agent for herpetic gingivostomatitis and fever blisters (Chapter 17).

Protozoa are also found in the mouth. They vary from 2 to almost 80 μm in length. **Protozoa**
The most common include *Entamoeba gingivalis*[40] and *Trichomonas.*

Of yeasts and molds the most frequently identified in the mouth is *Candida albicans.* **Yeasts and**
*Candida* may appear as round or oval bodies. In infections of the oral mucous mem- **molds**
branes and other organs, they may grow predominantly as filamentous forms,
producing a mycelium. Such infections are seen frequently in patients with reduced resistance (e.g., patients with AIDS) or in case of extended therapy with antibiotics, especially penicillin and tetracyclines. As the microbial flora is suppressed,
*Candida albicans* tends to proliferate. With increasing use of antibiotics, yeasts are
increasingly noted in plaque.

Dental stains occurring as adherent deposits constitute an esthetic problem. Some **Stains**
of the extrinsic stains are acellular pellicles discolored by food pigments (tea, coffee)
or by tobacco tar (e.g., that seen in smokers). Some stains in children and nonsmokers
are believed to be plaque colored by the activity of chromogenic bacteria (brown, black,
green, and orange stain).[10,41,42] Black stain on deciduous teeth consists of plaque with
a special microflora predominated by gram-positive rods that contains mineral crystals
like dental calculus.[43] Metal salts (e.g., silver nitrate) when used as medication may
also cause unsightly stains.[44] Antimicrobial agents such as topically applied chlorhexidine and systemically administered antibiotics will produce brown-stained pellicles.
Intrinsic stains fall outside the range of discussion of this text, except for reasons of
differential diagnosis.

## Historical perspective

The search for the microbial etiologic agents of destructive periodontal diseases **Early**
has been in progress for about 100 years. During this time there have been periods of **search**
great intensity in the search, followed by cycles in which interest in etiologic agents
diminished. The late 1800s and early 1900s were marked by a period of great activity.
Different groups of investigators in this era suggested three distinct groups of microorganisms as possible etiologic agents. Their choices of agents seemed to be the result
in part of the nature of the techniques employed.

Certain investigators sought the presence of amebae in stained smears of bacterial **Amebae**
plaque. They found higher proportions of amebae in lesions of destructive periodontal disease than in samples taken from sites in healthy mouths or mouths with gingivitis.[45-47] On the basis of this association with destructive lesions, they suggested therapies
directed at controlling amebae. Local therapies included the use of dyes or other
antiseptic agents to decrease the numbers of amebae in the oral cavity. Other approaches employed systemically administered agents such as emitin.[47] This agent was
thought to be a specific amebicide that could eliminate the amebae from the oral cavity.
Investigators using either method claimed great success for both the local and systemic
therapies. Emitin, however, is an emetic—that is, a drug that causes severe nausea
and vomiting. This compound was not an amebicide as originally thought but did
appear to have some antiinflammatory properties, which may have diminished the
severity of gingivitis. The role of amebae in periodontal disease has been questioned
since because amebae have been found in sites with minimal or no disease and can
not be detected in many sites with destructive disease.[48-50]

Other investigators used wet mount preparations for the examination of samples **Spirochetes**
of dental plaque. These preparations were viewed by either phase-contrast or dark-
field microscopy. They reported a higher proportion of spirochetes ( Fig. 8-9) and other
motile forms in lesions of destructive periodontal disease when compared with control
sites.[51-53] This finding suggested that spirochetes may have been the etiologic agents

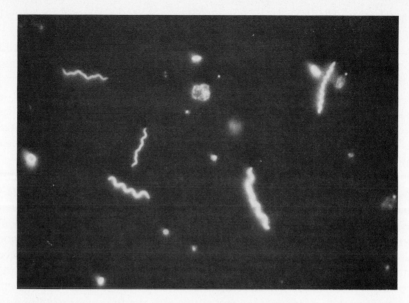

**Fig. 8-9.** Dark-field photomicrograph of diluted suspension of subgingival microorganisms from an untreated lesion of destructive periodontitis in an adult. Spirochetes of varying sizes are prominent morphotypes. (×1500.) (From Listgarten, M.A., and Helldén, L.: J. Clin. Periodontol. **5:**115, 1978, Munksgaard International.)

of destructive periodontal disease. Therapies were proposed that sought to control disease by the elimination or suppression of these microorganisms. In a classic example of this type of approach, the systemic administration of the then newly discovered antimicrobial agent, neosalvarsan (compound 606), coupled with subgingival scaling, was suggested.[52] Neosalvarsan was developed by Ehrlich and co-workers for the control of the spirochetal infection, syphilis. This agent appeared to have similar effects on oral spirochetes. Success in controlling advanced destructive periodontal disease by combining local and systemic therapy was claimed. Others questioned the relationship of this organism to periodontal diseases.[54,55]

**Streptococi**　　The third group of microorganisms proposed as etiologic agents were the streptococci. These microorganisms were incriminated on the basis of cultural examination of samples from subgingival sites of periodontal disease. The selection of the streptococci may have been decided by the fact that cultural techniques at that time were less effective than those available today. For example, approximately 0.5% of the microorganisms that could be counted microscopically could be cultivated with the techniques available at that time.[56] Currently, better than 70% of the microorganisms enumerated microscopically can be cultivated from supra- and subgingival plaque samples.[23,57] Thus when samples were taken from destructive periodontal lesions, only the organisms that were most easily cultivated would consistently be detected. Among this group, the streptococci would probably have been most prominent.[58-61] There were no methods available at the time for the specific control of streptococci. Neosalvarsan did not affect these microorganisms and antibiotics, such as penicillin, had not been developed. Thus workers turned to nonspecific agents such as mercury[62,63] or to the use of vaccines for the control of periodontal diseases.

**Vaccines**　　In this era, vaccines were commonly employed in attempts to control bacterial infections. Three types of vaccines were employed for the control of periodontal diseases. These included vaccines prepared from pure cultures of streptococci and other oral organisms,[48,64-72] autogenous vaccines, and stock vaccines such as Van Cott's vaccine[68] or Inava Endocorps vaccine.[69] Inava Endocorps was made of a mixture of seven microorganisms, including *Staphylococcus aureus, Escherichia coli*, and *Klebsiella pneumonia*. Autogenous vaccines were prepared from the dental plaque of patients with destructive periodontal disease. Plaque samples were removed from the diseased site, "sterilized" by immersion in iodine or formalin solutions, and then reinjected into the same patient, either in the local periodontal lesion or systemically.[52,73-78] Proponents of all three techniques claimed great efficacy for each of the vaccination methods, while others using the same techniques were skeptical.[49,79,80]

It is revealing that three completely different groups of bacteria were proposed as etiologic agents of periodontal disease. In retrospect the proposal of these agents was influenced by the nature of the laboratory techniques available. Workers employing stains specific for amebae were only able to focus on amebae as possible etiologic agents. In a similar fashion, the cultural microbiologists concentrated on the microorganisms that they could cultivate, primarily the streptococci. Finally, workers using wet mount preparations were attracted to the morphologically distinct spirochetes as possible etiologic agents of disease. The search for the etiologic agents of periodontal disease ended inconclusively, and, in retrospect, we can understand why. Probably the most important reason for the failure was the inability to conduct adequately controlled clinical trials and experiments. Some of the problems can be summarized as follows:

Comment

1. There were *no control groups* for any of the therapies employed. Thus similar improvements might have been observed in subjects treated by other methods or not treated at all.

2. There were *no objective measurements* of periodontal disease. The individuals did not report changes in bone level, attachment level, probing depth, or clinical indices. Their evaluations of the efficacy of therapy were based on their "clinical impressions," which of course were and still are highly subjective.

3. There was *no random assignment of patients into groups*. Often the patients were preselected to fit certain rather extreme, or even unfair, categories. For example, Hirschfeld[79] performed a test of Inava Endocorps vaccine on a group of patients who were preselected for not responding to conventional therapy. This does not seem to be a fair test of the efficacy of this treatment modality, since such patients might have been resistant to any other form of therapy.

4. The measurements, or evaluations, of periodontal disease were *not carried out "blind."* This means that the observers knew how the patients in an experimental group were being treated. Thus they were more likely to be influenced by their personal bias, particularly since in most instances the therapist and the evaluator were the same individual. If the individual believed in the therapy, it was likely that a "beneficial" effect would be observed, whereas opponents of the method would be more likely to observe no effect, or even a harmful effect on the patient.

5. There was virtually *no recognition of different forms of periodontal disease*. Thus a single modality of therapy was expected to control all forms of what was then considered to be a single disease.

The initial enthusiasm in the hunt for microbial etiologic agents slowly subsided, and by the mid-1930s few were involved in this quest.[81] From the mid-1920s to the early 1960s, attitudes toward the etiology of periodontal disease changed. In the first two decades of this period it was thought that periodontal disease was due to either some constitutional defect in the patient or to trauma from occlusion or to some combination.[82-84] Bacteria were thought to be secondary invaders in this process, or at most contributors to the inflammation observed in association with tissue destruction.

Declining interest in microorganisms

In the early 1960s, emphasis again was placed on the role of bacteria in the etiology of periodontal disease. Their role was considered to be as a nonspecific causative agent. According to this "nonspecific plaque" hypothesis, any accumulation of microorganisms at or below the gingival margin would be an irritant leading to inflammation. The inflammation in turn was thought to destroy periodontal tissues. The species of

Nonspecific plaque hypothesis

microorganisms accumulated on the teeth was not considered to be particularly significant, provided there were sufficiently large numbers to trigger a destructive process.

**Mixed anaerobic infections**

Beginning in the 1930s, microbiologists began to work on an aspect of the hypothesis of nonspecific infection. These investigators believed that periodontal disease was the result of "mixed infections." This hypothesis had been considered since the late 1800s, when microscopic observations by Vincent suggested that certain forms of periodontal disease—particularly acute necrotizing ulcerative gingivitis (ANUG)—were caused by a complex of microorganisms dominated by fusiforms and spirochetes and were known as fusospirochetal infections. In the early 1930s, Smith[85] and Proske and Sayers[86,87] found that mixtures of microorganisms taken from lung infections or from subgingival plaque could induce lesions when injected subcutaneously into experimental animals. Both groups of workers reported that a combination of a fusiform, a spirochete, an anaerobic vibrio, and an α-hemolytic streptococcus could cause transmissible mixed infections in the guinea pig (Fig. 8-10). Rosebury and co-workers[88-90] failed to reproduce their results, either with the above combination of microorganisms or with many other combinations. They did demonstrate, however, that mixed infections were caused by bacteria (rather than a virus). Mixtures of microorganisms from dental plaque retained infectivity for the guinea pig after 10 serial transfers on blood agar plates. However, these workers were unsuccessful in identifying specific combinations of pure cultures that would cause *transmissible* mixed infections. On the other hand, Macdonald and co-workers[91] were later able to produce transmissible mixed

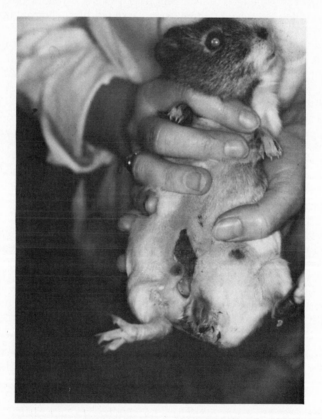

**Fig. 8-10.** Infection induced in a guinea pig by the subcutaneous injection of subgingival plaque from a subject with periodontitis. The microorganisms were introduced in the groin region and the animal was photographed 5 days after injection. Note that the infection spread along the abdominal wall and perforated, causing the observed open lesion.

infections using combinations of pure cultures. The critical mixture of four organisms included a *Bacteroides melaninogenicus* strain, a gram-positive anaerobic rod, and two other gram-negative anaerobic rods. This combination of organisms was completely different from those used by Smith[85] and Proske and Sayers[86,87] to cause transmissible infections. These results lead to the concept that mixed infections might be bacteriologically nonspecific but biochemically specific. In other words, any combination of microorganisms capable of producing an array of destructive metabolites could lead to transmissible infections in animals and, by extension, to destructive periodontal infections in humans. Later experiments suggested that members of the *B. melaninogenicus* group were the key species in these mixed infections. Other organisms could be substituted for the gram-positive and gram-negative rods as long as the *B. melaninogenicus* strains were present.[92] Macdonald and co-workers[91] proceeded to set up a germ-free rat colony with the express purpose of testing the relative importance

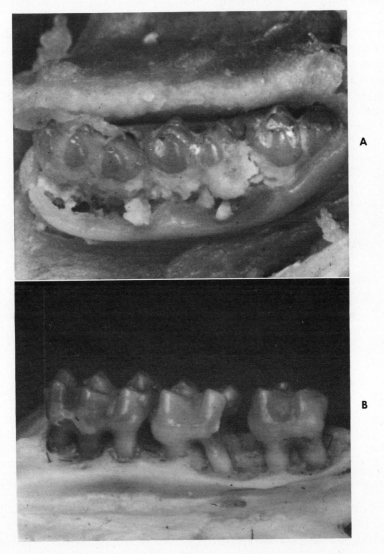

**Fig. 8-11.**  Destructive periodontal disease induced in a hamster by *Actinomyces viscosus*. The animal was maintained on a high sucrose diet for 90 days. **A,** Occlusal view of periodontitis. Note the masses of plaque and matera alba. **B,** Bone destruction in same animal following removal of gingiva.

of spirochetes and members of the *B. melaninogenicus* group, alone and in combination with other organisms, as infective agents for the periodontium of the rat. Virtually the only organisms that they were unsuccessful in establishing in this animal model system were spirochetes and members of the *B. melaninogenicus* group. Therefore the importance of these microorganisms as potential periodontal pathogens could not be established at that time by this technique.

**Transmissibility of hamster periodontal disease**

In the 1960s, interest in the specific microbial etiology of periodontal disease was rekindled.[93,94] Keyes and Jordan[93] demonstrated that periodontal disease could be transmitted in the hamster from animals with periodontal disease to animals without periodontal disease by caging them together (Fig. 8-11). They then demonstrated that swabs of plaque or feces from diseased animals were effective in transmitting the disease to animals free of disease. Finally, it was demonstrated that a pure culture of an organism, which later became known as *Actinomyces viscosus*, was capable of causing destructive periodontal disease in hamsters free of disease.[94] Other species isolated from the plaques of hamsters with periodontal disease did not have this capability.

**Invasion in acute necrotizing ulcerative gingivitis (ANUG)**

At about the same time, Listgarten[95] demonstrated that spirochetes can be detected in practically pure masses within the connective tissue and within the adjacent epithelium (Fig. 8-12) in lesions of acute necrotizing ulcerative gingivitis (ANUG). The spirochetes in these lesions are relatively homogeneous with respect to cell size, ultrastructural characteristics of their outer envelope, as well as number of axial fibrils (endoflagella). Control tissue taken from healthy individuals and individuals with other forms of periodontal disease did not exhibit a similar tissue invasion.

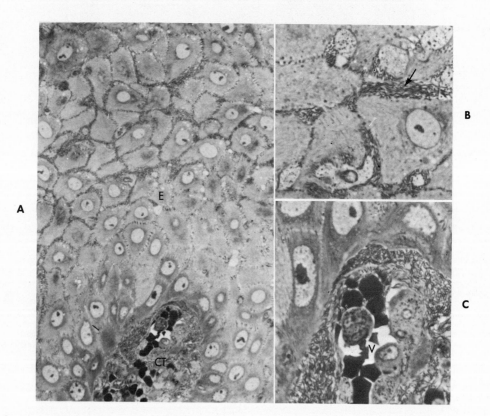

**Fig. 8-12.** **A,** Histologic section of gingiva adjacent to an ulcerative lesion in a patient with acute necrotizing ulcerative gingivitis. Both the epithelium (*E*) and connective tissue (*CT*) are infiltrated with spirochetes. (×660.) **B,** Magnified section of epithelium with spirochetes (*arrow*) within the intercellular spaces. (×1680.) **C,** Magnified section from **A** with dense infiltrate of spirochetes in the connective tissue. *V,* vessel containing blood cells. (×1680.)

Such findings suggested that there might be more specificity to the microbial etiology of periodontal disease than had been accepted for the previous four decades. Of all the hamster species tested, only *A. viscosus* was capable of transmitting periodontal disease in the hamster, while lesions of ANUG were characterized by the presence of large numbers of a spirochete not observed in samples from healthy periodontal tissues. Thus at least two forms of periodontal disease were clearly associated with specific microorganisms. It should be noted that the importance of these observations was not completely realized at that time. Indeed, the emphasis in the 1960s was on the mechanical control of bacterial plaque accumulation. This ap-

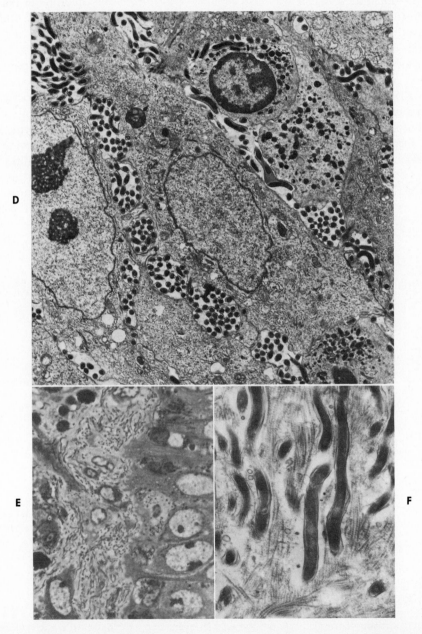

**Fig. 8-12, cont'd.   D,** Electron micrograph of spirochetes invading intercellular spaces of epithelium. (×7000). **E,** Spirochetes in gingival connective tissue. (×1680.) **F,** Electron micrograph of spirochetes invading connective tissue. (×24,000.) (**D** and **F** from Listgarten, M.A.: J. Periodontol. **36:**328, 1965.)

proach was consistent with the prevailing concept of the nonspecific plaque etiology of periodontal disease. This concept is still very much in evidence today and still serves as the basis of preventive techniques in most dental practices. It is also clear that nonspecific plaque control measures, while effective in most instances, are not able to prevent all forms of periodontal disease.

**Plaque-forming microorganisms as etiologic agents of periodontal disease**

The findings of Keyes and Jordan[93] stimulated the development of a new concept of the etiology of periodontal diseases. The organisms that were responsible for the destruction observed in the hamster clearly differed from other organisms in their ability to form large amounts of bacterial plaque both in the hamster and in in vitro test systems. Parallel studies of *Streptococcus mutans*, a prime etiologic agent of dental caries, demonstrated that it was also capable of forming large amounts of plaque in the hamster model system as well as large amounts of plaque, dental caries, and, most importantly, periodontal destruction in gnotobiotic rat systems.[96,97] Thus a concept emerged that microorganisms that were capable of forming large amounts of plaque in vitro and in vivo should be considered as prime suspects in the etiology of periodontal diseases. In vitro test systems were devised to seek plaque-forming microorganisms (Fig. 8-13). These included tests based on adhesion of pure cultures of microorganisms to the walls of culture vessels or to nichrome wires suspended in culture broth. Certain groups of microorganisms demonstrated this property. *Streptococcus mutans*, for example, formed abundant amounts of plaque in in vitro systems when provided with large amounts of sucrose, but not other carbohydrates, in the culture medium. *Actinomyces*, particularly *Actinomyces viscosus* and *Actinomyces naeslundii*, also demonstrated the property of in vitro plaque formation but would do so in the presence of sucrose as well as many other carbohydrates. Tests of the pathogenesis of these mi-

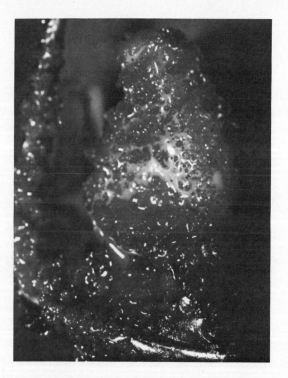

**Fig. 8-13.** In vitro plaque formation by a strain of *Streptococcus mutans*. The plaque, formed during 3 days of incubation in a sucrose-containing broth, was stained with erythrocin dye. Note that the plaque adhered to the extracted tooth as well as to the suspending wire. Strains of *A. viscosus* and *A. naeslundii* form similar in vitro plaques.

croorganisms in hamster or gnotobiotic rat systems demonstrated that the plaque formation seen in vitro could also be observed in vivo. Furthermore, in vivo plaque formation was associated with loss of periodontal support in the animal model systems (Fig. 8-14). These findings reinforced the concept that organisms that formed abundant plaque were responsible for destructive periodontal disease. Unfortunately, later research findings revealed major discrepancies in this hypothesis.

## Changing concepts of the microbial etiology of periodontal diseases

By the end of the 1960s it was generally accepted that dental plaque was in some way associated with human periodontal disease. It was believed that the presence of bacterial plaque initiated a series of as yet undefined events that led to the destruction of the periodontium. The composition of plaque was thought to be relatively similar from patient to patient and from site to site within patients. Variability was recognized, but the true extent of differences in bacterial composition was not appreciated. It was thought that the major event triggering destructive periodontal disease was an increase in mass of bacterial plaque, possibly accompanied by a diminution in host resistance. Indeed, in the mid 1960s the classic studies of Löe and co-workers[98-100] convincingly demonstrated that plaque accumulation directly preceded and initiated gingivitis. Many investigators believed that gingivitis was harmful and led to the eventual destruction of the periodontal tissues, probably by host-mediated events.

Yet, certain discrepancies continued to baffle clinicians and research workers alike. If all plaques were more or less alike and induced a particular systemic response in the host, why was periodontal destruction localized, taking place adjacent to one tooth but not another? If plaque mass was a prime trigger for periodontal tissue destruction, why did certain subjects accumulate much plaque, frequently accompanied by gingivitis, but fail, even after many years, to develop destruction of the supporting structures? On the other hand, why did some individuals with little detectable plaque or clinical inflammation develop rapid periodontal tissue destruction? If inflammation

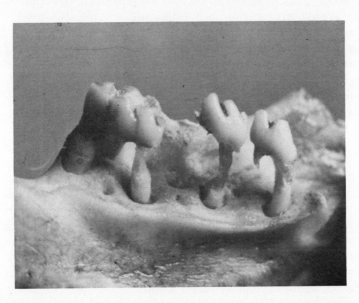

**Fig. 8-14.** Periodontal destruction induced in a germ-free rat by a pure culture of a human strain of *Actinomyces viscosus*. The animal was maintained on a high sucrose diet for 130 days. The extensive root caries and alveolar bone loss induced by this organism can be readily observed.

was the main mediator of tissue destruction, why were so many teeth retained in the presence of continual gingivitis? One explanation may have been the inconsistencies in the host response or the superimposition of local factors such as trauma from occlusion, overhanging fillings, etc. Other explanations can be derived from more recent studies of the microbiology of periodontal diseases. These studies, which have markedly altered our concepts of the etiology of periodontal diseases, are based largely on a better understanding of the structure and composition of the bacterial plaques associated with gingival and periodontal tissues.

Earlier considerations of plaque suggested that it was a heterogeneous bacterial mass that would lead to disease when allowed to overgrow. Recent studies have revealed that a relatively simple microbiota consisting of coccoid and short rod forms is associated with healthy periodontal sites. Distinctly different microbiotas have been shown to be associated with disease. Even more interesting has been the observation that characteristic microbial populations may be associated with clinically different periodontal diseases. Before considering the differences in microbiotas associated with different forms of periodontal disease, it is worth examining the evidence that bacteria are the etiologic agents of periodontal disease.

**Evidence for primary role of bacteria in etiology of periodontal disease**

Data gathered over the last 20 years indicate that the major mechanisms of destruction of the periodontium are mediated by bacteria. The evidence to support this contention has been extensively documented in a number of reviews[101-105] and is briefly summarized here. The acute phase of certain human forms of periodontal disease, such as acute necrotizing ulcerative gingivitis (ANUG) or (trench mouth) can be alleviated by any of a number of antibiotics, clearly indicating that microorganisms are the etiologic agents of this periodontal disease.[106-109] There is a positive correlation between the amount of bacterial plaque, the severity of gingivitis,[110-112] and amount of bone loss[113-114] in cross-sectional studies of human populations, although this correlation does not demonstrate whether the bacteria cause the diseases or the diseases favor the accumulation of bacteria. However the longitudinal studies of Löe and associates[98,100] demonstrated that intensive plaque control procedures essentially eradicated clinical gingivitis. Withdrawal of such procedures resulted in an increase in bacterial plaque, which was soon followed by the development of gingivitis. Clinical gingivitis could also be controlled by means of antibiotics[99,115,116] or antiseptic agents[117-121] such as chlorhexidine. Since the spectrum of activity of these agents is primarily directed toward microorganisms, the relevance of antimicrobial therapy to the prevention of gingivitis is obvious.

More recently, Lindhe and Nyman[122] and Rosling and associates[123,124] demonstrated that the progress of destructive periodontitis could be halted and partially reversed by surgical procedures accompanied by twice monthly professional tooth cleaning. These studies indicated that suppression of the total microbiota could be effective in controlling both gingivitis and destructive periodontitis in humans. What the studies did not and could not indicate is whether all or only segments of the microbiota were responsible for the observed clinical response. The success of antibiotic therapy in controlling the acute phase of ANUG[106-109,125,126] and in the therapy of juvenile periodontitis[127-129] underlines the etiologic role of microorganisms in these forms of human periodontal disease. Since only some of the species resident in bacterial plaque are sensitive to a given antibiotic and bacterial plaque returns after therapy, it appears that only some of the organisms are responsible for the diseases.

**Pathogenic mechanisms**

The studies of Waerhaug[130-134] and Rovin and co-workers[135] demonstrated that mechanical irritants were of relatively minor significance when compared to the accumulation of dental plaque. These studies as well as studies of ligature-induced disease in rats, beagles, and monkeys[136,137] also demonstrated the physical localization of inflammatory changes in direct proximity to massive accumulations of bacteria. Bacterial invasion, a comparatively rare event, may be triggered by experimentally induced depression of the natural host resistance (Fig. 8-15). Calculus can be regarded as a naturally occurring mechanical irritant. Calculus will form in germfree animals in abundant amounts.[96,138] Yet despite the presence of extensive accumulations of calculus, there is little evidence of inflammation, pocket formation, or destruction. Only when certain microorganisms are introduced into animals with calculus formation, does accelerated periodontal destruction occur.

Human bacterial plaque has demonstrated pathogenic potential when implanted into extraoral sites such as subcutaneous locations in humans[139,140] or experimental animals.[88-90,141,142] A number of toxic products can be detected in dental plaques— including endotoxins,[143-145] cell wall mucopeptides,[146] fatty and organic acids,[147-150] hy-

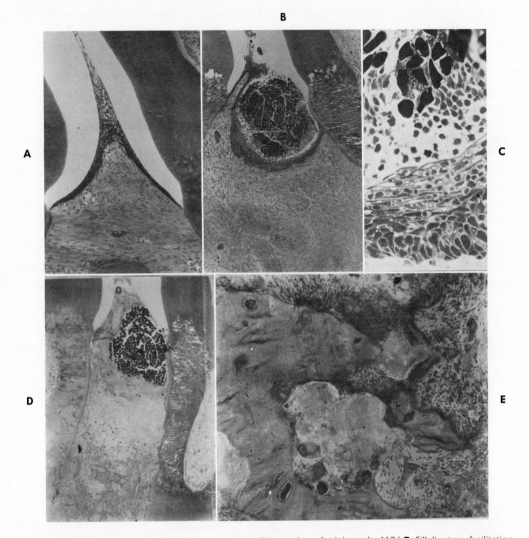

**Fig. 8-15.** **A,** Control interdental region between maxillary molars of adult rat. (× 112.) **B,** Silk ligature, facilitating the retention of microorganisms, results in marked inflammatory changes in gingival tissues. Note distortion of normal gingival anatomy but retention of an intact epithelial barrier. (× 70.) **C,** Higher magnification of **B.** Note numerous inflammatory cells in the epithelium. **D,** Ligated molar in a rat treated with cyclophosphamide to suppress host resistance. Also note absence of an intact epithelial barrier. (× 70.) **E,** Magnified view of crestal region of **D.** The connective tissue adjacent to the alveolar crest is invaded by a mass of gram-negative rods of homogeneous morphology. Bacterial invasion was not observed in animals in which the host resistance was not altered. (× 850.) (**A** to **E** from Sanavi, F., et al.: J. Periodontol. **56:**273, 1985.)

drogen sulfide,[151,152] ammonia,[153,154] indole,[155] amines,[152] leukotoxin,[156,157] and so on. In addition, enzymes have been shown to be produced by whole plaque or individual microorganisms from plaque, which can be demonstrated to hydrolyze a wide variety of tissue constituents.[158-165] Finally, it must be pointed out that the bacterial masses that accumulate at or in the gingival sulcus possess an array of antigens and possibly polyclonal activators capable of triggering sequences of host-mediated events that have been postulated as mechanisms of tissue destruction.

Studies in experimental animals have added considerable support to the hypothesis of the significant role of microorganisms in the etiology of periodontal disease. The use of antibiotics or antiseptics in a variety of animal model systems[166-177] controlled the soft tissue pathology and most of the hard tissue destruction in these animals. Periodontal disease can be transmitted from an animal harboring the disease to one initially free of it by caging diseased and disease-free animals together, or by the implantation of plaque or specific microorganisms derived from the plaques of diseased animals.[93,94,178,179] In addition, certain microorganisms isolated from human periodontal pockets can initiate periodontal destruction in several animal model systems.[97,180-182]

It should be pointed out that germfree animals are essentially free of periodontal destruction. Minimal observable inflammation of pocket formation and only minor amounts of bone loss are associated mainly with the impaction of hair, food, or bedding. However with the introduction of specific human or animal plaque isolates, severe periodontal pathology develops.

Studies in the beagle and monkey have indicated that daily removal of bacterial plaque can prevent the onset of gingivitis and destructive periodontal diseases even though gingivitis and destructive periodontal disease occurred in control sites.[183] Antibiotic or antiseptic administration without mechanical debridement also controlled gingivitis and retarded attachment loss.[172,177] Placement of a ligature in subgingival sites of beagles and monkeys results in massive plaque accumulation, inflammation, pocketing and loss of the attachment apparatus, including the alveolar bone.[184-187] These events occur rapidly, usually within 60 days (Fig. 8-16), and it is reported that the attachment loss can be prevented by administration of systemic tetracycline.[136]

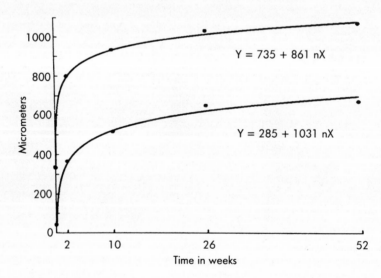

**Fig. 8-16.** Attachment loss in the squirrel monkey induced by ligature placement on mandibular bicuspids and first molars. The y axis indicates the number of micrometers from the cementoenamel junction (CEJ) to the alveolar crest in the top curve and from the CEJ to the junctional epithelium in the lower curve. The logarithmic functions of attachment loss versus time in weeks were fitted by Marquardt's least squares. (Data redrawn from Kennedy and Polson (1973) with permission; from Socransky, S.S.: J. Clin. Periodontol. **11:**21, 1984, Munksgaard International.)

Thus there is abundant evidence to implicate microorganisms as the primary etiologic agents of various forms of periodontal disease in man and experimental animals. The question is no longer whether organisms cause periodontal diseases, but rather what specific organisms are responsible for specific disease forms.

Recent evidence from a number of laboratories suggests that different forms of periodontal disease may have specific microbial etiologies. Examination of the microbiota associated with healthy tissues and tissues with different forms of disease revealed previously unsuspected major differences in microbial composition. The once prevalent view that dental plaque composition was reasonably consistent from individual to individual and site to site is clearly invalid. It is of interest that this misconception persisted for close to four decades.

**Microbial composition of plaques associated with periodontal tissues**

The impression that plaques were reasonably similar in composition was derived in part from studies of the infectious potential of plaque when injected subcutaneously into experimental animals and partly because investigators examined the microbial composition of pooled dental plaques with inadequate cultural methods. Experimental abscess studies indicated that the pathogenic potential of plaque taken from healthy individuals or individuals with different gingival and periodontal diseases was approximately equal (on a wet weight basis) when subcutaneously injected into experimental animals.[141,163] It was assumed that pathogenic potential mirrored microbial composition and thus the studies indirectly suggested similarities in microbial composition. Earlier cultural studies of the microbial composition of plaque usually employed samples of plaque pooled from several sites. Site-to-site differences in the subgingival microbiota were thus obscured by the simple act of combining the samples. Furthermore, investigators often removed supragingival and subgingival samples from several teeth. Since supragingival plaque is usually more abundant (and more easily removed) than subgingival plaque, the samples often reflected organisms that were dominant in the supragingival sites. Finally, some microorganisms (e.g., streptococci) proliferate more readily in vitro than some gram-negative anaerobes, such as spirochetes or the recently described *Bacteroides forsythus*. Thus the impression was gained of a relatively uniform plaque composition dominated by streptococci.

Differential growth of microorganisms in vitro is due in large part to problems that are technical in nature. These include problems in dispersion of plaque samples (while maintaining cell viability) and recovery of microorganisms that are often oxygen sensitive or fastidious in their growth requirements. Technical and conceptual advances in the last decade have permitted a more realistic view of dental plaque. Such advances include the routine use of continuous anaerobiosis techniques, better techniques of sample-taking and dispersion, as well as improvements in culture media and methods of identification of organisms.

Microbiologic sampling from discrete sites and microscopy of sections of *in situ* human plaque have proven to be synergistic approaches that have permitted a clearer understanding of the localization and patterns of colonization of possible subgingival pathogens. Much of this work is relatively recent, technically difficult to carry out, and as yet has not been used on large numbers of samples or a wide range of disease types. Thus information is currently more limited than one would hope. The descriptions of plaque composition summarized below are synthesized from a large number of recent articles that employed morphologic, immunofluorescent, or cultural techniques to determine the structural relationships and/or numbers of organisms in plaques associated with periodontal tissues in various states of health or disease.[95,100,188-228] A brief summary of such information will be helpful in understanding the concepts emerging from contemporary studies of the microbiology of periodontal diseases. It should be made clear, however, that different bacteriologic methods can produce apparent differences in results. Only careful compilation and comparison of data derived using different methods that are complementary will permit the drawing of comprehensive and realistic conclusions.

**Supragingival plaque at normal sites**

Supragingival plaque associated with healthy tissues appears to be relatively thin (approximately 1 to 20 cells in thickness) and consists predominantly of gram-positive, coccal-shaped microorganisms (Fig. 8-17). These organisms often include *Streptococcus sanguis*, types I and II; *Streptococcus mitis; Actinomyces viscosus; Actinomyces naeslundii; Staphylococcus epidermidis;* and *Rothia dentocariosa.* Gram-negative organisms, usually *Veillonella parvula,* may be detected in low numbers.*

**Plaque associated with gingivitis**

In experimental gingivitis, there is an increase in the total mass of plaque and the number of cell layers, which often extends to 100 to 300 cells in thickness (Fig. 8-18). The predominant supragingival cultivable microbiota in developing gingivitis plaques is almost entirely gram-positive and appears to represent an overgrowth of some of the forms found in plaques associated with healthy sites.[188,194,211,214] The increase in plaque mass is accompanied by an increase in proportions of members of the genus, *Actinomyces.* This group of organisms tends to be the dominant genus associated with supragingival plaque, frequently comprising 50% or more of the isolates. Subgingival plaque samples from experimental gingivitis also have elevated proportions of *A. viscosus,* as well as *A. naeslundii.* In addition, increases in the gram-negative species, *F. nucleatum, V. parvula,* and *Treponema* species, are observed.[225] In chronic gingivitis, approximately 25% of the microbiota may be gram-negative.[195] The gram-negative organisms may include large filaments that grow into the dental plaque from the surface[194] or members of *Fusobacterium, Campylobacter, Veillonella,*[195] and *B. intermedius.*[222] One interesting configuration often observed on the external surface of supragingival plaques is the "corncob" or *"Leptothrix racemosa"*

*See references 100, 188, 194, 197, 201, 207, 214, 219, and 229.

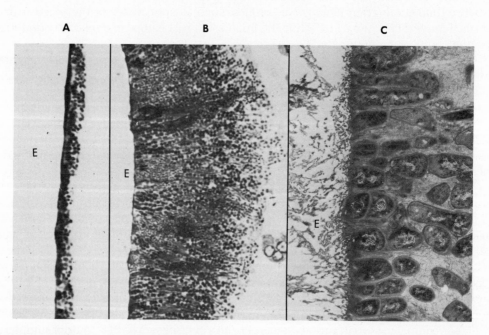

**Fig. 8-17.** **A,** Relatively thin layer of coccoid cells on an enamel surface adjacent to a healthy gingiva. *E,* enamel space. (×2000). **B,** Relatively thick layer of predominantly coccoid cells on an enamel surface adjacent to a healthy gingiva. (×2000.) **C,** Electron micrograph of a section of **A** showing coccoid cells with cell walls of the gram-positive type in contact with subsurface pellicle of enamel *(E).* (×11,000.) (**B** from Listgarten, M.A.: J. Periodontol. **47:**1, 1976.)

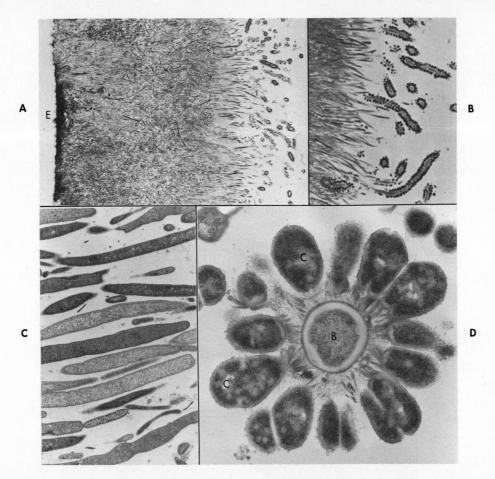

**Fig. 8-18.** **A,** Filamentous supragingival dental plaque on enamel *(E),* with "corncob" formations at the surface, previously adjacent to an inflamed marginal gingiva. (×950.) **B,** Magnified view of "corncob" formations on the surface of the predominantly filamentous microbial layer. (×2000.) **C,** The adherent microbial mass contains many gram-negative filamentous forms. (×7000.) **D,** "Corncob" formations consist of coccoid cells *(C)* attached to a central filamentous bacterium *(B).* (×23,000.) (**A** and **C** from Listgarten, M.A.: J. Periodontol. **47:**1, 1976; **D** from Listgarten, M.A.: J. Periodontol. **46:**10, 1975.)

arrangement[194] (Figs. 8-18 and 8-19). This consists of a central filament, often *Bacterionema matruchotii* covered with cocci such as *Streptococcus sanguis.* The dominant feature, however, of most supragingival plaques associated with gingivitis may well be the presence of large numbers of actinomycetes.

Ultrastructural studies of ANUG were critical in the investigation of this disease, since they demonstrated actual invasion of the host connective tissues by large numbers of spirochetes with a characteristic ultrastructural morphology[95] (see Fig. 8-12). This clinical condition appears to be the only periodontal disease in which invasion of microorganisms is a prominent feature. The spirochetes involved were of the intermediate type usually having more than six axial fibrils originating from each end.[230,231] Additional organisms, particularly fusiform-shaped bacteria, could be seen in necrotic zones immediately superficial to the spirochetal infiltration zone.[95] These intermediate-sized spirochetes cannot be routinely cultivated and thus their pathogenic potential cannot be accurately assessed. Circumstantial evidence appears to indict (although not convict) them as etiologic agents in this disease. Cultural studies of samples from ANUG lesions revealed an increase in proportions of *B. intermedius*[224] (Table 8-1).

**Acute necrotizing ulcerative gingivitis (ANUG)**

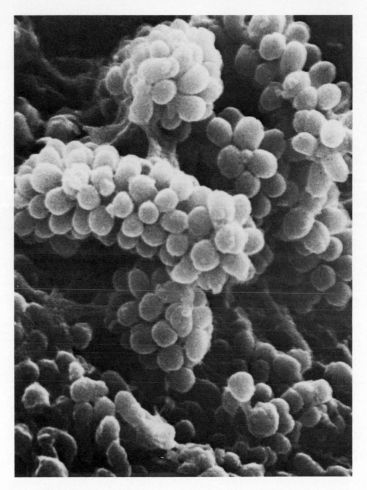

**Fig. 8-19.** Scanning electron photomicrograph of "corncob" formation in human supragingival plaque. The adherence of cocci to the underlying rod forms provides this configuration. (×4000.)

**Microbiota associated with juvenile periodontitis (periodontosis)**

The patient with localized juvenile periodontitis (classic "molar-incisor" periodontosis) generally exhibits minimal plaque accumulation, calculus, or clinically evident gingivitis. Such individuals have a relatively thin attached bacterial plaque at the orifice (Fig. 8-20) of their pockets and little if any plaque attached to the tooth surface in deep subgingival sites. Small accumulations of microorganisms may be observed in the subgingival area[208] but not necessarily attached to the tooth or epithelium.[188] Clusters of *Actinobacillus actinomycetemcomitans,* a large gram-negative coccobacillary cell, may be surrounded by cuticular material that accumulates on the root surface. The subgingival accumulations are often surrounded by disintegrating polymorphonuclear leukocytes.[188] Organisms in the subgingival accumulations are dominated by gram-negative forms.[196,200,206] In contrast, isolates from healthy sites in the same patients show a gram-positive microbiota typical of that seen in healthy individuals.

The predominant cultivable organisms found in the diseased lesions were not previously associated with periodontal disease, and several species had not been described. One of the organisms most frequently isolated, and in highest numbers, is a gram-negative, fusiform-shaped rod that can glide on agar surfaces and is called *Capnocytophaga*[232] (Fig. 8-21).

A second dominant species, *Actinobacillus actinomycetemcomitans,* has been im-

**Table 8-1**   Microorganisms associated with various forms of periodontal disease

| Clinical condition | By cultural techniques | By microscopic techniques | By antibody response |
|---|---|---|---|
| Health | *Actinomyces naeslundii* *Actinomyces viscosus* *Rothia dentocariosa* *Streptococcus mitis* *Streptococcus sanguis* *Streptococcus uberis* *Veillonella parvula* | Gram-positive and coccal forms, few spirochetes or motile rods | |
| Experimental gingivitis (supragingival) | *Actinomyces israelii* *Actinomyces viscosus* | Gram-positive, mainly coccoid forms, filaments, and fusiforms | |
| Experimental gingivitis (subgingival) | *Actinomyces naeslundii* *Actinomyces viscosus* *Fusobacterium nucleatum* *Lactobacillus* sp. *Streptococcus anginosus* *Treponema* sp. *Veillonella parvula* | Gram-positive and gram-negative forms, some spirochetes and motile rods | |
| Chronic gingivitis | *Actinomyces israelii* *Actinomyces naeslundii* *Actinomyces viscosus* *Bacteroides intermedius* *Campylobacter sputorum* *Capnocytophaga gingivalis* *Capnocytophaga ochracea* *Fusobacterium nucleatum* *Streptococcus sanguis* *Streptococcus uberis* *Veillonella parvula* | Mainly gram-positive forms, about 25% gram-negative cells, few motile rods or spirochetes | |
| Acute necrotizing ulcerative gingivitis (ANUG) | *Bacteroides intermedius* | Intermediate spirochetes invading tissue | |
| Localized juvenile periodontitis | *Actinobacillus actinomycetemcomitans* *Bacteroides intermedius* *Capnocytophaga ochracea* *Eikenella corrodens* | Short rods and fusiforms | *Actinobacillus actinomycetemcomitans* Sometimes depressed response to *Capnocytophaga sputigena* |
| Adult periodontitis | *Bacteroides capillus* *Bacteroides forsythus* *Bacteroides gingivalis* *Bacteroides intermedius* *Eikenella corrodens* *Eubacterium brachy* *Eubacterium nodatum* *Eubacterium timidum* *Fusobacterium nucleatum* *Lactobacillus minitus* *Selenomonas sputigena* *Streptococcus intermedius* *Wolinella recta* | Complex microbiota including coccoid, rod, and spiral forms with motile forms prominent | *Bacteroides gingivalis* *Bacteroides intermedius* *Fusobacterium nucleatum* *Selenomonas sputigena* *Wolinella recta* |

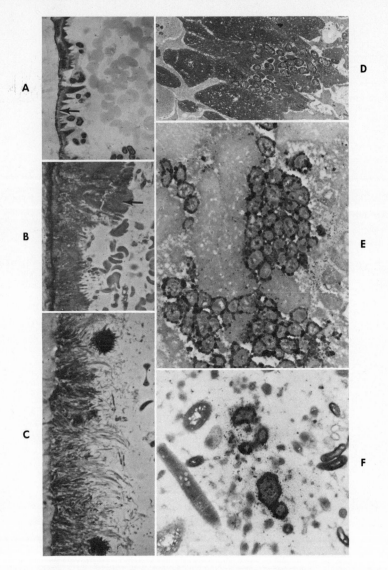

**Fig. 8-20. A** and **B,** In localized juvenile periodontitis, an irregularly shaped organic cuticle *(arrow)* frequently covers the root surface of affected teeth. (×1100.) **C,** A sparse, gram-negative microbial layer containing thin filamentous microorganisms may be present. (×1500.) **D,** Gram-negative coccoid cells in clusters may be located within the organic cuticle. (×3,500.) **E,** These cells can be labelled immunocytochemically with antibody against *Actinobacillus actinomycetemcomitans.* (×7500.) **F,** Horseradish peroxidase–labelled *Actinobacillus* in dental plaque covering the root of a tooth affected by localized juvenile periodontitis. (×9000.) (**A** to **D** from Listgarten, M.A.: J. Periodontol. **47**:1, 1976; **E** and **F** from Berthold, P., and Listgarten, M.A., J. Periodont. Res. **21**:473, 1986.)

plicated as a possible etiologic agent of juvenile periodontitis (Fig. 8-20). The organism has been recovered with greater frequency and in higher numbers from lesions of juvenile periodontitis than from healthy sites in the same individuals or from lesions of gingivitis or periodontitis.[129,213,221,223,233] Serum antibody titers of this microorganism are more frequently elevated in patients with juvenile periodontitis when compared to healthy individuals and individuals with other forms of periodontal disease.[129,234-241] Strains of *A. actinomycetemcomitans* produce a toxin capable of lysing polymorphonuclear leukocytes.[153,154,242] Antibodies for this leukotoxin that are protective against the toxin's lytic effect may be detected in the sera of juvenile periodontitis patients.[154]

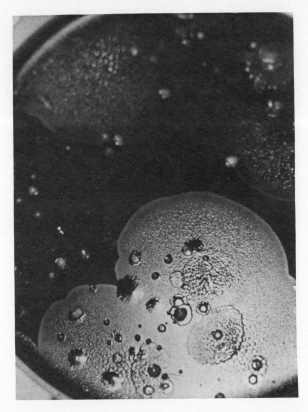

**Fig. 8-21.**  Primary isolation plate of a subgingival plaque sample from a lesion of localized juvenile periodontitis. The gliding *Capnocytophaga* strains are readily apparent as large spreading colonies on the surface of the blood agar plates. The plates were incubated anaerobically for 5 days at 35° C.

Strains of *A. actinomycetemcomitans* have been shown to accelerate alveolar bone loss in gnotobiotic rats[243] (Fig. 8-22). *A. actinomycetemcomitans* does not appear to be a numerically dominant member of the microbiota of individuals without adolescent destructive disease[213,221] but can attain proportions as high as 70% of the cultivable microbiota in sites of advanced destruction.[129] These data suggest at the very least an association and most likely an etiologic role for the species in adolescent destructive periodontal diseases.

Subgingival plaque associated with advanced periodontitis in adult patients may vary in amount from relatively scanty to extremely massive. In general, different organisms are detected in "scanty" plaques from those that predominate in the more massive plaques. In many individuals with evidence of recent active disease, the microbiota in the depths of the pocket appear to be dominated (greater than 85%) by gram-negative forms.[244] The types of gram-negative organisms appear to vary from individual to individual and site to site, although the range of gram-negative organisms appears relatively finite. The magnitude of this variation is as yet unknown.

Structural studies of *in situ* plaque associated with rapid progressing periodontitis have revealed a more complex picture of bacterial types than those observed in juvenile periodontitis[188] (Fig. 8-23). Periodontitis plaque is usually more abundant and often consists in part of a zone of primarily gram-positive organisms that apparently attach to the tooth surface. Between this zone and the epithelium, one finds a zone of loosely "packed" gram-negative organisms and spirochetes. This loose zone extends to the apical portion of the pocket.[188,215]

**Subgingival microbiota associated with advanced periodontitis**

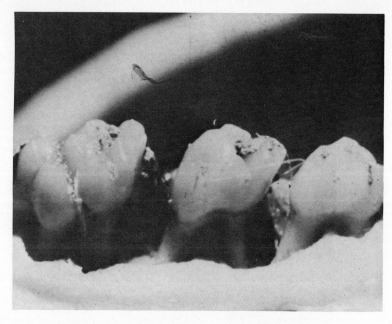

**Fig. 8-22.** Periodontal destruction induced in a germ-free rat by a pure culture of *Actinobacillus actinomycetem-comitans.* The animal was maintained for 90 days on a high sucrose diet. Interproximal alveolar bone loss may be observed but there is no evidence of root caries. (Reprinted with permission from Irving, J.T., et al., Arch. Oral Biol. **20:**219, 1975, Pergamon Press, Ltd.)

In adult forms of periodontal disease, *Bacteroides gingivalis* (formerly known as *B. melaninogenicus* and later as *B. asaccharolyticus*)[245] has been associated with markedly advanced and/or highly inflamed destructive lesions. In humans, *B. gingivalis* is present in higher proportions in many but not all lesions than it is in healthy sites or sites with other forms of periodontal disease.[202,216-218,246] Antibody titers to this organism are elevated in some, but not all, cases of advanced periodontitis in adults and generalized juvenile periodontitis in adolescents.[236] Treatment by mechanical débridement and antibiotics decreases the proportions of this species[204,205,217] and appears to slow or control progress of disease. Members of the *B. melaninogenicus* group were initially implicated as key pathogens in experimental mixed anaerobic infections in guinea pigs.[92] *B. gingivalis* can cause alveolar bone loss when implanted as a monocontaminant in gnotobiotic rats.[247] Furthermore, *B. gingivalis*-like organisms have been associated with bone loss in natural[248] and ligature-induced[137] periodontal disease in the beagle. Ligature-induced periodontitis in monkeys is also associated with an overgrowth of *B. gingivalis*-like strains and a *Haemophilus* species closely resembling *A. actinomyce-temcomitans.*[136]

Evidence implicating other species is not as conclusive. Association with certain types of advanced lesions has been shown for *Eikenella corrodens; B. intermedius, Wolinella recta* and *Fusobacterium nucleatum;*[218,228,246] *Bacteroides capillus;*[220] *Eubacterium nodatum; Eubacterium timidum; Eubacterium brachy; Lactobacillus minutus;* and *Peptostreptococcus micros.*[227,228,246] Elevated antibody titers to *Wolinella recta* and *Selenomonas sputigena* have been shown in adult patients and relatively lower antibody levels to *Capnocytophaga* in juvenile periodontitis patients.[236,249] The pathogenic potential of certain species has been shown by implanting them as monocontaminants in gnotobiotic rats (Fig. 8-24). These include *Eikenella corrodens,*[250] *Capnocytophaga* and *Fusobacterium nucleatum,*[251] and *Bacteroides forsythus* ("fusiform" *Bacteroides*).[252]

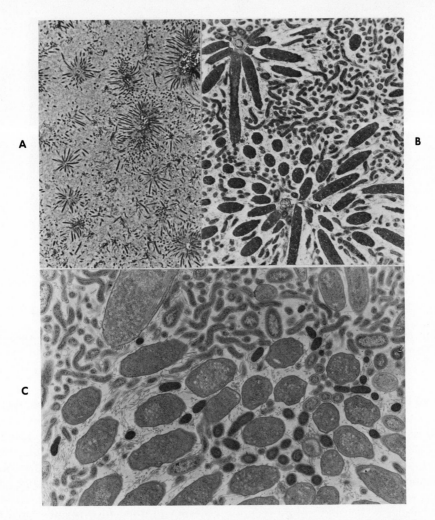

**Fig. 8-23.** **A,** Subgingival plaque from rapidly progressing periodontitis lesion in young adult. The flora contains predominantly gram-negative bacteria with many spirochetes, flagellated bacteria, and "test-tube–brush" formations. (×700.) **B,** Electron micrograph of previous field. Section through two "test-tube–brush" formations. Spirochetes predominate in the background. (×4500.) **C,** Note predominance of gram-negative, frequently flagellated morphotypes. (×15,000.) (From Listgarten, M.A.: J. Periodontol. **47:**1, 1976.)

Studies of periodontal disease in animals suggest a degree of specificity in the nature of organisms responsible for periodontal destruction. Many species of conventional animals maintained on a variety of diets do not demonstrate periodontal destruction, even though they harbor a reasonably complex microbiota; however, the addition of specific organisms from diseased animals can produce "disease." As discussed earlier, only *Actinomyces viscosus* could transmit the periodontal syndrome in the hamster.[94] The rice rat periodontal syndrome is also transmissible[178] and has a specific microbial etiology.[253] **Animal model systems**

Data from animal pathogenicity testing have been interesting but far from conclusive in clarifying the etiologic agents of human destructive periodontal disease. In general, it has been extremely difficult to establish human oral organisms in the oral cavity of conventional animals. Thus pathogenicity testing of human oral isolates has been largely confined to gnotobiotic animal systems. Early studies seeking etiologic

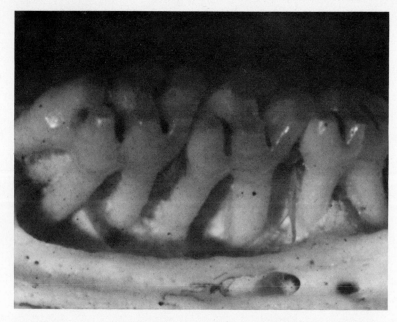

**Fig. 8-24.** Periodontal destruction induced in a germ-free rat by a pure culture of *Fusobacterium nucleatum*. The animal was maintained for 90 days on a high sucrose diet. An unusual pattern of palatal alveolar bone loss may be observed. (From Tanner, A.C.R., Ph.D. Thesis, University of London, 1981, p. 146.)

agents of hamster or rice rat disease revealed that certain gram-positive microorganisms, including *Actinomyces viscosus*, were capable of transmitting destructive periodontal disease from animal to animal.[93,94,253] Initial studies of the pathogenic potential of human isolates in gnotobiotic rat systems revealed that certain gram-positive organisms, which would form plaque in vivo on high sucrose diets, could accelerate destruction of alveolar bone. Such organisms include *Streptococcus mutans*, *Streptococcus salivarius*, *Actinomyces naeslundii*, *Actinomyces viscosus*, *Bacillus*, and *Nocardia* species.[97,180-182,254,255] More recently, certain gram-negative isolates have been shown to accelerate alveolar bone loss when implanted as monocontaminants in gnotobiotic rats. These include *A. actinomycetemcomitans* strains isolated from juvenile periodontitis; *Capnocytophaga* strains isolated from juvenile periodontitis and periodontitis; *Eikenella corrodens*, *Bacteroides gingivalis*, *Fusobacterium nucleatum*, and *Selenomonas sputigena* strains from periodontitis.[243,247,251,252]

The gram-positive and gram-negative experimental infections differed on a clinical and histopathologic basis. Disease induced by gram-positive organisms tends to exhibit root caries, more plaque, and less abundant osteoclastic responses than disease induced by gram-negative organisms.[243,247,251,255] Disease induced by either group of organisms demonstrated a minimal inflammatory response, with polymorphonuclear leukocytes present in the pocket, but with few white blood cells present in the underlying connective tissue. Lymphocytes or plasma cells were limited or absent in sections of tissue at sites of destruction.

It is difficult to interpret the animal pathogenicity testing data that have employed human subgingival isolates. Destruction induced by an organism may reveal the potential of the organism to lead to loss of periodontal tissues. However the gnotobiotic animal is a somewhat artificial situation in that the animal is exposed to a pure culture of a human isolate without the possible ameliorating effects resulting from competition with other microorganisms. In addition, the host response, at least histologically, is not typical of that detected in human lesions in which lymphocytes and plasma cells are quite numerous.

More recently, the microbiology of periodontal disease has been studied in larger animals including the beagle dog and monkeys. Experiments in naturally occurring periodontal disease in dogs maintained on soft diets revealed that periodontal destruction was accompanied by an overgrowth of gram-negative species; particularly a gram-negative rod that formed pigmented colonies on blood agar plates.[214,217,248] This last organism was similar in many biochemical characteristics to *B. gingivalis*. Ligature-induced disease in beagles[137] and monkeys[136,187] was also associated with increased proportions of gram-negative forms; usually small, round-ended rods (often surface translocating) as well as an increase in proportions of *B. gingivalis*-like organisms.

## The nature of destructive periodontal diseases: disease activity

The concept of chronic destructive periodontal disease as a continuously progressive infection has been prevalent for many decades. Evidence to support this belief is based on epidemiologic studies of human populations and on experimental periodontal disease in animals. From epidemiologic studies, there is a clear indication that periodontal diseases increase in severity with age in any human population.[256-260] The rates of attachment loss differ, but the cumulative effect is the same. Since in most studies, periodontal indices or mean values of attachment loss are employed, the data can be interpreted in at least two ways. The loss can be considered to be primarily because of a slowly worsening situation in diseased sites coupled with the introduction of some new sites into the continuous destructive disease pattern. Alternatively, the cumulative loss can be interpreted as being caused primarily by introduction of new diseased sites into individuals with prior evidence of disease as well as individuals previously free of disease. In addition, there can be further destruction resulting from new activity in some of the already diseased sites. The first interpretation seems to be the more widely accepted.

Studies of natural or experimental periodontal disease in animals appear to follow the same pattern as that observed in the human.[261] Mean changes in attachment level or other measures of periodontal disease indicate increasing destruction in groups of untreated animals monitored longitudinally. Assuming the model to be correct, it is interesting to examine the mean annual attachment loss in various populations. A mean annual loss of about 0.1 mm is a fairly consistent finding in untreated human populations.[262] This average figure gives the impression of a slow, continuously progressive disease. What is not clear from such data is how individual sites behave. Conceivably, all diseased sites could continue to break down at a more or less constant rate and, in time, new sites could be affected by this inexorable destructive process.

There are other models of destructive periodontal disease that may better explain the epidemiologic and experimental animal data. Before examining such models it is worth considering what is wrong with the continuous destructive disease model or what is the evidence that destructive periodontal diseases are not continuous. Probably the most compelling data is derived from longitudinal monitoring of individual sites in groups of patients with prior evidence of destructive periodontal disease.

Sequential attachment level measurements made at monthly intervals for a year demonstrated significant increases in probeable attachment level in 5.7% of 1155 sites monitored in 22 subjects.[263] Haffajee and associates,[264] using pairs of attachment level measurements made at 2-month intervals for 1 year at 3414 sites in a different group of 22 subjects, detected significant increase in probeable attachment loss in 2.8% of sites by the "tolerance method." The magnitude of the changes that took place in both studies was usually between 2 to 5 mm. Rates of change of this magnitude are not consistent with a continuous disease process. Furthermore, it has been[265] suggested that cycles may occur in the activity of destructive periodontal disease. Increases followed by decreases in "probing attachment level" have been demonstrated in certain sites. Changes in alveolar bone levels in humans appear to follow the same episodic pattern. Longitudinal monitoring of alveolar bone by $^{125}$I absorptiometry demonstrated periods of remission following bone loss in humans with periodontal disease.[266,267] Measurement of alveolar bone height in bite-wing radiographs taken at various time intervals over a 10-year period indicate that the annual rate of alveolar bone loss fluctuated in the majority of sites monitored.[268]

If periodontal disease is continuous, the monitored rate of destruction (i.e., the rate occurring between two sets of clinical measurements or two sets of radiographs) should be compatible with estimates of the prior rate of destruction based on extent of periodontal destruction on initial examination. This is often not the case. On occasion, observations may show a static or improved periodontal status following minimal or no treatment.[269]

Animal models of destructive periodontal disease also suggest that periodontal destruction may not be continuous. Ligature-induced periodontal disease in beagles or monkeys shows a rapid burst of attachment loss followed by a slowing or a remission of the process [184-186] (see Fig. 8-16). While one may question the relevance of the ligature-induced animal periodontitis to human periodontitis, we should be open to the possibility that this type of rapid destruction followed by a rapidly imposed homeostasis could also occur in human disease. Naturally occurring destructive periodontal disease in the beagle dog also demonstrates differences in lesion activity. Technetium-99m-tin-diphosphonate has been used to "predict" bone loss in beagles[270] when lesions were separated into "active" and "inactive" based on isotope uptake. Lesions where the isotope localized developed radiographic evidence of alveolar bone loss at a later time. However not all lesions progressed over the 2-year monitoring period, suggesting episodic attack. Similar conclusions were also reached by Listgarten and Levin[271] and Listgarten and associates[272] while monitoring patients previously treated for adult periodontitis.

Thus there are four lines of evidence to suggest that the model of continuous destructive periodontal disease is incorrect. First, there are attachment loss rates that are too fast or too slow to be consistent with the observed loss of attachment in individual subjects. Second, there are a large number of sites (with or without prior attachment loss) that do not appear to be changing, which seems inconsistent with the view of a slowly progressive destructive periodontal disease.[263-265] Third, data from animal studies indicate that the disease does not progress in all lesions.[183] Finally, even severe perturbations at a site, which induce rapidly destructive disease are soon brought under control by as yet unknown mechanisms.[136,184-186,273-277] Alternative models of destructive periodontal diseases have been suggested.[262]

The consequences of proposing and accepting an incorrect disease model are considerable both in terms of research design and patient care. If disease activity occurs in bursts, and sites with prior loss of attachment are studied as if they all were currently active, we have little hope of determining microbial pathogens or host-contributing or controlling factors. Since recent studies suggest that the majority of sites with prior evidence of disease are currently not "active," then pooling data from such sites with those from truly active sites could mask any meaningful differences.

Until recently, there have been few attempts at measuring destructive periodontal disease activity clinically and, in the absence of clinical validation, doubt must be cast on existing laboratory measurements of disease activity.[276,277] At this time, only two "primary standards" appear to be available to evaluate destructive disease activity: measurement of changes in attachment level by probing or measurement of changes in level of alveolar bone by radiographic techniques.

**Detection of destructive periodontal disease activity**

One method used to analyze attachment level changes is the "tolerance method."[264] In brief, the difference between means of pairs of measurements at each site taken at 2-month intervals is compared to see if it surpasses those of three sets of standards (1) population measurement error, (2) subject measurement error, and (3) pooled standard deviation of the measurements at that site. If the difference exceeds these standards, the site is considered to be "actively breaking down."

There are many problems, however, associated with probing. The probe tip may fall short of the junctional epithelium in a healthy site and may pass well beyond the junctional epithelial attachment in an inflamed pocket. The force that is applied to a probe also affects the position of the probe tip. Other difficulties associated with probing include angulation of the probe, shape of the tooth, subgingival deposits, and cooperation of the patient. Despite these shortcomings, probing from a fixed reference point appears to be the best estimator of changes in periodontal attachment levels. The error may no greater than 1.5 mm when compared with histologic measurements.[278]

Clinicians have employed certain clinical parameters as indicators of active, destructive disease; for example, bleeding on probing and suppuration. Pocket depths over certain thresholds have also been considered to have a high probability of demonstrating further destruction in the immediate future. For this reason, it is worth testing such parameters for their ability to diagnose and predict destructive disease activity.[279] In fairness, the clinical parameters chosen were not initially meant to indicate active destructive periodontal disease. Redness, plaque, and bleeding on probing have been used as measures of gingivitis and reflections of supragingival plaque accumulation. Suppuration provides a measure of polymorphonuclear leukocyte accumulations in pockets, which may well be associated with changes in gingival structures rather than overt pathology affecting the periodontal ligament and alveolar bone. Attachment level measurements, bone loss and, to some extent, pocket depth reflect the prior loss of attachment and as such measure the extent of prior but not necessarily current destruction. Each of the clinical parameters examined at one visit may provide information concerning the extent of previous disease or current periodontal status. Unfortunately, none of the parameters alone or in combination reflect the status of destructive periodontal disease *activity* at the individual site.[279]

**Microbiota associated with active and inactive periodontal lesions**

Phase-contrast or dark-field microscopic observations of wet mount preparations of plaque samples have been used to diagnose destructive periodontal disease activity. It was felt that increased proportions of spirochetes and/or motile rods were indicative of active periodontal breakdown at a site. However, dark-field examinations of plaque samples taken from sites of active periodontal destruction, as determined by changes in the attachment level measurement, when compared with samples taken from inactive sites in the same individuals do not support this hypothesis. Figs. 8-25 and 8-26 show the proportions of spirochetes, motile rods, and all motile organisms in samples from active sites and inactive sites as obtained by a scaler and by a flushing technique.[280] The differences in proportions in the motile groups were not particularly striking and were not statistically significant.

Fig. 8-27 demonstrates a receiver operating curve of the proportions of spirochetes, motile rods, and nonmotile rods used as a diagnostic test for the detection of disease activity. The sensitivity is a measure of the proportion of sites that are active and are

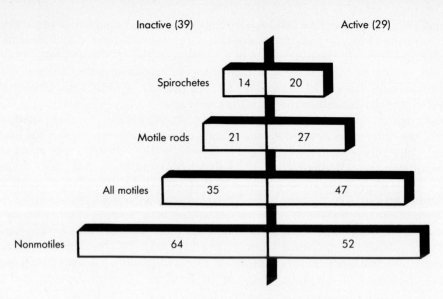

**Fig. 8-25.** Mean percentages of dark-field microbial groups in active and inactive sites sampled with a scaler. Disease activity was determined by changes in repeated attachment level measurements and the "tolerance" method of analysis. The number of sites sampled are indicated in parentheses and the mean percentages are indicated within the bars.

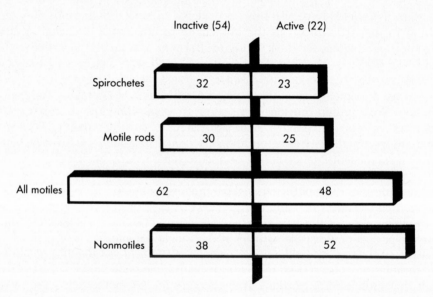

**Fig. 8-26.** Mean percentages of dark-field microbial groups in active and inactive sites sampled by means of a flushing technique. Disease activity was determined by changes in repeated attachment level measurements and the "tolerance" method of analysis. The number of sites sampled are indicated in parentheses and the mean percentages are indicated within the bars.

detected diagnostically by a given threshold of microorganisms in the plaque samples (Fig. 8-28). The specificity is the proportion of sites that are diagnostically negative to the test and are not active. The ideal diagnostic test is indicated by the X in Fig. 8-27. For a test to be diagnostically useful it should have a specificity and sensitivity greater than 0.9. Specificity and sensitivity are measures that indicate the proportion of false positives and negatives and true positives and negatives in diagnosis. If one assumes that 3% of sites are actively breaking down in a population, then the probability

**Table 8-2**   Predominant cultivable microbiota in inactive and active sites (% of species averaging >1% of isolates)

| Organisms | Inactive (%) | Active (%) |
|---|---|---|
| S. intermedius | 3.9 | 4.8 |
| S. mitis | 1.1 | 1.7 |
| S. morbillorum | 0.8 | 1.0 |
| S. sanguis I | 1.3 | 1.0 |
| S. sanguis II | 2.9* | 1.6 |
| S. uberis | 2.3 | 2.2 |
| Actinomyces, Group 1 | 2.8* | 0.6 |
| Actinomyces, Group 8 | 2.3 | 1.4 |
| Actinomyces, Group 31 | 1.5 | 0.5 |
| Actinomyces, Group 50 | 1.3* | 0.3 |
| A. actinomycetemcomitans | 0.4 | 1.6* |
| B. gingivalis | 1.1 | 2.1 |
| B. intermedius | 2.3 | 3.9 |
| B. forsythus | 0.0 | 2.4* |
| C. gingivalis | 1.5 | 0.9 |
| C. ochracea | 4.5 | 2.9 |
| E. corrodens | 1.4 | 2.1 |
| F. nucleatum | 7.7 | 9.7 |
| V. parvula | 2.1* | 0.5 |
| W. recta | 1.4 | 3.2* |
| Number of isolates | 5150 | 3450 |
| Number of sites | 103 | 69 |

*Significantly elevated at p <0.05.

**Table 8-3**   Significantly elevated species in 25 subjects

| Organisms | Inactive | Active |
|---|---|---|
| W. recta | 1* | 8 |
| B. intermedius | 0 | 5 |
| B. forsythus | 0 | 3 |
| B. gingivalis | 0 | 2 |
| A. actinomycetemcomitans | 0 | 2 |
| F. nucleatum | 3 | 3 |
| E. corrodens | 2 | 3 |
| C. gingivalis | 1 | 3 |
| V. parvula | 0 | 2 |
| Actinomyces, Group 1 | 1 | 5 |
| Actinomyces, Group 8 | 0 | 2 |
| Actinomyces, Group 50 | 0 | 3 |
| S. sanguis II | 0 | 4 |
| C. ochracea | 1 | 5 |

*Number of subjects.

*Fusobacterium nucleatum, Capnocytophaga gingivalis,* and *Eikenella corrodens* were found in significantly increased proportions in active sites of some subjects and inactive sites of others.[282] In a similar fashion, *A. actinomycetemcomitans* and *E. corrodens* were found to be significantly elevated in the actively breaking down lesions of eight patients with juvenile periodontitis.[283]

The recent interest in bursts of destructive periodontal disease activity has raised questions concerning etiology. The nature of changes that would account for such rapid destruction followed by prolonged remission is only speculative at this time. It

**Bacterial invasion of periodontal tissues**

would seem likely that the process is initiated by a proliferation of one or more members of the subgingival microbiota in the local site leading to the destructive process. This process may eventually be controlled by the host or other members of the microbiota. The speed of the process, however, does not seem consistent with disease induced at long range by microorganisms confined within the periodontal pocket. Thus the renewed interest in active invasion by microorganisms seems warranted.[284-289] Overt invasion by one or more species followed by a rapidly imposed host control, perhaps by local antibody synthesis or macrophage ingestion seems temptingly consistent with the apparent kinetics of destructive disease activity.

It is important, however, to distinguish between the presence of bacteria within tissues resulting from the translocation of bacteria from the pocket environment by mechanical means (such as chewing with a loose tooth or various oral hygiene measures) and bacterial invasion. The latter, which may result from increased bacterial virulence or decreased host resistance, is associated with proliferation as well as spread of the bacteria within the tissues. Where bacterial invasion may be expected to show microcolonies or spreading masses of selected bacteria, translocation is more likely to result in a heterogeneous mixture of bacterial morphotypes within the affected tissues.[290]

**Chemotherapeutic approaches for the control of periodontal diseases**

Since the destructive periodontal diseases are caused by bacteria, it is not surprising that there is a growing interest in the use of antibiotics and other antimicrobial agents for their control. Tetracycline is the most commonly used antibiotic for the treatment of certain forms of destructive periodontal disease. Recent reports[129,203,229,291] indicate that tetracycline, in combination with mechanical debridement, can have a major effect on the composition of subgingival microbiota and influence the clinical parameters of periodontal disease. Controlled clinical trials comparing efficacy of therapy with and without antibiotics have been relatively few in number. The progress of lesions in patients with classic "molar-incisor" juvenile periodontitis can be effectively stopped by a combination of systemically administered tetracycline and scaling[128] or surgery.[127]

The efficacy of tetracycline in the treatment of juvenile periodontitis may be related to at least three factors: the sensitivity of most *Actinobacillus* isolates to the antibiotic,[292,293] the increased concentration of tetracycline in crevicular fluid,[116,294-296] and the establishment in pockets after therapy of organisms that inhibit the growth of *A. actinomycetemcomitans*.[297] It is anticipated that the use of antibiotics as adjuncts in the treatment of periodontal disease will continue to grow. The choice of appropriate agents should depend on (1) the nature of the microorganisms that cause the patient's disease, (2) the levels of agent achieved at the site of disease, and (3) the nature of the microbiota that colonize after therapy. The establishment of microbiologic diagnostic laboratories will facilitate the task of detecting assorted pathogens and monitoring their disappearance following appropriate treatments.

## Summary

The search for the etiologic agents of periodontal diseases continues. It seems that microbiologists and immunologists continually propose new agents or mechanisms that "potentially may play a role" in the etiology or pathogenesis of destructive periodontal diseases. The list of microorganisms, mechanisms, or host responses "that may play a role" continues to grow at a fast pace but no one suggests taking organisms or mechanisms off the list. Interest in the suggested organism or metabolite merely fades as new and temporarily more exciting organisms or mechanisms are proposed. It seems essential to strengthen the association or lack thereof of certain organisms with destructive periodontal diseases. Obviously not all subgingival microorganisms are pathogenic. All microorganisms cannot have an equal potential to cause periodontal destruction. There is no known organ system for which all microbial species are equally pathogenic. The vast majority of infectious diseases of any organ system is caused by a handful of pathogens, with the remaining cases being caused by a somewhat wider range of less common etiologic agents. A similar relationship may be expected in destructive periodontal diseases. Thus our expectation in examining large numbers of cases of destructive periodontal disease would be to encounter similar "probable pathogens" in more than half of the cases and some less frequently encountered forms in a smaller number of cases.

Discrimination between pathogenic and nonpathogenic species will not be easy. Some species, such as *Actinobacillus actinomycetemcomitans, Bacteroides forsythus,* and *Wolinella recta* will fall easily into groups. Others will defy easy categorization. The problem of discrimination of pathogens is compounded by the fact that so many species reside in the pocket, most of which are taking advantage of the ecologic niche in which they may live in quiet compatibility with the host for years. To differentiate these commensals from the pathogens is an essential task. Knowledge of pathogenic organisms will permit (1) a precise classification of destructive periodontal diseases, (2) the potential for a precise diagnostic test, (3) a target for therapeutic procedures, (4) a monitoring tool for efficacy of therapy, and (5) a point of departure to test the feasibility and utility of potential vaccines. For organisms with relatively low virulence, host resistance may play a key role in determining whether the organisms will or will not act as pathogens.

The existence of periods of disease activity affects our concepts of destructive periodontal diseases and, hence, should have an effect on the way we monitor, choose sample sites and times, and treat periodontal patients. If we develop the ability to detect periods of disease activity, such information could be used to identify patients who require therapy. Therapy of individuals with inactive lesions may be a waste of time and money if the therapy does not lead to a reduction in the incidence of disease. Whether the treatment of such individuals should take place at all might be the subject of considerable debate! However it seems reasonable from both the clinicians' and the patients' point of view that if treatment is necessary, it should be carried out at the appropriate time.

Table 8-1 provides a list of microorganisms which, at this point in time, are most likely to be associated with different forms of periodontal disease or periodontal health. In the clinical condition of juvenile periodontitis, there are relatively few suspected pathogens. In contrast, large numbers of microorganisms appear in the list of suspected pathogens of destructive periodontitis. This list is extensive primarily because there may be different destructive periodontal diseases. The possible agents of these various forms of destructive periodontitis have been pooled into this rather lengthy list. It should also be noted that there is a relatively lengthy list of organisms that are compatible with health or at least do not appear to play a role in the destructive forms of periodontal disease. Some of these organisms may be protective to the host and control recolonization by pathogens after therapy. Organisms such as *Streptococcus sanguis* and some of the gram-positive rods may colonize after successful periodontal therapy and produce substances antagonistic to the return of the pathogens.

Where does this all lead? When a patient presents with evidence of periodontal disease, we would like to be able to take samples of plaque, crevicular fluid, and blood in order to determine if the individual has active periodontal disease, the nature of the etiologic species, and the adequacy of the host response. Sites that are actively breaking down could be detected and sites harboring specific pathogens identified. Knowledge of the activity of lesions and etiologic organisms would help in choosing the optimal therapy. The efficacy of therapy could be monitored by determining whether disease activity has stopped, whether the host resistance to the organism has increased, and by failure to detect the organism in new plaque samples. Thus the goals in the immediate future are to determine which organisms cause specific diseases, to develop tools for the measurement of activity, etiology, and host response, and to optimize therapy of the common forms of periodontal infections.

## REFERENCES

1. Löe, H., Theilade, E., and Jensen, S.B.: Experimental gingivitis in man, J. Periodontol. **36:**177, 1965.
2. Theilade, E., et al.: Experimental gingivitis in man. II. A longitudinal, clinical and bacteriologic investigation, J. Periodont. Res. **1:**1, 1966.
3. Krygier, G., et al.: Experimental gingivitis in *Macaca speciosa* monkeys: clinical, bacteriologic and histologic similarities to human gingivitis, J. Periodontol. **44:**454, 1973.
4. Socransky, S.S., and Crawford, A.C.R.: Recent advances in the microbiology of periodontal disease. In Goldman, H.M., et al., editors: Current therapy in dentistry, vol. 6, St. Louis, 1977, The C.V. Mosby Co.
5. Socransky, S.S.: Microbiology of periodontal disease—present status and future considerations, J. Periodontol. **48:**497, 1977.
6. Socransky, S.S., and Manganiello, S.D.: the oral microbiota of man from birth to senility, J. Periodontol. **42:**485, 1971.
7. McCarthy, C., Snyder, M.L., and Parker, R.B.: The indigenous oral flora of man. I. The newborn to the 1-year-old infant, Arch. Oral Biol. **10:**61, 1965.
8. de Araujo, W.C., and MacDonald, J.B.: Gingival crevice microbiota of preschool children, Arch. Oral Biol. **9:**227, 1964.
9. Dawes, C., Jenkins, G.N., and Tonge, C.H.: The nomenclature of the integuments of the enamel of teeth, Br. Dent. J. **115:**65, 1963.
9a. Listgarten, M.A.: Structure of surface coatings on teeth: A review, J. Periodontol. **47:**139, 1976.
10. Mandel, I.D.: Indices for measurement of soft accumulations in clinical studies of oral hygiene and periodontal disease, J. Periodont. Res. Suppl. **14:**7, 1974.
11. Lie, T.: Scanning and transmission electron microscope study of pellicle morphogenesis, Scand. J. Dent. Res. **85:**217, 1977.
12. Fine, D.H., et al.: Studies on plaque pathogenecity. I. Plaque collection and limulus lysate screening of adherent and loosely adherent plaque, J. Periodont. Res. **13:**17, 1978.
13. Tinanoff, N., Gross, A., and Brady, J.M.: Development of plaque on enamel. Parallel investigations, J. Periodont. Res. **11:**197, 1976.
14. Theilade, E., and Theilade, J.: Bacteriological and ultrastructural studies of developing dental plaque. In McHugh, W.D., editor: Dental plaque, Edinburgh, 1970, E. & S. Livingstone Ltd.
15. Gibbons, R.J., and van Houte, J.: On the formation of dental plaques, J. Periodontol. **44:**347, 1973.
16. Carlsson, J.: Plaque formation and streptococcal colonization on teeth, Odont. Rev. **19**(suppl. 14), 1968.
17. Ritz, H.L.: Microbial population shifts in developing human dental plaque, Arch. Oral Biol. **12:**1561, 1967.
18. Hardie, J.M., and Bowden, G.H.: The microbial flora of dental plaque: bacterial succession and isolation considerations. In Stiles, H.M., Loesche, W.J., and O'Brien, T.C., editors: Proceedings: Microbial aspects of dental caries, Sp. Suppl. Microbiol. Abstr. **1:**63, 1976.
18a. Lindhe, J., and Wicén, P.-O.: The effects on the gingivae of chewing fibrous foods, J. Periodont. Res. **4:**193, 1969.
19. Wade, A.B.: Effect on dental plaque of chewing apples, Dent. Pract. **21:**194, 1971.
20. Wilcox, C.E., and Everett, F.G.: Friction on the teeth and the gingiva during mastication, J. Am. Dent. Assoc. **66:**513, 1963.
21. Listgarten, M.A., Mayo, H.E., and Tremblay, R.: Development of dental plaque on epoxy resin crowns in man: a light and electron microscopic study, J. Periodontol. **46:**10, 1975.
22. Tanzer, J.M.: Current status of microbiology of periodontal diseases, World Workshop III, International Conference on Research in the Biology of Periodontal Diseases, Chicago, June 12-15, 1977.
23. Socransky, S.S., et al.: Bacteriological studies of developing supragingival dental plaque, J. Periodont. Res. **12:**90, 1977.
24. Manganiello, A.D., et al.: Attempts to increase viable count recovery of human supragingival dental plaque, J. Periodont. Res. **12:**107, 1977.
25. Listgarten, M.A.: Structure of the microbial flora associated with periodontal disease and health in man: a light and electron microscopic study, J. Periodontol. **47:**1, 1976.
26. Holt, R.L., and Mestecky, J.: Studies on human dental plaque. II. Immunochemical characteristics, J. Oral Pathol. **4:**86, 1975.
27. Hay, D.I., Gibbons, R.J., and Spinell, D.M.: Characteristics of some high molecular weight constituents with bacterial aggregating activity from whole saliva and dental plaque, Caries Res. **5:**111, 1971.
28. Critchley, P., et al.: The polymerisation of dietary sugars by dental plaque, Caries Res. **1:**112, 1967.

29. Newbrun, E.: Polysaccharide synthesis in plaque. In Stiles, H.M., Loesche, W.J., and O'Brien, T.C., editors: Proceedings: Microbial aspects of dental caries, Sp. Suppl. Microbiol. Abstr. **3:**649, 1976.

30. Littleton, N.W., McCabe, R.M., and Carter, C.H.: Studies of oral health in persons nourished by stomach tube. II. Acidogenic properties and selected bacterial components of plaque material, Arch. Oral Biol. **12:**601, 1967.

31. Socransky, S.S.: Relationship of bacteria to the etiology of periodontal disease, J. Dent. Res. **49:**203, 1970.

32. Kelstrup, J., and Theilade, E.: Microbes and periodontal disease, J. Clin. Periodontol. **1:**15, 1974.

33. van Palenstein Helderman, W.H., and Hoogeveen, C.J.C.M.: Bacterial enzymes and viable counts in crevices of noninflamed and inflamed gingiva, J. Periodont. Res. **11:**25, 1976.

34. Johnson, D.A., et al.: Role of bacterial products in periodontitis. I. Endotoxin content and immunogenicity of human plaque, J. Periodont. Res. **11:**349, 1976.

35. Shapiro, L., et al.: Endotoxin determinations in gingival inflammation, J. Periodontol. **43:**591, 1972.

36. Schwartz, J., Stinson, F.L., and Parker, R.B.: The passage of tritiated bacterial endotoxin across intact gingival crevicular epithelium, J. Periodontol. **43:**270, 1972.

37. Kraal, J.H., and Loesche, W.J.: Rabbit polymorphonuclear leukocyte migration in vitro in response to dental plaque, J. Periodont. Res. **9:**1, 1974.

38. Mergenhagen, S.E., Tempel, T.R., and Snyderman, R.: Immunologic reactions and periodontal inflammation, J. Dent. Res. **49:**256, 1970.

39. Tsai, C.-C, et al.: Interaction of inflammatory cells and oral microorganisms. VI. Exocytosis of PMN lysosomes in response to gram-negative bacteria, J. Periodont. Res. **13:**504, 1978.

40. Gottlieb, S.D., and Miller, L.H.: *Entamoeba gingivalis* in periodontal disease, J. Periodontol. **42:**412, 1971.

41. Bartels, H.A.: A note on chromogenic microorganisms from an orange colored deposit of the teeth, Am. J. Orthod. **25:**795, 1939.

42. Bowen, W.H., et al.: The microbiology and biochemistry of plaque, saliva and drinking water from two communities in Colombia, J. Dent. Res. **56:**632, 1977.

43. Theilade, J., Slots, J., and Fejerskov, O.: The ultrastructure of black stain on human primary teeth, Scand. J. Dent. Res. **81:**528, 1973.

44. Theilade, E., and Theilade, J.: Role of plaque in the etiology of periodontal disease and caries, Oral Sci. Rev. **9:**23, 1976.

45. Barrett, M.T.: Clinical report upon amoebic pyorrhea, Dent. Cosmos **56:**1345, 1914.

46. Le Clear, T.: Method of identification of endamoebae in dry smears, Dent. Cosmos **57:**1313, 1915.

47. Smith, T.S.: The emetin hydrochloride question in the treatment of pyorrhea alveolaris, Dent. Cosmos **57:**1313, 1915.

48. Howe, P.R.: The endamoebae and pyorrhea alveolaris, Dent. Cosmos **58:**369, 1916.

49. Medalia, L.S.: The present status of alveolar osteomyelitis pyorrhea alveolaris: its causes and treatment and vaccines, Dent. Cosmos **58:**1000-1012, 1916.

50. Merritt, A.: The irrationality of bacterial vaccines in the treatment of pyorrhea alveolaris, Dent. Cosmos **58:**62, 1916.

51. Kolle, W.: Spirochätenbefunde und Salvarsan bei Alveolar-pyorrhoe. Medizin. Klin. **3:**59, 1917.

52. Kritchevsky, B., and Seguin, P.: The pathogenesis and treatment of pyorrhea alveolaris, Dent. Cosmos **60:**781, 1918.

53. Kritchevsky, B., and Seguin, P.: The unity of spirochetoses in the mouth, Dent. Cosmos **66:**511, 1924.

54. Stafne, E.C.: *Spirochaetaceae* and *Fusiformis dentium* in the mouth, Dent. Cosmos **70:**493, 1928.

55. Hotchkiss, M.: Presence of fusiform bacilli and spirochetes in the mouths of a group of young adults, Dent. Cosmos **73:**728, 1931.

56. Kligler, I.J.: A biochemical study and differentiation of oral bacteria with special reference to dental caries. II. Experimental, J. Allied Dent. Soc. **10:**282, 1915.

57. Olsen, I., and Socransky, S.S.: Ultrasonic dispersion of pure cultures of plaque bacteria and plaque, Scand. J. Dent. Res. **89:**307, 1981.

58. Goadby, K.W.: The Eramus Wilson Lecture on pyorrhea alveolaris, Lancet **1:**633, 1907.

59. Glynn, E.E.: The organisms found in the periodontal infections, and their relation to the "toxaemia," Br. Dent. J. **44:**601, 681, 1923.

60. Fisher, J.H.: Pyorrhea alveolaris: the role of certain microorganisms found in the lesions, Dent. Cosmos **69:**851, 1927.

61. Lazarus-Barlow, P.: A bacteriological examination of the alveolar bone in relation to pyorrhea, Dent. Cosmos **70:**652, 1928.

62. White, P.G.: Deep muscular injections of succinimid of mercury in pyorrhea alveolaris, Dent. Cosmos **57:**405, 1915.

63. Wright, B.L.: The treatment of pyorrhea alveolaris and its secondary systemic infections by deep muscular injections of mercury, Dent. Cosmos. **57:**1003, 1915.

64. Darcissac, M., and Legrain, P.: La vaccinothérapie de la pyorrhée par le pansement microbien à demeure sous gouttière porte-vaccin, Rev. de Stomatol. **27:**1161, 1925.

65. Frey: 37 cas de pyorrhée vraie traités par un pansement gélo-bactérien, L'Odontologie **64:**699, 1926.

66. Nikolaewa, E.: Essai d'application des vaccins d'après Besredka dans des cas d'inflammations locales, aigües et chroniques, Ann. de L'Inst. Pasteur **10:**869, 1926.

67. Ottolenghi: L'antivirus Besredka nel trettamento delle malattie della cavita orale, La Stomatol. **28:**112, 1930.

68. McGehee, W.H.O.: Stock vaccines in the treatment of pyorrhea alveolaris, Dent. Cosmos **54:**997, 1912.

69. Casto, T.D.: The treatment of periodontoclasia with a polyvalent vaccine (Goldenberg's Inava Endocorps vaccine), Dent. Cosmos **67:**689, 1925.

70. McCall, J.O.: Minority report on vaccine treatment in periodontia, Am. Dent. Assoc. **13:**1624, 1926.

71. Centeno, G.A.R.: La vacunoterapia en odontologia, Rev. Odontol. Enero, 1-36, 1929.

72. Gaubert, P.: Le traitement vaccinal antipyorrhéique, L'Odontologie **68:**174, 1930.

73. Kritchevsky, B., and Seguin, P.: Local and general spirochaetosis, Dent. Cosmos **63:**888, 1921.

74. Hoffman, G.M.: Pyorrhea and autogeneous vaccines, Dent. Cosmos **61:**1095, 1919.

75. Briggs, H.F.: Local vaccine treatment of pyorrhea alveolaris, Dent. Cosmos **66:**697, 1924.

76. Kolmer, J.A. (1924) Infection, immunity and biologic therapy, 3rd edition, Philadelphia, 1924, W.B. Saunders Co.

77. Patterson, T.B.: Presidential address, B. Dent. J. **49:**459, 1928.

78. Lose, G.D., and Foure, J.R.: Observations on periodontoclasia, with special reference to the use of autogenous vaccine and surgical intervention, Dent. Cosmos **77:**868, 1935.

79. Hirschfeld, I.: An investigation of Inava Endocorps vaccine, J. Am. Dent. Assoc. **13:**1613, 1926.

80. Appleton, J.L.T.: The use of vaccines, antivirus, bacteriophage and non-specific protein therapy in mouth infections, Dent. Cosmos **72:**1276, 1930.

81. Belding, P.H., and Belding, L.J.: Bacteria: dental orphans, Dent. Cosmos **78:**506, 1936.

82. Bunting, R.W.: Is pyorrhea a local or constitutional disease? Dent. Cosmos **64:**731, 1922.

83. Prinz, H.: A few aphorisms concerning pyorrhea alveolaris, Dent. Cosmos **66:**127, 1924.

84. Prinz, H.: The etiology of pyorrhea alveolaris, Dent. Cosmos **68:**1, 1926.

85. Smith, D.T.: Fusospirocheta disease of the lungs produced with cultures from Vincent's angina, J. Infect. Dis. **46:**303, 1930.

86. Proske, H.O., and Sayers, R.R.: Pulmonary infections in pneumoconiosis. I. A bacteriologic and experimental study, Public Health Rep. **29:**839, 1934.

87. Proske, H.O., and Sayers, R.R.: Pulmonary infection in pneumoconiosis. II. Fuso-spirochetal infection: experiments in guinea pigs, Public Health Rep. **29:**1212, 1934.

88. Rosebury, T., et al.: Studies of fusospirochetal infection. I. Pathogenicity for guinea pigs of individual and combined cultures of spirochetes and other anaerobic bacteria derived from the human mouth, J. Infect. Dis. **87:**217, 1950.

89. Rosebury, T., et al.: Studies of fusospirochetal infection. II. Analysis and attempted quantitive recombination of the flora of fusospirochetal infection after repeated guinea pig passage, J. Infect. Dis. **87:**226, 1950.

90. Rosebury, T., et al.: Studies of fusobacterial infection. III. Further studies of a guinea pig passage strain of fusospirochetal infection, including the infectivity of sterile exudates, of mixed cultures through ten transfers, and of recombined pure cultures, J. Infect. Dis. **87:**234, 1950.

91. MacDonald, J.B., et al.: The pathogenic components of an experimental mixed infection, J. Infect. Dis. **98:**15, 1956.

92. Socransky, S.S., and Gibbons, R.J.: Required role of *Bacteroides melaninogenicus* in mixed anaerobic infections, J. Infect. Dis. **115:**247, 1965.

93. Keyes, P.H., and Jordan, H.V.: Periodontal lesions in the Syrian hamster. III. Findings related to an infectious and transmissable component, Arch. Oral Biol. **9:**377, 1964.

94. Jordan, H.V., and Keyes, P.H.: Aerobic, gram-positive, filamentous bacteria as etiologic agents of experimental periodontal disease in hamsters, Arch. Oral Biol. **9:**401, 1964.

95. Listgarten, M.A.: Electron microscopic observations of the bacterial flora of acute necrotizing ulcerative gingivitis, J. Periodontol. **36:**328, 1965.

96. Fitzgerald, R.J., and McDaniel, E.G.: Dental calculus in germfree rats, Arch. Oral Biol. **2:**239, 1960.

97. Gibbons, R.J., et al.: Dental caries and alveolar bone loss in gnotobiotic rats infected with capsule-forming streptococci of human origin, Arch. Oral Biol. **11:**549, 1966.

98. Löe, H., Theilade, E., and Jensen, S.B.: Experimental gingivitis in man, J. Periodontol. **36:**177, 1965.

99. Löe, H., et al.: Experimental gingivitis in man. III. The influence of antibiotics on gingival plaque development, J. Periodont. Res. **2:**282, 1967.

100. Theilade, E., et al.: Experimental gingivitis in man. II. A longitudinal clinical and bacteriological investigation, J. Periodont. Res. **1:**1, 1966.

101. Genco, R.J., Evans, R.T., and Ellison, S.A.: Dental research in microbiology with em-

phasis on periodontal disease, J. Am. Dent. Assoc. **78:**1016, 1969.

102. Ellison, S.A.: Oral bacteria and periodontal disease, J. Dent. Res. **49:**198, 1970.

103. Keyes, P.H.: Are periodontal pathoses caused by bacterial infections on cervicoradicular surfaces of teeth? J. Dent. Res. **49:**223, 1970.

104. Socransky, S.S.: Relationship of bacteria to the etiology of periodontal disease, J. Dent. Res. **49:**203, 1970.

105. Socransky, S.S.: Microbiology of periodontal disease: present status and future considerations, J. Periodontol. **48:**497, 1977.

106. Schuessler, C.F., Fairchild, J.M., and Stranksy, I.M.: Penicillin in the treatment of Vincent's infection, J. Am. Dent. Assoc. **32:**551, 1945.

107. Goldhaber, P., and Giddon, D.B.: Present concepts concerning the etiology and treatment of acute necrotizing ulcerative gingivitis, Int. Dent. J. **14:**468, 1964.

108. Mitchell, D.F., and Baker, B.R.: Topical antibiotic control of necrotizing ulcerative gingivitis, J. Periodontol. **39:**81, 1968.

109. Lozdan, J., et al.: The use of nitrimidazine in the treatment of acute ulcerative gingivitis: a double-blind controlled trial, Br. Dent. J. **130:**294, 1971.

110. Arno, A., et al.: Incidence of gingivitis as related to sex, occupation, tobacco consumption, toothbrushing and age, Oral Surg. **11:**587, 1958.

111. O'Leary, T.J., Shannon, I.L., and Prigmore, J.R.: Clinical correlations and systemic status in periodontal disease, South. Calif. Dent. J. **30:**47, 1962.

112. Ash, M.M., Jr., Gitlin, B.N., and Smith, W.A.: Correlation between plaque and periodontal disease, J. Periodontol. **35:**424, 1964.

113. Lövdal, A., et al.: Tooth mobility and alveolar bone resorption as a function of occlusal stress and oral hygiene and age, Acta Odontol. Scand. **17:**61, 1959.

114. Schei, O., et al.: Alveolar bone loss as related to oral hygiene and age, J. Periodontol. **30:**7, 1959.

115. Volpe, A.R.: Antimicrobial control of bacterial plaque and calculus and the effects of these agents on oral flora, J. Dent. Res. **48:**832, 1969.

116. Ciancio, S.G., Mather, M.L., and McMullen, J.A.: An evaluation of minocycline in patients with periodontal disease, J. Periodontol. **51:**530, 1980.

117. Davies, R.M., et al.: The effect of topical application of chlorhexidine on the bacterial colonization of the teeth and gingiva, J. Periodont. Res. **5:**96, 1970.

118. Gjermo, P., Baastad, K.L., and Rölla, C.: The plaque-inhibiting capacity of 11 antibacterial compounds, J. Periodont. Res. **5:**102, 1970.

119. Löe, H., and Schiott, C.R.: The effect of mouthrinses and topical application of chlorhexidine on the development of dental plaque and gingivitis in man, J. Periodont. Res. **5:**79, 1970.

120. Schiott, C.R., et al.: The effect of chlorhexidine mouth rinses on the human oral flora, J. Periodont. Res. **5:**84, 1970.

121. Löe, H., et al.: Two years oral use of chlorhexidine in man. I. General design and clinical effects, J. Periodont. Res. **11:**135, 1976.

122. Lindhe, J., and Nyman, S.: The effect of plaque control and surgical pocket elimination on the establishment and maintenance of periodontal health: a longitudinal study of periodontal therapy in cases of advanced periodontitis, J. Clin. Periodontol. **2:**67, 1975.

123. Rosling, B., Nyman, S., and Lindhe, J.: The effect of systematic plaque control on bone regeneration in infrabony pockets, J. Clin. Periodontol. **3:**38, 1976.

124. Rosling, B., et al.: The healing potential of the periodontal tissues following different techniques of periodontal surgery in plaque-free dentitions, J. Clin. Periodontol. **3:**233, 1976.

125. Strock, A.E.: The treatment of acute ulcerative gingivostomatitis (Vincent's infection) with penicillin, N.Y. J. Dent. **15:**263, 1945.

126. Shinn, D.L.S.: Metronidazole in acute ulcerative gingivitis, Lancet **1:**1191, 1962.

127. Liljenberg, B., and Lindhe, J.: Juvenile periodontitis: some microbiological, histopathological and clinical characteristic, J. Clin. Periodontol. **7:**48, 1980.

128. Genco, R.J., Cianciola, L.J., and Rosling, B.: Treatment of localized juvenile periodontitis: J. Dent. Res. **60A:**527, 1981.

129. Haffajee, A.D., et al.: Clinical, microbiological and immunological features associated with the treatment of active periodontosis lesions, J. Clin. Periodontol. **11:**600, 1983.

130. Waerhaug, J.: Effect of rough surfaces upon gingival tissue, J. Dent. Res. **35:**323, 1956.

131. Waerhaug, J.: Effect of zinc phosphate cement fillings on gingival tissues, J. Periodontol. **27:**284, 1956.

132. Waerhaug, J.: Observations on replanted teeth plated with gold foil: reaction to pure gold; mode of epithelial attachment to gold; expulsion of foreign bodies from pockets, Oral Surg. **9:**780, 1956.

133. Waerhaug, J.: Tissue reaction to metal wires in healthy gingival pockets, J. Periodontol. **28:**239, 1957.

134. Waerhaug, J.: Histological considerations which govern where the margins of restorations should be located in relation to the gingiva, Dent. Clin. North Am. p. 161, 1960.

135. Rovin, S., Costich, E.R., and Gordon, H.A.: The influence of bacteria and irritation on the initiation of periodontal disease in germfree

and conventional rats, J. Periodont. Res. **1:**193, 1966.

136. Slots, J., and Hausmann, E.: Longitudinal study of experimentally induced periodontal disease in *Macaca arctoides:* relationship between microflora and alveolar bone loss, Infect. Immun. **23:**260, 1979.

137. Siegrist, B., et al.: Microbiology of ligature-induced gingivitis in beagle dogs, J. Dent. Res. **59A:**387, 1980.

138. Gustafsson, B.E., and Krasse, B.: Dental calculus in germfree rats, Acta Odontol. Scand. **20:**135, 1962.

139. McMaster, P.E.: Human bite infection, Am. J. Surg. **45:**60, 1939.

140. Fritzell, K.E.: Infections of hand due to human mouth organisms, Lancet **60:**135, 1940.

141. Foley, G., and Rosebury, T.: Comparative infectivity for guinea pigs of fusospirochetal exudates from different diseases, J. Dent. Res. **21:**375, 1942.

142. Shpuntoff, H., and Rosebury, T.: Infectivity of fusospirochetal exudate for guinea pigs, hamsters, mice and chick embryos by several routes of inoculation, J. Dent. Res. **28:**7, 1949.

143. Mergenhagen, S.E.: Endotoxic properties of oral bacteria as revealed by the local Schwartzman reaction, J. Dent. Res. **39:**267, 1960.

144. Mergenhagen, S.E., Hampp, E.G., and Scherp, H.W.: Preparation and biological activities of endotoxins from oral bacteria, J. Infect. Dis. **108:**304, 1961.

145. Hofstad, T.: Antibodies reacting with lipopolysaccharides from *Bacteroides melaninogenicus, Bacteroides fragilis* and *Fusobacterium nucleatum* in serum from normal human subjects, J. Infect. Dis. **129:**349, 1974.

146. Schuster, G.S., Hayashi, J.A., and Bahn, A.N.: Toxic properties of the cell wall of gram-positive bacteria, J. Bacteriol. **93:**47, 1967.

147. Loesche, W.J., Socransky, S.S., and Gibbons, R.J.: *Bacteroides oralis:* proposed new species isolated from the oral cavity of man, J. Bacteriol. **88:**1329, 1964.

148. Loesche, W.J., and Gibbons, R.J.: Amino acid fermentation by *Fusobacterium nucleatum,* Arch. Oral Biol. **13:**191, 1968.

149. Socransky, S.S., et al.: Morphological and biochemical differentiation of three types of small oral spirochetes, J. Bacteriol. **98:**878, 1969.

150. Wahren, A., and Gibbons, R.J.: Amino acid fermentation by *Bacteroides melaninogenicus,* Antonie Van Leeuwenhoek **36:**149, 1970.

151. Macdonald, J.B., Gibbons, R.J., and Socransky, S.S.: Bacterial mechanisms in periodontal disease, Ann. N.Y. Acad. Sci. **85:**467, 1960.

152. Rizzo, A.A.: The possible role of hydrogen sulfide in human periodontal disease. I. Hydrogen sulfide production in periodontal pockets, Periodontics **5:**233, 1967.

153. Macdonald, J.B., and Gibbons, R.J.: The relationship of indigenous bacteria to periodontal disease, J. Dent. Res. **41:**320, 1962.

154. Rizzo, A.A.: Rabbit corneal irrigation as a model system for studies on the relative toxicity of bacterial products implicated in periodontal disease: the toxicity of neutralized ammonia solutions, J. Periodontol. **38:**491, 1967.

155. Socransky, S.S., et al.: Dependency of *Treponema microdentium* on other oral organisms for isobutyrate, polyamines, and a controlled oxidation-reduction potential, J. Bacteriol. **88:**200, 1964.

156. Baehni, P., et al.: Leukotoxicity of various *Actinobacillus actinomycetemcomitans* isolates, J. Dent. Res. **59A:**323, 1980.

157. McArthur, W., et al.: Leukotoxic effects of *Actinobacillus actinomycetemcomitans* (Y4): modulation by serum components, J. Periodont. Res. **16:**159, 1981.

158. Schultz-Haudt, S., Bruce, M.A., and Bibby, B.G.: Bacterial factors in nonspecific gingivitis, J. Dent. Res. **33:**454, 1954.

158a. Schultz-Haudt, S., and Scherp, H.W.: Lysis of collagen by human gingival bacteria, Proc. Soc. Exp. Biol. Med. **89:**697, 1955.

158b. Schultz-Haudt, S., and Scherp, H.W.: Production of hyaluronidase by *viridans* streptococci isolated from gingival crevices, J. Dent. Res. **34:**924, 1955.

158c. Schultz-Haudt, S., and Scherp, H.W.: Production of chondrosulfatase by microorganisms isolated from human gingival crevices, J. Dent. Res. **35:**299, 1956.

159. Dewar, M.R.: Bacterial enzymes and periodontal disease, J. Dent. Res. **37:**100, 1958.

160. Hampp, E.G., Mergenhagen, S.E., and Omata, R.R.: Studies of mucopolysaccharase activity on oral spirochetes, J. Dent. Res. **38:**979, 1959.

161. Gibbons, R.J., and Macdonald, J.B.: Degradation of collagenous substrates by *Bacteroides melaninogenicus,* J. Bacteriol. **81:**614, 1961.

162. Rosan, B., and Williams, N.B.: Hyaluronidase production by oral enterococci, Arch. Oral Biol. **9:**291, 1964.

163. Courant, P.R., Paunio, I., and Gibbons, R.J.: Infectivity and hyaluronidase activity of debris from healthy and diseased gingiva, Arch. Oral Biol. **10:**119, 1965.

164. Thonard, J.C., Hefflin, C.M., and Steinberg, A.I.: Neuraminidase activity in mixed culture supernatant fluids of human oral bacteria, J. Bacteriol. **89:**924, 1965.

165. Söder, P.O., and Frostell, G.: Proteolytic activity of dental plaque material on Azocoll, casein and gelatin, Acta Odontol. Scand. **24:**501, 1966.

USC
DENTAL BOOK STORE

09/10/93

0 #
101 #
BOOKS        73.10 K
6.03 TAX

CHECK      TL      79.13

THANK YOU

166. Mitchell, D.F., and Johnson, M.: The nature of the gingival plaque in the hamster: production, prevention and removal, J. Dent. Res. **35:**651, 1956.

167. Gupta, O.P., Auskaps, A.M., and Shaw, J.H.: Periodontal disease in the rice rat. IV. The effects of antibiotics on the incidence of periodontal lesions, Oral Surg. **10:**1169, 1957.

168. Shaw, J.H., Griffiths, D., and Auskaps, A.M.: The influence of antibiotics on the periodontal syndrome in the rice rat, J. Dent. Res. **40:**511, 1961.

169. Keyes, P.H., et al.: The effect of various drugs on caries and periodontal disease in albino hamsters, Proceedings of the 9th O.R.C.A. Congress, 1963, pp. 159-177.

170. Keyes, P.H., et al.: Bio-assays of medicaments for the control of dentobacterial plaque, dental caries and periodontal lesions in Syrian hamsters, J. Oral Ther. **3:**157, 1966.

171. Shaw, J.H.: Further studies on the sensitivity of the periodontal syndrome in the rice rat to dietary antibiotics, J. Dent. Res. **44:**431, 1965.

172. Lindhe, J., et al.: Influence of topical application of chlorhexidine on chronic gingivitis and gingival wound healing in the dog, Scand. J. Dent. Res. **78:**471, 1970.

173. Johnson, N.W., and Kenney, E.B.: Effects of topical application of chlorhexidine on plaque and gingivitis in monkeys, J. Periodont. Res. **7:**180, 1972.

174. Listgarten, M.A., and Ellegaard, B.: Experimental gingivitis in the monkey: relationship of leukocyte counts in junctional epithelium, sulcus depth, and connective tissue inflammation scores, J. Periodont. Res. **8:**199, 1973.

175. Heijl, L., and Lindhe, J.: The effect of metronidazole on the development of plaque and gingivitis in the beagle dog, J. Clin. Periodontol. **6:**197, 1979.

176. Listgarten, M.A., Lindhe, J., and Parodi, R.: The effect of systemic antimicrobial therapy on plaque and gingivitis in dogs, J. Periodont. Res. **14:**65, 1979.

177. Briner, W.W., et al.: Effect of chlorhexidine on plaque, gingivitis and alveolar bone loss in beagle dogs after seven years of treatment, J. Periodont. Res. **15:**390, 1980.

178. Dick, D.S., and Shaw, J.H.: The infectious and transmissible nature of the periodontal syndrome of the rice rat, Arch. Oral Biol. **11:**1095, 1966.

179. Baer, P.N., Keyes, P.H., and White, C.L.: Studies on experimental calculus formation in the rat. XII. On the transmissibility of factors affecting dental calculus, J. Periodontol. **39:**86, 1968.

180. Gibbons, R.J., and Banghart, S.: Induction of dental caries in gnotobiotic rats with a levan-forming streptococcus and a streptococcus isolated from subacute bacterial endocarditis, Arch. Oral Biol. **13:**297, 1968.

181. Socransky, S.S., Hubersak, C., and Propas, D.: Induction of periodontal destruction in gnotobiotic rats by a human actinomycete, Arch. Oral Biol. **15:**993, 1970.

182. Jordan, H.V., Keyes, P.H., and Bellack, S.: Periodontal lesions in hamsters and gnotobiotic rats infected with actinomyces of human origin, J. Periodont. Res. **7:**21-28, 1972.

183. Lindhe, J., Hamp, S.-E, and Löe, H.: Plaque-induced periodontal disease in beagle dogs: a 4-year clinical, roentgenographical and histometrical study. J. Periodont. Res. **10:**243, 1975.

184. Kennedy, J.E., and Polson, A.M.: Experimental marginal periodonitis in squirrel monkeys, J. Periodontol. **44:**140, 1973.

185. Schroeder, H.E., and Lindhe, J.: Conversion of a stable established gingivitis in the dog to destructive periodontitis, Arch. Oral Biol. **20:**775, 1975.

186. Schroeder, H.E., and Lindhe, J.: Conditions and pathological features of rapidly destructive, experimental periodontitis in dogs, J. Periodontol. **51:**6, 1980.

187. Kornman, K.S., Holt, S.C., and Robertson, P.B.: Subgingival microflora associated with the conversion of gingivitis to periodontitis in monkeys, J. Dent. Res. **59A:**388, 1980.

188. Listgarten, M.A.: Structure of the microbial flora associated with periodontal health and disease in man: a light and electron microscopic study, J. Periodontol. **47:**1, 1976.

189. Listgarten, M.A., and Lewis, D.W.: The distribution of spirochetes in the lesion of acute necrotizing ulcerative gingivitis: an electron microscopic and statistical survey, J. Periodontol. **38:**379, 1967.

190. Ritz, H.L.: Microbial population shifts in developing human dental plaque, Arch. Oral Biol. **12:**1561, 1967.

191. Dwyer, D.M., and Socransky, S.S.: Predominant cultivable microorganisms inhabiting periodontal pockets, Br. Dent. J. **124:**560, 1968.

192. Handleman, S.L., and Hess, C.: Bacterial populations of selected tooth surface sites, J. Dent. Res. **48:**67, 1969.

193. Salkind, A., Oshrain, H.I., and Mandel, I.D.: Bacteriological aspects of developing supragingival and subgingival plaque, J. Periodontol. **42:**706, 1971.

194. Listgarten, M.A., Mayo, H.E., and Tremblay, R.: Development of dental plaque on epoxy resin crowns in man: a light and electron microscopic study, J. Periodontol. **46:**10, 1975.

195. van Palenstein Helderman, W.H.: Total viable count and differential count of *Vibrio (Campylobacter) sputorum, Fusobacterium nucleatum, Selenomonas sputigena, Bacteroides ochraceus* and *Veillonella* in the inflamed and uninflamed human gingival crevice, J. Periodont. Res. **10:**294, 1975.

196. Newman, M.G., et al.: Studies of the microbiology of periodontosis, J. Periodontol. **47:**373, 1976.

197. Newman, M.G., et al.: Predominant microbiota associated with periodontal health in the aged, J. Periodontol. **49:**553, 1978.

198. Österberg, S.K.-A., Sudo, S.Z., and Folke, L.E.A.: Microbial succession in subgingival plaque of man, J. Periodont. Res. **11:**243, 1976.

199. Österberg, S.K.-A., Williams, B.L., and Jorgensen, J.: Long-term effects of tetracycline on the subgingival flora, J. Clin. Periodontol. **6:**133, 1979.

200. Slots, J.: The predominant cultivable organisms in juvenile periodontitis, Scand. J. Dent. Res. **84:**1, 1976.

201. Slots, J.: Microflora in the healthy gingival sulcus in man, Sand. J. Dent. Res. **85:**247, 1977.

202. Slots, J.: The predominant cultivable microflora of advanced periodontitis, Scand. J. Dent. Res. **85:**114, 1977.

203. Slots, J.: Subgingival microflora and periodontal disease, J. Clin. Periodontol. **6:**351, 1979.

204. Williams, B.L., Pantalone, R.M., and Sherris, J.C.: Subgingival microflora and periodontitis, J. Periodont. Res. **11:**1, 1976.

205. Williams, B.L., Osterberg, S.K., and Jorgensen, J.: Subgingival microflora of periodontal patients on tetracycline therapy, J. Clin. Periodontol. **6:**210, 1979.

206. Newman, M.G., and Socransky, S.S.: Predominant cultivable microbiota in periodontosis, J. Periodont. Res. **12:**120, 1977.

207. Socransky, S.S., et al.: Bacteriological studies of developing supragingival dental plaque, J. Periodont. Res. **12:**90, 1977.

208. Allen, A.L., and Brady, J.M.: Periodontosis: a case report with scanning electron microscopic observations, J. Periodontol. **49:**415, 1978.

209. Darwish, S., Hyppa, T., and Socransky, S.S.: Studies of the predominant cultivable microbiota of early periodontitis, J. Periodont. Res. **13:**1, 1978.

210. Listgarten, M.A., and Helldén, L.: Relative distribution of bacteria at clinically healthy and periodontally diseased sites in humans, J. Clin. Periodontol. **5:**115, 1978.

211. Loesche, W.J., and Syed, S.A.: Bacteriology of human experimental gingivitis: effect of plaque and gingivitis score, Infect. Immun. **21:**830, 1978.

212. Slots, J., et al.: Microbiota of gingivitis in man, Scand. J. Dent. Res. **86:**174, 1978.

213. Slots, J., Reynolds, H.S., and Genco, R.J.: *Actinobacillus actinomycetemcomitans* in human periodontal disease: a cross-sectional microbiological investigation, Infect. Immun. **29:**1013, 1980.

214. Syed, S.A., and Loesche, W.J.: Bacteriology of human experimental gingivitis: effect of plaque age, Infect. Immun. **21:**821, 1978.

215. Westergaard, J., Frandsen, A., and Slots, J.: Ultrastructure of the subgingival microflora in juvenile periodontitis, Scand. J. Dent. Res. **86:**421, 1978.

216. Spiegel, C.A., et al.: Black-pigmented bacteroides from clinically characterized periodontal sites, J. Periodont. Res. **14:**376, 1979.

217. Syed, S.A., Loesche, W.J., and Morrison, E.: Proportions of *Bacteroides asaccharolyticus* in the pocket plaques of untreated humans and beagle dogs with periodontitis, Washington, D.C., 1979, American Society for Microbiology, Abstract C(H)25.

218. Tanner, A.C.R., et al.: A study of the bacteria associated with advancing periodontal disease in man, J. Clin. Periodontol. **6:**278, 1979.

219. Lindhe, J., Liljenberg, B., and Listgarten, M.: Some microbiological and histopathological features of periodontal disease in man, J. Periodontol. **51:**264, 1980.

220. Kornman, K.S., and Holt, S.C.: Physiological and ultrastructural characterization of a new *Bacteroides* species (*Bacteroides capillus*) isolated from severe localized periodontitis, J. Periodont. Res. **16:**542, 1981.

221. Mandell, R.L., and Socransky, S.S.: A selective medium for *Actinobacillus actinomycetemcomitans* and the incidence of the organism in juvenile periodontitis, J. Periodontol. **52:**593, 1981.

222. White, D., and Mayrand, D.: Association of oral *Bacteroides* with gingivitis and adult periodontitis, J. Periodont. Res. **16:**259, 1981.

223. Zambon, J.J., Reynolds, H.S., and Slots, J.: Black-pigmented *Bacteroides* spp. in the human oral cavity, Infect. Immun. **32:**198, 1981.

224. Loesche, W.J., et al.: The bacteriology of acute necrotizing ulcerative gingivitis, J. Periodontol. **53:**223, 1982.

225. Moore, W.E.C., et al.: Bacteriology of experimental gingivitis in young adult humans, Infect. Immun. **38:**651, 1982.

226. Moore, W.E.C., Ranney, R.R., and Holdeman, L.V.: Subgingival microflora in periodontal disease: cultural studies. In Genco, R.J., and Mergenhagen, S.E., editors: Host-parasite interactions in periodontal diseases, Washington, D.C., 1982, American Society for Microbiology, pp. 13-26.

227. Moore, W.E.C., et al.: Bacteriology of severe periodontitis in young adult humans, Infect. Immun. **38:**1137, 1982.

228. Moore, W.E.C., et al.: Bacteriology of moderate (chronic) periodontitis in mature adult humans, Infect. Immun. **42:**510, 1983.

229. Listgarten, M.A., Lindhe, J., and Helldén, L.: Effect of tetracycline and/or scaling on human periodontal disease: clinical microbio-

logical and histological observation, J. Clin. Periodontol. **5:**246, 1978.

230. Listgarten, M.A., and Socransky, S.S.: Ultrastructural characteristics of a spirochete in lesions of acute necrotizing ulcerative gingivostomatitis (Vincent's infection), Arch. Oral Biol. **9:**95, 1964.

231. Listgarten, M.A., and Socransky, S.S.: Electron microscopy as an aid in the taxonomic differentiation of oral spirochetes, Arch. Oral Biol. **10:**127, 1965.

232. Leadbetter, E.R., Holt, S.C., and Socransky, S.S.: *Capnocytophaga:* new genus of gram-negative gliding bacteria. I. General characteristics, taxonomic considerations and significance, Arch. Microbiol. **122:**9, 1979.

233. Savitt, E.D., and Socransky, S.S.: Distribution of certain subgingival species in selected periodontal conditions, J. Periodont. Res. **19:**111, 1984.

234. Ebersole, J.L., et al.: An ELISA for measuring serum antibodies to *A. actinomycetemcomitans,* J. Periodont. Res. **15:**621, 1980.

235. Ebersole, J.L., et al.: Human immune responses to oral microorganisms. I. Association of localized juvenile periodontitis (LJP) with serum antibody responses to *Actinobacillus actinomycetemcomitans,* Clin. Exp. Immunol. **47:**43, 1982.

236. Ebersole, J.L., et al.: Humoral immune responses and diagnosis of periodontal disease, J. Periodont. Res. **17:**471, 1982.

237. Ebersole, J.L., et al.: Human immune responses to oral microorganisms. II. Serum antibody responses to antigens from *Actinobacillus actinomycetemcomitans* and the correlation with localized juvenile periodontitis, J. Clin. Immunol. **3:**321, 1983.

238. Genco, R.J., Taichman, N.A., and Sadowski, C.A.: Precipitating antibodies to *Actinobacillus actinomycetemcomitans* in localized juvenile periodontitis, J. Dent. Res. **59A:**329, 1980.

239. Lai, C.-H., and Listgarten, M.A.: Circulating antibody titers to *Actinobacillus actinomycetemcomitans* in patients with periodontal disease, J. Dent. Res. **59A:**513, 1980.

240. Murray, P.A., and Genco, R.J.: Serum and gingival fluid antibodies to *Actinobacillus actinomycetemcomitans* in localized juvenile periodontitis, J. Dent. Res. **59A:**329, 1980.

241. Listgarten, M.A., Lai, C.-H., and Evian, C.I.: Comparative antibody titers to *Actinobacillus actinomycetemcomitans* in juvenile periodontitis, chronic periodontitis and periodontally healthy subjects, J. Clin. Periodontol. **8:**155, 1981.

242. Baehni, P., et al.: Interaction of inflammatory cells and oral microorganisms. VIII. Detection of leukotoxic activity of a plaque-derived gram-negative microorganism, Infect. Immun. **24:**233, 1979.

243. Irving, J.T., et al.: Histologic changes in experimental periodontal disease in rats monoinfected with a gram-negative organism, Arch. Oral Biol. **20:**217, 1975.

244. Haffajee, A.D., et al.: Multidisciplinary research in periodontal diseases. I. Clinical and microbiological findings, J. Dent. Res. **62:**197, 1983.

245. Coykendall, A.L., Kaczmarek, F.S., and Slots, J.: Genetic heterogeneity in *Bacteroides asaccharolyticus* (Holdeman and Moore 1970) Finegold and Barnes (1977) (Approved Lists, 1980) and proposal of *Bacteroides gingivalis* sp. nov., and *Bacteroides macacae* (Slots and Genco), Int. J. System. Bacteriol. **30:**559, 1980.

246. Moore, W.E.C., et al.: Comparative bacteriology of juvenile periodontitis, Infect. Immun. **48:**507, 1985.

247. Crawford, A.C.R., et al.: Pathogenicity testing of oral isolates in gnotobiotic rats, J. Dent. Res. **56B:**120, 1977.

248. Svanberg, G.K., Syed, S.A., and Scott, B.W., Jr.: Relationship of subgingival plaque organisms to the severity of periodontal disease in beagles, J. Dent. Res. **59A:**387, 1980.

249. Ebersole, J.L., et al.: Human immune responses to periodontal organisms: *Capnocytophaga* and *Wolinella,* J. Dent. Res. **60A:**497, 1981.

250. Johnson, D.A., et al.: Role of bacterial products in periodontitis: immune response in gnotobiotic rats monoinfected with *Eikenella corrodens,* Infect. Immun. **19:**246, 1978.

251. Irving, J.T., Socransky, S.S., and Tanner, A.C.R.: Histological changes in experimental periodontal disease in rats monoinfected with gram-negative organisms, J. Periodont. Res. **13:**326, 1978.

252. Tanner, A.C.R.: A study of the bacteria associated with advancing periodontitis in man, Ph.D. Thesis, 1981, University of London.

253. Dick, D.S., Shaw, J.H., and Socransky, S.S.: Further studies on the microbial agent or agents responsible for the periodontal syndrome in the rice rat, Arch. Oral Biol. **13:**215, 1968.

254. Kelstrup, J., and Gibbons, R.J.: Induction of dental caries and alveolar bone loss by a human isolate resembling *Streptococcus salivarius,* Caries Res. **4:**360, 1970.

255. Irving, J.T., Socransky, S.S., and Heeley, J.D.: Histologic changes in experimental periodontal disease in gnotobiotic rats and conventional hamsters, J. Periodont. Res. **9:**73, 1974.

256. Scherp, H.: Current concepts in periodontal research: epidemiological contributions, J. Am. Dent. Assoc. **68:**667, 1964.

257. Russell, A.L.: Epidemiology of periodontal disease, Int. Dent. J. **17:**282, 1967.

258. Axelsson, P., and Lindhe, J.: Effect of controlled oral hygiene procedures on caries and

periodontal disease in adults, J. Clin. Periodontol. **5:**133, 1978.

259. Axelsson, P. and Lindhe, J.: The significance of maintenance care in the treatment of periodontal disease, J. Clin. Periodontol. **8:**281, 1981.

260. Löe, H., et al.: The natural history of periodontal disease in man: the rate of periodontal destruction before 40 years of age, J. Periodontol. **49:**607, 1978.

261. Saxe, S.R., et al.: Oral debris, calculus and periodontal disease in the beagle dog, Periodontics **5:**217, 1967.

262. Socransky, S.S., et al.: New concepts of destructive periodontal disease, J. Clin. Periodontol. **11:**21, 1984.

263. Goodson, J.M., et al.: Patterns of progression and regression of advanced destructive periodontal disease, J. Clin. Periodontol. **9:**472, 1982.

264. Haffajee, A.D., Socransky, S.S., and Goodson, J.M.: Comparison of different data analyses for detecting changes in attachment level, J. Clin. Periodontol. **10:**513, 1983.

265. Goodson, J.M., et al.: Evidence for episodic periodontal disease activity, J. Dent. Res. **60A:**387, 1981.

266. McHenry, K.R., et al. [125]I absorptiometry: alveolar bone mass measurements in untreated periodontal patients, J. Dent. Res. **60A:**387, 1981.

267. Hausmann, E., and McHenry, K.R.: Alveolar bone mass measurements by [125]I absorptiometry in untreated periodontal patients. In Menczel, et al., editors: Osteoporosis, New York, 1982, John Wiley & Sons, pp., 126-131.

268. Selikowitz, H-S., et al.: Retrospective longitudinal study of the rate of alveolar bone loss in humans using bite-wing radiographs, J. Clin. Periodontol. **8:**431, 1981.

269. Moskow, B.S.: Spontaneous arrest of advanced periodontal disease without treatment: an interesting case, J. Periodontol. **49:**465, 1978.

270. Jeffcoat, M.K., Kaplan, M.L., and Goldhaber, P.: Predicting alveolar bone loss in beagles using bone-seeking radiopharmaceutical uptake, J. Dent. Res. **59:**844, 1980.

271. Listgarten, M.A., and Levin, S.: Positive correlation between the proportions of subgingival spirochetes and motile bacteria and susceptibility of human subjects to periodontal deterioration, J. Clin. Periodontol. **8:**122, 1981.

272. Listgarten, M.A., et al.: Comparative longitudinal study of two methods of scheduling maintenance visits: two-year data, J. Clin. Periodontol. **13:**692, 1986.

273. Hausmann, E., Ortman, L.F., and Sedransk, N.: Experimental alveolar bone loss in the monkey evaluated by [125]I absorptiometry, Calc. Tissue Int. **29:**133, 1979.

274. Lindhe, J., and Ericsson, I.: Effect of ligature placement and dental plaque on periodontal tissue breakdown in the dog, J. Periodontol. **49:**343, 1979.

275. Rifkin, B.R., and Heijl, L.: The occurrence of mononuclear cells at sites of osteoclastic bone resorption in experimental periodontitis, J. Periodontol. **50:**636, 1979.

276. Hurt, W.C.: Periodontal diagnosis—1977, J. Periodontol. **48:**533, 1977.

277. Hancock, E.B.: Determination of periodontal disease activity, J. Periodontol. **52:**492, 1981.

278. Listgarten, M.A.: Periodontal probing: What does it mean? J. Clin. Periodontol. **7:**165, 1980.

279. Haffajee, A.D., Socransky, S.S., and Goodson, J.M.: Clinical parameters as predictors of destructive periodontal disease activity, J. Clin. Periodontol. **10:**527, 1983.

280. Dunham, S.L., et al.: Failure of darkfield microbiologic parameters to predict periodontal disease activity at periodontal sites, J. Dent. Res. **64A:**359, 1985.

281. Listgarten, M.A.: A perspective on periodontal diagnosis, J. Clin. Periodontol. **13:**175, 1986.

282. Dzink, J.L., et al.: Gram negative species associated with active destructive periodontal lesions, J. Clin. Periodontol. **12:**648, 1985.

283. Mandell, R.L.: A longitudinal microbiological investigation of *Actinobacillus actinomycetemcomitans* and *Eikenella corrodens* in juvenile periodontitis, Infect. Immun. **45:**778, 1984.

284. Frank, R.M., and Voegel, J.C.: Bacterial bone resorption in advanced cases of human periodontitis, J. Periodontol Res. **13:**251, 1978.

285. Allenspach-Petrzilka, G.E., and Guggenheim, B.: *Bacteroides melaninogenicus* subspecies *intermedius* invades rat gingival tissue, J. Dent. Res. **61:**259, 1982.

286. Fillery, E.D., and Pekovic, D.D.: Identification of microorganisms in immunopathological mechanisms on human gingivitis, J. Dent. Res. **61:**253, 1982.

287. Gillett, R., and Johnson, N.W.: Bacterial invasion of the periodontium in a case of juvenile periodontitis, J. Clin. Periodontol. **9:**93, 1982.

288. Newman, M.G., Saglie, R., and Carranza, F.A.: Pocket epithelium–associated plaque in human periodontal disease, J. Dent. Res. **61:**290, 1982.

289. Saglie, F., et al.: Identification of tissue-invading bacteria in human periodontal disease, J. Periodont. Res. **17:**452, 1982.

290. Sanavi, F., et al.: The colonization and establishment of invading bacteria in periodontium of ligature-treated immunosuppressed rats, J. Periodontol. **56:**273, 1985.

291. Slots, J., et al.: Periodontal therapy in humans. I. Microbiological and clinical effects

of a single course of periodontal scaling and root planing, and of adjunctive tetracycline therapy, J. Periodontol. **50:**495, 1979.

292. Slots, J., et al.: In vitro antimicrobial susceptibility of *Actinobacillus actinomycetemcomitans,* Antimicrob. Agents Chemother. **18:**9, 1980.

293. Walker, C.B., et al.: In vitro susceptibilities of bacteria from human periodontal pockets to 13 antimicrobial agents. In Nelson, J.D., and Grassi, C., editors: vol. 1, Current chemotherapy and infectious disease, Washington, D.C., 1980, American Society for Microbiology, pp. 508-511.

294. Gordon, J.M., et al.: Sensitive assay for measuring tetracyline levels in gingival crevice fluid, Antimicrob. Agents Chemother. **17:** 193, 1980.

295. Gordon, J.M.: et al.: Concentration of tetracyline in human gingival fluid after single doses. J. Clin. Periodontol. **8:**117, 1981.

296. Gordon, J.M., et al.: Tetracycline: levels achievable in gingival crevice fluid and *in vitro* effect on subgingival organisms. I. Concentrations in crevicular fluid after repeated doses, J. Periodontol. **52:**609, 1981.

297. Hillman, J.D., and Socransky, S.S.: Bacterial interference in the oral ecology of *Actinobacillus actinomycetemcomitans* and its relationship to human periodontosis, Arch. Oral Biol. **27:**75, 1982.

## ADDITIONAL SELECTED READING

Listgarten, M.A., et al.: Failure of a microbial assay to reliably predict disease recurrence in a treated periodontitis population receiving regularly scheduled prophylaxes, J. Clin. Periodontol. **13:**768, 1986.

Slots, J.: Bacterial specificity in adult periodontitis—a summary of recent work, J. Clin. Periodontol. **13:**912, 1986.

Slots, J., and Genco, R.J.: Black-pigmented *Bacteroides* species, *Capnocytophaga* species, and *Actinobacillus actinomycetemcomitans* in human periodontal disease: virulence factors in colonization, survival and tissue destruction, J. Dent. Res. **63:**412, 1984.

Slots, J., et al.: The occurrence of *Actinobacillus actinomycetemcomitans, Bacteroides gingivalis* and *Bacteroides intermedius* in destructive periodontal disease in adults, J. Clin. Periodontol. **13:**570, 1986.

# CHAPTER 9

# Calculus

**Classification**
Supragingival calculus
Subgingival calculus
Similarities and dissimilarities

**Formation**
Mode of attachment
Mineralization
Theories of mineralization
Deficiencies in proposed hypotheses
Inhibition with drugs

**Conclusion**

---

The role of calcified and uncalcified plaque on teeth as a primary etiologic factor in inflammatory periodontal disease has been demonstrated by epidemiologic, experimental, and clinical research.[1-12] Dental plaque has been demonstrated to be the major initiating factor in the development of gingivitis, but the presence of dental calculus is of equal concern to the therapist. These hard deposits play a role in maintaining and promoting the formation of plaque.[6,7,9,12-14] Soft deposits have been discussed in detail. This chapter will be concerned with dental calculus.

**Definition**    When dental plaque calcifies, the resulting deposit is called dental calculus. These calcified deposits occur as hard, firmly adhering masses on the clinical crowns* of teeth. They may also form on dentures and other oral appliances. The surface of dental calculus is always covered with uncalcified plaque. This coating consists of microorganisms of many types, desquamated epithelial cells, and leukocytes that have migrated through the sulcular epithelium, all held together by a sticky matrix.

What is the significance of calculus in periodontal disease? (1) Calculus is rough, porous,[15,16] and facilitates the retention of dental plaque with which it is always covered. (2) Calculus is permeable and may adsorb and absorb toxic products. Therefore calculus may be harmful both physically and chemically to the adjacent gingiva. Where calculus contacts the gingiva, the gingiva is inflamed.[1,17] Experience has shown that the removal of calculus reduces or eliminates gingival inflammation. Consequently the clinician must be versed in the art of calculus removal and the smoothing of root surfaces by careful instrumentation. The intimate relationship of the calcified deposit to the tooth (Figs. 9-1 and 9-2) must be fully appreciated by the dentist.[16,18]

---

*The clinical crown is the part of the tooth exposed to the oral cavity, including the tooth wall of the pocket.

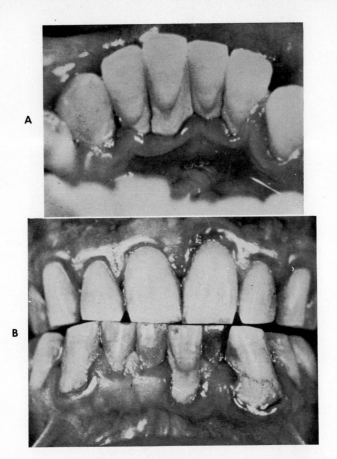

**Fig. 9-1.** **A,** Supragingival calculus on the oral (lingual) surface of the mandibular anterior teeth. **B,** Large masses of supragingival calculus on the vestibular (labial) surfaces of the mandibular anterior teeth.

## Classification

With the free gingival margin as a reference, calculus may be classified clinically as supragingival or subgingival. This classification refers to the location of the calculus at the time of examination.

### SUPRAGINGIVAL CALCULUS

Supragingival deposits are usually most abundant opposite the openings of major salivary glands, that is, on the oral surfaces of the lower anterior teeth and the vestibular surfaces of the upper first molars. Most adults acquire varying amounts of supragingival calculus. Inadequate oral hygiene, malposition of teeth, rough surfaces, or existing deposits favor the deposition of this material. Supragingival calculus usually is creamy white or yellowish in color (Fig. 9-1) unless it is stained by tobacco or other pigments. The consistency varies from moderately to very hard. Recurrence after removal may be rapid in some individuals.

### SUBGINGIVAL CALCULUS

Subgingival calculus may be found in periodontal pockets on any tooth in the mouth. However, subgingival calculus is most often found on the approximal surfaces and with less frequency on the buccal surfaces.[1,17] These deposits are more dense than supragingival calculus. Old subgingival calculus may be harder than cementum or

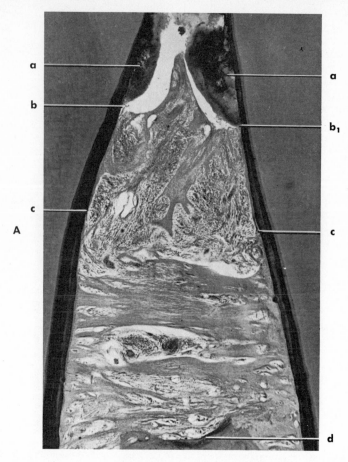

**Fig. 9-2.** **A,** Interdental space showing large masses of supragingival and subgingival calculus. The deposits extend to the bottom of the pockets. *a,* Calculus; *b* and *b₁,* bottom of the pocket; *c,* apical end of the junctional epithelium; *d,* alveolar crest. Note the inflammatory infiltrate in the subjacent connective tissue.

dentin.[19] It is usually dark brown to black and is found as a concretion on the tooth within the gingival sulcus or periodontal pocket. The extent of its deposition approximates the depth of the pocket. Deposits always extend to the base of the pocket, but the most apical part is always uncalcified plaque. This is demonstrated by microscopic studies[20] (Fig. 9-2). The space often seen in microscopic specimens between the deposit and the soft tissue wall of the pocket is an artifact caused by shrinkage during preparation for microscopic observation.

## SIMILARITIES AND DISSIMILARITIES

Supragingival calculus and subgingival calculus, although similar in their histology, chemistry, and microbiology,[21-24] exhibit differences[15] and some of their constituents are probably derived from different sources. It is likely that supragingival calculus has elements derived from saliva, whereas subgingival calculus has elements derived from gingival pocket exudate and saliva.[23,28-38]

**Morphology of subgingival calculus**

Subgingival calculus may take the following forms:

1. Crusty, spiny, or nodular (Fig. 9-3, *A*)
2. Ringlike or ledgelike formations encircling the tooth (Fig. 9-3, *B*)
3. Veneer type consisting of a thin, glassy, smooth layer
4. Fingerlike or fernlike extensions toward the bottom of the pocket (Fig. 9-3, *C* and *D*)

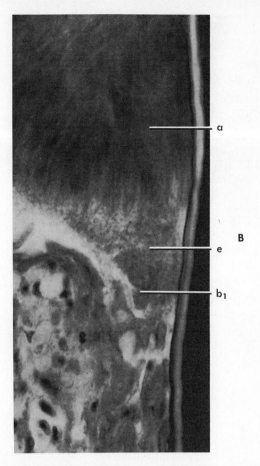

**Fig. 9-2, cont'd.    B,** *Higher magnification of the bottom of the pocket (b₁ in **A**). The unmineralized surface layer of plaque (e) extends to the bottom of the pocket. The pocket epithelium is extremely thin and shows transmigrating inflammatory cells. The space is an artifact resulting from shrinkage of tissue during histologic preparation.*

5. Individual islands or spots
6. Combinations of these forms

As the gingiva recedes, subgingival deposits may become supragingival and may be covered by the supragingival variety.

Subgingival calcified deposits are often seen in roentgenograms as irregularly shaped nodules or as ledges (Figs. 9-4 and 9-5). They do not indicate the depth of the pocket because the most apical part of the calculus may not be calcified enough to be radio-opaque. Supragingival calculus presents a somewhat different view radiographically (Fig. 9-6). The presence of calculus can be diagnosed from the x ray. Its absence cannot be confirmed by x ray because only a profile of the tooth is seen, and only well-calcified deposits of sufficient bulk are readily discernible. Old deposits, particularly of the subgingival type, sometimes have a radiopacity similar to that of tooth structure (Figs. 9-4 and 9-5). **Appearance of calculus in roentgenogram**

Dental calculus has been studied by chemical and physical analytic methodology (histochemistry, polarization microscopy, spectroscopy, x-ray diffraction,[27,39-46] and neutron activation analysis.[39,40] Since calculus is calcified plaque, the composition of its organic fraction[37,38,41,47,48] (Fig. 9-7) corresponds to that of dental plaque.

The inorganic components consist mainly of calcium and phosphates with small amounts of magnesium and carbonate. Traces of numerous other elements may also be found.[23,27,39,40] **Inorganic components**

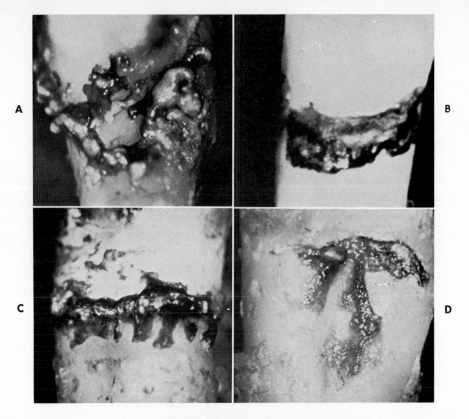

**Fig. 9-3.** Different forms of subgingival calculus. **A,** Nodular deposit on ring. **B,** Ringlike deposit. **C,** Fingerlike deposit on ring. **D,** Fernlike deposit.

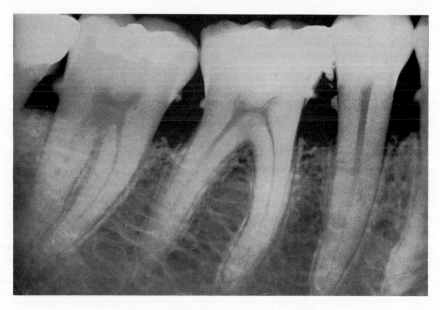

**Fig. 9-4.** Ledgelike subgingival calculus.

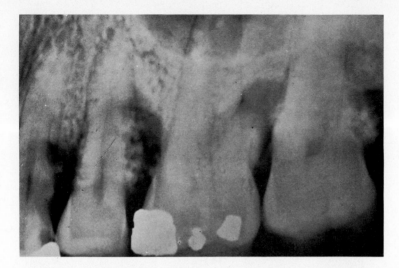

**Fig. 9-5.**   Heavy, nodular subgingival calculus deposits. Submarginal calculus may sometimes reach an opacity exceeding that of the tooth substance; this signifies a thoroughly calcified and probably old deposit.

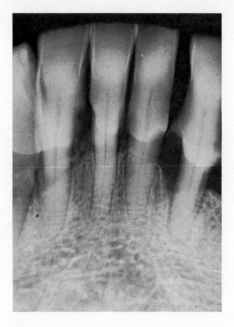

**Fig. 9-6.**   Radiograph of supragingival calculus, with a scalloped outline. The marginal gingiva fits around the deposits which extend to or close to the bottom of the pockets.


Most of the inorganic components are present in various types of calcium phosphate crystals. The principal types found are hydroxyapatite ($Ca_{10}[PO_4]_6$ $[OH]_2$), whitlockite ($Ca_{21}[PO_4]_{14}$), octocalcium phosphate ($Ca_8H_2[PO_4]_6, 6H_2O$), and brushite ($CaHPO_4 \cdot 2H_2O$).[18,26,27] Whereas brushite is the simple secondary calcium phosphate crystal, the other types mentioned have complex crystal lattices.

A compositional analysis of the percentage of inorganic constituents for calculus is surprisingly similar to that of other hard tissues of the body, although the sources of the minerals may vary.[32]

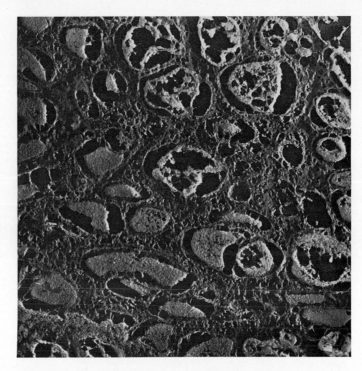

**Fig. 9-7.** Electron micrograph of decalcified calculus. The round ovoid structures are crosscut microorganisms. The interbacterial matrix is evident. (×26,000.) (Courtesy J. Theilade, Aarhus, Denmark, and M.U. Nylen and D.B. Scott, Bethesda, Maryland.)

## Formation

The formation of calculus has been studied by the examination of deposits of known age collected on plastic strips fastened temporarily to the teeth of calculus formers[46,49-54] (Fig. 9-8). The formation of calculus can be divided into three phases: (1) the initial attachment of bacteria to a tooth via the salivary pellicle, (2) the growth and organization of plaque, and (3) the mineralization of plaque. The first two stages were discussed in the chapters on saliva and microbiology.

Understanding the mode of attachment of well-established calculus is important for the successful removal of calculus during treatment and for subsequent maintenance (Figs. 9-9 and 9-10).

### MODE OF ATTACHMENT

Investigations by light and electron microscopy have revealed various modes of attachment of calculus to enamel, cementum, and exposed dentin[51,52,54-60]: (1) The calculus attachment may be mediated through an organic pellicle or cuticle.[61] This type of attachment seems to predominate on enamel and is also observed when calculus forms on plastic strips; it occurs only infrequently on cementum. (2) Calculus may be attached directly to the tooth surface through the organic calculus matrix adherent to the tooth surface or penetrating into cementum. (3) Finally, the attachment may occur by calculus matrix penetrating surface irregularities such as cracks, resorption lacunae, and carious defects.[56]

In experiments performed with plastic strips, the mineralization of the plaque starts when the deposit is from 1 to a few days old (Figs. 9-8 and 9-11, *A* and *B*). Concomitantly with the onset of mineralization, histochemical changes occur in isolated areas

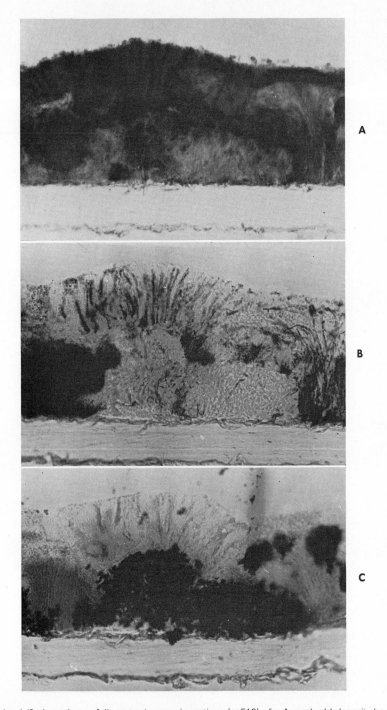

**Fig. 9-8.**   *Undecalcified specimen. Adjacent microscopic sections (×510) of a 4-week-old deposit show areas of mineralization and nonmineralization that have been stained as follows:* **A,** *Hematoxylin and eosin stain. Note the morphology of the deposit.* **B,** *Gram stain for bacteria. Note organisms circumscribing central area of mineralization.* **C,** *von Kossa stain to visualize areas of mineralization. A polyester strip had been ligated to a tooth and was removed after 4 weeks to study calculus deposition. (Courtesy S.P. Hazen, Washington, D.C.)*

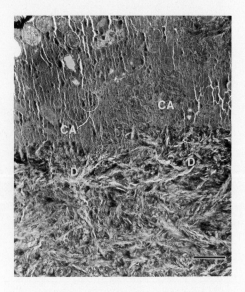

**Fig. 9-9.** Calculus *(CA)* in immediate contact with dentin *(D)*, exposed following root planing. Calcified bacteria appear as circular profiles. The accretion contains crystals that are smaller and more densely packed than those of the dentin. The intimate connection between calculus and underlying hard tissue can be seen. (×9000.) (From Selvig, K.A.: J. Periodont. Res. **5:**8, 1970.)

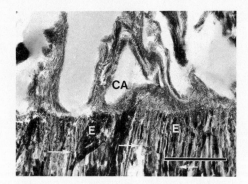

**Fig. 9-10.** Calculus *(CA)* attached to enamel *(E)*. Small crystals, similar to those in the accretion, can be seen between the larger crystals of the enamel to the depth indicated by arrows. (×16,000.) (From Selvig, K.A.: J. Periodont. Res. **5:**8, 1970.)

in the plaque, usually close to the tooth surface.[49,52,62] Before mineralization, structural changes of the intermicrobial matrix have been observed ultrastructurally.*

## MINERALIZATION

The minerals deposited may be observed in ground sections. Two modes of mineralization, type A and type B centers, have been distinguished ultrastructurally (Figs. 9-11 and 9-12). Type A mineralization centers are formed only in the presence and in association with microorganisms. Type B mineralization centers are apparently not related to microorganisms but have at least one common border with the Type A centers and included microorganisms.[64] Matrix can be demonstrated.[18] In the electron microscope the individual crystals appear as needlelike structures from 5 to 10 μm long (Figs. 9-9 to 9-13). In addition, platelike and ribbonlike crystals may be seen. The

---

*See references 18, 24, 50, 53, 58, and 63.

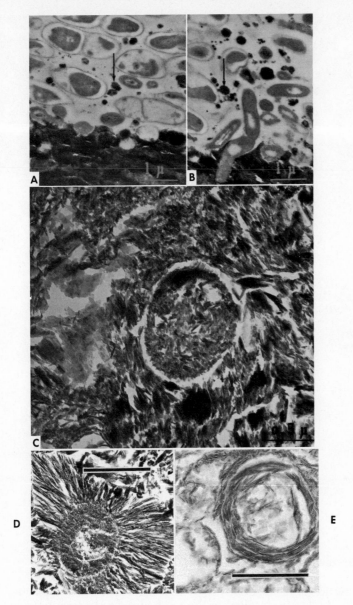

**Fig. 9-11.** **A,** and **B,** Electron micrographs of the surface of calculus; unmineralized plaque is seen toward the top of the illustrations. **C,** Electron micrograph of old calculus from which the organic matrix has been removed. Note the crystals of varying form and size outside as well as inside the round structure in the middle of the illustration, which represents a crosscut mineralized microorganism. ($\times 43,500$.) **D,** Microorganisms permeated with needle-shaped crystals in type B centers of mineralization. **E,** Microorganisms surrounded by a ring of platelet-shaped crystals oriented along the former cell membrane. (**A** and **B** courtesy J. Theilade, Aarhus, Denmark; **C** courtesy J. Theilade, Aarhus, Denmark, and M.U. Nylen and D.B. Scott, Bethesda, Maryland; **D** and **E** courtesy H.E. Schroeder, Zurich, Switzerland.)

specific type of calcium phosphate that these crystals represent has not yet been determined.[18] Scanning electron microscopy confirms two calcification patterns.[65] The crystals associated with type A have been identified as hydroxyapatite by x-ray diffraction. It is speculated that the crystal patterns in type B centers may be other forms such as octocalcium phosphate, whitlockite, and brushite. Mineralization of plaque microorganisms may occur at intracellular or extracellular sites.[22,66,67]

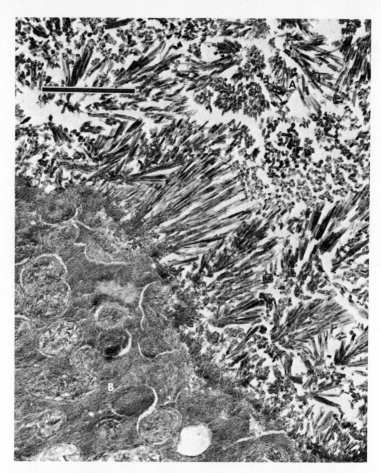

**Fig. 9-12.**  Borders show A and B types of centers of mineralization in old supragingival calculus (from which the organic material has been extracted with ethylenediamine). The B center in the right upper corner consists of hexagonal crystal columns, which grow in lanciform bunches. The A center in the lower left is densely packed with small needle-shaped or in part platelet-shaped crystals, including calcified microorganisms. (×31,000.) (From Schroeder, H.E.: Formation and inhibition of dental calculus, Berne, 1971, Hans Huber Medical Publisher.)

## THEORIES OF MINERALIZATION

There is no general agreement on the factors responsible for the deposition of inorganic salts in plaque attached to the tooth surface. Various hypotheses have emphasized the following:

1. Metabolism and degeneration of plaque bacteria[22,66-70]
2. Loss of carbon dioxide from saliva at the time of its secretion[23,71]
3. Epitaxis[21,71-73]

**Bacterial theory**

The role of bacteria in the formation of calculus may include microbial metabolic products, which produce local changes leading to the deposition of calcium salts or to physical characteristics favoring crystal nucleation.[73]

The finding of calculus in germ-free animals argues against a primary role for bacteria in the formation of calculus[74-80] but does not exclude other mechanisms for calculus deposition in which bacteria participate.

**$CO_2$ theory**

Saliva in the major salivary ducts is secreted at a high $CO_2$ tension, about 54 to 65 mm Hg, whereas the $CO_2$ pressure in atmospheric air is only about 0.3 mm Hg. Saliva emerging from the salivary ducts is believed to lose $CO_2$ to the atmosphere as a result

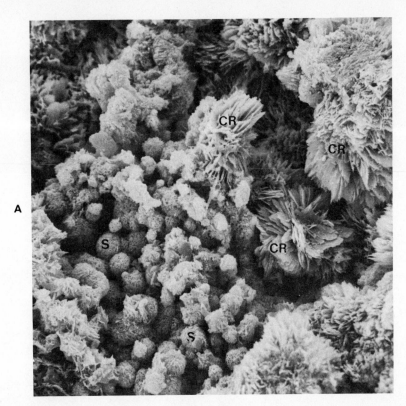

**Fig. 9-13.    A,** Configuration of platelet or needlelike crystal growths (CR) bordering a cluster of spheric growths (S). (×500.)                                                                                                     *Continued.*

of this large difference in $CO_2$ tension. Since the pH in saliva depends largely on the ratio between bicarbonate and free carbonic acid, the pH in saliva will increase when $CO_2$ escapes. Furthermore, the dissociation of phosphoric acid increases with a rise in alkalinity so that the concentration of less soluble secondary and tertiary phosphate ions increases. This increase in phosphate ions presumably leads to a situation in which the solubility product of calcium phosphate is exceeded and crystals form. Carbonic anhydrase, present in the saliva, may be one of the biochemical mechanisms of this reaction.[70]

**Epitaxis theory**

According to another hypothesis, calculus formation may be initiated through epitaxis by organic complexes in the matrix. Epitaxis refers to crystal formation (e.g., hydroxyapatite) through seeding by another compound not identified with it. The second compound has a special molecular configuration that is similar to the crystal lattice of hydroxyapatite so that calcium salts precipitate onto it from the metastable solution in saliva. The organic matrix of plaque is assumed to provide sites with molecular configurations capable of inducing an oriented precipitation of a hydroxyapatite not requiring the solubility product for hydroxyapatite to be surpassed.[72] Although this hypothesis was first advanced in the 1950s, it remains unproved. Other reports point to a more likely seeding of hydroxyapatite by transformation from brushite and octocalcium phosphate.[18,21,27]

Hydroxyapatite does not crystalize spontaneously in the saliva of patients with cystic fibrosis or in the saliva of light and heavy calculus formers. Although plaque is constantly bathed in saliva, there is no evidence that preformed mineral is present in saliva and can be deposited in plaque.

Attention has also been centered around the significance of the lipid component

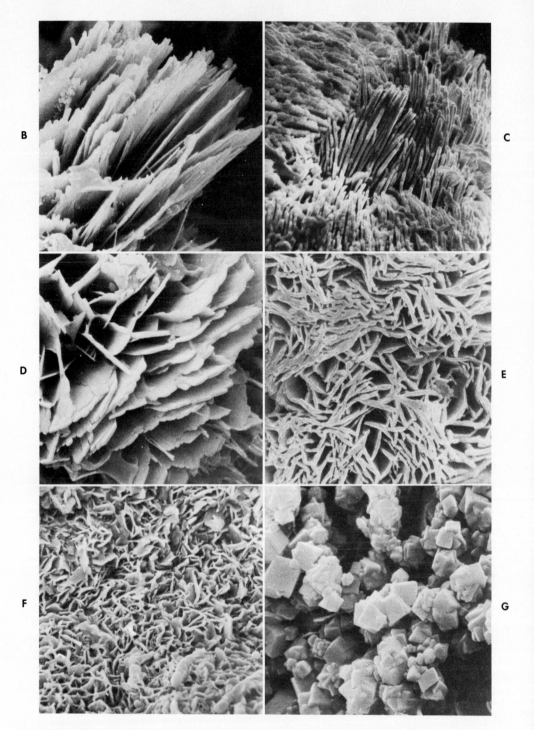

**Fig. 9-13, cont'd.** **B** to **G,** Various forms of crystal growths: **B** and **C,** Needlelike shapes or elongated shapes. **D** to **F,** Different shapes and sizes of platelet forms. (× 5000.) **G,** Cuboidal crystals. (× 10,000.) (From Lustmann, J., Lewin-Epstein, J., and Shteyer, A.: Calcif. Tissue Res. **21:**47, 1976.)

of the organic matrix for the mineralization of plaque, since in vitro experiments with decalcified calculus reveal that extraction of the lipid component prevents remineralization of the calculus matrix.[81]

Finally it is possible that mineralization may be promoted by increased concentrations of phosphate in the immediate environment where calculus formation starts. A number of phosphatases have been described both in saliva as well as gingival sulcular fluid.[35] The neutrophils, which are continuously migrating into the gingival sulcus of inflamed gingiva, are known to possess both acid and alkaline phosphatase activity. The enzyme activity could theoretically raise the local phosphate levels sufficiently to cause calcium phosphate precipitation. It has been reported that calculus formation is positively correlated with the level of certain salivary enzymes, including esterase and phosphatase activity.[82] The esterified mucin could bind available calcium ions and phosphate to form a "seeded" mucin that could promote calculus formation.

## DEFICIENCIES IN PROPOSED HYPOTHESES

The foregoing theories not only lack qualitative confirmation and demonstration of their quantitative importance but also fail to account for the distribution of calculus in the population and the preferential sites for the deposition of supragingival calculus in the oral cavity. Additionally, the question remains why many children[83] and some adults are free of calculus.

Dental plaque is almost always found on teeth, yet supragingival calculus forms most extensively near the orifices of the salivary gland ducts.[84,85] The bacterial theory does not explain this preferential location of supragingival calculus, whereas the $CO_2$ theory readily explains it.

Location of calculus

Whereas calculus may promote the onset and progression of plaque-associated periodontal diseases, it is also likely that the inflammation of the tissues may predispose to the formation of subgingival calculus—for example, through the increased concentration of phosphatase activity in the inflamed sulci and pockets. This mechanism might explain why subgingival calculus may originate throughout the mouth, wherever gingival inflammation occurs, whereas supragingival calculus tends to be related to the orifices of the major salivary glands.

There are few chemical and no bacterial studies in which calculus-immune and calculus-susceptible persons are compared.[86] Saliva from calculus-free and calculus-susceptible individuals has been analyzed for calcium, inorganic phosphate, protein, and pH.[87] The only statistically demonstrable difference is the higher concentration of calcium in the saliva of individuals who form calculus. Rapid calculus formers have more phosphorus and less potassium than the average amount in newly formed deposits. Mineralization is followed by an increase in calcium and phosphorus and a decrease in the proportion of potassium.[88,89] Individuals with a high viscosity of saliva seem to have a lower calculus formation rate than do those with a low viscosity.[18]

Calculus-free versus calculus-susceptible individuals

The relegation of calculus to the scientific "ash heap" is inconsistent with the fact that there are differences in the calcium and phosphorus levels of calculus produced by heavy and light formers. Mineralization appears to be associated with loss of carbohydrates. The heavy formers have higher levels of calcium and phosphorus and lower levels of potassium, methylpentose, and hexosamine than the light formers.[86,89]

## INHIBITION WITH DRUGS

Prevention or suppression of calculus formation by means of chemicals has often been attempted.[90-102] Complexing drugs such as hexametaphosphate or chelating agents have been recommended for the control of calculus formation.[98] Of the so-called calculus solvents, many are nothing more than dilute (and sometimes not so dilute) acids. Since composition of calculus closely resembles that of the calcified structures of teeth, destruction of teeth is inevitable when acids are applied. Of the calculus solvents, both sodium hexametaphosphate and the chelating agents should probably be considered skeptically for similar reasons.[30]

**Antimicrobial agents**

Since the microbial plaque provides the bulk of the organic matrix in calculus, a number of antimicrobial compounds have been tested for their capacity to reduce plaque formation or to inhibit its mineralization.[18,90-100] Enzyme preparations have been employed to liberate the inorganic constituents of calculus by degradation of the organic matrix or to inhibit the formation of the matrix necessary for mineralization.[95,97] Similarly, experiments designed to reduce calculus formation through the application of a crystal growth inhibitor have been performed.[101,102]

In fact, a reduction in calculus formation may not greatly benefit the state of gingival health, unless there is an accompanying alteration in the local microbiota that is compatible with gingival health. Chemical inhibition of plaque is discussed further in Chapter 31.

## Conclusion

Clinicians have observed that patients with periodontal disease who form calculus have progressively less trouble from these deposits if they follow a regimen of good oral hygiene and regular recall care. This improvement seems to result primarily from improved plaque control by toothbrushing and flossing. A change in the oral flora subsequent to the improved oral hygiene may also result and may be significant.

Removal of calculus is beneficial, first, because calculus acts as a retentive site for microbial plaque and interferes with the regular removal of plaque by the patient as part of normal plaque control measures. This calculus removal serves both a preventive goal as well as a necessary step in the initiation of therapy. The second benefit of calculus removal is related to therapeutic measures aimed at gaining new attachment. For new attachment to occur a calculus-free surface is essential and thorough calculus removal must be accomplished through the use of nonsurgical or surgical therapeutic procedures, or both.

Calcification of dental plaque can be demonstrated if the material is left undisturbed in the mouth for as short a time as 1 day. If the plaque is removed from the teeth every day by brushing, the rate of formation of calculus can be reduced. The safest, most effective and practical method for calculus control is still optimal oral hygiene and appropriately timed prophylaxes.

**REFERENCES**

1. Lövdal, A., Arno, A., and Waerhaug, J.: Incidence of clinical manifestations of periodontal disease in light of oral hygiene and calculus formation, J. Am. Dent. Assoc. **56:**21, 1958.
2. Schei, O., et al.: Alveolar bones loss as related to oral hygiene and age, J. Periodontol. **30:**7, 1959.
3. Theilade, J., and Schroeder, H.E.: Recent results in dental calculus research, Int. Dent. J. **16:**205, 1966.
4. Löe, H., Theilade, E., and Jensen, S.B.: Experimental gingivitis in man, J. Periodontol. **36:**177, 1965.
5. Theilade, E., et al.: Experimental gingivitis in man. II. A longitudinal clinical and bacteriological investigation, J. Periodont. Res. **1:**1, 1966.
6. Russell, A.L.: International nutrition surveys: a summary of preliminary dental findings, J. Dent. Res. **42:**233, 1963.
7. Greene, J.C.: Periodontal disease in India: report of an epidemiological study, J. Dent. Res. **39:**302, 1960.
8. Ramfjord, S.P.: The periodontal status of boys 11 to 17 years old in Bombay, India, J. Periodontol. **32:**237, 1961.
9. Baumhammers, A., and Rohrbaugh, E.A.: Permeability of human and rat dental calculus, J. Periodontol. **41:**279, 1970.
10. Löe, H.: Epidemiology of periodontal disease. An evaluation of the relative significance of the etiological factors in the light of recent epidemiological research, Odont. Tidskr. **71:**479, 1963.
11. Lövdal, A., et al.: Combined effects of subgingival scaling and controlled oral hygiene on

the incidence of gingivitis, Acta Odontol. Scand. **19:**537, 1961.

12. Moskow, B.S., et al.: What is the role of subgingival calculus in the etiology and progression of periodontal disease? J. Periodontol. **41:**283, 1970.

13. Theilade, J., et al.: What is the relationship between bacterial plaque and calculus formation? Periodont. Abstr. **15:**53, 1967.

14. Allen, D.L., and Kerr, D.A.: Tissue response in the guinea pig to sterile and nonsterile calculus, J. Periodontol. **36:**121, 1965.

15. Friskopp, J., and Hammarström, L.: A comparative, scanning electron microscopic study of supragingival and subgingival calculus, J. Periodontol. **51:**553, 1980.

16. Jones, S.S.: Morphology of calculus on the human tooth surface, Proc. R. Soc. Med. **65:**903, 1972.

17. Alexander, A.G.: A study of the distribution of supra- and subgingival calculus, bacterial plaque and gingival inflammation in the mouth of 400 individuals, J. Periodontol. **42:**21, 1971.

18. Schroeder, H.E.: Formation and inhibition of dental calculus, Berne, 1969, Hans Huber Medical Publisher.

19. Rautiola, C.A., and Craig, R.G.: The microhardness of cementum and underlying dentin of normal teeth and teeth exposed to periodontal disease, J. Periodontol. **32:**113, 1961.

20. Orban, B., and Manella, V.B.: A macroscopic and microscopic study of instruments designed for root planing, J. Periodontol. **27:**120, 1956.

21. Barone, J.P., and Nancollas, G.H.: The seeded growth of calcium phosphates: the kinetics of growth of dicalcium phosphate dihydrate on enamel dentin and calculus, J. Dent. Res. **57:**153, 1978.

22. Ennever, J., Streckfuss, J.L., and Goldschmidt, M.D.: Calcifiability comparison among selected microorganisms, J. Dent. Res. **60:**1793, 1981.

23. Leung, S.W.: Calculus formation. Salivary factors, Dent. Clin. North Am., p. 723, Nov. 1960.

24. Friskopp, J.: Ultrastructure of nondecalcified supragingival and subgingival calculus, J. Periodontol. **54:**542, 1983.

25. Little, M.F., and Hazen, S.P.: Dental calculus composition. II. Subgingival calculus: ash, calcium, phosphorus, and sodium, J. Dent. Res. **43:**645, 1964.

26. Legeros, R.Z., and Shannon, I.L.: The crystalline components of dental calculi: human vs. dog, J. Dent. Res. **58:**2371, 1979.

27. Kani, T., et al.: Microbeam x-ray diffraction analysis of dental calculus, J. Periodontol. **62:**92, 1983.

28. Lundberg, M., Söremark, R., and Thilander, H.: Analysis of some elements in supra

and subgingival calculus, J. Periodont. Res. **1:**245, 1966.

29. Ruzicka, F.: Structure of sub- and supragingival dental calculus in human periodontitis: an electron microscopic study, J. Periodont. Res. **19:**317, 1984.

30. Everett, F.G.: Calculus, J. Dent. Hygienist Assoc. **30:**121, 1956.

31. Brill, N., and Krasse, B.: The passage of tissue fluid into the clinically healthy gingival pocket, Acta Odontol. Scand. **16:**233, 1958.

32. Waerhaug, J.: The source of mineral salts in subgingival calculus, J. Dent. Res. **34:**563, 1955.

33. Mandel, I.D.: Dental plaque: nature, formation and effects, J. Periodontol. **37:**357, 1966.

34. Salkind, A., Oshrain, H.I., and Mandel, I.D.: Observations on gingival pocket fluid, Periodontics **1:**196, 1963.

35. Cimasoni, G.: The crevicular fluid, Basel, Switzerland, 1974, S. Karger.

36. Mathis, H.: Der supragingivale Zahnstein, Dtsch. Zahn. Mund. Kieferheilkd. **5:**114, 1938.

37. Little, M.F., Casciani, C., and Lensky, S.: The organic matrix of dental calculus, J. Dent. Res. **40:**753, 1961.

38. Mandel, I.D., Hampar, B., and Ellison, S.A.: Carbohydrate components of supragingival salivary calculus, Proc. Soc. Exp. Biol. Med. **110:**301, 1962.

39. Retief, D.H., et al.: Quantitative analysis of Mg, Na, Cl, Al, and Ca in human dental calculus by neutron activation analysis and high-resolution gamma spectrometry, J. Dent. Res. **51:**807, 1972.

40. Retief, D.H., et al.: The quantitative analysis of Sb, Ag, Zn, Co, and Fe in human dental calculus by neutron activation analysis and high-resolution gamma spectrometry, J. Periodont. Res. **8:**263, 1973.

41. Mandel, I.D.: Histochemical and biochemical aspects of calculus formation, Periodontics **1:**43, 1963.

42. Little, M.G., Casciani, C.A., and Rowley, J.: Dental calculus composition. I. Supragingival calculus: ash, calcium, phosphorus, sodium, and density, J. Dent. Res. **42:**78, 1963.

43. Kinoshita, S., et al.: Origin of fluoride in early dental calculus, Helv. Odont. Acta **9:**141, 1965.

44. Grøn, P., Van Campen, G.J., and Lindström, I.: Human dental calculus: inorganic chemical and crystallographic composition, Arch. Oral Biol. **12:**829, 1967.

45. Grøn, P., and Van Campen, G.J.: Mineral composition of human dental calculus, Helv. Odont. Acta **11:**71, 1967.

46. Mandel, I.D., Levy, B.M., and Wasserman, B.H.: Histochemistry of calculus formation, J. Periodontol. **28:**132, 1957.

47. Stanford, J.W.: Analysis of the organic portion of dental calculus, J. Dent. Res. **45:**128, 1966.

48. Slomiany, B.L., et al.: Lipids of supragingival calculus, J. Periodontol. **63:**862, 1983.

49. Theilade, J.: Electron microscopic structure of calculus attachment to smooth surfaces, Acta Odontol. Scand. **22:**379, 1964.

50. Zander, H.A., Hazen, S.P., and Scott, D.B.: Mineralization of dental calculus, Proc. Soc. Exp. Biol. Med. **103:**257, 1960.

51. Mühlemann, H.R., and Schroeder, H.E.: Dynamics of supragingival calculus formation, Adv. Oral Biol. **1:**175, 1964.

52. Oshrain, H.I., Salkind, A., and Mandel, I.D.: A method for collection of subgingival plaque and calculus, J. Periodontol. **39:**322, 1968.

53. Schroeder, H.E., Lenz, H., and Mühlemann, H.R.: Microstructures and mineralization of early dental calculus, Helv. Odont. Acta **8:**1, 1964.

54. Canis, M.F., Kramer, G.M., and Pameijer, C.M.: Calculus attachment: review of the literature and new findings, J. Periodontol. **50:**406, 1979.

55. Mislowsky, W.J., and Mazzella, W.J.: Supragingival and subgingival plaque and calculus formation in humans, J. Periodontol. **45:**822, 1974.

56. Zander, H.A.: The attachment of calculus to root surfaces, J. Periodontol. **24:**16, 1953.

57. Voreadis, E.G., and Zander, H.A.: Cuticular calculus attachment, Oral Surg. **11:**1120, 1958.

58. Selvig, K.A.: Attachment of plaque and calculus to tooth surfaces, J. Periodont. Res. **5:**8, 1970.

59. Kopczyk, R.A., and Conroy, C.W.: The attachment of calculus to root planed surfaces, Periodontics **6:**78, 1968.

60. Moskow, B.S.: Calculus attachment in cemental separations, J. Periodontol. **40:**125, 1969.

61. Eide, B., Lie, T., and Selvig, K.A.: Surface coatings on dental cementum incident to periodontal disease. I. A scanning electron microscopic study, J. Clin. Periodontol. **10:**157, 1983.

62. Mühlemann, H.R., and Schneider, U.K.: Early calculus formation, Helv. Odont. Acta **3:**22, 1959.

63. Lustmann, J., and Shteyer, A.: Salivary calculi: ultrastructural morphology and bacterial etiology, J. Dent. Res. **60:**1386, 1981.

64. Takazoe, I., Kurahashi, Y., and Takuma, S.: Electron microscopy in intercellular mineralization of oral filamentous microorganisms in vitro, J. Dent. Res. **42:**681, 1963.

65. Lustmann, J., Lewin-Epstein, J., and Shteyer, A.: Scanning electron microscopy of dental calculus, Calcif. Tissue Res. **21:**47, 1976.

66. Sidaway, D.A.: A microbial study of dental calculus. IV. An electron microscopic study of in vitro calcified organisms, J. Periodont. Res. **15:**240, 1980.

67. Lie, T., and Selvig, K.A.: Calcification of oral bacteria: an ultrastructural study of two strains of *Bacterionema matruchotii*, Scand. J. Dent. Res. **82:**8, 1974.

68. Sidaway, D.A.: A microbiological study of dental calculus. I. The microbial flora of mature calculus, J. Periodont. Res. **13:**349, 1978.

69. Sidaway, D.A.: A microbiological study of dental calculus. II. The in vitro calcification of microorganisms from dental calculus, J. Periodont. Res. **13:**360, 1978.

70. Sidaway, D.A.: A microbiological study of dental calculus. III. A comparison of the in vitro calcification of viable and non-viable microorganisms, J. Periodont. Res. **14:**167, 1979.

71. Rapp, G.W.: The biochemistry of oral calculus. I. Conditions predisposing to oral calculus deposition, J. Am. Dent. Assoc. **32:**1368, 1945.

72. Takazoe, I., Vogel, J., and Ennever, J.: Calcium hydroxide apatite nucleation by lipid extract of *Bacterionema matruchotii*, J. Dent. Res. **49:**395, 1970.

73. Ennever, J., et al.: Characterization of calculus matrix calcification nucleator, J. Dent. Res. **58:**619, 1979.

74. Baer, P.N., and Newton, W.L.: The occurrence of periodontal disease in germfree mice, J. Dent. Res. **38:**1238, 1959.

75. Fitzgerald, R.J., and McDaniel, E.G.: Dental calculus in the germfree rat, Arch. Oral Biol. **2:**239, 1960.

76. Glas, J.E., and Krasse, B.: Biophysical studies on dental calculus from germfree and conventional rats, Acta Odontol. Scand. **20:**127, 1962.

77. Gustafsson, B.E., and Krasse, B.: Dental calculus in germfree rats, Acta Odontol. Scand. **20:**135, 1962.

78. Theilade, J., et al.: Electron microscopic observations of dental calculus in germfree and conventional rats, Arch. Oral Biol. **9:**97, 1964.

79. Listgarten, M.A., and Heneghan, J.B.: Observations on the periodontium and acquired pellicle of adult germ-free dogs, J. Periodontol. **44:**85, 1973.

80. Frank, R.M., and Voegel, J.C.: Etude ultrastructurale de dépôts calcifiés coronaires au niveau de molaire de rats gnotobiotes, J. Biol. Bucc. **3:**167, 1975.

81. Ennever, J., Vogel, J., and Benson, L.A.: Lipid and calculus matrix calcification in vitro, J. Dent. Res. **52:**1056, 1973.

82. Draus, F.J., Tarbet, W.J., and Miklos, F.L.: Salivary enzymes and calculus formation, J. Periodont. Res. **3:**232, 1968.

83. Everett, F.G., Tuchler, H., and Lu, K.H.: Occurrence of calculus in grade school children in Portland, Oregon, J. Periodontol. **34:**54, 1963.

84. Leung, S.W.: The uneven distribution of cal-

culus in the mouth, J. Periodontol. **22:**7, 1951.

85. Everett, F.G.: The uneven distribution of salivary calculus in the mouth, J. Periodontol. **27:**50, 1956.

86. Mandel, I.: Biochemical aspects of calculus formation. Comparative studies of plaque in heavy and light calculus formers, J. Periodont. Res. **9:**10; 211, 1974.

87. Tenenbaum, B., and Karshan, M.: The composition and formation of salivary calculus, J. Periodontol. **15:**72, 1944.

88. Mandel, I.D.: Biochemical aspects of calculus formation, J. Periodont. Res. Suppl. **4:**7, 1969.

89. McGaughey, C., et al.: Relations between early dental calculus production and calcium and phosphate parameters of salivary fractions, J. Periodontol. **46:**681, 1975.

90. Theilade, J., and Fitzgerald, R.J.: Dental calculus in the rat: effect of diet and erythromycin, Acta Odontol. Scand. **21:**571, 1963.

91. Mitchell, D.F., and Holmes, L.A.: Topical antibiotics control of dentogingival plaque, J. Periodontol. **36:**202, 1965.

92. Müller, E., Schroeder, H.E., and Mühlemann, H.R.: The effect of two oral antiseptics on early calculus formation, Helv. Odont. Acta **6:**42, 1962.

93. Dossenbach, W.F., and Mühlemann, H.R.: Effect of penicillin and ricinoleate on early calculus formation, Helv. Odont. Acta **5:**25, 1961.

94. Jensen, A.L.: Use of dehydrated pancreas in oral hygiene, J. Am. Dent. Assoc. **59:**923, 1959.

95. Ennever, J., and Sturzenberger, O.P.: Inhibition of dental calculus formation by use of an enzyme chewing gum, J. Periodontol. **32:**331, 1961.

96. Aleece, A.A., and Forscher, B.K.: Calculus reduction with a mucinase dentifrice, J. Periodontol. **25:**122, 1954.

97. Löe, H., et al.: The effect of mouthrinses and topical application of chlorhexidine on calculus formation in man, J. Periodont. Res. **6:**312, 1971.

98. Weinstein, E., and Mandel, I.D.: The present status of anti-calculus agents, J. Oral Ther. **1:**327, 1964.

99. Stallard, R.E., Volpe, A.R., and Orban, J.E.: The effect of an antimicrobial mouth rinse on dental plaque, calculus and gingivitis, J. Periodontol. **40:**683, 1969.

100. McNeal, D.R.: Anticalculus agents for the treatment, control, and prevention of periodontal disease, J. Public Health Dent. **29:**138, 1969.

101. Sturzenberger, O.P., Swancer, J.R., and Reiter, G.: Reduction of dental calculus in humans through the use of a dentifrice containing a crystal growth inhibitor, J. Periodontol. **42:**416, 1971.

102. Picozzi, A., et al.: Calculus inhibition in humans, J. Periodontol. **43:**692, 1972.

# CHAPTER 10

# The epidemiology, etiology, and public health aspects of periodontal disease

Epidemiology is the science concerned with the factors and conditions that determine the occurrence and distribution of health, disease, defects, disability, and death among *groups* of individuals.[1] The science of epidemiology is also concerned with the determination of the factors that favor the origin and spread of a disease process or a physiologic state in a community. It is further concerned with elaborating ways and means of preventing and controlling the spread of disease with the ultimate aim being complete elimination of the disease.

The principal distinction between epidemiology and clinical practice is that an epidemiologist observes *groups of individuals* and makes observations pertinent to the *whole group,* both the affected and the nonaffected, whereas a clinician is concerned with the *individual patient.* The epidemiologist studies mass phenomena in terms of type, extent, and frequency of occurrence in relation to such factors as age, sex, race, occupation, heredity, and socioeconomic status.

To discover factors and conditions of the origin and spread of a disease process, the epidemiologist must study three important epidemiologic constants: the *disease agents,* the *environment of the host,* and the *host itself.* The epidemiologist is aware that disease production takes place only when there is an interaction among the agent, the host, and the environment. Once the epidemiologist has thoroughly studied the environmental factors, the disease agents, and the human host factors, he/she may be able to identify the causes of the disease process and take appropriate measures to intercept these causes to prevent the occurrence of the disease in a community. This goal is different from the concerns and goals of the therapist in the treatment of a single individual.

The first step in an epidemiologic investigation is to discover the *prevalence* and severity of the disease and the composition of the population affected.[2] The prevalence refers to the number of events or defects in an individual or a population at a specified time. *Incidence* refers to the number of defects that may occur during a given period of time. The data on prevalence and incidence indicate the extent and occurrence of the problem. This information is used for searching out the nature and causes of the disease. The data obtained by epidemiologists must be quantitative and easily reproducible by any trained examiner with little effort. It is not to be confused with the thorough examination required to make a clinical diagnosis in the treatment of a single individual.

**Prevalence and incidence**

The public health aspects of periodontal disease require a different perspective on periodontal diseases and their treatment than that generally used by practitioners concerned with the care of private patients. From a public health viewpoint, achieving the most good for the entire population with the least cost in time, personnel, and equipment is considered the optimal approach to the management of a particular disease. The public health dentist is concerned with dental health management for populations rather than the individual and cost-effectiveness is a major concern. This necessitates the avoidance of time-consuming or expensive therapeutic techniques that on an individual basis may conceivably yield better results. Whereas in public health, pain relief and retention of teeth may be the chief goals of prevention and therapy, the treatment of private patients also involves esthetic and other considerations. These play a minor role or no role at all in public health. To a great extent, this chapter reflects the point of view of the epidemiologist concerned with public dental health. Consequently the judgments about the need to treat or not treat certain conditions may not apply to the care of patients in a private practice.

There is no question, however, that the information obtained from epidemiologic studies of periodontal diseases must be translated into preventive and corrective practices that will affect the periodontist in a private practice as well as the public health dentist. It is only by keeping our minds alert to new factual information that our ability to prevent and treat periodontal diseases will improve. This chapter, therefore, provides a valuable foil to established, yet somewhat dogmatic, concepts that still pervade periodontal therapy.

Evidence from epidemiologic research has led to a reappraisal of the extent of the periodontal disease problem, the natural history of the disease, and the need for treatment.[3] It has become clear that periodontal disease is not a major public health problem and that although many people have gingival inflammation, the probability of the inflammation progressing to severe loss of periodontal attachment is not great. Tooth loss because of periodontal disease alone is not common; periodontal disease appears to lead to the loss of large numbers of teeth in a relatively small percentage of the population.[3]

Periodontal disease is a social disease. It is affected by age, gender, ethnicity, income, social class, and educational status. These social factors affect the accumulation and retention of dental bacterial plaque—the major etiologic factor in periodontal disease. Epidemiology provides a systematic means of describing what is known about the etiology and the natural history of a disease. The main uses of epidemiology in the study of periodontal disease are[4]:

**Uses**

1. To study historically the rise and fall of diseases in populations
2. To diagnose community problems of health and disease by study and analysis of the incidence, prevalence, and morbidity

3. To estimate the individual's risk and chances of developing the disease
4. To help complete the clinical picture and natural history of disease by group analyses
5. To identify clinical syndromes by observation of group behavior
6. To evaluate the need and effectiveness of health services
7. To search for causes of disease and of health by observation of group habits, customs, and models of life

Epidemiologic studies dealing with periodontal disease frequently do not differentiate between gingivitis and the more destructive forms of the disease. Most indices are based on the thesis of a gingivitis-periodontitis continuum. Recent studies dispute this concept. Therefore some epidemiologic studies that fail to differentiate between gingivitis and periodontitis may offer conclusions applicable to gingivitis but which do not pertain to periodontitis and vice versa.

## Secular variations in periodontal disease

Anthropologic evidence indicates that severe periodontal disease was present in our ancestors. The severity of periodontal disease appears to be decreasing in a number of industrialized societies (Table 10-1).[5] For example, in the United States 57.1% of women and 45.3% of men were periodontally healthy in 1971-1974 as compared to 31% and 20.9% respectively in 1960-1962.[5]

## Community diagnosis

One of the aims of epidemiology is to describe the distribution and size of disease problems in human populations. Thus objectives for reducing the problems can be established and alternative strategies can be proposed to achieve the objectives. Decisions on the care of a patient require an accurate clinical diagnosis based on history, examination, and other special tests. Care of disease in the community as a whole requires a community diagnosis that rests on epidemiologic information. Community diagnosis is the essential first step in the planning cycle. It is expressed in terms of rates that relate data on disease to data on the whole population.

**Prevalence rates**

Prevalence rates in general usage have become synonymous with what were once called *point-prevalence* rates. Such prevalence rates define the proportion of people affected by a disease at any particular time. The prevalence of gingival inflammation in U.S. schoolchildren aged 5 to 17 years was 95% in 1979-1980.[6] The severity of the disease ranged from mild or moderate gingival inflammation affecting less than half the teeth to true periodontal pocketing. Only 4.4% of children had no gingival inflammation; 64.5% had inflammation affecting less than half their teeth, 28.1% had half or more teeth affected, and 2.5% had severe gingivitis around one or more teeth. True periodontal pockets were detected in 0.5% of the children.

**Table 10-1** Periodontal status of U.S. adults 18 to 79 years—percentages by sex and year of survey

| Sex | Without disease | | Disease without pockets | | Disease with pockets | |
|---|---|---|---|---|---|---|
| | 1960-62 | 1971-74 | 1960-62 | 1971-74 | 1960-62 | 1971-74 |
| Men | 20.9 | 45.3 | 49.0 | 28.1 | 30.1 | 26.6 |
| Women | 31.0 | 57.1 | 47.9 | 22.5 | 20.1 | 20.4 |

From Douglass, C.W., et al.: National trends in the prevalence and severity of periodontal disease, J. Am. Dent. Assoc. **107:**403, 1983. Copyright by the American Dental Association. Reprinted by permission.

The interpretation of data such as these provided for U.S. schoolchildren must be carried out with caution because the presence of gingival inflammation does not imply the need for treatment if mild inflammation affects only one or two teeth. Most surveys of the prevalence of periodontal disease have scored as positive any individual with one or more inflamed gingival units. The number of gingival units affected or whether true pockets are present is very seldom presented. This shortcoming should be borne in mind when interpreting prevalence data.

A better understanding of the pattern of severity and distribution of periodontal disease can be obtained by examining epidemiologic data in more detail. From a survey of three groups of New Zealand adults, aged 15-19, 25-29, and 35-44 years, Cutress, Hunter, and Hoskins[3] found that less than 4% of the population were free of gingivitis. While most people had some gingival inflammation or pocketing, the range of involvement was wide. At age 15-19 (Periodontal Index), 20% were periodontally healthy, 79% were scored as having gingivitis, and 1% had periodontitis. If the data, however, are presented by the number and percentage of teeth affected in that age group, 65.3% of dental units were inflammation free, 34.4% had gingival inflammation, and 0.4% had periodontitis.

Cutress and associates[3] found that although the prevalence of periodontal disease was 91.9% in the total population surveyed, only 2.6% of teeth had periodontal pockets, an average of 1.3 teeth per person. These values are deceptive since many individuals may have pockets requiring treatment, although some subjects may have had more pockets than others. While this may not be perceived as a public health problem, the affected individuals have a problem. In any case, these data suggest that periodontal disease may not be an important public health problem in New Zealand and possibly in other industrialized countries such as the United States, Sweden and The Netherlands. However, the maintenance of a functional, acceptable dentition for the lifetime of individuals, nevertheless, is a reasonable public health goal.

Between 1971 and 1974 in the United States, Douglass and co-workers[7] reported that 46.9% of men and 35.8% of women aged 55-64 had periodontal disease with pockets (see Table 10-8). The percentages of men and women with pockets increased to 58.9% and 42.8% respectively when this age group (65-74 years) was re-examined in 1971-1974. However, of the cohort born around the turn of the century who were 55 to 64 years old during the 1960 to 1962 survey, only 39.1% of the men had gingivitis. Twelve years later during the 1971 to 1974 survey that same cohort was in the 65 to 74 year age group. Only 13.1% of the males had gingivitis. Douglass and associates[7] did not consider that the downward trend in gingivitis was affected by the decrease in the number of persons and teeth at risk to the disease. The decline in the prevalence and severity of periodontal disease in the United States was attributed to the improved oral hygiene status that had occurred since 1960. The Simplified Oral Hygiene Index (OHI-S) decreased from 1.9 to 1.3 between 1960 and 1974 in white men aged 55-64 years and from 2.5 to 1.6 in those aged 65-74 years.[7]

Whereas there was a decline in gingivitis in all age groups (see Table 10-8) and in the prevalence of periodontal pocketing in the younger age groups, the prevalence of pocketing was similar in U.S. adults aged 55-64 years examined in 1960 and in 1974. The prevalence increased in women aged 65-74 years (from 32.8% to 42.8%) but not much in men. The increase in prevalence of pocketing among women is most likely the result of an increase in the number of teeth present in the later cohort due to improved dental status. Douglass and co-workers[7] concluded that there was a significant improvement in the periodontal health of older people but this improvement was limited to the substantial decrease in those who had gingivitis rather than periodontitis or pocketing. This improvement in periodontal health reported in the United

States was not found in black Americans. Their Periodontal Index increased from 3.31 to 3.68 between 1960 and 1974 in 55-64 year olds (Table 10-2).

Similar trends in improving periodontal health have been reported by Hugoson and Jordan[8] in Sweden. They found a marked decrease in the percentage of tooth surfaces with gingival inflammation between 1973 and 1978. Their survey was based on a statistical sample of individuals aged 3-70 years who were examined clinically and radiographically. In 1973, Hugoson and Koch[9] found that 4.8% of 3-year-olds had gingival inflammation. At 10 years of age the percentage affected had increased to 26.3% and at 20 years a further increase was noted. In 1975 the percentages affected in the above-mentioned age groups were 3.5%, 13.3%, and 13.1%, respectively. The percentages of tooth surfaces with plaque also decreased from 33.9% to 19.9% in 10-year-olds and from 29.1% to 17.9% in 20-year-olds.

The Swedish report[8] used an interesting method of grouping individuals according to the severity of periodontal disease to assess the extent of the periodontal problem in the community. The assessment was based on a full-mouth clinical and radiographic examination. Individuals were grouped according to the following classification.

*Group 1.* Healthy to mild gingivitis. Up to 12 bleeding gingival units in the premolar-molar region were considered acceptable. No periodontal pockets; normal periodontal bone height.

*Group 2.* Gingivitis present. Up to 12 pathologically deepened pockets with probing depths of 4 mm or less in the premolar-molar region were accepted. Reduced bone density in the marginal alveolar bone could be detected but without any detectable change in the normal bone height.

*Group 3.* Gingivitis present plus pathologically deepened pockets (periodontitis). General marginal bone loss up to one third of normal bone height.

*Group 4.* Gingivitis present plus pathologically deepened pockets (periodontitis). General marginal bone loss affecting between one third and two thirds of normal bone height. Furcation involvements—degrees I and II.

*Group 5.* Gingivitis present plus pathologically deepened periodontal pockets (periodontitis). General bone loss affecting more than two thirds of normal bone height and/or infrabony pockets. Furcation involvements—degrees II and III.

Using this classification on the findings from the survey carried out in 1973, they found strikingly few people with severe periodontal breakdown (Table 10-3).

Results from this study apparently indicate that periodontitis remains stable, but this is equivocal. Those in the older age groups who became edentulous as a result of periodontitis would not have qualified for this study. Some teeth with severe periodontitis may have been extracted, leaving the subject with a reduced number of teeth in relative good health or with mild or moderate periodontal disease. Apparently, there is little disease progression in those over 65 years of age.

Theoretically, it should be possible to divide individuals into groups with different levels of disease. Most of the populations in industrialized countries have gingivitis

**Table 10-2**   Mean Periodontal Index* of older black Americans by age and sex

| Sex | Age | 1960-1962 | 1971-1974 |
| --- | --- | --- | --- |
| Men | 55-64 | 3.31 | 3.68 |
| | 65-74 | 2.83 | 4.06 |
| Women | 55-64 | 2.90 | 2.59 |
| | 65-74 | 2.03 | 3.34 |

From Douglass, C.W., et al.: National trends in the prevalence and and severity of periodontal disease, J. Am. Dent. Assoc. **107**:403, 1983. Copyright by the American Dental Association. Reprinted by permission.
*None of the differences in mean Periodontal Index (PI) between surveys is statistically significant.

and some periodontitis; however, the rate of progress of the disease is very slow. A small group in any population with severe periodontal destruction are at risk and require intensive periodontal therapy. Schaub[10] concluded that the high risk group was 10%-15% of dentate Dutch adults. They are likely to develop severe periodontal disease and lose teeth because of the disease.

In developing countries, on the other hand, the prevalence and severity of periodontal disease has been reported to be high. Littleton[11] reported that 97% of Ethiopians aged 5-84 years had periodontal disease and Greene[12] found that 97% of Indian males had the disease. The severity of the disease is generally reported to be greater in people from developing than from industrialized countries. Despite the high levels of periodontal disease, tooth loss from the disease is not common in developing countries. For example, in Nigeria where the severity of periodontal disease is high, persons aged 50 and over had lost on an average only 4 teeth per person.[13] In Tanzania, Lembariti[14] found a high prevalence of periodontal disease in adults. Their oral cleanliness was poor; heavy calculus and plaque deposits were present. Nevertheless, very few adults had deep pockets and tooth loss was uncommon.

These findings suggest that the rate of progression from periodontitis to tooth loss is slow in both industrialized and developing countries and may be compatible with maintaining sufficient periodontal support to retain many teeth for the lifetime of most individuals. In fact, periodontal disease in some developing countries, while prevalent, frequently appears to be limited to gingivitis and marginal periodontitis, which progress slowly. On the other hand, some populations are affected by rapidly progressing periodontitis that is untreated because of the lack of dental services. This lack of dental care may result in some lost teeth and the retention of many severely diseased teeth.[15] Therefore tooth loss, per se, may not be an adequate criterion for treatment needs. Other considerations include quality of function and esthetics.

The diverse figures obtained in epidemiologic studies and their interpretations illustrate the difficulties in describing dental health. Morbidity means what it is defined to mean: whether it is a subjective complaint, measurable evidence of disorder, or a pathology diagnosed by a health professional. The difficulty in defining dental health has implications for the assessment of the need for periodontal care.

Naturally the broader the scope of the definition of disease the more healthy people will be included within disease parameters. However, the narrower the definition of disease (e.g., periodontitis is present when pockets are greater than 7 mm) the healthier

**Table 10-3**  Number of people with natural teeth grouped by age and periodontal status

| Age group | Number of people with natural teeth | Periodontal grouping by severity*<br>Number of people | | | | |
|---|---|---|---|---|---|---|
| | | Group 1 | Group 2 | Group 3 | Group 4 | Group 5 |
| 20 | 100 | 28 | 68 | 4 | 0 | 0 |
| 30 | 100 | 16 | 69 | 15 | 0 | 0 |
| 40 | 99 | 5 | 51 | 41 | 0 | 2 |
| 50 | 95 | 0 | 36 | 56 | 2 | 1 |
| 60 | 80 | 0 | 9 | 65 | 2 | 4 |
| 70 | 63 | 0 | 7 | 52 | 4 | 0 |
| TOTAL | 537 | 49 | 240 | 233 | 8 | 7 |

From Hugoson, A., and Jordan, T.: Frequency distribution of individuals aged 20-70 years according to severity of periodontal disease, Community Dent. Oral Epidemiol. **10:**187, 1982; Munksgaard International.
*For description of severity groups, see text, p. 220.

the population would appear since some diseased people would be missed. For instance, group 2 in Table 10-3 counts less than 11 pockets as being healthy; such a definition skew the data so that some diseased people are counted as healthy (see discussion of sensitivity and specificity of diagnostic tests in Chapter 48).

## ASSESSING THE NEED FOR THERAPY

Most treatment need systems are based on a general assumption that everyone with disease would want treatment if it were available, affordable, and without inconvenience and discomfort. As can be seen from the data cited, most patients are capable of maintaining their dentitions (however incomplete) into an old age. Most periodontal treatment is efficacious, and only a small minority of all people require intensive treatment. Total tooth loss occurs in a relatively small number of periodontally diseased patients. Clinical experience indicates that careful periodic monitoring of the patient at risk may assist in the interception or prevention of periodic bouts of infection.

However, the assumption that there should be periodic monitoring of the patient at risk may not be completely valid. First, not all plaque bacteria are pathogenic and some plaque may be compatible with periodontal health.[16] Second, plaque reforms soon after a prophylaxis and with one exception[17] plaque and gingivitis resulting from plaque are not eliminated for more than 30 days.[18] Third, the sensitivity and specificity of diagnostic tests for early gingivitis and intra- and inter-examiner reproducibility are not good.[19] Finally, not everyone with the disease would want treatment if it were available. Consequently some patients at risk may not be properly identified.

Ramfjord[20] defined periodontal needs in terms of certain other criteria:

1. The number of people needing treatment and the extent of such treatment
2. The number of people needing preventive procedures or periodontal health care
3. The number and educational qualifications of personnel needed to perform the services that would be required to treat periodontal disease and maintain periodontal health

In countries, states, and communities where cost effectiveness is the prime concern, triage (the choosing of those to be sacrificed) or compromise must be employed because financial, political, ethical, social and cultural considerations of the population and the nation concerned determine the extent to which treatment needs will be met.

Bellini[21] in laying down requirements for measuring periodontal treatment needs, added three other useful parameters. He suggested that therapeutic procedures should be (1) classified and (2) related to the time and costs involved in carrying out the treatment. In addition, (3) the methods of examination should be *simple* and *quick*.

Two general approaches have been used to estimate periodontal treatment needs: a direct measurement of need[22-24] and converting prevalence data into treatment needs.[25,26] The *direct measurement systems* categorize people's mouths, or segments of their mouths, into those needing no treatment, oral hygiene instruction alone or in combination with scaling and removal of overhanging restorations, and those requiring surgery. The main differences between the different direct measurement systems are the levels of disease or local irritants in each of the four or five treatment categories and the specificity of the type of treatment required. For example, whereas McPhee[24] recommends oral hygiene instruction and prophylaxis plus gingivectomy for simple pockets, Bowden and associates[22] state that children with loss of attachment of at least 2 mm on at least one tooth require review by a dentist. Johansen, Gjermo, and Bellini[23] go further and specify that a mouth quadrant having a tooth with a periodontal pocket of more than 5 mm deep requires surgery.

The *converting prevalence data methods* that convert periodontal disease indices into treatment needs categorize people by ranges on the Periodontal Index (PI) or the Gingival and Plaque Indices.[27] Russell[28] has used his index to decide which people require a simple prophylaxis (PI = 0.1-1.0), minimal periodontal treatment (PI = 0.5-1.9), elaborate and protracted treatment (PI = 1.5-5.0), or full-mouth extractions (PI = 4.0-8.0). Scheinin, Honka, and Kankkunen[29] using the Gingival and Plaque Indices divided students into those with healthy mouths, gingivitis, and severe gingivitis on the basis of index scores.

Some of these systems have incorporated timings into their categories of treatment. Scheinin, Honka, and Kankkunen[29] assigned 20 minutes of oral hygiene instruction to persons with a Plaque Index of 0.00-0.19 and 60 minutes of instruction plus scaling to those with an index of 0.20-0.99. Johansen, Gjermo, and Bellini,[23] after assessing the actual time taken to treat patients, categorized patients according to clinical criteria, estimating that 60 minutes of oral hygiene instruction was required for those requiring oral hygiene instruction—30 minutes per quadrant for scaling and overhangs and 60 minutes per quadrant for periodontal surgery. They then proceeded to estimate the manpower and costs required to treat a group of industrial workers.[30]

To calculate the time and personnel required to treat a population, decisions must be made on the methods and types of personnel to be used in the treatment. Estimations of the time required to carry out each treatment method should be made under the circumstances in which the care is to be provided.[32] These timings can be applied to the findings and the total number of hours of care can be calculated and categorized by hours required for oral hygiene instruction, hours for scaling, and hours for more complex periodontal treatment per 1000 people. The estimates can then be extrapolated to the population.

Some of the systems for assessing periodontal treatment needs, such as the Community Periodontal Index of Treatment Needs (CPITN) (see Fig. 10-1 and the box on p. 225), have good elements, but none are satisfactory. The principal shortcomings are:

1. The criteria are too subjective and their sensitivity and specificity is questionable
2. The criteria for surgical treatment have not been scientifically tested
3. The criteria for treatment are insufficiently flexible; they do not allow for variations in treatment philosophies; they do not comply with many current practices
4. None of the systems include demographic or behavioral criteria
5. The systems have not been adequately tested in longitudinal studies

## ESTIMATES OF RISKS AND CHANCES

The risks of individuals in industrialized countries such as the United States, Sweden, Holland, and Great Britain developing advanced periodontal disease are relatively small. In a stratified statewide survey in Iowa, Beck and associates[33] found that a very small proportion (2%) of people aged 20 years and older had pockets 6 mm or deeper. The highest percentage occurred in the 45-54 age group; 6.8% of them had deep pockets. This latter figure is most likely to be more relevant because severe periodontal disease is relatively uncommon below that age and after that age the rate will be affected by the loss of teeth. In Sweden[8] 2.8% of people aged 20-70 years had severe periodontal disease and in Holland[34] 10% of adults had one or more pockets 6 mm or more deep. However, not all teeth nor all sites on the teeth are at similar risk. Of 4097 sites in the Swedish study reexamined at 3 and 6 years in subjects with mild to moderate periodontal attachment loss, 523 sites (11.6%) showed attachment loss of more than 2 mm. Sites with more advanced attachment loss were not more prone to additional loss but are not exempt from it.[8]

## The natural history of periodontal disease

The natural history of periodontal disease progression is not as simple as has been suggested. The common model of periodontal disease accepts the progression of gingivitis to periodontitis; then the loss of attachment and its bony support progresses continuously until the tooth is nonfunctional. This model is supported superficially by graphs showing an increasing severity of disease with increasing age. The acceptance of such a model has important implications for research on periodontal disease and on clinical treatment. It suggests that once a person has periodontal disease only continuous preventive care will prevent the inevitable progress of the destructive lesion. There is little evidence to support this model when the pattern of disease in individual sites is examined.

Recent evidence indicates that there are a number of models and different diseases.[35,36] The random burst model of Goodson and associates[35] and Socransky and coworkers[36] differs from the continuous disease model. In the random burst model, certain gingival sites could be free of destructive periodontal disease for a lifetime. Other sites might experience a brief burst of destructive disease followed by a period of remission or repair. The remission may be permanent or intermittent. The model suggests that a past history of severe gingivitis or periodontal destruction is not predictive of future destructive activity. This model explains the inactivity in sites with "contained gingivitis"[37] and why in some individuals, at some point, stable lesions become converted into slowly progressive destructive lesions for reasons that are not currently clear.[38-41] The main finding in the studies that leads to the proposed new model is the large number of periodontal sites which show no change, plus the finding that some sites are affected by rapidly destructive disease.

A third model, the asynchronous multiple burst model, has also been suggested by these authors.[35,36] Certain sites remain free of destructive disease. Others have bursts of destruction occurring asynchronously. The main difference between this model and the preceding one is that multiple sites break down within a short period and then go into prolonged periods of remission.

Socransky and associates[36] present four arguments against the continuous destructive disease model of periodontal disease. First, the attachment loss rates on individual surfaces are either too fast or too slow to be consistent with the observed mean loss

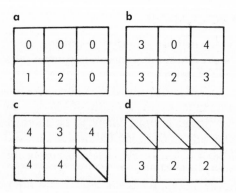

**Fig. 10-1.** Examples of CPITN recordings. Patient "a" needs scaling in the mandibular anterior sextant and oral hygiene instructions for the bleeding on the right posterior sextants. In patient "b" complex treatment is needed in 1 and scaling in all but one sextant. The possibility of juvenile periodontitis should be considered in young patients. Patient "c" needs complex treatment in four sextants and scaling in all but the edentulous mandibular left sextant. In patient "d" the maxilla is edentulous (or only one tooth remains). The mandibular teeth require scaling in all three sextants. In addition, patients "b," "c," "d" all require oral hygiene instruction as well.

### Community Periodontal Index of Treatment Needs (CPITN)

The most widely recommended system for estimating periodontal treatment needs is the Community Periodontal Index of Treatment Needs (CPITN).[31] The periodontal treatment needs are recorded for sextants, that is, sixths of the dentition. Third molars are not included except where they are functioning in the place of second molars. The sextants contain the following teeth (World Health Organization [WHO] numbering):

| | | |
|---|---|---|
| 17-14 | 13-23 | 24-27 |
| 47-44 | 43-33 | 34-37 |

American equivalent systems of tooth numbering are:

| | | |
|---|---|---|
| 2-5 | 6-11 | 12-15 |
| 31-28 | 27-22 | 21-18 |

The treatment need in a sextant is recorded only when two or more teeth are present and not indicated for extraction. The indication for extraction because of periodontal involvement is vertical mobility and discomfort. If only one functioning tooth remains in a sextant, it is included in the adjoining sextant. For example if only two teeth remained in the maxilla, the jaw would be recorded as one sextant. Missing sextants are indicated with a diagonal line through the appropriate box.

When assessing the periodontal treatment needs of a population, the recordings per sextant are based on findings from specified index teeth. The index teeth to be examined are:

| *WHO numbering* | | | *American equivalent* | | |
|---|---|---|---|---|---|
| 17, 16 | 11 | 26, 27 | 2, 3 | 8 | 14, 15 |
| 47, 46 | 31 | 36, 37 | 31, 30 | 25 | 18, 19 |

Although 10 index teeth are examined only six recordings, one relating to each sextant, are made. When both or one of the designated molars are present, the worst findings from these tooth surfaces are recorded for the sextant. If no index teeth are present in a sextant, all the remaining teeth in the sextant are examined and the worst score recorded (Fig. 10-1).

In oral screening examinations for the determination of treatment needs of individuals, where partial recording using index teeth may be considered insufficient, the recording for each sextant is based on the worst finding from all the teeth in that sextant.

A special probe is used for the CPITN. The pocket depth is measured through color coding with a black mark starting at 3.5 mm and ending at 5.5 mm. The probe has a ball tip of 0.5 mm diameter that allows easy detection of subgingival calculus and reduces the tendency to over-measure pockets by penetrating into the connective tissue. A force of no more than 25 g should be used when inserting the probe. When inserting the probe into the gingival sulcus, the ball tip should follow the anatomic configuration of the surface of the tooth root.

In assessing treatment needs, the presence of the following is determined for each sextant in the sequence indicated below:

*Code 4*   Pathologic pockets 6 mm or more
*Code 3*   Pathologic pockets 4.0-5.5 mm
*Code 2*   Supra or subgingival calculus
*Code 1*   Gingival bleeding after probing
*Code 0*   None of above signs present

A subject or a sextant are classified according to periodontal treatment need into one of the following categories:

  0 = No treatment (*Code 0*)
  I = Improvement in personal oral hygiene (*Code 1*)
 II = I + scaling (*Codes 2 and 3*)
III = I + II + complex treatment (*Code 4*)

of attachment in particular individuals. Second, there are a large number of gingival sites, with or without prior loss of periodontal attachment, which remain stable. Third, studies indicate that progression does not occur in all lesions. Fourth, even sites with severe rapidly destructive disease may go into remission and possibly undergo repair and regeneration, for unknown reasons.

So there may be at least three models of destructive periodontal disease. Regardless of the models, not all subjects, not all teeth, and not all surfaces are equally susceptible to loss of attachment. The bilateral symmetry of disease distribution indicates that the incidence of disease cannot be based on a completely random model. Furthermore, the concept of a mean annual rate of loss of attachment is meaningless and possibly misleading (Table 10-4). For example, if periodontal disease is a slow continuous disease with an annual rate of loss of only 0.05-0.10 mm, then the need for treating the disease is unclear. Because most people will die before the age of 85 years, then all that would be necessary would be the maintenance of at least shortened upper and lower arches for life (shortening being due to the loss of some teeth from the arch).[42]

If either of the burst models is correct then the rationale for treatment of affected sites is the reduction or decrease of the intensity of the burst or the prevention of future bursts of disease activity since rapidly progressive disease could cause selective tooth loss.

While the retention of some teeth and the loss of others may be acceptable from a public health viewpoint, it is nevertheless essential to maximize the number of teeth retained, their state of health, and their appearance. The extent to which this can be done will vary from one geographic region to another and given the other factors mentioned earlier (see p. 222).

## Identification of syndromes

Epidemiologic methods assist in the identification of syndromes by analyzing the recurrent patterns of symptoms, signs, onset, course, prognosis, and pathology. For example, Baer[43] defined periodontosis in relation to age of onset (between 11 and 13 years), sex ratio (women/men ratio 3:1), familial background, lack of positive relation between local etiologic factors and presence of deep periodontal pockets, distinctive radiographic pattern of alveolar bone loss, rate of progression, lack of involvement of primary teeth. Later it was suggested that the term *juvenile periodontitis* should replace periodontosis and that there were two different forms of the disease: the localized form limited to first molars and/or incisors and the generalized form in which additional teeth may be affected. A characteristic microbiota has been associated with the localized form of the disease.

Epidemiologic surveys of white populations indicate that juvenile periodontitis is uncommon. It occurs in one in a thousand 16-year-olds (0.1%-0.95%, confidence limits 0.06% and 0.26%). The girl/boy sex ratio is 16:12.[44] The higher rate in women decreases with increasing age, indicating that the disease may occur at an earlier age in

**Table 10-4** Mean annual periodontal attachment loss in untreated populations

| Population | Age | Mean annual rate (mm) |
| --- | --- | --- |
| American | 18-40 | $-0.11^{38}$ |
| American | 19-59 | $-0.13^{39}$ |
| Norwegian | 17-37+ | $-0.08^{40}$ |
| Sri Lankan | 15-37+ | $-0.24^{40}$ |
| British | adults | $-0.03$ to $-0.06^{41}$ |

women than men.[45] There is a strong positive correlation between age and the number of teeth involved and between the prevalence of gingival bleeding and the generalization of the disease.[46] It can be concluded that juvenile periodontitis may start with bone destruction localized to first molars and/or incisors and develops into a more generalized form where almost the whole dentition is involved.

## A search for causes of periodontal disease

A principal use of epidemiology is to discover causes of disease. Periodontal disease is associated mainly with dental bacterial plaque, but the response of the periodontal tissues to the presence of plaque is influenced by the composition of the dental plaque and by ill-defined systemic factors.[37] In assessing the local and systemic factors that have been suggested as causes of periodontal disease, consideration should be given to the statement by Sir Bradford Hill[47] that before deciding whether an association between two variables shows a cause-and-effect relationship, the association must have strength, consistency, specificity, and temporality. It must reveal a biologic gradient and have biologic plausability. Finally, the relationship must be a coherent one. Associations should be studied from these viewpoints but none of them can bring indisputable evidence for or against the cause-and-effect hypothesis and none can be required as a sine qua non. The strongest support for any causation hypothesis cannot be obtained from association but can be obtained only by experimental proof.

Numerous studies have shown that bacterial plaque is the major cause of periodontal disease. There is a positive association between the severity of periodontal disease on the one hand and age, plaque, and calculus on the other (r = +0.76).[48] Russell[28,49] found that the combined effect of age, plaque, and calculus were strongly correlated with the severity of periodontal disease (r = +0.95). He clearly summed up the relationship when he concluded that less than 10% of the variance in group periodontal scores remain to be explained after the combined influence of age and mouth cleanliness has been considered. A residual factor, *wholly independent* of age or hygiene, therefore, can have little effect on periodontal disease. It should be pointed out, however, that Russell did not separate gingivitis from periodontitis and considered these entities to be part of a disease continuum. Russell correlated plaque and calculus with severity of disease but did not separate gingivitis from periodontitis but considered these entities to be part of a continuum.

The severity of periodontal disease is greater in persons with larger amounts of plaque and calculus. There is a level of plaque which is compatible with no progression of periodontal disease.[50] Up to that level the rate of progression increases with increasing levels of plaque, but beyond a certain level, which may differ from one population to another, no further increase in severity will occur. Sheiham[47] has shown that a Debris Index of 0.6 is compatible with nonprogression of gingivitis in adults. Burt, Ismail, and Eklund[51] concluded that a simplified Oral Hygiene Index (OHI-S) of 0.3-0.6 might be compatible with virtual absence of destructive periodontal disease for most people. Slightly higher levels of OHI-S (0.7-1.3) were associated with low-to-moderate levels of periodontal disease.

However, the relationship of plaque and calculus to severity of periodontal disease is not as clearcut as Russell's[28] data would indicate. In juvenile periodontitis, plaque and calculus are often notable by their absence. Disease progression may be associated with the presence of a specific microbial infection. Likewise, in certain populations, high levels of plaque and calculus are prevalent, yet periodontitis is reported to be rare. However, little is known about plaque composition in these populations or the host factors that may increase their resistance to periodontitis.

The relationship between bacterial plaque and periodontal disease is biologically plausible as plaque contains large numbers of bacteria. However, only some of these bacteria have been associated with inflammatory changes or attachment loss.

Extensive experimental evidence exists for the relationship between bacterial plaque and gingivitis. Löe and associates[17] have shown that if, by stopping all active methods of oral hygiene, plaque is allowed to accumulate on the teeth of persons with healthy gingiva, gingivitis will develop. Gingivitis developed in different individuals at different times ranging from 10 to 21 days. Gingival inflammation resolved 1 week after starting oral hygiene again. Additional supporting evidence of the relationship between plaque and periodontal disease has been presented by Axelsson and Lindhe.[52] In a number of studies on children and adults they demonstrated that frequent control of plaque by dental professionals leads to the elimination or reduction of gingivitis in children and adults.[53]

The crucial role of bacterial plaque in gingivitis has been demonstrated by the analysis of the factors affecting the differences in levels of gingivitis between men and women, blacks and whites, different socioeconomic groups, smokers and nonsmokers, and children with various levels of malocclusion. Virtually no differences in levels of periodontal disease were found when the groups were standardized by level of oral cleanliness.[48,54,55]

The commonly used measure of oral cleanliness, the OHI-S,[56] has plaque and calculus components. Statistically the Calculus Index has been shown to have a higher correlation with gingivitis than the Debris Index (Table 10-5). A fallacious conclusion— that calculus is more important than plaque—may be deduced from the data. Calculus is calcified bacterial plaque covered by noncalcified plaque. The plaque on the surface of calculus causes changes in the gingival tissues. This relationship illustrates the fact that association does not necessarily imply causation. The high correlation between calculus and periodontal disease may indicate that people with high calculus scores clean their teeth ineffectively, thus allowing plaque to calcify more readily.

## LOCAL FACTORS AND PERIODONTAL DISEASE

Local factors such as malocclusion; iatrogenic factors such as overhanging restorations, poorly fitted dentures, crowns and bridges, and orthodontic appliances; cigarette smoking and betel nut chewing; and trauma from occlusion have been implicated as etiologic factors in periodontal disease.[57,58]

The relationship between malocclusion and periodontal disease is equivocal.[59] Some studies have demonstrated a relationship, whereas others have not. The differences in findings may be accounted for by the different methods used. In particular, plaque and malocclusion scores were frequently recorded as averages of whole mouth scores and individual tooth irregularities have not been taken into account.[55] Ainamo[60] has suggested that at the extremes of oral hygiene scores, the effect of tooth malposition on periodontal health is masked.

**Table 10-5** Simple linear correlation matrix for four selected independent variables, with periodontal index as the dependent variable—Ecuador and Montana civilians

| | | Variable | | | |
|---|---|---|---|---|---|
| Variable | Age | Debris index | Calculus index | Oral hygiene index-S | Periodontal index |
| Age | 1.0 | 0.22 | 0.68 | 0.56 | 0.66 |
| Debris index | | 1.00 | 0.43 | 0.80 | 0.41 |
| Calculus index | | | 1.00 | 0.89 | 0.71 |
| Simplified oral hygiene index | | | | 1.00 | 0.69 |

From Greene, J.C.: Oral hygiene and periodontal disease, Am. J. Public Health, **55:**913, 1963.

Malpositioned teeth accumulate more plaque than well-aligned teeth.[59] The degree of malalignment correlates with plaque accumulation and gingivitis only in subjects with low plaque scores.[55,60] However the amount of plaque that accumulates on a group of teeth depends more on the position of the segment than the presence or absence of malaligned teeth in the segment. For example, the amount of plaque in the anterior segments, whether well- or malaligned, correlates with the total mouth plaque scores. Nevertheless, upper well-or malaligned anterior segments had less plaque than the mouth overall, whereas lower segments had higher plaque scores than the mouth overall.[55] The position of the mouth segment has an overriding effect on the amount of plaque that accumulates and is more important than the effect of malaligned teeth in the segment. It should be noted that the correlation of gingivitis to plaque is much better than the correlation of periodontitis to plaque.

Some aspects of dental treatment have iatrogenic consequences for the periodontal tissues.[37] The extent of the damage has not been quantified. Poorly finished and badly positioned dental restorations are etiologic factors in periodontal disease.[61] Removable dentures and fixed appliance orthodontic treatment are associated with more severe periodontal disease. Periodontal disease is also associated with the use of tobacco in any of several forms.[54,62] Smokers generally have more severe periodontal disease than nonsmokers. All the studies that associate tobacco smoking with more severe periodontal disease also report that smokers have higher plaque and calculus scores than nonsmokers. Smokers and nonsmokers with similar plaque and calculus scores have similar levels of periodontal disease. There is a gradient of oral cleanliness and severity of periodontal disease from low in nonsmokers to high in smokers of 11 or more cigarettes per day. Persons who smoked 1 to 10 cigarettes per day had less severe periodontal disease and cleaner mouths than those who smoked more.[54]

There is consistent epidemiologic evidence against a relationship between traumatic occlusion and inflammatory periodontal disease.[63-66] This finding is not in complete agreement with experimental data.

## SYSTEMIC FACTORS AND PERIODONTAL DISEASE

There is no epidemiologic evidence that systemic factors are a significant primary cause of chronic periodontal disease. Some hormonal, metabolic, genetic, and nutritional variables may modify the progress of the disease. Hormonal changes during puberty, pregnancy, and menopause or brought on by drug therapy are related to gingivitis. Certain groups of people with genetic or immunologic anomalies, leukocyte dysfunction or with acquired or inborn errors of metabolism, such as diabetes, trisomy G syndrome, or Papillon-Lefèvre syndrome, show a high susceptibility to severe periodontal diseases.[37]

The interaction of nutritional deficiencies with periodontal disease is not clearly defined because, although specific nutritional deficiencies have been shown to affect the components of the periodontium of experimental animals, the effect in humans is not clear. Periodontal disease is not a manifestation of specific nutritional deficiency.[67] Nevertheless, nonspecific depletion of a combination of nutrients may increase the rate of the disease. Russell and associates[68] found that there was a tendency for South Vietnamese villagers on a low intake of calories, protein, carbohydrates, riboflavin, and iron to have a higher Periodontal Index (PI) than villagers living on an adequate diet. Waerhaug[15] found a positive correlation between clinical signs of vitamin B deficiency (such as angular stomatitis, cheilosis, and erosion and fissuring of the tongue) and the severity of periodontal disease in persons examined in Sri Lanka. Compared to the effect of dental plaque, however, the effect of the deficiency was small.

Some investigators have reported that persons with low levels of certain nutrients such as riboflavin and vitamin C have less severe periodontal disease than those with normal levels. Providing vitamin C–deficient patients with therapeutic doses of ascorbic acid did not improve their gingival condition.[69] There is no support for using more than recommended intakes of ascorbic acid in the prevention or treatment of periodontal diseases because only a weak association was found between periodontal disease and ascorbic acid levels in a representative sample of the U.S. population.[70] The highest prevalence and severity of periodontal disease occurs in populations where malnutrition is common, so the possibility exists that general malnutrition does affect the severity of disease.

Most of the epidemiologic surveys on the relationship between nutritional factors and periodontal disease are based on biochemical estimates of nutrients. Cautious inferences should be drawn from comparisons between the nutritional status of a population on a specific day and the accumulated lifetime experience of oral diseases. Dietary, biochemical, and clinical measurements assess different chronologic aspects of nutritional status: the dietary measurement is made at the time of the survey, the biochemical measurement shows the relatively recent past, while the clinical changes require a longer period for exhaustion of tissue stores of the particular nutrient. Similarly, once a lesion is produced, it may require much time to revert to normal; some lesions may be irreversible and therefore permanent. It is, therefore, important to compare the biochemical estimates of nutritional deficiency with the dietary and clinical findings. When this is done the relationship between nutrition and periodontal health is more positive than it first appears to be. For example, signs of scorbutic gingivitis do occur in persons with low ascorbic acid dietary intakes but the gingival condition is not positively related with plasma ascorbic acid levels.[71] In Vietnamese villagers[68] there was a tendency for more severe periodontal disease to occur in those with low dietary intakes of calories, protein, carbohydrates, riboflavin, and iron. Nevertheless, there was only a weak and statistically insignificant correlation between the severity of periodontal disease and serum total protein values, urinary riboflavin, hemoglobin levels, and clinical signs of nutritional deficiency. These findings indicate that information obtained from dietary and biochemical findings are not necessarily interchangeable.[71] In addition the biochemical results obtained in the studies on which the main nutrition and periodontal disease data are based suffer from errors of sampling and the average values employed restrict their usefulness in depicting variations in the nutritional status of the population. Biochemical analyses were carried out for only a small subsample of persons who were examined dentally. For example, in the survey conducted by Russell and associates,[68] 2474 persons had dental examinations while only 456 had one or more biochemical analysis; the data for only 90 of these 456 were complete for all the estimates. It was on the results of these 90 persons that a multiple correlation analysis was compiled to assess the correlation between periodontal disease and various levels of nutrients.

It appears that the reports supporting the hypothesis that specific nutritional deficiencies are not strongly associated with the severity of periodontal disease are based on small numbers of biochemical estimates. These estimates suffer from errors of sampling. Therefore the relationship between the biochemical estimates of nutritional status and the clinical nutritional status are questionable.

## Some important epidemiologic variables in periodontal disease

In descriptive and analytic epidemiologic studies certain basic variables and attributes such as age, sex, ethnic group, occupation, socioeconomic status, and geography are related to the severity of periodontal disease.

## AGE

Periodontal disease increases in prevalence and severity with increasing age.[4,40] The increase may be the result of a cumulative effect of episodes of periodontal destruction or a gradual increase in severity of destruction caused either by a deterioration in oral cleanliness or by a change in host response and/or plaque composition with increasing age. The increase in severity with increasing age may be the result of at least two factors.[1] More gingival units become inflamed or the frequency of destructive lesions increases in a proportion of the dentate population or there may be an additional factor of some units with gingivitis progressing to periodontitis. Another factor is the age-cohort phenomenon.

Although the proportion of people with periodontal disease increases with age, approximately one third of U.S. adults aged 65-74 years have no periodontal disease and 50.6% have one or more pockets.[51,72] Of those with pockets approximately 25% have one to three pockets per person and the remainder (25%) have four or more pockets (Table 10-6). However, the average number of teeth present in the group studied was 17.2. This means that they lost 10.8 teeth per person for unknown causes that could have been periodontal. Of the 65- to 74-year-olds, only 21.6% still had 25 or more teeth.[51] Those with 25 or more teeth had a low Periodontal Index (PI) (men, 1.4; women, 0.9), indicating that a large number of teeth can be retained into older age with minor changes in the periodontium but only by a small proportion of people. However, this is only true for one fifth of the population in this age bracket. In data from the statewide survey in Iowa,[33] the percentage with bleeding on probing increased from 26.1% at 5-11 years to 46.9% at 65+ and the percentage with pockets of 3-6 mm increased from 3.3% to 31.9% at 65+. A very small proportion (2.1%) of the oldest age group had pockets of 6 mm + (Table 10-7).[33] However, no data was given on teeth lost because of periodontal or other causes.

**Table 10-6**  Percent distribution of men and women by periodontal classification, United States 1971-1974, according to age

| Age | No disease | | Gingivitis | | 1-3 Pockets | | 4 Pockets or more | |
|---|---|---|---|---|---|---|---|---|
|  | Male | Female | Male | Female | Male | Female | Male | Female |
| 6-11 | 83.3 | 89.0 | 16.4 | 10.7 | 0.3 | 0.3 | 0.0 | 0.0 |
| 12-17 | 60.9 | 72.0 | 37.3 | 27.0 | 0.8 | 0.4 | 0.9 | 0.6 |
| 18-44 | 49.8 | 62.7 | 33.2 | 24.5 | 4.7 | 4.3 | 12.3 | 8.5 |
| 45-64 | 38.8 | 47.8 | 19.8 | 20.1 | 8.7 | 9.8 | 32.7 | 22.3 |
| 65-74 | 27.8 | 43.2 | 13.1 | 13.8 | 11.5 | 9.7 | 47.6 | 33.2 |

From Kelly, J.E., and Harney, C.R.: Basic data on dental examination findings of persons 1-74 years: United States, 1971-74, D.H.E.W. Pub. No. (PHS) 79-1662, Ser. 11, No. 214, Washington, D.C., 1979, U.S. Government Printing Office.

**Table 10-7**  Percent distribution of Iowans by periodontal status—1980

| Age Group* | With bleeding | With pockets 3-6 mm | With pockets 6 mm+ |
|---|---|---|---|
|  | % | % | % |
| 5-11 | 26.1 | 3.3 | 0.0 |
| 35-44 | 38.9 | 24.2 | 1.7 |
| 55-64 | 44.8 | 31.2 | 2.1 |
| 65+ | 46.9 | 31.9 | 2.1 |

From Beck, J.D.: Risk factors for various levels of periodontal disease and treatment needs, Community Dent. Oral Epidemiol. **12:**12, 1984, Munksgaard International.
*No data is given on number of teeth lost.

In a national survey in New Zealand, the PI increased from 0.89 to 1.21 in persons aged 35 and 64 years. The percentages in these age groups requiring either extractions for periodontal disease or periodontal surgery increased from 3% to 15% (extractions) and 9% to 22% (surgery). Not all teeth were affected. The increase in PI was the result of a larger number of teeth being affected by mild gingivitis rather than an increase in periodontitis.[73]

In people who have gingival sites with pockets, the loss of periodontal attachment does progress, albeit on an average very slowly with increasing age. In a long-term study on the natural history of periodontal disease in Norway and Sri Lanka,[40] half of the 17-year-olds experienced no loss of periodontal attachment. At that age 99% of all root surfaces had 0 or 1 mm loss of attachment. Each age group showed a very slow mean increase in loss of attachment over a 6-year period. At 37+ years the mean loss was 1.66 mm; 46.5% of surfaces still had 0 or 1 mm loss and 46% measured between 2 and 4 mm of loss. The mean annual rate of loss of attachment did not increase significantly with increasing age. The rate ranged from 0.07 to 0.11 mm a year. At that rate, about 6 mm of attachment would be lost by age 80 assuming an equal rate of progression of attachment loss on all surfaces, an assumption that has been shown to be incorrect in this and other studies.

Not all periodontal lesions progress. In the United States, the 65- to 74-year-olds who retained more than 25 or more teeth had low oral hygiene scores. Population samples with low plaque scores do not appear to develop periodontal disease readily, whatever their age.[72]

The second factor that may account for the apparent increase in periodontal disease with increasing age is the age-cohort phenomenon. Within a population, people of approximately the same age form an age-cohort who share a similar environment from birth to death. Fewer of the present groups of older Americans have periodontal disease than those examined in 1960-62 and there has been a substantial decrease in the proportion with gingivitis[4,7] (Table 10-8). However, there has been no change in periodontitis. The proportion with pockets remained unchanged despite the fact that the percentage of edentulous subjects had decreased and the numbers of teeth per dentate person increased. Each age-specific group of younger adults is experiencing better periodontal health than their predecessors.[7] It appears that the higher periodontal disease scores in older people may result as much from their generational experience as from the physical conditions of older age.[74] Age is an indicator of generation, reflecting the impact of a unique combination of historic circumstances on the health, values, attitudes, and behavior patterns of individuals. The Americans who were 65-74 in 1960-62 experienced different economic, social, and educational circumstances than the younger age groups who reached the same age one or two decades later.

**Table 10-8**  Proportion of U.S. adults aged 55-64 and 65-74 years with periodontal disease by sex and year of survey

| Age | Year of examination | Without disease | | Disease without pockets | | Disease with pockets | |
|---|---|---|---|---|---|---|---|
| | | Men | Women | Men | Women | Men | Women |
| 55-64 | 1960-62 | 15.3 | 20.8 | 39.1 | 43.6 | 45.6 | 35.5 |
| | 1971-74 | 37.8 | 46.1 | 15.3 | 18.1 | 46.9 | 35.8 |
| 65-74 | 1960-62 | 5.6 | 15.2 | 36.0 | 52.0 | 58.4 | 32.8 |
| | 1971-74 | 27.9 | 43.3 | 13.1 | 13.8 | 58.9 | 42.8 |

From Douglass, C., et al.: The potential for increase in the periodontal diseases of the aged population, J. Periodontol. **54:**721, 1983.

## SEX

Variations between the sexes in disease frequency and severity can be the result of physiologic or behavioral differences. Women have less severe periodontal disease than men and fewer women have the disease. The sex difference in periodontal disease can be ascribed to the superior oral cleanliness of women. For example, in a study of employed British persons, Sheiham[75] found that women had an Oral Hygiene Index (OHI) of 2.92 compared to 4.42 in men. Thirty-one percent of women had low OHI scores compared to 6.6% of men. When women and men of similar oral cleanliness levels were matched, there was no difference in the levels of periodontal disease. These observations do not apply to juvenile periodontitis, for example.

## SOCIAL FACTORS

Black Americans have more severe periodontal disease than whites.[4] The difference results primarily from a better level of oral hygiene in one group than in the other. In a study in Birmingham, Alabama in which education, occupation, race, relative need for restorative dental care, and presence or absence of dental plaque were considered simultaneously, it was found that plaque accounted for the differences in incidence of disease between blacks and whites. Poorer oral cleanliness scores among blacks was related to their poorer socioeconomic status.[76] When blacks and whites of similar oral cleanliness were matched, no differences in periodontal disease was found.[48] However, in some diseases, such as juvenile periodontitis, racial differences may exist which cannot be explained by plaque scores alone.

Despite the higher levels of periodontal disease in U.S. blacks, they retain more teeth than whites and fewer blacks are edentulous. The increased number of teeth in blacks may account for their higher periodontal scores but that is unlikely because the differences in periodontal disease occur in the younger age groups. There is a poor relationship between the severity of periodontal disease and tooth loss, which remains unexplained. It may be that more diseased teeth are retained because of less dental care and, therefore, fewer extractions.

Periodontal disease is more prevalent in Asia and Africa than in Europe, Australia, and the United States. When the data are standardized for oral hygiene status, education, and economic level, it is clear that the differences in periodontal disease severity cannot be attributed to ethnic groupings but depends on socioeconomic factors.[77] The higher the standard of living and educational level, the lower the severity of periodontal disease and the better the level of oral cleanliness.

## Public health aspects of periodontal diseases

Compared to debilitating or life-threatening diseases, chronic periodontal diseases are not important public health problems, but they do constitute an important public dental health problem. Although periodontal diseases are relatively common, pain and distress from bleeding gums and gingival recession and tooth loss because of the diseases are relatively infrequent. It is the effect on tooth loss that elevated periodontal disease to importance in public dental health. However, the popular statement that periodontal disease is the most common cause of tooth loss after age 35 has not been critically evaluated.[10] The most frequently quoted study on tooth loss was by Pelton, Pennell, and Druzina in 1954.[78] The population studied consisted of Navy personnel, prisoners, and prison officers. Data were abstracted from record cards, but no description of the criteria used were given. The relationship between age and cause of tooth extraction was calculated on a unidentified subgroup.

The most important shortcoming of all studies on causes of tooth loss is the assumption that periodontal disease is the major cause of tooth loss after age 35. This assumption is based on numbers of teeth extracted after age 35 instead of being based on the population of patients.[10] In a recent study in Sweden, periodontal disease was no more important than caries as a cause of tooth loss for any age group.[79]

## Components of strategies for controlling periodontal disease

The current practice of periodontics is strongly influenced by theories of specific etiology and by a manipulative approach to the restoration of periodontal health. Such an approach suggests that people's periodontal health can be influenced mainly by dental intervention and education.

This model of periodontal care differs from the socially oriented model, which does not define health as the absence of disease but as a state of positive well-being. Such a concept questions the implicit goal that all clinically detectable periodontal disease should be eliminated and the idea that periodontal health is the absence of gingivitis, no progressive loss of attachment, and esthetically acceptable gingival contours.

Many social and educational variables influence oral cleaning behavior. One of the most important is socialization—the process whereby informal knowledge, values, attitudes, and routines are transmitted to individuals through social interaction.[80] Young children copy the mouth-cleaning habits of their parents and teachers. In adolescence, brushing one's teeth is an integral part of personal hygiene and grooming behavior, both of which are influenced by family and peers. Thus tooth-brushing behavior is not primarily health-directed in most people. The majority of people clean their teeth regularly because tooth cleaning is associated with grooming and personal hygiene.

The adoption of the social model, with its orientation towards lay competence, interrelatedness of health behavior, and primary and secondary socialization, involves three conceptual reorientations[81]:

1. From dental orientation to lay competence
2. From authoritarian health education to supportive health education
3. From individualistic behavior modification to a systematic population strategy using public health approaches

The social model of periodontal health has important implications for the future of periodontics, particularly because the dominant models of periodontal diseases are currently being questioned.

What are the possible effects of this new concept in deciding on strategies for controlling periodontal disease? The most consistent finding in periodontal research is that people with more plaque have more severe periodontal disease. At a community level there is a level of plaque which is compatible with no progress of periodontal disease, but, even within populations and mouths with low plaque scores, some people or periodontal sites develop severe periodontal disease that may lead to advanced loss of tooth support by the age of 50. These findings suggest the following plan for achieving the objective of maintaining a natural functioning dentition for life, including all the social and biologic functions such as self-esteem, esthetic appearance, speech, chewing, taste, and absence of discomfort. This objective does not imply that all 32 teeth will have physiologically and anatomically perfect periodontal support with the attachment at the cemento-enamel junction. A certain level of structural change can be tolerated. Some change in periodontal support is acceptable if that change does not affect the functioning of the dentition and can be tolerated by the patient and peers and does not deteriorate further.

The plan for controlling peridontal disease has three components: This plan is in agreement with current trends in periodontics.

1. A population strategy for altering life practices and in particular oral cleaning effectiveness to reduce the dental plaque level of the community
2. A secondary preventive strategy to detect and treat people with destructive periodontal disease
3. A high-risk strategy for bringing preventive and therapeutic care to individuals at special risk

## POPULATION STRATEGY

The population strategy is most likely to benefit the periodontal health of the majority of people because a small reduction in the overall plaque index per year will reduce the general level of periodontal disease, mainly gingivitis. This should lead to the extraction of fewer teeth than if the bulk of resources is concentrated on a small number of high-risk people. This was recognized by the WHO Expert Committee on Periodontal Disease.[37] They indicated that the dentist-patient approach to reducing tooth loss from periodontal disease is largely ineffective at a community level. Public health education and prevention must be undertaken to achieve the goals of keeping teeth for life and eliminating suffering, pain, and loss of function from periodontal disease.

A reduction in plaque in the general population can be achieved by using the information on factors affecting tooth-cleaning behavior. The most important factor is socialization. Because tooth cleaning is associated with grooming and personal hygiene and religious beliefs, most people do clean their teeth regularly. The objective of health education is to improve the effectiveness of tooth-cleaning behavior. Since tooth cleaning is part of general hygiene behavior, programs directed at improving tooth cleanliness should be incorporated in health education directed at improving body cleanliness and grooming. These programs should emphasize lay competence, be supportive and non-mystifying, and should not "blame the victim."

The programs should contain the following components:

1. A community-wide approach incorporating the principles of integrating oral hygiene practices with general health education, diversity of educational approaches, and community participation in planning and implementation
2. Community leader education to improve health behavior through the better understanding and involvement of leaders of public opinion; they should act as role models and their management and organizational skills should help to implement preventive strategies
3. Public education to increase awareness and knowledge of good hygiene behavior by educating all age groups in a continuing and consistent program
4. Mass-media methods to increase community awareness of body hygiene and tooth cleanliness, the availability of oral hygiene aids, and existence of plaque-disclosing agents that can be used for feedback
5. Environmental changes—the encouragement of health-promoting behavior by modifying the environment, that is, instituting improvements in hygiene at schools and in the workplace as well as providing washing facilities and introducing marketing practices that encourage the sale of good oral hygiene aids at low cost
6. Professional education to improve tooth-cleaning instruction by professional personnel; teachers, nursery school attendants, health visitors, nurses, doctors, dentists, and other dental personnel and health educators should be provided with specific oral hygiene education so that they will provide accurate information and set good examples

## SECONDARY PREVENTION STRATEGY

In those people known to have the disease, applying measures to influence the course of detected periodontitis will help to reduce tooth loss. The principal therapeutic strategy is to reduce the amount of dental plaque. There are effective simple methods of encouraging people to improve the level of tooth cleanliness. For example, Glavind, Zeuner, and Attström[82] have matched levels of periodontal health achieved in elaborate comprehensive preventive programs by Axelsson and Lindhe[52] using relatively simple feedback methods.

On the other hand, most of the current methods of plaque control being used by dentists and by researchers comparing plaque control, scaling, and root planing regimens have major shortcomings. Among these is the failure to recognize that the methods are more appropriate to treating acute disease that requires a high rate of short-term compliance, whereas long-term health behavior change is required for controlling a chronic condition like periodontal disease. If the acute phases could be identified, such methods might be appropriate. If patients think that the treatment will lead to permanent cure, they may relapse to their former cleaning pattern when they feel the disease is cured. In addition, the commonly used methods of oral hygiene instruction are based on an incorrect theory of behavioral change—that knowledge is a prerequisite for attitude and behavior change. Furthermore, the frequent repetition and exhortation to improve tooth-cleaning may have a dampening effect on motivation for both the patients and the educators, thus reducing the possible effects of the instruction.

## HIGH-RISK STRATEGY

There are a small number of people who will have severe progressive destructive periodontal disease despite effective tooth-cleaning practices. In these cases, appropriate antimicrobial therapy could be used to change the bacterial flora in the pockets. At the present time, evidence incriminating the immune response is equivocal, and immunotherapy is not a currently effective method of treatment.

The other groups of people who require a high-risk strategy are those with medical or sociopsychologic conditions that are affected by periodontal disease. Some day, the periodontal and the medical high-risk groups may be assessed by sociopsychologic as well as clinical and bacteriologic methods because there is growing evidence that psychologic states can affect the immune response and alter the bacterial flora of the mouth. The established subgingival flora can be affected in the short term but is remarkably robust in the long term.

It is apparent that a combination of population strategy, secondary prevention strategy, and high-risk strategy is essential to achieve the objective of maintaining a functionally, esthetically, and socially acceptable natural dentition for the lifespan of most people. The balance of effort should be heavily weighed toward the population strategy. If that strategy is adopted, the need for treatment will be reduced and treatment will be more successful.

**Summary of preventive strategies**

The adoption of a population strategy is socially and economically more acceptable for a number of reasons. First, periodontal disease is not considered an important public health problem. Epidemiologic evidence supports such consideration. Hugoson and Jordan[8] reported "strikingly few cases of severe destructive periodontitis among a random selection of individuals aged 20-70 years." In Norway and the United States, Robertson and associates[83] reported low rates of attachment loss among young adults. In the Netherlands, Schaub[10] concluded that "the low prevalence of severe symptoms of periodontal disease is a reason to rethink the nature and extent of periodontal disease as a public health problem," a conclusion supported by the European Economic Community (EEC) Workshop on Periodontal Disease.[84] These conclusions are relevant to some underdeveloped countries because, although gingivitis and shallow pocketing are common, few people lose teeth because of periodontal diseases. There is no doubt that inflammatory changes of the periodontum are widespread in most populations but the need to aggressively treat every inflamed periodontal site must be questioned.

Second, the dentist-based approach is very expensive. It would take 160 days per year of chair-time to treat 1000 patients using the conventional approaches that are currently taught in British and Scandinavian dental schools.[85] Third, the population strategy approach can be incorporated into health education programs concerned with controlling chronic diseases such as cardiovascular and lung diseases and school-based education programs on personal hygiene. Therefore the cost will be low and the effectiveness may be high. Fourth, the strategy will be continuous and will not rely on campaigns and fear-arousing victim-blaming methods.

The most important implication from the analysis of relevant strategies for controlling periodontal diseases is that, since the diseases are bacterial diseases and can be altered by improvements in general body cleanliness, efforts should be integrated with general hygiene programs carried out by primary health workers and teachers.

## Screening for periodontal disease

Relatively scant attention has been paid to the concept of screening for periodontal disease. The failure to apply principles of screening[86] to the detection of cases requiring treatment for periodontal disease may be related to the conceptual differences between screening for medical conditions and screening for periodontal diseases. These differences are important and require a full evaluation. *The principal difference is that screening of individuals for periodontal disease is not primarily concerned with identification of diseased individuals in order that they may immediately receive treatment, the important medical screening objective. Instead, screening for periodontal disease is mainly directed at obtaining a statistical estimate of the quantity of periodontal treatment a population is likely to need.* Identifying individual treatment needs appears to be of secondary importance and is rarely done by screening. Most dental studies are primarily concerned with estimating the relative proportions of people requiring periodontal treatment of varying complexity so that an administrative decision could be made about the types of cases that could be treated with the available resources.

However, screening for periodontal disease and medical screening are similar in one important feature: both are concerned with identifying the diseased population. The difference arises when what happens after identification is considered. In most medical screening surveys, patients with a disease are referred for treatment, whereas in periodontal screening this may not necessarily occur. Instead the data are used for planning of treatment services. This difference is not important because, as stated earlier, most dentate people have periodontal disease and the results of a survey to screen for those with different levels of disease are frequently publicized in the press. This creates an awareness among the public and an expressed demand for treatment.

Further differences between medical and periodontal screening methods are apparent when evaluating whether screening for periodontal disease conforms to the principles of screening enunciated by Wilson and Jungner.[86]

1. The condition being sought should be an important health problem for the individual and the community
2. There should be an acceptable form of treatment for patients with recognizable disease
3. Facilities for diagnosis and treatment should be available
4. There should be a recognizable latent or early symptomatic stage
5. There should be a suitable test for examination
6. The test should be acceptable to the population
7. The natural history of the condition, including development from latent to declared disease, should be adequately understood
8. There should be an agreed policy on whom to treat as patients
9. The cost of casefinding (including diagnosis and treatment of patients diagnosed) should be economically balanced in relation to possible expenditure on medical care as a whole
10. Casefinding should be a continuing process and not a "once and for all project."

McKeown[87] formulated a more precise scheme but covered the same ground as Wilson and Jungner. They were concerned with definition of the problem, review of the position before screening, and review of the evidence concerning the screening procedures (including effectiveness of treatment). They added three more principles: (1) conclusions concerning the state of evidence on the problem as a whole, (2) proposals for acquisition of further evidence, and (3) proposals for initial applications. Holland[88] in "taking stock" of the screening position restated the principles giving more emphasis to the natural history of the disease, its public health importance, and its acceptability, sensitivity, specificity, and precision.

The prime objective of screening is to detect disease at an earlier stage than would normally occur with people having the illness, on the assumption that earlier treatment would "alter the natural history of the disease in a significant proportion." Therefore well-substantiated evidence indicating the effectiveness of treating the stages of the disease must be available before deciding on screening or the screening methods. While emphasizing this objective, Sackett[89] has added a further criterion, namely that the therapy must favorably alter the natural history of the condition, not simply by advancing the point in time at which diagnosis occurs, but by improving survival, function, or both. The modification of "risk factors" is not sufficient evidence of effectiveness, nor is the fact that the proposed therapy is "commonly accepted."

Although screening can be used, periodontal disease does not fulfil many of the requirements for a condition suitable for population screening. It is true that the disease is easily defined; gingivitis and periodontitis can be easily detected and diagnosed; the examinations are acceptable, rapid, and cheap; and sections of the population with a high proportion of affected individuals can be identified. On the other hand, there is no reliable evidence that earlier detection of the disease alters the natural history of the disease. This lack of evidence on efficacy is not surprising as the natural history of the disease is not fully known and there have been few well-documented clinical trials to assess the patterns of disease occurrence in patients undergoing the common periodontal therapies.

Periodontal conditions have been defined but the diagnostic importance of various clinical signs has not been established. We do not know whether screening tests are likely to have an important impact on periodontal health. For example, does gingivitis evidenced as redness progress to periodontitis? Is bleeding an important sign of destructive periodontal disease? What level of periodontal disease is compatible with a rate of bone loss that will leave sufficient periodontal support for the teeth for the life of the individual? Finally, since periodontal disease occurs at discrete sites and may be episodic, will current screening methods suffice in place of absolute clinical tests?

Three further problems require elucidation before screening surveys are done. First, is the benefit of earlier detection and treatment merely a shift of the starting point for the measurement backward—a common error in assessing the effectiveness of earlier diagnosis and treatment of chronic and malignant diseases. This error occurs in the following manner. If two groups of patients, one diagnosed and treated 1 year earlier than the other because of earlier detection of disease following screening, are compared to see the benefits of earlier treatment, the group treated earlier appears to have benefited if the assessment is made at a stated period—for instance, 5 years—from the commencement of treatment. However, if the assessment of the group detected earlier were made 1 year later, 6 years after commencement of treatment, then the level of disease may be similar to that of the group diagnosed a year later. Thus "lead time" does not necessarily improve the outcome of treatment.

The second problem relates to the level of periodontal disease that dental practitioners recognize as disease. Little will be gained by carrying out a screening examination and referring persons with disease for treatment if dentists do not agree that treatment is required. There are marked differences in the signs of periodontal disease that dentists consider as indicators of the need for periodontal treatment.

Finally, what are the prospects that people will comply with therapeutic regimens initiated as a result of screening programs? Compliance with dental therapeutic regimens in patients who complain about bleeding gums, gingival recession, and mobility may not be very good. Can we expect persons who are asymptomatic to be as compliant as those who have symptoms? Screening studies should not be undertaken until the answer to that question is in the affirmative.

It is apparent that major gaps exist in our knowledge about important features of periodontal disease and its treatment. Similar gaps exist for dental caries, certain cancers, diabetes, the fetus at risk, cardiovascular disease, and psychiatric disorders. In order that a more systematic approach may be adopted to acquire the requisite information, a scheme is proposed that is a modification of one outlined by McKeown[87] (Table 10-9). After evaluating the procedure, further evidence may be necessary. The logistics and cost of obtaining the evidence must be carefully assessed.

## The measurement of periodontal diseases

As with all scientific observation, the results of an epidemiologic study must be amenable to evaluation by persons other than the investigator. It is therefore necessary for the investigator to define and standardize the precision with which the observations are made. Standardized methods of observation and recording are essential in epidemiology. Before commencing any study it is necessary to:

1. Decide what observations to make
2. Choose a suitable technique
3. Train personnel to use the technique
4. Test the technique

### DEFINING THE OBSERVATIONS TO BE MADE

When requested by a patient, a dentist must carry out every clinical test necessary to diagnose the disease. However, when confronted by a community, the dental epidemiologist must carry out the minimum number of tests necessary to measure the occurrence and severity of periodontal disease with a degree of accuracy sufficient for the purpose. In epidemiologic studies, it is often unnecessary to make measurements with the same precision as that required for clinical work, but it is essential that the degree of imprecision can at least be approximately specified.

**Table 10-9** Scheme for evaluation of prescriptive screening procedures

| Definition of problem | Review of position before screening |
| --- | --- |
| What abnormality of dental significance is to be detected? | Evidence regarding the prevalence, natural history, and dental or medical significance with conclusions on the adequacy of the evidence |
| What prevention or therapy is to be offered? | Evidence concerning effectiveness of previous methods of prevention and treatment; comparison of effectiveness with treatment following conventional diagnosis |
| Which group(s) is to be screened? | Applicability to group(s) proposed |
| At what stage(s) is detection aimed? | Is the stage(s) clearly defined? Evidence on life history; reversibility of disease at detection stage |
| What investigation and tests are proposed? | Evidence concerning the effectiveness of the proposed diagnostic method(s); error rates, applicability, cost |

From McKeown, T.: Validation of screening procedures. In Lord Cohen, Williams, E.T., and McLochlan, G., editors: Screening in Medical Care, Oxford, 1968, Oxford University Press.

The most important considerations when choosing a technique for measuring periodontal diseases is that it is valid and standardized. Only in that way can results obtained in one study be compared with those in others.

There are four types of epidemiologic investigations. Each type may require different methods of measuring periodontal diseases. The types of studies are[90]:

1. Surveys on prevalence, severity, and incidence
2. Longitudinal experimental studies to evaluate the life-history of the disease or prophylactic and/or therapeutic measures in populations
3. Controlled clinical trials on small well-controlled groups
4. Surveys to assess periodontal treatment needs

## Indices

There are a number of indices for the epidemiologic study of periodontal diseases and etiologic factors. The choice of index should relate to the type and objectives of the study. As mentioned previously, there are four types of studies in which periodontal indices are used. Table 10-10 shows the types of studies and the index recommended for each type of study.

Before these indices are discussed, however, it is important to understand how an index functions. An index is a numeric value describing the relative status of a population on a graduated scale with definite upper and lower limits, which is designed to permit and facilitate comparison with other populations classified by the same criteria and methods.[91] Ideally, an index should possess the following characteristics:[92]

1. *Validity*. It must measure what it is intended to measure, so it should correspond with clinical stages of the disease under study at each point. A valid measure of disease should

**Table 10-10**  Recommended indices for periodontal studies

| Factor assessed | Surveys | Longitudinal studies | Controlled trials | Treatment needs |
|---|---|---|---|---|
| | | **Type of study** | | |
| Plaque | OHI-S,[56] PlI[93] Yes/No | PDI,[105,110] PlI, QHT[94] | PlI, plaque weight, QHT | |
| Calculus | OHI-S Yes/No | CSI,[96] VM,[97] MLC[98] | CSI, VM, MLC | CPITN[31] |
| Gingivitis | GI,[27] PBI,[100] bleeding[99] | GI, PBI | GI | Bleeding, CPITN |
| Loss of periodontium | PI,[25] PDI, probing | Probing,[106] radiographs[63,111] | Probing, radiographs | Probing, CPITN |
| Mobility | Miller index[107] Yes/No | Periodontometry[108,109] | Periodontometry, Miller index | |

OHI-S—Simplified Oral Hygiene Index.
PlI—Plaque Index.
PDI—Periodontal Disease Index (Ramfjord).
QHT—Quigley, Hein, and Turesky Plaque Index.
CSI—Calculus Surface Index.
VM—Volpe Manhold Probe Method.
MLC—Marginal Line Calculus Index.
CPITN—Community Periodontal Index of Treatment Needs.
GI—Gingival Index.
PBI—Papillary Bleeding Index.
PI—Periodontal Index (Russell).
Miller Index of Tooth Mobility.

be both sensitive and specific. *Sensitivity* refers to ability to detect a high proportion of true cases, that is, to yield few false negative results. *Specificity* is the reverse: a specific test is one that correctly identifies the true negatives and hence yields few false positive verdicts.

2. *Practicality.* Use of the technique should be practical in the particular circumstances of the survey, and it should be sufficiently simple and inexpensive to use to permit study of large numbers of persons.

3. *Reliability.* The index should measure consistently at different times and under varied conditions. The term *reliability* is almost synonymous with reproducibility, which means the ability of the examiner or different examiners to interpret and use the index in the same way.

4. *Quantifiability.* The index should be amenable to statistical analysis, so that the status of a group can be expressed by a number that corresponds to a relative position on a scale from zero to the upper limit.

5. *Sensitivity.* The index should be able to detect reasonably small shifts in condition, in either direction. It should be equally sensitive throughout and indicate in a meaningful way the clinical stages of the disease process.

6. *Clarity, simplicity, and objectivity.* The examiner should be able to remember the criteria easily. It should be easy to apply and the criteria should be clear and unambiguous with mutually exclusive categories to promote accuracy and reproducibility.

7. *Acceptability.* The use of the index should not be painful or embarrassing to the subject.

An index measures either prevalence (absence/presence) or severity. If a severity grading is used then four scales of measurement can be applied: nominal, ordinal, interval, and ratio. A *nominal scale* separates subjects into mutually exclusive separate classes so that all in a single class are equivalent with respect to some attribute. A name or a number is assigned to each class. Scales with increasing or decreasing numbers denote a greater or smaller presence of an attribute or property are called *ordinal scales*. The intervals between the numbers are not necessary equal. For example, there can be categorization of gingival status as good, fair, poor with the assignment of numbers 3, 2, 1 to these categories. This indicates that people with a good (3) status have healthier mouths than those with fair status. Scales in which the differences in the amount of a characteristic may be distinguished but, in addition, all differences between categories are of equal magnitude are called *interval measurements*. *Ratio scales* differ from interval scales in that the zero point is not arbitrary but indicates an absence of the property measured.

## MEASUREMENT OF PLAQUE AND DEBRIS

Five indices to measure plaque are the Simplified Oral Hygiene Index; the Plaque Index (Silness and Löe); the Quigley, Hein, and Turesky Plaque Index; the Navy Plaque Index; and plaque weight.

### Simplified Oral Hygiene Index (OHI-S)

The Simplified Oral Hygiene Index (OHI-S) of Greene and Vermillion[56] is a numeric index for area.

0 = No debris or stain
1 = Soft debris covering up to one third of the tooth surface or extrinsic stain without debris
2 = Soft debris covering one third to two thirds of the tooth surface
3 = Soft debris covering more than two thirds of the tooth surface

The surfaces and teeth examined are the buccal aspects of the upper first molars, the lingual aspects of the lower first molars, and the labial aspects of the upper right and lower left incisors.

The index has two components: the plaque or debris index (DI-S) and the calculus index (CI-S). Each of these indices in turn is based on numeric determinations representing the amount of debris or calculus found on six preselected tooth surfaces. The six surfaces examined for the OHI-S are selected from four posterior and two anterior teeth. In the posterior portion of the dentition, the first fully erupted tooth distal to the second premolar, usually the first molar, is examined on each side of each arch. The vestibular surfaces of the selected upper molars and the oral surfaces of the selected lower molars are inspected. In the anterior portion of the mouth, the vestibular surfaces of the upper right and the lower left central incisors are scored. In the absence of either of these anterior teeth, the central incisor on the opposite side is substituted. Plaque and calculus are graded on a numeric scale from 0 to 3, depending on the severity and extent of the deposits. The debris scores are totaled and divided by the number of surfaces scored for each individual. The score for a group of individuals is obtained by computing the average of the individual scores, which is the DI-S; the same methods are used to obtain the CI-S. The average individual or group DI-S and CI-S scores are combined to obtain the simplified oral hygiene index (OHI-S).

## Plaque Index (Silness and Löe) (PlI)

There is no universally accepted index for the assessment of plaque. However, such an assessment can be made with the DI-S of Greene and Vermillion as well as the oral hygiene component of Ramfjord's Periodontal Index. A specific index for scoring plaque has been adapted by Löe[27] and Silness and Löe[93] from the PMA index of Schour and Massler. It is based on an assessment of the severity and location of soft debris aggregates in terms of scores of 0, 1, 2, and 3.

In this system the most stress is placed on the thickness of the plaque at the gingival margin area on all four surfaces of each tooth. The plaque index is computed for all surfaces—mesial, distal, oral, and vestibular—on all or selected teeth or on specific areas of all or selected teeth. This index may be employed for large-scale epidemiologic studies as well as for clinical studies of smaller groups. The assessment of the index requires a light source, gentle drying of the teeth and gingiva, a mirror, and a probe. If optimal conditions and chairside assistance are provided, *approximately 5 minutes* should be sufficient time to score all the teeth. The scores of all four areas of all the teeth can then be added and divided by the number of teeth.

The Plaque Index (PlI) scores only differences in thickness of the soft deposits in the gingival area of the tooth surfaces. The index can be scored for all surfaces or selected teeth or for selected surfaces of all or selected teeth. By adding the indexes for the individual teeth and dividing by the number of teeth examined, the PlI for the individual is obtained.

0 = Gingival area of tooth free of plaque; the surface is tested by running a probe across the tooth surface; if no soft material adheres, then the area is considered plaque free

1 = No plaque observed in situ by the unaided eye, but plaque is made visible on the point of a probe after the probe has been moved over the tooth surface at the entrance of the gingival crevice

2 = Gingival area covered by a thin to moderately thick layer of plaque visible to the naked eye

3 = Heavy accumulation of soft matter, the thickness of which fills the crevice produced by the gingival margin and the tooth surface

## Quigley, Hein, and Turesky Plaque Index

The Quigley, Hein, and Turesky Plaque Index (QHT)[94] gives greater attention to the gingival third of the tooth. The scoring technique can be used on all labial, buccal, and lingual surfaces. Disclosing agents can be used to stain the plaque.

0 = No plaque
1 = Separate flecks of plaque at the cervical margin of the tooth
2 = A thin continuous band of plaque (up to 1 mm) at the cervical margin
3 = A band of plaque thicker than 1 mm but covering less than one third of the crown
4 = Plaque covering two thirds or more of the crown

## Navy Plaque Index

The Navy Plaque Index (NPI)[95] was designed to assess the plaque control status of a patient and to measure any subsequent changes.

The plaque index is obtained by scoring the amount of plaque found on six teeth: maxillary right first molar, left central incisor, and left first premolar and mandibular left first molar, right central incisor, and right first premolar. The facial and lingual surfaces of each of the six teeth are divided into three major areas: a gingival area (G), mesial proximal area (M), and distal proximal area (D). These areas are apical to an imaginary line connecting the contact area or height of contour, depending on the presence or absence of adjacent teeth. To be scored in these areas, stained plaque must be in contact with the gingival tissue. Stained plaque in contact with the gingiva is scored as follows: area M is scored 3; area G, 2; and area D, 3. When plaque is not in contact with gingival tissue but is found on any tooth surface, one point is added to the facial or lingual score. The highest total for any of the six teeth scored is the patient's Navy Plaque Index score. Scores of all teeth are added to give the total NPI score.

## Plaque weight

Sandblasted standardized mylar foils attached to the lingual surface of lower anterior teeth are weighed on removal after a set time. Removal of plaque directly from the tooth and subsequent weighing is less precise but simpler than the foil technique.

## MEASUREMENT OF CALCULUS

There are four indices used in the measurement of calculus.

## Simplified Oral Hygiene Index (CI-S)

The selection of teeth to be measured for calculus by the Simplified Oral Hygiene Index (Cl-S)[56] has been described previously.

0 = No calculus
1 = Supragingival calculus covering not more than one third of surface
2 = Supragingival calculus covering one third to two thirds of the surface or flecks of subgingival calculus
3 = Supragingival calculus covering over two thirds of surface or a continuous heavy band of subgingival calculus

## Calculus Surface Index (CSI)

The Calculus Surface Index (CSI)[96] method uses four mandibular incisor teeth. Calculus is considered present if any amount of supra- or subgingival calculus can be detected either visually or by touch. Each of the lower anterior teeth are considered on the basis of four surfaces: two proximals and one labial and one lingual. The number of surfaces on which calculus is detected is the subject's calculus score. The Calculus Surface Severity Index (CSSI) is a measure of the quantity of calculus present on the four surfaces of the four mandibular incisors.

0 = No calculus
1 = Calculus not exceeding 0.5 mm in width and/or thickness
2 = Calculus not exceeding 1.0 mm in width and/or thickness
3 = Calculus exceeding 1.0 mm in width and/or thickness

## Volpe Manhold Probe Method

In the Volpe Manhold Probe Method (VM)[97] a probe, graduated in millimeters and tape-colored to facilitate reading, is used to measure supragingival calculus on the lingual surface of the six mandibular anterior teeth by bisecting the surfaces and recording the calculus in mm. There are three readings for each lingual surface—one for the vertical, second for the distal, and third for the mesial measurements.

### Marginal Line Calculus Index (MLC)

The Marginal Line Calculus Index (MLC)[98] only scores supragingival calculus formed in the cervical area along the marginal gingivae on the lingual side of the four mandibular incisors. The cervical band paralleling the free gingiva is divided into two parts by an axial plane that bisects the incisal edge of the incisors and is directed toward the most apical position of the marginal gingiva. The resulting mesial and distal parts of the band or line are scored separately by estimating the percentage of the distance covered by calculus deposits. Only 0, 12.5, 25, 50, 75 and 100 percentages are used.

### MEASUREMENT OF GINGIVAL INFLAMMATION

Four indices that are commonly used to measure gingival inflammation are the Bleeding Index,[99] Papillary Bleeding Index,[100] the Gingival Index,[27] and gingival crevicular fluid flow. The Bleeding Index described by Ainamo and Bay[99] records only presence or absence of bleeding on gentle probing of the gingivae.

### The Papillary Bleeding Index (PBI)

The Papillary Bleeding Index (PBI)[100] uses the following ranking for measurement of gingival inflammation.

0 = No bleeding
1 = Bleeding some seconds after probing
2 = Bleeding immediately after probing
3 = Bleeding on probing spreading towards the marginal gingiva

### The Gingival Index (GI)

In the Gingival Index (GI)[27] each gingival unit—buccal, lingual, mesial and distal—of the individual tooth is scored. Scores for the four areas are added and then divided by four to equal the GI for the tooth. Scores for the individual teeth are added and divided by the number of teeth examined to give the GI for the subject.

0 = Absence of inflammation
1 = Mild inflammation; there is slight change in color and little change in texture; no bleeding on probing
2 = Moderate inflammation; there is moderate glazing, redness, edema and hypertrophy; bleeding on probing
3 = Severe inflammation; there is marked redness and hypertrophy; tendency to spontaneous bleeding; ulceration.

### Gingival Crevicular Fluid Flow (GCF)

A number of studies have related the severity of gingival inflammation to the flow of gingival crevicular fluid.[101,102] The flow rate of GCF may provide an objective and sensitive measure of early gingival inflammation. The GCF may be measured on standardized filter paper strips that are stained or measured electronically with a special apparatus. The flow is expressed in volume/unit of time. Specific contents of the gingival crevicular fluid may be measured biochemically.

## OTHER INDICES

There are a number of methods for the measurement and assessment of periodontal disease.

### Periodontal Index (Russell)

In Russell's Periodontal Index (PI)[25] the condition of both the gingiva and the bone is estimated individually for each tooth in the mouth. A progressive scale that gives relatively little weight to gingival inflammation and relatively much weight to alveolar bone resorption is used for scoring. The scores from each tooth are added together, and the total is divided by the number of teeth present in the mouth. The result gives the periodontal disease index of the patient, which reflects the average status of periodontal disease in a given mouth without reference to the type or causes of the disease (Table 10-11). The community's score is the arithmetic average of individual scores of persons examined. Such scoring tends to blur individual distinction.

### PMA Index (Schour and Massler)

The PMA Index[103] is used for recording the prevalence and severity of gingivitis in schoolchildren. The presence or absence of gingivitis is noted in each of three areas: the gingival papillae (P), the gingival margin (M), and the attached gingiva (A). Each of these areas is scored according to the presence or absence of inflammation as 1 or 0, respectively. PMA values are totaled separately, added together, and then expressed in one figure (the PMA Index). When the values for papillae are between 1 and 4 and those for margins between 0 and 2, the cases are termed mild; if values are 4 to 8 for papillae and 2 to 4 for margins, the cases are called moderate. If values of more than 9 for papillae and more than 4 for margins are assigned, the patients are classified as having severe inflammation. Whenever the attached gingiva is involved, the case is always considered one of severe inflammation. The index is computed from findings in the anterior ten teeth; it has been found to represent 82% to 85% of the gingival inflammation in the entire mouth. The average PMA for the group is determined by totaling the number of units affected and dividing by the number of cases under study. This index is used infrequently by epidemiologists at the present time.

**Table 10-11**   Scoring and criteria for the Periodontal Index

| Score | Criteria |
|---|---|
| 0 | *Negative*—there is neither overt inflammation in the investing tissues nor loss of function because of destruction of supporting tissue |
| 1 | *Mild gingivitis*—there is an overt area of inflammation in the free gingiva circumscribing the tooth |
| 2 | *Gingivitis*—inflammation completely circumscribes the tooth but probing depth is within normal limits |
| 6 | *Gingivitis with pocket formation*—there is a pocket (not merely a deepened gingival sulcus because of swelling of the free gingivae), there is no interference with normal masticatory function; the tooth is firm in its socket and has not drifted |
| 8 | *Advanced destruction with loss of masticatory function*—the tooth may be loose, may have drifted; may sound dull on percussion with a metallic instrument and may be depressible in its socket |

Modified from Russell, A.L.: A system of classification and scoring for prevalence surveys of periodontal disease, J. Dent. Res. **35**:350, 1956.

## Gingiva-Bone Count (Dunning and Leach)

The Gingiva-Bone (GB) Count[104] permits differential recording of both gingival and bone conditions. Subjective measurement of gingivitis is made on an arbitrary scale of 0 to 3 for each tooth, and proportionate measurement of bone loss is made on a 0 to 5 scale. Scores of the entire mouth are then added to obtain the Gingiva-Bone (GB) Count. This count weighs gingivitis and bone loss on an arbitrary relation of a 3 to 5 basis (Table 10-12). Estimation of bone loss by radiographs is affected by a number of variables in technique and reproducibility. In addition, needless radiation should be avoided.

## Periodontal Disease Index (Ramfjord)

For the Periodontal Disease Index (Ramfjord)[105] a thorough clinical examination of the periodontal status of six teeth—maxillary right first molar, left central incisor, and left first premolar and mandibular left first molar, right central incisor, and right first premolar—is made. The following factors are evaluated: gingival condition, pocket depth, calculus and plaque deposits, attrition, mobility, and lack of contact. The gingivitis is graded on a numeric scale from 0 to 3, depending on the severity and extent of the inflammation. The pocket depth is measured in millimeters on the mesial, vestibular, distal, and oral aspects of each tooth examined. The pocket depths are measured from the cementoenamel junction as a reference point. A numeric score is tabulated for each of the examined teeth. If the gingival sulcus in none of the four measured areas extends apical to the cementoenamel junction, the recorded score for gingivitis is the score for periodontal disease for that tooth. If the gingival sulcus in any of the four measured areas extends beyond the cementoenamel junction but not more than 3 mm in any area, the tooth is assigned a score of 4. When periodontal

**Table 10-12** Gingiva-bone–count index

| Observation | Score |
|---|---|
| **Gingivitis** | |
| (One score assigned for each tooth studied, and a mean computed for whole mouth) | |
| Negative | 0 |
| Mild gingivitis involving free gingiva (margin, papilla, or both) | 1 |
| Moderate gingivitis (involving both free and attached gingiva) | 2 |
| Severe gingivitis with hypertrophy and easy hemorrhage | 3 |
| Maximum score | 3 |
| **Bone loss** | |
| (One score assigned for each tooth studied visually or by x-ray film, and a mean computed for whole mouth) | |
| Negative | 0 |
| Incipient (not greater than 2 mm) bone loss or notching of alveolar crest | 1 |
| Bone loss approximating one fourth of root length or pocket formation one side not over one half of root length | 2 |
| Bone loss approximating one half of root length or pocket formation one side not over three fourths of root length; mobility slight* | 3 |
| Bone loss approximating three fourths of root length or pocket formation one side to apex; mobility moderate* | 4 |
| Bone loss complete; mobility marked* | 5 |
| Maximum score | 5 |
| Maximum GB count per person | 8 |

Modified from Dunning, J.M., and Leach, L.B.: Gingival bone count: a method for epidemiological study of periodontal disease, J. Dent. Res. **39:**506, 1960.
*If mobility varies considerably from that to be expected with the bone loss seen, the score may be altered up or down one point.

disease exists, the score for gingivitis for that tooth is disregarded in the final index. If the gingival sulcus in any of the four recorded areas of the tooth extends apically from 3 to 6 mm beyond the cementoenamel junction, the tooth is assigned a score of 5. If the gingival sulcus extends more than 6 mm apically beyond the cementoenamel junction in any of the measured areas of the tooth, a score of 6 is given. The scores of individual teeth are added and divided by the number of teeth examined, which yields Ramfjord's Periodontal Disease Index.

## Navy Periodontal Disease Index

The Navy Periodontal Disease Index (NPDI)[95] is a combination of the gingival and pocket scores of six teeth: maxillary right first molar, left central incisor, and left first premolar and mandibular left first molar, right central incisor, and right first premolar. The gingival scores are determined by examining the gingival tissues, and the pocket scores by probing sulcular or pocket depth. The gingival examination is for color, consistency, contour, and bleeding. The pocket examination includes six probing measurements of the depth of the gingival sulcus (or pocket) on each of the six designated teeth. These measurements are taken on the mesial, middle, and distal areas of both facial and lingual surfaces. The mesial and distal areas are measured at the facial and lingual line angles. The greatest single measurement determines the pocket score for the tooth. The following gingival and pocket scores are added to give the NPDI:

### Gingival score

0 = Gingival tissue is of normal color, has firm consistency, and no exudate is present
1 = Inflammatory changes are present but do not completely encircle the tooth; changes may include any color change, loss of normal density and consistency, slight enlargement and/or blunting of papilla or gingiva, and tendency to bleed on palpation
2 = Inflammatory changes listed above completely encircle the tooth

### Pocket score

0 = Probing depth not over 3 mm
5 = Probing depth greater than 3 mm but not over 5 mm
8 = Probing depth greater than 5 mm

## MEASUREMENT OF LOSS OF PERIODONTAL ATTACHMENT

Evaluation of the loss of supporting structures of the periodontium (probing from a fixed reference point) is best performed by the actual measurement of the distances from the cementum-enamel junction or margins of restorations to the bottom of the probeable periodontal sulcus. Probes with a millimeter scale are used. It was assumed that periodontal probing provided the actual depth of the sulcus or pocket. However, it is apparent that probing generally overestimates pocket depth because of penetration of the tissue by the probe. The extent of penetration is related to the thickness of the probe, pressure applied, contour of the tooth surface, degree of inflammation, and the loss of collagen fibers.[106] The tip of the probe stops at the level of intact connective tissue fibers, about 0.25-0.40 mm apical to the termination of the junctional epithelium. If the junctional epithelium is infiltrated with inflammatory cells or the connective tissue has lost a fair amount of collagen fibers that have been replaced by inflammatory cells, the probe will encounter little resistance. But the pathologically altered tissues should not be considered as being continuous with and part of the periodontal pocket. The magnitude of the difference in probing depths could range from a fraction of a millimeter to several millimeters[106] Despite these qualifications about the interpretation of probing measurement, the periodontal probe is a relatively reliable means of evaluating relative periodontal status.

## MOBILITY

Miller[107] described the most commonly used clinical method in which the tooth is held firmly between two instruments and moved back and forth. Mobility is scored 0 to 3. A score of 0 means that there is no detectable movement when force is applied. A score of 1 indicates barely distinguishable tooth movement. When the crown of the tooth moves up to 1 mm in any direction, mobility is scored as 2, and movement of more than 1 mm in any direction is scored as 3. Teeth that can be depressed or rotated in their sockets are also given a score of 3. The system used in this text is a more sensitive modification of the Miller Index.

The method of assessing mobility in some clinical trials uses a periodontometer,[108,109] an instrument attached to the dental arches, which supports a dial test indicator. The teeth are deflected with a standard force. The measurements obtained are more precise and objective than with the Miller Index, but this instrument is not practical for large-scale surveys involving many subjects and teeth.

## MEASUREMENT OF TREATMENT NEEDS

Several epidemiologic methods for determining treatment needs in populations have been developed. The method recommended by WHO is the Community Periodontal Index of Treatment Needs (CPITN).[31] The criteria to assess the levels of disease appear to be satisfactory but the treatment philosophies may have to be evaluated depending on individual circumstances (see box on p. 225 and Fig. 10-1 for details).

## SUMMARY

The principal purpose of indices is to provide a more objective estimate of disease severity or treatment needs than might be obtained by the use of simple descriptive language. They are used whenever direct measurement using a continuous scale cannot be readily performed. The data obtained from indices permit research workers to analyze their findings statistically for the purpose of providing descriptive statistics or testing various hypotheses.

Although they were not developed for the purpose, certain indices, notably those measuring plaque and gingivitis, have been adapted to serve as motivators for patients in active treatment and in long-term recall programs. By means of serial index scores, patients can be made more aware of their efficiency in plaque removal and may be motivated to maximize their efforts.

### REFERENCES

1. Leavell, H.R., and Clark, E.G.: Preventive medicine for the doctor in his community, New York, 1965, McGraw-Hill Book Co.
2. Ellen, R.P.: Microbiological assays for dental caries and periodontal disease susceptibility, Oral Sci. Rev. **8**:3, 1976.
3. Cutress, T.W., Hunter, P.B.V., and Hoskins, D.I.H.: Adult oral health in New Zealand 1976-1982, Wellington, 1983, Dental Research Unit, Medical Research Council of New Zealand.
4. Morris, J.N.: Uses of epidemiology, ed. 3, Edinburgh, 1976, Churchill Livingstone, Inc.
5. Douglass, C.W., et al.: National trends in the prevalence and severity of periodontal disease, J. Am. Dent. Assoc. **107**:403, 1983.
6. U.S. Department of Health and Human Services: Dental treatment needs of United States children 1979-1980, The National Dental Caries Prevalence Survey, National Institutes of Health, N.I.H. Pub. No. 83-2246, Washington, D.C., 1982, U.S. Government Printing Office.
7. Douglass, C., et al.: The potential for increase in the periodontal diseases of the aged population, J. Periodontol. **54**:721, 1983.
8. Hugoson, A., and Jordan, T.: Frequency distribution of individuals aged 20-70 years according to severity of periodontal disease, Community Dent. Oral Epidemiol. **10**:187, 1982.
9. Hugoson, A., and Koch, G.: Oral health in 1000 individuals aged 3-70 years in the community of Jonkoping, Sweden, Swed. Dent. J. **3**:69, 1979.
10. Schaub, R.M.H.: Barriers to effective periodontal care, Groningen, Netherlands, 1984, Riyksuniversiteit Te Groningen.

11. Littleton, N.W.: Dental caries and periodontal diseases among Ethiopian civilians, Public Health Rep. **78:**631, 1963.
12. Greene, J.C.: Periodontal disease in India: report of an epidemiological study, J. Dent. Res. **39:**302, 1960.
13. Sheiham, A.: The prevalence of dental caries in Nigerian populations, Br. Dent. J. **123:**144, 1967.
14. Lembariti, B.S.: Periodontal diseases in urban and rural populations in Tanzania, Dar es Salaam, University Press, Tanzania, 1983.
15. Waerhaug, J.: Prevalence of periodontal disease in Ceylon, Acta Odontol. Scand. **25:**205, 1967.
16. Lang, M.P., Cumming, B.R., and Löe, H.: Toothbrushing frequency as it relates to plaque development and gingival health, J. Periodontol. **44:**396, 1973.
17. Löe, H., Theilade, E., and Jensen, S.B.: Experimental gingivitis in man, J. Periodontol. **36:**177, 1965.
18. Rosling, B., et al.: The healing potential of the periodontal tissues following different techniques of periodontal surgery in plaque-free dentitions, J. Clin. Periodontol. **3:**233, 1976.
19. Thorner, R.M., and Remein, Q.R.: Principles and procedures in the evaluation of screening for disease, Public Health Service Monograph No. 67, PHS Pub. No. 846, Washington, D.C., 1721, U.S. Government Printing Office.
20. Ramfjord, S.P.: Methodology for determining periodontal needs. In O'Leary, T.J., editor: The periodontal needs of the United States population, Workshop Report, Chicago, 1967, American Academy of Periodontology.
21. Bellini, H.T.: A system to determine the periodontal needs of a population, Oslo, 1973, Universitetsforlaget.
22. Bowden, D.E.J., et al.: A treatment need survey of a 15-year-old population, Br. Dent. J. **134:**375, 1973.
23. Johansen, J.R., Gjermo, P., and Bellini, H.T.: A system to classify the need for periodontal treatment, Acta Odontol. Scand. **31:**297, 1973.
24. McPhee, I.T.: Periodontal scoring—a simple method as a basis for treatment planning in teaching hospitals and in general practice, Dent. Practitioner, **17:**269, 1967.
25. Russell, A.L.: A system of classification and scoring for prevalence surveys of periodontal disease, J. Dent. Res. **35:**350, 1956.
26. Heloe, L.A.: Oral health status and treatment needs in a disadvantaged rural population in Norway, Comm. Dent. Oral Epidemiol. **1:**94, 1973.
27. Löe, H.: The Gingival Index, the Plaque Index and the Retention Index Systems, J. Periodontol. **38:**610, 1967.
28. Russell, A.L.: Periodontal disease incidence in the United States. In O'Leary, T.J., editor: The periodontal needs of the United States population, Workshop Report, Chicago, 1967, American Academy of Periodontology.
29. Scheinin, U., Honka, K., and Kankkunen, S.: Dental conditions and need for dental treatment among university students in Turku: periodontal, orthodontic, surgical, prosthetic and prophylactic treatments, Acta Odontol. Scand. **28:**523, 1970.
30. Bellini, H.T., and Gjermo, P.: Application of the periodontal treatment need system (PTNS) in a group of Norwegian industrial employees, Community Dent. Oral Epidemiol. **1:**22, 1973.
31. Ainamo, J., et al.: Development of the World Health Organization (WHO) Community Periodontal Index of Treatment Needs (CPITN), Int. Dent. J. **32:**281, 1982.
32. Ekanayaka, A.N.I., and Sheiham, A.: Estimating the time and personnel required to treat periodontal disease, J. Clin. Periodontol. **5:**85, 1978.
33. Beck, J.D., et al.: Risk factors for various levels of periodontal disease and treatment needs in Iowa, Community Dent. Oral Epidemiol. **12:**17, 1984.
34. Plasschaert, A.J.M., et al.: An epidemiologic survey of periodontal disease in Dutch adults, Community Dent. Oral Epidemiol. **6:**65, 1978.
35. Goodson, J.M., et al.: Patterns of progression and regression of advanced destructive periodontal disease, J. Clin. Periodontol. **9:**472, 1982.
36. Socransky, S.S., et al.: New concepts of destructive periodontal disease, J. Clin. Periodontol. **11:**21, 1984.
37. World Health Organization: Epidemiology, etiology and prevention of periodontal diseases, Report of a WHO Scientific Group, World Health Organization Technical Rep. Series 621, Geneva, 1978, World Health Organization.
38. Suomi, J.D., et al.: The effect of controlled oral hygiene procedures on the progression of periodontal disease in adults: results after third and final year, J. Periodontol. **42:**152, 1971.
39. Haffajee, A.D., Socransky, S.S., and Goodson, J.M.: Comparison of different data analyses for detecting changes in attachment level, J. Clin. Periodontol. **10:**298, 1983.
40. Löe, H., et al.: The natural history of periodontal disease in man, J. Periodontol. **49:**607, 1978.
41. Selikowitz, H.S., et al.: Retrospective longitudinal study of the rate of alveolar bone loss in humans using bite-wing radiogroups, J. Clin. Periodontol. **8:**431, 1981.
42. Kayser, A.F.: Shortened dental arches and oral function, J. Oral Rehabil. **8:**457, 1981.
43. Baer, P.N.: The case for periodontosis as a clinical entity, J. Periodontol. **42:**516, 1971.

44. Saxén, L.: Juvenile periodontitis, J. Clin. Periodontol. **7:**1, 1980.

45. Hørmand, J., and Frandsen, A.: Juvenile periodontitis: localization of bone loss in relation to age, sex and teeth, J. Clin. Periodontol. **6:**407, 1979.

46. Sáxen, L., and Murtomaa, H.: Age-related expression of juvenile periodontitis, J. Clin. Periodontol. **12:**21, 1985.

47. Hill, A.B.: The environment and disease: association or causation? Proc. R. Soc. Med. **58:**295, 1965.

48. Greene, J.C.: Oral hygiene and periodontal disease, Am. J. Public Health **53:**913, 1963.

49. Russell, A.L.: International Nutrition Surveys: a summary of preliminary dental findings, J. Dent. Res. **42:**233, 1963.

50. Sheiham, A.: Current concepts in health education, In Shanley, D.B., editor: Efficacy of treatment procedures in periodontics, Chicago, 1980, Quintessence Publishing Co., Inc.

51. Burt, B.A., Ismail, A.I., and Eklund, S.A.: Periodontal disease, tooth loss and oral hygiene among older Americans, Community Dent. Oral Epidemiol. **13:**93, 1985.

52. Axelsson, P., and Lindhe, J.: Effect of controlled oral hygiene procedures on caries and periodontal disease in adults, J. Clin. Periodontol. **5:**133, 1978.

53. Axelsson, P., Lindhe, J., and Waseby, J.: The effect of various plaque control measures on gingivitis and caries in schoolchildren, Community Dent. Oral Epidemiol. **4:**232, 1976.

54. Sheiham, A.: Periodontal disease and oral cleanliness in tobacco smokers, J. Periodontol. **42:**259, 1971.

55. Griffiths, G.S., and Addy, N.: Effects of malalignment of teeth in the anterior segments on plaque accumulation, J. Clin. Periodontol. **8:**481, 1981.

56. Greene, J.C., and Vermillion, J.R.: The Simplified Oral Hygiene Index, J. Am. Dent. Assoc. **68:**7, 1964.

57. Glass, R.L., et al.: Analyses of components of periodontal disease, J. Dent. Res. **52:**1238, 1973.

58. Tersin, J.: Studies of gingival conditions in relation to orthodontic treatment. II. Changes in amounts of gingival exudate in relation to orthodontic treatment, Swed. Dent. J. **68:**201, 1975.

59. Shaw, W.C., Addy, M., and Ray, C.: Dental and social effects of malocclusion and effectiveness of orthodontic treatment: a review, Community Dent. Oral Epidemiol. **8:**36, 1980.

60. Ainamo, J.: Relationship between malalignment of the teeth and periodontal disease, Scand. J. Dent. Res. **80:**104, 1972.

61. Than, A., Duguid, R., and McKendrick, A.J.W.: Relationship between restorations and the level of the periodontal attachment, J. Clin. Periodontol. **9:**193, 1982.

62. Summers, C.J., and Oberman, A.: Association of oral disease with 12 selected variables. I. Periodontal disease, J. Dent. Res. **47:**457, 1968.

63. Schei, O., et al.: Alveolar bone loss as related to oral hygiene and age, J. Periodontol. **30:**7, 1959.

64. Lovdal, A., et al.: Tooth mobility and alveolar bone resorption as a function of occlusal stress and oral hygiene, Acta Odontol. Scand. **17:**61, 1959.

65. Rateitschak, K.H.: The therapeutic effect of local treatment on periodontal disease assessed upon evaluation of different diagnostic criteria: changes in tooth mobility, J. Periodontol. **34:**540, 1963.

66. Gilmore, N.D., and Russell, A.L.: A clinical epidemiological study of vertical osseous defects of the periodontium, J. Periodontol. Res. **10:**(suppl.)17, 1972.

67. Russell, A.L.: World epidemiology and oral health. In Kreshover, S.J., and McClure, F.S., editors: Environmental variables in oral disease, Washington, 1966, American Association for the Advancement of Science.

68. Russell, A.L., et al.: Periodontal disease and nutrition in South Vietnam, J. Dent. Res. **44:**775, 1965.

69. Parfitt, G.J., and Hand, C.D.: Reduced plasma ascorbic acid levels and gingival health, J. Periodontol. **34:**347, 1963.

70. Ismail, A.I., Burt, B.A., and Eklund, S.A.: Relation between ascorbic acid intake and periodontal disease in the United States, J. Am. Dent. Assoc. **107:**927, 1983.

71. Plough, I.C., and Bridgeforth, E.B.: Relations of clinical and dietary findings in nutrition surveys, Public Health Rep. **75:**699, 1960.

72. Kelly, J.E., and Harvey, C.R.: Basic data on dental examination findings of persons 1-74 years, United States, 1971-74, D.H.E.W. Pub. No. (PHS) 79-1662, Ser. 11, No. 214, Washington, D.C., 1979, U.S. Government Printing Office.

73. Cutress, T.W., et al.: Adult oral health and attitudes to dentistry in New Zealand 1976, Wellington, 1979, Medical Research Council of New Zealand.

74. Davis, P.: The social context of dentistry, London, 1980, Croom Helm, Ltd.

75. Sheiham, A.: Dental cleanliness and chronic periodontal disease. Br. Dent. J. **129:**413, 1970.

76. Anderson, R., et al., editors: Equity in health services: empirical analyses in social policy, Cambridge, MA, 1975, Ballinger Publishing Co.

77. Kelly, J.E., and Van Kirk, L.E.: Periodontal disease in adults, United States 1960-62, Vital and Health Statistics PHS Pub. No. 1000,

Ser. 11, No. 12, Washington, D.C., 1965, U.S. Government Printing Office.

78. Pelton, W.F., Pennell, E.H., and Druzina, A.: Tooth morbidity experiences of adults, J. Am. Dent. Assoc. **49:**439, 1954.

79. Lundquist, C.: Tooth mortality in Sweden: a statistical survey of tooth loss in the Swedish population, Acta Odontol. Scand. **25:**289, 1967.

80. Sheiham, A.: Promoting periodontal health—effective programmes of education and promotion, Int. Dent. J. **33:**182, 1983.

81. Kickbusch, I.: Involvement in health: a social concept of health education, Int. J. Health Educ. **14**(suppl. 3):1981.

82. Glavind, L., Zeuner, E., and Attström, R.: Evaluation of various feed-back mechanisms in relation to compliance by adult patients with oral home care instructions, J. Clin. Periodontol. **10:**57, 1983.

83. Robertson, P.B., et al.: Periodontal diseases in young adults. II. Gingivitis and loss of attachment (abstract), J. Dent. Res. **62:**827, 1983.

84. Frandsen, A., editor: Public health aspects of periodontal disease, Chicago, 1984, Quintessence Publishing Co.

85. Sheiham, A., and Smales, F.C.: Some results from a computer model for predicting the long-term effects of periodontal therapy upon tooth loss in large populations, J. Periodont. Res. **14:**248, 1979.

86. Wilson, J.M.G., and Jungner, G.: Principles and practice of screening for disease, Public Health Papers No. 34, Geneva, 1968, World Health Organization.

87. McKeown, T.: Validation of screening procedures. In Lord Cohen, Williams, E.T., and McLachlan, G., editors: Screening in medical care Oxford, 1968, Oxford University Press.

88. Holland, W.W.: Taking stock. In Screening for disease, Lancet, Adam Street, 1974.

89. Sackett, D.L.: Cardiovascular disease, In Screening for disease, Lancet, Adam Street, 1974.

90. Gjermo, P.: Formal discussion of paper by S.P. Hazen, J. Periodont. Res. **9**(suppl. 14):70, 1974.

91. Russell, A.L.: Epidemiology and the rational bases of dental public health and dental practice. In Young, W.O., and Striffler, D.F., editors: The dentist, his practice, and his community, ed. 2, Philadelphia, 1969, W.B. Saunders Co.

92. Burt, B.A.: Methods for assessing the distribution of oral diseases. In Striffler, D.F., Young, W.O., and Burt, B.A., editors: Dentistry, dental practice, and the community, ed. 3, Philadelphia, 1983, W.B. Saunders Co.

93. Silness, J., and Löe, H.: Periodontal disease in pregnancy. II. Correlation between oral hygiene and periodontal condition, Acta Odontol. Scand. **22:**121, 1964.

94. Turesky, S., Gilmore, N.D., and Glickman, I.: Reduced plaque formation by the chloromethyl analogue of Vitamin C, J. Periodontol. **41:**41, 1970.

95. Grossman, F.D., and Fedi, P.F.: Navy Periodontal Screening Examination, J. Am. Soc. Prev. Dent. **3:**41, 1974.

96. Ennever, J., Sturzenberger, O.P., and Radike, A.W.: The Calculus Surface Index method of scoring clinical calculus studies, J. Periodontol. **32:**54, 1961.

97. Manhold, J.H., et al.: In vivo calculus assessment. II. A comparison of scoring techniques, J. Periodontol. **36:**299, 1965.

98. Muhlemann, H.R., and Villa, P.: The Marginal Line Calculus Index, Helv. Odontol. Acta **11:**175, 1967.

99. Ainamo, J., and Bay, I.: Problems and proposals for recording gingivitis and plaque, Int. Dent. J. **25:**229, 1975.

100. Saxer, U.P., and Muhlemann, H.R.: Motwation und aufklarung, Schweiz, Monatsschr. Zahnheilk. **85:**905, 1975.

101. Golub, L.M., and Kleinberg, I.: Gingival crevicular fluid: a new diagnostic aid in managing the periodontal patient, Oral Sci. Rev. **8:**49, 1976.

102. Cimasoni, G.: The crevicular fluid. Basel, 1974, S. Karger.

103. Massler, M., Schour, I., and Chopra, B.: Occurrence of gingivitis in suburban Chicago school children, J. Periodontol. **21:**146, 1950.

104. Dunning, J.M., and Leach, L.B.: Gingival bone count: a method for epidemiological study of periodontal disease, J. Dent. Res. **39:**506, 1960.

105. Ramfjord, S.P.: Indices for prevalence and incidence of periodontal disease, J. Periodontol. **30:**51, 1959.

106. Listgarten, M.A.: Periodontal probing: what does it mean? J. Clin. Periodontol. **7:**165, 1980.

107. Miller, S.C.: Textbook of periodontia, ed. 3, Philadelphia, 1950, The Blakeston Co.

108. Mühlemann, H.R.: Periodontometry: a method for measuring tooth mobility, Oral Surg. **4:**1220, 1951.

109. O'Leary, T.J., and Rudd, K.D.: An instrument for measuring horizontal tooth mobility, Periodontics **1:**249, 1963.

110. Ramfjord, S.P.: Design of studies or clinical trials to evaluate the effectiveness of agents or procedures for the prevention, or treatment, of loss of the periodontium, J. Periodont. Res. **9**(suppl. 14):78, 1974.

111. Bjorn, H., and Holmberg, K.: Radiographic determination of periodontal bone destruction in epidemiological research. Odont. Rev. **17:**232, 1966.

# CHAPTER 11

# Host response: inflammation

## Inflammation
### CHARACTERISTICS

**Definition**    Inflammation may be defined as the normal response of living tissue to a sublethal injury. It is characterized by specific physiologic and biochemical alterations. The inflammatory process mobilizes the resources of the body at the site of injury as a defense against microbes and microbial products.

**History**    The cardinal signs of inflammation are redness and swelling, with heat and pain (Celsus, first century AD) and loss of function (Galen, first century AD). The changes and processes of inflammation were not well understood until 1882, when Cohnheim gave his classical description of the vascular events. Metchnikoff in 1905 outlined the cellular events, including phagocytosis.

**Gross stages**    Following are the gross stages in the inflammatory process[1]:

1. Injurious stimuli that initiate the reaction
2. Hyperemia (dilatation of capillaries and venules)
3. Increased vascular permeability and the accumulation of inflammatory exudate (containing polymorphonuclear leukocytes, macrophages, and lymphocytes)
4. Neutralization, dilution, and destruction of the irritant
5. Containment of inflammation (circumscribing the area by young, fibrous connective tissue)
6. Initiation of repair

### PHYSIOLOGIC AND HISTOPATHOLOGIC FACTORS

Cell injury provokes inflammation, which may be induced by external noxious stimuli or by the activation of various endogenous systems (e.g., complement).[2] These specific endogenous compounds are called *mediators*.[2]

Healing and repair are brought about primarily by connective tissue elements. Macrophages appear and digest precipitated fibrin and engulf debris. Capillaries, accompanied by fibroblasts, invade the area. In 3 to 4 weeks, the area is vascularized, and maturation of collagen proceeds.

Inflammation involves two basic sequences: *vascular alterations* and *cellular phenomena*.[3] These appear to develop separately: the vascular alterations occur early in the inflammatory process, whereas the cellular phenomena usually appear later and progress more slowly. Each event may be mediated by different endogenous compounds.

## VASCULAR ALTERATIONS

The initial changes occur in the microcirculation and exhibit three major features: a brief transient vasoconstriction of arterioles followed by prolonged vasodilatation and augmented blood flow, increased vascular permeability, and, somewhat later, emigration of neutrophilic leukocytes.[3]

The microcirculation consists of the arterioles, venules, capillaries, and metarterioles.[4] Capillaries arise from both metarterioles and terminal arterioles. Metarterioles act as shunts or thoroughfare channels leading directly from the arterioles to the venules. The flow of blood through the metarteriolar shunts, in turn, governs capillary blood flow by bypassing the terminal capillary bed. The terminal capillary bed can be opened or closed according to functional demands. When increased blood flow is required, as in exercise, the terminal capillary bed is opened. Most often the major blood flow is by means of the metarteriolar shunt.

*Microcir-culation*

The precapillary sphincter, a ring of smooth muscle found at the junction of a capillary and a metarteriole, is involved in the local regulation of capillary blood flow. Vasomotion is the local humoral control of blood flow to tissues beyond the precapillary sphincters. All vessels are controlled by sympathetic vasoconstrictor tone. However, tissue cells have final determination through humoral factors. For example, during exercise, the accumulation of metabolic products (lactic acid, carbon dioxide, other metabolites) produces a direct relaxation of the smooth muscle of blood vessels. The precapillary sphincters are apparently sensitive to these factors and relax to permit increased blood flow to the tissues involved.

*Precapillary sphincter*

Under normal circumstances fluid leaves the vessel at the precapillary end of the terminal vascular bed and enters interstitial spaces. The postcapillary vessels have decreased luminal pressure, which favors the return of fluid to the vasculature from interstitial spaces. In inflammation an increase in postcapillary intraluminal pressure causes a shift in equilibrium so that fluid return is impeded and so accumulates in the tissue. The result is edema.

Capillaries and venules are made up of a mosaic of flattened endothelial cells. Although these cells are closely adjacent, intercellular junctions of 150 to 200 Å occur between them. A mucoprotein material present in these junctions acts as both an intercellular cement and a differential filter for passive transport. The endothelial cells also contain pinocytotic vesicles at both the basal and luminal surfaces, indicative of active transport.

Substances leave vessels by two mechanisms: (1) diffusion of low molecular–weight substances through the intercellular junctions and (2) ferrying of larger molecules across the endothelial cells by way of pinocytotic vesicles.

In inflammation there is a transient arteriolar constriction that lasts from 10 seconds to several minutes and is rapidly followed by a prolonged vasodilatation of the arterioles, metarterioles, and venules. Capillary sphincters then become relaxed, and engorgement of the capillaries follows. Blood flow through the metarterioles increases greatly at first; venular dilatation lags behind arteriolar dilatation, resulting in an increase in hydrostatic pressure of the vascular bed. Endothelial cells of the venules become spherical, and large openings form at the intercellular junctions. This results in in-

*Alteration of microcir-culation*

creased vascular permeability. Leakage of plasma proteins into the interstitial spaces results in a concentration of 1 to 6 gm of protein per 100 ml of exudate. The increased hydrostatic pressure also contributes secondarily to the loss of fluid from the vascular compartment. Blood flow, which was at first quickened through the vasodilation, now becomes sluggish and finally static because of the increased viscosity of the blood resulting from the loss of fluid from the vascular compartment. Some margination of polymorphonuclear (PMN) leukocytes can be seen during this time, but emigration occurs mainly during the prolonged late phase of vascular alterations.[5]

During the prolonged late phase of the acute inflammatory reaction, alterations in the affected tissues and vessels result in sludging and thrombus formation by way of platelet aggregation and the formation of fibrin. If these alterations are sufficiently severe, ischemia, tissue anoxia, acidosis, and finally necrosis of the involved vessels and tissue follow.

Resolution

If the defense reaction of tissue in the acute phase of the inflammatory response is successful, acute inflammation subsides and healing results. The alternative is the production of a chronic inflammatory reaction and possibly permanent tissue damage.

Lymphatics

Lymphatics play an important part in inflammation. Lymphatic capillaries differ in their histologic makeup from blood capillaries. They lack a distinct basal lamina, and

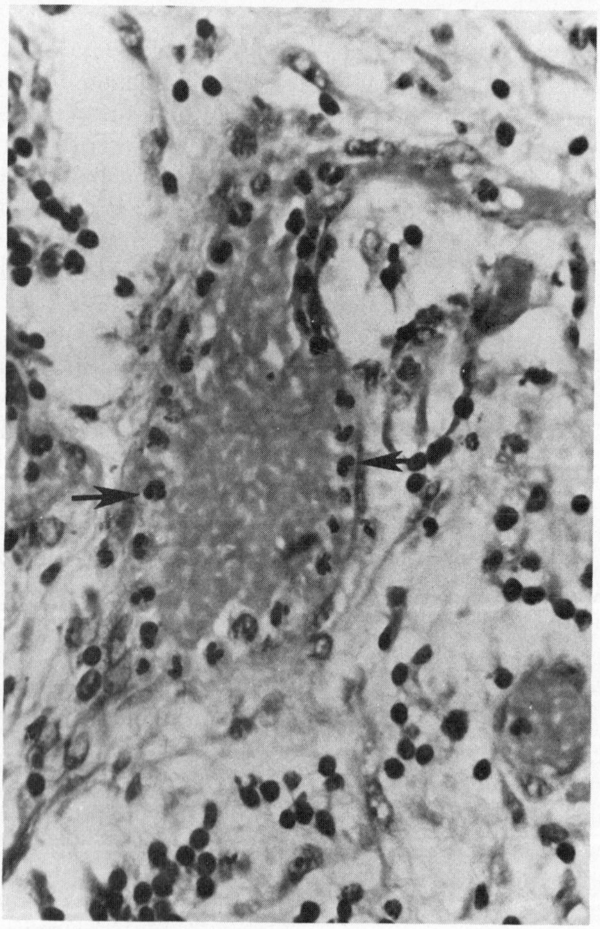

**Fig. 11-1.** Acute inflammation—margination. A dilated and congested capillary *(arrow)* is shown in which polymorphonuclear leukocytes are arranged around the periphery in contact with the endothelium. (From Cawson, R.A., McCracken, A.W., and Marcus, P.B.: Pathologic mechanisms in human disease, St. Louis, 1982, The C.V. Mosby Co.)

contiguous cells may be separated by junctions of 1500 to 2000 Å.[6] Lymph capillaries, because of their wide intercellular spaces, permit the entry of large molecular–weight proteins, blood cells, and macrophages. Lymphatic flow is increased in the presence of inflammation.[3,7] In cases of severe infection, an inflammation of the large lymphatic vessels (*lymphangitis*) or lymph nodes (*lymphadenopathy*) may result.

The severity of gingival inflammation is concomitant with the quantity of fluid passing through the sulcular epithelium.[8] Topical application of bacterial endotoxin produces marked leakage of subsulcular vessels.[9]

In healthy gingiva there is a layered arrangement of anastomosing vessels (plexus) just beneath the sulcular epithelium. In chronically inflamed gingiva the regular plexus of vessels is replaced by enlarged tufts of looping vessels. The overall number of vessels also appears to be increased.[10]

## CELLULAR ALTERATIONS

During the late phase of permeability, white blood cells adhere to venular walls (*pavementing*) (Fig. 11-1) and then emigrate (*diapedesis*) (Fig. 11-2). The polymorphonuclear leukocytes are the first to emigrate. However, other white cells and platelets also emigrate.

Monocytic emigration begins in 2 or 3 days. These large, phagocytic cells (15 to

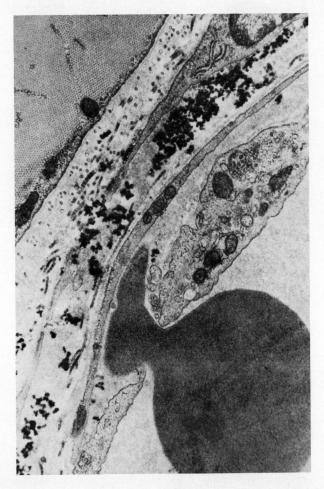

**Fig. 11-2.** Diapedesis. A red cell is passively squeezed through a preexisting endothelial gap. (From Cawson, R.A.: Aspects of acute inflammation, Kalamazoo, Mich., 1969, The Upjohn Co.)

80 μm) move more slowly than PMN leukocytes. In the early stages of inflammation the exudate contains PMN leukocytes principally, and in later stages, monocytes.

Neutrophils and monocytes have the faculty of migrating toward attractants (*chemotaxis*) (Fig. 11-3). These attractants can be bacterial products, antigen-antibody complexes, and other substances. A group of antibodies, the *opsonins*, attach to the surface of bacteria and aid in their ingestion by PMNs and macrophages (tissue monocytes).

Neutrophils also produce a kininlike peptide that may function as an endogenous inflammatory mediator during the late phase of acute inflammation (Fig. 11-4). Other protein- and carbohydrate-dissolving lysosomal enzymes and fibrinolytic systems (Fig. 11-5) are involved in the degeneration of connective tissue. In the Shwartzmann reaction,* for example, the release of lysosomal enzymes is believed to be involved in the production of the hemorrhagic necrotizing reaction.

Neutrophils are found in large numbers in the gingiva and in the gingival sulcus in

---

*"If a filtrate of *Bacillus typhosis* is injected into the skin of a rabbit, it produces relatively little reaction. If this is followed 24 hours later by an intravenous challenge with the same bacterial filtrate, a hemorrhagic and often necrotic lesion is produced at the original site of intradermal injection." (From Zweifach, B.W., Grant, L., and McCluskey, R.T., editors: The inflammatory process, New York, 1965, Academic Press, Inc., p. 13.)

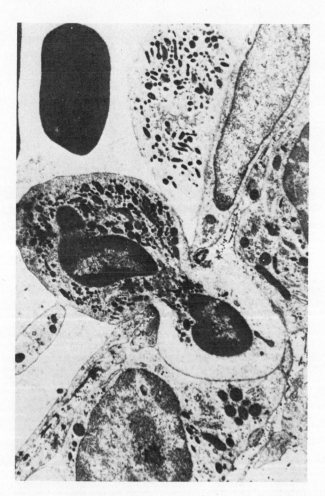

**Fig. 11-3.** Leukocyte emigration. A neutrophil is squeezing through an endothelial gap. The leading edge is devoid of granules. (From Cawson, R.A.: Aspects of acute inflammation, Kalamazoo, Mich., 1969, The Upjohn Co.)

inflammation. Their numbers are increased with increasing severity,[11] which may be a result of the chemotactic properties of plaque.[12] The numbers of leukocytes and concentration of lysosomal enzymes in the sulcus may be correlated with degree of damage.[13] Reducing the number of leukocytes by inducing leukopenia in animals reduces the levels of lysosomal enzymes in the sulcus,[14] and the sulcular fluid flow is reduced.[14,15]

Eosinophils, which may function in hypersensitivity reactions[16]; plasma cells and lymphocytes, which typify the chronic reaction; and mast cells, which may be involved in some acute reactions, are also found in inflammation.

Changes in intracellular and extracellular pH toward the acidic range influence the activity of PMN leukocytes, macrophages, and inflammatory mediators.

## ENDOGENOUS MEDIATORS

At present, the following groups are thought to be chemical mediators of inflammation[17,18]:

1. *Vasoactive amines.* Histamine and 5-hydroxytryptamine, as well as their natural liberators, and enzymes that inactivate normally occurring vasoconstrictor substances
2. *Proteases.* Plasmin, kallikrein, Hageman factor, various permeability factors, and enzymes of the complement sequence

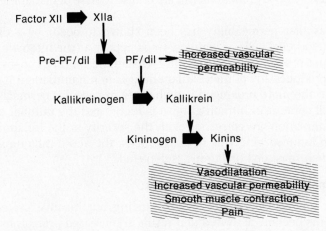

**Fig. 11-4.**  Kallikrein-kinin system. *PF/dil,* dilute permeability factor. (From Cawson, R.A., McCracken, A.W., and Marcus, P.B.: Pathologic mechanisms in human disease, St. Louis, 1982, The C.V. Mosby Co.)

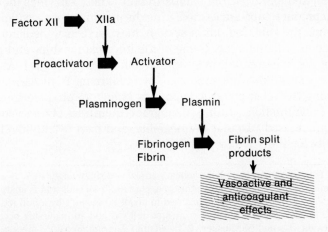

**Fig. 11-5.**  The fibrinolytic system in relation to inflammation. (From Cawson, R.A., McCracken, A.W., and Marcus, P.B.: Pathologic mechanisms in human disease, St. Louis, 1982, The C.V. Mosby Co.)

3. *Polypeptides.* Bradykinin, kallidin, other kinin peptides, and other basic and acidic polypeptides
4. *Nucleic acids and derivatives.* Lymph node permeability factor (LNPF)
5. *Lipid-soluble acids.* Lysolecithin, slow-reacting–substance anaphylaxis (SRS-A), and prostaglandins
6. *Lysosome contents.* Lysosomal enzymes, proteases, and other constituents
7. *Lymphokines.* Generic name for nonimmunoglobulin materials released by stimulated lymphocytes

## Vasoactive amines

Histamine mediates the early phase of the permeability response of the acute inflammatory reaction. Histamine is released from cells of the skin by injury and certain immune reactions. The triple response,* occurring from mild injury to the skin, is due to histamine release.[19]

Histamine is formed by the action of the enzyme histidine decarboxylase and is inactivated by the enzyme histaminase. Except for the large quantities of histamine present in the parietal cells of the stomach, the major storage sites for histamine are mast cells, platelets, and basophils. Mast cell histamine is released when tissues are damaged. Antigen-antibody reactions can also cause release of histamine through mast cell lysis.

Increased vascular permeability has been shown to occur by a direct action of histamine on endothelial cells of venules. Gaps appear at the intercellular junctions; leakage of plasma protein and fluid results. Histamine neither causes emigration of leukocytes nor produces any of the cellular changes of inflammation. It does not seem to be involved in the more prolonged late changes in vascular permeability.

The mast cell content in human gingiva is high[20] and the number of plasma cells in gingival inflammation are correlated with the severity of the inflammation.[21,22]

In endotoxin-induced gingivitis in beagle dogs, the acute inflammatory reactions are inhibited when mast cell histamine is depleted.[23]

## Protease enzymes and polypeptide products

It has been suggested that normally occurring but inactive proteolytic enzyme (protease) systems become activated and result in increased proteolysis.[24] In fact, the acute inflammatory reaction may be described as a sequence of events resulting from the initial release of intracellular and intravascular protease and esterase systems into the extracellular and extravascular compartments. These enzymes then act on various substrates that produce substances mediating the inflammatory reaction.[25] One of these protease systems, the kallikrein-kinin system, may serve as a mediator prolonging the late phase of acute inflammation. Some of the interrelationships and probable means of activation of the kallikrein-kinin system are shown in Fig. 11-4. At least four polypeptides, known as kinins, are produced by kallikreins from various sources.[19,26-28] These are among the most potent compounds known to produce some of the classic signs of acute inflammation. Minute (nanogram) quantities of these compounds cause vasodilatation, increased vascular permeability, and pain.[28,29] Kallikrein exhibits chemotactic activity for PMN leukocytes.[30]

---

*"Triple response is the reaction that follows a heavy stroke of a sharp edge (such as a ruler edge) across the skin. First there is a dull red line that begins to appear in 20 seconds and is sharply demarcated and corresponds to the line of pressure. This is followed in about 30 seconds by a dull red halo (axon reflex) and, last, after 70 seconds by a wheal that is at first dull red and subsequently becomes pale." (From Zweifach, B.W., Grant, L., and McCluskey, R.T., editors: The inflammatory process, New York, 1965, Academic Press, Inc., p. 26.)

Some of the highly active kininase enzymes (which inactivate kinin peptides) are inhibited by the slightly acidic pH (6) attained at inflammatory sites. Therefore, the activity of the kinins is likely to be increased in inflammation. Inhibition of kallikrein activity prevents the increase in vascular permeability seen during the late phase of acute inflammation. In some experimentally induced inflammatory reactions, a sequential release of histamine, followed by kinin activation and lastly by prostaglandin release, has been proposed as being responsible for acute inflammation. Each compound mediates specific phases of the acute inflammatory reaction.[31,32] A number of anti-inflammatory drugs (salicylates, glucocorticosteroids) may exert their antiphlogistic action by preventing the formation of kinin peptides whereas others may inhibit prostaglandin synthesis.

The kallikrein-kinin system plays a role in mediating certain aspects of gingival inflammation. Kallikrein-kinin activities have been found in fluid taken from the gingival pockets of patients with periodontal disease.[33] Likewise, a definite relationship has been shown between the degree of gingival inflammation observed histologically and the presence of kinin activity[34] (see Fig. 11-4).

Topically applied human plaque extracts and bacterial endotoxins produce an inflammatory gingival vascular permeability and an increased sulcular fluid. The extent of increase corresponds with the kallikrein-kinin activities present in the exudate.[35-39] The acute gingival inflammatory response to both bacterial endotoxins and other products can be inhibited by kallikrein/protease inhibitors.[40,41] Depletion of kininogen, the substrate for kinin formation, likewise prevents the gingival inflammatory response to endotoxin.[23] Histamine depletion also inhibits endotoxin-induced gingivitis.[23]

## Lipid-soluble acids: prostaglandins

The prostaglandins (E series) are partially unsaturated, long-chain fatty acids containing a saturated cyclopentane ring. They are present in many tissues. Prostaglandin $E_2$ ($PGE_2$) produces effects characteristic of the inflammatory reaction. Some of the F series (PGF) and some of the E series (PGE) may exhibit anti-inflammatory activity.[2,42] Their actions may be related to alterations in cyclic adenosine monophosphate (AMP) and cyclic guanosine 5'-phosphoric acid (GMP) within the tissue cells.[42] Some nonsteroid anti-inflammatory drugs such as indomethacin act by inhibiting the synthesis of prostaglandins.[2,43] Elevations in PGE levels have been demonstrated both in experimentally induced[44,45] and spontaneously occurring inflammation.[46,47] Levels of $PGE_2$ are increased in human gingival tissue and in purulent periodontal exudates.[48] The highest levels found are comparable to the amounts needed to maximally stimulate bone resorption in vitro.[49] These findings suggests a role for these agents in periodontal disease.

## Lysosomal enzymes

A lysosome is a subcellular organelle containing proteases and other enzymes. These enzymes are ordinarily discharged into phagocytic vesicles but can be released extracellularly during the death and lysis of leukocytes. It is currently recognized that lysosomes in PMN leukocytes, macrophages, and possibly mast cells are important in producing some of the changes observed in acute inflammation because they release inflammatory mediators.[17,50] The lysosomal and extralysosomal fractions of PMN leukocytes contain enzymes for both the formation and the degradation of kininlike peptides.[17,28] Thus a mechanism is provided by which the leukocytes emigrating to the inflamed area can contribute to the formation and destruction of inflammatory mediators.[50]

In addition, lysosomal enzymes may cause tissue damage since they degrade proteins and carbohydrates. They contain collagenase, hyaluronidase, proteases, esterases, phosphatases, arylsulfatases, and other enzymes. The presence of enzymes similar to those found in lysosomes (collagenase, protease, hyaluronidase, acid phosphatase, and β-glucuronidase) has been demonstrated in gingival debris, suggesting that lysosomal enzymes are released in the area of inflamed gingiva.[51] Plaque extracts and oral bacteria have been shown to release lysosomal enzymes from macrophages[52] and neutrophils.[53] Plaque bacteria also produce enzymes similar to, but distinct from, those found in lysosomes.

## Release and activation of mediators through immune reactions

It has been stated previously that all or some of the classic components of the inflammatory response (increased vascular permeability, chemotactic response, diapedesis of leukocytes) can be initiated through immunologic reactions. Inflammatory responses thus may be triggered by various types of insults to the tissues as well as by beneficial (e.g., homografts) or harmless (e.g., ragweed pollen) substances.

The immunologic capability of humans is believed to include (1) the recognition of certain nonself substances by antigen-recognizing lymphocytes, (2) the subsequent generation of specific effector capabilities such as the complement system (Fig. 11-6), and (3) the generation of specific immunologic memory. Antigen recognition is the domain of small lymphocytes belonging to two interactive but distinct groups, the so-called thymus-dependent (T cell) and the thymus-independent (B cell) populations.[54-56]

## Initiators of periodontal inflammation

The majority of periodontal diseases are inflammatory. There is a dense cellular infiltrate in the connective tissue subjacent to the pocket. An exudate, which contains polymorphonuclear leukocytes and inflammatory serum components, emanates from the pocket. Although the inflammatory reaction of the gingiva exhibits the same characteristic pattern as inflammation elsewhere, the periodontium possesses certain unique features:

1. The soft tissue is in intimate contact with the tooth on which plaque accumulates.
2. The junctional epithelium is nonkeratinized and has wide intercellular spaces.

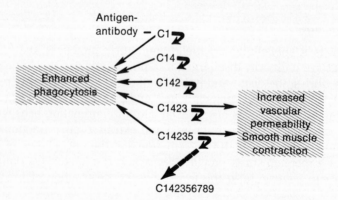

**Fig. 11-6.** Relationship of the complement system to inflammation. (From Cawson, R.A., McCracken, A.W., and Marcus, P.B.: Pathologic mechanisms in human disease, St. Louis, 1982, The C.V. Mosby Co.)

3. An extensive microvasculature is subjacent to the sulcus. Plaque-bacterial products appear to have access to it.
4. These plaque-bacterial products can provoke increased permeability and exudation. The quantity of fluid exudate is directly related to the degree of gingival inflammation.
5. The crevicular fluid contains inflammatory components and mediators.
6. The initial phases of periodontal disease appear to involve preferential diffusion through the junctional epithelium.

## ENDOTOXINS

The cytotoxic compounds produced by plaque bacteria[57] include the endotoxins. Both endotoxins and foreign proteins permeate the clinically normal,[9,58,59] as well as the ulcerated,[60] sulcular epithelium. Although the exact mechanism of entrance is conjectural, topically applied endotoxin produces changes in the intercellular integrity of junctional epithelium.[61] The next change apparently occurs in the microvasculature. A vasculitis (inflammation of the vessel wall or endothelium) precedes the other changes. Endotoxin is a good candidate as an initiator of these changes.

Endotoxins are multipotential initiators of gingival inflammation, exhibiting (1) "primary" toxicity, (2) ability to activate complement beginning at the C3 component, and (3) ability to serve as an antigen. A close correlation exists between the levels of endotoxin activity in subgingival plaque and the degree of gingival inflammation.

## ENZYMES

The enzymes produced by plaque bacteria comprise another means by which periodontal disease may be initiated. Plaque bacteria produce a battery of enzymes, including hyaluronidase, collagenase, chondroitin sulfatase, elastase, proteases, and proteolytic enzymes, that activate endogenous mediator systems. These may act against the host's cells, producing inflammation and tissue destruction directly, or they may act by compromising the integrity of the junctional epithelium, increasing its permeability and enhancing the penetration of other active plaque components.

**Plaque bacterial enzymes**

# Involvement of polymorphonuclear leukocytes in periodontal diseases

There is evidence indicating that polymorphonuclear (PMN) leukocytes are involved in the pathogenesis of periodontal diseases. Although PMNs are found in sulcular fluid and in biopsies of clinically healthy human gingiva, there is a rapid increase in number during the earliest stages of gingivitis that persists throughout the subsequent disease process.[11,14,15,62,63] The PMNs emigrate from venules, then pass through the connective tissue and junctional epithelial cells to reach the gingival sulcus, where they are shed into the saliva. The rate of migration has been correlated with the severity of gingival inflammation.[64,65] The greater the severity of the inflammation, the larger the number of PMNs that enter the saliva.

The increased PMN emigration in periodontal diseases reflects the chemotactic activity of dental plaque products.[66-69] Induction of PMN chemotaxis by dental plaque products may occur through elaboration of low molecular–weight peptides that are directly chemotactic. Alternatively sequential activation of the complement pathways (classical and alternate pathways) by dental plaque,[70] bacterial endotoxins,[69] and immune complexes[71] may release chemotactic complement peptides. PMN lysosomal proteases can also generate chemotactic peptides from complement substrates.[72]

Others have proposed that PMN leukocytes exert some protective influence in normal individuals against periodontal diseases. This concept has been investigated by examining individuals with compromised PMN functions. In PMN disorders such

**Table 11-1**   Sequence of the main events in acute inflammation and their mediators

| Events | Mediated by |
| --- | --- |
| Injury | |
| Transient arteriolar constriction | Antidromal nerve reflex |
| Vasodilatation, endothelial separation, and increased permeability of venules | Amines, kinins, prostaglandins |
| Similar changes in capillaries | Monoamine oxidase, lysolecithin(?) |
| Slowing of local circulation | Disturbance of laminar flow |
| Margination and pavementing leukocytes | Alteration in leukocyte cell membrane |
| Leukocyte emigration ( ± red cell diapedesis) and aggregation | Chemotactic factors including complement complexes, fibrin split products, and kallikrein |
| Phagocytosis | Attachment between leukocytes, bacteria, and foreign materials |
| Pus formation | Leukocyte proteolytic enzymes |

From Cawson, R.A., McCracken, A.W., and Marcus, P.B.: Pathologic mechanisms and human disease, St. Louis, 1982, The C.V. Mosby Co.

as agranulocytosis,[73-75] cyclic neutropenia,[75] congenital neutropenia,[76] and Chédiak-Higashi syndrome,[77-78] unusually aggressive periodontal disease occurs with severe loss of supporting alveolar bone.[73-78] Other PMN abnormalities such as lazy leukocyte syndrome[79] and infantile hereditary agranulocytosis[80] have been associated with the early onset of gingivitis. These clinical studies support the hypothesis that PMNs exert a protective influence and PMN dysfunction leads to increased susceptibility to periodontal disease.

Recently, PMNs from patients with juvenile periodontitis were found to have markedly reduced bacterial phagocytic activity compared to PMNs from age- and sex-matched controls.[81,82] In addition, neutrophils from these patients have decreased chemotactic responses to bacterial chemotactic factor and endotoxin-activated serum complement chemotactic peptides. These characteristics may be unique to this particular form of juvenile periodontitis since the majority of adults with periodontal disease do not have similar neutrophil dysfunction.

## Summary

A variety of possible interactions of host with bacterial factors has been reviewed. Most trigger one or more aspects of the inflammatory response either directly or indirectly (Table 11-1). Evidence shows that humans mount a variety of responses to the continued presence of sulcular and pocket microflora.

It seems probable that inflammatory responses present early in the development of gingivitis as well as a part of the inflammation seen in established gingivitis and periodontitis result from the nonimmunologic effects of endotoxins, chemotactic materials, and other plaque products. It appears, however, that soon after plaque accumulation, immunologic sensitization develops to a variety of antigens associated with the oral microflora. Continued and possibly progressing antigenic challenge at the plaque-host interface would then be expected to trigger a variety of local inflammatory responses, leading to progressive tissue destruction.

**REFERENCES**

1. Bhaskar, S.N.: Synopsis of oral pathology, ed. 5, St. Louis, 1977, The C.V. Mosby Co.
2. Rocha e Silva, M., and Leme, G.: Chemical mediators of the acute inflammatory reaction, New York, 1972, Pergamon Press, Inc.
3. Zweifach, B.W.: Microvascular aspects of tissue injury. In Zweifach, B.W., Grant, L., and McCluskey, R.T., editors: The inflammatory process, vol. II, ed. 2, New York, 1973, Academic Press, Inc.
4. Zweifach, B.W.: Functional behavior of the mi-

crocirculation, Springfield, Ill., 1961, Charles C Thomas, Publisher.

5. Thomas, L., Uhr, J.W., and Grant, L.: Injury, inflammation and immunity, Baltimore, 1964, Williams & Wilkins.

6. Palay, S.L., and Karlin, L.J.: An electron microscopic study of the intestinal villus, J. Biophys. Biochem. Cytol. **5:**373, 1959.

7. Pullinger, B.H., and Florey, H.W.: Some observations on structure and function of lymphatics, Br. J. Exp. Pathol. **16:**49, 1935.

8. Cimasoni, G.: The crevicular fluid. In Meyers, H.M., editor: Monographs in oral science, vol. 3, New York, 1974, S. Karger.

9. Ranney, R.R., and Montgomery, E.H.: Vascular leakage resulting from topical application of endotoxin to the gingiva of the beagle dog, Arch. Oral Biol. **18:**963, 1973.

10. Egelberg, J.: The blood vessels of the dentogingival junction, J. Periodont. Res. **1:**163, 1966.

11. Attström, R.: Presence of leukocytes within the crevices of healthy and chronically inflamed gingiva. J. Periodont. Res. **5:**42, 1970.

12. Helldén, L., and Lindhe, J.: Enhanced emigration of crevicular leukocytes mediated by factors in human dental plaque, Scand. J. Dent. Res. **81:**123, 1973.

13. Bang, J., Cimasoni, G., and Held, A.J.: β-glucuronidase correlated with inflammation in the exudate from human gingiva, Arch. Oral Biol. **15:**445, 1970.

14. Attström, R., and Egelberg, J.: Effect of experimental leukopenia on chronic gingival inflammation in dogs. I. Induction of leukopenia by nitrogen mustard, J. Periodont. Res. **6:**194, 1971.

15. Attström, R., Tynelius-Bratthall, G., and Egelberg, J.: Effect of experimental leukopenia on chronic gingival inflammation in dogs. II. Induction of leukopenia by heterologous antineutrophil serum, J. Periodont. Res. **6:**200, 1971.

16. Hirsch, J.G.: Neutrophil and eosinophil leukocytes. In Zweifach, B.W., Grant, L., and McCluskey, R.T., editors: The inflammatory process, New York, 1965, Academic Press, Inc.

17. Movat, H.Z.: Inflammation, immunity and hypersensitivity, New York, 1971, Harper & Row, Publishers.

18. Weissman, G.: Introduction. In Weissman, G., editor: Mediators of inflammation, New York, 1974, Plenum Press.

19. Lewis, T.: The blood vessels of the human skin and their responses, London, 1927, Shaw & Sons Ltd.

20. Zachrisson, B.U., and Schultz-Haudt, S.D.: Biologically active substances of the mast cell, J. Periodont. Res. **2:**21, 1967.

21. Shelton, L.E., and Hall, W.B.: Human gingival mast cells: effects on chronic inflammation, J. Periodont. Res. **3:**214, 1968.

22. Zachrisson, B.U.: Mast cells of the human gingiva, J. Periodont. Res. **3:**136, 1968.

23. Ranney, R.R., and Montgomery, E.M.: Vascular leakage resulting from topical application of endotoxin to the gingival of the beagle dog, Arch. Oral Biol. **18:**963, 1973.

24. Ungar, G.: The fibrinolytic system and inflammation. In Jasminin, G., and Robert, A., editors: The mechanism of inflammation, Montreal, 1953, Acta, Inc.

25. Houck, J.C.: A personal overview of inflammation. In Forscher, B.K., editor: Chemical biology of inflammation, New York, 1968, Pergamon Press, Inc.

26. Erdos, E.G.: Hypotensive peptides: bradykinin, kallidin, and eledoisin, Adv. Pharmacol. **4:**1, 1966.

27. Rocha e Silva, M.: Kinin hormones, Springfield, Ill., 1970, Charles C Thomas, Publisher.

28. Spragg, J.: The plasma kinin-forming system. In Weissman, G., editor: Mediators of inflammation, New York, 1974, Plenum Press.

29. Erdos, E.G.: Chemical biology of inflammation, New York, 1968, Pergamon Press, Inc.

30. Kaplan, A.P., Kay, A.B., and Austen, K.F.: A prealbumin activator of prekallikrein. III. Appearance of chemotactic activity for human neutrophils by the conversion of human prekallikrein to kallikrein, J. Exp. Med. **135:**81, 1972.

31. Di Rosa, M., Giroud, J.P., and Willoughby, D.A.: Studies of the mediators of the acute inflammatory response induced in rats in different sites by carrageenin and turpentine, J. Pathol. **104:**15, 1971.

32. Willoughby, D.A.: Recent advances in inflammation. In Eastoe, J.E., Picton, D.C. A., and Alexander, A.G., editors: The prevention of periodontal disease, London, 1971, Henry Kimpton Publishers.

33. Kroeger, D.C., and Weatherred, J.G.: Plasma kinins and oral physiology, Adv. Oral Biol. **2:**31, 1966.

34. Rodin, H.A., et al.: The relationship of gingival bradykinin activity to chronic gingivitis and periodontitis, J. Periodontol. **43:**476, 1972.

35. Willoughby, D.A.: The inflammatory response, J. Dent. Res. **51:**226, 1972.

36. Kellermeyer, R.W., and Graham, R.C.: Kinins, possible physiologic and pathologic roles in man, N. Engl. J. Med. **279:**754, 1968.

37. Collier, H.O.S.: Actions of kinins and prostaglandins, Proc. Royal Soc. Med. **64:**1, 1971.

38. Montgomery, E.H.: Assessment of initiators and endogenous mediators of acute inflammation with a new model, Tex. Rep. Biol. Med. **31:**103, 1973.

39. Montgomery, E.H., and White, R.R.: Kinin generation in the gingival inflammatory response to topically applied bacterial lipopolysaccharide, J. Dent. Res. **65:**113, 1986.

40. Helldén, L., and Lindhe, J.: Enhanced emigration of crevicular leukocytes mediated by factors in human dental plaque, Scand. J. Dent. Res. **81:**123, 1973.

41. Kohanberg, K.E., Lindhe, J., and Helldén, L.: Initial gingivitis induced by topical application of plaque extract, J. Periodont. Res. **11:**218, 1976.

42. Zurier, R.B.: Prostaglandins. In Weissman, G., editor: Mediators of inflammation, New York, 1974, Plenum Press, Inc.

43. Willoughby, D.A.: Mediation of increased vascular permeability. In Zweifach, B.W., Grant, L. and McCluskey, R.T., editors: The inflammatory process, ed. 2, vol. II, New York, 1973, Academic Press, Inc.

44. Willis, A.L.: Identification of prostaglandin $E_2$ in rat inflammatory exudate, Pharmacol. Res. Commun. **2:**297, 1970.

45. Arthurson, G., Hamberg, M., and Johnson, C.E.: Prostaglandins in human burn blister fluid, Acta Physiol. Scand. **87:**270, 1973.

46. Greaves, M.W., Søndergaard, J., and McDonald-Gibson, W.: Recovery of prostaglandins in human cutaneous inflammation, Br. Med. J. **2:**258, 1971.

47. Eakins, K.E., et al.: Prostaglandin-like activity in ocular inflammation, Br. Med. J. **3:**452, 1972.

48. Goodson, J.M., Dewhirst, F.E., and Brunetti, A.: Prostaglandin $E_2$ levels and human periodontal disease, Prostaglandins **6:**81, 1974.

49. Klein, D.C., and Raisz, L.G.: Prostaglandins: stimulation of bone resorption in tissue culture, Endocrinology **86:**1436, 1970.

50. Taichman, N.S.: Mediation of inflammation by the polymorphonuclear leukocyte as a sequela of immune reactions, J. Periodontol. **41:**228, 1970.

51. Tynelius-Bratthall, G., and Attström, R.: Acid phosphatase, hyaluronidase, and protease in crevices of healthy and chronically inflamed gingiva in dogs, J. Dent. Res. Suppl. **51:**279, 1972.

52. Page, R.C., Davies, P., and Allison, A.C.: Plaque-induced production and release of lysosomal hydrolases by macrophages in culture, J. Dent. Res. **52**(special issue):99, Abstract no. 161, 1973.

53. Ellegaard, B., Borregaard, N., and Ellegaard, J.: Neutrophil chemotaxis and phagocytosis in juvenile periodontitis, J. Periodont. Res. **19:**261, 1984.

54. Cooper, M.D., et al.: The function of the thymus system and bursa system in the chicken, J. Exp. Med. **123:**75, 1966.

55. Miller, J.F.A.P., and Mitchell, G.F.: Thymus and antigen-reactive cells, Transplant. Rev. **1:**3, 1969.

56. Greaves, M.F., Owen, J.J.T., and Raff, M.C.: T and B lymphocytes, New York, 1974, American Elsevier Publishing Co., Inc.

57. Kelstrup, J., and Theilade, E.: Microbes and periodontal disease, J. Clin. Periodontol. **1:**15, 1974.

58. Schwartz, J., Stinson, F.L., and Parker, R.B.: The passage of tritiated bacterial endotoxin across intact gingival crevicular epithelium, J. Periodontol. **43:**270, 1972.

59. Ranney, R.R.: Specific antibody in gingiva and submandibular nodes of monkeys with allergic periodontal diseases, J. Periodont. Res. **5:**1, 1970.

60. Rizzo, A.A.: Histologic and immunologic evaluation of antigen penetration into oral tissues after topical application, J. Periodontol. **41:**210, 1970.

61. Fulton, R.S., et al.: Ultrastructural changes in gingiva following topical application of endotoxin, J. Dent. Res. **54**(special issue):96, Abstract no. 207, 1975.

62. Schroeder, H.E.: The structure and relationship of plaque to the hard and soft tissues: electron microscopic determination, Int. Dent. J. **20:**353, 1970.

63. Wilton, J.M.A., Renggli, H.H., and Lehner, T.: A functional comparison of blood and gingival inflammatory polymorphonuclear leukocytes in man, Clin. Exp. Immunol. **27:**152, 1977.

64. Klinkhamer, J.: Quantitative evaluation of gingivitis and periodontal disease. I. The orogranulocytic migratory rate, Periodontics **6:**207, 1968.

65. Lantzman, E., and Michman, J.: Leukocyte counts in the saliva of adults before and after extraction of teeth, Oral Surg. **30:**766, 1970.

66. Lindhe, J., and Helldén, L.: Neutrophil chemotactic activity elaborated by human dental plaque, J. Periodont. Res. **7:**297, 1972.

67. Kahnberg, K.E., Lindhe, J., and Helldén, L.: Initial gingivitis induced by topical application of plaque extract, J. Periodont. Res. **11:**218, 1976.

68. Mergenhagen, S.E., Tempel, T.R., and Snyderman, R.: Immunologic reactions and periodontal inflammation, J. Dent. Res. **49:**256, 1970.

69. Tempel, T.R., et al.: Factors in saliva and oral bacteria, chemotactic for polymorphonuclear leukocytes: their possible role in gingival inflammation, J. Periodontol. **41:**71, 1970.

70. Allison, A.C., and Schorlemmer, H.U.: Activation of complement by the alternate pathway as a factor in the pathogenesis of periodontal disease, Lancet **2:**1001, 1976.

71. Genco, R.J., et al.: Antibody-mediated effects on the periodontium, J. Periodontol. **45:**330, 1974.

72. Ward, P.A., and Hill, J.H.: C5 chemotactic fragments produced by an enzyme in lysosomal granules of neutrophils, J. Immunol. **104:**535, 1970.

73. Bauer, W.H.: The supporting tissues of the tooth in acute secondary agranulocytosis (ar-

sphenamin neutropenia), J. Dent. Res. **25:**501, 1946.

74. Davey, K.W., and Konchak, P.A.: Agranulocytosis, Oral Surg. **28:**166, 1961.

75. Cohen, D.W., and Morris, A.L.: A periodontal manifestation of cyclic neutropenia, J. Periodontol. **32:**159, 1961.

76. Levine, S.: Chronic familial neutropenia with marked periodontal lesions: report of a case, Oral Surg. **12:**310, 1959.

77. Hamilton, R.E., and Giansanti, J.S.: The Chédiak-Higashi syndrome, Oral Surg. **37:**754, 1974.

78. Tempel, T.R., et al.: Host factors in periodontal disease: periodontal manifestation of Chédiak-Higashi syndrome, J. Periodont. Res. Suppl. **10:**26, 1972.

79. Miller, M.E., Oski, F.A., and Harris, M.B.: Lazy-leucocyte syndrome: a new disorder of neutrophil function, Lancet **1:**665, 1971.

80. Kostman, R.: Infantile genetic agranulocytosis, Acta Paediatr. Scand. **64:**362, 1975.

81. Cianciola, L.J., et al.: Defective polymorphonuclear leukocyte function in a human periodontal disease, Nature **265:**445, 1977.

82. Suzuki, J.B., et al.: Immunologic profile of localized and generalized juvenile periodontitis. II. Neutrophil chemotaxis, phagocytosis, and intracellular spore germination, J. Periodontol. **55:**461, 1984.

# CHAPTER 12

# Immunology of periodontal diseases

## Introduction

The immune system—a complex series of integrated biologic mechanisms—participates in the host response. For that reason an understanding of the nature of immunocompetent cells, their interaction with each other, and their interactions with bacterial plaque is necessary. Activation of the immune responses is primarily protective in nature, contributing to the host response to disease although immune responses can also be destructive to the host. The reaction, be it destructive or protective, is carried out by cellular and humoral (antibody) immune mechanisms.

It is proposed that immune mechanisms may be a major factor in the pathogenesis of some periodontal lesions. Dysfunctions of immune mechanisms, such as impaired neutrophil chemotaxis or depressed autologous mixed lymphocyte reactions, also appear to play a role (Fig. 12-1).

## Direct bacterial tissue damage

Tissue destruction in periodontal disease may occur as a direct result of bacterial products or bacterial action.[1-5] Bacterial products can be broadly classified into two major groups based upon whether they cause direct or indirect tissue destruction:

| Direct tissue destruction | Indirect tissue destruction |
|---|---|
| Endotoxins (lipopolysaccharides) | Antigens |
| Exotoxins | Mitogens |
| Hydrolytic and proteolytic enzymes | Other bacterial products |

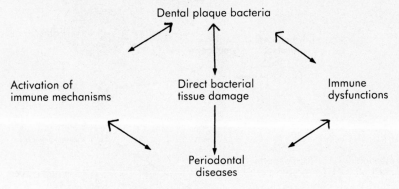

**Fig. 12-1.** *Pathogenic mechanisms of periodontal diseases.*

Several hydrolytic and proteolytic enzymes as well as assorted cytotoxic substances from plaque microorganisms have been identified and can directly disrupt the integrity of tissues and cells. They are:

| Enzymes | Cytotoxic molecules |
|---|---|
| Chondroitin sulfatase | Ammonia |
| Collagenase | Endotoxin |
| Deoxyribonuclease | Hydrogen sulfate |
| Hyaluronidase | Mucopeptides |
| Neuraminidase | Organic |
| Proteases | Toxic amines |
| Ribonuclease | |
| Others | |

The destructive role of endotoxins (lipopolysaccharides), exotoxins, and hydrolytic and proteolytic enzymes in the periodontal diseases is self-evident.[6,7] Bacterial products that cause indirect tissue destruction include antigens, mitogens, and other bacterial products.

Bacteria have been reported to directly invade periodontal tissues.[8-10] However, these reports may have other interpretations. The presence of bacteria in epithelial or connective tissues may damage the tissues and alter cells of the immune response.[11-13]

Microorganisms contain various antigens, mitogens, and other products that may differ between genus and species.[14] The molecules may modify the cellular and biochemical activities of fibroblasts, epithelial cells, and immunocompetent cells of the periodontium. For example, leukotoxin secreted by *Actinobacillus actinomycetemcomitans*, a bacterium found in patients with juvenile periodontitis, is toxic to neutrophils.[11,13] Another genus associated with juvenile periodontitis, *Capnocytophaga*, has been reported to cause systemic depression of neutrophil responses.[15] Spirochetes in dental plaque impair lymphocytic response to known activators of neutrophils.[16]

## Mechanisms of immunologic injury to tissue

### ANTIGENS

Immune reactions responsible for the destruction of tissue are induced by molecular structures called *antigens*. Antigens may be soluble proteins, polysaccharides, or combinations of these or particulate moieties like viruses and bacteria. On exposure to or immunization with antigen, circulating antibody (humoral) responses or cell-mediated (delayed) responses may be elicited. Antigens rarely induce a single isolated in vivo

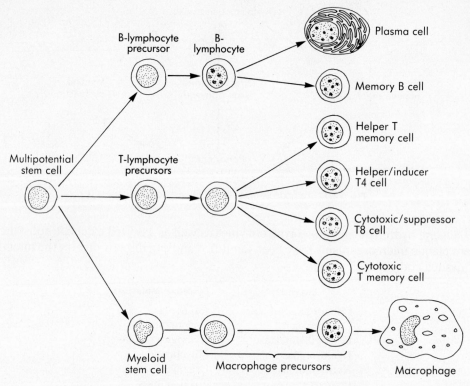

**Fig. 12-2.** Multipotential stem cells in the bone marrow give rise to B- and T-lymphocytes and macrophages as well as other blood cells. These cells have many interactions. B-lymphocytes appropriately stimulated by antigen develop into antibody-producing plasma cells and memory B-lymphocytes specific for the antigen. T-lymphocyte precursors develop into T-4 lymphocytes with helper/inducer functions and T-8 lymphocytes with suppressor and killer cell functions. Macrophages engulf and process antigen and present the processed antigen to T-lymphocytes. They also release interleukin 1, which stimulates T-lymphocytes to divide. Helper T-lymphocytes bind to B-lymphocytes and release an interleukin (B-cell growth factor) that helps B cells to divide and mature. Helper T-lymphocytes also secrete interferon, which binds with receptors on macrophages and increases macrophage activity.

response; normally, a multiplicity of antibodies of different immunoglobulin classes and immune lymphocytes capable of different cellular effector functions are induced. A specific disease often involves the expression of various immune responses whose mechanisms are responsible for tissue destruction. In later parts of this chapter these various immune responses and mechanisms of tissue destruction will be explored along with their relationship to periodontal disease.

**Immuno-genicity**

*Immunogenicity* is the capacity to induce a detectable immune response such as the production of antibodies (immunoglobulins) or the stimulation of cellular immunity. Usually, both antibody (humoral) and cellular responses are elicited when antigens are foreign to the host. Immunogenicity of an antigen occurs in a host when the antigen has a sufficient molecular size, has a rather complex chemical structure, and is foreign. In addition, other factors such as the genetic constitution of the host and the method of antigenic challenge to the host influence immunogenicity.

**Antigenicity**

The second property of an antigen is antigenicity. *Antigenicity* is the capacity of the foreign agent to combine with or be recognized by metabolites or products of the immune response. The site of the molecule where combination occurs is called an *antigenic determinant*. When a region of an antigen molecule has the ability to serve as an antigenic determinant and induce the formation of antibodies, it is referred to as immunopotent. Factors influencing immunopotency are accessibility to immunocompetent cells and genetic factors. Antigens usually stimulate less than 0.01% of immunocompetent cells.

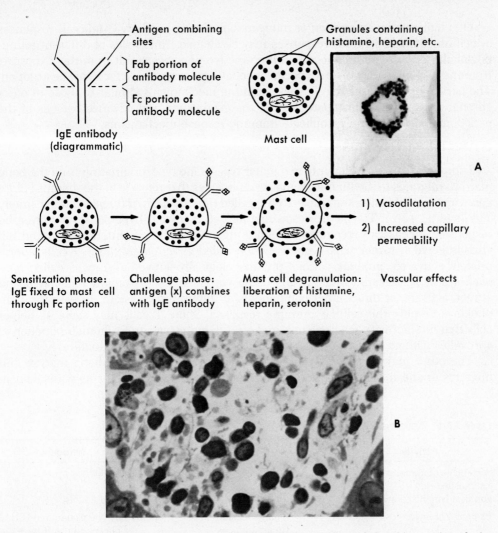

**Fig. 12-3.  A,** Degranulation of mast cells. Mast cell degranulation can also be induced by a variety of other stimuli such as complement-derived anaphylatoxins. *Inset,* Mast cell. **B,** Histologic section from gingiva of patient with periodontitis showing mast cells. (*Inset,* courtesy R.T. Ferris, Altamonte Springs, Florida, and S.N. Bhaskar, Monterey, California.)

The two main types of lymphocytes, T- and B-lymphocytes, are distinguished by differences in development and maturation of cell lines (Fig. 12-2) and by differences in immune functions. T- and B-lymphocytes recognize specific determinants on antigen molecules. A *carrier* is a part of the antigen molecule recognized by T-lymphocytes. A *hapten* is a part of the antigen molecule recognized by B-lymphocytes.

## MITOGENS

Some foreign molecules may be immunogenic without the involvement of T-lymphocytes. These foreign molecules stimulate B-lymphoctyes (antibody-producing cells), resulting in antibody formation. This class of foreign molecules, which usually has a repetition of chemical structural units such as bacterial polysaccharides and lipopolysaccharides, is called a *mitogen.*

Mitogens have the potential of inducing antibody production and stimulating blastogenesis or mitosis of resting lymphocytes. Mitogens usually stimulate 3% to 70% of immunocompetent cells. The major differences between antigens and mitogens are summarized in Table 12-1.

On challenge by an antigen or mitogen, circulating antibody (humoral) responses or cell-mnediated (delayed) responses may be elicited. Antibodies of different immunoglobulin classes are produced and immune lymphocytes result from this exposure. Immune responses may involve specific mechanisms responsible for tissue destruction. The periodontal diseases may involve immune mechanisms similar to those in other chronic diseases. The histopathology of the established and advanced stages of the periodontal lesion strongly implicate immune resonse mechanisms.

## T- AND B-LYMPHOCYTES

Lymphocytes are divided into two major types. One type, originating from the bone marrow, migrates to the thymus gland. Lymphocytes that migrate to the thymus before going on to circulate through the body are called *thymus-derived lymphocytes* or simply *T cells* (Fig. 12-2). T cells are resonsible for cell mediated hypersensitivity immune responses. T cells can recognize foreign antigens and directly interact with and kill virus infected or tumor cells, a phenomenon called *direct cytotoxicity*. T cells, appropriately activated, produce various pharmacologically active substances called *lymphokines* or *mediators* (Table 12-2). These lymphokines are rapidly elaborated and attract, activate, or direct other components of the immune system. In essence, lymphokines amplify the cellular immune response. Some T cells may serve as helper cells that interact with macrophages and other lymphocytes to facilitate production of antibodies. Others act as suppressor cells that inhibit antibody production.

The other major type of lymphocyte also originates from the bone marrow but migrates to and matures in the Bursa of Fabricius (in chickens) or its equivalent in

**Table 12-1**   Antigens and mitogens

| Activity | Antigens | Mitogens |
|---|---|---|
| Percentage of immune cells stimulated | 0.01% | 3%-70% |
| Forms of lymphocytes activated | T and B cells | T and B cells |
| Examples of molecules | Tetanus toxoid | Phytohemagglutinin (PHA) |
| | Tumor antigens | Concanavalin A (Con A) |
| | Herpes simplex viruses | Pokeweed mitogen (PWM) |

**Table 12-2**   Physical and biological properties of selected lymphokines and other effective molecules of T-lymphocytes

| T-lymphocyte products | Molecular weight | Physical properties |
|---|---|---|
| Chemotactic factors | 60,000 | |
| MIF (macrophage migration inhibition factor) | 25,000-55,000 | Heat stable Nondialyzable |
| Lymphotoxin(s) | 80,000-150,000 | Heat labile Nondialyzable |
| Skin reactive factor(s) | 70,000 | |
| Transfer factor(s) | 10,000(?) | Heat labile Dialyzable polypeptide Nondialyzable |
| Mitogenic factors | 25,000 | |
| Osteoclast-activating factor | 25,000 | |
| Interferon | 25,000 | Heat stable |

humans, probably the bone marrow or gut-associated lymphoid tissue. These lymphocytes are referred to as *bursa-derived lymphocytes* or simply *B cells* ( Fig. 12-2). B cells have specific receptors for antigens that, on interaction with an antigen, induce immune B cells to differentiate into plasma cells and produce antibodies. Plasma cells are differentiated B cells that can produce large quantities of antibodies during their short lifetime of 5 to 10 days. In addition, activated B cells can produce lymphokines physicochemically identical to those produced by T cells.

## MAST CELLS

Mast cells are found randomly distributed in the junctional epithelium and perivascularly in the connective tissue of the periodontium. Histologically, mast cells have prominent electron dense granules that contain histamine, serotonin, heparin, and proteases. Mast cells secrete when the cells are activated by antigens in the presence of serum IgE. Endotoxins, exotoxins, or other bacterial substances may serve as antigens, causing activation of mast cells.

**Mast cells**

IgE antibody combines with receptors on the surface of mast cells. When antibody-carrying mast cells combine with specific antigens, granules within the mast cell release their contents.[17] This reaction is referred to as type I (IgE or reagin-dependent type) hypersensitivity (anaphylaxis), discussed in the following section ( Fig. 12-3).

# Immune mechanisms of tissue injury

Histologic studies of diseased periodontium consistently demonstrate an increased number of lymphocytes and plasma cells with increasing clinical severity of periodontal disease.[17-19] The cellular infiltrate in the early stage of the periodontal lesion is composed primarily of neutrophils and lymphocytes.[20,21] The infiltrates are believed to be protective in nature. Neutrophils continue to be present throughout all stages of periodontal pathogenesis and appear to be the first line of defense against plaque microorganisms. Plasma cells are present in established and advanced stages and produce antibodies within locally infiltrated tissues, primarily as a protective mechanism.

Other immunocompetent cells present are macrophages and T-lymphocytes. The macrophages participate in phagocytosis of bacteria and processing of antigens. The T-lymphocytes secrete lymphokines capable of recruiting and maintaining inflammatory cells at a tissue site. It is believed that these cells function to maintain periodontal health.

| Activities | |
|---|---|
| **In vitro** | **In vivo** |
| Attracts PMNs and macrophages | Untested |
| Prevents random migration of macrophages; may activate macrophages | Accumulation of macrophages; may increase phagocytosis |
| Target cell injury | May destroy target cells |
| | Localized cutaneous reaction |
| Unknown | Transfer of reactivity to uncommitted lymphocytes |
| Lymphocyte transformation | |
| Nonspecific lymphocyte transformation | Untested |
| Bone resorption | Untested |
| Inhibits viral replication | Inhibits viral replication |

However, if the activities of these cells are inappropriately directed or are impaired, periodontal lesions may develop at a faster rate (e.g., rapidly progressive periodontitis) or may be initated at an earlier age (prepubertal or juvenile periodontitis).

**Early gingivitis**

Immunopathologic studies have shown that early gingivitis lesions contain primarily lymphocytes without membrane-associated immunoglobulins and Fc receptors for IgG.[22,23] Lymphocytes lacking these membrane markers are normally characterized as T-lymphocytes (thymus derived). Therefore early gingivitis lesions contain predominantly T-lymphocytes. However early gingivitis lesions may also contain small numbers of B-lymphocytes and plasma cells clustered in foci near the junctional epithelium–connective tissue interface.

T-lymphocyte predominance in the early gingivitis lesion lends support to the suggestion that T-lymphocytes stimulated by dental plaque antigen play a role in the progression of early periodontal lesions. T-lymphocytes stimulated by antigens produce pharmacologically active chemicals known as *lymphokines*.[24,25] The physical and biologic properties of selected lymphokines and other effector molecules of T-lymphocytes are listed in Table 12-2.

**Advanced gingivitis**

As the disease progresses to advanced gingivitis, increased numbers of B-lymphocytes are seen near the junctional epithelium–connective tissue interface. Immunoglobulin-bearing lymphocytes and plasma cells spread throughout the inflamed gingiva.[22,23] Approximately half of the lymphocytes have membrane-associated IgG, primarily of the IgG-1 and IgG-3 subclasses. Studies of isolated lymphocytes from moderate to advanced gingivitis reveal equivalent numbers of T- and B-cells. In early gingivitis T-lymphocytes predominate and in advanced gingivitis B-lymphocytes predominate.

Immune responses initiated by the combination of antibody with antigen are called *antibody-mediated* and are part of *humoral immunity*. Antibody mediated (immediate-type) hypersensitivity is initiated by the combination of antigen with specific antibody (Table 12-3). Responses effected by T-lymphocyte activities or products are examples of cell-mediated (cellular) immunity. In the hypersensitive or allergic condition, tissue damage (often localized by inflammation) is induced in the immunized (sensitized) host by subsequent contact with specific antigen. Cell-mediated (delayed-type) hypersensitivity results from the interaction of T-lymphocytes with antigen.[26]

## Four immune mechanisms of tissue injury

There are four types of immune reactions[26]:

| Type | Manifestation |
|------|---------------|
| I | Reagin type (anaphylaxis, atopy) |
| II | Cytotoxic (complement fixing) |
| III | Antibody-mediated (immediate, Arthus phenomenon) hypersensitivity |
| IV | Cell-mediated (delayed) hypersensitivity |

Although, as previously discussed, immune reactions are usually beneficial to the host, they may also produce tissue destruction.

### TYPE I REACTIONS: IgE OR REAGIN-DEPENDENT HYPERSENSITIVITY (ATOPY)

Exposure to an antigen may provoke a unique antibody production (IgE or reagin) by plasma cells. This antibody binds with receptors on mast cells, basophils, and platelets. A subsequent exposure to the same antigen causes the antibody bound to the cell surfaces to combine with the antigen to form an antibody-antigen complex. This complex results in degranulation of mast cells associated with IgE antibody ( Fig.

12-3, *A*). Degranulation of mast cells (or basophils and platelets) results in histamine release, which causes vasodilatation of blood vessels, increased permeability, and shock (Table 12-4). Smooth muscle contractions may occur at two target sites: the bronchi of the lungs and the liver. Generalized anaphylaxis is a state similar to shock and occurs within minutes of exposure to an offending antigen.

Other chemical mediators of anaphylaxis (Table 12-4) include a slow-reacting substance of anaphylaxis (SRS-A), an acidic lipoprotein having a prolonged constrictive effect on smooth muscle; eosinophil chemotactic factor of anaphylaxis (ECF-A), an acidic peptide causing an influx of eosinophils into the site of tissue injury; bradykinin, a nonapeptide (nine amino acid peptide chain) split by the enzyme kallikrein from serum precursors causing a prolonged contraction of smooth muscle; and serotonin (5-hydroxytryptamine), which is not a significant mediator in humans.

The target cells of IgE-mediated allergic reactions are mast cells, basophils, and platelets. Mast cells are observed histologically in healthy periodontal connective tissues and junctional epithelium and increase in number with inflammation. These observations suggest a role for these cells in the periodontal diseases. Antigens may induce degranulation of mast cells associated with cell-borne (cytophilic) IgE antibody. The mast cells, in turn, release histamine and other vasoactive substances that have a pronounced effect on increasing permeability.

IgE antibody can become fixed or bound to the surfaces of various cells. The ability to become fixed to cell surfaces is controlled through a specific receptor site on the Fc component of the antibody molecule, a crystallizable fragment composed of the C-terminal half of the molecule's two heavy chains. Such fixation does not involve the Fab portion. The Fab portion is a fragment that contains the combining sites for antigens. The reaction of an antigen with a specific IgE antibody bound to the surfaces of mast cells leads to the degranulation of the affected mast cell (Fig. 12-3).

IgE is present in low concentrations in the serum (1 μg antibody protein/ml) in healthy individuals but may be elevated in patients with allergic reactions to different antigens or allergens. The anaphylactic reaction in allergic patients is marked by

**Table 12-3** Differences between antibody-mediated (humoral, immediate type) hypersensitivity and cell-mediated (cellular, delayed type) hypersensitivity

| Activity | Antibody mediated | Cell mediated |
|---|---|---|
| Sensitizing molecules | Proteins, polysaccharides, lipids | Proteins, haptens |
| Molecule/cell interaction | Combination of antibody and antigen | Stimulation of lymphocytes with antigen |
| Response time | Immediate (minutes to hours) | Delayed (24-72 hours) |
| Transfer | Circulating serum antibody | Cells and cell-derived transfer factors |
| Effector factors | Complement, vasoactive amines | Secreted soluble chemical |

**Table 12-4** Chemical mediators of anaphylaxis

| Mediator | Action |
|---|---|
| Histamine | Vasodilation |
| | Increased permeability of blood vessels |
| | Shock |
| Slow-reacting substance of anaphylaxis (SRS-A) | Prolonged constriction of smooth muscle |
| Eosinophil chemotactic factor of anaphylaxis (ECF-A) | Influx of eosinophils |
| Bradykinin | Slow, prolonged contraction of smooth muscle |
| Serotonin (5-hydoxytryptamine) | Not significant in humans |

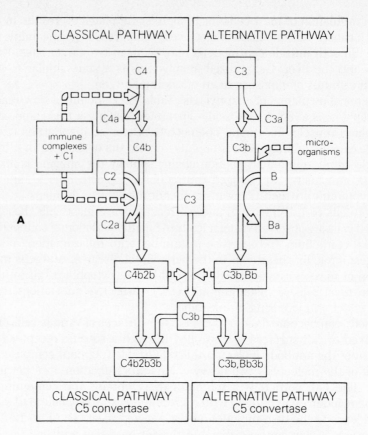

**Fig. 12-4. A,** Activation of the complement cascade.

extravasation of plasma proteins into the surrounding tissue and diapedesis of leukocytes from blood vessels.

A few studies suggest that IgE (reagin) type (anaphylactic) hypersensitivity may play a role in periodontal disease. IgE is localized in periodontal tissues.[27,28] Morphometric studies[29,30] have shown that the quantity of mast cells increases with the severity of periodontal inflammation. Mast cells were primarily associated with plasma cells and were not seen near aggregates of lymphocytes. Degranulation of mast cells could contribute to inflammatory periodontal disease through the release of prostaglandins capable of enhancing bone resorption.[31] In addition to prostaglandins and histamine, mast cells contain a substance that may participate in collagen degradation.[32,33]

Other mast cell functions have also been implicated in the initiation and pathogenesis of periodontal diseases. IgG-4, a subclass of IgG in periodontitis lesions, has been observed to bind to mast cells and cause degranulation and release of prostaglandins.[34] The C3a and C5a components of the complement cascade also cause mast cell degranulation and inflammation.[35]

## TYPE II REACTIONS: CYTOTOXIC (COMPLEMENT-FIXING)

Type II reactions, or cytotoxic reactions, are antibody dependent and involve the binding of IgM or IgG antibodies to cell surface determinants or tissue antigens. There are three components of type II reactions: antibody binding (Fab portion) to cell or tissue antigens, antibody-dependent cell activity, and activation of complement via the Fc portion of the antibody molecule.

Complement plays a role in the lysis of the antibody-coated cells. The lytic function

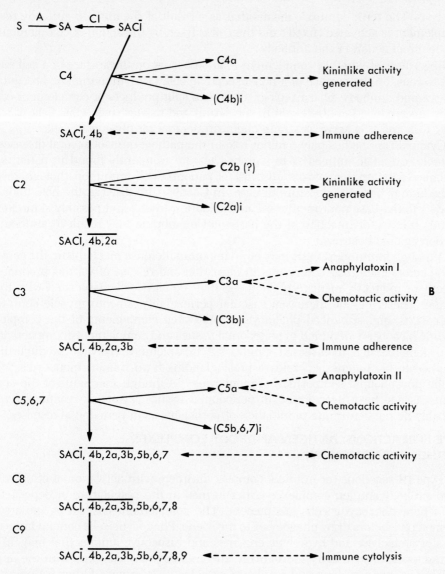

**Fig. 12-4, cont'd.    B,** In the sequential activation of the complement system, a number of substances with pharmacologic activity are produced (right column). (**A** from Roitt, I.M., Brostoff, J., and Male, D.K.: Immunology, New York, 1985, Gower Medical Publishing, distributed by C.V. Mosby Co.; **B** based on data from H.R. Creamer, Portland, Oregon.)

of complement may be involved in killing of plaque bacteria. Antibody- and complement-enhanced phagocytosis and killing are important mechanisms in the elimination of gram-positive bacteria. Complement-dependent lysis without phagocytosis is effective in killing some gram-negative organisms. Both mechanisms may be involved in maintaining periodontal health in the presence of plaque.

Complement-dependent lysis of susceptible cells requires the activation or fixation of complement on the surface of the affected cell (Fig. 12-4, *A* and *B*). Fixation or activation refers to the sequential involvement of a multitude of blood proteins and is classically triggered by the union of antibody with antigen. Receptor sites on the Fc components of bound IgG or IgM antibody molecules react with C1 and initiate the complement cascade. Complement fixation through C9 occurs on the surface membranes of a variety of bacterial and mammalian cell types and leads to cytotoxicity and cell lysis. The term *cytotoxic* means that as a result of the antigen-antibody reaction complement is activated (fixed) and the cell is lysed by the action of complement (not by the direct action of the antibody).

Regardless of whether complement fixation occurs on the surface of a cell susceptible to lysis, on the surface of a nonsusceptible cell, or in an inanimate precipitate of antigen and antibody, pharmacologically active split products of complement components are produced and released in the serum and tissues (e.g., C2b, C4a, C3a, and C5a). C3a and C5a serve as strong chemoattractants for phagocytic cells.

Cytotoxic antibodies play a minor role in the pathogenesis of several diseases. For example, cytotoxic antibodies to lymphocytes are frequently found in patients with systemic lupus erythematosus. Also 5% of patients with immunopathologic diseases of the kidney have Goodpasture disease. In Goodpasture disease, the host makes antibodies to the basement membrane of the kidney, lungs, and possibly skin. Noxious agents, trauma, or infection of the basement membrane may result in antibody production against host tissues.

Although immunocytolysis may be an important defense mechanism, the activation of the complement cascade results in formation and release of various products that directly or indirectly mediate phenomena that are classically associated with inflammation. These include increased vascular permeability, smooth muscle contraction, chemotaxis, and enhanced phagocytosis. Activated components of the complement cascade have been identified in periodontal tissues and complement-fixing activity has been demonstrated in diseased gingiva.[36-38] Complement cleavage products inhibit lymphocyte blastogenesis,[37] release prostaglandins from human monocytes,[39,40] and inhibit phospholipid composition of monocytes.[41] Although fragments of the complement cascade have been found in periodontal tissues, cytotoxic reactions (type II) probably do not contribute to initiation or pathogenesis of periodontal diseases.

## TYPE III REACTIONS: ANTIGEN-ANTIBODY COMPLEXES (ARTHUS PHENOMENON)

Type III reactions (or immune complex disorders with activation of effector cells) have antibody-antigen complexes either formed in the vasculature or deposited in a site where phagocytic cells are present. The complement cascade is initiated and chemotactic factors draw phagocytes to the scene. Phagocytic cells contain large quantities of proteolytic and hydrolytic enzymes and vasoactive amines that may, in turn, lead to tissue destruction. Alternatively, the antibody may combine with the antigen, which does not circulate, and results in pathologic alterations. Other factors that influence the severity of the tissue alterations in type III reactions include: persistence and amount of antigen, class and affinity of antibody involved, ratio of antibody to antigen complexes, activation of the classic or alternate complement pathways, neutrophilic and phagocytic infiltration of tissues, and genetic susceptibility of the host.

The classic example of tissue damage triggered by the deposition of immune complexes is a type III reaction. Repeated injections of horse serum into the skin of a rabbit produces a hemorrhagic and necrotic reaction. At first, there is a rapid development of a wheal with erythema but this reaction subsides quickly. After each succeeding injection, the reaction becomes more intense until a necrotic lesion is produced. The intensity of this reaction (known as the Arthus phenomenon) is related to the level of circulating specific antibody.[28] The precipitation of a soluble antigen (e.g., foreign albumin) by complement-fixing antibody in the walls of venules and in tissue spaces leads to activation of complement, subsequent chemotactic attraction of phagocytic cells, and destruction of local tissue resulting from activities of the phagocytic cells. The phenomenon demonstrates how the precipitation of antigen-antibody complexes (themselves innocuous) at a site leads to tissue damage through the intense, localized inflammatory response instigated by cleaved products of complement.

Arthus hypersensitivity refers to the presence of high levels of circulating antibodies of any immunoglobulin class that precipitates antigen by forming antigen-antibody immune complexes.[42] The precipitation of antigen by circulating antibody is probably responsible for the normal clearance of antigen. However, these immune complexes can also result in tissue damage. A classic example is the deposition of immune complexes and concomitant activation of the complement pathway on the epithelial side of the glomerular basement membranes in glomerulonephritis.

If the classic complement pathway is activated by immune complexes, a number of biologically active mediators are produced. These biologically active substances may induce increased vascular permeability, platelet aggregation, phagocyte chemotaxis, opsonization and engulfment of bacteria and antigens, and killing of bacteria. Complement activation is associated with the release of lysosomal enzymes from phagocytes, resulting in local damage of tissue. If activation of the alternative complement pathway occurs, a similar reaction to that induced by the classical pathway may result. Substances such as lipopolysaccharides, peptidoglycans, and other plaque bacterial products have the potential of activating the alternative complement pathway.[43] Activation of both pathways of the complement system may occur concomitantly.

Localized inflammatory responses may be initiated by immune complexes that fix complement and release numerous peptides (e.g., C2b, C3a, C4a, and C5a) capable of inducing secondary inflammatory effects. Several of these peptides are inflammatory as well as chemotactic for PMN leukocytes. In addition, platelets may be aggregated through immune adherence to these complexes and undergo lysis, releasing vasoactive substances (kinins). These kinins help facilitate the accumulation of neutrophils, which is a distinctive feature of the Arthus lesion. The phagocytized immune complexes may cause neutrophils to undergo degranulation, releasing enzymes such as cathepsins, peptidases, lipases, nucleases, proteases, lysozymes, and phosphatases. These enzymes are capable of damaging tissue and enhance the inflammatory lesion first initiated by immune complexes. The same pathologic process may be produced by activation of complement by bacterial endotoxins commonly found in dental plaque.[44] These endotoxins are potent inflammatory agents and are presumed to contribute to the inflammation associated with periodontal disease.

Periodontal patients frequently have circulating antibodies to the oral bacteria that have been associated with gingival inflammation.[45,46] Nearly all patients with periodontal disease have antibodies to *Actinomyces* species.[47] Serum titers, however, may not correlate with the severity of periodontal disease. Two thirds of periodontal patients have anti-*Leptotrichia buccalis* antibodies and one fourth have anti-*Bacteroides melaninogenicus* antibodies.[48] Indirect immunofluorescence indicates that these antibodies are principally of the IgG and IgM class and that the titers increase with age. Serum antibodies in juvenile periodontitis frequently are elevated.[49]

Inflamed gingiva has higher concentrations of immunoglobulins than normal gingiva.[50] Gingival immunoglobulins specific for *Fusobacterium* and *Veillonella* are found.[51]

Other investigators have analyzed the increased flow of crevicular fluid associated with gingival inflammation and have observed increased concentrations of IgG.[52] Increased levels of immunoglobulin and complement (C3) are found in gingival fluid.[53] Other components of the complement system have also been found in periodontal pockets.[54]

Large molecular weight immune complexes have not been detected in periodontal tissues. However, because plaque antigens are present in periodontal tissues and antibodies are produced by the B-lymphocyte series of cells, immune complexes may play a role in the pathogenesis of periodontal disease. Direct immunofluorescent stain-

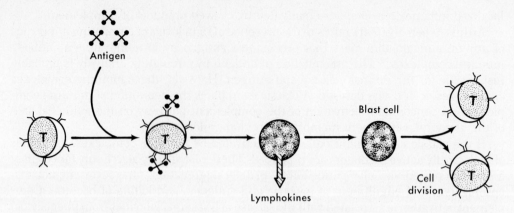

**Fig. 12-5.** Antigen activation of immune thymus-derived lymphocytes (T) (transformation or blastogenesis).

ing for immunoglobulin and the C3 complement component[38] suggests that complement is activated by antibody-antigen complexes. Also, gingival crevicular neutrophils have membrane bound IgG, IgM and C3 and C3b.

## TYPE IV REACTIONS: CELL-MEDIATED (DELAYED) HYPERSENSITIVITY

Type IV reactions or cell-mediated (delayed) hypersensitivity involves the stimulation of T- and B-cell lymphocytes by antigens. Plaque antigens may stimulate this lymphocyte proliferation. Cell-mediated reactions can involve lymphocyte contact with a target cell that is injured or killed by lymphocyte product(s). Antibody or complement may also participate in these reactions.

A classic example of cell-mediated hypersensitivity is the delayed skin reaction to antigenic stimulation. A characteristic mononuclear infiltrate develops 24 to 72 hours after stimulation. A relatively small number (less than 0.1%) of the lymphocytes secrete lymphokines or mediators promoting an increasingly dense inflammatory infiltrate. The inflammatory cells, which are immunocompetent, may become activated to become bactericidal, fungicidal, viracidal, or tumoricidal.

Antigen recognition by small lymphocytes, especially by T cells, results in the generation and release of nonimmunoglobulin products that affect lymphocytes and other cell types. The factors, known as lymphokines,[55,56] are nonspecific in action (i.e., they affect cells of normal as well as sensitized animals). They apparently orchestrate many of the cellular events occurring during the development of the inflammatory response (and tissue damage) characteristic of cell-mediated immunity (delayed-type hypersensitivity).[57,58] Such phenomena as the allergy of infection (e.g., tuberculin sensitivity), contact allergy (e.g., poison ivy), and transplantation immunity (e.g., homograft rejection) are examples of cell-mediated immunity.

A wide variety of factors (lymphokines), have been described and named on the basis of their activity in test systems (Table 12-5). Because of multiple activities more than one name may exist for the same factor. However it appears that several are distinct entities: (1) chemotactic factor (CF), which is chemotactic for macrophages (monocytes); (2) activation factor, which induces an increased level of metabolic and functional activity in affected macrophages; (3) migration inhibition factor (MIF), a nontoxic glycoprotein that inhibits the migration of macrophages and theoretically leads to their accumulation at the reaction site; (4) lymphotoxin (LT), a factor that can lead to the death of fibroblasts in culture; and (5) blastogenic factor (several individual factors causing nonspecific lymphocyte transformation).

These and similar lymphokines apparently act by concentrating lymphocytes, mono-

**Table 12-5**   Selected lymphokines: properties and biologic actions

| Lymphokine | Effect |
| --- | --- |
| Antifungal factor | Inhibits growth of yeast in vitro |
| Cell cooperation factor | Increases the number or rate of formation for antibody-producing cells |
| Cloning inhibition factor | Inhibits proliferation of clones of cultured cells |
| Inhibition factor | Inhibits neutrophil function |
| Interferon | Prevents replication of viruses |
| Lymphotoxin | Nonspecifically kills cultured cells |
| Potentiating factor | Potentiates lymphocyte blastogenesis |
| Proliferation inhibition factor | Inhibits proliferation of cultured cells |
| Macrophage-activating factor | Induces macrophage activation |
| Macrophage aggregation factor | Causes macrophage aggregation |
| Macrophage chemotactic factor | Produces chemotactic effect on macrophages |
| Macrophage disappearance factor | Enhances macrophage adherence to peritoneal wall |
| Macrophage fusion factor | Causes macrophage fusion and giant cell formation |
| Migration inhibitory factor | Inhibits macrophage migration |
| Mitogenic factor | Induces lymphocyte blastogenesis |

cytes, and granulocytes at the site of antigenic challenge, affecting vascular permeability, activating macrophages and lymphocytes, and possibly killing or damaging resident cells in the area. Products released by T cells may enhance inflammation at the site of antigenic challenge in the sensitized animal.

The pathologic tissue alterations observed in many chronic diseases including periodontitis may result from the activities of leukocytes responding to bacterial antigens or mitogens.[59] The blastogenic response of peripheral blood lymphoid cells to antigens has been considered to be an in vitro correlate of specific immunologic sensitization.

When lymphocytes from an individual sensitive to an antigen or mitogen (e.g., tuberculin) are cultured in vitro with the agent, the lymphocytes undergo a proliferative response, termed blastogenesis or transformation ( Fig. 12-5). Such proliferative responses are presumed to represent an expansion of a clone of immunocompetent lymphocytes capable of memory, regulatory, or effector functions. Antigen-induced lymphocyte transformation has traditionally been considered an in vitro correlate of cell-mediated immunity.

Experiments using in vitro culture systems aimed at determining whether patients with gingivitis and periodontitis are sensitized to antigens present in the bacteria associated with these diseases[24,60-65] produce results indicative of lymphocyte blastogenesis ( Fig. 12-6). A positive correlation between in vitro responsiveness of peripheral blood leukocytes and gingivitis and periodontitis has been reported.[24,60-65]

Employing this in vitro approach, extracts of *Actinomyces viscosus, Veillonella alcalescens, Bacteroides melaninogenicus,* and *Fusobacterium fusiforme* induce lymphocyte transformation of cells from patients with various degrees of periodontal disease.[63,64] Autologous dental plaque also induces lymphocyte blastogenic responses.

Other laboratories have been unable to demonstrate a direct quantitative relationship.[66-69]

Lymphocytes from patients with severe periodontal disease may have negligible levels of transformation[64,70,71] suggesting that they may lack immune responsiveness to dental plaque antigens. This lack of plaque-induced transformation may be caused by the presence of serum inhibitory factors modulating lymphocyte responses by specifically binding dental plaque antigens.

Both sensitized T- and B-lymphocytes from patients with periodontal disease may

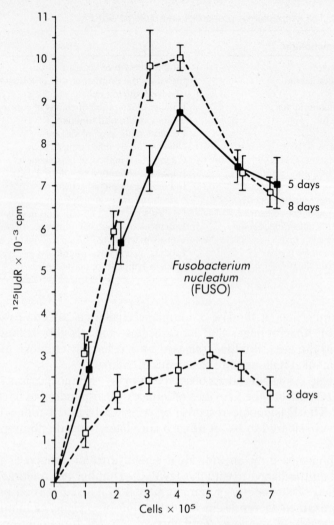

**Fig. 12-6.**  Results of a typical experiment using a range of concentrations of cells harvested from a normal donor, activated with *Fusobacterium nucleatum* (FUSO) and incubated for 3.5 and 8 days before pulse labelling with $^{125}$Iododeoxyuridine. (From Suzuki, J.B., Sims, T., and Page, R.C.: J. Periodontol. **54:**408, 1983.)

undergo blastogenesis.[61] The immune B-cell activation may be mediated by cooperation with a few T-helper cells or by potentiation of B cells through their complement receptors.

The interpretation of lymphocyte blastogenesis data has been clouded by large variations in responsiveness from time to time. In most of the experiments, lymphocytes from some individuals who were clinically normal responded (Fig. 12-6), although lymphocytes from many patients with gingivitis or periodontitis did not. Other reports indicate that responsiveness of lymphocytes from patients do not differ from those of healthy controls.[67-69]

Similarly, lymphocyte blastogenesis studies in juvenile periodontitis are not in agreement. Peripheral blood lymphocyte blast transformation from such patients was impaired when stimulated by dental plaque and selected gram-negative bacteria.[72] These results implicate a selective, cell-mediated immunodeficiency. On the other hand, reports indicate significantly higher lymphocyte blastogenesis to selected bacterial antigens and mitogens in juvenile periodontitis than in normal subjects or adult periodontitis patients.[73] Furthermore, the mitogenic and antigenic responses of cells from juvenile periodontitis patients were less suppressed by prostaglandins than were those in healthy subjects or adult patients.[73]

Evaluation of the blastogenic response of peripheral blood lymphocytes stimulated by putative periodontal pathogens shows no significant differences between juvenile periodontitis patients compared to age-matched healthy subjects.[74]

Factors other than periodontal status appear to influence lymphocyte blastogenesis assays in vitro.[75-77] These variables include cell concentration, shape of the culture microtest well, presence of bacterial and lymphoid cell inhibitors of thymidine incorporation, and time of incubation in establishing lymphocyte cultures. Cells from healthy adult subjects and nonresponding adult periodontitis patients can be made to undergo blastogenesis to bacterial preparations when these variables are controlled. Recent evidence also demonstrates lymphocyte blastogenesis to bacterial preparations in young and healthy adults.[67,76,78,79] Thus authorities do not agree on the usefulness of lymphocyte blastogenesis testing either for diagnostic or epidemiologic purposes. At this time it is not clinically useful.

Recent studies report that unstimulated peripheral blood lymphocytes in culture from young patients with severe periodontitis had lower background counts.[78-81] Background counts measure the incorporation of labelled DNA precursors (e.g., $^3$H-thymidine or $^{125}$Iododeoxyuridine) into the DNA of unstimulated lymphocytes. The proliferation of lymphocytes in culture in the absence of any known exogenous stimulant reflects the autologous mixed lymphocyte reaction (AMLR). The AMLR is defined as the stimulation of T cells when cocultured with autologous non–T cells. This reaction shows specificity and memory and hence has an immunologic basis.[82,83] The decreased incorporation of $^3$H-thymidine by unstimulated lymphocytes in culture in severe, rapidly progressive, and adult periodontitis patients indicates a suppressed AMLR.[79,84] Impairment of the AMLR may reflect an aberrant T-cell responsiveness and regulatory function.[85-87] Diseases such as systemic lupus erythematosus, Hodgkin disease, and mixed connective tissue disease have a decreased AMLR and display defects in induced suppressor T-cell function.[88-91]

Periodontal therapy in patients with generalized periodontal disease appears to restore the spontaneous lymphocyte response to the range of healthy subjects but has little effect on spontaneous lymphocyte responses of juvenile periodontitis patients. A depressed response of lymphocytes from severe and rapidly progressive periodontitis patients may reflect improper regulation of B cells by T cells. A variety of suppressor cells may be produced during the AMLR culture.[92] If AMLR responses are caused by regulatory mechanisms of B cells by T cells, then the reduced AMLR response seen with rapidly progressive patients indicates a regulatory T-cell defect. A paucity of suppressor T cells during in vitro culture may explain the B-cell hyperresponsiveness to staphylococcal protein A.[93] The apparent restoration of the AMLR with successful periodontal therapy suggests that AMLR is related to periodontal disease activity.[80] Therapy of several systemic diseases (systemic lupus erythematosus, mixed connective tissue disease) also has a significant influence on decreased AMLR values and returns the AMLR to normal.[86,91]

**Autologous mixed lymphocyte reaction**

## Neutrophils and periodontal disease

Neutrophil dysfunctions in chemotaxis and in phagocytosis have been reported in juvenile periodontitis patients.[94-98] Reports also indicate that a neutrophil dysfunction in chemotaxis is seen in patients with severe, generalized forms of periodontitis.[84,96,97,99]

## NEUTROPHIL FUNCTION

Neutrophils comprise between 50% to 70% of the peripheral circulating leukocytes in humans. These phagocytic cells generally migrate to sites of bacterial challenge and tissue injury. Their numbers usually increase during infectious states. These cells serve as a primary defense of the periodontium against oral microorganisms. At the same time however, neutrophils may be destructive to the periodontium. Dysfunctions of neutrophils have been associated with severe early-onset forms of periodontal disease.

The influx of neutrophils into extravascular periodontal tissues is consistent with acute inflammation and is a host response against microorganisms. Although lysosomal enzymes are partially responsible for tissue destruction in periodontal disease, recent evidence has shown that the neutrophil response to oral microorganisms is primarily protective.

## NEUTROPHIL DEVELOPMENT

Myeloblasts are immature cells of the granulocyte series and are produced in bone marrow. They differentiate into promyelocytes and then into neutrophilic myelocytes. Neutrophilic myelocytes undergo several divisions and when they no longer divide are called *metamyelocytes*. These cells differentiate into neutrophils in the bone marrow and are then released into the peripheral circulation. The half-life of a circulating neutrophil is approximately 8 hours.

## CHEMOTAXIS

Mobility and phagocytosis of neutrophils is a protection against infection. The innate mechanisms of phagocytosis have been known since the turn of the century.[100] This phenomenon was soon recognized as an important defense mechanism against a wide variety of bacteria, fungi, and protozoa. It included the leukocyte's ability to ingest and kill bacteria.[101-104] Exceptions to this observation have been reported. In rare instances, phagocytic cells do not kill bacteria but may promote an infection when they are overcome by ingested bacteria.[105-113]

Cellular mobility toward an attractant similar to ameboid movement is known as *chemotaxis*. The intracellular cytoplasmic network of actin and myosin filaments produce the movement.[114,115] When neutrophil chemotaxis is stimulated by a chemical attractant, the movement is "directed."

*Random migration* is the nondirected movement of neutrophils. Bacterial plaque contains chemical factors that are chemotactic for neutrophils.[116] Chemotaxis of neutrophils and monocytes from the blood vasculature and connective tissue to gingival sulci and pockets is an early host response to bacterial plaque.[117]

Neutrophils are present during all four stages of the pathogenesis of the periodontal lesion and increase in number during the development of disease.[21] Neutrophil abnormalities in juvenile and rapidly progressive periodontitis and in diabetes have been documented.[94-96,118-120]

Bacterial plaque development on teeth and in gingival sulci and pockets provides chemical mediators of inflammation such as antigens, mitogens, enzymes, and chemotactic molecules. Many of these chemical mediators can diffuse through junctional epithelium[121] and enter the connective tissues. Chemotactic agents derived from bacteria in plaque enhance directed chemotaxis of neutrophils.

In general, neutrophils move from an area of lower concentration of chemoattractant to an area of higher concentration, that is, from connective tissue to periodontal sulci or pockets.[122,123] This chemotactic movement of neutrophils appears to be an early host response to bacterial plaque invasion of tissues.

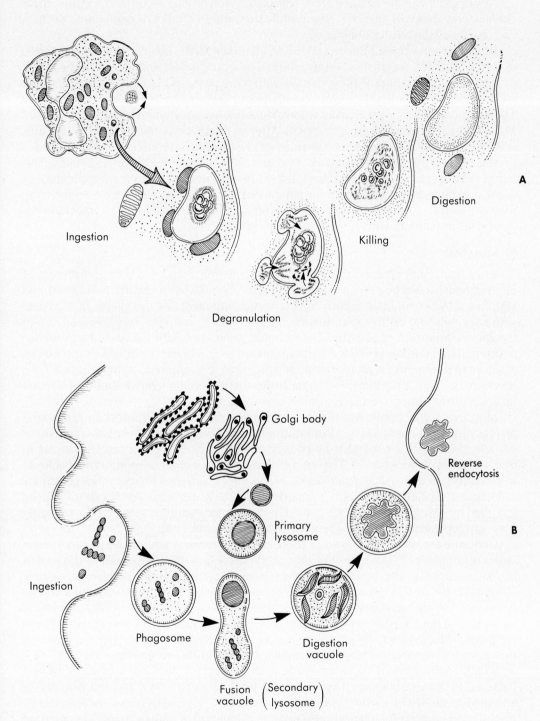

Ingestion

Degranulation

Killing

Digestion

**A**

Golgi body

Reverse endocytosis

Primary lysosome

Ingestion

Phagosome

Fusion vacuole (Secondary lysosome)

Digestion vacuole

**B**

**Fig. 12-7.** Diagram of neutrophil phagocytosis. **A,** From endocytosis through digestion. **B,** Showing intracellular organelles involved in the process.

## Chemotaxis testing in the laboratory

Neutrophils can be isolated from the peripheral venous blood and examined for chemotactic ability in vitro.[97,98] Neutrophils from gingival sulci or periodontal pockets can also be evaluated for chemotaxis in vivo.[124]

In vitro testing uses a Boyden diffusion chamber. Cells, usually at a concentration of $2 \times 10^5/0.1$ ml, are suspended in minimal essential media and placed in the upper compartment. A membrane filter, usually with 5 μm pores, is placed between the upper and lower compartments. The lower compartment contains a chemoattractant solution. The chemoattractants are usually n-formyl-methionylleucylphenylalanine ($10^{-7}$-$10^{-9}$ M), endotoxin-activated serum, or casein. After an incubation time of 30 to 120 minutes at 37° C, the filter is removed and the number of cells that have migrated to the opposite (lower) side of the filter is counted. A control from a healthy individual is used. Differences between patient and control individuals are evaluated. Defective chemotaxis is considered to be two standard deviations below control values. Receptors for complement factors on the neutrophil membrane may be responsible for chemotactic defects seen in patients with juvenile periodontitis.

## Phagocytosis

After neutrophil chemotaxis in vivo, the process of phagocytosis or engulfment of microorganisms begins. Phagocytosis, and also chemotaxis, is greatly influenced and stimulated by activation of serum complement components by the classic or alternate pathways. Specific antibodies enhance phagocytosis[125] and play an important role in the intracellular fate of bacteria. For example, tubercle bacilli fail to multiply within neutrophils of animals protected with antibodies.[126,127] However antibodies are not an absolute requirement for phagocytosis because they are acquired relatively slowly (i.e., several days after infection).[128] Phagocytosis then prevents overwhelming microbial invasion during the pre-antibody phase of acute infection.

Monocytes and tissue macrophages behave similarly with respect to neutrophil phagocytosis and chemotaxis. After neutrophil chemotaxis toward a microorganism or particle, pseudopodia enclose it by endocytosis (Fig. 12-7, A),[129] a process similar to that observed in amebae.[129] The engulfed particle occupies a membrane enclosed intracellular vacuole called a *phagocytic vacuole* or *phagosome*. Phagocytosis continues as particles challenge the cell. As many as 25 to 50 particles (or bacteria) can be engulfed by a single cell (Fig. 12-7, B). The energy for engulfment is derived primarily from glycolysis that results in the accumulation of lactic acid.[107,125,130]

Concomitant with this ingestion process, the lysosomes within the phagocyte decrease in number.[131] The extent of this degranulation is directly related to the extent of phagocytosis. In postengulfment activity, lysosomes fuse with the phagocytic vacuole (Fig. 12-7, B). At this point, the hydrolytic and proteolytic enzymes contained within lysosomes are able to digest the bacteria. The efficiency of phagocytic engulfment of bacteria or of foreign particles can be measured in the laboratory. Four primary methods for testing phagocytosis employ light microscopy, electron microscopy, culture, and radioisotopes. Reverse endocytosis completes postengulfment activity (Fig. 12-7, B).

Traditionally, stained slides are made from in vitro incubations of neutrophils and bacteria. Prepared slides are then observed by light microscopy and the number of engulfed intracellular particles per cell are counted.[132,133] Electron microscopy of neutrophils and bacteria incubations also permits evaluation of phagocytosis. This method is tedious, expensive, time-consuming, and is not commonly used to assess phagocytosis. Culture methods using dilutions of neutrophil-bacteria suspensions show a decrease with time in cultivatable microflora during successful phagocytosis.

More sophisticated methods use bacteria labeled with a radiosotope, usually $^3$H, $^{14}$C, or $^{45}$Ca. Incubations of labeled bacteria and neutrophils are separated after phagocytosis proceeds, usually for 2 to 15 minutes. Unengulfed labeled bacteria are separated from neutrophil-engulfed bacteria by differential centrifugation or by membrane filtration.[113,134,135]

Phagocytosis of plaque bacteria is an important host defense. Deficiencies of neutrophil phagocytosis have been reported in patients with juvenile periodontitis.[94,98] These observations, however, are not in agreement with findings of other laboratories.[136]

### Energy metabolism during neutrophil degradation of bacteria

In postengulfment stages, and concurrent with lysosome degranulation, neutrophil oxygen uptake is stimulated and glycolysis and the pentose phosphate pathway (hexose monophosphate shunt) is increased.[125,137-139] Lactic acid produced by glycolysis results in an acidic pH of 3.0 to 4.5. This may be bacteriocidal for some bacteria.

Hydrogen peroxide is formed during the oxidation of glucose by glycolysis and the pentose phosphate pathway. Specifically, hydrogen peroxide results from the action of NADPH oxidase on NADPH as a metabolite of the pentose phosphate pathway.[140-143] Hydrogen peroxide may be bacteriocidal for several bacteria[144,145] but usually acts in concert with myeloperoxidase and iodine to form a more potent killing mechanism.[146-151]

In summary, most bacteria, including those found in plaque, emit chemotactic agents that attract increasing numbers of neutrophils to the site of plaque colonization and bacterial challenge. Phagocytosis of bacteria occurs and, along with lysosome degranulation, cellular metabolism generates killing agents such as hydrogen peroxide and lactic acid.[129]

### Bacterial degradation

The outcome of each encounter between bacteria and neutrophils depends on normal chemotaxis, normal phagocytosis, opsonization or presence of antibody, normal intracellular mechanisms for bacterial degradation, and properties of microorganisms denying or inhibiting neutrophil function. Finally, after neutrophil action has been completed or the bacterial challenge overwhelms the cell, the neutrophil itself may undergo autolysis.

### Neutrophils and periodontal destruction

After neutrophil autolysis following phagocytosis of bacteria or particulate matter or after neutrophil cell death, extracellular lysosomal enzyme release may result in tissue damage to the host. Secretion of enzymes from neutrophils not directly related to phagocytosis may also occur and cause periodontal destruction. Collagenase, hyaluronidase, acid hydrolases, elastase, and chondrotin sulfatase are a few of the lysosomal enzymes with potential for tissue destruction.[152-155]

Other factors contained within neutrophil lysosomes have the potential for periodontal destruction and amplifying the inflammatory response. Factors have been identified that induce capillary permeability, monocyte chemotactic agents, complement-cleaving enzymes,[156] neutral proteinases, and modifiers of immediate and delayed hypersensitivity.[157-159]

## Immunologic profile of periodontitis patients

Lymphocytes from patients with gingivitis and periodontitis may have greater in vitro responsiveness to bacteria than do those of controls,[57,61,63-65,160-163] although recent evidence has questioned the validity of these correlations.[66,69,164-167] However, the possibility of using immunologic markers as indicators of periodontal disease activity is intriguing.

**Table 12-6**  Immunologic prolife of periodontitis

| Periodontitis group | Neutrophil function | | Cellular immunity (blastogenesis) | Autologous mixed lymphocyte response | Serum antibodies |
|---|---|---|---|---|---|
| | Chemotaxis | Phagocytosis | | | |
| Adult | Normal | Normal | Normal | Normal | Elevated |
| Rapidly progressive | Depressed (55%-65%)* | Normal | Normal | Depressed | Elevated |
| Juvenile | Depressed (65%-100%) | Depressed/normal | Normal | Normal† | Elevated |
| Prepubertal | Depressed | ? | ? | ? | Elevated |

*Percentage of patients with a defect greater than 2 standard deviations from a healthy donor.
†AMLR within range of cells from healthy donors but tendency toward elevated values.

Four major types of periodontitis have been described:[167] adult, rapidly progressive, juvenile, and prepubertal. The immunologic features of each are summarized in Table 12-6. The majority of adult periodontitis patients do not have neutrophil defects in chemotaxis or phagocytosis.

Although there are no significant differences in lymphocyte blastogenic response to various bacterial preparations,[78] some patients with adult periodontitis have a depressed autologous mixed lymphocyte reaction (AMLR). A depressed AMLR indicates that immunologic mechanisms may not be optimal in selected patients with adult periodontitis. Serum antibody levels in adult periodontitis are elevated to specific microorganisms.

Rapidly progressive and juvenile periodontitis patients have no significant differences in lymphocyte blastogenesis to bacterial preparations.[74,81,168] Several laboratories have confirmed a significantly depressed AMLR for young patients with rapidly progressive disease.[79,81,84,168] Many rapidly progressive and juvenile periodontitis patients also have a defect in neutrophil chemotaxis.[95-98] Defects of neutrophil phagocytosis in juvenile periodontitis patients have also been reported.[94,98,169,170]

Little information has been published regarding the immunologic profiles of prepubertal periodontitis patients (Table 12-6).

**REFERENCES**

1. Socransky, S.S.: Relationship of bacteria to the etiology of periodontal disease, J. Dent. Res. **49**:203, 1970.
2. Socransky, S.S.: Microbiology of periodontal disease—present status and future considerations, J. Periodontol. **48**:497, 1977.
3. Schwartz, J., Stinson, F.L., and Parker, R.B.: The passage of tritiated bacterial endotoxin across intact gingival crevicular epithelium, J. Periodontol. **43**:270, 1972.
4. Rizzo, A.A.: Histologic and immunologic evaluations of antigen penetration into oral tissues after topical application, J. Periodontol. **41**:210, 1970.
5. Fulton, R.S., et al.: Ultrastructural changes in gingiva following topical application of endotoxin, J. Dent. Res. **54**(special issue):96, Abstract no. 207, 1975.
6. Slots, J.: Importance of black-pigmented bacteroides in human periodontal disease. In Genco, R.J., and Mergenhagen, S.E. editors: Host-parasite interactions in periodontal diseases, Washington, D.C., 1982, American Society for Microbiology.
7. Robertson, P.B., et al.: Collagenolytic activity associated with *Bacteroides* species and *Actinobacillus actinomycetemcomitans,* J. Periodont. Res. **17**:275, 1982.
8. Saglie, R., et al.: Bacterial invasion of gingiva in advanced periodontitis in humans, J. Periodontol. **53**:217, 1982.
9. Carranza, F.A., Jr., et al.: Scanning and transmission electron microscopic study of tissue invading microorganisms in localized juvenile periodontitis, J. Periodontol. **54**:598, 1983.
10. Frank, R.M.: Bacterial penetration in the apical pocket wall of advanced human periodontitis, J. Periodont. Res. **15**:563, 1980.
11. Shenker, B.J., MacArthur, W.P., and Tsai, C.C.: Immune suppression induced by *Actinobacillus actinomycetemcomitans.* I. Effects on human peripheral blood lymphocyte responses to mitogens and antigens, J. Immunol. **128**:148, 1982.
12. Schwab, J.H.: Suppression of the immune response by microorganisms, Bacteriol. Rev. **39**:121, 1975.

13. Baehni, P., et al.: Interaction of inflammatory cells and oral microorganisms. VIII. Detection of leukotoxic activity of a plaque-derived gram-negative microorganism, Infect. Immun. **24:**233, 1979.

14. van Palenstein Helderman, W.H.: Microbial etiology of periodontal disease, J. Clin. Periodontol. **8:**261, 1981.

15. Shurin, S.B., et al.: A neutrophil disorder induced by *Capnocytophaga,* a dental microorganism, New Engl. J. Med. **301:**849, 1979.

16. Loesche, W.J., and Laughon, B.E.: Role of spirochetes in periodontal disease. In Genco, R.J., and Mergenhagen, S.E., editors: Host-parasite interactions in periodontal disease. Washington, D.C., 1982, American Society for Microbiology.

17. Zachrisson, B.U., and Schultz-Haudt, S.D.: Biologically active substances of the mast cell, J. Periodont. Res. **2:**21, 1967.

18. Zachinsky, L.: Range of histologic variation in clinically normal gingiva, J. Dent. Res. **33:**580, 1954.

19. Wittmer, J.W., Deckler, E.H., and Toto, P.D.: Comparative frequencies of plasma cells and lymphocytes in gingivitis, J. Periodontol. **40:**274, 1969.

20. Payne, W.A., et al.: Histopathologic features of the initial and early stages of experimental gingivitis in man, J. Periodont. Res. **10:**51, 1975.

21. Page, R.C., and Schroeder, H.E.: Pathogenesis of inflammatory periodontal disease, Lab. Invest. **34:**235, 1976.

22. Mackler, B.F., et al.: IgG subclasses in human periodontal disease. I. Distribution and incidence of IgG subclass bearing lymphocytes and plasma cells, J. Periodont. Res. **13:**109, 1978.

23. Mackler, B.F., et al.: IgG subclasses in human periodontal disease. II. Cytophilic and membrane IgG subclasses immunoglublins, J. Periodont. Res. **13:**433, 1978.

24. Ivanyi, L., Wilton, J.M.A., and Lehner, T.: Cell-mediated immunity in periodontal disease; cytotoxicity, migration inhibition and lymphocyte transformation studies, Immunology **22:**141, 1972.

25. Horton, J.E., et al.: Bone resorbing activity in supernatant fluid from cultured human peripheral blood leukocytes, Science **177:**793, 1972.

26. Coombs, R.R.A., and Gell, P.G.H.: Classification of allergic reactions, responsible for clinical hypersensitivity and disease. In Gell, P.G.H., Coombs, R.R.A., and Lachmann, P.J., editors: Clinical aspects of immunology, ed. 3, Oxford, England, 1975, Blackwell Scientific Publications Ltd.

27. Nisengard, R.J., Beutner, E.H., and Gauto, M.: Immunofluorescent studies of IgE in periodontal disease, Ann. NY Acad. Sci. **177:**39, 1971.

28. Nisengard, R., and Jarret, C.: Coating of subgingival bacteria with immunoglobulin and complement, J. Periodontol. **47:**518, 1976.

29. Angelopoulas, A.P.: Studies of mast cells in the human gingiva, J. Periodont. Res. **8:**314, 1973.

30. Dienstein, B., Ratcliff, P.A., and Williams, R.K.: Mast cell density and distribution in gingival biopsies: a quantitative study, J. Periodontol. **38:**198, 1967.

31. Goldhaber, P.: Heparin enhancement of factors stimulating bone resorption in tissue culture, Science **147:**407, 1965.

32. Taylor, A.C.: Collagenolysis in cultured tissue. I. Digestion of mesenteric fibers by enzymes from explanted gingival tissue, J. Dent. Res. **50:**1294, 1971.

33. Taylor, A.C.: Collagenolysis in cultured tissue. II. Role of mast cells, J. Dent. Res. **50:**1301, 1971.

34. Vijay, H.M., and Perlmutter, L.: Reagin-mediated histamine release from human leukocytes by human IgG-4, Fed. Proc. **34:**1045, 1975.

35. Muller-Eberhard, H.J.: Complement, Ann. Rev. Biochem. **44:**697, 1975.

36. Schonfeld, S.E., Drury, G.I., and Herbs, S.M.: Complement fixing activity in diseased human gingival tissues, J. Periodont. Res. **16:**574, 1981.

37. Schenkein, H., and Genco, R.: Inhibition of lymphocyte blastogenesis by C3 and C3d, J. Immunol. **122:**1126, 1979.

38. Suzuki, J.B., Gargiulo, A.W., and Toto, P.D.: Immunoglobulins and complement in gingiva from human periodontal disease. In Underkofler, L.A., editor: Developments in industrial microbiology, Vol. 20, Washington, D.C., 1979, American Institute of Biological Sciences.

39. Schenkein, H., and Rutherford, B.: C3-mediated release of prostoglandin from human monocytes: behaviour in short-term culture, Immunology **51:**83, 1984.

40. Schenkein, H., and Rutherford, B.: Effects of serum on C3b-stimulated release of prostaglandins and thromboxane B2 from human monocytes, Immunopharmacology **8:**79, 1984.

41. Kennett, F., et al.: Phospholipid composition of human monocytes and alterations occurring due to culture and stimulation by C3b, Biochim. Biophys. Acta, **804:**301, 1984.

42. Inman, R.D., and Day, N.K.: Immunologic and clinical aspects of immune complex disease, Am. J. Med. **70:**1097, 1981.

43. Williams, R.C.: Immune complexes: a clinical perspective, Am. J. Med. **71:**743, 1981.

44. Mergenhagen, S.E.: Complement as a mediator of inflammation: formation of biologically active products after interaction of serum complement with endotoxin and anti-

gen-antibody complexes, J. Periodontol. **41:** 202, 1970.

45. Vincent, J.W., et al.: Reaction of human sera for juvenile periodontitis, rapidly progressive periodontitis, and adult periodontitis with selected periodontopathogens, J. Periodontol. **56:**464, 1985.

46. Gilmour, M.N., and Nisengard, R.J.: Interactions between serum titers to filamentous bacteria and their relationship to human periodontal disease, Arch. Oral Biol. **19:**959, 1974.

47. Nisengard, R.J., and Beutner, E.H.: Immunology studies of periodontal disease. V. IgG type antibodies and skin test responses to *Actinomyces* and mixed oral flora, J. Periodontol. **41:**149, 1970.

48. Mashimo, P.A., Genco, R.J., and Ellison, S.A.: Antibodies reactive with *Leptotrichia buccalis* in human serum from infancy to adulthood, Arch. Oral Biol. **21:**277, 1976.

49. Vincent, J., et al.: Reaction of human sera from juvenile periodontitis (JP) patients following therapy. J. Dent. Res. **55:**762, 1985.

50. Byers, C.W., Toto, P.D., and Garguilo, A.W.: Levels of immunoglobulins IgG, IgA and IgM in the human inflamed gingiva, J. Periodontol. **46:**387, 1975.

51. Berglund, S.E.: Immunoglobulins in human gingiva with specificity for oral bacteria. J. Periodontol. **42:**546, 1971.

52. Holmberg, L., and Killander, J.: Quantitative determination of immunoglobulin (IgG, IgA and IgM) and identification of IgA-type in the gingival fluid, J. Periodont. Res. **6:**1, 1971.

53. Shillitoe, E.J., and Lehner, T.: Immunoglobulins and complement in crevicular fluid, serum and saliva in man, Arch. Oral. Biol. **17:**241, 1972.

54. Attström, R., et al.: Complement factors in gingival crevice material from healthy and inflamed gingiva in humans, J. Periodont. Res. **10:**19, 1975.

55. Dumonde, D.C., et al.: "Lymphokines": non-antibody mediators of cellular immunity generated by lymphocyte activation, Nature **224:**38, 1969.

56. Pick, E., and Turk, J.L.: The biological activities of soluble lymphocyte products, Clin. Exp. Immunol. **10:**1, 1972.

57. Bloom, B.R.: In vitro approaches to the mechanism of cell-mediated immune reactions, Adv. Immunol. **13:**101, 1971.

58. Pierce, C.W., and Benacerraf, B.: The cellular basis of immune responses. In Miescher, P.A., and Muller-Eberhard, H.J., editors: Textbook of immunopathology, vol. 1, ed. 2, New York, 1976, Grune & Stratton, Inc.

59. Miller, D.R., Lamster, I.B., and Chasens, A.I.: Role of the polymorphonuclear leukocyte in periodontal health and disease, J. Clin. Periodontol. **11:**1, 1984.

60. Horton, J.E., Oppenheim, J.J., and Mergenhagen, S.E.: Elaboration of lymphotoxin by cultured human peripheral blood leukocytes stimulated with dental plaque deposits, Clin. Exp. Immunol. **13:**383, 1973.

61. Mackler, B.R., et al.: Blastogenesis and lymphokine synthesis by T- and B-lymphocytes from patients with periodontal disease, Infect. Immun. **10:**844, 1974.

62. Baker, J.J., et al.: Importance of *Actinomyces* and certain gram-negative anaerobic organisms in the transformation of lymphocytes from patients with periodontal disease, Infect. Immun. **13:**1363, 1976.

63. Ivanyi, L., and Lehner, T.: Stimulation of lymphocyte transformation by bacterial antigens in patients with periodontal disease, Arch. Oral Biol. **15:**1089, 1970.

64. Ivanyi, L., and Lehner, T.: Lymphocyte transformation by sonicates of dental plaque in human periodontal disease, Arch. Oral Biol. **16:**1117, 1971.

65. Patters, M.R., et al.: Blastogenic response of human lymphocytes to oral bacterial antigens: comparison of individuals with periodontal disease to normal and edentulous individuals. Infec. Immun. **14:**1213, 1976.

66. Kiger, R.D., Wright, W.H., and Creamer, H.R.: The significance of lymphocyte transformation responses to various microbial stimulants, J. Periodontol. **45:**780, 1974.

67. Donaldson, S.L., et al.: Blastogenic responses by lymphocytes from periodontally healthy populations induced by periodontitis associated bacteria. J. Periodontol. **53:**743, 1982.

68. Suzuki, J.B., et al.: Influence of cell proximity on the blastogenic response of lymphocytes, J. Dent. Res. **59:**251(Abstract), 1980.

69. Suzuki, J.B., Sims, T., and Page, R.C.: Effect of factors other than pathologic status on responsiveness of peripheral blood mononuclear cells from patients with chronic periodontitis. J. Periodontol. **54:**408, 1983.

70. Ivanyi, L., et al.: Cell-mediated immunity in periodontal disease: cytotoxicity, migration inhibition, and lymphocyte transformation, Immunology **22:**141, 1972.

71. Guillo, B., and Chaput, A.: Test dé transformation lymphoblastique et états cliniques du parodonte, Rev. Fr. Odontostomatol. **19:**315, 1972.

72. Lehner, T., et al.: Immunological aspects of juvenile periodontitis (periodontosis), J. Periodont. Res. **9:**261, 1974.

73. Sims, T., Clagett, J.A., and Page, R.C.: Effects of cell concentration and exogenous prostaglandin on the interaction and responsiveness of human peripheral blood lymphocytes, Clin. Immunol. Immunopathol. **12:** 150, 1978.

74. Suzuki, J.B., Park, S., and Falkler, W.A., Jr.: Immunologic profile of localized and gener-

alized juvenile periodontitis. I. Lymphocyte blastogenesis and the autologous mixed lymphocyte response, J. Periodontol. **55:**453, 1984.

75. Suzuki, J.B., Sims, T., and Page, R.C.: In vitro assessment of lymphocyte responsiveness in patients with periodontitis, J. Dent. Res. **60:**749, 1981.

76. Suzuki, J.B., et al.: Lymphocyte blastogenesis and the mixed lymphocyte reaction in periodontitis, Annual Meeting of the American Society for Microbiology Abstract No. E73, p. 114, New Orleans, LA, 1983.

77. Sims, T., and Page, R.C.: Effects of endogenous and exogenous inhibitors on the incorporation of labeled precursors into DNA by human mononuclear cells, Infec. Immun. **38:**502, 1982.

78. Suzuki, J.B., et al.: Blastogenic responsiveness of human lymphoid cells to mitogens and to homogenates of periodontal pocket bacteria, J. Periodont. Res. **19:**352, 1984.

79. Ranney, R.R., Debski, B.F., and Tew, J.G.: Pathogenesis of gingivitis and periodontal disease in children and young adults, Pediat. Dent. **3:**89 (Special Issue), 1981.

80. Suzuki, J., et al.: Effect of periodontal therapy on spontaneous lymphocyte response and neutrophil chemotaxis in localized and generalized juvenile periodontitis patients, J. Clin. Periodont. **12:**124, 1985.

81. Tew, J.G., et al.: Immunological studies of young adults with severe periodontitis. II. Cellular factors, J. Periodont. Res. **16:**403, 1981.

82. Opelz, G., et al.: Autologous stimulation of human lymphocyte subpopulation, J. Exp. Med. **142:**1327, 1975.

83. Weksler, M.E., and Kozak, R.: Lymphocyte transformation induced by autologous cells. V. Generation of immunologic memory and specificity during the autologous mixed lymphocyte reaction, J. Exp. Med. **146:**1833, 1977.

84. Suzuki, J.B., et al.: Effect of therapy on immunologic profile in juvenile periodontitis, J. Periodontol. **55,**301, 1984.

85. Abdou, N.I., et al.: Suppressor T-cell abnormality in idiopathic systemic lupus erythematosus, Clin. Immunol. Immunopathol. **6:**192, 1976.

86. Sakane, T., Steinberg, A.D., and Green, I: Failure of autologous mixed lymphocyte reactions between T and non T–cells in patients with systemic lupus erythematosus, Proc. Natl. Sci. (USA) **75:**3464, 1978.

87. Sakane, T., Steinberg, A.D., and Green, I.: Studies of immune functions of patients with systemic lupus erythematosus. V. T-cell suppressor function and autologous mixed lymphocyte reaction during active and inactive phases, Arthr. Rheum. **23:**225, 1980.

88. Fauci, A.A., et al.: Immunoregulatory aberrations in systemic lupus erythematosus, J. Immunol. **121:**1473, 1978.

89. Kuntz, M.M., Innes, J.B., and Weksler, M.E.: The cellular basis of the impaired autologous mixed lymphocyte reaction in patients with systemic lupus erythematosus, J. Clin. Invest. **63:**151, 1979.

90. Engleman, E.G., et al.: Suppressor cells of the mixed lymphocyte reaction in patients with Hodgkin's disease, Transplant. Proc. **11:**1827, 1979.

91. Palacios, R. and Alarcon-Segovia, D.: Human post-thymic precursor cells in health disease. VI. Effect of serum thymic factor on the response of cells from patients with systemic lupus erythematosus or mixed connective tissue disease in autologous mixed lymphocyte reaction, Clin. Immunol. Immunopathol. **18:**362, 1981.

92. Goeken, N.E., and Thompson, J.S.: Suppressor cells induced in the human mixed lymphocyte reaction. Hum. Immunol. **4:**37, 1982.

93. Smith, S., et al.: Polyclonal B-cell activation: severe periodontal disease in young adults, Clin. Immunol. Immunopathol. **16:**354, 1980.

94. Cianciola, L.J., et al.: Defective polymorphonuclear leukocyte function in a human periodontal disease, Nature (London) **265:**445, 1977.

95. Clark, R.A., Page, R.C., and Wilde, G.: Defective neutrophil chemotaxis in juvenile periodontitis. Infec. Immun. **13:**694, 1977.

96. Lavine, W.S., et al.: Impaired neutrophil chemotaxis in patients with juvenile and rapidly progressing periodontitis, J. Periodont. Res. **14:**10, 1979.

97. Van Dyke, T.E., et al.: Neutrophil chemotaxis dysfunction in human periodontitis, Infec. Immun. **27:**124, 1980.

98. Suzuki, J.B., et al.: Immunologic profile of localized and generalized juvenile periodontitis. II. Neutrophil chemotaxis, phagocytosis, and intracellular spore germination, J. Periodontal. **55:**461, 1984.

99. Van Dyke, T.E., et al: Periodontal disease and neutrophil abnormalities. In Genco, R.J., and Mergenhagen, S.E., editors, Host-parasite interactions in periodontal diseases, Washington, D.C., 1982, American Society for Microbiology.

100. Metchnikoff, E.: Lectures on the comparative pathology of inflammation, Kegan Paul, Trench, Truber, & Co., London, 1905.

101. Suter, E.: Interaction between phagocytes and pathogenic microorganism, Bacteriol. Rev. **20:**94, 1956.

102. Hirsch, J.G.: Antimicrobial factors in tissues and phagocytic cells, Bacteriol. Rev. **24:**133, 1960.

103. Rowley, D.: Phagocytosis, Adv. Immunol. **2:**241, 1962.

104. Suter, E., and Ramseier, H.: Cellular reactions in infection, Adv. Immunol. **4:**117, 1964.

105. Fothergill, L.D., Chandler, C.A., and Dingle, J.H.: The survival of virulent *H. influenzae* in phagocytes, J. Immunol. **32:**335, 1937.

106. Adams, J.W.: Intracellular bacilli in intestinal and mesenteric lesions of typhoid fever, Am. J. Pathol. **15:**561, 1939.

107. Martin, S.P., et al: The effect of tubercle bacilli on the polymorphonuclear leukocytes of normal animals, J. Exp. Med. **91:**381, 1950.

108. Braude, A.I.: Studies in the pathology and pathogenesis of experimental brucellosis: I. A comparison of the pathogenicity of *Brucella abortus, Brucella melitensis,* and *Brucella suis* for guinea pigs, J. Infec. Dis. **89:**76, 1951.

109. Braude, A.I.: Studies in the pathology and pathogenesis of experimental brucellosis. II. The formation of the hepatic granuloma and its evolution, J. Infec. Dis. **89:**87, 1951.

110. Suter, E.: The multiplication of tubercle bacilli within normal macrophages in tissue culture, J. Exp. Med. **94:**137, 1952.

111. Suter, E.: Multiplication of tubercle bacilli within mononuclear phogocytes in tissue cultures derived from normal animals vaccinated with BCG, J. Exp. Med. **97:**235, 1953.

112. Pomales-Lebron, A., and Stinebring, W.R.: Intracellular multiplication of *Brucella abortus* in normal and immune mononuclear phagocytes, Proc. Soc. Exp. Biol. Med. **94:**78, 1957.

113. Suzuki, J.B., Booth, R., and Grecz, N.: Evaluation of phagocytic activity by ingestion of labeled bacteria, J. Infec. Dis. **123:**93, 1971.

114. Stossel, T.P.: Phagocytosis, N. Engl. J. Med. **290:**713, 1974.

115. Garant, P.R., and Mulvihill, J.E.: The ultrastructure of leukocyte emigration through the sulcular epithelium in the beagle dog, J. Periodont. Res. **6:**266, 1971.

116. Garant, P.R.: Plaque-neutrophil interaction in mono-infected rats as visualized by transmission electron microscopy, J. Periodontol. **47:**132, 1976.

117. Attström, R., and Egelberg, J.: Emigration of blood neutrophils and monocytes into gingival crevices, J. Periodont. Res. **5:**48, 1970.

118. McMullen, J.A., et al.: Neutrophil chemotaxis in individuals with advanced periodontal disease and a genetic predisposition to diabetes mellitus, J. Periodontol. **52:**167, 1981.

119. Mowat, A.G., and Baum, J.: Chemotaxis of polymorphonuclear leukocytes from patients with diabetes mellitus, N. Engl. J. Med. **284:**621, 1971.

120. Manouchehr-Pour, M., et al.: Comparison of neutrophil chemotactic response in diabetic patients with mild and severe periodontal disease, J. Periodontol. **52:**410, 1981.

121. Rizzo, A.A., and Mitchell, C.T.: Chronic allergic inflammation induced by repeated deposition of antigen in rabbit gingival pockets, Periodontics **4:**5, 1966.

122. Lindhe, J., and Helldén, L.: Neutrophil chemotactic activity elaborated by human dental plaque, J. Periodontal Res. **7:**297, 1972.

123. Marchesi, V.T., and Florey, H.W.: Electron micrographic observations on the emigration of leukocytes, Quant. J. Exper. Physiol. **45:**343, 1960.

124. Golub, L.M., et al.: The response of human sulcular leukocytes to a chemotactic challenge, J. Periodont. Res. **16:**171, 1981.

125. Cohn, Z.A., and Morse, S.I.: Functional and metabolic properties of polymorphonuclear leukocytes, J. Exp. Med. **111:**667, 1960.

126. Lurie, M.B.: The correlation between the histological changes and the fate of living tubercle bacilli in the organs of tuberculous rabbits. J. Exp. Med. **55:**31, 1932.

127. Lurie, M.B.: The correlation between the histological changes and the fate of living tubercle bacilli in the organs of reinfected rabbits, J. Exp. Med. **57:**181, 1933.

128. Shayegani, M.: Failure of immune sera to enhance significantly phagocytosis of *Staphylococcus aureus:* non-specific adsorption of phagocytosis-promoting factors, Infect. Immun. **2:**742, 1970.

129. Suzuki, J.B., and Grecz, N.: A study of metabolic factors involved in the intracellular germination of *Clostidium botulinum* spores after phagocytosis, J. Med. Microbiol. **5:**381, 1972.

130. Sbarra, A.J., and M.L. Karnovsky: The biochemical basis of phagocytosis. I. Metabolic changes during the ingestion of particles by polymorphonuclear leukocytes, J. Biol. Chem. **234:**1355, 1959.

131. Hirsch, J.G., and Cohn, Z.A.: Degranulation of polymorphonuclear leukocytes following phagocytosis of microorganisms, J. Exp. Med. **112:**1005, 1960.

132. Schneerson, A.N.: Phagocytic activity of leukocytes of rabbits and guinea pigs toward *C. perfringens*, J. Microbiol. Epidem. Immun. (U.S.S.R.) **28:**547, 1957.

133. Ozmidova, I.V.: The phagocytic index as an index of the special features of the reaction of sensitized dogs to hypothermia, J. Microbiol. Epidem. Immun. (U.S.S.R.) **32:**119, 1961.

134. Downey, R.J., and Diedrich, B.F.: A new method for assessing particle ingestion by phagocytic cells, Exp. Cell. Res. **50:**483, 1968.

135. Brzuchowska, W.: Use of radioactive isotopes in studies on phagocytosis in vitro, Nature (London) **212:**210, 1966.

136. Ellegaard, B., Borregaard, N., and Ellegaard, J.: Neutrophil chemotaxis and phagocytosis in juvenile peridontitis, J. Periodont. Res. **19:**261, 1984.

137. Stahelin, H., Suter, E., and Karnovsky, M.L.: Studies on the interaction between phagocytes and tubercle bacilli, J. Exp. Med. **104:**121, 1956.

138. Evans, D.G., and Myrvik, Q.N.: Phagocytosis and stimulation of the hexosemonophosphate shunt in alveolar macrophages, J. Reticuloendothelial Soc. **3:**330, 1966.

139. Stahelin, H., et al.: Studies on the interaction between phagocytes and tubercle bacilli. III. Some metabolic effects in guinea pigs associated with injection with tubercle bacilli, J. Exp. Med. **105,**265, 1957.

140. Paul, B., et al.: Effect of phagocytosis on myeloperoxidase and NADPH oxidase, J. Reticuloendothel. Soc. **7:**644, 1970.

141. Paul, B., and Sbarra, A.J.: The role of the phagocyte in host-parasite interactions. XIII. The direct quantitative estimation of $H_2O_2$ in phagocytizing cells, Biochim. Biophys. Acta **156:**168, 1968.

142. McRipley, R.J., and Sbarra, A.J.: Role of the phagocyte in host-parasite interactions. XI. Relationship between stimulated oxidative metabolism and $H_2O_2$ formation, and intracellular killing, J. Bacteriol. **94:**1417, 1967.

143. Iyer, G.Y., Islan, M.F., and Quastel, J.H.: Biochemical aspects of phagocytosis, Nature **192:**535, 1961.

144. Zatti, M., Rossi, F., and Meneghelli, V.: Metabolic and morphological changes of polymorphonuclear leukocytes during phagocytosis, Brit. J. Exp. Pathol. **46:**227, 1965.

145. Zatti, M., Rossi, F., and Patriarca, P.: The $H_2O_2$ production by polymorphonuclear leukocytes during phagocytosis, Experimentia **24:**699, 1968.

146. Klebanoff, S.J.: Myeloperoxidase: contribution to the microbicidal activity of intact leukocytes, Science **169:**1095, 1970.

147. Klebanoff, S.J.: Myeloperoxidase-halide-$H_2O_2$ antibacterial system, J. Bacteriol **95:**2131, 1968.

148. Klebanoff, S.J.: Iodination of bacteria: a bactericidal mechanism, J. Exp. Med. **126:**1063, 1967.

149. Paul, B., et al.: Function of $H_2O_2$, myeloperoxidase, and hexose monophosphate shunt enzymes in phagocytizing cells from different species, Infec. Immun. **1:**338, 1970.

150. McRipley, R.J., and Sbarra, A.J.: Role of the phagocyte in host-parasite interactions. XI. Relationship between stimulated oxidative metabolism and $H_2O_2$ formation, and intracellular killing, J. Bacteriol. **94:**1417, 1967.

151. McRipley, R.J., and Sbarra, A.J.: Role of the phagocyte in host-parasite interactions. XII. $H_2O_2$-myeloperoxidase bactericidal system in the phagocyte, J. Bacteriol. **94:**1425, 1967.

152. Ohlsson, K., Olsson, I., and Tynelius-Bratthall, G.: Neutrophyil leukocyte collagenase, elastase, and serum protease inhibitors in human gingival crevices, Acta Odontol. Scandinav. **32:**51, 1974.

153. Passo, S.A., et al.: Interaction of inflammatory cells and oral microorganisms. IX. The bactericidal effects of human polymorphonuclear leukocytes on isolated plaque microorganisms, J. Periodont. Res. **15:**470, 1980.

154. Kowashi, Y., Jaccard, F., and Cimasoni, G.: Increase of free collagenase and neutral protease activities in the gingival crevice during experimental gingivitis in man, Arch. Oral Biol. **24:**645, 1979.

155. Goldstein, I.M.: Polymorphonuclear leukocyte lysosomes and immune tissue injury, Progr. Allergy **20:**301, 1976.

156. Genco, R., and Mergenhagen, S.: Host-parasite interactions in periodontal disease, Publications, Washington, D.C., 1982, American Society of Microbiology.

157. Baggiolini, M., et al.: The polymorphonuclear leukocyte, Agents Actions **8:**3, 1978.

158. Kamster, I.B., et al.: Modification of in vitro and in vivo immune function by acute inflammatory cells, Transplantation **30:**2, 1980.

159. Rodrick, M.L., et al.: Effects of supernatants of polymorphonuclear neutrophils recruited by different inflammatory substances on mitogen responses of lymphocytes, Inflammation **6:**1, 1982.

160. Horton, J.E., Leikin, S., and Oppenheim, J.J.: Human lymphoproliferative reaction to saliva and dental plaque-deposits: an in vitro correlation with periodontal disease, J. Periodontol. **43:**522, 1972.

161. Lang, N.P., and Smith, F.N.: Lymphocyte blastogenesis to plaque antigens in human periodontal disease. I. Populations of varying severities of disease. J. Periodont. Res. **12:**298, 1977.

162. Patters, M.R., Sedransk, N., and Genco, R.J.: The lympho-proliferative response during human experimental gingivitis, J. Periodont. Res. **14:**269, 1979.

163. Smith, F.N., Lang, N.P., and Löe, H.: Cell mediated immune responses to plaque antigens during experimental gingivitis in man, J. Periodont. Res. **13:**232, 1978.

164. Sims, T., Clagett, J.A., and Page, R.C.: Effects of cell concentration and exogenous prostaglandin on the interaction and responsiveness of human peripheral blood lymphocytes, Clin. Immunol. Immunopathol. **12:**150, 1978.

165. Budtz-Jorgensen, J., et al.: Leukocyte migration inhibition by bacterial antigens in patients with periodontal disease, J. Periodontol. Res. **12:**21, 1977.

166. Osterberg, S.K., et al.: Blastogenic respon-

siveness of peripheral blood mononuclear cells from individuals with various forms of periodontitis and effects of treatment, J. Clin. Periodontol. **10:**72, 1983.

167. Page, R.C., and Schroeder, H.: Periodontitis in man and other animals, Zurich, 1982, S. Karger.

168. Tew, J.G., et al.: Immunological studies of young adults with severe periodontitis. II. Cellular factors, J. Periodont. Res. **16:**403, 1981.

169. Genco, R.J. and Mergenhagen, S.E.: Summary of a workshop on leukocyte function in bacterial diseases with an emphasis on periodontal disease. J. Infect. Dis. **139:**604, 1979.

170. Murphy, P.: The neutrophil, New York, 1976, Plenum Publishing Corp.

# CHAPTER 13

# Diet and nutrition

## Introduction

In the developing areas of the world, such factors as illiteracy, overpopulation, low soil productivity, and low levels of industrialization account for the nutritional problems of public health concern.

In contrast, nutritional problems in the industrialized nations are quite often conditioned malnutrition. This type is often secondary to mental, physical, physiologic, and habitual stress or occurs as a complication of other diseases. Some studies, nevertheless, have uncovered areas in the United States where primary nutritional problems approximate situations present in underdeveloped countries.[1-3] In addition, the aged represent a group of special concern since they may have altered tasted function, xerostomia, and diminished income all compounding malnutrition.

The pattern and distribution of periodontal diseases among various population groups involve both the disease-producing agents and the possible contribution of various host factors. Host resistance is an important factor modifying the severity of a disease. Tissue resistance is modified in turn by physical and emotional stress, nutritional status, and various systemic conditions. The course and severity of most infections are exaggerated in malnutrition.[4-6]

Nutrition may influence the growth, development, and metabolic activities of the periodontium. Malnutrition can modify the expression of the primary etiologic factors whereas diet may influence the progression of periodontal lesions. Tissues with a rapid rate of cell renewal, such as the periodontium, depend on the ready availability of essential nutrients for the maintenance of their activities. They are therefore susceptible to the effects of malnutrition.[7,8]

## Primary nutrient deficiencies

Severe nutritional deficiency appears to play a role in the etiologic history of periodontal diseases. Protein-calorie malnutrition is a common problem in developing coun-

*Marginal notes:*

**Primary malnutrition**

**Conditioned malnutrition**

**Host resistance**

**Inter-relationships**

**Protein-calorie malnutrition**

tries. It promotes the development of acute periodontal lesions in children and in adults. Protein-calorie malnutrition (kwashiorkor) is by far the most widespread nutritional disorder in underdeveloped countries and is usually complicated by concurrent deficiencies of other essential nutrients.[4,9-10] It is primarily a disease of infants and young children, with a peak age incidence of 1 to 3 years. Poor lactation because of maternal malnutrition and inadequacy of the diets of weaned children are major causative factors.[11,12] Lesions of the buccal mucosa may be observed in this disease.[13] Buccal scrapings show typical histologic changes when compared with normal scrapings.[14,15] Significant generalized osteoporosis has been demonstrated,[16] and there is evidence of alveolar bone loss.[17] Epidemiologic studies reveal that children suffering from kwashiorkor show significant differences in their oral hygiene index (OHI) scores and demonstrate more periodontal pathologic conditions when compared with children of similar ages drawn from a higher socioeconomic level.[18,19] Well-fed Nigerian children enjoy a better state of periodontal health than do their age counterparts in poor rural areas, regardless of local factors.[18] These observations are supported by studies of malnutrition in experimental animals that show degeneration of the connective tissue fibers in the gingiva and periodontal ligament, pronounced osteoporosis of the alveolar bone, and marked retardation in deposition of cementum.[20-25] There is evidence that the younger the animal, the more profound the effects of protein malnutrition on the periodontium.[26]

**NUG**

Of particular interest are the severity and age distribution patterns of certain oral diseases in protein-calorie–deficient populations. Necrotizing ulcerative gingivitis (NUG) is rarely seen in children in developed countries[27,28] but assumes a different age distribution pattern in poor nations. More than half the cases seen in India are reported in children under 10 years of age.[29,30] Protein-calorie–malnourished children have a higher incidence of NUG than do well-fed age controls in the same country.[19,31,32] Fig. 13-1 shows a case of NUG in a 3-year-old Nigerian village child. Examination of children from high and low socioeconomic groups in Nigeria revealed no case of NUG in the high group.[33] In the low socioeconomic group, drawn from a village with high incidence of protein malnutrition, eighty-seven cases of NUG were observed in a period of 15 months, and all but two were in children 1 to 10 years old. The peak incidence was at 2 to 3 years of age, which corresponded with the immediate post-weaning period. In some cases the NUG extended into adjacent tissues, producing extensive necrosis and destruction of orofacial tissues (Fig. 13-2). This condition, known as

**Noma**

*noma* or cancrum oris, is extremely rare in developed countries except during famines. It is commonly encountered in poor nations[34-36] and is closely associated with malnutrition and states of debilitation.[34-37] Jelliffe reported fifty-three cases in which the ages of the patients varied from 2 to 5 years.[34] He noted that all had had protein-deficient diets for periods of 6 months to 2 years. On the rare occasion when noma is encountered in developed countries, the patient almost invariably is nutritionally deprived.[38] Thus cancrum oris, essentially a socioeconomic disease, represents an outcome of the synergism between malnutrition and infection, probably mediated by impaired immune function.

## Conditioned, marginal nutrient deficiencies

Conditioned, marginal nutrient deficiencies are common and may play a role in the etiology of periodontitis.[39] Marginal nutrient deficiencies may be "conditioned" by a number of factors and social habits. These marginal deficiencies do not manifest the clinical signs and symptoms associated with classical, frank deficiency. Factors that contribute to marginal nutrient deficiencies include increased use of drugs, learned taste aversions, alcoholism, and food faddism. Increased use of a variety of drugs by apparently healthy people can contribute to nutritional problems. These drugs need

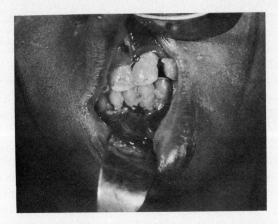

**Fig. 13-1.** Necrotizing ulcerative gingivitis in a 3-year-old Nigerian girl. The typical ulcerations, gingival craters, pseudomembranous slough, and oral debris are seen around the mandibular incisors. (From Enwonwu. C.O.: Nutrition and dental health: epidemiological study of dental growth and dental diseases in western Nigerian children in relation to socio-economic status. Doctoral thesis, Bristol University, England, 1966; courtesy C.O. Enwonwu, Nashville, Tennessee.)

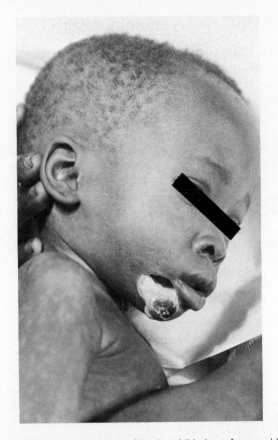

**Fig. 13-2.** Noma (cancrum oris) in a malnourished Nigerian child about 4 years old. (From Enwonwu. C.O.: Nutrition and dental health: epidemiological study of dental growth and dental diseases in western Nigerian children in relation to socio-economic status. Doctoral thesis, Bristol University, England, 1966; courtesy C.O. Enwonwu, Nashville, Tennessee.)

**Contraceptive
steroids**

**Cathartics**

not be "street drugs" or powerful cardiovascular or psychotropic agents to exert a nutritional effect. Contraceptive steroids may condition marginal nutrient deficiencies by increasing requirements for folate, ascorbate, and pyridoxine. Similarly, mineral oil and magnesium salt cathartics result in impaired absorption of fat-soluble vitamins and calcium. Calcium and magnesium deficiencies can also be conditioned by the consumption of aluminum-containing antacids. Thus seemingly innocuous over-the-counter drug preparations should not be ignored in the etiology of marginal nutrient deficiencies. In addition, one should be cognizant of the dual effects of alcoholism on nutritional status. The alcoholic who takes in 1200 or more calories each day from ethanol has proportionally less opportunity to consume the additional nutrients required for a balanced diet. Furthermore, as alcoholism progresses, altered liver and digestive functions can result with specific deficiencies of thiamine and folate.

**Alcohol**

Learned taste aversions may develop when an individual becomes ill after consuming a type of food. For instance, taste aversions to citrus fruits may contribute to ascorbate deficiency. Deprivation of vitamin C will lead to scurvy.[40] Learned taste aversions are paralleled in effect by food faddism. Some people avoid all food except grains (Zen Macrobiotics), whereas others avoid poultry skin because of its cholesterol content. Although food faddism can result in severe primary nutrient deficiencies, most individuals are not sufficiently diligent in their adherence to the diet, so only marginal deficiencies result. The mechanisms by which chronic marginal nutrient deficiencies can affect the periodontal tissues are only beginning to be elucidated.

**Food faddism**

## Local effects of food on periodontal health

**Bacteria**

It is apparent that the composition of the diet can have a local effect altering the distribution and metabolism of bacteria in plaque. Virtually all these changes occur in supragingival plaque, which has ready access to nutrients.[41] Subgingival plaque[30]—important in the genesis of periodontal inflammation—is relatively shielded from direct dietary modification because of its location. Diet probably affects the subgingival microflora primarily by its systemic absorption and distribution in serum, rather than directly. Nevertheless, water-soluble extracts of certain foods acting as mediators have been shown to initiate a cellular immune response.[42] Gingival inflammation in gnotobiotic rat gingiva is believed to be related to immune responses to food.

**Mediators**

**Consistency of
diet**

The physical consistency of the diet—that is, a firm, fibrous diet—is believed to promote cleanliness of the teeth. This appears to be true only in animal model systems[43,44] in which firm foods promote gingival keratinization. Nevertheless, the consumption of a fibrous diet may promote optimal salivary gland function (Table 13-1) with consequent benefit to oral health.

**Keratinization**

## Carbohydrates and fats

Although studies in various experimental animals indicate that high-carbohydrate diets are conducive to the development of severe periodontal lesions, such experiments are difficult to interpret.[45-48] For instance, it is difficult to separate effects resulting from the high carbohydrate content from those attributable to the low protein content of such diets. It is also dangerous to consider the quantity of food in diets in isolation from the composition or quality of the food.[49] Animals eat to satisfy their energy requirements primarily and in the absence of force-feeding will not ingest enough protein from a predominantly carbohydrate diet to meet these requirements. In addition, many of the high-carbohydrate diets employed in such studies are of powdery consistency. This factor introduces a major variable with regard to retention of food particles in the mouth. Also there is sufficient evidence that ingestion of liquid or powdered food has

**Table 13-1**  Summary of the effect of the physical consistency of food on the sulcular complex and the salivary glands

| Diet | Sulcular complex | | Salivary glands (saliva) | |
|------|------------------|-------------------|------------------|--------------|
| | **Animals** | **Human** | **Animals** | **Human** |
| Soft | Dogs: increase in plaque and gingival fluid; gingivitis; bacterial flora move to fusiforms and spirochetes<br>Rat, hamster: Consistent with above | Insufficient evidence to draw any conclusion | Rats (parotid gland): disuse atrophy; decreased flow; decreased expulsion and synthesis of secretory products; decrease in growth, differentiation, and maturation of acinar cells | Reduction in flow (volume), total protein, and amylase activity of stimulated saliva |
| Hard | Dogs: prevention of above<br>Rat, hamster: destruction of interdental papilla; probably because of presence of coarse particles in food | Bulk of evidence suggests mastication of fibrous foods has no effect on formation of plaque, volume of gingival fluid, or degree of gingival inflammation; more evidence needed | Reverse of changes listed above | Reverse of changes listed above |

From Sreebny, L.M.: Food consistency and periodontal disease. In Hazen, S.P., editor: Diet, nutrition and periodontal disease, Chicago, 1975, American Society for Preventive Dentistry.

an adverse effect on the structure and function of the salivary glands,[50-52] attributable to reduced masticatory function.[50]

Changes in the periodontium have also been reported in rats fed either a fat-free or a high-fat diet. More detailed, adequately controlled studies are necessary before any meaningful extrapolations of these findings can be made.

## Vitamins

The absence of vitamins from diets results in deficiency diseases. The vitamins are generally considered under two major subdivisions: water-soluble and fat-soluble.

### WATER-SOLUBLE VITAMINS

**Vitamin C (ascorbic acid)**

The body stores of ascorbic acid in healthy, well-fed men approximate 1500 mg and are used at an average daily rate of 3% of the existing pool. Dietary deprivation of vitamin C for 3 months precedes marked depletion of the body stores; at this stage the amount available for daily catabolism is not enough to prevent scurvy.[53] Many of the signs of deficiency may appear during the first month of dietary deprivation. There is still some controversy regarding the human daily dietary requirement of vitamin C. Although 30 mg/day is the recommended intake for normal persons, a daily intake of 10 mg is believed to be necessary to prevent scurvy in healthy adults.[54] This opinion is supported by the observation that a daily dose of only 6.5 mg of ascorbic acid produces remarkable improvement in experimentally induced scurvy in adult males.[53] On the contrary, Berry and Schaefer found a close association between the prevalence of gingival pathologic conditions and dietary intake of 15 to 23 mg of ascorbic acid per day.[54]

The main sources of dietary vitamin C are fresh fruits. Diagnosis of vitamin C deficiency is often based on the plasma ascorbic acid level, and there is good evidence that this test lacks precision.[53] The absence of measurable vitamin C in serum or plasma is compatible with scurvy; but it is not diagnostic, since zero levels have also been reported in persons without any clinical manifestations of scurvy.[53-56] This occurs because plasma vitamin C is labile and varies with the recent dietary intake as well as with other conditions (e.g., infections). Values below 0.2 mg/100 ml of serum are indicative of marked ascorbic acid deficiency,[57] but experimental studies have shown obvious scurvy when serum levels were above 0.2 mg/100 ml.[53]

Among the signs and symptoms often observed in marked ascorbic acid depletion are ocular hemorrhages, xerostomia, femoral neuropathy, impaired vascular reactivity or poor responses to stimuli that normally activate the vasomotor adaptive mechanisms, psychologic disturbances, scorbutic arthritis, and gingivitis.

Gingivitis is a common classical manifestation of frank scurvy,[58] although some investigators believe that local irritation must be present for acute deficiency of vitamin C to cause gingivitis and periodontitis.[59-61] Among the oral manifestations of scurvy are intense gingival reddening, attributable to engorgement of the underlying blood vessels, and fiery red, smooth, glazed, swollen gingiva devoid of normal stippling. The gingival lesions usually start in the interdental area and spread to involve the marginal gingiva. Secondary infection of the gingiva occurs frequently, with ulceration, necrosis, and sloughing.[58] Gingival lesions of scurvy rarely occur in the absence of teeth.

Fig. 13-3, *A*, demonstrates some of the oral lesions in a case of infantile scurvy in a 3-year-old child in western Nigeria. The child had had an attack of measles; later the mother noticed the child's inability to stand erect for an appreciable length of time. The knee joints were very tender on examination. The gingiva was hemorrhagic and hypertrophied, the teeth were mobile, and the mandibular right deciduous central incisor had been exfoliated. Roentgenographic examination showed separation of the epiphyses of the femur and tibia of the left knee, together with calcification in the large hematoma around the lower femoral diaphysis (Fig. 13-3, *B*).

Blood examination showed a serum ascorbic acid level of 0.07 mg/100 ml, which was compatible with the diagnosis of scurvy. Treatment with 30 mg of ascorbic acid daily produced marked remission of the oral lesions in a week.

Among the prominent features of scorbutic gingivitis are a periodontal ligament widened by resorption of surrounding bone and a breakdown of collagen fibers in the periodontium.[62]

Vitamin C deficiency affects fibroblasts, osteoblasts, and odontoblasts. The cells fail to produce normal collagen, osteoid, and dentin; the ability of the cells to form epithelial and vascular basement membranes is also restricted.[63] Vitamin C deficiency impairs the hydroxylation of proline. Severe vitamin C deficiency is characterized by hemorrhagic tendencies, impaired wound healing, and osteoporosis.

**Wound healing**

The principal cell involved in wound healing and repair is the fibroblast. Among the prominent alterations in this cell in vitamin C deficiency are the following: vacuolization of the cisternae of the ergastoplasm with loss of the characteristic configuration of membrane-bound polyribosomes; increase in the number of free ribosomes; and presence of large numbers of lipid deposits in the cytoplasm.[64,65] These features reflect reduced protein biosynthesis.[66,67] The extracellular space shows fewer collagen bundles, although individual fibrils of indeterminate nature are present.[65] Vitamin C may also be involved in the metabolism of mucopolysaccharides.[68]

**Niacin (nicotinamide)**

Deficiency of niacin or of tryptophan (which could be metabolized inefficiently to niacin) is responsible for pellagra. Gingivitis, attributable to deficiency of niacin, is characterized by extremely painful, wedge-shaped, punched-out ulcers involving the interdental papillae and marginal gingiva.[58] The lesions in humans are necrotic, exudative, and foul smelling. In dogs severe inflammatory changes in the oral mucosa, including the sulcular epithelium, capillary dilatation, and osteoporosis of the alveolar bone, have been reported.[69]

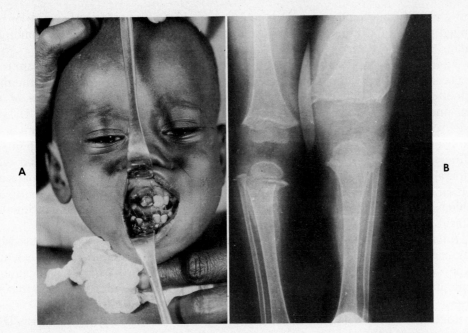

**Fig. 13-3. A,** Oral lesions of scurvy. **B,** Roentgenographic appearance of skeletal alterations in infantile scurvy. Nigerian child aged 3 years. (From Enwonwu, C.O.: Nutrition and dental health: epidemiological study of dental growth and dental diseases in western Nigerian children in relation to socio-economic status. Doctoral thesis, Bristol University, England, 1966; courtesy C.O. Enwonwu, Nashville, Tennessee.)

Riboflavin is a constituent of the flavoproteins, which are important in tissue oxidation. Deficiency of riboflavin causes glossitis and angular cheilosis, although these lesions are not specific for riboflavin deficiency. Epithelial atrophy is a basic feature, which may account for the association of this condition with gingivitis in monkeys.[70,71] **Riboflavin**

The important food sources of folic acid are liver, kidney, yeast, and mushrooms. Folic acid deficiency is characterized by lesions in cells with rapid rate of renewal, which demonstrates the importance of this vitamin in the synthesis of DNA.[72] In folic acid deficiency, there is impairment of keratinization with increased susceptibility to ulceration and secondary infections.[73,74] Severe gingivitis and necrosis of oral and gingival mucosa have been reported in folic acid–deficient monkeys.[58,70,71,75] **Folic acid (pteroylglutamic acid)**

The relationship of the remaining water-soluble vitamins to periodontal pathology in humans has not been adequately studied. **Other water-soluble vitamins**

## FAT-SOLUBLE VITAMINS

Vitamin A occurs in the animal kingdom, especially in marine fish liver oils, liver fat, fat of dairy products, and eggs. The provitamins (carotenoid precursors) are found in green vegetables, carrots, etc. Proformed vitamin A is deposited primarily in the liver and kidneys. In view of this storage, to produce clinical and biochemical manifestations of deficiency, there must be a prolonged period of deprivation. **Vitamin A**

Deficiency of vitamin A produces marked retardation in growth; alterations in epithelial and nervous tissues, cartilage, and bone; and severe interference with vision and reproduction. Hyperplasia and keratinization in mucous membranes are characteristic features. Evidence is inconclusive for participation of vitamin A depletion in human periodontal disease.[76]

Ingestion of excessive amounts of vitamin A (more than a hundred times required amount) is just as deleterious to health as dietary deprivation of the vitamin. Among the features observed in hypervitaminosis A are mucous dysplasia of epithelium, thickening of skin and suppression of keratinization, bleeding tendency because of prolonged prothrombin time, and increased absorption of bone with loss of chondroitin sulfate.

**Vitamin D**

Vitamin D is represented by a group of steroid alcohols, primarily vitamin $D_2$ (ergocalciferol) and vitamin $D_3$ (cholecalciferol). The latter is believed to be the most potent of the D vitamins, and its relative importance varies with the species of animal under consideration. Among the precursors are ergosterol (provitamin $D_2$) and 7-dehydrocholesterol (provitamin $D_3$). The main food sources of the D vitamins are the liver oils of many fishes. Vitamin D is stored by mammals in small amounts. It influences absorption and excretion of calcium, phosphate, magnesium, and other minerals; it also plays an important role in the ossification of cartilage. In humans and certain animal species severe vitamin D deficiency produces rickets in the young and osteomalacia in the old; these lesions are characterized by defective mineralization of osteoid.

Information on the role of vitamin D deficiency in human periodontal disease is fragmentary and often contradictory. Feeding young rats a diet that has a high calcium-to-phosphorus ratio but is deficient in vitamin D results in defective calcification of cementum and alveolar bone with hyaline degeneration of connective tissue in some cases.[77-79]

Ingestion of excessive amounts of all forms of vitamin D (hypervitaminosis D) is dangerous, and the characteristic features of the syndrome are hypercalcemia and deposition of calcium phosphate in any matrix containing mucoproteins. The calcinosis is widespread, affecting the kidneys, myocardium, endocrine glands, arteries, gastrointestinal tract, joints, cornea, and several other tissues. Advanced stages of hypervitaminosis D often show demineralization of bones. Little is known regarding involvement of the human periodontal tissues in this syndrome. Among the outstanding features seen in young rats subjected to hypervitaminosis D are large numbers of enlarged osteocytes engaged in lacunar resorption, enlarged cementocytes with the presence of cementoid, and increased amounts of connective tissue fibers of the periodontium (resulting in an enlargement of the interdental papillae).[79] Calcification of periodontal ligament fibers and ankylosis were noted in rats fed excessive amounts of vitamin D.[80]

**Vitamin E**

Vitamin E is represented by the compounds known as tocopherols. Vegetable oils are the most important sources of this vitamin. The clinical features of vitamin E deficiency show marked variability in different animal species. The prominent deficiency sign in the human is increased tendency to hemolysis. Vitamin E deficiency is believed to affect the cross-linking of collagen.[68]

**Vitamin K**

The main sources of naturally occurring K vitamins (2-methyl-1,4-naphthoquinone derivatives) are green plants and bacteria. Vitamin K is necessary for prevention of the hemorrhagic condition associated with insufficient ability of the blood to coagulate. The defect in coagulation may result from inadequate biosynthesis of proconvertin, prothrombin, and other plasmatic factors involved in the blood-clotting system. Vitamin K deficiency can be induced by administration of antagonists like coumarin and other related compounds. Avitaminosis K promotes a hemorrhagic diathesis.

## Minerals

Maintenance of life and optimal health requires the availability of several inorganic elements, of which some (calcium, phosphorus, magnesium) are present in the body in macroquantities and others (iron, copper, cobalt, iodine, sulfur, manganese, zinc, fluorine, sodium, potassium, chlorine) are required in relatively trace amounts.[81] These nutrients participate in essential metabolic processes in the body, functioning in a complex and interrelated manner with one another and with the major food nutrients and the endocrine and enzyme systems. Prolonged ingestion of foods that are imbalanced, deficient, or high in these elements produces physiologic and biochemical defects as well as structural alterations in various tissues and organs, depending on the elements involved.

**Calcium and phosphorus**

There is general agreement that dietary deficiency of phosphorus hardly exists in humans. Nordin[82] is of the opinion that some forms of osteoporosis can be explained on the basis of malabsorption of calcium or dietary lack of the element. The latter view is now adequately substantiated only in experimental animal studies.[80] Among the findings in calcium-deficient young rats and cats are osteoporosis of alveolar bone, reduction in amount of secondary cementum, and reduction in size and number of the periodontal fibers. In rats fed diets deficient in phosphorus, slight rachitic and osteomalacic alterations were observed in the young and adult animals.[79,83,84] A deficiency in calcium or an excess of phosphorus may lead to metabolic bone loss. A nutritional secondary hyperparathyroidism (NSH) occurs to maintain serum calcium levels in the presence of altered $C_2/P$ rates. Calcium is removed from bone to maintain serum levels. Evidence that such disease is related to alveolar bone loss in periodontitis is not convincing.[85-90]

**Magnesium**

Simple uncomplicated deficiency of magnesium rarely occurs in humans but is a frequent complication of protein-calorie malnutrition resulting from gastrointestinal losses of the ion during chronic diarrhea and vomiting[91] and renal losses after intensive intravenous administration of magnesium-free electrolyte and glucose solutions.[92] Skin and oral lesions have been described in magnesium-deficient rats.[93] In studies of 67 seriously malnourished Nigerian children with orofacial lesions of cancrum oris, Caddell[94] found magnesium-supplemented therapy superior to therapy without magnesium supplementation.

**Iron and other minerals**

Few studies have been undertaken to establish the role of iron and other elements in the maintenance of good periodontal health. Abnormalities of the mouth such as angular stomatitis and atrophic changes on the dorsum of the tongue and the buccal mucosa have been noted in iron deficiency.[95-97] It is also worthy to note that one of the two enzymes intimately involved with the antimicrobial activities of the phagocytic cell is an iron-containing enzyme called myeloperoxidase.[98] Higashi and co-workers[99] showed that patients with iron deficiency have a deficiency of this enzyme and a consequent decrease in bactericidal activity. The possible effects of such a situation in terms of the defense of the periodontal tissues against plaque microorganisms should not be overlooked.

**Fluoride**

There are conflicting reports on the role of fluoride in periodontal health.[79] Studies in humans have failed to show a beneficial or detrimental effect of ingested fluoride on periodontal health.[100]

Many essential metabolic functions are carried out by microelements, and thus more information on their relevance to dental health is needed.

## Summary

The effect of foodstuffs on teeth are related to their cleansing action on the tooth surface and to their potential for enhancing or retarding plaque deposition.[101-104] Another effect of diet is the production of erosion produced by ingesting acidic foods or beverages,[105] or by the acidity of vomitus in bulimic people[106] after engaging in a food-eating binge.

There can be no doubt that malnutrition produces abnormalities in metabolism. On the other hand, inflammatory periodontal disease is not a primary nutritional deficiency disease. There is no significant evidence that diet and nutrition are primary causal agents of periodontal disease. Nutritional inadequacies may predispose to periodontal disease or may possibly modify the course of the disease.[107-119] Such deficiencies do not cause bacterially induced periodontal disease (gingivitis and periodontitis), but they can condition the response of the periodontium to disease so that an individual's response is less than normal.

A most alarming view held by some is that (bacterially induced, inflammatory) periodontal disease can be treated by dietary manipulation. There has never been a demonstration in a carefully controlled study of a dietary cure for such a disease. On the other hand, careful evaluation of the epidemiologic data produces some useful insights.

## Epidemiologic considerations

Although periodontal disease is not a manifestation of specific nutritional deficiency,[117] nonspecific depletion of a combination of nutrients may increase the rate of the disease.[118]

Some investigators have reported that persons with low levels of certain nutrients such as riboflavin and vitamin C have less severe periodontal disease than those with normal levels. Providing vitamin C–deficient patients with therapeutic doses of ascorbic acid does not improve their gingival condition.[120] There is no support for using more than recommended intakes of ascorbic acid in the prevention or treatment of periodontal diseases because only a weak association has been found between periodontal disease and ascorbic acid levels in a representative sample of the U.S. population.[121] The highest prevalence and severity of periodontal disease occurs in populations where malnutrition is common, so the possibility exists that general malnutrition does affect the severity of disease.

Most of the epidemiologic surveys on the relationship between nutritional factors and periodontal disease are based on biochemical estimates of nutrients. Cautious inferences should be drawn from comparisons between the nutritional status of a population on a specific day and the accumulated lifetime experience of oral diseases. Dietary, biochemical, and clinical measurements assess different chronologic aspects of nutritional status: the dietary measurement is made at the time of the survey, the biochemical measurement shows the relatively recent past, while the clinical changes require a longer period for exhaustion of tissue stores of the particular nutrient. Similarly, once a lesion is produced it may require much time to revert to normal; some lesions may be irreversible and therefore permanent. It is therefore important to compare the biochemical estimates of nutritional deficiency with the dietary and clinical findings. When this is done, the relationship between nutrition and periodontal health is more positive. For example, signs of scorbutic gingivitis do occur in persons with low ascorbic acid dietary intakes but the gingival condition is not positively related with plasma ascorbic acid levels.[121]

The hypotheses that specific nutritional deficiencies are or are not strongly associated with the severity of periodontal disease[122] are based on small numbers of biochemical estimates. These estimates suffer from errors of sampling, and the relationship between the biochemical estimates of nutritional status and the clinical nutritional status is questionable.

**REFERENCES**

1. Mayer, J.: White House Conference on Food, Nutrition and Health, final report, Publication no. 0-378-473, U.S. Department of Health, Education, and Welfare, Washington, D.C., 1970, U.S. Government Printing Office.

2. American Academy of Pediatrics Committee Statement: The Ten-State Nutrition Survey: a pediatric perspective, Pediatrics **51:**1095, 1975.

3. Abraham, S., Lowenstein. F.W., and Johnson, C.L.: Preliminary findings of the first

Health and Nutrition Examination Survey, United States, 1971-1972: dietary intake and biochemical findings, U.S. Department of Health, Education and Welfare, Washington, D.C., 1974, U.S. Government Printing Office.

4. Scrimshaw, N.S.: Ecological factors in nutritional disease, Am. J. Clin. Nutr. **14:**112, 1964.

5. Scrimshaw, N.S., Taylor, C.E., and Gordon, J.E.: Interactions of nutrition and infection, Geneva, 1968, World Health Organization.

6. Gontzea, I.: Nutrition and anti-infectious defense, Basel, Switzerland, 1974, S. Karger.

7. Ramalingaswami, V.: Perspectives in protein malnutrition, Nature **201:**546, 1964.

8. Winick, M., and Noble, A.: Quantitative changes in DNA, RNA and protein during prenatal and postnatal growth in the rat, Dev. Biol. **12:**451, 1965.

9. Scrimshaw, N.S., and Waterlow, J.C.: The concept of kwashiorkor from a public health point of view, Bull. WHO **16:**458, 1957.

10. Scrimshaw, N.S.: World-wide importance of protein malnutrition and progress toward its prevention, Am. J. Public Health **53:**1781, 1963.

11. Platt, B.S.: Infant-feeding practices: breast feeding and the prevention of infant malnutrition, Proc. Nutr. Soc. **13:**94, 1954.

12. Behar, M., and Scrimshaw, N.S.: Effect of environment on nutritional status, Arch. Environ. Health **5:**257, 1962.

13. Trowell, H.C., Davies, J.N.P., and Dean, R.F.A.: Kwashiorkor, London, 1954, Edward Arnold & Co.

14. Squires, B.T.: Observations upon the oral mucosa of the African, Cent. Afr. J. Med. **4:**104, 1958.

15. Squires, B.T.: Differential staining of buccal epithelial smears as an indicator of poor nutritional status due to protein-calorie deficiency, J. Pediatr. **66:**891, 1965.

16. Garn, S.M., et al.: Compact bone deficiency in protein-calorie malnutrition, Science **145:**1444, 1964.

17. Owens, P.D.A.: The effects of undernutrition and rehabilitation on the jaws and teeth of pigs. In McCance, R.A., and Widdowson, E.M., editors: Calorie deficiencies and protein deficiencies, Boston, 1968, Little, Brown & Co.

18. Enwonwu, C.O., and Edozien, J.C.: Epidemiology of periodontal disease in western Nigerians in relation to socio-economic status. Arch. Oral Biol. **15:**1231, 1970.

19. Pindborg, J.J., Bhat, M., and Roed-Petersen, B.: Oral changes in South Indian children with severe protein deficiency, J. Periodontol. **38:**218, 1967.

20. Stahl, S.S.: Response of the periodontium to protein-calorie malnutrition, J. Oral Med. **21:**146, 1966.

21. Stahl, S.S.: Host resistance and periodontal disease, J. Dent. Res. Suppl. **49:**248, 1970.

22. Stein, G., and Ziskin, D.E.: The effect of a protein-free diet on the teeth and periodontium of the albino rat. J. Dent. Res. **28:**529, 1949.

23. Chawla, T.N., and Glickman, I.: Protein deprivation and the periodontal structures of the albino rat, Oral Surg. **4:**578, 1951.

24. Stahl, S.S., Sandler, H.C., and Cahn, L.: The effects of protein deprivation upon the oral tissues of the rat, and particularly upon periodontal structures under irritation, Oral Surg. **8:**760, 1955.

25. Carranza, F.A., Jr., et al.: Histometric analysis of interradicular bone in protein deficient animals, J. Periodont. Res. **4:**292, 1969.

26. Goldman, H.M.: The effects of dietary protein deprivation and of age on the periodontal tissues of the rat and spider monkey, J. Periodontal. **25:**87, 1954.

27. Manson, J.D., and Rand, H.: Recurrent Vincent's disease (a survey of 61 cases), Br. Dent. J. **110:**386, 1961.

28. Skach, M., Zabrodsky, S., and Mrklas, L.: A study of the effect of age and season on the incidence of ulcerative gingivitis, J. Periodont. Res. **5:**187, 1970.

29. Miglani, D.C., and Sharma, O.P.: Incidence of acute necrotizing gingivitis and periodontosis among cases seen at the Government Hospital, Madras, J. All India Dent. Assoc. **37:**183, 1965.

30. Pindborg, J.J., et al.: Occurrence of acute necrotizing gingivitis in South Indian children, J. Periodontol. **37:**14, 1966.

31. Sheiham, A.: An epidemiological study of oral disease in Nigerians, J. Dent. Res. **44:**1184, 1965.

32. Malberger, E.: Acute infectious oral necrosis among young children in the Gambia, West Africa, J. Periodont. Res. **2:**154, 1967.

33. Emslie, R.D.: Cancrum oris, Dent. Pract. **13:**481, 1963.

34. Jelliffe, D.B.: Infective gangrene of the mouth (cancrum oris), Pediatrics **9:**544, 1952.

35. Pahn-Dinh-Tuan: Noma in Vietnam, Indian J. Pediatr. **29:**367, 1962.

36. Tempest, M.N.: Cancrum oris, Br. J. Surg. **53:**949, 1966.

37. Agnew, R.G.: Cancrum oris, J. Periodontol. **18:**22, 1947.

38. Ruben, M.P., and Miller, M.: Noma: its association with nutritional deprivation and physical debilitation: report of a case, Oral Surg. **18:**167, 1964.

39. Alfano, M.C.: Prospects for improving the prevention of inflammatory periodontal disease, J. Prev. Dent. **5:**26, 1978.

40. Hodges, R.E.: What's new about scurvy? Am. J. Clin. Nutr. **24:**383, 1971.

41. Morhart, R., and Fitzgerald, R.: Nutritional determinants of the ecology of the oral flora, Dent. Clin. North Am. **20:**473, 1976.

42. Radentz, W.H., et al.: Human lymphoproliferative reaction to food products: possible role in periodontal inflammation, J. Periodontol. **46:**562, 1975.

43. Sreebny, L.M.: Effect of physical consistency of food on the "crevicular complex" and the salivary glands, Int. Dent. J. **22:**394, 1972.

44. Sreebny, L.M.: Food consistency and periodontal disease. In Hazen, S.P., editor: Diet, nutrition and periodontal disease, Chicago, 1975, American Society for Preventive Dentistry.

45. Keyes, P.H., and Likins, R.C.: Plaque formation, periodontal disease, and dental caries in Syrian hamsters, abstracted, J. Dent. Res. **25:**166, 1946.

46. Auskaps, A.M., Gupta, O.P., and Shaw, J.H.: Periodontal disease in the rice rat. III. Survey of dietary influences, J. Nutr. **63:**325, 1957.

47. Shaw, J.H., and Griffiths, D.: Relation of protein, carbohydrate, and fat intake to the periodontal syndrome, J. Dent. Res. **40:**614, 1961.

48. Keyes, P.H., and Jordan, H.V.: Periodontal lesions in the Syrian hamster. III. Findings related to an infective and transmissible component. Arch. Oral Biol. **9:**377, 1964.

49. Food and Agriculture Organization of the United Nations: Calorie requirements, FAO nutritional studies no. 15, Rome, 1957, Food and Agriculture Organization.

50. Hall, H.D., and Schneyer, C.A.: Salivary gland atrophy in rat induced by liquid diet, Proc. Soc. Exp. Biol. Med. **117:**789, 1964.

51. Sreebny, L.M., and Johnson, D.A.: Effect of food consistency and decreased food intake on rat parotid and pancreas, Am. J. Physiol. **215:**455, 1968.

52. Wilborn, W.H., and Schneyer, C.A.: Ultrastructural changes of rat parotid glands induced by a diet of liquid Metrecal, Z. Zellforsch. **103:**1, 1970.

53. British Medical Research Council: Vitamin C requirements in human adults, Special Report Series of the Medical Research Council, no. 280, London, 1953, Her Majesty's Stationery Office.

54. Berry, F.B., and Schaefer, A.: Nutrition surveys in the Near and Far East, Report of the Interdepartmental Committee on Nutrition for National Defense, N.I.H., Am. J. Clin. Nutr. **6:**342, 1958.

55. Pauling, L.: Vitamin C and the common cold, San Francisco, 1970, W.H. Freeman & Co. Publishers.

56. Vilter, R.W., Woolford, R., and Spies, T.D.S.: Severe scurvy: a clinical and hematologic study, J. Lab. Clin. Med. **31:**609, 1946.

57. Pearson, W.N.: Biochemcial appraisal of the vitamin nutritional status in man, JAMA **180:**49, 1962.

58. Dreizen, A.: Oral indications of the deficiency states, Postgrad. Med. **49:**97, 1971.

59. Glickman, I.: Acute vitamin C deficiency and periodontal disease. II. The effect of acute vitamin C deficiency upon the response of the periodontal tissues of the guinea pig to artificially induced inflammation, J. Dent. Res. **27:**201, 1948.

60. Glickman, I.: Nutrition in the prevention and treatment of gingival and periodontal diseases, J. Dent. Med. **19:**179, 1964.

61. El-Ashiry, G.M., Ringsdorf, W.M., Jr., and Cheraskin, E.: Local and systemic influences in periodontal disease. II. Effect of prophylaxis and natural versus synthetic vitamin C upon gingivitis, J. Periodontol. **35:**250, 1964.

62. Dreizen, S., Levy, B.M., and Bernick, S.: Studies on the biology of the periodontium of marmosets. VII. The effect of vitamin C deficiency on the marmoset periodontium, J. Periodont. Res. **4:**274, 1969.

63. Priest, R.E.: Formation of epithelial basement membrane is restricted by scurvy in vitro and is stimulated by vitamin C, Nature **225:**744, 1970.

64. Ross, R., and Benditt, E.P.: Wound healing in components of guinea pig skin wounds observed in the electron microscope, J. Biophys. Biochem. Cytol. **11:**677, 1961.

65. Ross, R., and Benditt, E.P.: Wound healing and collagen formation. IV. Distortion of ribosomal patterns of fibroblasts in scurvy, J. Cell Biol. **22:**365, 1964.

66. Enwonwu, C.O., and Sreebny, L.M.: Experimental protein-calorie malnutrition in rats: biochemical and ultrastructural studies, Exp. Mol. Pathol. **12:**332, 1970.

67. Enwonwu, C.O., and Sreebny, L.M.: Studies of hepatic lesions in experimental protein-calorie malnutrition in rats and immediate effects of refeeding on an adequate protein diet, J. Nutr. **101:**501, 1971.

68. Gould, B.S.: The role of certain vitamins in collagen formation. In Gould, B.S., editor: Biology of collagen, vol. 2, New York, 1968, Academic Press, Inc.

69. Becks, H., Wainright, W.W., and Morgan, A.F.: Comparative study of oral changes in dogs due to pantothenic acid, nicotinic acid and unknowns of the B vitamin complex, Am. J. Orthod. **29:**183, 1943.

70. Topping, N.N., and Fraser, H.F.: Mouth lesions associated with dietary deficiencies in monkeys, Public Health Rep. **54:**416, 1939.

71. Chapman, O.D., and Harris, A.E.: Oral lesions associated with dietary deficiencies in monkeys, J. Infect. Dis. **69:**7, 1941.

72. O'Brien, J.A.: The role of the folate coenzymes in cellular division: a review, Cancer Res. **22:**267, 1962.

73. Langston, W.C., et al.: Nutritional cytopenia (vitamin M deficiency) in the monkey, J. Exp. Med. **69:**923, 1938.

74. Shaw, J.H.: The relation of nutrition to periodontal disease, J. Dent. Res. **41:**264, 1962.

75. Dreizen, S., Levy, B.M., and Bernick, S.: Studies on the biology of the periodontium of marmosets. VIII. The effect of folic acid deficiency on the marmoset oral mucosa, J. Dent. Res. **49:**616, 1970.

76. Jolly, M.: Vitamin A deficiency: a review. II. J. Oral Ther. **3:**439, 1967.

77. Oliver, W.M.: The effect of deficiencies of calcium, vitamin D or calcium and vitamin D and or variations in the source of dietary protein on the supporting tissues of the rat molar, J. Periodont. Res. **4:**56, 1969.

78. Ferguson, H.W., and Hertles, R.L.: The effect of vitamin D on the dentine of the incisor teeth and on the alveolar bone of young rats maintained on diets deficient in calcium or phosphorus, Arch. Oral Biol. **9:**447, 1964.

79. Ferguson, H.W.: Effect of nutrition on the periodontium. In Melcher, A.H., and Bowen, W.H., editors: Biology of the periodontium, New York, 1969, Academic Press, Inc.

80. Bernick, S., Ershoff, B.H., and Lal, J.B.: Effect of hypervitaminosis D on bones and teeth of rats, Int. J. Nutr. Res. **41:**480, 1971.

81. Harris, R.S.: Macrominerals: calcium, phosphorus, magnesium and calcification; iron and micro elements. In Nizel, A.E., editor: The science of nutrition and its application in clinical dentistry, Philadelphia, 1966, W.B. Saunders Co.

82. Nordin, B.E.C.: Osteomalacia, osteoporosis and calcium deficiency, Clin. Orthop. **17:**235, 1960.

83. Ferguson, H.W., and Hertles, R.L.: The effects of diets deficient in calcium or phosphorus in the presence and absence of supplements of vitamin D on the secondary cementum and alveolar bone of young rats, Arch. Oral Biol. **9:**647, 1964.

84. Ferguson, H.W., and Hertles, R.L.: The effect of diets deficient in calcium or phosphorus in the presence and absence of supplements of vitamin D on the incisor teeth and bone of adult rats, Arch. Oral Biol. **11:**1345, 1966.

85. Henrikson, P.: Periodontal disease and calcium deficiency: An experimental study in the dog, Acta Odontol. Scand. **26**(suppl. 50), 1968.

86. Krook, L., et al.: Bone flow, Rev. Can. Biol. **29:**157, 1970.

87. Krook, L., et al.: Human periodontal disease: Morphology and response to calcium therapy, Cornell Vet. **63:**32, 1972.

88. Krook, L., et al.: Human periodontal disease and osteoporosis, Cornell Vet. **63:**371, 1972.

89. Lesser, G.V., and Krook, L.: Bone physiology and periodontal disease, Ann. Dent. **33:**7, 1974.

90. Krook, L., et al.: Experimental studies on osteoporosis, Methods Achiev. Exp. Pathol. **7:**72, 1976.

91. Thorén, L.: Magnesium deficiency in gastrointestinal fluid loss, Acta Chir. Scand. Suppl. **188:**306, 1963.

92. Flink, E.B., et al.: Evidences for clinical magnesium deficiency, Ann. Intern. Med. **47:**956, 1957.

93. Klein, H., Orent, E.R., and McCollum, E.V.: The effects of magnesium deficiency on the teeth and their supporting structures in rats, Am. J. Physiol. **112:**256, 1935.

94. Caddell, J.L.: Magnesium in the therapy of orofacial lesions of severe protein-calorie malnutrition, Br. J. Surg. **56:**826, 1969.

95. Beveridge, B.T., et al.: Hypochromic anaemia: a retrospective study of follow-up of 378 inpatients, Q.J. Med. **34:**145, 1965.

96. Jacobs, A.: Carbohydrates and sulphur-containing compounds in the anaemic buccal epithelium, J. Clin. Pathol. **14:**610, 1961.

97. Jacobs, A.: Iron-containing enzymes in the buccal epithelium, Lancet **2:**1331, 1961.

98. Sbarra, A.J., et al.: The biochemical and antimicrobial activities of phagocytozing cells, Am. J. Clin. Nutr. **24:**272, 1971.

99. Higashi, O., et al.: Mean cellular peroxidase (MCP) of leukocytes in iron deficiency anemia, Tohoku J. Exp. Med. **93:**105, 1967.

100. Russell, A.L., and White, C.L.: In Muhler, J.C., and Hine, M.K., editors: Fluorine and dental health, London, 1960, Staples Press.

101. Rateitschak-Plüss, E.M., and Guggenheim, B.: Effects of a carbohydrate-free diet and sugar substitutes on dental plaque accumulation, J. Clin. Periodontol. **9:**239, 1982.

102. Sidi, A.D., and Ashley, F.P.: Influence of frequent sugar intakes on experimental gingivitis, J. Periodontol. **55:**419, 1984.

103. Jalil, R.A., Cornick, D.E.R., and Waite, I.M.: Effect of variation in dietary sucrose intake on plaque removal by mechanical means, J. Clin. Periodontol. **10:**389, 1983.

104. Savoff, K., and Rateitschak, K.H.: Influence of eating frequency upon plaque formation and periodontal bone loss, J. Clin. Periodontol. **7:**374, 1980.

105. Mueninghoff, L.A., and Johnson, M.H.: Erosion: a case caused by unusual diet, J. Am. Dent. Assoc. **104:**51, 1982.

106. Wolcott, R.B., Yager, J., and Gordon, G.: Dental sequelae to the binge-purge syndrome (bulimia): report of cases, J. Am. Dent. Assoc. **109:**723, 1984.

107. Enwonwu, C.O.: Nutrition and periodontal disease. In Grant, D.A., Stern, I.B., and Everett, F.G., editors: Orban's periodontics: a concept—theory and practice, ed. 4, St. Louis, 1972, The C.V. Mosby Co.

108. Enwonwu, C.O.: Role of biochemistry and nutrition in preventive dentistry, J. Am. Soc. Prev. Dent. **4:**6, 1974.

109. Ferguson, H.W.: Effect of nutrition on the periodontium. In Melcher, A.H., and Bowen, W.H., editors: Biology of the periodontium, New York, 1969, Academic Press, Inc.

110. Glickman, I.: Nutrition in the prevention and treatment of gingival and periodontal disease, J. Dent. Med. **19:**179, 1964.

111. Stahl, S.S.: Nutritional influences on periodontal disease, World Rev. Nutr. Diet. **13:**277, 1971.

112. DePaola, D.P., and Alfano, M.C.: Diet and oral health, Nutr. Today **12:**6, 1977.

113. Alfano, M.C.: Controversies, perspectives, and clinical implications of nutrition in periodontal disease, Dent. Clin. North Am. **20:**519, 1976.

114. Oliver, R.C.: Critique of workshop on diet, nutrition and periodontal disease. In Hazen, S.P., editor: Diet, nutrition and periodontal disease, Chicago, 1975, American Society for Preventive Dentistry.

115. Stepnick, R.J.: Is nutrition relevant to periodontal disease? J. Am. Soc. Prev. Dent. **5:**16, 1975.

116. Stone, H.: A practical view of the periodontal patient. In Hazen, S.P., editor: Diet, nutrition and periodontal disease, Chicago, 1975, American Society for Preventive Dentistry.

117. Russell: World epidemiology and oral health. In Kreshover, S.J., and McClure, F.S., editors: Environmental variables in oral disease, Washington, 1966, American Association for the Advancement of Science.

118. Russell, A.L., et al.: Periodontal disease and nutrition in South Vietnam, J. Dent. Res. **44:**775, 1965.

119. Waerhaug, J.: Prevalence of periodontal disease in Ceylon, Acta Odontol. Scand. **25:**205, 1967.

120. Parfitt, G.J., and Hand, C.D.: Reduced plasma ascorbic acid levels and gingival health, J. Periodontol. **34:**347, 1963.

121. Ismail, A.I., Burt, B.A., and Eklund, S.A.: Relation between ascorbic acid intake and periodontal disease in the United States, J. Am. Dent. Assoc. **107:**927, 1983.

122. Plough, I.C., and Bridgeforth, E.B.: Relations of clinical and dietary findings in nutrition surveys, Public Health Rep. **75:**699, 1960.

# CHAPTER 14

# Other contributory etiologic factors

**Contributory and modulating influences**
Other predisposing factors
Traumatic factors

## Contributory and modulating influences

Microbiology and host responses in the pathogenesis of inflammatory periodontal diseases have been discussed in detail in previous chapters. Their effect is modulated by other systemic and local factors.[1-10]

Neglected or improper oral hygiene contributes to and modulates the largest percentage of gingivitis and periodontitis[1-4] (Fig. 14-1). Bacteria, calculus, and food debris collected along gingival margins and in sulci combine to provoke the destructive changes that follow. Bacteria and plaque-coated calcified deposits both contribute to periodontitis and tooth loss. They are the prime etiologic factors in inflammatory periodontal disease.[5]

**Oral hygiene and calcified and uncalcified deposits**

Soft or sticky foods that tend to collect on the teeth predispose to bacterial adhesion by providing a substrate for sticky capsule formation.[6,8]

**Composition of diet**

Irregularities of tooth position or inclination, overlapping, malposed, and tilted teeth are conducive to harboring bacteria (Fig. 14-2). In addition, cavities, poorly designed restorations, or defects such as bell-shaped crowns may also become plaque harbors.[9] A significant statistical relationship was found between defects in margins of dental restorations and reduced bone height.[10]

**Tooth position, contour, margins, and food impaction**

The essential components of the periodontal disease process are infection and the response of the host tissues. The infective process includes: (1) the bacterial colonization of the tooth surface, (2) the proliferation of bacteria, (3) the destructive phase involving bacterial metabolites (enzymes, endotoxins, antigenic components, and so on) and the possible bacterial invasion of periodontal tissues, and (4) a host response to the local microbiota.

Nevertheless, the reason why gingivitis in many cases fails to progress to periodontitis is unanswered.

The presence of a pathogen does not necessarily result in disease. Additional factors such as the presence of other organisms, their number, and location, environmental conditions, and host susceptibility influence the pathologic sequelae. Consequently the host may harbor the pathogenic microbiota during quiescent intermittent periods without ill effect because of the absence of one or more additional factors needed to produce disease.

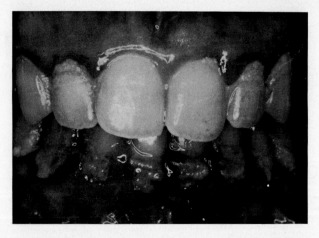

**Fig. 14-1.** Poor oral hygiene and the accumulation of plaque and calcified deposits are evident in a 34-year-old woman.

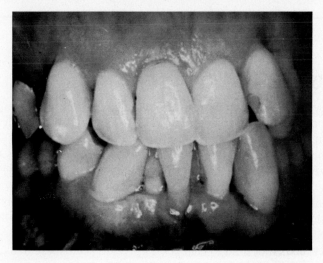

**Fig. 14-2.** Overlapping malposed teeth in a 45-year-old woman encourage plaque retention and food impaction and make good oral hygiene difficult to achieve.

## OTHER PREDISPOSING FACTORS

There are predisposing factors in the etiology of bacterially induced inflammatory periodontal disease. For instance there may be poor patient compliance in matters of plaque removal. When the patient is unwilling or unable to remove plaque on a daily basis, bacterial numbers will increase. If calcified deposits are not removed, bacterial colonization over calculus is rapid.

**Inadequate dental treatment**   Inadequate dental treatment such as overhang or deficient margins, open contact, and improperly designed prostheses can contribute to periodontal disease (Fig. 14-3). There is a direct correlation between surface roughness or marginal irregularities of a tooth and the retention of plaque.

**Orthodontic appliances**   Orthodontic appliances contribute to plaque retention and interfere with the performance of good oral hygiene[11] (Fig. 14-4).

The careless use of home care implements may damage tissues and thus lower host resistance to bacterial insult. Mouth breathing or incomplete lip closure tends to impart a glossy erythematous appearance to the gingiva because of drying.

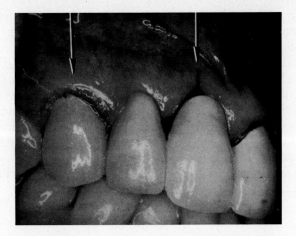

**Fig. 14-3.**   A gingival cleft is present over the right central incisor, and inflammation can be seen over the canine, caused by plaque retention at the crown margins.

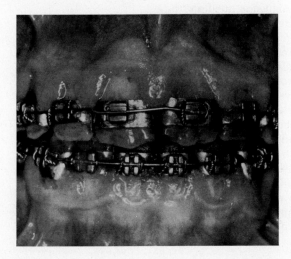

**Fig. 14-4.**   Orthodontic appliances can act as plaque harbors and make proper oral hygiene difficult. An inflammatory hyperplasia is evident.

Anatomic factors that may predispose to disease include aberrations inherent in the form of soft tissues. High frena or muscle attachments can encourage the collection of debris along gingival margins or impede home dental care. Shallow vestibules or narrow inadequate zones of gingiva may also predispose to disease by promoting plaque retention along gingival margins. Thin, finely textured gingiva may be easily injured during mastication or brushing, and recession of gingival margins may follow.    **Anatomy of soft tissues**

Injuries from improper brushing, flossing, and stimulating may produce abrasions of oral mucous membranes. Injurious oral habits, such as biting threads, pipestems, fingernails, or pencils may contribute to breakdown or may alter tooth position (Fig. 14-5). Tongue thrusting may contribute to tooth malposition, open bite, and gingival recession.    **Habits**

## TRAUMATIC FACTORS

Occlusal trauma factors can produce lesions resulting in a widened periodontal ligament and tooth mobility. The trigger is the force of the musculature transmitted by way of tooth-to-tooth contact to the periodontal ligament and the alveolar bone. The    **Anatomy of soft tissues** greatest forces are produced by parafunctional muscular contraction such as in bruxism, clenching, and clamping. The forces exerted in mastication, deglutition, and speech rarely produce traumatic effects.

The periodontium adapts to all these forces but can be damaged when the forces exceed physiologic limits. Naturally in situations in which traumatic factors are coupled with bacterially induced inflammatory factors, the rate of breakdown may be increased. With increasing bone loss and mobility, the tooth may no longer be maintainable. Such teeth are sometimes salvageable by periodontal treatment and splinting or prosthesis, but at other times diminished support, or loading of partial prosthesis can contribute to the pathologic course of the disease.

Following is a summary outline of contributory factors in periodontal disease:

I. Contributing local factors
  A. Plaque retention factors
    1. Calculus
    2. Food impaction and retention
    3. Open and loose contacts
    4. Overhanging margins of restorations
    5. Poorly designed or fitted prostheses
    6. Soft or sticky consistency of diet
    7. Mouth breathing; incomplete lip closure
  B. Anatomic predisposing
    1. Tooth malalignment, malposition, altered anatomy
    2. High frena or muscle attachments
    3. Shallow vestibule
    4. Insufficient gingival width
    5. Thin, finely textured gingiva
    6. Thick, bulbous gingival margins
  C. Tissue trauma
    1. Toothbrush trauma
    2. Injurious habits (toothpicks)
    3. Improper dental treatment methods
    4. Other injury
  D. Functional: periodontal trauma
    1. Muscle hypertonicity
    2. Bruxism

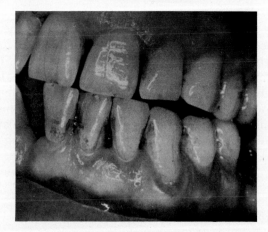

**Fig. 14-5.** Habitual biting on a pipestem has caused an open bite to occur in the canine region. Plaque was found around the necks of the teeth used to grasp the pipestem. This may have been caused by the altered position of the teeth, interfering with oral hygiene methods.

    3. Clenching and clamping
    4. Excessive loads on abutment teeth
    5. Unfavorable crown-root ratio
    6. Plunger cusps
    7. Mobility
    8. Drifting of teeth

II. Contributing host factors
  A. Immunologic defects (including polymorphonuclear cell defects)
    1. Chédiak-Higashi syndrome
    2. Down syndrome
    3. Lazy leukocyte syndrome
    4. Juvenile periodontitis
  B. Endocrine dysfunctions
    1. Pubertal
    2. Pregnancy
    3. Postmenopausal
    4. Hyperthyroidism
    5. Hypothyroidism
    6. Juvenile diabetes
  C. Metabolic, genetically transmitted diseases
    1. Diabetes
    2. Hyperkeratosis palmoplantaris
    3. Hereditary agranulocytosis
    4. Hypophosphatasia
  D. Psychosomatic or emotional disorders
    1. Fatigue
    2. Stress
  E. Drugs and metallic poisons
    1. Phenytoin (Dilantin), etc.
    2. Corticosteroids
    3. Smoking
  F. Nutrition and diet
    1. Hypervitaminosis A and D
    2. Protein-calorie malnutrition
    3. Scurvy

**REFERENCES**

1. Berg, M., Burrill, D.Y., and Fosdick, L.S.: Chemical studies in periodontal disease. IV. Putrefaction rate as an index of periodontal disease. J. Dent. Res. **26:**67, 1947.
2. Bernier, J.L.: The role of inflammation in periodontal disease, Oral Surg. **2:**583, 1949.
3. Löe, H., Theilade, E., and Jensen, S.B.: Experimental gingivitis in man, J. Periodontol. **36:**177, 1965.
4. Ramfjord, S.: Local factors in periodontal disease, J. Am. Dent. Assoc. **44:**647, 1952.
5. Björby, A., and Löe, H.: The relative significance of different local factors in the initiation and development of peridontal inflammation, J. Periodont. Res. **2:**76, 1967.
6. Mitchell, D.F.: The production of periodontal disease in the hamster as related to diet, coprophagy, and maintenance factors, J. Dent. Res. **29:**732, 1950.
7. Sognnaes, R.F.: Experimental production of periodontal disease in animals fed on a purified nutritionally adequate diet, J. Dent. Res. **26:**475, 1947.
8. King, J.D., and Glover, R.E.: The relative effects of dietary constituents and other factors upon calculus and gingival disease in the ferret, J. Pathol. Bacteriol. **57:**353, 1945.
9. Romine, E.R.: Relation of operative and prosthetic dentistry to periodontal disease, J. Am. Dent. Assoc. **44:**742, 1952.
10. Bjorn, A.L., Bjorn, H., and Grcovic, B.: Marginal fit of restorations and its relation to periodontal bone level, Odont. Rev. **20:**311, 1969.
11. Morris, M.L.: Orthodontic-periodontic relationship. In Horowitz, S.L., and Hixon, E.H.: The nature of orthodontic diagnosis, St. Louis, 1966, The C.V. Mosby Co.

**ADDITIONAL SUGGESTED READING**

Baumhammers, A., and Rohrbaugh, E.A.: Permeability of human and rat dental calculus, J. Periodontol. **41:**279, 1970.

Egelberg, J.: Local effect of diet on plaque formation and development of gingivitis in dogs, Odontol. Rev. **16:**50, 1965.

Frostell, G., and Söder, P.: The proteolytic activity of plaque and its relation to soft tissue pathology, Int. Dent. J. **20:**436, 1970.

Newman, M.G.: Current concepts of the pathogenesis of periodontal disease, J. Periodontol. **56:**734, 1985.

Pennel, B.M., and Keagle, J.G.: Predisposing factors in the etiology of chronic inflammatory disease, J. Periodontol. **48:**517, 1977.

Weinmann, J.P.: Periodontitis: etiology, pathology, symptomatology, J. Am. Dent. Assoc. **44:**701, 1952.

# PART THREE

## Periodontal Diseases

# Gingivitis

## Definition

Gingivitis is an inflammation of the gingiva. It fluctuates in intensity and is reversible.[1,2] This disease has characteristics that may be described on clinical,[3-5] microscopic,[3-6] ultrastructural,[7-10] biochemical,[11-19] and physiologic levels.[3,20]

Clinically, gingivitis is recognized by the well-known signs of inflammation: redness, swelling, bleeding, exudation, and less frequently, by pain,[2,3,5] as seen in Plates 4 and 5.

**Clinical signs**

Acute gingivitis has a sudden onset, the affected gingiva may show a dramatic bright red color, and the patient feels pain. Acute gingivitis is most often seen as a result of injury or as acute necrotizing ulcerative gingivitis (Vincent's). Less frequently, it is seen in patients with immunodeficiencies, in those taking immunosuppresive drugs, and in infrequent, diffuse bacterial infections, scurvy, allergic and autoimmune reactions.

**Acute gingivitis**

Gingivitis most often occurs as a chronic or recurrent disease. Chronic gingivitis is a persistent, long-lasting gingival inflammation, which is usually painless.

**Chronic gingivitis**

Tissue destruction and tissue repair take place concurrently or alternately in chronic gingivitis. This interaction of destruction and repair affects the clinical appearance of the gingiva. Thus the gingiva may vary in color from slightly red to a more brilliant red to magenta. The color may be influenced by keratinization of the tissue, vascularity, the amount of fibrous tissue overlying the dilated vessels, and the degree of blood flow through the tissues. The shape of the gingiva may be influenced by alternating episodes of collagen fiber destruction and repair. When much of the collagenous framework has been lost, the gingiva may be soft or boggy in texture. When collagen synthesis during phases of repair produces new fibers—sometimes in excessive amounts (fibrosis)—the gingiva may become very firm with rolled or blunted margins.

**Gingival pocket**

**Pseudopocket**

Gingival margins may become enlarged either by edema or fibrosis. The inflammation can cause enlargement of the gingival margin, resulting in a deepened sulcus without any apical migration of the sulcus bottom. A deepened sulcus with inflammatory changes in the adjacent gingiva is called a *gingival pocket*. When the pocket is the result of gingival enlargement rather than apical displacement of the sulcus bottom, it is called a *pseudopocket*. A *true pocket* is caused by apical displacement of junctional epithelium and the sulcus bottom.

When the gingiva is thin, gingival recession may result from inflammatory changes. Loss of collagen combined with epithelial proliferation and ulceration can destroy the marginal gingiva, resulting in recession, often with little or no probing depth.

The clinical characteristics of gingivitis, which may vary in the same mouth and in different patients, may be described by the following observations:

**Clinical characteristics**

**Extent of Lesion**

Localized
Generalized

**Distribution of Lesions**

Papillary
Marginal
Gingival (entire zone)

**State of Inflammation**

Acute
Chronic

**Clinical Features**

Color
Edematous enlargement
Fibrous enlargement
Recession
Ulceration
Necrosis
Formation of pseudomembranes
Purulent exudation
Serous exudation
Hemorrhage

## Microscopic characteristics

Microscopically, gingivitis is characterized by the following features. Plaque and calcified deposits are found adherent to the tooth surface and in intimate contact with the sulcular epithelium (Fig. 15-1). There is an exudate of inflammatory cells in the gingival lamina propria.[3,21-28] Gingival fibers have been lysed. The junctional and sulcular epithelia have proliferated into the inflamed lamina propria. Leukocytes have migrated from vessels in the lamina propria through the junctional epithelium into the sulcus[22,23,29] (Figs. 15-2, *A* and *B*, and 15-3). The inflamed lamina propria is filled with enlarged blood vessels[3,21,25,30-32] (Fig. 15-4). The blood vessels are surrounded by a perivascular inflammatory infiltrate[3,22] (Figs. 15-2, *A* and *C*, and 15-4).

The changes seen in gingivitis are believed to be tissue responses caused by antigenic and chemotactic factors in bacterial plaque.[29,33-39] Other extrinsic and intrinsic[40-55] factors may affect the resistance and susceptibility of the host and also the character of host response—for example, whether the gingiva is enlarged or receded, edematous or fibrotic.

## Ultrastructural characteristics

**Junctional and sulcular epithelium**

Ultrastructural changes in gingivitis have been described in both the epithelial and connective tissue compartments of the gingiva.[7-10] The intercellular spaces of epithelial cells are widened with some loss of intercellular junctions (Figs. 15-5 and 15-6). The volume of intercellular fluid is increased, and polymorphonuclear (PMN) leukocytes (Fig. 15-7) and, occasionally, lymphocytes (Fig. 15-8) and plasma cells (Fig. 15-9) may enter the widened intercellular spaces.[10,18,22-30]

**Lamina propria**

The following changes are seen to varying degrees in the gingival lamina propria. Perivascular collagen is lysed (Plate 4, 2C, p. 339). The fibroblasts in the area of

*Text continued on p. 324.*

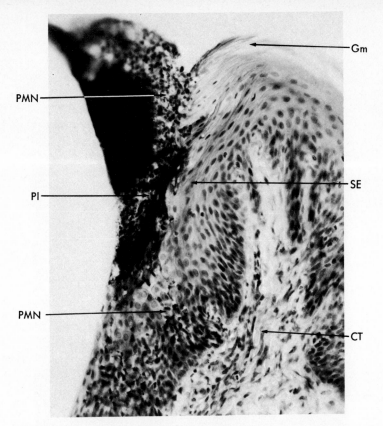

**Fig. 15-1.** Plaque and a neutrophil-filled inflammatory fluid are in intimate contact with the sulcular (pocket) epithelium in this gingivitis in a marmoset. Polymorphonuclear leukocytes are migrating through the junctional epithelium toward the sulcus (pocket). *Pl*, Plaque; *PMN*, polymorphonuclear leukocytes; *SE*, sulcular epithelium; *Gm*, parakeratinized gingival margin; *CT*, connective tissue of gingival lamina propria.

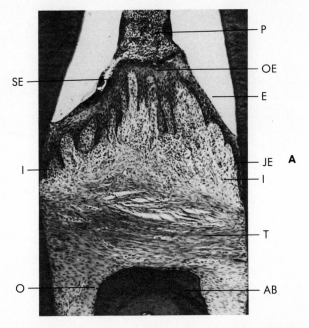

**Fig. 15-2.** **A,** Gingivitis in a marmoset. A shallow pocket ends on enamel and junctional epithelium has proliferated onto cementum. A sparse inflammatory infiltrate, principally of mononuclear cells, like lymphocytes, is congregated adjacent to the junctional and sulcular epithelium and beneath proliferating epithelial rete ridges from oral epithelium at the tip of the papilla. The infiltrate is also formed perivascularly within the transseptal fiber group. The alveolar crest is lined by osteoblasts, showing incremental bone apposition with no evidence of resorption. *P*, plaque; *I*, inflammatory infiltrate; *JE*, junctional epithelium; *OE*, oral epithelium; *SE*, sulcular epithelium; *AB*, alveolar crest; *E*, enamel space; *T*, transseptal fibers; *O*, osteoblasts.

*Continued.*

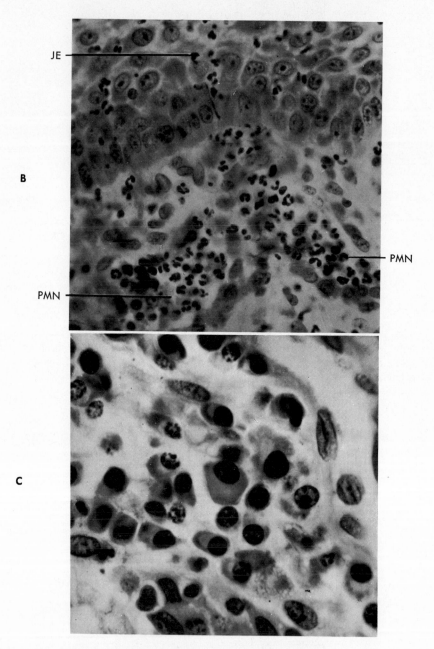

**Fig. 15-2, cont'd.** **B,** High magnification in human specimen showing dilated blood vessels filled with leukocytes *(PMN)*. Some PMNs are migrating through the junctional epithelium *(JE)*. **C,** Plasma cells are congregated perivascularly in chronic gingivitis. Capillaries are thin.

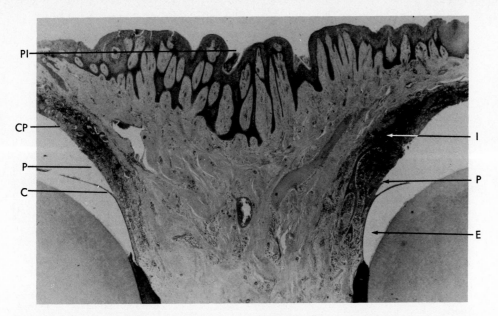

**Fig. 15-3.** Gingivitis in a cross section through two human teeth. The interdental papilla is stippled, and the lamina propria free of inflammatory cells. The inflammation with dense accumulation of plasma cells, lymphocytes, and neutrophils is located in a narrow band of connective tissue on the buccal surface. *E,* Enamel space; *C,* cuticle; *I,* inflammatory infiltrate; *Pl,* stippled interdental papilla. (From the collection of A. Lufkin.)

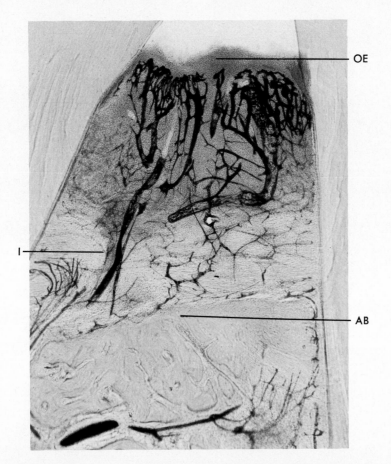

**Fig. 15-4.** Carbon perfusion of blood vessels shows the enlarged character of the vessels in this gingivitis in a spider monkey. The shaded area indicates the extent of inflammation and collagen fiber loss. Note the perivascular location of the infiltrate near bone. *OE,* Epithelial margin of interdental papilla; *AB,* alveolar bone crest; *I,* perivascular course of infiltrate near bone.

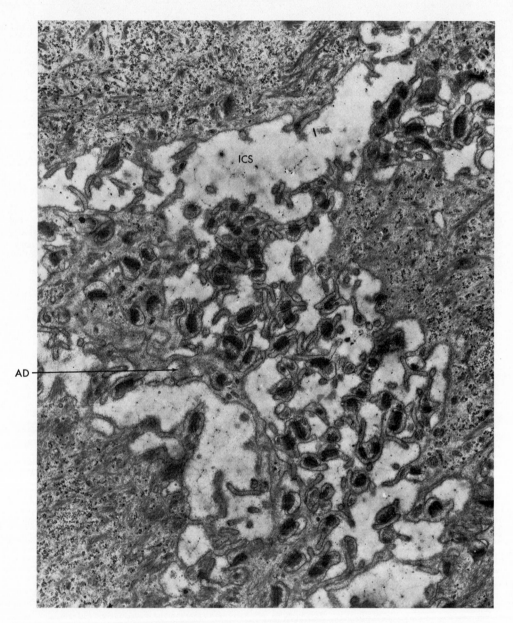

**Fig. 15-5.** Gingivitis. Widened intercellular spaces *(ICS)* with amorphous deposits *(AD)* on both the plasma membrane and intercellularly. (×19,500.) (Courtesy P. Toto, Chicago, Illinois.)

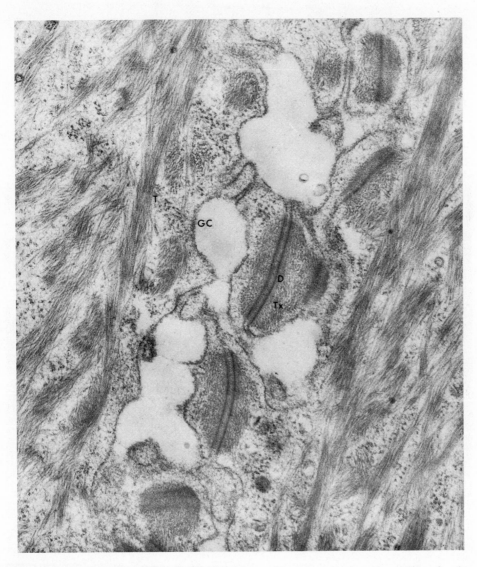

**Fig. 15-6.**   Gingivitis. Higher magnification of intercellular space. The plasma membrane is coated by a fine deposit (glycocalyx, GC). *T* and *Tx,* Tonofilaments; *D,* desmosome.

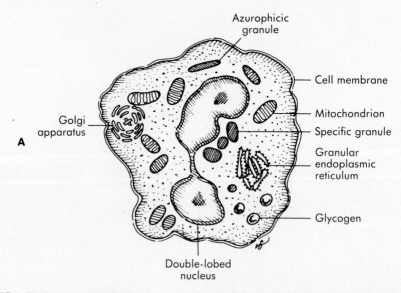

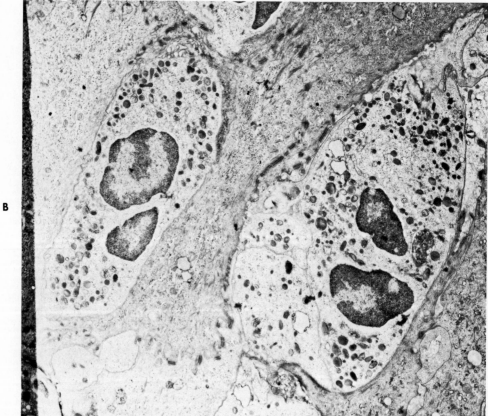

**Fig. 15-7. A,** Neutrophil morphology. **B,** Two polymorphonuclear leukocytes in the epithelium. These cells are recognizable by their multilobed nuclei and lysosomal bodies (granules). The epithelial cells are darker and contain tonofilaments. The granulocytes have no desmosomes and fill the intercellular space.

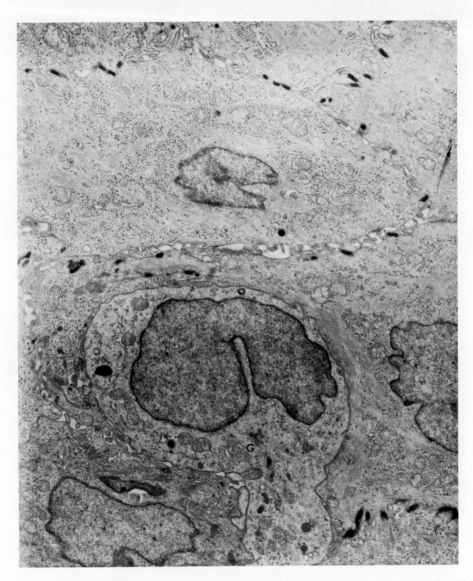

**Fig. 15-8.** Lymphocyte migrating through the epithelium, recognizable by indented nucleus, opposite which is the Golgi apparatus, *G*. There are no tonofilaments surrounding the lymphocytes or desmosomes. The rough-surfaced endoplasmic reticulum is sparse. The epithelial cells have typical desmosomes.

PIC

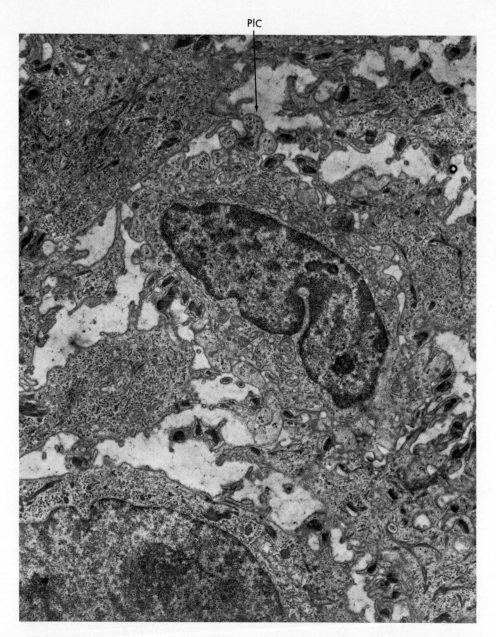

**Fig. 15-9.** Plasma cell *(PIC)* migrating through epithelium. The cell has many protoplasmic processes and a well-developed rough endoplasmic reticulum. The surrounding epithelial cells have typical desmosomes and tonofilaments.

inflammation show degenerative changes,[56-58] which may include significant cytoplasmic swelling. Their endoplasmic reticulum is reduced, and the cisternae may be enlarged. The mitochondria frequently exhibit loss of cristae. The plasma membrane may be ruptured. These cytopathic changes appear to be associated with lymphocytic activity, since the altered fibroblasts are often seen in intimate contact with lymphocytes[57,58] In the incipient stage of developing gingivitis, the loss of perivascular collagen is more easily discerned in electron micrographs.[8,9] Lymphocytes (see Fig. 15-8) and plasma cells[8] are found in areas of collagen destruction and appear in chronologic sequences indicative of the stage of inflammation.[59] Mast cells, PMN

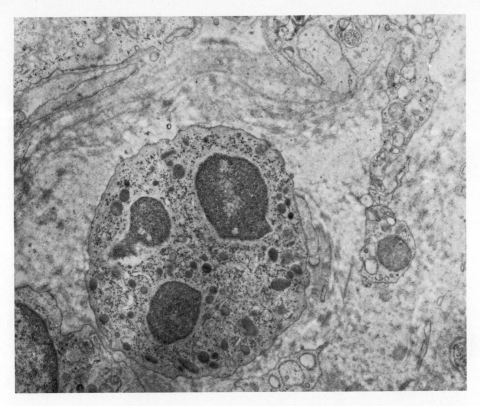

**Fig. 15-10.**   Granulocyte in gingival lamina propria.

leukocytes, and macrophages (Figs. 15-10 and 15-11) are frequently found.

Bone resorption at the crest is not characteristic of gingivitis; however, fibrosis of the endosseous marrow spaces may take place and may occur early in the sequential development of the lesions. A fatty endosseous marrow is characteristic of alveolar bone (in health) in adults. Conversion of the fatty marrow to a fibrous marrow is seen in inflammation and may be a sequela of disease.

**Microscopic features in bone**

## Biochemical and physiologic characteristics

The widened intercellular spaces in the junctional epithelium (see Figs. 15-5 and 15-6) are probably related to the increased fluid content and may be accompanied by a disaggregation of mucopolysaccharide both between epithelial cells and in the basement membrane. These events in turn may be related to the increased motility of epithelial cells that migrate into areas of collagen destruction as proliferating epithelial rete strands.

The widened intercellular spaces in the junctional epithelium are associated with more extensive leukocytic migration and exudation, as demonstrated by the increased quantity of sulcular fluid and numbers of crevicular leukocytes. PMN leukocytes contain lysosomes which produce digestive enzymes such as collagenase[60] and carbohydrases.[61] Degranulating PMN leukocytes may release these enzymes as well as other proteolytic enzymes into the tissues where they can contribute to further tissue damage.[7]

Peripheral blood lymphocytes from patients with inflammatory periodontal disease have been shown to be sensitized to antigenic substances in human dental plaque.

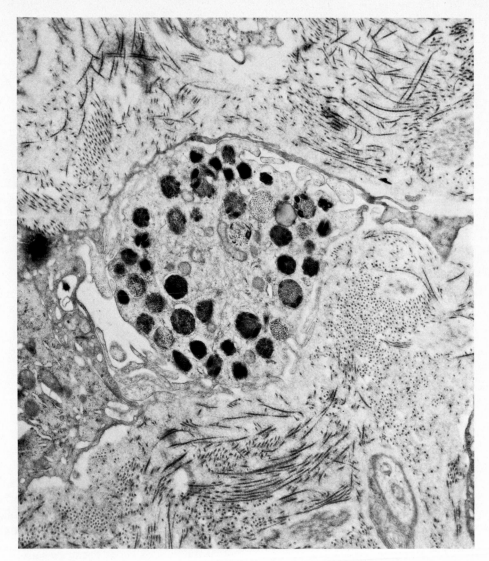

**Fig. 15-11.** *Mast cell in gingival lamina propria.*

These cells undergo blast transformation when cultured in vitro with plaque antigens. Fluids from such cultures have a cytotoxic effect on gingival fibroblasts.[62-64] Thus a relationship is suggested between these in vitro events and those seen in vivo in the early stages of gingivitis.

The loss of collagen fibers and their replacement by a fluid and cellular infiltrate and the proliferation of blood vessels contribute to redness of the gingiva,[65] blunting of its margins, gingival enlargement, and easy retractibility of the gingival tissue.

## Development

**Experimental gingivitis**

The development of gingivitis in individuals with healthy gingiva is best seen in experimental situations.[2,31,66] When carefully controlled experiments are made to create gingivitis, a sequential series of changes occurs that parallels the classic events seen in inflammation. Some of these events are not discernible morphologically, since the earliest happenings in the hemodynamics of inflammation are not readily seen in fixed

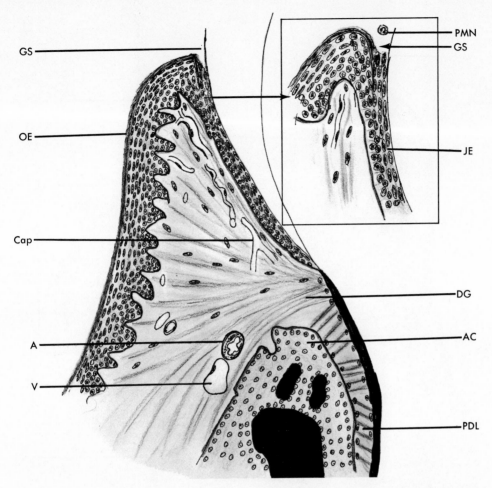

**Fig. 15-12.** *Schema of the healthy marginal gingiva in an orofacial section of a tooth. Inset illustrates the shallow gingival sulcus near the gingival margin. A single polymorphonuclear leukocyte has migrated into the sulcus. GS, Gingival sulcus; JE, junctional epithelium; PMN, polymorphonuclear leukocyte; OE, oral epithelium; Cap, capillary; V, venule; A, arteriole; DG, dentogingival and dentoperiosteal fibers; AC, alveolar crest; PDL, periodontal ligament.*

microscopic specimens. Other events, such as the margination (pavementing) of leukocytes in the subepithelial vascular plexus, occur later in the hemodynamic sequence but are seen as an early change in the microscopic sequence.

Although the changes from health to inflammation are an interrelated, rapidly changing series of events, they may be arbitrarily divided into a healthy stage[67] (Fig. 15-12) and three stages of disease. These stages have been described as the (1) *initial*, (2) *early*, and (3) *established* lesions of inflammatory periodontal disease.[68] It should be noted that while the chronologic development of an experimentally induced gingivitis may well be progressive and follow the above nomenclature, the episodic nature of naturally occurring gingivitis results in the *development* as well as the *reversal* of these stages. In addition, lesions in any stage of development may remain relatively stable for an indeterminate length of time. Therefore use of the above terminology to describe the inflammatory lesions must take into account the complex dynamics of gingivitis. The characteristic features of health (Fig. 15-12) and of initial, early, and established lesions of gingivitis are illustrated in Figs. 15-13 to 15-15.

**Stages**

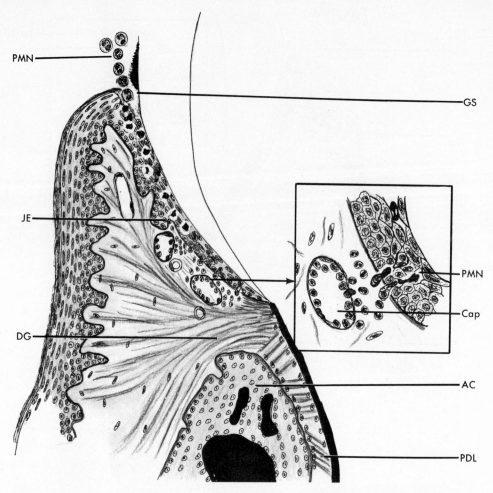

**Fig. 15-13.** Schema of the initial lesion in gingivitis the lesion is localized subjacent to the junctional epithelium. Inset illustrates margination and diapedesis of polymorphonuclear leukocytes in venules subjacent to the junctional epithelium. Leukocytes are migrating from the vessels and entering the widened intercellular spaces of the junctional epithelium. *GS*, Gingival sulcus; *PMN*, polymorphonuclear leukocytes; *JE*, junctional eipthelium; *Cap*, capillary; *AC*, alveolar crest; *PDL*, periodontal ligament; *DG*, dentogingival and dentoperiosteal fibers.

## HEALTHY GINGIVA

When one examines disease-free gingiva histologically[10,67] (see Fig. 15-11), a small number of PMN leukocytes, a few macrophages, and blast-transforming lymphocytes may be seen in the junctional epithelium and in the lamina propria.[68] The perivascular collagen may be intact or a small portion may be lysed, with the space becoming occupied by fluid serum proteins (especially fibrin) and the inflammatory cells.

**Development of gingivitis**

Immunoglobulins, especially IgG and complement, are probably present in the extravascular tissues[69-72] in response to the bacterial flora on the tooth or in the sulcus.[22,68] Chemotactic and antigenic properties of the bacteria or their products are probably responsible for the round cell and immunoglobulin presence.[22,39] The round cells may be regarded as resident defense cells. With an increase in bacterial population, a significant increase in the levels of leukocyte migration and fluid exudation occurs by the second day in experimental gingivitis in dogs. The quantity of sulcular fluid appears to vary with the size of the reaction site in connective tissue.[30]

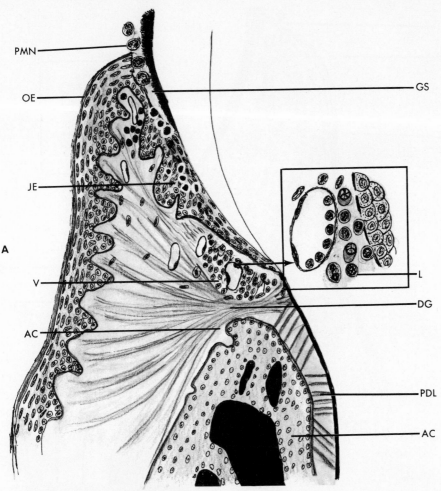

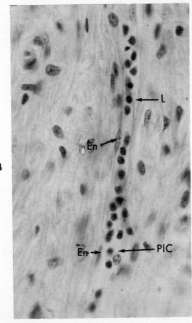

**Fig. 15-14.** **A,** Schema of the early lesion. An enlarged area of collagen destruction is present subjacent to the junctional epithelium. An increased flow of gingival fluid with polymorphonuclear leukocytes is exiting from the gingival sulcus. *Inset,* Margination of leukocytes in a vessel close to the junctional epithelium. The inflammatory infiltrate consists principally of lymphocytes *(L)* with lesser numbers of PMNs and few plasma cells. *PMN,* Polymorphonuclear leukocytes; *GS,* gingival sulcus; *OE,* oral epithelium; *DG,* dentogingival and dentoperiosteal fibers; *V,* blood vessel; *JE,* junctional epithelium; *PDL,* periodontal ligament; *AC,* alveolar crest. **B,** Lymphatic vessel located lateral to an infiltrate. There is an accumulation of lymphocytes and plasma cells within the lumen of this vessel. *En,* Endothelial cell; *L,* lymphocytes; *PIC,* plasma cells. (Iron hematoxylin; × 250.) (**B** from Bernick, S., and Grant, D.A.: J. Dent. Res. **57:**810, 1978.)

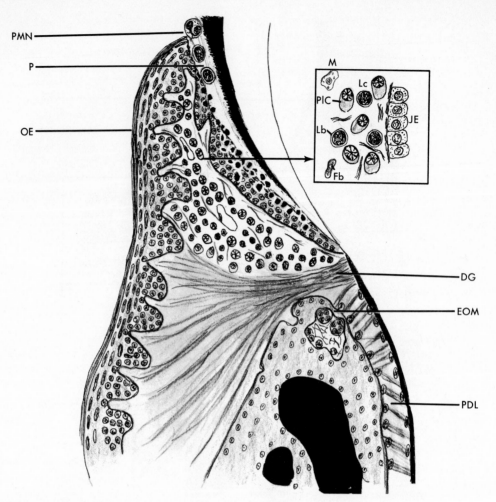

**Fig. 15-15.** Schema of the established lesion (chronic gingivitis). The area of collagen destruction is enlarged, with few remnants of collagen fibers remaining in the area of inflammation. Plasma cells predominate, with fewer lymphocytes undergoing blast transformation. Neutrophils (PMNs) are migrating through the junctional epithelium into a developing pocket, where plaque and calculus are present. A marrow space at the alveolar crest is now fibrotic, and osteoclasts are destroying bone. *Inset,* Some cells of the inflammatory infiltrate next to the junctional epithelium; *PMN,* polymorphonuclear leukocyte; *PIC,* plasma cell; *Lb,* lymphoblast; *Lc,* lymphocyte; *M,* macrophage; *Fb,* fibroblasts; *OE,* oral epithelium; *P,* pocket; *JE,* junctional epithelium; *DG,* dentogingival and dentoperiosteal fibers; *EOM,* fibrous endosseous marrow space with osteoclasts in alveolar bone; *PDL,* periodontal ligament.

## INITIAL LESION

Within 2 to 4 days after cessation of oral hygiene, the earliest changes in experimental gingivitis are visible in microscopic specimens. These consist of a margination of leukocytes in vessels close to the junctional epithelium. Some destruction of perivascular collagen accompanies the emigration of leukocytes. Sloughed epithelial cells and bacteria are found in the gingival sulcus. There is little or no proliferation of junctional epithelium laterally (rete pegs). Thus, the change from the clinically normal to the inflamed gingiva is gradual (see Fig. 15-13 and Plate 4, *1A*).

## EARLY LESION

The initial lesion may be transitory and may be quickly repaired after removal of plaque. However if bacterial plaque is permitted to accumulate and remain in contact with the marginal gingiva, further changes take place that accentuate the lesion (see Fig. 15-14, *A,* and Plate 4, *2A*). The area of collagen destruction becomes larger and is occupied by fluid that contains serum proteins; fibrin; immunoglobulins,[69] especially IgG; complement; and inflamatory cells, principally lymphocytes. Fibroblasts near the inflamed area show cytopathic alterations.

In early inflammation, distended lymphatic vessels are demonstrable. These vessels have structural characteristics typical of lymphatic vessels; thin walls, irregular shapes, valves, and lymphocytes and plasma cells within their lumina[73] (see Fig. 15-14, *B*). **Lymphatics**

The dilated lymph vessels provide a drainage system for the continuous removal of interstitial materials (excessive fluid, proteins, cells, debris, and other particulates) from the site of inflammation. This mechanism probably assists healing and may help to confine the inflammatory process to the gingiva. In more intensive inflammation, lymph vessels are difficult to demonstrate and may be collapsed.[73]

## ESTABLISHED LESION

In chronic gingivitis (see Fig. 15-15) the cytologic characteristics of the inflammatory infiltrate in the gingival lamina propria are changed. In the early stage, lymphocytes were the predominant cell; now, plasma cells predominate. They are seen close to the junctional and sulcular epithelium and either perivascularly in localized areas or throughout the lamina propria. The plasma cells, some of which are degenerating,[7,74] may be seen in large numbers in areas of collagen destruction, or alternatively the areas may be occupied by a fluid exudate with a few cells. IgG is produced by most of the plasma cells, with a few cells present containing IgA. IgM-containing cells are rarely seen.

Significant levels of immunoglobulins are found in both epithelial and connective tissue compartments.[69,75,76] Although severe periodontal disease has been reported in individuals suffering abnormalities in neutrophil function or neutropenia,[75] increased or more severe periodontal disease has not been reported in young persons in which other immune functions are compromised, such as T- and B-cell deficient states.[47] This latter observation is equivocal, since some of the same individuals in the study were receiving antibiotics and were of an age group (6 years) in which severe periodontal disease is seen infrequently. **Immunoglobulins**

Migrating leukocytes are found in the junctional epithelium, within widened intercellular spaces. Bacteria, shed epithelial cells, calcified deposits, and leukocytes are seen in the pocket and at the gingival margin. The oral gingival epithelium may show increased keratinization with mild inflammation. Keratinization may disappear with increasing severity of the inflammation.[77] Proliferating epithelial rete ridges are seen in areas of collagen destruction; junctional epithelium may begin to migrate apically onto cementum. Bleeding may be provoked at the gingival margin and within the diseased sulcus (pocket). **Epithelial changes**

*True pocket* formation may begin at this stage of gingivitis. It is charactized by the appearance of *pocket epithelium* lining the deepened sulcus.[78] Pocket epithelium is most likely derived from junctional epithelium, which is heavily infiltrated with inflammatory cells and may be easily split. This epithelial lining may become extremely thin and may exhibit microulcerations. Epithelial proliferation produces finger-like projections extending into the fiber-poor, cell-rich, or cell-poor connective tissue subjacent to the pocket. Pocket epithelium is typically located between the sulcular epithelium close to the marginal gingiva and the junctional epithelium, which gradually migrates apically.

Antigens of bacterial plaque may penetrate epithelium of inflamed gingiva and sensitize immune effector cells. Tissue damage in gingivitis and in periodontitis could therefore be the result of responses of sensitized immune effector cells to bacterial **Lymphocyte blastogenic response** antigens. Using blastogeneses of peripheral lymphocytes as an in vitro correlate of cell-mediated immunity, it has been demonstrated that lymphocytes of individuals with inflammatory periodontal disease are reactive to microbial dental plaque.[79-84] This lymphocyte blastogenic response is also found in naturally occurring gingivitis. Its magnitude is directly related to the severity of gingival inflammation and diminishes with improvement in gingival health.[85]

**Vascular events**

Extensive vascular proliferation may occur. Vessels become enlarged and vascular loops (varicosities) develop in connective tissue papillae[86] (see Figs. 15-3 and 15-4). An inflammatory infiltrate is congregated around vascular channels[86,87] (see Fig. 15-13 and Plate 4, 2C). Complement and antigen-antibody complexes may be present around blood vessels.[34]

This chronic stage of gingivitis (see Fig. 15-15 and Plates 4 to 6) may persist for years in some humans and animals, with reparative phenomena counterbalancing the destructive potential of the inflammation.[87-91] In others, bone destruction may take place at the crest, signaling the onset of periodontitis.[92]

## Contributory pathogenetic factors

### EXTRINSIC FACTORS

Plaque-induced effector mechanisms play a major role in the pathogenesis of gingivitis. Cellular and humoral pathways have been implicated in periodontal inflammation, but other extrinsic and intrinsic factors may combine with the bacterial and immunologic factors to influence the clinical and microscopic character of the host response. Extrinsic factors frequently seen are tissue injury (trauma) and mouth breathing or incomplete lip closure.

Injury to the gingiva, such as that from a toothbrush, toothpick, or hard food, may provoke infection from the ever-present oral flora, with accompanying redness and swelling.[93] This injury may be a transient event that heals readily. When the injury is repeated or persistent, such as when the incisal edges of mandibular incisors traumatize the palatal marginal gingiva or maxillary gingiva, the injury and resultant inflammation may persist, resulting in a swollen, inflamed gingiva (Fig. 15-16).

**Mouth breathing and incomplete lip closure**

Enlarged gingival margins that are red, shiny, and erythematous are often found in mouth breathers and those with incomplete lip closure.[94] The affected area frequently is clearly demarcated and follows the lip outline bordering the gingiva when the mouth is open or lips incompletely closed (Fig. 15-17). Treatment should include not only effective regular removal of plaque by the patient but measures to cope with the mouth breathing.

### SYSTEMIC FACTORS

The inflammatory response may be conditioned by systemic factors such as disease affecting host immune response,[95] hormonal changes in puberty and pregnancy,[96-100] hormonal contraceptives,[101-104] nutritional deficiencies,[105-106] diabetes mellitus,[107,108] allergy,[109] and metal poisoning.

**Puberty**

A notable statistical increase in the incidence and in the severity of gingivitis occurs at about the time of puberty. Altered sex hormone levels may explain the exaggerated inflammatory and proliferative response sometimes seen clinically (Fig. 15-18). However gingivitis in puberty responds readily to measures of plaque and calculus removal, with a consequent reduction in redness and swelling.

**Oral contraceptives**

The effect of oral contraceptives on the incidence of gingivitis is controversial. Some studies report no differences in gingivitis levels with use of hormonal contraceptives, whereas another study reports periodontal destruction in women taking hormonal contraceptives for more than 18 months.[101-104]

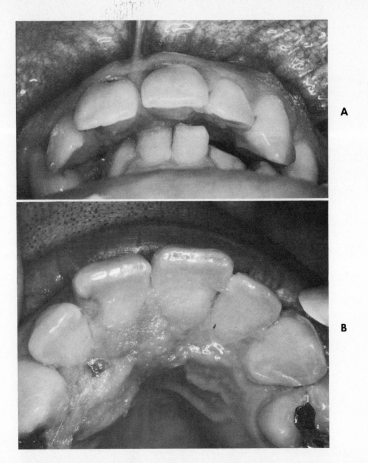

**Fig. 15-16.** **A,** The interdental papilla between the maxillary central incisors is swollen, edematous, and ulcerated at the tip. The lesion resulted from a direct traumatic injury caused by mandibular incisors in a deep overbite (traumatic gingivitis). **B,** Oral view of the maxillary incisors. The interdental papilla is swollen and the tip necrotic because of direct traumatic injury by the mandibular incisors (deep overbite).

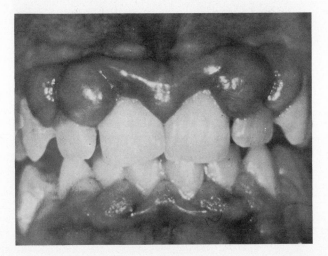

**Fig. 15-17.** Hyperplastic gingivitis in an adolescent girl. Mouth breathing and poor hygiene aggravated the condition. The lip line is clearly indicated by the outline of the hyperplastic tissue.

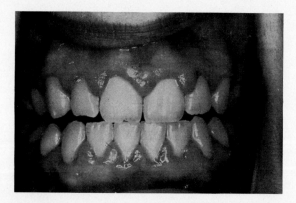

**Fig. 15-18.** Chronic, marginal, papillary hyperplastic gingivitis in a 15-year-old girl.

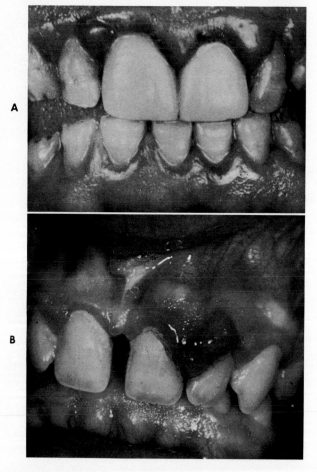

**Fig. 15-19. A,** Gingivitis in a pregnant woman. Papillae are enlarged and prominent, and gingival margins irregular and fringed. **B,** Epulis-like enlargement of the gingiva in a pregnant woman (pregnancy tumor).

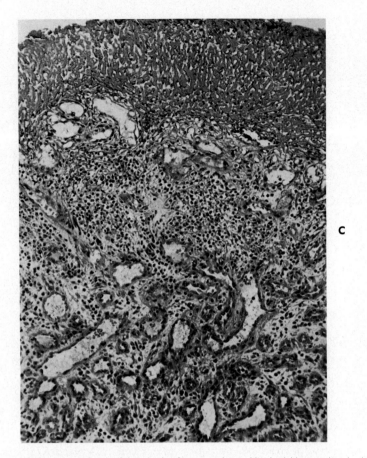

C

**Fig. 15-19, cont'd.   C,** Biopsy specimen of the gingiva from a patient with gingivitis associated with pregnancy. The microscopic picture resembles that of a pyogenic granuloma.

The severity of gingivitis is increased in pregnancy from the first trimester until parturition.[97-100] About half of all pregnant women show such increased severity of inflammation. The proliferation of connective tissue elements, particularly endothelium, leads to hyperplastic changes in the gingival margins and papillae (Fig. 15-19, *A*). Tumorlike enlargements of the gingiva are frequently seen (Fig. 15-19, *B*). Histologically, such tumors are indistinguishable from pyogenic granulomas (Fig. 15-19, *C*). Pregnancy tumors and the increased severity of gingivitis tend to regress after parturition but may recur in subsequent pregnancies. **Pregnancy**

Nutritional deficiencies manifesting themselves in periodontal tissues are rare in industrialized nations[105,106] but are more frequently found in developing countries, where starvation is sometimes endemic. **Nutritional deficiencies**

Scorbutic gingivitis[105] was once common but now occurs infrequently except in areas of famine, during warfare, and rarely because of dietary habits. Symptoms include hemorrhage in joints, muscles, and skin and difficulty in walking. The gingiva is bright red with a generalized marginal and papillary gingivitis. The gingival margins may be hyperplastic, ulcerated, and hemorrhagic (Fig. 15-20). **Scorbutic gingivitis**

Microscopically a highly edematous, acutely inflamed gingiva is seen with ulcerations in the pocket walls. The blood vessels are dilated, and microscopic hemorrhages are evident throughout the gingiva (Fig. 15-20, *C*). At higher magnification, many macrophages filled with hemosiderin crystals may be seen. The disappearance of collagen fibers from the gingival lamina propria (Fig. 15-20, *C*) is not unique to scurvy

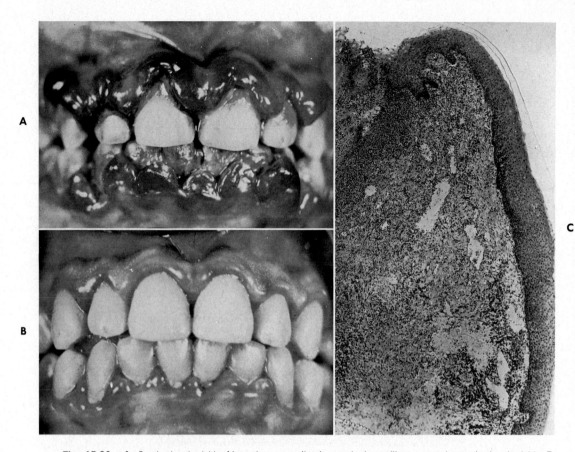

**Fig. 15-20. A,** Scorbutic gingivitis. Note the generalized, marginal, papillary, acute hyperplastic gingivitis. **B,** Improvement, without débridement, after 3 months of vitamin C therapy, is evident. A marginal gingivitis, still present as a result of plaque irritation, requires additional treatment. **C,** Biopsy specimen, prior to treatment, of gingiva in the patient with scorbutus (scurvy) shown in **A.** There was acutely inflamed, edematous tissue with almost complete disappearance of collagen fibers. With appropriate stains, hemosiderin crystals could be seen.

but may be observed in many severely inflamed gingival biopsies.[92] With appropriate treatment, which may include mechanical débridement as well as dietary supplementation, organized collagen fiber bundles will reappear (Fig. 15-20, *D* and *E*).

Therapy of 1500 mg ascorbic acid daily for a week, reduced to 500 mg daily for 4 weeks, then 300 mg daily for a month, and 100 mg daily thereafter can resolve the scorbutic symptoms. Plaque-induced inflammation may persist, however, if calculus remains and plaque control is inadequate.

## Correlation of clinical and microscopic characteristics

The clinical and microscopic tissue changes in gingivitis may be viewed as a spectrum beginning with the earliest deviation from healthy gingiva, which may be seen only on careful examination, to extensive inflammatory changes that are easily discerned. The rate of development of the inflammatory reaction, its intensity, and other characteristics depend on the quantity as well as the quality (composition) of the microbiota, the host response, and the anatomy of the periodontal tissues (e.g., if the tissues are thick or thin). These factors may vary considerably from subject to subject. A construction of sequential changes may be seen on Plate 4.

**Incipient gingivitis**

The first clinical sign may be a change in color from coral pink to light red. A slight blunting or edema of the interdental papilla may be seen (Plate 4, *1A*). Microscopically

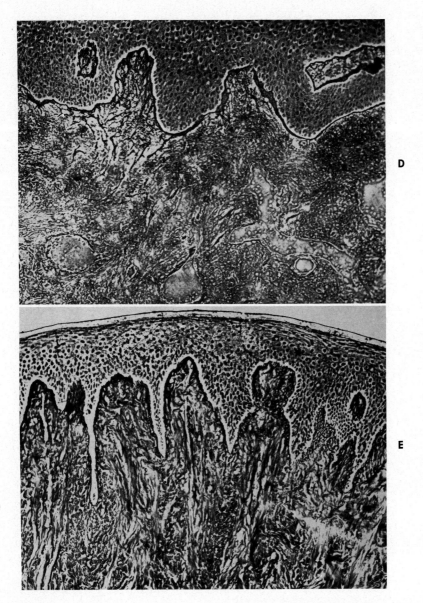

**Fig. 15-20, cont'd.** Biopsy specimens of gingiva of the patient with scrobutus shown in **A** (prior to treatment) and **B** (following treatment). (Silver stain.) **D,** After 3 months of vitamin C therapy, regeneration of collagen fibers has occurred. **E,** The collagen fibers are replaced by a fine, argyrophilic network of fibrils.

this may be correlated with the presence of a sparse inflammatory infiltrate close to the junctional epithelium (*1B*) and migration of PMN leukocytes into the surrounding connective tissue and then through the junctional and sulcular epithelia (*1C*) into the sulcus (*1D*). This initial stage may be immediately succeeded by the next stage, in which the gingiva may be slightly redder or more edematous (Plate 4, *2A*). Microscopically a sparse round cell infiltrate, consisting of lymphocytes and other mononuclear cells, is found congregated close to the junctional and sulcular epithelium. Coronally, plaque and calculus are in contact with the gingival margin and pocket (sulcular) epithelium, and leukocytes have migrated into the pocket toward the plaque (*2B*). Apically, some lysis of dentogingival fibers has taken place, and a pathologic alteration of fibro-

*Text continued on p. 342.*

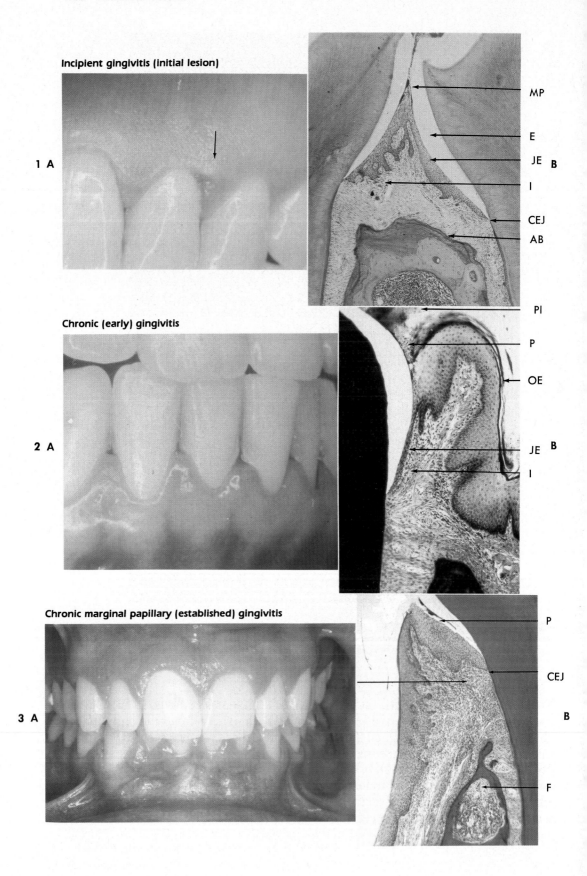

### Incipient gingivitis (initial lesion)

1 A

MP
E
JE  B
I
CEJ
AB

### Chronic (early) gingivitis

2 A

PI
P
OE
JE  B
I

### Chronic marginal papillary (established) gingivitis

3 A

P
CEJ
B
F

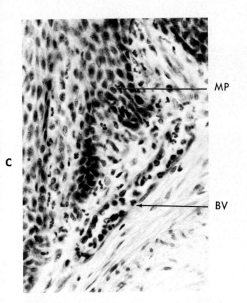

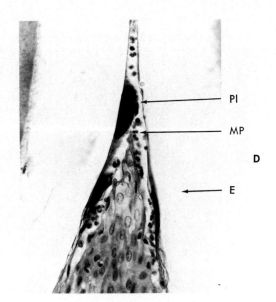

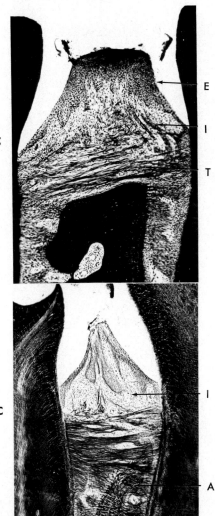

**Plate 4.** *AB,* Alveolar bone; *CEJ,* cementoenamel junction; *E,* enamel space; *I,* inflammatory infiltrate; *JE,* junctional epithelium; *MP,* migrating PMN; *P,* pocket; *BP,* bottom of pocket; *PI,* plaque; *F,* fibrous tissue in endosseous marrow space; *T,* transseptal fibers; *B,* red blood cells and leukocytes on ulcerated surface of pocket epithelium; *BV,* dilated blood vessels filled with leukocytes; *PIC,* plasma cells. **1A,** Incipient gingivitis. Arrow indicates reddened edematous marginal papillary gingivae. **1B,** Incipient gingivitis in a marmoset. Plaque is found astride the tip of the interdental papilla. A sparse inflammatory infiltrate is subjacent to the junctional epithelium. Lateral to this the gingival fibers are intact. Bone is not resorbed. Endosseous marrow spaces are filled with hematopoietic marrow. **1C,** High magnification of area subjacent to the junctional epithelium. PMNs are clustered along the vessel wall (pavementing), migrating from the vessel toward and into the junctional epithelium. **1D,** PMNs migrating from oral epithelium toward plaque found in sulcus and interdentally. **2A,** Chronic (developing) gingivitis (early lesion). Papillae are enlarged and edematous. Marginal and papillary gingivae are reddened. **2B,** Chronic (developing) gingivitis (early lesion) in a marmoset. The area of collagen destruction is larger than in **1A.** The inflammatory infiltrate is both cellular and fluid in character. Proliferation of junctional and sulcular epithelium laterally has taken place. The alveolar crest is intact, **2C,** Chronic (developing) gingivitis (early lesion) in a marmoset. Dentogingival fibers have been lysed and replaced by an inflammatory infiltrate. Epithelial rete pegs have proliferated into the inflamed lamina propria. Transseptal fibers demarcate the inflammatory infiltrate superiorly. Alveolar bone is rounded, without resorption. **3A,** Chronic marginal papillary gingivitis. Gingival margins and papillae are enlarged and edematous. **3B,** Chronic gingivitis (established lesion) in a marmoset. Papilla is enlarged and filled with a cellular inflammatory infiltrate. The junctional epithelium ends at the cementoenamel junction. Alveolar bone shows no resorption at the crest. Endosteal bone resorption has occurred near the crest. The coronal third of one marrow space contains fibrous tissue. **3C,** Marmoset. A slight proliferation of junctional epithelium onto cementum has occurred. The area of collagen loss, filled with an inflammatory infiltrate, a few remnants of dentogingival fibers, and proliferating rete ridges, is demarcated by transseptal fibers. Sharpey's fibers can be seen in the intact alveolar crest.

**Chronic marginal (established) papillary gingivitis**

4 A

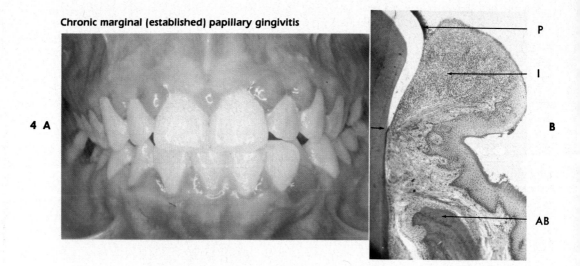

**Chronic marginal (established) papillary gingivitis**

5 A

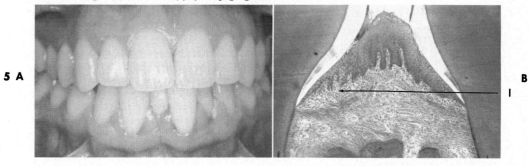

**Bleeding on probing in gingivitis**

6 A

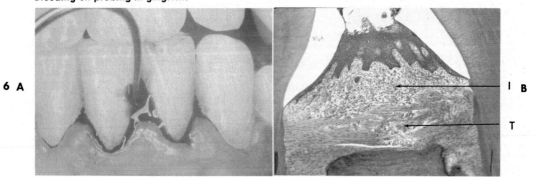

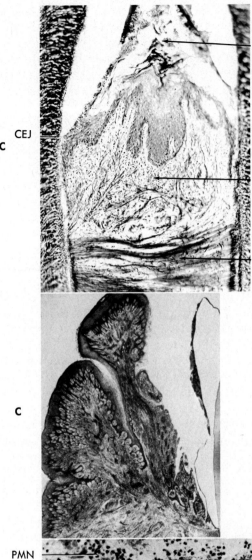

PI

CEJ

C

I

T

**Plate 5.** **4A,** Chronic marginal, papillary gingivitis. Grossly enlarged papillae and blunted gingival margins can be seen. **4B,** Marmoset. A dense cellular inflammatory infiltrate fills the coronal two thirds of the enlarged marginal gingiva. Plaque fills the shallow pocket. The junctional epithelium ends at the cementoenamel junction. No bone destruction has taken place at the crest. **4C,** The papilla and shallow pockets are covered by plaque. Epithelial rete ridges have proliferated into the inflamed lamina propria filled with round cells and collagen fiber fragments. The inflammation is bounded inferiorly by transseptal fibers. **5A,** Chronic papillary, marginal gingivitis. Mandibular papillae are fibrous and enlarged. **5B,** Marmoset. Hyperplastic oral sulcular and junctional epithelia contain an inflammatory infiltrate bounded by dense collagen fibers. The junctional epithelium ends at the cementoenamel junction. **5C,** Histologic section of hyperplastic gingivitis with epithelial and connective tissue proliferation. **6A,** Bleeding is easily provoked or may be spontaneous in gingivitis. **6B,** Epithelial cells are shed from the tip of the papilla. Proliferating rete ridges invade the inflamed lamina propria. The inflammatory infiltrate is bounded by transseptal fibers. The alveolar crest is intact. **6C,** Biopsy specimen of gingival pocket. In the connective tissue, close to the surface, dilated blood vessels, *BV,* filled with leukocytes are prominent. In the deeper layer, plasma cells, *PIC,* are numerous. The leukocytes migrate through pocket epithelium, *EP,* to the surface, which is covered by red blood cells and leukocytes, *PMN.* (**5C** from the collection of B. Gottlieb; color courtesy The John Butler Toothbrush Co., Chicago, Illinois.)

C

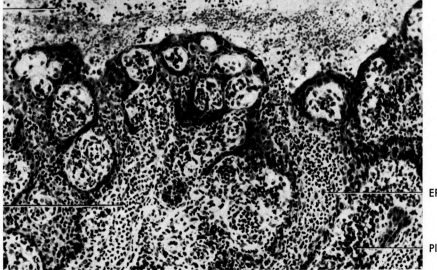

PMN

C

BV

EP

PIC

blasts has occurred, but the inflammatory infiltrate is contained by intact transseptal fibers. No bone destruction has occurred at the crest (2C). Microscopically an incipient gingivitis is likely to exhibit features typically observed in the initial or early lesion.

**Developing gingivitis**

As the intensity of the gingivitis progresses further, the color change may be intense, becoming brighter red or magenta. The lesions may be generalized or localized (Plate 4, 3A). The gingival margins may be blunted, receded, hyperplastic, or edematous. Bleeding may be easily elicited (see Plate 5, 6A). Microscopically this progression can be correlated with an increased inflammatory infiltrate, at first consisting mostly of lymphocytes (early lesion, 3B), but with time predominantly consisting of plasma cells (established lesion), with a slight increase in pocket depth (3B), the presence of pus or hemorrhage, and sometimes a slight apical proliferation of junctional epithelium (3C). Fibroplasia may be seen bordering the inflamed area. However the bottom of the pocket remains on enamel, and there is no bone loss at the alveolar crest (3C). This lesion is widespread in some humans and animals and may persist at this stage for years. In other animals and humans, the disease may progress in severity quite rapidly.

**Chronic gingivitis**

With increasing severity and with time, the gingiva may appear redder or magenta in color. Gingival margins may become enlarged by edema or fibrosis or a combination of these (Plate 5, 4A). Microscopically one may see extensive collagenolysis in the gingival lamina propria with an extensive inflammatory infiltrate sometimes appearing like an abscess (4B) and laterally with plasma cells and lymphocytes in the area of fiber

**Hyperplastic gingivitis**

loss (4C); clinically, the gingiva may be enlarged (Plate 5, 5A), and gingival corium may be inflamed in the region of the pocket (5B). Fibrosis and inflammation contribute to the enlargement (5C). Fibrosis lateral to the inflammation is characterized by proliferation of the connective tissue, probably in a reparative phase, resulting in the gingival enlargement (5C).

**Bleeding**

Bleeding may be easily provoked (Plate 5, 6A) or may be spontaneous. The gingival corium is inflamed (6B), and ulceration of pocket epithelium permits exudation of blood and leukocytes (6C).

## Summary

Gingivitis is primarily plaque induced. Its characteristics have been described.[3-20] It is caused by substances derived from microbial plaque that collect in and around the gingival sulcus.[110-115] Other local and systemic influences may enhance the susceptibility of gingival tissues to disease or may promote the growth or the retention of the microbiota.[93-109] The early lesion is characterized by an infiltrate dominated by T lymphocytes.[115-117] With progression, the established lesion appears, dominated by B lymphocytes and plasma cells.[117-119] Lesions may remain stable, revert, or progress.[120-122] While most lesions are transient or stable, there is evidence to suggest a quantitative relationship between gingivitis and periodontitis. The conversion of gingivitis to periodontitis has been demonstrated in animal models,[122-123] and such progression is seen clinically in humans.[88-90] It appears to be associated with alterations in the composition of the periodontal microbiota.[83] Gingivitis and periodontitis may be a continuum. They may also be separate disease entities that share common inflammatory responses to inciting bacterial infections.[124]

**REFERENCES**

1. Hoover, D.R., and Lefkowitz, W.: Fluctuation in marginal gingivitis, J. Periodontol. **36:**310, 1965.
2. Löe, H., Theilade, E., and Jensen, S.B.: Experimental gingivitis in man, J. Periodontol. **36:**177, 1965.
3. Orban, B.J.: Gingivitis, J. Periodontol. **26:**173, 1955.
4. Rüdin, H.J., Overdiek, H.F., and Rateitschak, K.H.: Correlation between sulcus fluid rate and clinical and histologic inflammation of the marginal gingiva, Helv. Odontol. Acta **14:**2126, 1970.
5. Hock, J.: A clinical study of gingivitis of deciduous and succedaneous permanent teeth in dogs, J. Periodont. Res. **13:**68, 1978.
6. Payne, W.A.: Histopathologic features of the initial and early stages of experimental gingivitis in man, J. Periodont. Res. **10:**51, 1975.
7. Freedman, H.L., Listgarten, M.A., and Taichman, N.S.: Electron microscopic features of chronically inflamed human gingiva, J. Periodont. Res. **3:**313, 1968.
8. Garant, P.R., and Mulvihill, J.E.: The fine structure of gingivitis in the beagle. III. Plasma cell infiltration of the subepithelial connective tissue, J. Periodont. Res. **7:**161, 1971.
9. Gavin, J.R.: Ultrastructural features of chronic marginal gingivitis, J. Periodont. Res. **5:**19, 1970.
10. Mazzella, W.J., and Vernick, S.H.: The ultrastructure of normal and pathologic human gingival epithelium, J. Periodontol. **39:**5, 1968.
11. Fullmer, H.M.: A histochemical study of periodontal disease in the maxillary alveolar processes of 135 autopsies, J. Periodontol. **32:**206, 1961.
12. Horton, J.E., Oppenheim, J.J., and Mergenhagen, S.E.: A role for cell mediated immunity in the pathogenesis of periodontal disease, J. Periodontol. **45:**351, 1974.
13. Lange, D., and Schroeder, H.E.: Cytochemistry and ultrastructure of gingival sulcus cells, Helv. Odontol. Acta **15**(suppl. 6):65, 1971.
14. Melcher, A.H.: Some histological and histochemical observations on the connective tissue of chronically inflamed human gingiva, J. Periodont. Res. **2:**127, 1967.
15. Mutschelknaus, R.: Das marginale Parodontium: Klinische, Histologische und histochemische Untersuchungen, Munich, 1968, C. Hanser Verlag.
16. Schroeder, H.E., Münzel-Pedrazzoli, S., and Page, R.E.: Correlated morphometric and biochemical analysis of gingival tissue in early chronic gingivitis in man, Arch. Oral Biol. **18:**899, 1973.
17. Toto, P.D., and Sicher, H.: The epithelial attachment, Periodontics **2:**154, 1964.
18. Toto, P.D., and Gargiulo, A.W.: Epithelial and connective tissue changes in periodontitis, J. Periodontol. **45:**587, 1970.
19. Toto, P.D., Gargiulo, A.W., and Kwan, H.W.: Immunoglobulins of intact epithelium, J. Dent. Res. **49:**179, 1970.
20. Löe, J.: Physiological aspects of the gingival pocket, Acta Odontol. Scand. **19:**387, 1961.
21. James, W.W., and Counsell, A.: A histologic investigation into "so-called pyorrhea alveolaris," Br. Dent. J. **48:**1237, 1927.
22. Grant, D.A., and Orban, B.: Leukocytes in the epithelial attachment, J. Periodontol. **31:**87, 1960.
23. Attström, R.: Studies on neutrophil polymorphonuclear leukocytes at the dentogingival junction in gingival health and disease, J. Periodont. Res. Suppl. **8:**1, 1971.
24. Schroeder, H.E., Graf-de Beer, M., and Attström, R.: Initial gingivitis in dogs, J. Periodont. Res. **10:**128, 1975.
25. Krygier, G., et al.: Experimental gingivitis in *Macaca speciosa* monkey: clinical, bacteriologic and histologic similarities to human gingivitis, J. Periodontol. **44:**435, 1973.
26. Hopps, R.M., and Johnson, N.W.: Cell dynamics of experimental gingivitis in macaques; cell proliferation within the inflammatory infiltrate, J. Periodont. Res. **11:**210, 1976.
27. Johnson, N.W., and Hopps, R.M.: Cell dynamics of experimental gingivitis in macaques; the nature of the cellular infiltrate with varying degrees of gingivitis, J. Periodont. Res. **10:**177, 1975.
28. Schroeder, H.E., and Graf-de Beer, M.: Stereologic analysis of chronic lymphoid cell infiltrates in human gingiva, Arch. Oral Biol. **21:**527, 1976.
29. Lindhe, J., and Helldén, L.: Neutrophilic chemotatic activity elaborated by dental plaque, J. Periodont. Res. **7:**297, 1972.
30. Lindhe, J., et al.: Clinical and stereologic analysis of the course of early gingivitis in dogs, J. Periodont. Res. **9:**314, 1974.
31. Listgarten, M.A., and Ellegaard, B.: Experimental gingivitis in rhesus monkeys, J. Periodont. Res. **8:**199, 1973.
32. Soderholm, G., and Attström, R.: Vascular permeability during initial gingivitis in dogs, J. Periodont. Res. **12:**395, 1977.
33. Levy, B.M., Robertson, P.B., and Dreizen, S.: Adjuvant induced destructive periodontitis in non-human primates; a comparative study, J. Periodont. Res. **11:**54, 1976.
34. Genco, R.J., et al.: Antibody-mediated effects on the periodontium, J. Periodontol. **45:**330, 1974.
35. Helldén, L., and Lindhe, J.: Enhanced emigration of crevicular leukocytes mediated by

factors in human dental plaque, Scand. J. Dent. Res. **81:**123, 1973.

36. Taichman, N.S., et al.: Interaction of inflammatory cells and oral microorganisms. IV. In vitro release of lysosomal constituents from polymorphonuclear leukocytes exposed to supragingival and subgingival bacterial plaque, Infect. Immun. **16:**1013, 1977.

37. Taichman, N.S., et al.: Conference on inflammation: polymorphonuclear leukocytic-bacterial interaction as a pathogenetic mechanism in periodontal disease, J. Endocrinol. **3:**292, 1977.

38. Kahnberg, K.E., Lindhe, J., and Helldén, L.: Initial gingivitis induced by topical application of plaque extraction, J. Periodont. Res. **11:**218, 1976.

39. Tempel, T.R., Snyderman, J., and Jordan, H.V.: Factors in saliva and oral bacteria, chemotactic for polymorphonuclear leukocytes: their possible role in gingival inflammation, J. Periodontol. **41:**71, 1970.

40. Bauer, W.H.: The supporting tissues of the tooth in acute secondary agranulocytosis (arsphenamine neutropenia), J. Dent. Res. **25:**501, 1946.

41. Cohen, D.W., and Morris, A.L.: A periodontal manifestation of cyclic neutropenia, J. Periodontol. **32:**159, 1961.

42. Tempel, T.R., et al.: Host factors in periodontal disease: periodontal manifestations of Chédiak-Higashi Syndrome, J. Periodont. Res. Suppl. **10:**26, 1972.

43. Lund, J.E., Padgett, G.A., and Ott, R.L.: Cyclic neutropenia in grey collie dogs, Blood **29:**452, 1967.

44. Lavine, W., Page, R.C., and Padgett, G.A.: The dental and periodontal status of mink and mice affected by Chédiak-Higashi syndrome, J. Periodontol. **47:**621, 1976.

45. Miller, M.E., Oski, F.A., and Harris, M.B.: Lazy-leucocyte syndrome: a new disorder of neutrophil function, Lancet **1:**665, 1971.

46. Kostman, R.: Infantile genetic agranulocytosis, Acta Paediatr. Scand. **64:**362, 1975.

47. Robertson, P.B., et al.: Oral status of patients with abnormalities of the immune system, Abstract no. 160, J. Dent. Res. **56:**B92, 1977.

48. Gilman, C., Bernstein, J., and van Oss, C.J.: Decreased phagocytosis associated with increased surface hydrophobicity of neutrophils of children with chronic infections, Fed. Proc. **35:**227, 1976.

49. Cianciola, L.J., et al.: Defective polymorphonuclear leukocyte function in a human periodontal disease, Nature **265:**445, 1977.

50. van Oss, C.J., Gilman, C.F., and Newman, A.W.: Phagocyte engulfment and cell adhesiveness, New York, 1975, Marcel Dekker, Inc.

51. Cianciola, L.J., et al.: A family study of neutrophil chemotaxis in idiopathic juvenile periodontitis (periodontosis), I.A.D.R. Abstract, 1977.

52. Molenaar, D.M., et al.: Leukocyte chemotaxis in diabetic patients and their non-diabetic first degree relatives, Diabetes **25:**880, 1976.

53. Kretschmer, R.R., Lopez-Osuna, M., and De la Rosa, L.: Leukocyte function in Down's syndrome: quantitative NBT reduction and bactericidal capacity, Clin. Immunol. Immunopathol. **2:**449, 1974.

54. Summers, C.J., and Oberman, A.: Association of oral disease with 12 selected variables. I. Periodontal disease, J. Dent. Res. **47:**457, 1968.

55. Tuckman, M.A., et al.: The relationship of glucose tolerance to periodontal status, J. Periodontol. **41:**27, 1970.

56. Schectman, L.R., et al.: Host tissue response in chronic periodontal disease. II. Histologic features of the normal periodontium, and histopathologic and ultrastructural manifestations of disease in the marmoset, J. Periodont. Res. **7:**195, 1972.

57. Simpson, D.M., and Avery, B.E.: Pathologically-altered fibroblasts within lymphoid infiltrates in early gingivitis, J. Dent. Res. **52:**1156, 1973.

58. Schroeder, H.E., and Page, R.C.: Lymphocyte-fibroblast interaction in the pathogenesis of inflammatory gingival disease, Experientia **28:**1228, 1972.

59. Kaslick, R.S., et al.: Investigation of periodontosis with periodontitis: ultra microanalysis of gingival fluid, gross examination of the periodontal ligament and approach to treatment, J. Periodontol. **42:**428, 1971.

60. Wahl, L.M., et al.: Collagenase production by lymphokine-activated macrophages, Science **187:**261, 1975.

61. White, R.R., and Montgomery, E.H.: Exocytosis of polymorphonuclear leukocyte lysosomal contents induced by dental plaque, Infect. Immun. **16:**934, 1977.

62. Horton, J.E., Leikin, S., and Oppenheim, J.J.: Human lymphoproliferative reaction to saliva and dental deposits: an *in vitro* correlation with periodontal disease, J. Periodontol. **43:**522, 1972.

63. Ivanyi, L., and Lehner, T.: Stimulation of lymphocyte transformation by bacterial antigens in patients with periodontal disease, Arch. Oral Biol. **15:**1089, 1970.

64. Kahnberg, K.E., Lindhe, J., and Attström, R.: The role of complement in initial gingivitis. I. The effect of decomplementation by cobra venom factor, J. Periodont. Res. **11:**269, 1976.

65. Dragoo, M., Grant, D., and Gutverg, M.: Root planing with and without chlorhexidine rinses, Int. J. Periodont. Rest. Dent. **4(3):**9, 1984.

66. Zachrisson, B.U.: A histological study of experimental gingivitis in man, J. Periodont. Res. **3:**11, 1969.

67. Attström, R., Graf-de Beer, M., and Schroeder, H.E.: Clinical and stereologic characteristics and normal gingiva, J. Periodont. Res. **10:**115, 1975.

68. Page, R.C., and Schroeder, H.E.: Pathogenesis of inflammatory periodontal disease: a summary of current work, Lab. Invest. **33:**235, 1976.

69. Byers, C.W., Toto, P.D., and Gargiulo, A.W.: Levels of immunoglobulins IgG, IgA, and IgM in the human inflamed gingiva, J. Periodontol. **48:**387, 1975.

70. Brandtzaeg, P.: Presence of J chain in human immunocytes containing various immunoglobulin classes, Nature **252:**418, 1974.

71. Lehner, T., et al.: Sequential cell-mediated responses in experimental gingivitis in man, Clin. Exp. Immunol. **16:**481, 1974.

72. Lang, N.P., and Smith, F.N.: Lymphocyte response to T-cell mitogen during experimental gingivitis in humans, Infect. Immun. **13:**108, 1976.

73. Bernick, S., and Grant, D.A.: Lymphatic vessels of healthy and inflamed gingiva, J. Dent. Res. **57:**810, 1978.

74. Simpson, D.M., and Avery, B.E.: Histopathologic and ultrastructural features of inflamed gingiva in the baboon, J. Periodontol. **45:**500, 1974.

75. Genco, R.J., et al.: Antibody-mediated effects on the periodontium, J. Periodontol. **45:**330, 1974.

76. Brandtzaeg, P.: Local formation and transport of immunoglobulins related to the oral cavity. In MacPhee, T., editor: Host resistance to commensal bacteria, Edinburgh, 1972, Churchill Livingstone, Inc.

77. Weiss, M.D., Weinmann, J.P., and Meyer, J.: Degree of keratinization and glycogen content in the uninflamed and inflamed gingiva and alveolar mucosa, J. Periodontol. **30:**208, 1959.

78. Schroeder, H.E., and Attström, R.: Pocket formation: an hypothesis. In Lehner, T., and Cimasoni, G., editors: The borderline between caries and periodontal disease, vol. 2, London, 1980, Academic Press, Inc.

79. Lehner, T., et al.: The relationship between serum and salivary antibodies and cell-mediated immunity in oral disease in man, Adv. Exp. Med. Biol. **45:**485, 1973.

80. Patters, M.R., et al.: Blastogenic response of human lymphocytes to oral bacterial antigens: comparison of individuals with periodontal disease to normal and edentulous subjects, Infect. Immun. **14:**1213, 1976.

81. Ivanyi, L., and Lehner, T.: Lymphocyte transformation by sonicates of dental plaque in human periodontal disease, Arch. Oral Biol. **6:**1117, 1971.

82. Gaumer, H.R., Holm-Pedersen, P., and Folke, L.E.A.: Indirect blastogenesis of peripheral blood leukocytes in experimental gingivitis, Infect. Immun. **13:**1347, 1976.

83. Baker, J.J., et al.: Importance of *Actinomyces* and certain gram-negative anaerobic organisms in the transformation of lymphocytes from patients with periodontal disease, Infect. Immun. **13:**1363, 1976.

84. Lang, N.P., and Smith, F.N.: Cellular immune response to plaque antigens in human periodontal disease, J. Dent. Res. **55B:**205, 1976.

85. Patters, M.R., Sedransk, N., and Genco, R.J.: Lymphoproliferative response during resolution and recurrence of naturally occurring gingivitis, J. Periodontol. **48:**373, 1978.

86. Grant, D.A., and Bernick, S.: Vascularity of crestal bone in periodonally healthy and diseased monkeys, I.A.D.R. Abstract no. 821, J. Dent. Res. **53:**260, 1974.

87. Grant, D., Chase, J., and Bernick, S.: Biology of the periodontium in primates of the Galago species, J. Periodontol. **44:**540, 1973.

88. Suomi, J.D., et al.: The effect of controlled oral hygiene procedures on the progression of periodontal disease in adults: results after two years, J. Periodontol. **40:**416, 1969.

89. Suomi, J.D., et al.: The effect of controlled oral hygiene procedures on the progression of periodontal disease in adults: results after third and final year, J. Periodontol. **42:**152, 1971.

90. Suomi, J.D., Leatherwood, E.C., and Chang, J.J.: A follow-up study of former participants in a controlled oral hygiene study, J. Periodontol. **44:**662, 1973.

91. Suomi, J.D., et al.: The effect of controlled oral hygiene procedures on the progression of periodontal disease in adults: radiographic findings, J. Periodontol. **42:**562, 1971.

92. Page, R.C., and Schroeder, H.E.: Periodontitis in man and other animals: a comparative review, Basel, 1982, S. Karger.

93. Meyer, J.: Abscesses of periodontal origin (abstr.), Actual. Odontostomatol. **117:**137, 1977.

94. Lite, T., Diucaio, D.J., and Burman, L.R.: Gingival pathosis in mouth breathers, Oral Surg. **8:**382, 1955.

95. Genco, R.J., and Cianciola, L.T.: Relationship of the neutrophile to host resistance in periodontal disease, Alpha Omegan **10:**31, 1977.

96. el-Ashiry, G.M., et al.: Effects of oral contraceptives on the gingiva, J. Periodontol. **42:**273, 1971.

97. Cohen, D.W., et al.: A longitudinal investigation of the periodontal changes during pregnancy, J. Periodontol. **40:**563, 1969.

98. Cohen, D.W., et al.: A longitudinal investigation of the periodontal changes during pregnancy and fifteen months postpartum. II. J. Periodontol. **42:**653, 1971.

99. Samant, A., et al.: Gingivitis and periodontal

disease in pregnancy, J. Periodontol. **47:**415, 1976.

100. Maier, A.W., and Orban, B.: Gingivitis in pregnancy, Oral Surg. **2:**334, 1949.

101. Knight, G.M., and Wade, H.B.: The effects of hormonal contraceptives on the human periodontium, J. Periodont. Res. **9:**18, 1974.

102. Sumner, C.F., and Baer, P.N.: Clinical observations of gingiva of patients on Norethynodrel therapy, J. Periodontol. **33:**344, 1962.

103. Lindhe, J., and Attström, R.: Gingival exudation during the menstrual cycle, J. Periodont. Res. **2:**194, 1967.

104. Lindhe, J., and Bjorn, A.: Influence of hormonal contraceptives on the gingiva of women, J. Periodont. Res. **2:**1, 1967.

105. Orban, B., Martin, W.B., and Hehn, R.M.: Histopathologic investigation of a case of scorbutic gingivitis, J. Periodontol. **18:**95, 1947.

106. Baer, P.N.: Relation of the physical character of the diet to the periodontium and periodontal disease, Oral Surg. **9:**839, 1956.

107. Belting, C.M., Hinniker, J.J., and Dummett, C.O.: Influence of diabetes mellitus on the severity of periodontal disease, J. Periodontol. **35:**476, 1964.

108. Cianciola, L.J., et al.: Prevalence of periodontal disease in insulin-dependent diabetes mellitus (juvenile diabetes), J. Am. Dent. Assoc. **104:**653, 1982.

109. Kerr, D.A., McClatchey, K.D., and Regezi, J.A.: Allergic gingivostomatitis (due to gum chewing), J. Periodontol. **42:**709, 1971.

110. Page, R.C.: Gingivitis, J. Clin. Periodontol. **13:**345, 1986.

111. Löe, H., Theilade, E., and Jensen, S.B.: Experimental gingivitis in man, J. Periodontol. **36:**177, 1965.

112. Lindhe, J., and Rylander, H.: Experimental gingivitis in young dogs: a morphometric study, Scand. J. Dent. Res. **83:**314, 1975.

113. Payne, W.A., et al.: Histopathologic features of the initial and early stages of experimental gingivitis in man, J. Periodont. Res. **10:**51, 1975.

114. Page, R.C., and Schroeder, H.E.: Pathogenesis of inflammatory periodontal disease, Lab. Investigations **33:**235, 1976.

115. Moore, W.E.C., et al.: Bacteriology of experimental gingivitis in young adult humans, Infection and Immunity **38:**651, 1982.

116. Schroeder, H.E., Münzel-Pedrazzoli, S., and Page, R.C.: Correlated morphometric and biochemical analysis of early chronic gingivitis in man, Arch. Oral Biol. **18:**899, 1973.

117. Seymour, G.J., and Greenspan, J.S.: The phenotypic characterization of lymphocyte subpopulations in established human periodontitis, J. Periodont. Res. **14:**39, 1979.

118. Schroeder, H.E., and Attström, R.: Effect of mechanical plaque control on development of subgingival plaque and initial gingivitis in neutropenic dogs, Scand. J. Dent. Res. **87:**279, 1979.

119. Mackler, B.F. et al.: Immunoglobulins bearing lymphocytes and plasma cells in human periodontal disease, J. Periodont. Res. **12:**37, 1977.

120. Mackler, B.F., et al.: IgG subclasses in human periodontal disease. I. Distribution and incidence of IgG subclass bearing lymphocytes and plasma cells, J. Periodont. Res. **13:**109, 1978.

121. Lovdal, A., Arno, A, and Waerhaug, J.: Incidence of manifestations of periodontal disease in light of oral hygiene and calculus formation, J. Am. Dent. Assoc. **56:**21, 1958.

122. Listgarten, M.A., Lindhe, J., and Helldén, L.: Effect of tetracycline and/or scaling on human periodontal disease: clinical, microbiological and histologic observations, J. Clin. Periodontol. **5:**246, 1978.

123. Schroeder, H.E., and Lindhe, J.: Conversion of established gingivitis in the dog into destructive periodontitis, Arch. Oral Biol. **20:**775, 1975.

124. Grant, D.A., Stern, I.B., and Everett, F.E.: Periodontics, ed. 5, St. Louis, 1979, The C.V. Mosby Co., p. 275.

## ADDITIONAL SUGGESTED READING

Abrams, K., Caton, J., and Polson, A.: Histologic comparisons of interproximal gingival tissues related to the presence or absence of bleeding, J. Periodontol. **55:**629, 1984.

Alfano, M.C.: The origin of crevicular fluid, J. Theor. Biol. **47:**127, 1974.

Allison, A.C., et al.: Activation of complement by the alternative pathway as a factor in the pathogenesis of periodontal disease, Lancet **2:**1001, 1976.

Appelgren, R., et al.: Gingivitis and eosinophils, J. Dent. Res. **56:**546, 1977.

Charbeneau, T.D., and Hurt, W.C.: Gingival findings in spontaneous scurvy: a case report, J. Periodontol. **54:**694, 1983.

Cooper, P.G., Caton, J.G., and Polson, A.M.: Cell populations associated with gingival bleeding, J. Periodontol. **54:**497, 1983.

Fine, A.S., et al.: Subcellular distribution of oxidative enzymes in human, inflamed and dilantin hyperplastic gingiva, Arch. Oral Biol. **19:**565, 1974.

Genco, R.J., and Slots, J.: Host responses in periodontal diseases, J. Dent. Res. **63:**441, 1984.

Golub, L.M., and Kleinberg, I.: Gingival crevicular fluid: a new diagnostic aid in managing the periodontal patient, Oral Sci. Rev. **8:**49, 1976.

Gusberti, F.A., et al.: Puberty gingivitis in insulin-dependent diabetic children. I. Cross sectional observations, J. Periodontol. **54:**71, 1983.

Hasegawa, K., Cimasoni, G., and Vuagnat, P.: Inflamed gingivae contain more free lysosomal enzyme, Experientia **31:**765, 1975.

Ivanyi, L., and Lehner, T.: Stimulation of human lymphocytes by B-cell mitogens, Clin. Exp. Immunol. **18:**347, 1974.

Kalkwarf, K.L.: Effect of oral contraceptive therapy on gingival inflammation in humans, J. Periodontol. **49:**560, 1978.

Klinge, B., Matsson, L., and Allström, R.: Histopathology of initial gingivitis in humans: a pilot study, J. Clin. Periodontol. **10:**364, 1983.

Lareau, D.E., Herzberg, M.C., and Nelson, R.D.: Human neutrophil migration under agarose to bacteria associated with the development of gingivitis, J. Periodontol. **55:**540, 1984.

Lehner, T.: Immunological aspects of dental caries and periodontal disease, Br. Med. Bull. **31:**125, 1975.

Listgarten, M.A.: A perspective on periodontal diagnosis, J. Clin. Periodontol. **13:**175, 1986.

Listgarten, M.A., Schifter, C.C., and Laster, L.: Three-year longitudinal study of the periodontal status of an adult population with gingivitis, J. Clin. Periodontol. **12:**225, 1985.

Matsson, L., and Goldberg, P.: Gingival inflammatory reaction in children at different ages, J. Clin. Periodontol. **12:**98, 1985.

Ramamurthy, N.S., and Golub, L.M.: Diabetes increases collagenase activity in extracts of rat gingiva and skin, J. Periodont. Res. **18:**23, 1983.

Seymour, G.J., et al.: Experimental gingivitis in humans: a histochemical and immunologic characterization of the lymphoid cell subpopulations, J. Periodont. Res. **18:**375, 1983.

Silverman, S., Jr., and Lozada, F.: An epilogue to plasma-cell gingivostomatitis (allergic gingivostomatitis), Oral Surg. **43:**211, 1977.

VanderVelder, J., Abbas, F., and Hart, A.A.M.: Experimental gingivitis in relation to susceptability to periodontal disease. I. Clinical observation, J. Clin. Periodontol. **12:**61, 1985.

# CHAPTER 16

# Periodontitis

**Definition**

**Clinical features**
Microscopic features
Pathogenesis
Periodontal pocket
Gingival pocket wall
Cytologic characteristics

**Progress of inflammation**
Perivascular pathway
Aggressive and nonaggressive lesions

**Bone destruction**
Suprabony pocket
Infrabony pocket

**Systemic factors**
Diabetes mellitus
Disseminated lesions
Endocrine dysfunction

**Occlusion**

**Summary**

## Definition

Periodontitis is an inflammatory disease of the gingiva and the deeper periodontal tissues. Periodontitis is preceded and accompanied by gingivitis. However, gingivitis may persist without progressing to periodontitis.

Periodontitis involves destruction of gingival and periodontal fibers, resorption of crestal bone, and apical proliferation of junctional epithelium.

In observing a spectrum of periodontal patients, a slow, progressive course that may proceed to the loss of teeth is suggested. However the disease may persist without progression, or it may proceed in episodic (cyclic) bouts in which localized areas

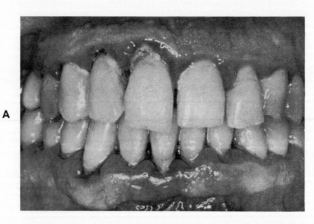

**Fig. 16-1. A,** Typical case of periodontitis in which plaque and signs of disease are apparent.

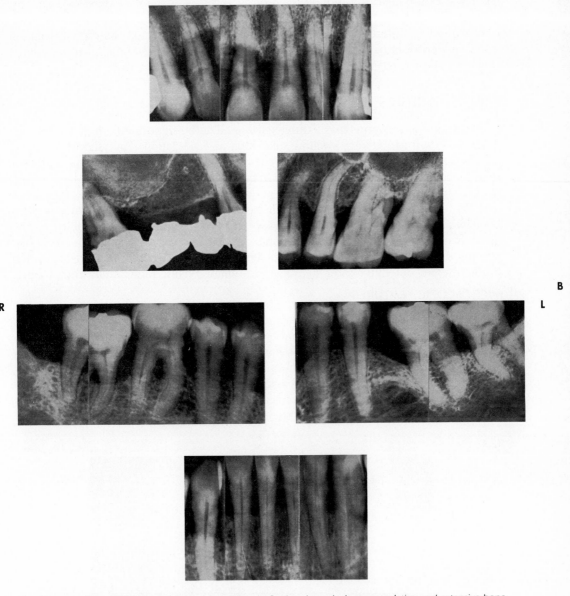

**Fig. 16-1, cont'd.  B,** Roentgenograms of the patient in **A,** showing calculus accumulation and extensive bone resorption. Several molars show furcation involvements. Alveolar crests are irregular.

undergo relatively rapid destruction in a limited time period. These episodes of relatively acute disease may last from several days to a few weeks and be separated by extended intervals of remission lasting from several weeks to several years. During the periods of remission, periodontal destruction does not progress and some repair may occur.[1-3]

The rate at which the disease progresses is partly related to the mass and composition of the microbiota and the ability of the host to deal with the microbial population.[4] It is also clear that not all teeth or all surfaces of the same tooth are equally susceptible to periodontitis. Maxillary molars, for example, are much more susceptible than canines.[5-7] Interdental surfaces are more severely affected than are vestibular surfaces. Periodontitis has characteristics that can be described on clinical,[8-20] microscopic,[8-20] ultrastructural,[21-28] biochemical,[29] and physiologic levels.[30,31]

## Clinical features

Clinically, periodontitis may exhibit some or all of the signs of inflammation seen in gingivitis, such as redness, swelling, bleeding, and exudation. The gingival margins may be enlarged and either fibrotic or edematous in texture. In other cases gingival margins may be blunted but unchanged in height. Principal clinical characteristics are pocket formation accompanied by resorption of bone at the alveolar crest (Figs. 16-1 and 16-2). In moderate and advanced disease, there is radiographic evidence of prior bone loss but the progression of the disease may not be evident. Tooth mobility may be an early or late symptom. In some patients, the presence of periodontitis is easily discernible (Fig. 16-1, *A*), whereas in others it may not be apparent on visual examination but is revealed only after careful clinical examination using radiographs and probing.

### MICROSCOPIC FEATURES

Microscopically periodontitis is characterized by bone destruction at the alveolar crest, apical proliferation of junctional epithelium onto cementum, and lysis of dentogingival, dentoperiosteal, and transseptal fibers. The area of collagen fiber loss is occupied by a cellular and fluid inflammatory infiltrate. Plasma cells usually predominate, with lymphocytes, macrophages, and polymorphonuclear leukocytes also present. Large amounts of immunoglobulins are found in the fluid infiltrate, and antigen-antibody complexes have been reported in the pocket wall and around blood ves-

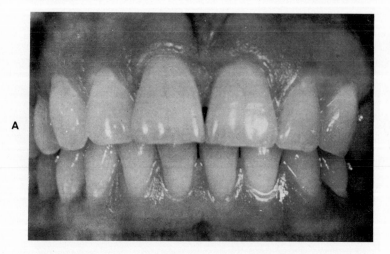

**Fig. 16-2. A,** Periodontitis in a dentition with relatively minimal plaque. The appearance of the tissues is relatively normal.

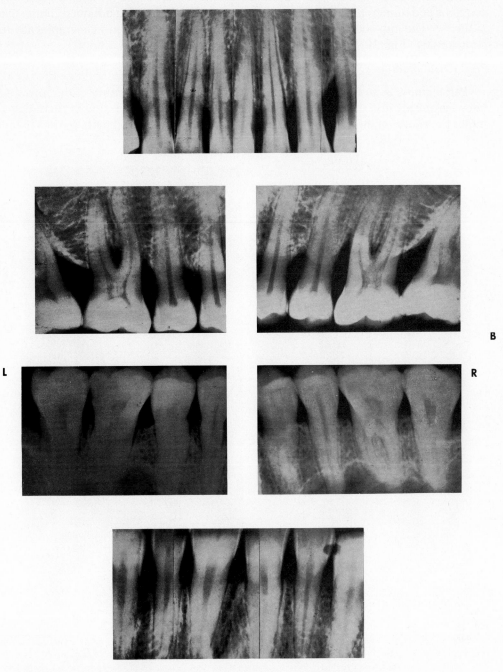

**Fig. 16-2, cont'd.** **B,** Roentgenograms of the same patient. Note the cup-shaped alveolar crests in the maxilla and the oblique inclination of the alveolar crests in the mandible.

**Pocket**

sels.[31-39] Continuing collagen loss can be observed in the area of infiltration; fiber regeneration may occur in areas bordering the inflamed area. Gingival sulcular depth is increased, and the deepened sulcus is now called a *pocket* (Fig. 16-3). The pocket typically is lined by pocket epithelium, an attenuated epithelial lining with microulcerations and numerous projections extending into the underlying inflamed connective tissue.[27,40] The cup-shaped form of alveolar crests sometimes seen radiographically in periodontitis (Fig. 16-4) reflects the histologic appearance (Fig. 16-3, *B*).

## PATHOGENESIS

Periodontitis is an infection of the periodontal tissues. The nature of the infecting microorganisms and the ability of host defense mechanisms to deal with them determines the course of the disease.[2-4,41-43] The difference between, and perhaps the change

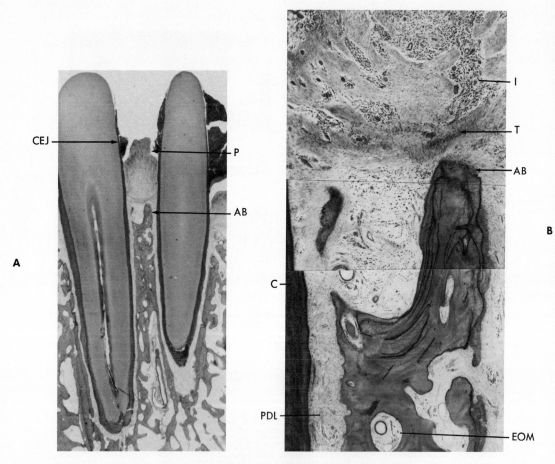

**Fig. 16-3. A,** Periodontitis in a human. The coronal thirds of the interdental septae have been destroyed in periodontitis. Viewing apically and moving coronally, endosseous marrow spaces are fibrotic. The alveolar crest is cup shaped due to bone resorption. The gingival lamina propria contains dense aggregates of inflammatory cells. The junctional epithelia are attached to cementum. Epithelial rete strands have proliferated into the lamina propria, where the orientation of fiber bundles is lost due to collagenolysis. Dense calcified deposits and plaque reside in the pocket and supragingivally. *AB,* Alveolar bone crest; *CEJ,* cementoenamel junction; *P,* pocket. **B,** Montage of higher magnification of alveolar crest area in **A.** Remnants of transseptal fibers above bone. Aggregates of inflammatory cells reside perivascularly and in areas of more extensive collagenolysis. An endosseous marrow space has been opened by bone destruction coronally to produce a cup-shaped crestal bone form. Endosseous marrow spaces are fibrotic. *AB,* Alveolar bone crest; *EOM,* fibrotic endosseous marrow space; *T,* transseptal fibers; *I,* inflammatory infiltrate; *C,* cementum; *PDL,* periodontal ligament.

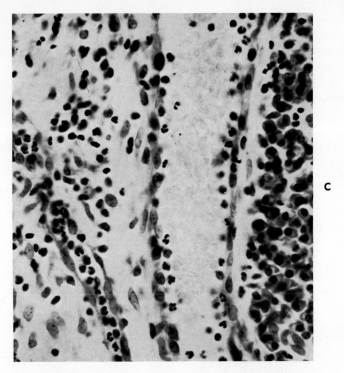

C

**Fig. 16-3, cont'd.** **C,** Polymorphonuclear leukocytes accumulate in blood vessels and migrate into the surrounding tissue. Plasma cells are clustered lateral to the blood vessels. (**A** and **B** from the collection of A. Lufkin.)

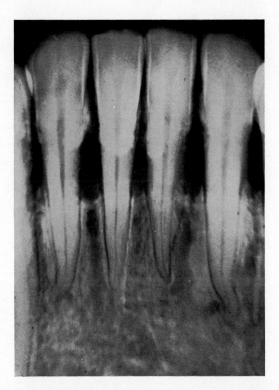

**Fig. 16-4.** Roentgenogram showing cup-shaped alveolar crests and widened nutrient canals in bone. These are suggestive of resorption caused by extension of the inflammation into the deeper tissues.

from, gingivitis to periodontitis may occur with alterations in the composition of the periodontal microbiota. It should be noted, however, that neither the microbial changes nor the parameters of host defense are sufficiently well defined at this time to warrant using these as exclusive diagnostic criteria.

**Diagnostic
criteria**

Whenever crestal bone and periodontal ligament fibers are destroyed and the junctional epithelium has proliferated onto cementum, a diagnosis of periodontitis can be made. The clinical end result of these pathologic events is the deepened pocket, which is a characteristic feature of periodontitis.[44-47] Pocket depth in periodontitis is primarily a reflection of intermittently progressive bone loss and apical migration of junctional epithelium, but it may also be accompanied by swelling and enlargement of the gingival margins, which can add to pocket depth. Thus the clinical diagnosis of periodontitis is based on gingival inflammation, pocket formation with or without exudation, destruction of periodontal ligament, and alveolar bone resorption. The disease is frequently painless. Pain may be a feature of abscesses and advanced mobility. Mobility may occur early or may be a late symptom after extensive bone loss; it is sometimes minimal even after extensive alveolar bone loss. The principal microscopic features of periodontitis are shown in Fig. 16-5. These features correspond to the *advanced lesion.*[48,49]

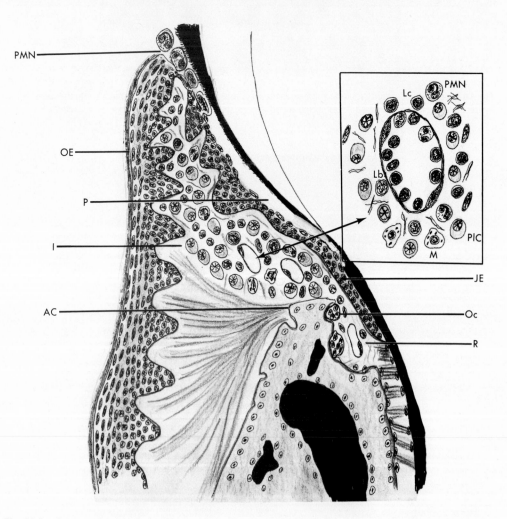

**Fig. 16-5.** *Schema of early periodontitis. Inset,* Magnification of inflammatory cells around a capillary; *I,* inflammatory infiltrate; *JE,* junctional epithelium; *P,* pocket; *R,* resorptive bone lacuna; *Oc,* osteoclasts; *AC,* alveolar crest; *PMN,* polymorphonuclear leukocytes; *PIC,* plasma cells; *Lc,* lymphocytes; *Lb,* lymphoblasts; *M,* macrophage; *OE,* oral epithelium.

## PERIODONTAL POCKET

The periodontal pocket is bordered on one side by loosely and firmly adherent plaque covering calcified deposits on the cementum and enamel.[11] The loosely adherent plaque is in direct contact with the gingival wall of the pocket (Fig. 16-6).

Shallow and deep periodontal pockets harbor a characteristic, though variable, microbiota.[50] The pathogenicity of both the adherent and loosely adherent bacterial plaque flora in shallow and deep periodontal pockets has been demonstrated.[51] Several entities have been identified as inducers of bone destruction in vitro, including (1) microorganisms and their products from dental plaque[52-54]; (2) substances extracted from inflamed gingiva, such as prostaglandins[55-66]; and (3) factors generated by activation of the host's immune system, including by-products of the complement cascade.[67-70]

## GINGIVAL POCKET WALL

The soft tissue wall of the pocket is lined by a thin epithelium, with microulcerations and epithelial strands that extend into the underlying connective tissue. Epithelial proliferation occurs whenever the inflammatory process results in loss of collagen fibers. It represents an unsuccessful attempt by the epithelium to restore the integrity of the tissues.

Vascular proliferation and stasis results in numerous engorged blood vessels close to the pocket wall. They are frequently filled with polymorphonuclear leukocytes in various stages of diapedesis. The cells migrate through the epithelium toward the

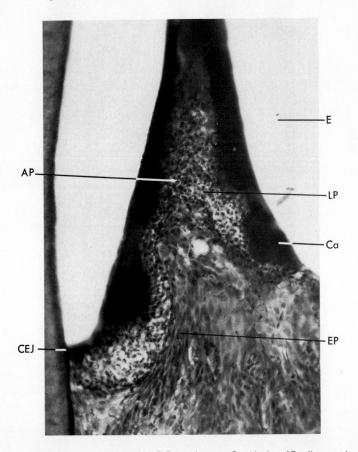

**Fig. 16-6.** Periodontal pocket in early periodontitis. *E*, Enamel space; *Ca*, calculus; *AP*, adherent plaque; *LP*, loosely adherent plaque; *EP*, pocket epithelium; *CEJ*, cementoenamel junction.

pocket where they accumulate as a distinct layer between the microbial mass in the pocket and the tissue wall. Periodontal probing readily elicits bleeding because of the proximity of the vessels to the tissue surface, their dilation, and tendency to leak[71] and the loss of a protective, dense collagenous matrix.

## CYTOLOGIC CHARACTERISTICS

The lamina propria may be sparsely or densely infiltrated by inflammatory cells (Figs. 16-7 and 16-8). Plasma cells usually predominate in the inflammatory lesion characteristic of periodontitis.[15,48,49] Lymphocytes, mast cells,[72] and macrophages are also present. Clusters of plasma cells and lymphocytes are found deep in connective tissue residing between remnants and fragments of fiber bundles and around blood vessels (see Fig. 16-3, *B* and *C*). The inflammation then may proceed laterally and apically, destroying the characteristic organization of dentogingival and dentoperiosteal fiber groups. Fragmentation of transseptal fibers also occurs although they reform at more apical levels (Fig. 16-9).

Bacterial cells may enter the pocket wall.[73-77] Reports of frequent bacteremias in subjects with periodontal disease[78-81] further supports the presence of bacterial penetration into the tissues.[82] These penetrations are reported to be a mixture of bacterial

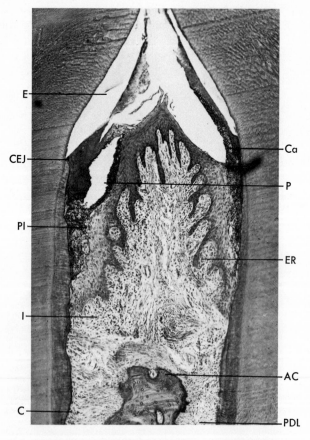

**Fig. 16-7.** Periodontitis in a marmoset. *E,* Enamel space; *CEJ,* cementoenamel junction; *P,* pocket; *Pl,* plaque in pocket; *Ca,* calculus; *ER,* proliferating epithelial rete ridges; *I,* inflammatory infiltrate; *AC,* alveolar crest; *C,* cementum; *PDL,* periodontal ligament.

morphotypes within the tissues rather than homogeneous populations of bacteria in single or multiple colonies. Presence of bacteria as mixtures of isolated cells would indicate that the bacteria have been passively introduced. Bacterial invasion, on the other hand, presupposes that the bacteria are actively proliferating within the tissues, a process which would be reflected by the presence of microbial aggregates of homogeneous cell types.

While bacterial invasion of the pocket wall cannot be excluded as a primary cause of the periodic exacerbations characteristic of periodontitis, demonstrations of bacterial cells in the pocket wall may not constitute definitive evidence of bacterial invasion. A distinction must be made between bacterial invasion, in which bacteria are actively proliferating and spreading within the tissues, and bacterial translocation (the passive introduction of bacteria) into the tissue through chewing on loose teeth, oral hygiene practices, or other tissue manipulations.

Periodontal pockets have been classified in several ways. Pockets are classified according to the relationship of the bottom of the pocket to bone. When the bottom of the pocket is coronal to the alveolar crest, it is called a *suprabony* or *supra-alveolar*

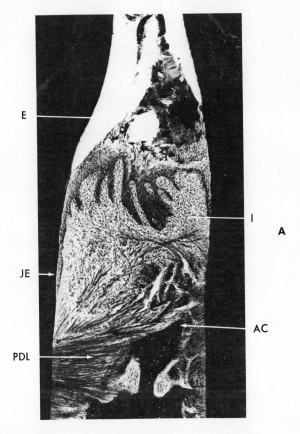

**Fig. 16-8. A,** Periodontitis in a spider monkey. Proliferating junctional epithelium is on cementum. The pocket and the interdental tooth structure are filled with plaque and calculus. The pocket epithelium is ulcerated, and rete strands have proliferated into the inflamed lamina propria. An extensive inflammatory infiltrate fills the gingival corium, where only fragments of fibers remain. Transseptal fibers are reformed apically, over the alveolar bone reduced by resorption. *E,* Enamel space; *I,* inflammatory infiltrate; *JE,* junctional epithelium; *AC,* alveolar crest; *PDL,* periodontal ligament. *Continued.*

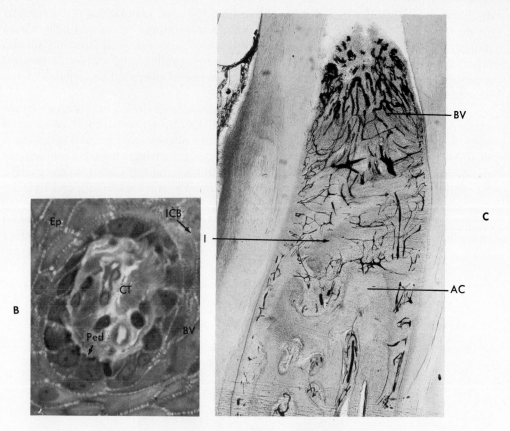

**Fig. 16-8, cont'd. B,** Connective tissue papilla with vessel in cross section. *Ep,* Epithelial cells; *ICB,* intercellular bridges; *Ped,* pedicles; *CT,* connective tissue; *BV,* blood vessel. **C,** In a perfused section, enlarged, proliferating blood vessels can be seen to fill the lamina propria and to extend to the ulcerated pocket surface. The shaded area in the lamina propria indicates that areas of collagen destruction are now occupied by an inflammatory infiltrate, which is extending perivascularly toward bone. *BV,* Blood vessels; *I,* inflammatory infiltrate; *AC,* alveolar crest.

*pocket.* When the bottom of the pocket is apical to the alveolar crest and bone is present lateral to the soft tissue pocket wall, the pocket is called an *infrabony* or *intrabony pocket.* When pocket depth is due to enlargement of the marginal gingiva and there has been no loss of attachment, the pocket is called a *pseudopocket.* Additionally, pockets in gingivitis have been called *gingival pockets,* while those in periodontitis have been called *periodontal pockets.*

## Progress of inflammation

### PERIVASCULAR PATHWAY

**Morphology of bone defects**

The destructive inflammatory lesion appears to extend perivascularly to bone; the resultant bony defect[11,59,60] reflects the morphologic distribution of the vessels (Fig. 16-10). If the vessels penetrate the alveolar crest at this center or if bone resorption has opened a marrow space (Fig. 16-11), the defect may appear cup shaped roentgenographically and cratered when a flap is reflected. If the vessels enter the gingiva

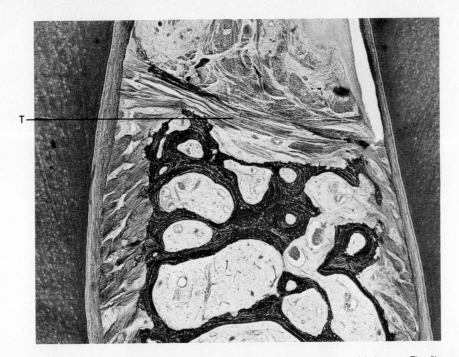

**Fig. 16-9.** Transseptal fiber group extends above the resorbed alveolar crest in an elderly man. The fiber group has reformed apical to its position in health. *T,* Transseptal fibers.

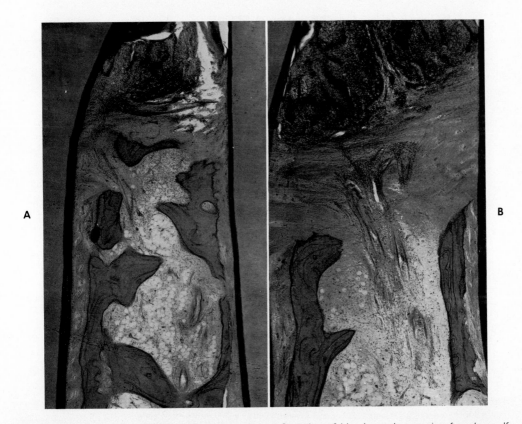

**Fig. 16-10.** Patterns of bone resorption. **A,** Y-shaped configuration of blood vessels emerging from bone. If resorption of the crest were to occur, the bony defect seen in **B** would be caused. At this time vessels appear to emerge from bone in the center at the crest. This may not have been so; rather the vascular morphologic characteristics seen in **A** may have been present. *Continued.*

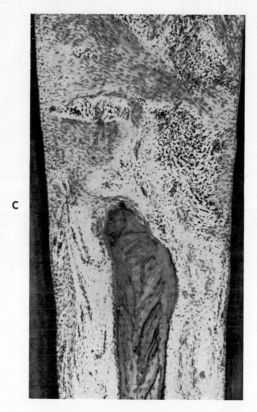

C

**Fig. 16-10, cont'd.   C,** High magnification of a narrow interdental space and a very thin alveolar crest. In this instance the inflammation extends into the periodontal ligament. (From the collection of J.P. Weinmann.)

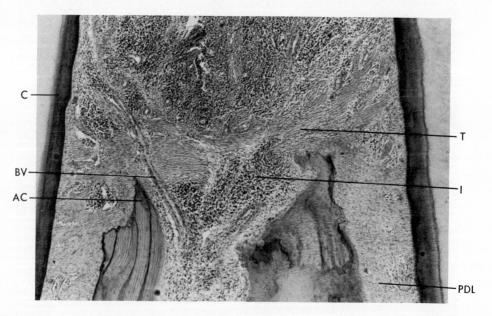

**Fig. 16-11.**   Cup-shaped bone deformity at the alveolar crest in a human. A dense inflammatory infiltrate is present coronal to fragmented transseptal fibers and extends perivascularly into a bony defect that probably was once a marrow space. The large blood vessel *(BV)* enters the bony defect from the corner. *T,* Transseptal fibers; *I,* inflammatory infiltrate; *AC,* alveolar crest; *PDL,* periodontal ligament; *C,* cementum.

from the corner of the crest or by way of the periodontal ligament, and if bone destruction is limited to one side or is greater on one side (see Fig. 16-10), the defect may be angular or infrabony in form (Fig. 16-12). (See Chapter 5 for vascular distribution at the alveolar crest.)

## AGGRESSIVE AND NONAGGRESSIVE LESIONS

Some lesions are aggressive and progress rapidly; others are nonaggressive and progress slowly or not at all. Periods of aggressive and nonaggressive behavior can occur in a single lesion and have been referred to as periods of exacerbation and quiescence.[1-3,49] These behaviors may account for the varying histopathologic features seen in different microscopic specimens.[11] In any lesion, both lytic and reparative phenomena take place. Periods of remission may be characterized by increased collagen deposition, which can result in a fibrotic, enlarged gingival margin (Fig. 16-13). Periods of exacerbation are marked by increased collagenolysis, bone destruction, and apical proliferation of junctional epithelium, which result in a deepened pocket. This cycle is likely to be repeated over a period of years in some individuals; in others, a more aggressive and rapid destructive pattern is seen clinically and is sometimes referred to as a *rapidly progressive* or *fulminating periodontitis*.[83]

Gingival and periodontal abscesses are a common occurrence in periodontitis. These acute events are often the principal reason for the patient's visit to the dentist. They can cause extensive tissue destruction in a short time.

## Bone destruction

A number of factors are incriminated in bone destruction seen in periodontitis: microorganisms[51-54] and their products, substances in inflamed gingiva,[55-67] and im-

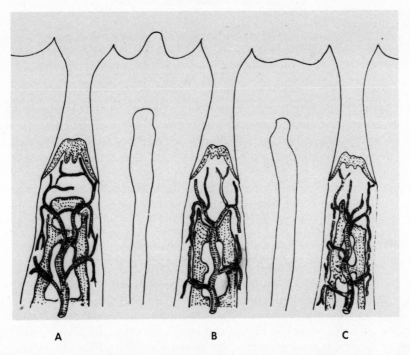

**Fig. 16-12.** *Schema to illustrate the relation of blood vessel location to bone resorption at the alveolar crest.* **A,** *Vessel configuration seen most frequently to emerge from bone.* **B,** *Resorption of the alveolar crest could produce a cratered defect. Note course of blood vessels.* **C,** *Resorption limited to one side or more rapid on one side can produce an angular bony defect.*

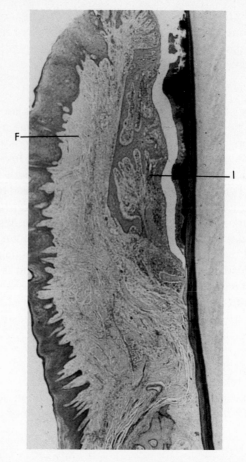

**Fig. 16-13.** Deposition of dense bundles of collagen fibers *(F)* has produced an enlarged, thick gingival margin. The outer surface of the gingiva is stippled, and the oral epithelium is regular. The surface appearance is one of health. Bordering the deep pocket is a dense aggregate of inflammatory cells *(I)* and proliferating epithelial strands, features characteristic of disease. The lateral fibrosis conceals the inflammation along the pocket.

mune responses.[43,48,51] The patterns of bone destruction are noted to be irregular. These are broadly categorized as "horizontal" and "vertical" bone destruction. In actuality, the patterns are more irregular and sometimes bizarre.[84,85] Available evidence indicates that the inflammatory lesion extends perivascularly, at least when destruction is not rapid and aggressive.[8,86]

In other cases periodontitis is complicated by the presence of other systemic diseases or by periodontal traumatism. Then the course of the disease may become more rapid and the pattern of bone loss more bizarre.

## SUPRABONY POCKET

Pockets have been classified according to the relationship of the pocket to alveolar bone. In a suprabony pocket, the bottom of the pocket is coronal to the alveolar crest. The bony defects in periodontitis are often irregular and the resulting crestal bone form is different from the "normal." The structural characteristics and relationships in the epithelial, soft connective tissue, and bony compartments may also differ markedly from known quantitative parameters in health[28,40,49,87] (Figs. 16-14 and 16-15). The "biologic width" may be different from that seen in health.[88] The junctional epithelium may be very long or as short as one cell in length. The distance between the

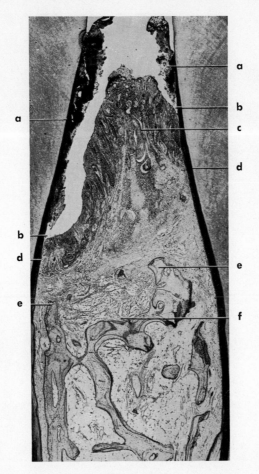

**Fig. 16-14.** Interdental area with inflammation from a periodontal pocket encroaching on the interdental alveolar septum. An osteitis is evident in the alveolar process. Bone is being resorbed. *a,* Calculus; *b,* bottom of the periodontal pocket; *c,* highly inflamed interdental gingiva; *d,* apical end of the epithelial attachment; *e,* alveolar bone; *f,* cup-shaped alveolar crest.

apical end of the junctional epithelium and the alveolar crest varies considerably and may be greater than 1 mm, or less. The distance between the bottom of the pocket and alveolar bone crest may be greater or less than 2 mm.

## INFRABONY POCKET

In an infrabony pocket, bone is found in the lateral wall of the pocket and at the bottom. The presumptive events in the formation of an infrabony pocket may be seen in Plate 6, *A*. The characteristic features of periodontitis are shown in Plate 6, *A*. A vascular bundle extends from the periodontal ligament on the right to course over the alveolar crest toward the junctional epithelium on the left. The inflammatory infiltrate, which is prominent subepithelially, extends apically and perivascularly toward bone. At higher magnification (Plate 6, *B*), the vascular bundle emerges from the periodontal ligament between tooth and bone and is surrounded by an infiltrate of mononuclear lymphocyte-like cells and some mast cells. In an alternate cut section the subepithelial and perivascular areas of fiber lysis, framed by remaining transseptal and periodontal ligament fiber bundles, are graphically illustrated (Plate 6, *C*). As the destruction continues, the alveolar crest is resorbed, in this instance resulting in an infrabony defect (Plate 6, *D*).

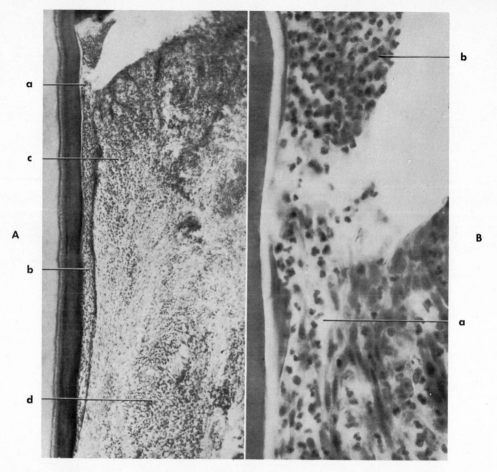

**Fig. 16-15. A,** Pocket area, *a,* and long junctional epithelium, *b,* in a case of periodontitis. Severe inflammation below the bottom of the pocket, *c,* extends to deeper areas, *d.* **B,** Higher magnification of the bottom of the pocket. Polymorphonuclear leukocytes migrate through the epithelium, *a,* into the pocket, forming pus, *b.* Note the dental cuticle on the surface of the tooth. (**A** and **B** from Grant, D., and Orban, B.: J. Periodontol. **31:**87, 1960.)

## Systemic factors

Systemic factors refers to a variety of host factors that may interact with local factors (bacteria, calculus) to influence the host-parasite balance and the resulting characteristics of the disease process. The relationship of different microbiotas to different forms of periodontitis is likely associated with different immunologic competencies.[43] At this time it is not clear how the immune response may influence the pathogenesis of periodontitis, that is to what extent it is protective of the host and to what extent it contributes to local tissue destruction.[89]

While genetic influences on the disease process are likely,[90] these factors are probably indirect. For example, the ability of a host to deal with infections may be controlled by genetic factors that influence specific mechanisms of host defense, such as leukocyte function or the ability to respond to bacterial and other antigens.

Pathogenic processes, such as those in diabetes mellitus and neoplastic diseases of the reticuloendothelial system, may influence the course of periodontitis. Individuals with defective immune responses[43] or defects in polymorphonuclear leukocyte functions (diabetes, lazy leukocyte syndrome, agranulocytosis, neutropenia, and Chédiak-Higashi syndrome) are notably susceptible to crestal alveolar bone loss and abscess formation.[91-105] Likewise uncontrolled diabetes mellitus may lead to an increased incidence and severity of periodontitis.[96,106,107]

## DIABETES MELLITUS

Diabetes mellitus includes a number of biochemical and anatomic abnormalities occurring with disturbed glucose utilization because of a pathologic condition in the beta cells (islets of Langerhans) of the pancreas. Diabetes mellitus leads to protein breakdown, degenerative processes, lowered resistance to infection, vascular changes, and an increase in the severity of inflammatory reactions. In turn the increased severity of diabetes when inflammation is present is the result of glucose formed locally at the inflammatory sites from the breakdown of protein and from the liberation of toxic or injurious exudates at these sites. The glucose acts on the liver, raising the level of the blood sugar (gluconeogenesis) and increasing insulin requirements.

Available evidence indicates that adult patients with periodontal disease who are uncontrolled diabetics will show more severe and rapid alveolar bone resorption, and they may incur periodontal abscesses more frequently.[107-118] The clinical appearance will be that of periodontitis (Fig. 16-16), usually indistinguishable from the periodontitis in patients who are not diabetic. The increased host susceptibility to inflammatory periodontal disease should be kept in mind throughout the clinical range of diabetes to include those with prediabetic, subclinical, latent, and overt states. However some poorly controlled or uncontrolled diabetics and juvenile diabetics show greater periodontal disease susceptibility.[106-118]

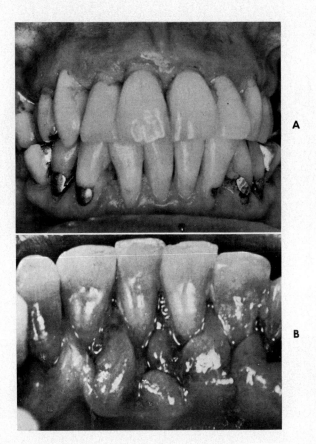

**Fig. 16-16. A,** Periodontitis in a diabetic patient. **B,** Hyperplastic tissue reaction on the oral (lingual) surface of the mandibular incisors in the same patient.

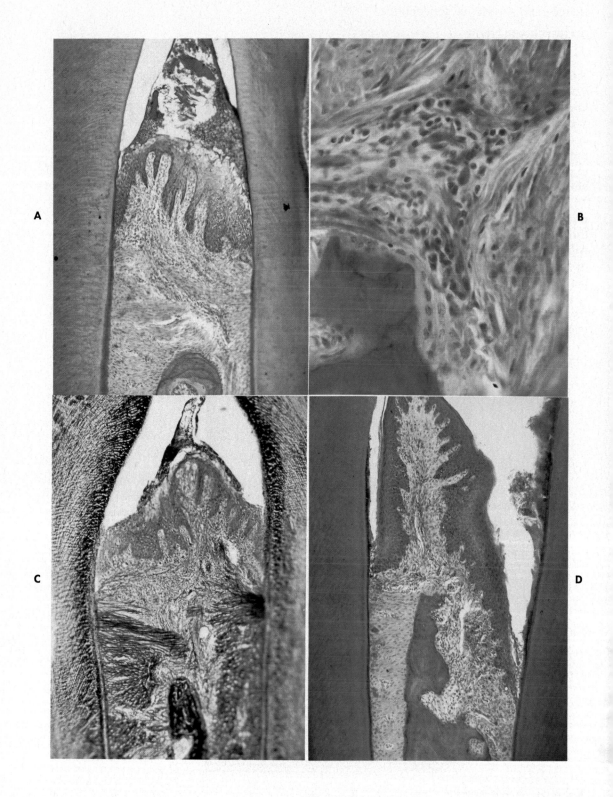

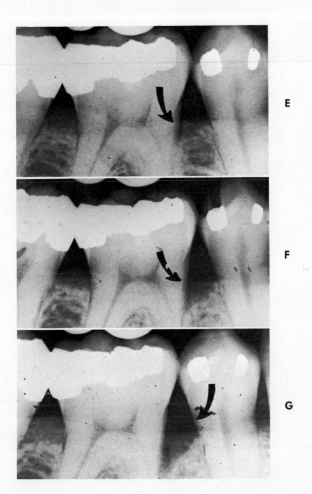

E

F

G

**Plate 6.** **A,** Periodontitis in a marmoset. A vascular bundle with a perivascular inflammatory infiltrate can be seen emerging from the periodontal ligament to course over the alveolar crest into the inflamed lamina propria. **B,** At higher magnification, the vascular bundle and the cellular perivascular infiltrate, with red-staining mast cells included, emerge from the periodontal ligament to course over the bony crest. **C,** In an alternate cut section stained with silver nitrate, the collagenolysis in the lamina propria and the apical inflammatory progression along perivascular pathways can be seen. **D,** If the inflammatory lesion and bone destruction seen in **A** and **C** were to proceed, one could construct the microscopic pathogeneisis of an infrabony pocket. **E** to **G,** Radiographic record of the progression of an infrabony pocket in a human. (**E** to **G** courtesy G. Tussing, Lincoln, Nebraska.)

The susceptibility of juvenile and some adult diabetics to periodontal disease is related to altered host defenses.[94,96,101,110] Phagocytosis is impaired in hyperglycemia and ketoacidosis. Chemotaxis of polymorphonuclear leukocytes is impaired in the absence of insulin.[95]

Vascular changes are prominent in diabetics. Small blood vessels in the gingiva show an increased positive fuchsinophilic reaction in the basement membrane, which may also appear thickened ultrastructurally.[119,120] The walls of small blood vessels are reported to be thickened.[115,119-124] Deep necrotic foci in gingival collagen are also reported (Fig. 16-17).

In general, caution is necessary in the treatment of diabetics. Efforts should be made to reduce emotional stress, especially during surgery. Where necessary, tran-

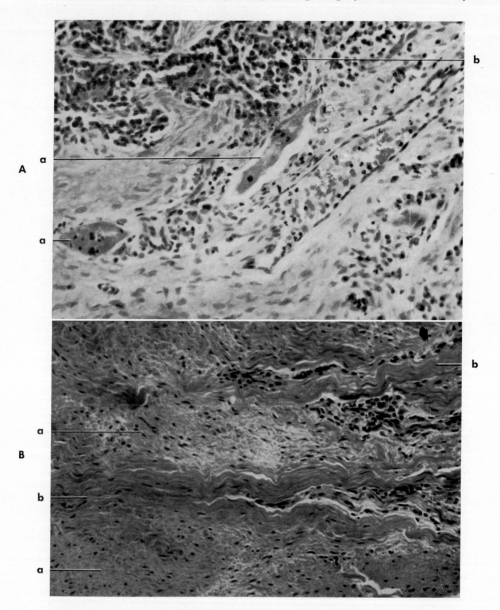

**Fig. 16-17.** **A,** Biopsy of the gingiva of the patient shown in Fig. 16-16. Histologic section shows, *a,* thrombosis of blood vessels and, *b,* chronic inflammatory infiltration. **B,** Biopsy of the gingiva in a diabetic patient with periodontitis. Degeneration of collagen, *a,* is observed between unchanged collagen fiber bundles, *b.*

quilizers or sedatives should be used. Carbohydrate intake is recommended just before appointments; the insulin-dependent patient should be treated before the peak action of the patient's type of insulin is reached. Preoperative and postoperative antibiotics should be prescribed to patients with histories of abscesses or increased susceptibility to infection.

A study of insulin-dependent diabetics has revealed a marked increase in the incidence of periodontitis lesions. When the young patients in the study reached the age of 14, the prevalence of periodontitis increased dramatically during the teens to affect 39% of the adolescents 19 years or older.[110] In addition to the increased susceptibility to periodontitis, the lesions preferentially affected the incisors and first molars in a pattern reminiscent of that seen in juvenile periodontitis (periodontosis) (see Chapter 17).

## DISSEMINATED LESIONS

Disseminated disease is sometimes observed in periodontal tissues. Tuberculosis may have periodontal manifestations. A clinical photograph and roentgenograms of a 26-year-old individual with acute, disseminated, miliary tuberculosis and diabetes are shown in Fig. 16-18. The teeth are extremely mobile. Numerous yellowish pinhead-

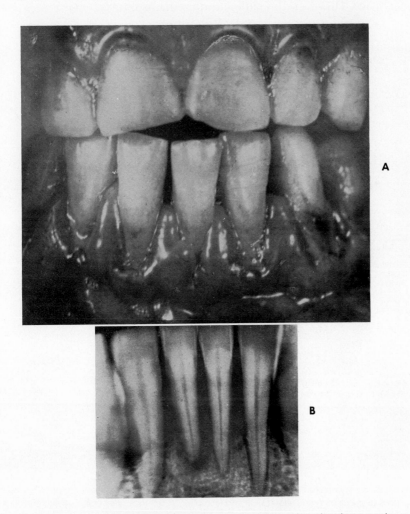

**Fig. 16-18.  A,** Tuberculous periodontitis. **B,** Roentgenogram of the same patient showing extensive resorption of bone.

sized tubercles can be seen on the mucous membranes, including the gingival margin. Some of the teeth have been extracted, and a considerable amount of soft, adherent granulomatous tissue was removed with them. The microscopic examination of this tissue reveals numerous tubercles in the periodontum (Fig. 16-19). The patient died of tuberculosis meningitis. The periodontal condition can be interpreted in part as the oral manifestation of an intrinsic disease.

Leukemic infiltrates frequently lead to marked swelling of the gingival tissues in affected patients as well as localized necrotic lesions that may affect the alveolar bone and periodontal ligament as well.

## ENDOCRINE DYSFUNCTION

In addition other endocrine dysfunctions may influence the pathogenesis of periodontitis by altering the manner in which the host is able to fight infection or repair damages of the periodontal tissues.

Hyperparathyroidism is a rather rare disease that is capable of causing a widening of the periodontal ligament space in addition to causing a disappearance of the lamina dura radiographically. It is not clear, however, that the rate of crestal alveolar bone resorption is increased. In scleroderma, there is a marked widening of the periodontal ligament space. However, the lamina dura remains intact.

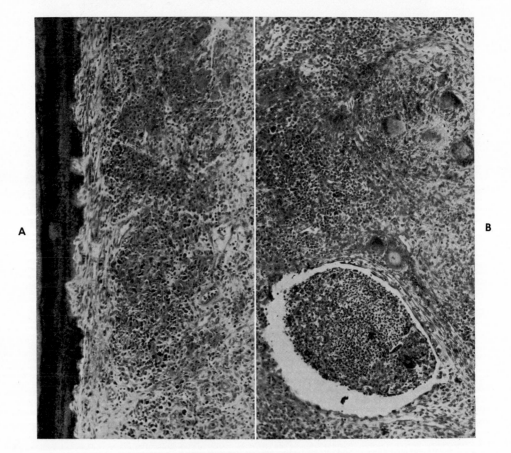

**Fig. 16-19.** **A,** Biopsy of a tooth and surrounding periodontal tissue of the patient shown in Fig. 16-18. Histologic section shows tuberculous granulation tissue and resorption of the root surface. **B,** Tuberculous granulation tissue with giant cells, epithelioid cells, and lymphocytic infiltration.

# Occlusion

The controversial role of occlusion (periodontal trauma) in the progression of periodontitis is discussed in Chapter 24.

# Summary

Periodontitis is an infection resulting in an inflammatory destruction of the periodontal tissues supporting the tooth—namely bone and periodontal ligament. It is preceded and accompanied by gingivitis. Its occurrence is episodic, with prolonged periods of remission interspersed with relatively short periods of exacerbation activity. If left untreated, periodontitis will lead to progressive loss of the supporting structures of the teeth. The rate of loss varies among subjects, types of teeth, and on individual tooth surfaces.

The primary cause of the disease is a bacterial infection produced by one or more of a limited number of microbial species. The tissue alterations are the result of a host-parasite interaction in which host response is unable to prevent the onset and progression of the pathology.

Treatment of periodontitis is aimed at controlling the microbial populations[125] that act as a primary etiologic agent and to encourage the replacement of the pathogenic microbiota with a flora that is compatible with periodontal health. Treatment is also aimed at eliminating the anatomic anomalies that are the result of recurrent episodes of active disease (e.g., pocket depth and loss of attachment) and where possible trying to restore lost periodontal structure. When the disease is treated, the periodontitis can be arrested and the superimposed gingivitis eliminated. The microscopic characteristics of periodontitis may change following treatment and vary with the treatment and with the depth of pockets. Following treatment, the pocket wall in shallow pockets may be almost entirely free of inflammatory cell aggregates and the lamina propria may exhibit dense regular fiber bundles free of inflammation. The gingival surface may be keratinized. In the presence of deeper pockets (5 mm or greater), cornification of the gingival margin may be seen on gingival surfaces accessible to plaque removal (see Fig. 16-13). A zone free of inflammatory cells may be evident directly beneath the oral epithelium. Inflammatory cell aggregates may be evident close to the junctional epithelium and close to the apical border of the sulcular or pocket epithelium. Dense aggregates of inflammatory cells intervene between intact, thick bundles of dentogingival, alveologingival, and transseptal fiber bundles.

The characteristics of periodontitis presented in this chapter should be related to the procedures in examination and diagnosis (Chapter 28).

### REFERENCES

1. Socransky, S.S., et al.: New concepts of destructive periodontal disease, J. Clin. Periodontol. **11:**21, 1984.
2. Goodson, J.M.: Acute exacerbation in chronic periodontal disease, J. Can. Dent. Assoc. **50:**380, 1984.
3. Listgarten, M.A.: A perspective on periodontal diagnosis, J. Clin. Periodontol. **13:**175, 1986.
4. Genco, R.J.: Pathogenesis of periodontal disease: new concepts, J. Can. Dent. Assoc. **50:**391, 1984.
5. Löe, H., et al.: The natural history of periodontal disease in man: the rate of periodontal destruction before 40 years of age, J. Periodontol. **49:**607, 1978.
6. Hirschfeld, L., and Wasserman, B.: A long-term survey of tooth loss in 600 treated periodontal patients, J. Periodontol. **49:**225, 1978.
7. Burmeister, J.A., et al.: Localized juvenile periodontitis and generalized severe periodontitis: clinical findings, J. Clin. Periodontol. **11:**181, 1984.
8. Weinmann, J.P.: Periodontitis: etiology, pathology, symptomatology, J. Am. Dent. Assoc. **44:**701, 1952.
9. Weinmann, J.P.: Progress of gingival inflam-

mation into the supporting structures of the teeth, J. Periodontol. **12:**71, 1941.

10. Toto, P.D. and Gargiulo, A.W.: Epithelial and connective tissue changes in peridonititis, J. Periodontol. **41:**587, 1970.

11. Ritchey, B., and Orban, B.: The periodontal pocket, J. Periodontol. **23:**199, 1952.

12. Grant, D.A., and Orban, B.: Leukocytes in the epithelial attachment, J. Periodontol. **31:**87, 1960.

13. Toto, P.D., Pollock, R.J., and Gargiulo, A.W.: Pathogenesis of periodontitis, Periodontics **2:**197, 1964.

14. Carvel, R.I., and Carr, R.F.: Clinico-pathologic correlation of 385 lesions of marginal destructive periodontitis, J. Periodontol. **53:** 328, 1982.

15. Davenport, R.H., Jr., Simpson, D.M., and Hassell, T.M.: Histometric comparison of active and inactive lesions of advanced periodontitis, J. Periodontol. **53:**285, 1982.

16. Karn, K.W., et al.: Topographic classification of deformities of the alveolar process, J. Periodontol. **55:**336, 1984.

17. Lane, J.J., and O'Neal, R.B.: The relationship between periodontitis and the maxillary sinus, J. Periodontol. **55:**477, 1984.

18. Lindhe, J., Liljenberg, B., and Listgarten, M.: Some microbiological and histopathological features of periodontal disease in man, J. Periodontol. **51:**264, 1980.

19. Waerhaug, J.: The infrabony pocket and its relationship to trauma from occlusion and subgingival plaque, J. Periodontol. **50:**355, 1979.

20. Waerhaug, J.: The furcation problem: etiology, pathogenesis, diagnosis, therapy and prognosis, J. Clin. Periodontol. **7:**73, 1980.

21. Takarada, H., et al.: Ultrastructural studies of human gingiva. I. The upper part of the pocket in chronic periodontitis. J. Periodontol. **45:**30, 1974.

22. Takarada, H., et al.: Ultrastructural studies of human gingiva. II. The lower part of pocket epithelium in chronic periodontitis, J. Periodontol. **45:**155, 1974.

23. Takarada, H., et al.: Ultrastructural studies of human gingiva. III. Changes of the basal lamina in chronic periodontitis, J. Periodontol. **45:**288, 1974.

24. Takarada, H., et al.: Ultrastructural studies of human gingiva. IV. Anchoring fibrils and perforations of the basal lamina in chronic periodontitis, J. Periodontol. **45:**810, 1974.

25. Takarada, J., Cattoni, M., and Rose, G.C.: Ultrastructural studies of human gingiva. V. Microfibrils of elastic nature and their direct penetration of the basal lamina in chronic periodontitis. J. Periodontol. **46:**293, 1975.

26. Kaplan, G.B., Ruben, M.P., and Pameijer, C.H.: Scanning electron microscopy of the periodontal pocket, J. Periodontol. **48:**634, 1977.

27. Müller-Glauser, W., and Schroeder, H.E.: The pocket epithelium: a light and electron-microscopic study, J. Periodontol. **53:**133, 1982.

28. Schroeder, H.E., and Rateitschak-Plüss, E.M.: Focal root resorption lacunae causing retention of subgingival plaque in periodontal pockets, Schweiz. Mschr. Zahnheilk. **93:** 1033, 1983.

29. Page, R.C., and Schroeder, H.E.: Biochemical aspects of connective tissue alterations in inflammatory gingival and periodontal disease, Int. Dent. J. **23:**455, 1973.

30. Glickman, I., Tueresky, S., and Hill R.: Determination of oxygen consumption in normal and inflamed human gingiva using the Waerhaug manometric technique, J. Dent. Res. **28:**83, 1949.

31. Valazza, A., et al.: Correlation between pocket fluid, gingival inflammation, pocket depths and bone loss, Schweiz. Mschr. Zahnheilk. **82:**824, 1972.

32. Genco, R.J., and Cianciola, L.J.: Relationship of the neutrophile to host resistance in periodontal disease, Alpha Omegan **10:**31, 1977.

33. Platt, D., Crosby, R.G., and Dalbow, M.H.: Evidence for the presence of immunoglobulins and circulating antibodies in inflamed periodontal tissues, J. Periodontol. **41:**215, 1970.

34. Brandtzaeg, P., and Kraus, F.W.: Autoimmunity and periodontal disease, Odontol. Tidsk. **73:**285, 1965.

35. Ranney, R.R.: Immunofluorescent localization of soluble dental plaque components in human gingiva affected by periodontitis, J. Periodont. Res. **13:**99, 1978.

36. Seymour, G.J., and Greenspan, J.S.: The phenotypic characterization of lymphocyte subpopulations in established human periodontal disease, J. Periodont. Res. **14:**39, 1979.

37. Van Swol, R.L., et al.: Immunoglobulins in periodontal tissues. II. Concentrations of immunoglobulins in granulation tissue from pockets of periodontosis and periodontitis patients, J. Periodontol. **51:**20, 1980.

38. Schonfeld, S.E., Drury, G.I., and Herles, S.M.: Complement-fixing activity in diseased human gingival tissues, J. Periodont. Res. **16:**574, 1981.

39. Schonfeld, S.E., and Kagan, J.M.: Specificity of gingival plasma cells for bacterial somatic antigens, J. Periodont. Res. **17:**60, 1982.

40. Schroeder, H.E., and Attström, R.: Pocket formation: an hypothesis. In Lehner, T., and Camasoni, G., editors: The borderland between caries and periodontal disease, vol. 2, London, 1980, Academic Press, Inc.

41. Loesche, W.J.: The bacterial etiology of dental decay and periodontal disease: the specific plaque hypothesis, Clin. Dent. **2:**1, 1982.

42. Socransky, S.S.: Microbiology of periodontal disease: present status and future considerations, J. Periodontol. **48:**497, 1977.

43. Genco, R.J., and Slots, J.: Host responses in periodontal diseases, J. Dent. Res. **63:**441, 1984.

44. Soames, J.V., Entwisle, D.N., and Davies, R.M.: The progression of gingivitis to periodontitis in the beagle dog: a histological and morphometric investigation, J. Periodontol. **47:**435, 1976.

45. Lindhe, J., Hamp, S.E., and Löe, H.: Experimental periodontitis in the beagle dog, J. Periodont. Res. **8:**1, 1973.

46. Schroeder, H.E., and Lindhe, J.: Conversion of a stable established gingivitis into periodontitis, Arch Oral Biol. **20:**775, 1975.

47. Akiyoshi, M., and Mori, K.: Marginal periodontitis: a histological study of the incipient stage, J. Periodontol. **38:**45, 1967.

48. Page, R.C., and Schroeder, H.E.: Pathogenesis of inflammatory periodontal disease: a summary of current work, Lab. Invest. **33:**235, 1976.

49. Page, R.C., and Schroeder, H.E.: Periodontitis in man and other animals: a comparative review, Basel, 1982, S. Karger.

50. Evian, C.I., Rosenberg, E.S., and Listgarten, M.A.: Bacterial variability within diseased periodontal sites, J. Periodontol. **53:**595, 1982.

51. Slots, J., and Genco, R.J.: Black-pigmented *Bacteroides* species, *Capnocytophaga* species, and *Actinobacillus actinomycetemcomitans* in human periodontal disease: virulence factors in colonization, survival, and tissue destruction, J. Dent. Res. **63:**412, 1984.

52. Hofstad, T.: Biological activities of endotoxin from *Bacteroides melaninogenicus,* Arch. Oral Biol. **15:**343, 1970.

53. Hausmann, E., Raisz, L.G., and Miller, W.A.: Endotoxin stimulation of bone resorption in tissue culture, Science **168:**862, 1970.

54. Sveen, K., and Skang, N.: Bone resorption stimulated by lipopolysaccharides from *Bacteroides, Fusobacterium,* and *Veillonella,* and by the lipid A and the polysaccharide part of *Fusobacterium* lipopolysaccharide, Scand. J. Dent. Res. **88:**535, 1980.

55. Caton, M.P.L.: Chemistry, structure and availability. In Cuthbert, M.F, editor: The prostaglandins: pharmacological and therapeutic advances, London, 1973, William Heinmann.

56. Dietrich, J.W., Goodson, J.M., and Raisz, L.G.: Stimulation of bone resorption by various prostaglandins in organ culture, Prostaglandins **10:**231, 1975.

57. Ferraris, V.A., et al.: Release of prostaglandins by mitogen—and antigen-stimulated leukocytes in culture, J. Clin. Invest. **54:**378, 1974.

58. Goldhaber, P., et al.: Bone resorption and tissue culture and its relevance to periodontal disease, J. Am. Dent. Assoc. **87:**1027, 1973.

59. Gomes, B., et al.: Prostaglandins: bone resorption stimulating factors released from monkey gingiva, Calcif. Tissue Res. **19:**285, 1976.

60. Goodson, J.M., Dewhirst, F.E., and Brunetti, A.: Prostaglandins $E_2$ levels and human periodontal disease, Prostaglandins **10:**81, 1974.

61. Goodson, J.M., McClatchy, K., and Revell, C.: Prostaglandin-induced resorption of the adult rat calvarium, J. Dent. Res. **53:**670, 1974.

62. Higgs, G.A., McCall, E., and Youlten, L.J.F.: A chemotactic role for prostaglandins released from polymorphonuclear leucocytes during phagocytosis, Br. J. Pharmacol. **53:**539, 1975.

63. Klein, D.C., and Raisz, L.G.: Prostaglandins: stimulation of bone resorption in tissue culture, Endocrinology **86:**436, 1970.

64. Kloeze, J.: Influence of prostaglandins on platelet adhesiveness and platelet aggregation. In Bergstrom, S., and Samuelsson, B., editors: Prostaglandins, Proceedings of the Second Nobel Symposium, London, 1966, Interscience, 1967.

65. Koopman, W.J., Orange, R.P., and Austen, K.F.: Prostaglandin inhibition of the immunologic release of slow reacting substance of anaphylaxis in the rat, Proc. Soc. Exp. Biol. Med. **137:**64, 1971.

66. Löning, T., et al.: Prostaglandin E and the local immune response in chronic periodontal disease: immunohistochemical and radioimmunological observations, J. Periodont. Res. **15:**525, 1980.

67. Mergenhagen, S.: Complement as a mediator of the inflammatory response: interaction of complement with mammalian and bacterial enzymes, J. Dent. Res. **51:**251, 1972.

68. Attström, R., et al.: Complement factors in gingival crevice material from healthy and inflamed gingiva in humans, J. Periodont. Res. **10:**19, 1975.

69. Okada, H., and Silverman, M.S.: Chemotactic activity in periodontal disease. I. The role of complement in monocyte chemotaxis, J. Periodont. Res. **14:**20, 1979.

70. Okada, H., and Silverman, M.S.: Chemotactic activity in periodontal disease. II. The generation of complement-derived chemotactic factors, J. Periodont. Res. **14:**147, 1979.

71. Hock, J., and Nuki, K.: Microvascular response to chronic inflammation in gingiva, Bibl. Anat. **13:**186, 1975.

72. Coleman, E.J., et al.: Mast cells and periodontal disease, J. Periodont. Res. **9:**366, 1974.

73. Frank, R.M., and Voegel, J.C.: Bacterial bone resorption in advanced cases of human periodontitis, J. Periodont. Res. **13:**251, 1978.

74. Frank, R.M.: Bacterial penetration in the api-

cal pocket wall of advanced human periodontitis in humans, J. Periodont. Res. **15:**563, 1980.

75. Saglie, R., et al. Bacterial invasion of gingiva in advanced periodontitis in humans, J. Periodontol. **53:**217, 1982.

76. Saglie, R., et al.: Identification of tissue-invading bacteria in human periodontal disease, J. Periodont. Res. **17:**452, 1982.

77. Manor, A., et al.: Bacterial invasion of periodontal tissues in advanced periodontitis in humans, J. Periodontol. **55:**567, 1984.

78. Sconyers, J.R., Crawford, J.J., and Moriarty, J.D.: Relationship of bacteremia to tooth brushing in patients with periodontitis, J. Am. Dent. Assoc. **87:**616, 1973.

79. Silver, J.G., Martin, A.W., and McBride, B.C.: Experimental transient bacteremias in human subjects with varying degrees of plaque accumulation and gingival inflammation, J. Clin. Periodontol. **4:**92, 1977.

80. Carroll, G.C., and Sebor, R.J.: Dental flossing and its relationship to transient bacteremia, J. Periodontol. **51:**691, 1980.

81. Guntheroth, W.G.: How important are dental procedures as a cause of infective endocarditis? Am. J. Cardiol. **54:**797, 1984.

82. Sanavi, F., et al.: The colonization and establishment of invading bacteria in periodontium of ligature-treated immunosuppressed rats, J. Periodontol. **56:**273, 1985.

83. Page, R.C., et al.: Rapidly progressive periodontitis, a distinct clinical condition, J. Periodontol. **54:**197, 1983.

84. Saari, J.T., Hurt, W.C., and Biggs, N.L.: Periodontal bony defects in the dry skull, J. Periodontol. **39:**278, 1968.

85. Ramirez, J.M., and Hurt, W.C.: Bone remodeling in periodontal lesions, J. Periodontol. **48:**74, 1977.

86. Grant, D.A., and Bernick, S.: Vascularity of crestal bone in periodontally healthy and diseased monkeys, I.A.D.R. Abstract no. 821, J. Dent. Res. **53,** 1974.

87. Attström, R., Graf de Beer, M., and Schroeder, H.E.: Clinical and stereologic characteristics of normal gingiva, J. Periodont. Res. **10:**115, 1975.

88. Gargiulo, A.W., Wentz, F.M., and Orban, B.J.: Dimensions and relations of the dentogingival junction in humans, J. Periodontol. **32:**261, 1961.

89. Taubman, M.A., et al.: Host response in experimental periodontal disease, J. Dent. Res. **63:**455, 1984.

90. Goteiner, D., and Goldman, M.J.: Human lymphocyte antigen haplotype and resistance to periodontitis, J. Periodontol. **55:**155, 1984.

91. Tempel, T.R., et al.: Host factors in periodontal disease: periodontal manifestations of Chédiak-Higashi syndrome, J. Periodont. Res. Suppl. **10:**26, 1972.

92. Lavine, W., Page, R.C., and Padgett, G.A.: The dental and periodontal status of mink and mice affected by Chédiak-Higashi syndrome, J. Periodontol. **47:**621, 1976.

93. Miller, M.E., Oski, F.A., and Harris, M.B.: Lazy-leucocyte syndrome: a new disorder of neutrophil function, Lancet **1:**665, 1971.

94. Gilman, C., Bernstein, J., and van Oss, C.J.: Decreased phagocytosis associated with increased surface hydrophobicity of neutrophils of children with chronic infections, Fed. Proc. **35:**227, 1976.

95. Cianciola, L.J., et al.: Defective polymorphonuclear leukocyte function in a human periodontal disease, Nature **265:**445, 1977.

96. Molenaar, D.M., et al.: Leukocyte chemotaxis in diabetic patients and their nondiabetic first-degree relatives, Diabetes **25:**880, 1976.

97. Kretschmer, R.R., Lopez-Osuna, M., and De la Rosa, L.: Leukocyte function in Down's syndrome: quantitative NBT reduction and bactericidal capacity, Clin. Immunol. Immunopathol. **2:**449, 1974.

98. Bauer, W.H.: The supporting tissues of the tooth in acute secondary agranulocytosis (arsphenamin neutropenia), J. Dent. Res. **25:**501, 1946.

99. Cohen, D.W., and Morris, A.L.: A periodontal manifestation of cyclic neutropenia, J. Periodontol. **32:**159, 1961.

100. Clark, R.A., and Kimball, H.R.: Defective granulocyte chemotaxis in the Chédiak-Higashi Syndrome, J. Clin. Invest. **50:**2645, 1971.

101. Golub, L.M., et al.: In vivo crevicular leukocyte response to a chemotactic challenge: inhibition by experimental diabetes, Infect. Immun. **37:**1013, 1982.

102. Miller, D.R., Lamster, I.B., and Chasens, H.I.: Role of the polymorphonuclear leukocyte in periodontal health and disease, J. Clin. Periodontol. **11:**1, 1984.

103. Vandesteen, G.E., Altman, L.C., and Page, R.C.: Peripheral blood leukocyte abnormalities and periodontal disease: a family study, J. Periodontol. **52:**174, 1981.

104. Lavine, W.S., et al.: Impaired neutrophil chemotaxis in patients with juvenile and rapidly progressing periodontitis, J. Periodont. Res. **14:**10, 1979.

105. Van Dyke, T., et al.: Neutrophil chemotaxis dysfunction in human periodontitis, Infect. Immun. **27:**124, 1980.

106. Benveniste, R., Bixler, D., and Conneally, P.M.: Periodontal disease in diabetics, J. Periodontol. **38:**271, 1967.

107. Belting, C.M., Hinniker, J.J., and Dummett, C.O.: Influence of diabetes mellitus on the severity of periodontal disease, J. Periodontol. **35:**476, 1964.

108. Bernick, S.M., et al.: Dental disease in children with diabetes mellitus, J. Periodontol. **46:**241 1975.

109. Campbell, M.J.A.: Epidemiology of periodontal disease in the diabetic and the non-diabetic, Aust. Dent. J. **17:**274, 1972.

110. Cianciola, L.J., et al.: Prevalence of periodontal disease in insulin-dependent diabetes mellitus (juvenile diabetes), J. Am. Dent. Assoc. **104:**653, 1982.

111. Nichols, C., Laster, L.L., and Bodak-Gyovai, L.Z.: Diabetes mellitus and periodontal disease, J. Periodontol. **49:**85, 1978.

112. Cohen, D.W., et al.: Diabetes mellitus and periodontal disease: two year longitudinal observations. J. Periodontol. **41:**709, 1970.

113. Glavind, L., Lund, B., and Löe, H.: The relationship between periodontal state and diabetes duration, insulin dosage and retinal changes, J. Periodont. Res. **4:**164, 1969.

114. Hove, K.A., and Stallard, R.E.: Diabetes and the periodontal patient, J. Peridontol. **41:**713, 1970.

115. McMullen, J.A., et al.: Microangiopathy within the gingival tissues of diabetic subjects with special reference to the prediabetic state, Periodontics, **5:**61, 1967.

116. Tuckman, M.A., et al.: The relationship of glucose tolerance to periodontal status, J. Periodontol. **41:**27, 1970.

117. Becker. W., Berg, L., and Becker, B.E.: Untreated periodontal disease: a longitudinal study, J. Periodontol. **50:**234, 1979.

118. Sznajder, N., et al.: Periodontal findings in diabetic and non-diabetic patients, J. Periodontol. **49:**445, 1978.

119. Keene, J.J., Jr.: Observations of small blood vessels in human non-diabetic and diabetic gingiva, J. Dent. Res. **48:**967, 1969.

120. McMullen, J., Gottsegen, R., and Camerini-Davalos, R.: PAS fuchsinophilic thickening of small blood vessels in diabetic gingiva due to accumulation in the periendothelial area, J. Periodontol. **5:**61, 1967.

121. Campbell, M.J.A.: An electron microscope study of the basement membrane of the small vessels from the gingival tissue of the diabetic and non-diabetic patient. J. Dent Res. **45:**1302, 1967.

122. Frantzis, T.G., Reeve, C.M., and Brown, J.R.: The ultrastructure of capillary basement membranes in the attached gingiva of diabetic and nondiabetic patients with periodontal disease, J. Periodontol. **42:**406 1971.

123. Listgarten, M.A., et al.: Vascular basement lamina thickness in the normal and inflamed gingiva of diabetics and non-diabletics, J. Periodontol. **45:**676, 1974.

124. Keene, J.J., Jr.: A histochemical evaluation for small vessel calcification in human non-diabetic and diabetic gingiva, J. Dent. Res. **48:**968, 1969.

125. Offenbacher, S. Odle, B., and vanDyke, T.: The microbial morphotypes associated with periodontal health and adult periodontitis: composition and distribution. J. Clin. Periodontol. **12:**736, 1984.

**ADDITIONAL SUGGESTED READING**

Latcham, N.L., et al.: A radiographic study of chronic periodontitis in 15-year-old Queensland children, J. Clin. Periodontol. **10:**37, 1983.

Makris, G.P. and Stoller, N.H.: Rapidly advancing periodontitis in a patient with sarcoidosis: a case report, J. Periodontol. **54:**690, 1983.

Manouchehr-Pour, M., and Bissada, N.: Periodontal disease in juvenile and adult diabetic patients: a review of the literature, J. Am. Dent. Assoc. **107:**766, 1983.

Movin, S.: Relationship between periodontal disease and cirrohosis of the liver in humans, J. Clin. Periodontol. **8:**450, 1981.

Newman, H.N., and Rule, D.C.: Plaque-host imbalance in severe periodontitis: a discussion based on two cases, J. Clin. Periodontol. **10:**137, 1983.

Tew, J.G., et al.: Immunologic studies of young adults with severe periodontitis. II. Cellular factors, J. Periodont. Res. **16:**403, 1981.

# CHAPTER 17

# Early-onset periodontitis

**Juvenile periodontitis**
Clinical features
Microscopic studies
Culture studies
Immunology
Neutrophil dysfunction
Treatment
Prognosis

**Prepubertal periodontitis**

**Rapidly progressive periodontitis**

---

Early-onset periodontitis (EOP) is a general category of periodontal diseases that begin typically in young individuals (children to young adults) and progress rapidly to cause severe loss of the alveolar bone and attachment apparatus. Early onset periodontitis can be subdivided into the following categories:

1. Juvenile periodontitis
2. Prepubertal periodontitis
3. Rapidly progressive periodontitis

These are relatively rare conditions. Of the three types listed, juvenile periodontitis has received the most attention and is the best defined entity.

## Juvenile periodontitis

Juvenile periodontitis (periodontosis) is a relatively rare form of periodontitis[1] characterized by a pattern of rapid vertical loss of alveolar bone around the permanent first molars and incisors. The rapidity and severity of the destruction are not proportional to the mass of plaque or calculus. The disease affects adolescents who otherwise appear healthy. It may be discovered in early adulthood. For practical purposes the clinical distribution of bone loss and age incidence are usually diagnostic.

**History**   Gottlieb[2,3] is credited with the initial description of the disease, which he referred to as diffuse atrophy of the alveolar bone. Wannenmacher[4] was the first to recognize the entity of a rapidly progressing form of periodontitis in young individuals that was characterized by bone loss around incisors and first molars. He named it *Paradentose* (paradontosis). Other early descriptions by Miller[5] and by Thoma and Goldman[6] appeared, and Orban and Weinmann[7] introduced the term *periodontosis*.

Periodontosis is described by Baer[8] as a disease of the periodontium that occurs in an otherwise healthy adolescent. It is characterized by a rapid loss of alveolar bone surrounding more than one tooth of the permanent dentition, little plaque, and little or no clinical inflammation. In the *localized* form the only teeth affected are the permanent first molars and incisors. In the *generalized* form, other teeth can also be affected. In recent years periodontosis has been referred to as *juvenile periodontitis*.[9]

## CLINICAL FEATURES

Juvenile periodontitis is rarely diagnosed in its incipiency when there are few signs and symptoms. Early diagnosis is sometimes made fortuitously on examination of routine oral roentgenograms. In these cases the gingiva is largely free of gross clinical signs of inflammation. Late clinical features of the disease are migration of teeth, with the formation of diastemata, and elongation of teeth. By the time the patient seeks help deep pockets are usually present.

Several distinctive features of this disease justify its classification as a discrete clinical entity separate from adult periodontitis[8]:

1. Age at onset
2. Sex ratio
3. Familial tendency
4. Lack of commensurate relationship between local (extrinsic) etiologic factors and severity of response (severe periodontal destruction)
5. Distinctive roentgenographic pattern of alveolar bone loss (Figs. 17-1 to 17-3)
6. Rate of progression
7. Microbiologic characteristics
8. Immunologic characteristics

## Onset

The onset of juvenile periodontitis is insidious and generally is first detected during the circumpubertal period, between the ages of 11 and 13 years. The alveolar bone appears to develop normally, with normal eruption of teeth. Subsequent to eruption, the bone undergoes resorptive changes (Fig. 17-3). Thus the alveolar bone loss does not seem to be the result of a developmental or congenital defect of the periodontal tissues.

The most striking feature of early juvenile periodontitis is the lack of clinical inflammation. Pocket formation, together with mobility and migration, about the incisors and first molars occurs later. Gingivitis may develop later.

Other symptoms of periodontal disease may arise. Root surfaces may become sensitive to thermal and tactile stimuli. Dull, radiating pain resulting from the mobility of

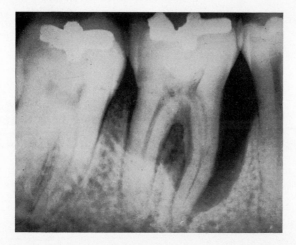

**Fig. 17-1.** Vertical type of bone resorption in juvenile periodontitis.

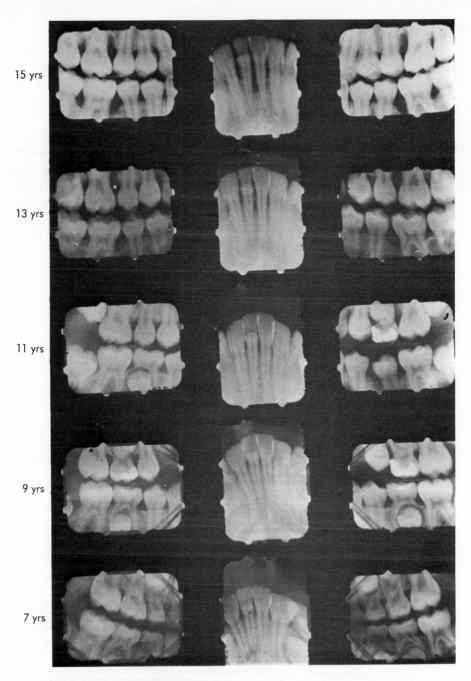

**Fig. 17-2.** The development of bone-destructive lesions of juvenile periodontitis in a girl between the ages of 7 and 15 years can be followed in the roentgenograms. (Courtesy G. Tussing, Lincoln, Nebraska.)

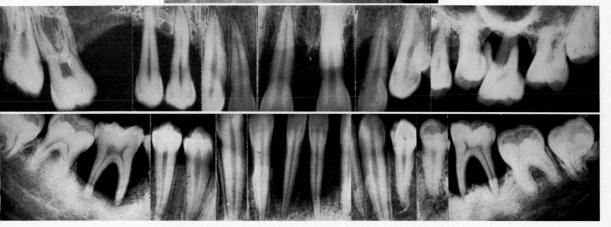

A

B

**Fig. 17-3.** Juvenile periodontitis in a 17-year-old girl. Note the migration of the teeth, the opening of diastemata, and the relative lack of plaque and calcified deposits. **B,** Roentgenograms of the same patient showing extensive bone destruction characteristic of localized juvenile periodontitis, which affects the first molars, incisors, and other teeth.

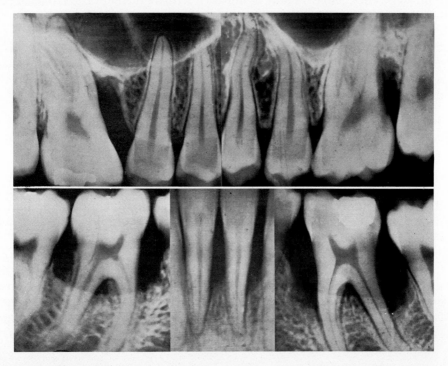

**Fig. 17-4.** Roentgenograms of the teeth of a 15-year-old girl. Extensive vertical bone resorption has occurred in the region of the mandibular first molars and incisors. (Courtesy C.L. Foss, San Diego, California.)

teeth and the impaction of food may occur during mastication. Periodontal abscesses may form. A high incidence of regional lymph node enlargement in affected individuals has been reported.[10]

## Epidemiology

**Incidence**

The prevalence of the disease has been reported to be between 0.1% and 15%, depending on the stringency of diagnostic criteria. It occurs less frequently in Scandinavia[11,12] than in the Mediterranean countries or the Far East.[13-15] In the United States it is more prevalent in blacks than in whites.[16,17]

The prevalence in the United States among whites is in excess of 0.1%. Among Native Americans the prevalence is higher.[8,18] Differences in prevalence may exist in other countries' populations.[11,12,15,19]

The variation in the reported prevalence[9] may be the result of errors in differentiation between adult and juvenile periodontitis. Despite this lack of uniformity certain patterns can be noted, and the prevalence in developed nations is probably less than 1% and in underdeveloped regions, in the range of 5%.[1,14,15]

**Sex ratio**

It has been reported that juvenile periodontitis affects three times as many females as males. Some report cases in both males and females,[19-22] while others report a primarily female distribution.[15] The sex ratio may be variable depending on age, with females predominating in the early teens and a ratio approaching equality in later years.

**Familial tendencies**

There are familial tendencies in juvenile periodontitis,[18] usually following the maternal side of the line.

## Genetics

The relatively few direct genetic analyses of juvenile periodontitis classify the disease into familial patterns and consanguinity determinations,[23,24] possibly involving HL-A antigens[25,26] and ABO blood groups.[25-29] The disease may be inherited as an X-linked, dominant trait[30] or as an autosomal recessive trait.[24,31,32]

The familial pattern of incidence suggests the possibility of (1) genetic predispositions to infection by specific groups of bacteria, (2) a genetically determined immunodeficiency, and (3) faulty or impaired formation and maintenance of periodontal tissue integrity.

The likelihood of a genetic component in the pathogenesis of juvenile periodontitis does not imply that the disease is necessarily of a congenital nature. The familial occurrence may be linked to a transmissible microbial agent. The acquisition of this agent and its ability to injure the host may be genetically modulated via specific differences in host defense mechanisms.

## Severity

The rapidity and severity of the disease process seem out of proportion to the intensity of the local factors.

Contrary to what occurs with intrinsic diseases (e.g., Down syndrome, cyclic neutropenia, hypophosphatasia, Papillon-Lefèvre syndrome), where the primary as well as the permanent dentitions are affected, in juvenile periodontitis the primary teeth are not affected and are not prematurely exfoliated. This disease seems to be entirely of the permanent dentition (Fig. 17-4).

**Roentgenographic findings**

The roentgenograms may show a cupped-out defect in the alveolar bone extending from the distal surface of the second bicuspid to the mesial surface of the second molar. This bone loss occurs bilaterally, and the two sides are generally mirror images of each other (Figs. 17-4 to 17-7). In some instances only the first molars are involved. Generally, the mesial surface has the bone loss, but in some cases the distal surface is involved. The degree and morphology of the bone loss generally depend on the stage

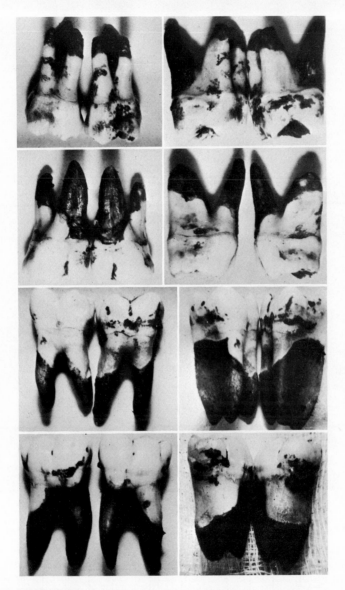

**Fig. 17-5.**   Stained extracted teeth from two patients with juvenile periodontitis exhibiting a mirror-image pathologic condition. (From Kaslick, R.S., and Chasens, A.I.: Oral Surg. **25:**327, 1968.)

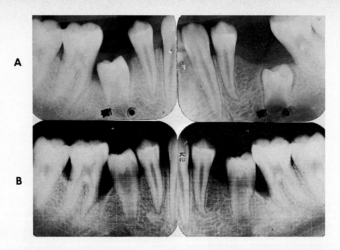

**Fig. 17-6. A,** Roentgenograms (June 1967) of a 14-year-old girl with juvenile periodontitis. (Black marks are artifacts.) Note the bilateral bone loss at the mesial aspect of the first molar before eruption of the second premolar. **B,** Same patient, May 1969. The defects now appear as typical vertical alveolar resorptions. No bone was lost in the area during the time between the two roentgenograms. Rather, new bone was added through the eruption of the second premolar.

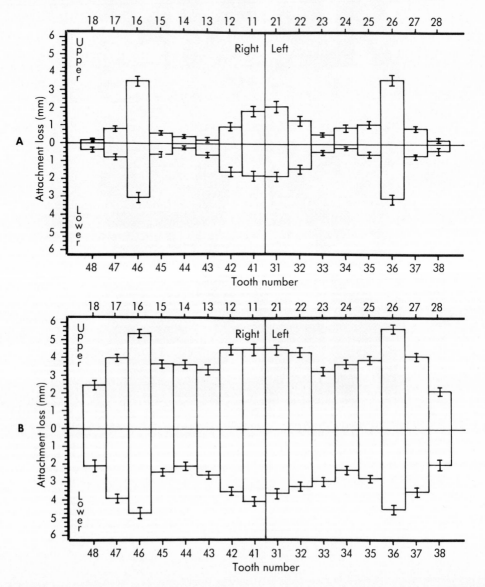

**Fig. 17-7. A,** Distribution of periodontal attachment loss in subjects with localized juvenile periodontitis as compared with, **B,** severe, more generalized periodontitis. In both groups incisors and first molars tend to be the most severely affected teeth. (From Burmeister, J.A., et al.: J. Clin. Periodontol. **11:**181, 1984, Munksgaard Int.)

of the disease at the time of diagnosis (early or advanced). Only the proximal surface of one first molar may be involved initially. As the disease progresses other molars may become affected. Since the buccal and lingual or palatal plates of alveolar bone are the last to resorb, the furcations of the molar teeth become involved as a later manifestation of the disease (see Fig. 17-3).

As the disease progresses the proximal contact areas of the first molars and incisors tend to open. Later, in addition to the formation of diastemata, rotation and elongation of individual teeth take place. Classically, there is a lateral and labial migration of the maxillary incisors with formation of diastemata (see Fig. 17-3). The lower incisors have less tendency to migrate. Occlusal patterns and tongue pressures influence the amount and type of migration noted. At this stage there is an apparent increase in size of the clinical crown, accumulation of plaque and calculus, and clinical inflammation.[33] In some cases, slender or short roots complicate the pathogenetic outcome. Enamel hypoplasia concurrent with the disease has been reported.[34]

### Distribution

It has been suggested that the bilateral and symmetric pattern of bone loss (Fig. 17-5) results from a genetically determined developmental defect. At one time the symmetric pattern was thought to be related to a genetic factor or to occlusal trauma. The disease was classified as degenerative since it seemed to lack a microbial etiology. Juvenile periodontitis is no longer considered to be a "degenerative" disease. Its development appears to be closely related to the acquisition of the microbial pathogen *Actinobacillus actinomycetemcomitans*, which is typically observed in subjects who exhibit defective neutrophil functions. The symmetric distribution of bone loss may be related to the eruption pattern of the affected teeth and consequently to the tooth surfaces that are available to colonization by the microbial pathogens if and when these are acquired by the host. The existence of a preexisting microbial population on erupted teeth may interfere with colonization of these surfaces by a newly acquired pathogen. Furthermore, prepubertal alterations in the host of an undefined nature may be needed for the establishment of the microbial pathogen. Thus the symmetric distribution of lesions on incisors and first molars may be related to specific events that make it possible for *A. actinomycetemcomitans* to colonize these teeth at a time when they erupt into the oral cavity. The predilection of lesions for mesial surfaces of the first molars may be caused by the absence of a protective (plaque-retentive) embrasure on the distal surface of the first molars for several years following their eruption. The microbiology of juvenile periodontitis will be discussed later. Since a multiplicity of factors may cause breakdown about a single tooth, roentgenographic findings of bone loss about a single tooth are not considered to be evidence of juvenile periodontitis.

The development of elevated antibody titers to *A. actinomycetemcomitans* in the serum of affected subjects may serve to protect the host, at least partially, against further tooth colonization and further tissue destruction.

The rate of tissue destruction in older subjects (ages 22 to 29 years) is slower than in younger subjects (ages 14 to 21 years). It has been suggested that only the younger patients should be classified as having juvenile periodontitis and that older subjects should be categorized as a "post-juvenile periodontitis" group.[10]

### Rate of bone destruction

Unlike adult periodontitis, which progresses at a slow rate, juvenile periodontitis progresses rapidly. The present available roentgenographic evidence indicates that an affected tooth can lose approximately three fourths of its alveolar bone around one or more of the involved root surfaces in a 5-year period or less. This is at least three to four times the rate of progression for adult periodontitis.[35]

A generalized form of periodontitis may occur in juveniles.[10] The disease process may affect most of the dentition instead of the molars and incisors (the localized form of the disease). It has been suggested that the generalized form of the disease is different from the localized form[33,36,37] although this view is not universal.[22]

**"Burn out"**

Sometimes sudden and unexplainable decreases in the rate of bone destruction occur, generally when the patient is in the middle and late twenties. Arrests of this kind have been referred to as "burn out."[38] These sudden remissions in the course of the disease may represent an altered host-parasite interaction.

**Other conditions**

Other specific conditions may produce clinical and histopathologic signs similar to those seen in juvenile periodontitis. These include faulty cementum, occlusal trauma, and local hemangiomas.[39]

Other systemic diseases and syndromes that have been related to juvenile periodontitis include cyclic neutropenia,[40-43] lazy leukocyte syndrome.[44] Chédiak-Higashi syndrome,[45] Papillon-Lefèvre syndrome,[46-49] Down syndrome,[50] diabetes mellitus,[51] gout, hypophosphatasia,[52] hypothyroidism,[53] and subclinical hypoadrenocorticoidism.[53,54] Some of these conditions are associated with *prepubertal periodontitis* and *rapidly progressive periodontitis* (see later discussion).

Despite the potential influence of systemic factors, most cases of juvenile periodontitis do not involve conditions readily detectable on routine medical laboratory tests.

**Case reports**

A typical case is of a 17-year-old girl (see Fig. 17-3). Wide diastemata suddenly appeared between the incisors. The roentgenograms (see Fig. 17-3, *B*) reveal severe bone loss, especially in the region of the incisors and first molars. One first molar was lost a week before the consultation. Medical history was noncontributory, and standard laboratory testing failed to reveal any pertinent systemic factors.

A similar but less extensive case in a 15-year-old girl is shown in the roentgenograms in Fig. 17-4. Resorption of bone is limited to the four first molars and to two mandibular incisors. The medical history was noncontributory. In neither of these cases were the patients tested for polymorphonuclear cell dysfunction, which is now known to be present in 70% of affected patients.

## MICROSCOPIC STUDIES

Light and electron microscopic observation of extracted teeth from patients diagnosed as having juvenile periodontitis reveals a minimum amount of attached bacterial plaque on the tooth surface near the apical portions of the pockets[21,55,56] (Fig. 17-8). When the plaque is attached to the tooth surface, it is usually located close to the cementoenamel junction. In addition, fewer morphologic forms are seen. Comparison can be made with the microbiota associated with gingivitis or periodontitis in which the plaque is complex, heterogeneous, and at least a portion appears to be firmly attached to the tooth surface. Organisms in the apical region of the lesions have cell wall structures consistent with those described for gram-negative organisms as determined by electron microscopy. In addition, an unusual cuticle-like structure may be present on the cemental surface of some involved teeth[55] (Fig. 17-9). The origin, composition, and significance of this structure are unclear at the present time.

The distribution of bacterial morphotypes in the pockets of patients with juvenile periodontitis, post-juvenile periodontitis, and adult periodontitis has been examined by means of differential dark-field microscopy.[57] A marked difference was noted between the flora of juvenile periodontitis, which consists primarily of coccoid cells and nonmotile rods, and the microbiota of adult and post-juvenile periodontitis, which consists of a large proportion of spirochetes and motile rods. These results confirm some earlier reports that were based on sectioned material but differ from other reports,[58] that nonetheless note major populations of spirochetes and motile rods.

The prevalence of *A. actinomycetemcomitans* as well as its proportion in the cultivable microbiota is substantially greater in juvenile periodontitis than in other periodontal conditions.[59-62] The data are compatible with the assessment of serum antibody levels to *A. actinomycetemcomitans* as reported in Table 17-2. Occasionally, high proportions of *A. actinomycetemcomitans* are also recovered in other conditions, such as rapidly progressive periodontitis in adults, prepubertal periodontitis, and juvenile diabetic periodontitis, an observation that suggests the involvement of this microorganism in more than one form of periodontal disease.[60,63-65]

It is conceivable that other microorganisms may participate as causative agents of juvenile periodontitis, although not as commonly as *A. actinomycetemcomitans*. Six of seven affected children in a single family were found to be infected with *Bacteroides gingivalis*, a microorganism more commonly associated with severe forms of periodontitis in adults.[63,66]

The presence of gram-negative bacteria has been described in the soft tissues adjacent to periodontal pockets in patients with juvenile periodontitis.[67,68] In contrast to similar reports in patients with adult periodontitis, the microorganisms often appeared in clusters of morphologically similar bacteria, suggesting that the organisms may be proliferating within the tissues. Thus there is some support for the assertion that bacterial invasion is a feature of the disease and that the presence of bacteria in these tissues is not merely the result of tissue manipulations that have introduced bacteria into the tissues.[69] *A. actinomycetemcomitans* is well suited to evade host defense mechanisms.[70] It is able to inhibit neutrophil chemotaxis,[71,72] use its leukotoxin to kill neutrophils and monocytes,[73-77] and resist the bactericidal activity of complement-activated serum.[78] It can cause tissue damage by inhibiting fibroblast activity[79,80] and by producing endotoxin,[81] collagenase,[82] and a bone-resorbing factor.[83,84] It may also act to inhibit the proliferation of stimulated lymphocytes, a key step in immune defense mechanisms.[85,86]

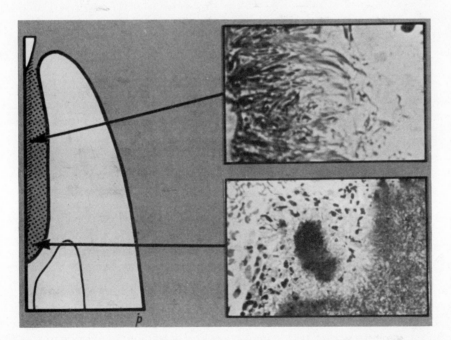

**Fig. 17-8.** Periodontosis. Artist's conception of lesion of juvenile periodontitis with approximate proportion of adherent *(diagonal lines* in sulcus adjacent to tooth) versus loosely adherent plaque *(dots)*. Histologic sections of plaque demonstrate the sparsely colonized tooth surface. The unattached plaque is surrounded by polymorphonuclear leukocytes from the adjacent soft tissue. (From Newman, M.G., et al.: J. Periodontol. **47:**377, 1976.)

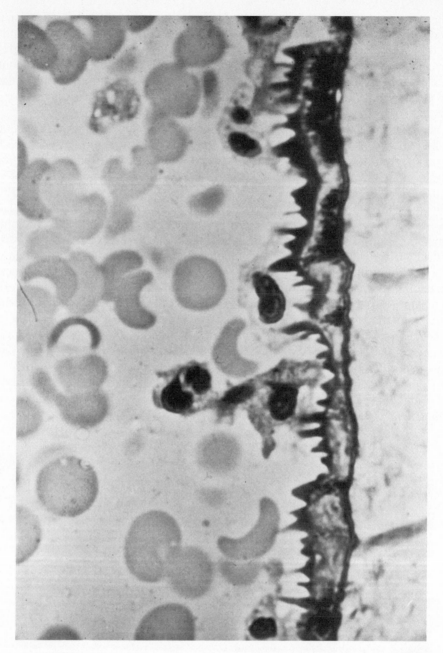

**Fig. 17-9.** Lobulated cuticle of amorphous material covering the root surface of a tooth with localized juvenile periodontitis.

## CULTURE STUDIES

Early studies of juvenile periodontitis[21,87] revealed the presence of various gram-negative rods, many of which belonged to the *Capnocytophaga*[88] and *Actinobacillus* species.[59,89] *Actinobacillus actinomycetemcomitans* was of particular interest because of its ability to cause severe periodontal bone loss in monoinfected rats, primarily by stimulating osteoclastic activity.[90] In vitro studies of the purified cell wall components of *A. actinomycetemcomitans* indicated that membranous vesicles[91,92] shed from the outer layer of the cell wall contained several biologically active components including endotoxin,[81,83,84,92] a bone-resorbing factor,[83] and a leukotoxic substance.[73,74,93] The leu-

**Table 17-1**    Prevalence of *A. actinomycetemcomitans* in human periodontal disease

| Patient group | Slots et al.[59] (1980) | Mandell & Socransky[61] (1981) | Mashimo et al.[115] (1983) | Zambon et al.[60] (1983) | Eisenmann et al.[62] (1983) |
|---|---|---|---|---|---|
| Normal juveniles | 2/10* | | | | |
| Localized juvenile periodontitis | 9/10 | 6/6 | | 28/29 | 12/12 |
| Diabetic juveniles | | | 3/14 | 5/98 | |
| Normal adults | 4/11 | | | 24/142 | |
| Adult gingivitis and periodontitis | 6/12 | 0/48 | | 28/134 | 6/10 |

From Zambon, J.J.: *Actinobacillus actinomycetemcomitans* in human periodontal disease, J. Clin. Periodontol. **12:**1, 1985, Munksgaard Int.
*Number of subjects with cultivable *A. actinomycetemcomitans*/total number examined.

**Table 17-2**    Proportions of periodontal patient groups with significantly elevated serum antibody titers to *A. actinomycetemcomitans*

| Patient group | Genco et al.[95] (1980)* | Ebersole et al.[98] (1982)† | Ranney et al.[100] (1982)* |
|---|---|---|---|
| Normal | 10% | 13% | 3% |
| Localized juvenile periodontitis | 69% | 90% | 77% |
| Generalized juvenile periodontitis | 25% | 54% | |
| Adult periodontitis | 15% | 26% | |
| Severe periodontitis | | | 40% |

From Zambon, J.J.: *Actinobacillus actinomycetemcomitans* in human periodontal disease, J. Clin. Periodontol. **12:**1, 1985, Munksgaard Int.
*Precipitating antibody to *A. actinomycetemcomitans* measured in agarose gel diffusion.
†Enzyme-linked immunosorbent assays of serum IgG.

kotoxin was found to be active against human monocytes[75] as well as polymorphonuclear leukocytes. Not all strains of *A. actinomycetemcomitans* are leukotoxic.[59,76] Currently, the species can be subdivided into three serotypes and ten biotypes.[59,60] This subdivision has been of particular value in confirming the intrafamilial spread of the organism since members of the same family tend to harbor the same biotype and serotype.[60] The finding also suggests that the organism is not readily transmissible and that close and repeated contact is necessary for infection.

The prevalence of *A. actinomycetemcomitans* in juvenile periodontitis as compared to other forms of periodontal disease is shown in Table 17-1.

## IMMUNOLOGY

Until recently there were few systematic reports directly concerned with the immunologic aspects of juvenile periodontitis. Cell-mediated and humoral immunologic investigations[94] were carried out in 23 patients diagnosed as having juvenile periodontitis. Patients with juvenile periodontitis had significantly increased concentrations of serum IgG, IgM, and IgA as compared with matched controls. The level of IgM was elevated to a relatively greater extent than that of IgG and IgA. It was postulated that the increase in IgM might reflect a recent response to gram-negative organisms. Whether the immunoglobulin response is induced by bacteria "causing" the disease or by microorganisms inhabiting the lesion sites subsequent to bone loss is not clear. In the study cited, lymphocytes from patients with juvenile periodontitis failed to respond to plaque and selected gram-negative bacteria (transform) in spite of intact macrophage migration inhibition. These and other findings led to the hypothesis of a selective cell-mediated immunodeficiency resulting in an abnormal defense reaction to specific bacteria.[94-95]

Significantly more patients with juvenile periodontitis (Table 17-2) exhibit detectable serum antibody levels to *A. actinomycetemcomitans,* and those levels tend to be higher in patients with juvenile periodontitis than in others (Table 17-3).[96-99]

Elevated antibody levels to three leukotoxic strains in patients with juvenile periodontitis have been reported[96] but not to a strain without leukotoxin activity. Leukotoxin-neutralizing activity in the serum of affected patients has been reported.[97] This activity was detected in 94% of patients with juvenile periodontitis. Other sera had an opposite effect, tending to enhance the leukotoxic effect. These findings suggest that leukotoxic strains may play a more important role in the active disease phase than nonleukotoxic strains.

## NEUTROPHIL DYSFUNCTION

Although neutrophils may be affected by bacterial products,[71,72] several reports have indicated that patients with juvenile periodontitis frequently exhibit intrinsic neutrophil dysfunctions, which affect chemotaxis primarily and phagocytosis to a lesser extent.[100-105] Monocytes may occasionally be affected as well.[104] The defect does not depend on serum for its expression, nor does it disappear after the lesions are treated.

Diagnostic tests based on microbiology, immunology, and neutrophil function of patients with juvenile periodontitis are still being developed. It is likely that in the next few years tests will become available that will provide the clinician with an added measure of reliability in the diagnosis and treatment of this condition.

## TREATMENT

The prognosis of juvenile periodontitis has been guarded.[106] However, recent studies suggest that the 5-year prognosis can be quite good.[107]

The efficacy of various treatments to eradicate the defects of the disease as well as prevent colonization by *A. actinomycetemcomitans* has been studied.[108] Scaling and root planing alone, with or without subgingival iodine irrigation, failed to influence the infection. The surgical treatment of the lesions was considerably more effective in eliminating *A. actinomycetemcomitans,* reducing the number of infected sites by 50%.[109] A 14-day course of tetracycline (1 gm/day intraorally) eliminated *A. actinomycetemcomitans* for a period of approximately 6 months.[108]

Successful results in the treatment of 16 patients with juvenile periodontitis followed for a 5-year period have been reported.[107] The patients, ranging in age from 14 to 18 years, were treated in parallel with 12 patients with adult periodontitis, ranging in age from 39 to 48 years. The treatment included surgical débridement of the defects, a 14-day course of systemic tetracycline (1 gm/day), 0.2% chlorhexidine oral rinses daily for 2 weeks, and professional prophylaxis monthly for the first 6 months and every 3 months thereafter. Good healing was observed in both groups of patients. However recurrent lesions developed at six sites in four subjects with juvenile periodontitis during the first 12-month period. After the sites were retreated, they healed

**Table 17-3** Relative serum antibody levels to *A. actinomycetemcomitans* in various subject groups

| Subject group | Listgarten et al.[96] (1981)* | Ebersole et al.[98] (1982)† |
|---|---|---|
| Localized juvenile periodontitis | 64 | 280 |
| Healthy periodontium/mild gingivitis | 1 | 12 |
| Adult periodontitis | 4 | 60 |

*Immunofluorescent antibody technique of serum IgG.
†Enzyme-linked immunosorbent assay of serum IgG.

well without further recurrence of disease. The results indicate that the prognosis for juvenile periodontitis lesions may be as good as that for adult periodontitis lesions. Ongoing studies are examining the need for tetracycline treatment if the lesions are treated surgically. Preliminary results indicate that surgical treatment alone is almost as effective in controlling the disease as surgery combined with tetracycline therapy.[110]

Although occlusal therapy may be indicated where occlusal disharmonies coexist with the disease,[106] routine treatment of the occlusion is not presently accepted. No evidence is available to show occlusal therapy in conjunction with mechanical débridement improves the results achieved by débridement alone (Figs. 17-10 and 17-11).

When juvenile periodontitis is diagnosed, it is often not known just when the bony changes have taken place; perhaps the disease is in a state of remission and the changes have been present for years. To assess the acuteness of the disease, examination of

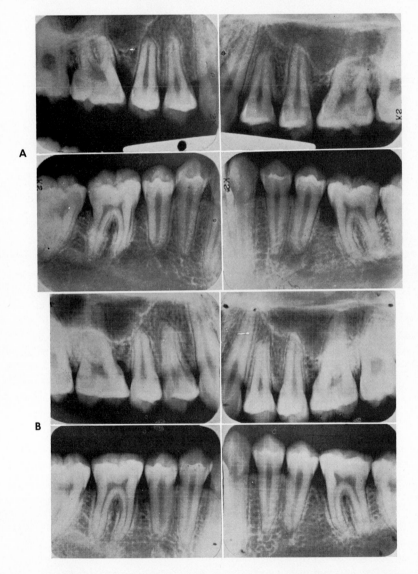

**Fig. 17-10.** Juvenile periodontitis in a 15-year-old girl. Roentgenograms show loss of bone on the mesial aspects of the four first molars. **B,** Roentgenograms taken a year later show considerable improvement in all but the lower right first molar, where the bone defect has remained more or less stable. Note the flattened molars, treated by shortening with occlusal grinding to enhance tooth eruption.

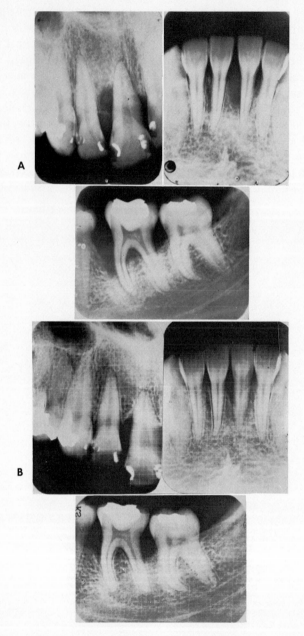

**Fig. 17-11.**  Juvenile periodontitis in a 19-year-old girl. A diastema is present on the lower left between the second premolar and the first molar, and another between the lower central incisors. **B,** Roentgenograms taken of the same area 3 years later. Note the spontaneous closure of the diastemata and the greatly improved appearance of the alveolar bone. The occlusal contour in the treated molars is flattened; they had been ground to promote tooth eruption. There has been not only bone apposition but also increased trabeculation.

older roentgenograms is helpful (see Fig. 17-6). When the destruction is advanced, the involved tooth may have to be sacrificed.

Following are various courses of treatment:

1. When loss of support has rendered restoration hopeless, extraction may be necessary. After extraction, healing and bone regeneration within the alveolus occur, and there may be no further evidence of the disease.
2. Tooth transplantation has also been used successfully (Fig. 17-12).

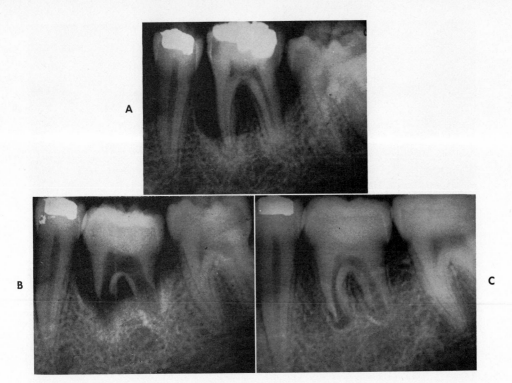

**Fig. 17-12.    A,** Preoperative view (July 1964). **B,** Third molar autotransplanted into first molar site (August 1964). **C,** Eighteen months after transplantation (February 1966). (Courtesy P.N. Baer, Stoney Brook, New York, and J.W. Gamble, Shreveport, Louisiana.)

3. Another approach involves variations of standard periodontal treatment, ranging from scaling and curettage supplemented with antibiotic therapy to surgical intervention (Figure 17-13). Success seems to depend on the level of destruction; less advanced lesions have a better prognosis (see Fig. 17-6). Good results have been reported with the use of autogenous marrow–cancellous bone autografts around involved teeth.[111].

4. Root amputation and hemisection in applicable cases of partly involved molars may be indicated.

5. Fixed splinting and orthodontic measures may be important for the aesthetic appearance of the patient and to prevent secondary occlusal trauma.[112] If occlusal traumatism is present, adjustment by selective grinding may be performed. Systematic and repeated grinding of the occlusal surfaces to permit the involved tooth to erupt is sometimes beneficial[113] (see Figs. 17-10 and 17-11).

Tooth transplantation has been tried by various investigators (Fig. 17-12) as a means of replacing first molars in particular. In transplantation the tooth is extracted, and the socket is prepared to receive the third molar germ.[111,114] The third molar germ is removed and transplanted to the first molar alveolus. The right time for this operation is the time when the bifurcation of the third molar germ has just formed. In the operative procedure the bony septum separating the roots of the first molar should be removed, and the transplanted tooth germ should be embedded in its new socket below the plane of occlusion; the flap is then sutured in place.

A few words of caution should be added about the rare occurrence of juvenile periodontitis during routine orthodontic therapy. Orthodontists who take a full-mouth roentgenogram when they begin treatment would be well advised to continue such complete surveys at regular intervals to avoid overlooking a developing juvenile periodontitis. It is next to impossible for the periodontist to convince parents that the

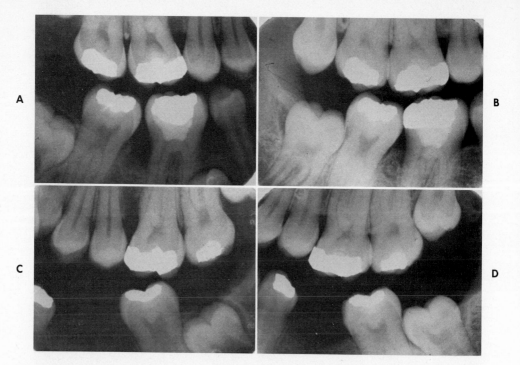

**Fig. 17-13.** Roentgenograms of a 15-year-old patient with juvenile periodontitis, before and after treatment. **A,** Moderate lesion around mandibular first molar and mesial surface of maxillary first molar. **B,** Demonstration of bone regeneration 4 years after treatment. **C** and **D,** Similar findings in patient's other maxillary first molar. Patient was treated by thorough root planing with access obtained through flap procedures and, at the time of surgery only, systemic administration of antibiotics.

destruction of periodontitis has occurred entirely independent of the orthodontic treatment.

## PROGNOSIS

It is now evident that, like most forms of periodontitis, juvenile periodontitis is an *infectious disease*. The association of *Actinobacillus actinomycetemcomitans* with the disease, the pathogenic potential of the organism, the immunologic response of the host to it, and its frequent disappearance after successful treatment strongly suggest that *A. actinomycetemcomitans* plays a key role in the etiology of the disease.

Although genetic influences on host defenses may modulate the interaction of this microorganism with the host, therapy directed at the elimination of this organism appears to be predictably successful. Surgical therapy with or without tetracycline coverage appears to offer the best approach to the control of this form of periodontal disease.

It is likely that in the next few years rapid tests for detecting the presence of *A. actinomycetemcomitans* will be developed and become available as a supplemental diagnostic tool for the therapist to permit monitoring this bacterium during and after active therapy.

## Prepubertal periodontitis

Prepubertal periodontitis (PPP)[37] occurs both in a *generalized* as well as a *localized* form.

*Generalized PPP* is a rare condition that affects both the primary and secondary dentition. It begins with the eruption of the primary teeth. The surrounding gingival tissues become markedly inflamed and bone loss follows. The teeth become loose and are lost in rapid succession.

The patients generally exhibit polymorphonuclear leukocyte *and* mononuclear leukocyte defects. They are frequently subject to other infections such as otitis media and upper respiratory infections. Treatment with or without antibiotics does not appear to have much impact on the progression of the disease.

*Localized PPP* is generally localized to only some of the primary teeth. Inflammation is less pronounced than in the generalized form. Leukocyte defects may involve either polymorphonuclear leukocytes *or* mononuclear cells, but not both. The rate of tissue destruction is less rapid than in the generalized form. The patients respond well to mechanical débridement coupled with antimicrobial therapy. Penicillin or erythromycin appear to be the drugs of choice. They are given in dosages of 250 mg q.i.d. for 3-week periods.

Unlike those with juvenile periodontitis, PPP patients *are not* infected with *A. actinomycetemcomitans* or *B. gingivalis*. *Selenomonas sputigena* and *Bacteroides intermedius* are frequently recovered in cultures. Serologic studies reveal elevated antibody titers to *Capnocytophaga sputigena*.

## Rapidly progressive periodontitis

Rapidly progressive periodontitis (RPP)[115] is seen most commonly in young adults in their twenties to early thirties. During phases of active destruction, the gingival tissues are markedly inflamed and bone loss occurs rapidly. The disease may have periods of spontaneous remission characterized by clinically normal gingiva in the presence of deep pockets and advanced bone loss. These patients exhibit defects in either neutrophil or monocyte chemotaxis. Some patients respond well to mechanical débridement and antimicrobial therapy, while others do not. It is not currently possible to distinguish diagnostically between these patients prior to treatment.

This disease category probably consists of several different diseases, all of which result in rapidly progressive destruction of the bone and periodontal ligament.

The following systemic diseases may predispose to or be related to RPP:

1. Diabetes mellitus (especially the insulin-dependent type)[116]
2. Down syndrome (mongolism)
3. Papillon-Lefèvre syndrome (hyperkeratosis palmaris et plantaris)
4. Crohn's disease (regional ileitis)
5. Neutropenia
6. Agranulocytosis
7. Lazy leukocyte syndrome
8. Chédiak-Higashi syndrome

The *generalized* form of juvenile periodontitis is considered by some to fit under this category.

### REFERENCES

1. Russell, A.L.: Epidemiology of periodontal disease, Int. Dent. J. **17:**1, 1967.
2. Gottlieb, B.: Zur Aetiologie und Therapie der Alveolarpyorrhoe, Z. Stomatol. **18:**59, 1920.
3. Gottlieb, B.: Die diffuse Atrophie des Alveolarknochens, Z. Stomatol. **21:**195, 1923.
4. Wannenmacher, E.: Umschau auf dem Gebiete der Paradentose, Dtsch. Zahnärztl. Mund. Kieferheilkd. **3:**81, 1938.
5. Miller, S.C.: Precocious advanced alveolar atrophy, J. Periodontol. **19:**146, 1948.
6. Thoma, K.H., and Goldman, H.M.: Wandering and elongation of the teeth and pocket formation in paradontosis, J. Am. Dent. Assoc. **27:**335, 1940.
7. Orban, B., and Weinmann, J.P.: Diffuse atrophy of the alveolar bone (periodontosis), J. Periodontol. **13:**31, 1942.
8. Baer, P.N.: The case for periodontosis as a clinical entity, J. Periodontol. **42:**516, 1971.

9. Petit, H.: Parodontite juvénile, Paris, 1970, Prelat.

10. Manson, J.D., and Lehner, T.: Clinical features of juvenile periodontitis (periodontosis), J. Periodontol. **45:**636, 1974.

11. Saxén, L.: Prevalence of juvenile periodontitis in Finland, J. Clin. Periodontol. **7:**177, 1980.

12. Hoover, J.N., Ellegaard, B., and Attström, R.: Radiographic and clinical examination of periodontal status of first molars in 15 to 16-year-old Danish school children, Scand. J. Dent. Res. **89:**260, 1981.

13. Marshall-Day, C.D.: Periodontal disease prevalence and incidence, J. Dent. Res. **33:**673, 1954.

14. Miglani, D.C.: Incidence of acute necrotizing ulcerative gingivitis and periodontosis among cases seen at the Government Hospital, Madras, J. All India Dent. Assoc. **37:**183, 1965.

15. Rao, S.S., and Tewani, S.V.: Prevalence of periodontosis among Indians, J. Periodontol. **37:**27, 1968.

16. Burmeister, J.A., et al.: Localized juvenile periodontitis and generalized severe periodontitis; clinical findings, J. Clin. Periodontol. **11:**181, 1984.

17. Kelley, J.E., and Van Kirk, L.E.: Periodontal disease in adults, Vital Health Stat. **12:**13, 1963.

18. Benjamin, S.D., and Baer, P.N.: Familial patterns of advanced alveolar bone loss in adolescence (periodontosis), Periodontics **34:**533, 1963.

19. Butler, J.H.: A familial pattern of juvenile periodontitis (periodontosis), J. Periodontol. **40:**51, 1969.

20. Emslie, R.D.: Periodontal disease in tropical Africa, Parodontopathies **18:**26, 1966.

21. Newman, M.G., and Socransky, S.S.: The microbiota of periodontosis, J. Periodont. Res. **12:**120, 1977.

22. Hormand, J., and Frandsen, A.: Juvenile periodontitis: localization of bone loss in relation to age, sex, and teeth, J. Clin. Periodontol. **6:**407, 1979.

23. Dekker, G., and Jansen, L.H.: Periodontosis in a child with hyperkeratosis palmo-plantaris, J. Periodontol. **29:**266, 1958.

24. Fourel, J.: Periodontosis: a periodontal syndrome, J. Periodontol. **43:**240, 1972.

25. Kaslick, R.S., et al.: Association between HL-A2 antigen and various periodontal diseases in young adults, J. Dent. Res. **54:**424, 1975.

26. Reinholdt, J., Bay, I., and Svejgaard, A.: Association between HLA antigens and periodontal disease, J. Dent. Res. **56:**1261, 1977.

27. Kaslick, R.S., et al.: Investigation of periodontosis with periodontitis: literature survey and findings based on ABO blood groups, J. Periodontol. **42:**420, 1971.

28. Cullinan, M.P., et al.: The distribution of HLA-A and -B antigens in patients and their families with periodontosis, J. Periodont. Res. **15:**177, 1980.

29. Saxén, L., and Koskimies, S.: Juvenile periodontitis—no linkage with HLA-antigens, J. Periodont. Res. **19:**441, 1984.

30. Melnick, M., Shields, E.D., and Bixler, D.: Periodontosis: a phenotypic and genetic analysis, Oral Surg. **42:**32, 1976.

31. Saxen, L.: Heredity of juvenile periodontitis, J. Clin. Periodontol. **7:**276, 1980.

32. Saxén, L., and Nevanlinna, H.R.: Autosomal recessive inheritance of juvenile periodontitis: test of a hypothesis, Clin. Genet. **25:**332, 1984.

33. Newman, M.G.: Periodontosis, J. West Soc. Periodont. **24:**5, 1976.

34. Grant, D., Stern, I.B., and Everett, F.G.: Orban's periodontics, ed. 2, St. Louis, 1963, The C.V. Mosby Co, pp. 180-182.

35. Grant, D.A., Stern, I.B., and Everett, F.G.: Orban's periodontics: a concept—theory and practice, ed. 4, St. Louis, 1972, The C.V. Mosby Co.

36. Fourel, J.: Periodontosis, juvenile periodontitis, or Gottlieb syndrome? Report of 4 cases, J. Periodontol. **45:**234, 1974.

37. Page, R.C., et al.: Prepubertal periodontitis. I. Definition of a clinical disease entity, J. Periodontol. **54:**257, 1983.

38. Baer, P.N., and Benjamin, S.: Periodontal disease in children and adolescents, Philadelphia, 1974, J.B. Lippincott Co.

39. Cawson, R.A.: Periodontosis associated with gingival lesions in a child, J. Periodontol. **30:**112, 1959.

40. Kaslick, R., and Kutscher, A.H.: Cyclic neutropenia, J. Clin. Stomatol. **4:**56, 1963.

41. Telsey, B., et al.: Oral manifestations of cyclic neutropenia associated with hypergammaglobulinemia, Oral Surg. **15:**540, 1962.

42. Cohen, D.W., and Morris, A.L.: Periodontal manifestation of cyclic neutropenia, J. Periodontol. **32:**159, 1961.

43. Bauer, W.H.: The supporting tissues of the tooth in acute secondary granulocytosis (arsphenamine neutropenia), J. Dent. Res. **25:**501, 1946.

44. Arnold, R.N., and Hoffman, D.L.: Oral management of lazy leukocyte syndrome: a case report, Quintessence Int. **10:**9, 1979.

45. Tempel, T.R., et al.: Host factors in periodontal disease: periodontal manifestations of Chédiak-Higashi syndrome, J. Periodont. Res. **7**(suppl.):26, 1972.

46. Gorlin, R.S., Sedano, H., and Anderson, V.E.: The syndromes of palmar-plantar hyperkeratosis and premature periodontal destruction of the teeth, J. Pediatr. **65:**895, 1964.

47. Ingle, J.I.: Papillon-Lefèvre syndrome: precocious periodontosis with associated epidermal lesions, J. Periodontol. **30:**230, 1959.

48. Galanter, D.R., and Stewart, B.: Hyperkeratosis palmoplantaris and periodontosis, J. Periodontol. **40,** 1969.

49. Martinez Lalis, R., Lopez Otero, R., and Carranza, F.A., Jr.: A case of Papillon-Lefèvre syndrome, Periodontics **3:**292, 1965.

50. Kisling, E., and Krebs, G.: Periodontal conditions in adult patients with mongolism (Down's syndrome), Acta Odontol. Scand. **21:**391, 1963.

51. Cianciola, J.L., et al.: Prevalence of periodontal disease in insulin-dependent diabetes mellitus (juvenile diabetes), J. Am. Dent. Assoc. **104:**653, 1982.

52. Bruckner, R.J., Rickles, N.H., and Porter, D.R.: Hypophosphatasia with premature shedding of teeth and aplasia of cementum, Oral Surg. **15:**1351, 1962.

53. Kerr, D.A.: Summary of systemic relations in periodontal disease, J. Periodontol. **22:**27, 1951.

54. Ross, L.F., et al.: Endocrine and laboratory studies of precocious advanced alveolar atrophy, Periodontics **12:**61, 1958.

55. Listgarten, M.A.: Structure of the microbial flora associated with periodontal health and disease in man, J. Periodontol. **47:**1, 1976.

56. Kaslick, R.S., and Chasens, A.I.: Periodontosis with periodontitis: a study involving young adult males, Oral Surg. **25:**327, 1968.

57. Liljenberg, B., and Lindhe, J.: Juvenile periodontitis: some microbiological, histopathological and clinical characteristics, J. Clin. Periodontol. **7:**48, 1980.

58. Westergaard, J., Frandsen, A., and Slots, J.: Ultrastructure of the subgingival microflora in juvenile periodontitis, Scand. J. Dent. Res. **86:**421, 1978.

59. Slots, J., Reynolds, H.S., and Genco, R.J.: *Actinobacillus actinomycetemcomitans* in human periodontal disease: a cross-sectional microbiological investigation, Infect. Immun. **29:**1013, 1980.

60. Zambon, J.J., Christersson, L.A., and Slots, J.: *Actinobacillus actinomycetemcomitans* in human periodontal disease: prevalence in patient groups and distribution of biotypes and serotypes within families, J. Periodontol. **54:**707, 1983.

61. Mandell, R.L., and Socransky, S.S.: A selective medium for *Actinobacillus actinomycetemcomitans* and the incidence of the organism juvenile periodontitis, J. Periodontol. **52:**593, 1981.

62. Eisenmann, A.C., et al.: Microbiological study of localized juvenile periodontitis in Panama, J. Periodontol. **54:**712, 1983.

63. Slots, J.: *Actinobacillus actinomycetemcomitans* and *Bacteroides gingivalis* in advanced periodontitis in man, Dtsch. Zahnärztl. Z. **39:**615, 1984.

64. Slots, J., et al.: *Actinobacillus actinomycetemcomitans* in human periodontal disease: association, serology, leukotoxicity, and treatment, J. Periodont. Res. **17:**447, 1982.

65. Mashimo, P.A., et al.: The periodontal microflora of juvenile diabetics: culture, immunofluorescence, and serum antibody studies, J. Periodontol. **54:**420, 1983.

66. Vandesteen, G.E., et al.: Clinical, microbiological and immunological studies of a family with a high prevalence of early-onset periodontitis, J. Periodontol. **55:**159, 1984.

67. Saglie, R., et al.: Identification of tissue-invading bacteria in human periodontal disease, J. Periodont. Res. **17:**452, 1982.

68. Christersson, L.A., et al.: Demonstration of *Actinobacillus actinomycetemcomitans* in gingiva of localized juvenile periodontitis lesions, J. Dent. Res. **62:**198, 1983. (Abstr. 255.)

69. Sanavi, F., et al.: The colonization and establishment of invading bacteria in periodontium of ligature-treated immunosuppressed rats, J. Periodontol. **56:**273, 1985.

70. Slots, J., and Genco, R.J.: Black-pigmented *Bacteroides* species, *Capnocytophaga* species, and *Actinobacillus actinomycetemcomitans* in human periodontal disease: virulence factors in colonization, survival and tissue destruction, J. Dent. Res. **63:**412, 1984.

71. Van Dyke, T.E., et al.: Inhibition of neutrophil chemotaxis by soluble bacterial products, J. Periodontol. **503:**502, 1982.

72. Van Dyke, T.E.: Neutrophil receptor modulation in the pathogenesis of periodontal diseases, J. Dent. Res. **63:**452, 1984.

73. Baehni, P., et al.: Interaction of inflammatory cells and oral microorganisms. VIII. Detection of leukotoxic activity of a plaque-derived gram-negative microorganism, Infect. Immun. **24:**233, 1979.

74. Tsai, C.-C., et al.: Extraction and partial characterization of a leukotoxin from a plaque-derived gram-negative microorganism, Infect. Immun. **25:**427, 1979.

75. Taichman, N.S., Dean, R.T., and Sanderson, C.J.: Biochemical and morphological characterization of the killing of human monocytes by a leukotoxin derived from *Actinobacillus actinomycetemcomitans*, Infect. Immun. **28:**258, 1980.

76. Baehni, P.C., et al.: Leukotoxic activity in different strains of the bacterium *Actinobacillus actinomycetemcomitans* isolated from juvenile periodontitis in man, Arch. Oral Biol. **26:**671, 1981.

77. Taichman, N.S., et al.: Cytopathic effects of *Actinobacillus actinomycetemcomitans* on monkey blood leukocytes, J. Periodont. Res. **19:**133, 1984.

78. Sundqvist, G., and Johansson, E.: Bactericidal effect of pooled human serum on *Bacteroides melaninogenicus, Bacteroides asac-*

*charolyticus* and *Actinobacillus actinomy-cetemcomitans,* Scand. J. Dent. Res. **90:**29, 1982.

79. Shenker, B.J., Kushner, M.E., and Tsai, C.-C.: Inhibition of fibroblast proliferation by *Actinobacillus actinomycetemcomitans,* Infect. Immun. **38:**986, 1982.

80. Stevens, R.H., Gatewood, C., and Hammond, B.F.: Cytotoxicity of the bacterium *Actinobacillus actinomycetemcomitans* extracts in human gingival fibroblasts, Arch. Oral Biol. **28:**981, 1983.

81. Kiley, P., and Holt, S.C.: Characterization of the lipopolysaccharide from *Actinobacillus actinomycetemcomitans* Y4 and N27, Infect. Immun. **30:**862, 1980.

82. Rozanis, J., et al.: Further studies on collagenase of *Actinobacillus actinomycetemcomitans,* Abstract No. 1177, J. Dent. Res. **62:**300, 1983.

83. Nowotny, A., et al.: Bone resorbing potential of endotoxin and its immunopharmacological modulations. In Agarwal, M.K., and Yoshida, M., editors: Immunopharmacology of endotoxicosis, Berlin, 1984, Walter de Gruyter and Co., p. 261.

84. Nowotny, A., et al.: Release of toxic microvesicles by *Actinobacillus actinomycetemcomitans,* Infect. Immun. **37:**151, 1982.

85. Shenker, B.J., McArthur, W.P., and Tsai, C.-C.: Immune suppression induced by *Actinobacillus actinomycetemcomitans.* I. Effects on human peripheral blood lymphocyte responses to mitogens and antigens, J. Immunol. **128:**148, 1982.

86. Shenker, B.J., Tsai, C.-C., and Taichman, N.S.: Suppression of lymphocyte responses by *Actinobacillus actinomycetemcomitans,* J. Periodont. Res. **17:**462, 1982.

87. Slots, J.: The predominant cultivable organisms in juvenile periodontitis, Scand. J. Dent. Res. **84:**1, 1976.

88. Socransky, S.S., et al.: *Capnocytophaga:* new genus of gram-negative gliding bacteria. III. Physiological characterization, Arch. Microbiol. **122:**29, 1979.

89. Tanner, A.C.R., et al.: A study of the bacteria associated with advancing periodontitis in man, J. Clin. Periodontol. **6:**278, 1979.

90. Irving, J.T., et al.: Histological changes in experimental periodontal disease in rats monoinfected with a gram-negative organism, Arch. Oral Biol. **20:**219, 1975.

91. Lai, C.-H., Listgarten, M.A., and Hammond, B.F.: Comparative ultrastructure of leukotoxic and non-leukotoxic strains of *Actinobacillus actinomycetemcomitans,* J. Periodont. Res. **16:**379, 1981.

92. Holt, S.C., Tanner, A.C.R., and Socransky, S.S.: Morphology and ultrastructure of oral strains of *Actinobacillus actinomycetemcomitans* and *Haemophilus aphrophilus,* Infect. Immun. **30:**588, 1980.

93. Baehni, P., et al.: Electron microscopic study of the interaction of oral microorganisms with polymorphonuclear leukocytes, Arch. Oral Biol. **22:**685, 1977.

94. Lehner, T., et al.: Immunologic aspects of juvenile periodontitis (periodontosis), J. Periodont. Res. **9:**261, 1974.

95. Genco, R.J., et al.: Systemic immune responses to oral anaerobic organisms. In Lambe, D.W., Jr., Genco, R.J., and Mayberry-Carson, K.J., editors: Anaerobic bacteria: selected topics, New York, 1980, Plenum Press, p. 277.

96. Listgarten, M.A., Lai, C.-H., and Evian, C.I.: Comparative antibody titers to *Actinobacillus actinomycetemcomitans* in juvenile periodontitis, chronic periodontitis and periodontally healthy subjects, J. Clin. Periodontol. **8:**155, 1981.

97. Tsai, C.-C., et al.: Serum neutralizing activity against *Actinobacillus actinomycetemcomitans* leukotoxin in juvenile periodontitis, J. Clin. Periodontol. **8:**338, 1981.

98. Ebersole, J.L., et al.: Human immune responses to oral microorganisms. I. Association of juvenile periodontitis (LJP) with serum antibody responses to *Actinobacillus actinomycetemcomitans,* Clin. Exp. Immunol. **47:**43, 1982.

99. Ebersole, J.L., et al.: Human immune responses to oral microorganisms. II. Serum antibody responses to antigens from *Actinobacillus actinomycetemcomitans* and the correlation with localized juvenile periodontitis, J. Clin. Immunol. **3:**321, 1983.

100. Ranney, R.R., et al.: Relationship between attachment loss and precipitating serum antibody to *Actinobacillus actinomycetemcomitans* in adolescents and young adults having severe periodontal destruction, J. Periodontol. **53:**1, 1982.

101. Cianciola, L.J., et al.: Defective polymorphonuclear leukocyte functions in a human periodontal disease, Nature **265:**445, 1977.

102. Clark, R.A., Page, R.C., and Wilde, G.: Defective neutrophil chemotaxis in juvenile periodontitis, Infect. Immun. **18:**694, 1977.

103. Lavine, W.S., et al.: Impaired neutrophil chemotaxis in patients with juvenile and rapidly progressing periodontitis, J. Periodont. Res. **14:**10, 1979.

104. Genco, R.J., et al.: Neutrophil chemotaxis impairment in juvenile periodontitis: evaluation of specificity, adherence, deformability and serum factors, J. Reticuloendothelial Soc. (Suppl.) **28:**81, 1980.

105. Ellegaard, B., Borregaard, N., and Ellegaard, J.: Neutrophil chemotaxis and phagocytosis in juvenile periodontitis, J. Periodont. Res. **19:**261, 1984.

106. Evian, C.I., Amsterdam, M., and Rosenberg, E.S.: Juvenile periodontitis: healing follow-

ing therapy to control inflammation and traumatic etiologic components of the disease, J. Clin. Periodontol. **9:**1, 1982.

107. Lindhe, J., and Liljenberg, B.: Treatment of localized juvenile periodontitis: results after 5 years, J. Clin. Periodontol. **11:**339, 1984.

108. Slots, J., and Rosling, B.G.: Suppression of the periodontopathic microflora in localized juvenile periodontitis by systemic tetracycline, J. Clin. Periodontol. **10:**465, 1983.

109. Christersson, L., et al.: Suppression of *Actinobacillus actinomycetemcomitans* in localized juvenile periodontitis, J. Dent. Res. **62:**198, 1983.

110. Christersson, L.A., et al.: Microbiological and clinical effects of surgical treatment of localized juvenile periodontitis, J. Clin. Periodontol. **12:**465, 1985.

111. Baer, P.N., and Gamble, J.W.: Autogenous dental transplants as a method of treating the osseous defect in periodontosis, Oral Surg. **22:**405, 1966.

112. Tenenbaum, B., et al.: Results of several types of treatment of periodontosis, J. Am. Dent. Assoc. **55:**651, 1957.

113. Everett, F.G., and Baer, P.N.: A preliminary report on the treatment of the osseous defect in periodontosis, J. Periodontol. **35:**429, 1964.

114. Borring-Moller, G., and Frandsen, A.: Autologous tooth transplantation to replace molars lost in patients with juvenile periodontitis, J. Clin. Periodontol. **5:**152, 1978.

115. Page, R.C., et al.: Rapidly progressive periodontitis: a distinct clinical condition, J. Periodontol. **54:**197, 1983.

116. Mashimo, P.A., et al.: The periodontal microflora of juvenile diabetics: culture, immunofluorescence, and serum antibody studies, J. Periodontol. **54:**420, 1983.

## ADDITIONAL SUGGESTED READING

Bowta, Y., et al.: Rapid identification of periodontal pathogens in subgingival plaque: comparison of indirect immunofluorescence microscopy with bacterial culture for detection of *Actinobacillus actinomycetemcomitans,* J. Dent. Res. **64:**793, 1985.

Christersson, L.A., et al.: Transmission and colonization of *Actinobacillus antinomycetemcomitans* in localized juvenile periodontitis patients, J. Periodontol. **56:**127, 1985.

Genco, R.J., Christersson, L.A., and Zambon, J.J.: Juvenile periodontitis, Internat. Dent. J. **36:**168, 1986.

Gjermo, P.: Chemotherapy in juvenile periodontitis, J. Clin. Periodontol. **13:**982, 1986.

Haffajee, A.D., et al.: Clinical, microbiological and immunological features associated with the treatment of active periodontosis lesions, J. Clin. Periodontol. **11:**600, 1984.

Jaffin, R.A., Greenstein, G., and Berman, C.L.: Treatment of juvenile periodontitis patients by control of infection and inflammation: four case reports, J. Periodontol. **55:**261, 1984.

Krill, D.B., and Fry, H.R.: Treatment of localized juvenile periodontitis (periodontosis), J. Periodontol. **58:**1, 1987.

Newman, M.G., et al.: Mycoplasma in periodontal disease: isolation in juvenile periodontitis, J. Periodontol. **55:**574, 1985.

Sandholm, L., and Tolo, K.: Serum antibody levels to 4 periodontal pathogens remain unaltered after mechanical therapy of juvenile periodontitis, J. Clin. Periodontol. **13:**646, 1986.

Saxén, L., and Murtomaa, H.: Age-related expression of juvenile periodontitis, J. Clin. Periodontol. **12:**21, 1985.

Saxén, L., et al.: Treatment of juvenile periodontitis without antibiotics: a follow-up study, J. Clin. Periodontol. **13:**714, 1986.

Spektor, M.D., Vandesteen, G.E., and Page, R.C.: Clinical studies of one family manifesting rapidly progressive, juvenile and prepubertal periodontitis, J. Periodontol. **56:**93, 1985.

Suzuki, J.B., Park, S.K., and Falkler, W.A., Jr.: Immunologic profile of juvenile periodontitis. I. Lymphocyte blastogenesis and the mixed lymphocyte response, J. Periodontol. **55:**453, 1984.

Suzuki, J.B., et al.: Immunologic profile of juvenile periodontitis. II. Neutrophil chemotaxis, phagocytosis and spore generation, J. Periodontol. **55:**461, 1984.

Suzuki, J.B., et al.: Effect of periodontal therapy on spontaneous lymphocyte response and neutrophil chemotaxis in localized and generalized juvenile periodontitis patients, J. Clin. Periodontol. **12:**124, 1985.

Zambon, J.J.: *Actinobacillus actinomycetemcomitans* in human periodontal disease, J. Clin. Periodontol. **12:**1, 1985.

Zambon, J.J., Christersson, L.A., and Genco, R.J.: Diagnosis and treatment of localized juvenile periodontitis, J. Am. Dent. Assoc. **113:**295, 1986.

# CHAPTER 18

# Necrotizing ulcerative gingivitis

**Diagnostic features**
Site and extent of involvement
Alterations in tissue form with repeated attacks
Recurrent NUG with bone loss—necrotizing ulcerative
   periodontitis
Histopathologic features
Differential diagnosis and concurrent conditions

**Prevalence**

**Etiology**
Bacteria
Extrinsic predisposing factors
Intrinsic predisposing factors
Psychogenic causes

**Treatment**
Reduction of acute symptoms
Elimination of predisposing factors
Correction of tissue deformities

---

Necrotizing ulcerative gingivitis (NUG) is an acute infection of the gingiva. It is also known as Vincent's infection (because of the description by Vincent of the organisms associated with the disease)[1] and trench mouth (because of the heavy incidence among soldiers in trenches during World War I). Actually, the disease has been known since ancient times under a variety of names.[2,3] The current name is derived from the key symptoms: necrosis, ulceration, and inflammation of the gingiva. Since similar symptoms may occur in other diseases (e.g., acute herpetic gingivostomatitis), NUG must be distinguished from them. NUG is generally a disease seen in adolescents and young adults; however, it has been reported in children and has been seen rarely in middle-aged adults.

## Diagnostic features

The classical signs and symptoms from which diagnosis may be made include the following[4,5]

1. Ulceration of the tips of interdental papillae
2. Bleeding
3. Apparent sudden onset
4. Pain
5. Foul odor (*fetor oris*)

**Recurrence**

In the earliest stages only two clinical signs may be apparent[5,6]: necrosis of the tips of the interdental papillae and the col[7,8] (Fig. 18-1) and a tendency toward easy gingival bleeding. At this early stage pain may be absent,[6,9] but probing will produce pain. At one time the disease was classified clinically into acute, subacute, and chronic forms. Such differentiation is based on the severity, duration, and onset of the infection and not on the type of inflammation. Subacute and chronic cases are due to recurring

**Necrotizing ulcerative periodontitis**

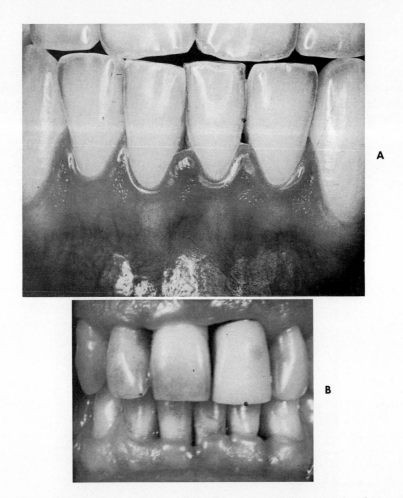

**Fig. 18-1.    A,** Early necrotizing ulcerative gingivitis. The initial signs are ulcerations at the tips of the papillae. Pain may be absent. **B,** Necrotizing ulcerative periodontitis. This patient, seen at an acute recurrence, suffered periodic bouts of NUG. Bone destruction and periodontitis ensued. (**A** from the collection of H.E. Grupe, Sr.; **B** courtesy A. Ariaudo, San Diego, California.)

acute episodes of the disease. With recurrent attacks bone loss may occur. Attacks of *acute necrotizing gingivitis* can be superimposed on periodontitis (Figs. 18-1, *B,* and 18-5).

Diagnosis rests on the clinical appearance of the lesions.[10] The interdental papillae may appear eroded, punched out, or clipped off because of the ulcerative destruction. The ulcerations may progress to include the marginal and, rarely, the attached gingivae. The lesions may be covered with a whitish, yellowish, or gray pseudomembrane. The gingiva around the ulcerations is an angry red color and bleeds easily when it is touched. The regional lymph nodes are seldom swollen in adolescents or young adults.[6] However lymphadenitis[5] has been reported, particularly in the cervical nodes of children with the disease. Children also tend to have elevated temperatures,[5] an infrequent observation in adolescents and young adults.[11] Ulcerative lesions, lymphadenitis, and elevated temperatures are typically found in primary herpetic gingivostomatitis, a viral infection that frequently occurs in children. It is important to differentiate between the two conditions when these clinical signs are observed in younger patients.

## SITE AND EXTENT OF INVOLVEMENT

The interdental cols and tips of the interdental papillae (Fig. 18-1) are characteristically affected first, although the disease may progressively involve the gingival margins. (Fig. 18-2). The gingiva of any area of the mouth may be affected, and the entire mouth or regions of the mouth may be involved. The distribution of the disease does not follow any consistent pattern and may differ from mouth to mouth. Initially, involvement of the incisor regions and third molar flaps seems to occur most frequently (Fig. 18-3). The infection may spread to other parts of the oral mucosa, although this rarely occurs. Direct contact may cause lip and tongue ulcers. Pharyngeal involvement (Vincent's angina) may also accompany the gingival infection (Fig. 18-4). Pain is usually the patient's main complaint. It may be so severe as to interfere with mastication and toothbrushing. The patient may state that his teeth feel as if they were separating or were wooden. The patient may also complain of increased salivation, of a metallic taste, and of a foul mouth odor.

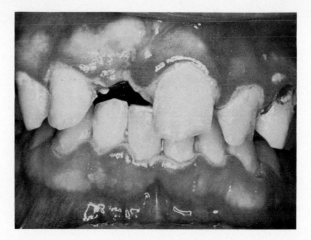

**Fig. 18-2.** The marginal and papillary gingivae are extensively involved, most severely in the anterior region.

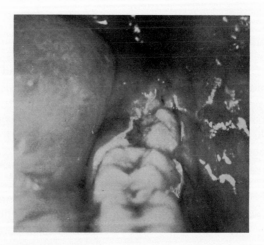

**Fig. 18-3.** Necrotizing ulcerative gingivitis. Note the ulceration of the third molar flap.

## ALTERATIONS IN TISSUE FORM WITH REPEATED ATTACKS

In time, slight proliferation of the gingiva adjacent to the necrotic area may take place (Fig. 18-5). With more extensive or repeated attacks, the interdental tissue may become cratered (Fig. 18-6). This combination of necrosis and proliferation can produce irregular outlines in the marginal and papillary gingivae (e.g., punched-out tips; flaplike, serpentine, and papilla-less types) (Figs. 18-5 and 18-6). These signs are usually indicative of repeated attacks.

When deep interdental craters occur and the tips of the papillae proliferate, the buccal and lingual portions of the papillae may form movable flaps. Such ulcerations remain hidden unless the flap of loose gingiva is reflected to reveal the cratered area.

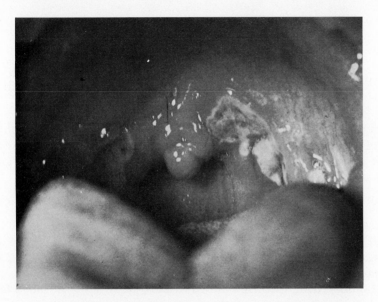

**Fig. 18-4.** Involvement of the tonsillar region in Vincent's angina. (From the collection of H.E. Grupe, Sr.)

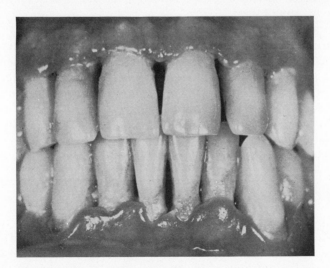

**Fig. 18-5.** Recurrent necrotizing ulcerative periodontitis. The repeated acute attacks have caused the loss of the interproximal gingiva, producing a reverse architecture. Interdental craters, troughs, and loss of crestal bone mark this destruction.

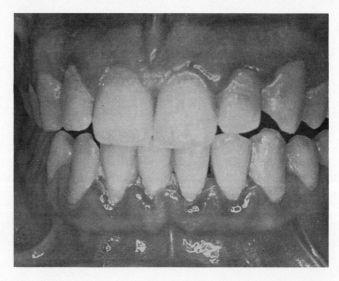

**Fig. 18-6.** *Acute necrotizing ulcerative gingivitis. There is necrosis of the tips of the gingival papillae and of cols; the gingiva shows inflammatory hyperplasia.*

When roots are closely approximated the septum may be lost, resulting in the formation of a deep cleft or reverse architecture. Even when the disease process is arrested the deformity of reverse architecture may remain. Such gingival and osseous deformities may require surgical correction.

### RECURRENT NUG WITH BONE LOSS—NECROTIZING ULCERATIVE PERIODONTITIS

The reasons for the recurrence of NUG are as incompletely known as the reasons for the primary appearance of the disease. Apparently, the acute phase can be brought under control by a variety of techniques and medications. Unfortunately, as soon as the symptoms abate many patients tend to discontinue treatment and proper oral hygiene. The underlying extrinsic, intrinsic, and psychogenic causative factors may then contribute to a relapse. Incomplete or insufficient treatment plays an important role in such recurrence. However, the tendency for the disease to recur is great regardless of the treatment used.

The patient and therapist must be aware that recurrence is likely.[10,11] The patient should be informed that easy bleeding is an early and significant sign of recurrence and that, on noticing this symptom, he/she must return for treatment regardless of the date of the next appointment. The practitioner should continue to observe the patient at regular intervals for at least a year after completion of treatment. Otherwise, treatment may have been terminated prematurely.

*Necrotizing ulcerative gingivitis leading to periodontitis*

Recurrent NUG may become a chronic condition in some patients. Acute exacerbations of the disease may lead to periodontitis. This periodontitis is characterized by severe interdental craters and gingival recession coapted with enlargement at the gingival margins (see Fig. 18-5).

### HISTOPATHOLOGIC FEATURES

The microscopic picture of NUG reveals an acute inflammatory process with ulceration and the formation of a pseudomembrane on the surface (Fig. 18-7). Leukocytes may be seen in the pseudomembrane (Fig. 18-8) and in the tissue (Fig. 18-9). In recurrent cases large masses of plasma cells may accumulate in the deeper layer, and tissue necrosis may become a prominent feature. Spirochetes can be seen invading the tissue (Fig. 18-10).

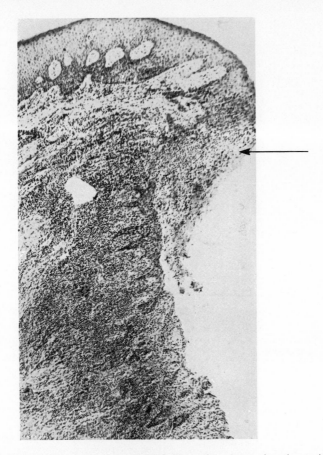

**Fig. 18-7.** Biopsy of the gingiva of a patient with NUG. The surface shows ulceration and a fragment of pseudomembrane *(arrow)*.

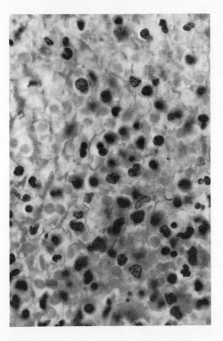

**Fig. 18-8.** High magnification of a pseudomembrane of a patient with NUG. The fibrinous network enmeshes erythrocytes, leukocytes, and macrophages.

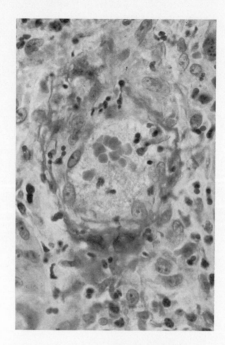

**Fig. 18-9.** Fibrinous exudate surrounding a capillary with migrating leukocytes in a case of NUG.

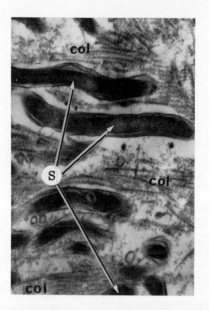

**Fig. 18-10.** Zone of spirochetal infiltration. *S,* Spirochetes infiltrating the connective tissue beneath the ulcerated lesion; *col,* collagen fibers. (From Listgarten, M.A.: J. Periodontol. **36:**328, 1965.)

## DIFFERENTIAL DIAGNOSIS AND CONCURRENT CONDITIONS

NUG may have to be differentiated[12] from herpetic gingivostomatitis, streptococcal stomatitis,[13] erythema multiforme, and infectious mononucleosis. The possibility that NUG may be superimposed on an underlying agranulocytosis[14] (malignant neutropenia), acute leukemia,[15] or heavy metal poisoning should not be ignored. These conditions may be accompanied by mild gingival swelling and ulceration and may become complicated by NUG. Whenever severe NUG does not improve in the first few days of treatment, a differential blood count is indicated. The possibility of missing the underlying disease is real. Any unusual complication warrants medical consultation and/or hospitalization.

## Prevalence

In the United States and in Europe acute NUG occurs primarily among adolescents and young adults. Reports of epidemics of NUG in the United States probably represent misdiagnoses.[16] Reports from other continents indicate that NUG may occur in children, particularly when they are malnourished. Noma (cancrum oris) may follow in conditions of famine[17-23] (see Fig. 13-2).

In a survey of close to 10,000 patients registered in a U.S. dental school clinic,[24] a 0.5% prevalence of NUG was reported. These patients had a mean age of 24 years (range, 14 to 33 years), compared to 35 years for the registered patient population. The prevalence increased to 1.4% if only patients 34 years of age and under were considered. In a population of 870 military recruits there was a reported prevalence of 2.2%.[6] This is close to the 2.5% reported in a population of 326 freshman college students.[25,26] A somewhat higher prevalence of 6% was noted in a group of Danish military recruits with NUG.[27,28] An incidence of 8.3% for NUG among 15- to 19-year-old patients attending a dental clinic serving a population of 10,000 patients was reported.[29] This study also reports a seasonal incidence with peak periods in September to October, December to January, and June.

An unusually high prevalence of NUG was noted in a population of 806 institutionalized, mentally retarded patients with Down syndrome.[30] Thirty-five percent of the patients with Down syndrome were affected as compared to 4% of the patients without Down syndrome. The mean age at onset for both groups was between 9 and 10 years of age. The rate of recurrence of NUG in patients with Down syndrome was almost double that of the non-Down–syndrome patients (49% vs. 27%).

In 218 cases of NUG, a predilection was noted for whites over nonwhites.[9] In another study 98% of patients with NUG were white even though only 59% of the clinic population was white; most of the rest were black.[24]

Smoking[5,16,24,31-33] and emotional stress appear to play an important role as predisposing factors in the onset of NUG. It has been postulated that smoking may act by interfering with normal leukocyte function.[32] Patients with NUG may have previously existing polymorphonuclear leukocytes with depressed chemotactic and phagocytic functions[33] so that smoking could conceivably further compromise already weakened host defense mechanisms.

Emotional stress also appears to act as a prominent predisposing factor.[24-26,34-40] The exact mechanism for this effect is not known. Stressful periods may be associated with elevated 17-hydroxycorticosteroid levels in patients with NUG.[38,39] These and other physiologic changes[41] may favor the overgrowth of potentially pathogenic microorganisms such as spirochetes, fusiform bacilli, and *Bacteroides intermedius*, which may lead to tissue destruction. In addition, stress may provoke certain individuals to smoking, a habit that may further compromise host resistance.

## Etiology

The causes of NUG are not fully understood. Bacteria and other extrinsic factors as well as intrinsic and psychogenic factors have all been incriminated.

### BACTERIA

NUG is believed to be an infectious disease that is characterized by elevated proportions of fusiform bacilli and medium-sized spirochetes, the latter capable of invading the gingival tissues. Since elevated proportions of these organisms also exist in other forms of periodontal disease, notably periodontitis, positive smears for these microbial forms cannot be considered as pathognomonic of NUG. However in conjunction with clinical observations, elevated numbers of spirochetes and fusiform bacilli may provide confirmatory evidence for a diagnosis of NUG.

*Fusobacterium nucleatum* is a gram-negative or weakly gram-positive anaerobic bacillus, 8 to 16 μm in length, occurring as straight or curved rods whose pointed outer ends give the characteristic cigar-shaped appearance to this bacterium (Fig. 18-11).

*Borrelia vincentii* is a loosely wound spirochete, 8 to 12 μm in length, with three to eight irregular shallow spirals.[42,43] It is gram negative.

Attempts to transmit the disease in humans have failed almost without exception.[44] There are reports of severe, foul-smelling infections associated with human bite wounds. These do not represent the same disease. The conclusion has been drawn that the disease is not communicable.[45] However evidence is, as yet, incomplete.[16]

**Microbiologic experimentation**

Experimentation, on the other hand, has yielded some interesting results. When mixed cultures obtained from acute cases are injected subcutaneously into the groins of guinea pigs, abscess formation and necrosis result.[45] Spirochetes and fusiform bacilli can be recovered from such lesions. This infection can be passed through several transfers. In experimental transmission into guinea pigs, the presence of *Bacteroides melaninogenicus* was found to be essential.[46,47] Hampp and Mergenhagen[48] insist that spirochetes cannot be dismissed as causative agents because abscesses can be produced in the guinea pig by injection of *Borrelia vincentii* and *B. buccalis*. These investigators[49] produced intracutaneous abscesses by injection of oral fusobacteria separately or in combination with a strain of oral spirochetes. Listgarten and Socransky[50] stress that the major spirochete in NUG is distinctly different from *Borrelia vincentii*. Spirochetes can be seen invading gingival epithelium and connective tissue subjacent to the lesion[51,52] (Fig. 18-12). An immunofluorescent study failed to show a significant rise in antibody titers against *Borrelia vincentii, Fusobacterium nucleatum,* and *Bacteroides melaninogenicus* in patients suffering from acute NUG.[53,54.]

Although these experiments are important the relationship to the clinical disease entity remains tenuous. None of the experiments has produced oral lesions typical of NUG. The weight of evidence, however, indicates that the organisms are in some way implicated. The administration of antibiotics is effective in treatment. Koch's first and second postulates are satisfied because the organisms are always present in the lesions and some can be isolated in pure culture. However, his third postulate is not satisfied because the disease cannot be reproduced in humans or animals in its typical clinical form. No single organism or combination has yet been proved to be the causative agent in NUG.

One recently described animal model may be of value in gaining additional information about NUG. Mikx and Van Campen[55,56] reported that a group of dogs treated with triamcinolone, a steroid drug, became infected with scrapings from NUG lesions and developed typical lesions.[57,58] Presumably, pretreatment with the glucocorticoid decreased the resistance of the dogs to infection, thereby allowing the spirochetes to gain a foothold and invade the tissues. Other organisms recovered included fusobacteria, spirilla, and *Bacteroides intermedius*,[59] organisms that are also found in human lesions.[60,61]

## EXTRINSIC PREDISPOSING FACTORS

In addition to the microbiologic factors other coincident or predisposing findings include poor oral hygiene, pericoronal flaps and crypts, and excessive smoking.[5,28,31] However, the disease may occur in the absence of any or all of these factors. NUG may occur in nonsmokers and in mouths that are scrupulously clean.[6] Since

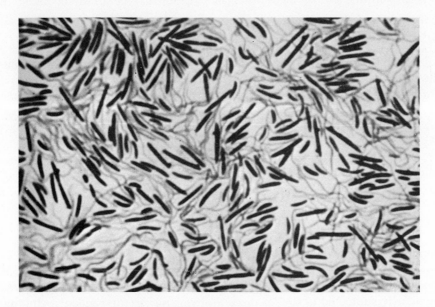

**Fig. 18-11.**   Oral smear from a patient with NUG demonstrating spirochetes and fusiform microorganisms. (From the collection of E.D. Coolidge.)

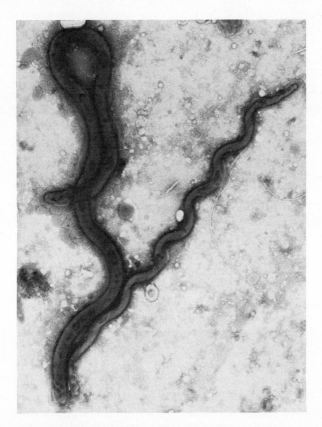

**Fig. 18-12.**   Small and medium size spirochetes from NUG lesion. (Negative-stained preparation, ×2300.) (From Listgarten, M.A., and Socransky, S.S.: J. Bacteriol. **88:**1087, 1964.)

brushing is painful for these patients, poor hygiene may be an effect rather than a cause.

## INTRINSIC PREDISPOSING FACTORS

Oral fusospirochetal infection occasionally follows acute febrile or debilitating diseases such as nutritional deficiency, leukemia, agranulocytosis, pernicious anemia, infectious mononucleosis, and erythema multiforme. These conditions may affect host resistance and repair potential. Should the patient fail to respond to local treatment, the possible presence of a systemic disease should be investigated.[62] Differences in the lymphocyte transformation were reported when NUG patients and controls were compared.[62,63] The results suggest that a cellular type of immune deficiency plays a role in this disease. Patients with NUG frequently exhibit depressed polymorphonuclear leukocyte phagocytic and chemotactic function.[63]

## PSYCHOGENIC CAUSES

A psychogenic origin has been suggested for NUG.[26,34,35] Psychogenic factors probably predispose to the disease by favoring bacterial overgrowth and/or weakening host resistance. Pseudoepidemics can be attributed to the fact that populations may be simultaneously subjected to similar disease-provoking circumstances, including war, military service, examinations in schools, divorce, and so on. 17-Hydroxycorticosteroids are elevated in NUG. Such elevation has been associated with stress. The resulting chemical changes may promote the selective proliferation of pathogenic organisms or may weaken the host, who in turn may become more susceptible to infection.

# Treatment

The objectives of treatment of NUG are (1) reduction of acute symptoms (elimination of the necrotizing process), (2) elimination of predisposing factors and (3) correction of tissue deformities by surgery. Initial treatment may be varied and/or supplemented according to the needs of the patient. A regular recall program should be instituted.

## REDUCTION OF ACUTE SYMPTOMS

The acute symptoms of NUG must be reduced. Medication (e.g. antibiotic therapy, antiseptic mouth rinses, oxygen-releasing rinses), débridement, and the institution of oral hygiene procedures may all be used for reduction of the acute symptoms. Medication alone may produce a temporary remission of symptoms without effecting a cure (see discussion of recurrent NUG earlier in the chapter). Medication is only one of several steps in the treatment of NUG.[64,65]

## ELIMINATION OF PREDISPOSING FACTORS

The extrinsic and intrinsic predisposing factors must be eliminated when possible. Otherwise, they may continue to promote recurrence of the disease. The patient should be placed in a generally healthful situation. Factors that could possibly lower tissue resistance, such as fatigue, alcoholism, and excessive smoking, should be reduced or eliminated. Bed rest may be advisable in extremely severe cases, especially if fever is present. Fever seldom exceeds 101° F (38.3° C), except in patients under the age of 14 years. The possible role of psychogenic stress should be mentioned and gently investigated.

The mouth is examined and a diagnosis made. The mouth is gently sprayed to remove slough. Preliminary débridement is performed. A topical anesthetic may be used if necessary. Ultrasonic débridement has a special place in the treatment of NUG.[66] Lavage is an asset in the débridement of bacteria and necrotic tissue.

**First appointment**

The patient is instructed in the use of hot-water rinses as a home treatment. A mouthful of water, as warm as the patient can stand, is forcefully swished back and forth between the teeth for several minutes. Rinsing should be performed several times a day. The necrotic slough will be loosened, and anaerobic organisms will be diminished in number. In 24 hours subjective and objective improvement should be noted.

Dilute hydrogen peroxide solution (1 part in 4 parts of warm water) may be used instead of hot water. The topical application of Gly-Oxide (a hydrogen peroxide–urea preparation in glycerin) also seems to be beneficial. Oxygenating drugs were originally introduced with the rationale that the causative organisms are anaerobic. The dentist should carefully supervise the use of oxgenating drugs and should discontinue their prescription after 2 weeks. Longer use may lead to the formation of black (hairy) tongue and tooth decalcification of tooth substance.

Antibiotics, either locally or systemically administered, may be employed in treatment. Most patients with NUG can be treated successfully without the use of antibiotics.[64] The organisms are sensitive to penicillin. The advantage of using antibiotics lies in the quick resolution of the ulcerative necrotizing process, thus minimizing permanent tissue damage. The symptoms diminish in 24 hours, but medication should be continued for 5 to 7 days. The disadvantage of using antibiotics lies in the possibility of sensitization of the patient to the drug. Antibiotics may cause changes in the oral flora and lead to candidiasis infection (thrush). However, this reaction is temporary. Metronidazole, used for the elimination of trichomonal infections of the vagina, has been used successfully in the treatment of NUG.[67]

The diet should be soft and bland for the first few days after an acute attack. Vitamin supplementation such as a preparation containing at least 150 mg of ascorbic acid, 50 mg of riboflavin, and double the minimal amounts of the other components of the B complex group may be prescribed twice daily.

In 24 to 48 hours the patient should be considerably improved. Pain should be greatly reduced or absent. Additional débridement and root planing is carried out under topical anesthesia. Instruction in oral hygiene procedures with a soft, multitufted toothbrush is given.

**Second appointment**

The patient should now be seen at least once a week. During these visits scaling and polishing of the teeth should be completed. Oral hygiene can be evaluated and altered according to the needs of the patient. Stim-U-Dents or similarly shaped toothpicks are useful for the maintenance of interdental areas.

**Subsequent appointments**

## CORRECTION OF TISSUE DEFORMITIES

Surgery performed at the height of the disease is contraindicated. Surgery and extractions are usually deferred until the acute phase of the disease is under control. The third molar flaps (see Fig. 18-3) and other nidi of infection should be eliminated. The disease may be superimposed on or lead to the development of periodontitis. In either event, gingival and osseous deformities may remain after the acute phase has been resolved. When the cratering is mild, rigorous application of oral hygiene and massaging procedures may lead to complete recovery of normal papillary form. When deformities persist, gingival and osseous surgery may be necessary; otherwise these deformities may predispose to recurrent NUG or periodontitis.

**Recovery of papillary form in mild cases**

## REFERENCES

1. Vincent, H.: Sur une forme particuliere d'angine diphteŕoide (angine à bacilles fusiformes), Arch. Int. Laryngol. **11**:44, 1898.
2. Hirschfeld, I., Beube, F., and Siegel, E.H.: The history of Vincent's infection, J. Periodontol. **11**:89, 1940.
3. Pickard, H.M.: Historical aspects of Vincent's disease, Proc. R. Soc. Med. **66**:695, 1973.
4. Schaffer, E.M.: Necrotizing ulcerative gingivitis, Northwest Dent. **33**:267, 1954.
5. Goldhaber, P., and Giddon, D.B.: Present concepts concerning the etiology and treatment of acute necrotizing ulcerative gingivitis, Int. Dent. J. **14**:468, 1964.
6. Grupe, H.E., and Wilder, L.S.: Observations of necrotizing gingivitis in 870 military trainees, J. Periodontol. **27**:255, 1956.
7. Plüss, E., and Rateitschak, K.H.: Die Initiallesion bei Gingivitis ulcerosa, Schweiz. Monatsschr. Zahnheilkd. **81**:499, 1971.
8. Kardachi, B.J.R., and Clarke, N.G.: Aetiology of acute necrotizing gingivitis, J. Periodontol. **45**:830, 1974.
9. Barnes, G.P., Bowles, W.F., and Carter, H.G.: Acute necrotizing ulcerative gingivitis, J. Periodontol. **44**:35, 1973.
10. Grant, D.A.: Necrotizing ulcerative gingivitis, J. South. Calif. Dent. Assoc. **23**:21, 1955.
11. Silver, J.G., Southcott, R.J., and Wade, A.B.: Acute necrotizing ulcerative gingivitis, J. Periodontol. **45**:308, 1974.
12. Knolle, G., and Strassburg, M.: Die ulzeröse Stomatitis und differentialdiagnostisch wichtige Krankheitbilder. In Hardt, E., editor: Deutscher Zahnärtzekalender 1972, Munich, 1971, Carl Hanser Verlag.
13. Blake, G.C., and Trott, J.R.: Acute streptococcal gingivitis, Dent. Pract. **10**:43, 1959.
14. Anday, G., and Orban, B.: Acute agranulocytosis, Arch. Pathol. **39**:369, 1945.
15. Lynch, M.A., and Ship, I.: Initial oral manifestations of leukemia, J. Am. Dent. Assoc. **75**:932, 1967.
16. Everett, F.G.: Necrotizing ulcerative gingivitis, a reportable disease? J. Periodontol. **27**:198, 1956.
17. Sheiham, A.: An epidemiological survey of acute ulcerative gingivitis in Nigerians, Arch. Oral Biol. **11**:937, 1966.
18. Emslie, R.D.: Periodontal disease in tropical Africa, Parodontopathies **18**:26, 1966.
19. Pindborg, J.J., et al.: Occurrence of acute necrotizing ulcerative gingivitis in South Indian children, J. Periodontol. **37**:14, 1966.
20. Zinserling, W.D.: Ueber die spirochetöse Gangrän und einige verwandte Prozesses vorzugsweise bei Kindern, Jena, East Germany, 1928, Gustav Fischer.
21. Jimenez, L.M., et al.: The familial occurrence of acute necrotizing gingivitis in children in Colombia, South America, J. Periodontol. **40**:414, 1969.
22. Reade, P.C.: Infantile acute ulcerative gingivitis, J. Periodontol. **34**:387, 1963.
23. Enwonwu, C.O.: Epidemiological and biochemical studies of necrotizing ulcerative gingivitis and noma (cancrum oris) in Nigerian children, Arch. Oral Biol. **17**:1357, 1971.
24. Stevens, A.W., Jr., et al.: Demographic and clinical data associated with acute necrotizing ulcerative gingivitis in a dental school population (ANUG—demographic and clinical data), J. Clin. Periodontol. **11**:487, 1984.
25. Giddon, D.B., Goldhaber, P., and Dunning, J.M.: Prevalence of reported cases of acute necrotizing ulcerative gingivitis in a university population, J. Periodontol. **34**:366, 1953.
26. Giddon, D.B., Zackin, S.J., and Goldhaber, P.: Acute necrotizing ulcerative gingivitis in college students. J. Am. Dent. Assoc. **68**:381, 1964.
27. Pindborg, J.: Gingivitis in military personnel with special reference to ulceromembranous gingivitis, Odontol. Rev. **59**:407, 1951.
28. Pindborg, J.: Influence of service in armed forces on incidence of gingivitis, J. Am. Dent. Assoc. **42**:517, 1951.
29. Skach, M., Zabrodsky, S., and Marklas, L.: A study of the effect of age and season on the incidence of ulcerative gingivitis, J. Periodont. Res. **5**:187, 1970.
30. Brown, R.H.: Necrotizing ulcerative gingivitis in mongoloid and non-mongoloid individuals, J. Periodont. Res. **8**:290, 1973.
31. Schwartz, D.M., and Baumhammers, A.: Smoking and periodontal disease, Periodont. Abstr. **20**:103, 1972.
32. Kenny, E.B., et al.: The effect of cigarette smoke on human oral polymorphonuclear leukocytes, J. Periodont. Res. **12**:227, 1977.
33. Pindborg, J.J.: The epidemiology of ulceromembraneous gingivitis showing the influence of service in the armed forces, Parodontologia **10**:114, 1956.
34. Moulton, R., Ewen, S., and Thieman, W.: Emotional factors in periodontal disease, Oral Surg. **5**:833, 1952.
35. Formicola, A.J., Witte, E.T., and Curran, P.M.: A study of personality traits and acute necrotizing ulcerative gingivitis, J. Periodontol. **41**:36, 1970.
36. Baker, E.G., Crook, G.H., and Schwabacher, E.D.: Personality correlates of periodontal disease, J. Dent. Res. **40**:396, 1961.
37. Davis, C.H, and Jenkins, C.D.: Mental stress and oral diseases, J. Dent. Res. **41**:1045, 1961.
38. Loving, R.H., Weber, T.B., and Mazzarella, M.A.: Blood serum 17-hydroxycorticosteroid levels in necrotizing ulcerative gingivitis, J. Dent. Res. **39**:663, 1960.
39. Maupin, C.C., and Bell, W.B.: The relationship

of 17-hydroxycorticosteroids to acute necrotizing ulcerative gingivitis, J. Periodontol. **46:**721, 1975.

40. Shannon, I.L., Kilgore, W.G., and O'Leary, T.J.: Stress as a predisposing factor in necrotizing gingivitis, J. Periodontol. **40:**240, 1969.

41. Clark, R.E., and Giddon, D.B.: Body geometry of patients who had recurrent attacks of acute necrotizing ulcerative gingivitis, Arch. Oral Biol. **16:**205, 1971.

42. Appleton, J.L.T.: Bacterial infection, ed. 4, Philadelphia, 1950, Lea & Febiger.

43. Hampp, E.G., Scott, D.B., and Wyckoff, R.W.: Morphological characteristics of certain cultured strains of oral spirochetes and *Treponema pallidum* as revealed by the electron microscope, J. Bacteriol. **56:**755, 1948.

44. King, J.D.: Nutritional and other factors in trench mouth with special reference to the nicotinic acid component of vitamin B complex, Br. Dent. J. **74:**113, 1943.

45. Rosebury, T.: The role of infection in periodontal disease, Oral Surg. **5:**363,, 1952.

46. MacDonald, J.B., Socransky, S.S., and Gibbons, R.J.: Aspects of mixed anaerobic infections of mucous membranes, J. Dent. Res. **42:**529, 1963.

47. Socransky, S.S.: Relationship of bacteria to periodontal disease, J. Dent. Res. **49:**203, 1970.

48. Hampp, E.G., and Mergenhagen, S.E.: Experimental infections with oral spirochetes, J. Infect. Dis. **109:**43, 1961.

49. Hampp, E.G., and Mergenhagen, S.E.: Experimental intracutaneous fusobacterial and fusospirochetal infections, J. Infect. Dis. **112:**84,, 1963.

50. Listgarten, M.A., and Socransky, S.S.: Ultrastructural characteristics of a spirochete in the lesion of acute necrotizing ulcerative gingivostomatitis (Vincent's infection). Arch. Oral Biol. **9:**95, 1964.

51. Listgarten, M.A.: Electron microscopic observations on the bacterial flora of acute necrotizing ulcerative gingivitis. J. Periodontol. **36:**328, 1965.

52. Listgarten, M.A., and Lewis, D.W.: The distribution of spirochetes in the lesion of acute necrotizing ulcerative gingivitis: an electron microscopic and statistical survey, J. Periodontol. **38:**379, 1967.

53. Lehner, T., and Clarry, E.D.: Acute ulcerative gingivitis, Br. Dent. J. **121:**366, 1966.

54. Dolby, A.E.: Acute ulcerative gingivitis: immune complex, J. Dent. Res. **51:**1639, 1972.

55. Mikx, F.H.M., and van Campen, G.J.: Preliminary evaluation of the microflora in spontaneous and induced necrotizing ulcerative gingivitis in the beagle dog, J. Periodont. Res. **17:**460, 1982.

56. Mikx, F.H.M., and van Campen, G.J.: Microscopical evaluation of the microflora in relation to necrotizing ulcerative gingivitis in the beagle dog, J. Periodont. Res. **17:**576,, 1982.

57. Hug, H.U., Maltha, J.C., and Mikx, F.H.M.: Necrotizing ulcerative gingivitis in beagle dogs. II. Histologic characteristics of NUG in relation to interproximal contacts, J. Periodont. Res. **19:**89, 1984.

58. Maltha, J.C., Mikx, F.H.M., and Kuijpers, F.J.: Necrotizing ulcerative gingivitis in beagle dogs. III. Distribution of spirochaetes in interdental gingival tissue, J. Periodont. Res. **20:**522, 1985.

59. Mikx, F.H.M., Hug, H.U., and Maltha, J.C.: Necrotizing ulcerative gingivitis in beagle dogs. I. Attempts at unilateral induction of and intraoral transmission of NUG, a microbiological and clinical study, J. Periodont. Res. **19:**76, 1984.

60. Hadi, A.W., and Russell, C.: Quantitative estimations of fusiforms in saliva from normal individuals and cases of acute ulcerative gingivitis, Arch. Oral Biol. **13:**1371, 1958.

61. Loesche, W.J., et al.: The bacteriology of acute necrotizing ulcerative gingivitis, J. Periodontol. **53:**223, 1982.

62. Wilton, J.M.A., Ivanyi, L., and Lehner, T.: Cell-mediated immunity in acute ulcerative gingivitis, J. Periodont. Res. **6:**9, 1971.

63. Cogen, R.B., et al.: Leukocyte function in the etiology of acute necrotizing ulcerative gingivitis, J. Periodontol. **54:**402, 1983.

64. Schaffer, E.M.: The effects of drugs in the treatment of necrotizing ulcerative gingivitis, J. Am. Dent. Assoc. **48:**279, 1954.

65. Stern, I.B.: Necrotizing ulcerative gingivitis. In Kutscher, A.H., Zegarelli, E.V., and Hyman, G.A., editors: Pharmacotherapeutics of oral disease, New York, 1964, McGraw-Hill Book Co.

66. Fitch, H.B., et al.: Acute necrotizing ulcerative gingivitis, J. Periodontol. **34:**422, 1963.

67. Proctor, D.B., and Baker, C.C.: Treatment of acute ulcerative gingivitis with metronidazole, J. Can. Dent. Assoc. **37:**376, 1971.

**ADDITIONAL SUGGESTED READING**

Brown, R.H.: Necrotizing ulcerative gingivitis in mongoloid and non-mongoloid individuals, J. Periodont. Res. **8:**290, 1973.

Chong, C.P., et al.: Bacterial IgG and IgM antibodies in acute necrotizing ulcerative gingivitis, J. Periodontol. **54:**557, 1983.

Courtois, G.J., III, Cobb, M.M., and Killoy, W.J.: Acute necrotizing ulcerative stomatitis: a transmission electron microscope study, J. Periodontol. **54:**671, 1983.

Emslie, R.D.: Cancrum oris, Dent. Pract. **13:**481, 1963.

Emslie, R.D.: Treatment of acute gingivitis, Br. Dent. J. **122:**307, 1967.

Fröhlich, E.: Die Pathologie der postulzerösen Zahnfleischnische und ihre Therapie, Dtsch. Zahnarztl. Z. **27:**284, 1972.

Hooper, P.A., and Seymour, G.J.: The histopathogenesis of acute ulcerative gingivitis, J. Periodontol. **50:**419, 1979.

Jimenez, M.L., and Baer, P.N.: Necrotizing ulcerative gingivitis in children: a 9-year clinical study, J. Periodontol. **46:**715, 1975.

Shields, W.B.: Acute ulcerative gingivitis: a study of the contributing factors and their validity in an army population, J. Periodontol. **48:**346, 1977.

CHAPTER **19**

# Viral infections

**Herpetic gingivostomatitis**

**Treatment**
Recurrent oral aphthae
Erythema multiforme
Herpangina
AIDS

---

## Herpetic gingivostomatitis

Herpetic gingivostomatitis (HGS) is an acute infection that can involve the gingiva, other oral tissues, the lips, and, occasionally, the face circumorally. A high temperature (103° to 104° F [39.5° to 40° C]), general malaise, dehydration, and generalized oral lesions are characteristic. Oral ulcerations are prominent, and the mouth is sore. HGS is not susceptible to antibiotics. It is seen most frequently in children but also occurs in adolescents and adults[1-3] (Fig. 19-1). Acute HGS runs its course in 2 weeks.

Primary infection with herpesvirus leads to acute herpetic gingivostomatitis. The **Herpesvirus** primary attack is believed to confer immunity, but some patients report a second primary attack. By age 60, most persons have antibodies against the herpesvirus. Thus most people have had a prior herpes simplex infection.

The herpes simplex virion is one of the largest known viruses with a size of approximately 100 to 200 $\mu$m (1000 to 2000 Å).[4,5] When fully formed it consists of a core containing the genetic material (DNA) surrounded by a capsule (capsid). The capsid is made of hexagonal particles called *capsomeres* (Figs. 19-2 and 19-3). The capsid in turn is surrounded by a membrane or envelope (Fig. 19-4). The herpes simplex virion is dermatotropic and neurotropic, meaning that the cells it attacks are those of the skin and the nervous system. The fully grown virion penetrates the cell membrane. Once inside the protoplasm the virion loses its coating. Later it gains entrance into the nucleus. When viewed under the light microscope the chromatic material of the nucleus of the infected cell forms round aggregates, called *inclusion bodies*.[6] In the nucleus the DNA of the virus subverts the host nucleus and codes the host DNA for the production of material necessary for viral replication. In subverting the host cell to its own uses, the virion inflicts severe damage to the cell, which ultimately lyses, due to liquefaction necrosis (hydropic degeneration). The hydropic degeneration gives rise to so-called balloon cells of Unna[7] (Fig. 19-5).

After exposure and infection have taken place there is a brief prodromal period of **Pathogenesis** slight fever and malaise. HGS begins with the formation of small vesicles or groups of vesicles in the mouth and sometimes on the skin (see Fig. 19-1). Oral vesicles break

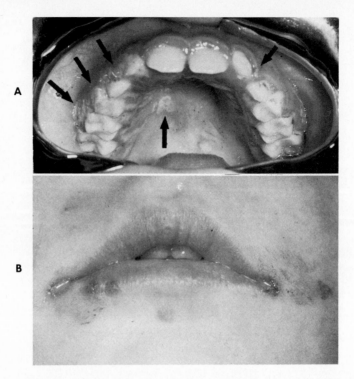

**Fig. 19-1.** **A,** Acute herpetic gingivostomatitis. The gingiva is swollen; ulceration is present in the gingiva and other parts of the oral mucosa *(arrows)*. **B,** Same 6-year-old patient. Note groups of blisters also on the facial skin.

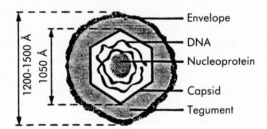

**Fig. 19-2.** The structure of this virus particle is typical of the group of herpesviruses. (From Rapp, F.: Am. Scientist **66:**670, 1978.)

very early and form yellowish gray shallow ulcers surrounded by a red halo. Although the vesicles occur in the gingiva they appear with equal frequency in other parts of the oral mucosa, including lips, cheeks, palate, pharynx, and tongue. Patients have a middle-to-high range of fever, pain (particularly on eating), and malaise. The breath becomes malodorous. The disease is self-limiting and runs its course in approximately 2 weeks.

The lesions of HGS are intraepithelial vesicles, the result of liquefaction necrosis (see Fig. 19-5). The vesicles contain fluid, degenerating cells, and herpesvirus. Herpes simplex is contagious; the mode of infection is by droplets or direct contact.

A patient who has suffered an attack of HGS carries humoral and possibly cellular antibodies throughout life.[8] After infection has taken place some virus survives in a latent stage in the nerve ganglion and may on provocation (exposure to sunlight, fever, colds, mechanical stretching of the lip) produce a recurrence (*secondary herpes labialis*, fever blister, cold sore). Herpesvirus may be shed intermittently, presumably

**Secondary herpes labialis**

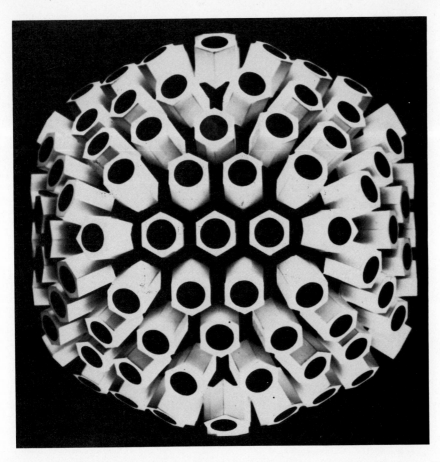

**Fig. 19-3.** Capsid of herpesvirion, composed of capsomeres. (Photograph courtesy Dr. R.W. Horne, Norwich, England; model constructed by Mrs. C.V. Waugh.)

even when the patient is apparently well. It may appear in conjunction with pharyngeal or pulmonary lesions, thus casting some question on the true latency of the virus.[9] The sulcular epithelium may act as a reservoir for the virus.[10,11]

The fever blister is a single vesicle or a group of vesicles on the vermilion border or other parts of the lip. Before an eruption occurs there is often a prodromal period of burning and tingling in the area. The blisters break after a few days and form a crust. The lesion heals after about 2 weeks. If crusts persist longer the clinician should consider an alternative diagnosis.

The location of the virus between the primary and secondary attacks of herpes is in the gasserian ganglion.[12] The virus may descend to the lip through the trigeminal nerve, which may explain why the location of the blister on the lip is usually the same. Resistance to recurrent attacks may depend on antibody, complement, and leukocytes. Deficiency in any of these three might lead to recurrence. It has also been suggested that such recurrent attacks may be associated with decreased interferon formation (a lymphokine produced by T-lymphocytes that is a nonspecific inhibitor of virus replication).

Antibodies to herpes simplex virus may be found in most people in the serum and in their gingival fluid.[8,11] However, the latent stage can be maintained in the absence of neutralizing antibody.[13] Thus animals and humans may harbor the virus without clinical signs of the disease (latency). Since latent infections persist in the ganglion for life[14] and peripheral lesions can recur periodically, vaccines are needed to protect

**Immunology**

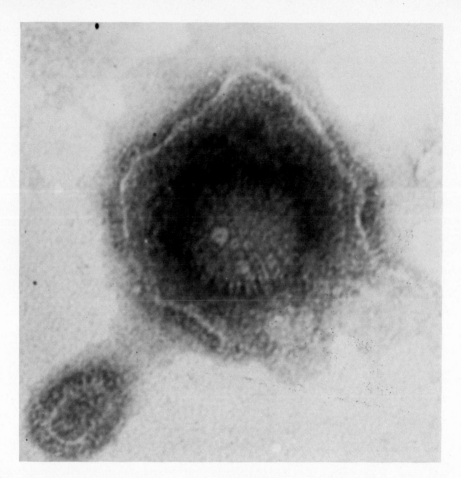

**Fig. 19-4.** Herpesvirion surrounded by envelope. (×280,000.) (Courtesy Dr. R.W. Horne, Norwich, England.)

against both primary and latent infections.[15] Efforts to produce such a vaccine are underway.[15]

**Transfer of infection**

Transfer of the herpesvirus may be by direct contact or by contact with contaminated materials or surfaces. The dental professional is at risk, and an infection occasionally occurs on the hand or finger (called *herpetic whitlow*). From such sites the virus may be transferred to patients,[16] to one's own eyes, and so on. Rubber gloves must be worn when patients present with primary or secondary herpetic lesions. Each infected individual serves as a permanent carrier who is intermittently infectious.

**Clinical diagnosis**

The clinical diagnosis of acute HGS can be made on the basis of symptoms and clinical appearance. The confirmatory diagnosis depends on one or more of the following laboratory tests: (a) inoculation of the virus from a suspected site to tissue culture,[17]

**Laboratory diagnosis**

a technique that takes 3 to 6 days; the virus can be distinguished as type 1 or 2; (b) fluorescent monoclonal antibody testing of scrapings[18]; and (c) serologic studies. The monoclonal antibody fluorescent test requires only 15 to 20 minutes to perform and thus represents a practical test. Such tests are 94% to 99% sensitive for culture confirmation and 85% to 90% sensitive for direct diagnosis of specimens smeared on microscope slides.[18] The role of serologic tests is uncertain. Primary infection can be diagnosed by seroconversion, but this requires both an acute and convalescent sample. Moreover, the high prevalence of antibody (50% or greater) in the adult population limits the usefulness of this test, and recurrent infections can produce an increase in antibody titer.

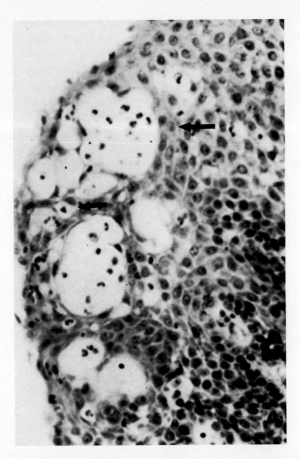

**Fig. 19-5.** Balloon cells *(small arrow)* and intraepithelial blisters *(large arrow)* created by fusion of balloon cells.

The herpesviruses have been classifed on the basis of common morphologic findings (see Fig. 19-2). Five members infect humans[19]: (1) herpesvirus type 1—oropharyngeal (responsible for acute HGS and cold sores), (2) herpesvirus type 2—genital (responsible for genital lesions), (3) cytomegalovirus (responsible for cytomegalic inclusion disease), (4) varicella-zoster virus (responsible for chickenpox and shingles), and (5) Epstein-Barr virus (responsible for infectious mononucleosis and Burkitt lymphoma). They are also responsible, but more rarely, for encephalitis, keratoconjunctivitis, and hepatitis. **Herpesvirus classification**

Although herpesvirus type 2 occurs in the genital area, it can occur orally, and the oral form can occur genitally. Twenty-five percent of the genital lesions are of type 1 herpesvirus. Both forms appear to have a cancer relatedness. Evidence for a viral etiology of cancer[20] includes Epstein-Barr virus for Burkitt lymphoma and nasopharyngeal carcinoma. It is strengthened by the association of herpes simplex viruses with cancer of the cervix.[19] Both types of herpesvirus can be transmitted during oral sex.[19]

Herpes simplex infection of the newborn is a serious health problem with a significant associated mortality.

## Treatment

Research using antiviral chemotherapy and chemoprophylaxis has led to the development of several antiviral compounds.[21] These have an effect on the acute manifestations of several herpesvirus infections but have little or no effect on the establishment or maintenance of latent infection. These antiviral compounds[21] are pyrimidine nucleoside analogues that inhibit virus DNA synthesis. They include intravenously administered *Vira-A* or *vidarabine,* which is used to treat infections of immunosuppressed patients, herpes zoster (shingles), herpes simplex encephalitis, and viral infections of the newborn. *Acyclovir* (Zovirax), administered cutaneously, can be used either topically or orally in patients at high risk. 5-Iodo-2'-deoxyuridine (IUDR) is restricted to the treatment of herpes simplex keratitis and phosphonofiate.[21]

Related drugs have been tested orally, but there is no ideal drug as yet. Ara-C or cytosine arabinoside is helpful in preventing lesions of recurrences when such recurrences can be anticipated.[22] Carbenoxolone sodium cream shortens the course of the infection.[23] Iodoxyuridine (IUDR) or acyclovir applied with iontophoresis (since the drugs do not otherwise penetrate the skin) produces major improvement within 1 day.[24] A lymphokine product of T-lymphocytes (interferon), which is a nonspecific inhibitor of virus replication, has yet to be tested in the treatment of HGS.

In the past herpes has been treated by painting with dyes (neutral red) and irradiating with ultraviolet light, which inactivates the virus. This treatment should be avoided since it may induce malignant transformation.[20]

**Supportive treatment**

The use of mild, soothing mouthwashes is helpful. Eating can be painful. Bland foods and liquid supplements (Metrecal, Slender, Nutrament) are recommended.

A helpful mouthwash is:

Warm water (⅔ tumbler)
White Karo syrup (⅓ tumbler)
Lidocaine (Xylocaine) viscous (2 tablespoons)
Sig: rinse before meals, on arising, and before retiring

Mucosal ointments (Orabase) can be applied to the lesions with a cotton swab for temporary relief.

When oral tissues are extremely ulcerated, the pressure of the tongue against the gingiva and palate is so painful that the patient would rather drool than swallow. In such cases placement of periodontal surgical dressing may afford relief. Infants and young children may require nasopharyngeal intubation. Hydrogen peroxide is irritating and contraindicated in HGS. Penicillin is ineffective for HGS and may protract the duration and aggravate the course of the disease.

**Mucosal ointments**

Treatment of herpes labialis (fever blisters) is symptomatic.[1] Pharmaceutic preparations such as Blistex, Stopcil, and Topcin may afford relief. Some patients report success in preventing recurrences with daily dosage of 500 mg of lysine.

## RECURRENT ORAL APHTHAE

The possible similarities and differences between HGS and necrotizing ulcerative gingivitis should be reviewed (Chapter 15). Other lesions that are sometimes confused with HGS include recurrent oral aphthae. These may occur in clusters. They may be related to steroid sex hormones and additional factors that regulate immune responses and play a secondary role.[25]

Isolated oral aphthae may cause varying degrees of painfulness, depending on number and location. The actual cause of oral aphthae is unknown.

There may be a variant of aphthous ulceration that resembles the herpetic lesion. These lesions are referred to as herpetiform ulceration. However the virus has not been recovered from the lesions in any of the patients studied.

## ERYTHEMA MULTIFORME

Erythema multiforme is another less common condition that may resemble HGS. The vesicles in erythema multiforme are larger and are usually accompanied by involvement of the skin and other mucous membranes. Thus erythema multiforme is a mucocutaneous disease with a variable pattern of recurrence. It can be limited to the oral cavity where it is characterized by multiple painful ulcers. It may be caused by an allergic reaction but is unrelated to herpesvirus.[26]

## HERPANGINA

Herpangina is a disease with lesions on the soft palate and the pharynx. It is caused by the coxsackie A virus, which can be isolated and identified. There may be manifestations of the coxsackievirus infection on the skin.

## AIDS

Acquired immune deficiency syndrome (AIDS) is another viral disease that may have oral symptoms. It is caused by human T cell lymphotropic virus type III (HTLV-III). This RNA virus shares features with retroviruses linked to leukemia in animals and HTLV-I–induced leukemia in man. HTLV-III produces a cytotoxic effect on helper T-lymphocytes, compromising the immunologic response since most of the T-helper cells are eliminated. Medical symptoms include fever (100° to 104° F), night sweats, a persistent dry cough, shortness of breath, loss of appetite and weight, diarrhea, lymphadenopathy, Kaposi sarcoma, monilial infections, leukopenia, and malaise. The dentist may encounter oral monilial infections (thrush),[27] enlargement of lymph nodes of the neck, and reddish brown or bluish spots in the mouth or on the facial skin that gradually enlarge rather than improve (Kaposi sarcoma) and hairy leukoplakia.[28]

Screening tests for the presence of HTLV-III antibody may indicate whether or not a person has been exposed to the virus but not whether the person has or will develop the disease. Five to twenty percent of those who test positive go on to develop AIDS. Whether or not those who test positive can transmit the disease is unknown, but it is presumed that those who carry the virus are potentially infectious to others. False positive test results are known to occur.

AIDS is transmitted by sexual contact, sharing nonsterile hypodermic syringes, or by transfusions of infected blood (the latter is now no longer probable because of screening tests).

The HTLV-III virus is readily killed by soap and disinfectants and is not easily transmitted. The patient with AIDS is more at risk (because of immunosuppression) of contracting other diseases.

The AIDS virus has been found in blood and less commonly in saliva, but the possibility that HTLV-III can be transmitted by saliva should be considered.[29] Precautions in the dental office[30] when treating known AIDS patients include double gloving and wearing of surgical mask and gown. Instruments should be disinfected before autoclaving, and dental equipment and adjacent surfaces should be wiped with disinfectants. The transmission of AIDS among dental personnel may be linked to patient care although this has not been confirmed.

### REFERENCES

1. Everett, F.G.: Aureomycin in the treatment of herpes simplex, J. Am. Dent. Assoc. **40:**555, 1950.
2. Hermann, D.: Gingivostomatitis herpetica bei Erwachsenen, Dtsch. Zahnärztl. Z. **27:**870, 1972.
3. Silverman, S., Jr., and Beumer. J., III: Primary herpetic gingivostomatitis of adult onset, Oral Surg. **36:**496, 1973.
4. Kaplan, A.S., editor: The herpes virus, New York, 1973, Academic Press, Inc.
5. Juel-Jensen, B.E., and MacCallum, F.O.: Herpes simplex, varicella and zoster, Philadelphia, 1972, J.B. Lippincott Co.
6. Lipschütz, B.: Untersuchungen über die Aetiologie der Krankheiten der Herpesgruppe, Arch. Dermatol. Syph. **136:**428, 1921.
7. Unna, P.G.: The histopathology of the diseases of the skin, transl. by N. Walker, Edinburgh, 1896, W.F. Clay.
8. Gordon, G.D., et al.: Studies of herpes simplex virus and interferon in human gingival cells, J. Periodontol. **46:**86, 1975.

9. Daniels, C.A., LeGoff, S.G., and Notkins, A.L.: Shedding of infectious virus/antibody complexes from vesicular lesions of patients with recurrent herpes labialis, Lancet **2:**524, 1975.

10. Zakay-Rones, Z., et al.: The sulcular epithelium as a reservoir for herpes simplex virus in man, J. Periodontol. **44:**779, 1973.

11. Hochman, N., et al.: Antibodies to herpes simplex virus in human gingival fluid, J. Periodontol. **52:**324, 1981.

12. Tenser, R.B., Miller, R.L., and Rapp, F.: Trigeminal ganglion infection by thymidine kinase–negative mutants of herpes simplex virus, Science **205:**915, 1979.

13. Sekizawa, T., et al.: Latency of herpes simplex virus in absence of neutralizing antibody: model for reactivation, Science **210:**1026, 1980.

14. Wigdahl, B.L., et al.: High efficiency latency and activation of herpes simplex virus in human cells, Science **217:**1145, 1982.

15. Cremer, K.J., et al.: Vaccinia virus recombinant expressing herpes simplex virus type I glycoprotein D prevents latent herpes in mice, Science **228:**737, 1985.

16. Manzella, J.P., et al.: An outbreak of herpes simplex virus type I gingivitis in a dental hygiene practice, JAMA **252:**2019, 1984.

17. Mintz, G.A., and Rose, S.L.: Diagnosis of oral herpes simplex virus infections: practical aspects of viral culture, Oral Surg. **58:**486, 1984.

18. Nowinski, R.C., et al.: Monoclonal antibodies for diagnosis of infectious diseases in humans, Science **219:**637, 1983.

19. Rapp, F.: Herpesvirus, venereal disease and cancer, Am. Scientist **66:**670, 1978.

20. Marx, J.L.: Viral carcinogenesis: role of DNA viruses, Science **183:**1066, 1974.

21. Dolin, R.: Antiviral chemotherapy and chemoprophylaxis, Science **227:**1296, 1985.

22. Kurtz, J.R.: Symposium: oral herpes simplex infection treatment, J. R. Soc. Med. **72:**134, 1979.

23. Partridge, M., and Poswillo, D.E.: Topical carbenoxolone sodium in the management of herpes simplex infextion, Br. J. Oral Maxillofac. Surg. **22:**138, 1984.

24. Henley-Cohn, J., and Hausfeld, J.N.: Iontophoretic treatment of oral herpes, Laryngoscope **94:**118, 1984.

25. Ferguson, M.M., Carter, J., and Boyle, P.: An epidemiological study of factors associated with recurrent aphthae in women, J. Oral Med. **39:**212, 1984.

26. Lozada-Nur, F., and Shillitoe, E.J.: Erytheme multiforme and herpes simplex virus, J. Dent. Res. **64:**930, 1983.

27. Wofford, D.T., and Miller, R.I.: Acquired immune deficiency syndrome (AIDS): disease characteristics and oral manifestation, J. Am. Dent. Assoc. **101:**258, 1985.

28. Greenspan, J.S., et al.: Replication of Epstein-Barr virus within the epithelial cells of oral "hairy" leukoplakia, an AIDS-associated lesion, New Engl. J. Med. **313:**1564, 1985.

29. Groopman, J.E., et al.: HTLV-III in saliva of people with AIDS-related complex and healthy homosexual men at risk for AIDS, Science **226:**447, 1984.

30. David, D.R., and Knapp, J.F.: The significance of AIDS to dentists and dental practice, J. Prosthet. Dent. **52:**736, 1984.

## ADDITIONAL SUGGESTED READING

Addy, M., and Dolby, A.: Aphthous ulceration: the antinuclear factor, J. Dent. Res. **51:**1594, 1972.

Brown, R.H.: Necrotizing ulcerative gingivitis in mongoloid and non-mongoloid individuals, J. Periodont. Res. **8:**290, 1973.

Nahmias, A.J., and Roizman, B.: Infection with herpes-simplex virus 1 and 2. I. to III., N. Engl. J. Med. **289:**667, 719, 781, 1973.

Sabin, A.B., and Tarro, G.: Herpes simplex and herpes genitalis viruses in etiology of some human cancers, Proc. Natl. Acad. Sci. U.S.A. **70:**3225, 1973.

# CHAPTER 20

# Pericoronitis

**Anatomic relationships**
*Signs and symptoms*

**Treatment**

**Prevention**

**Complications**

---

Pericoronitis is an acute infection with accompanying inflammation of gingival and **Definition**
contiguous soft tissues about the crown of an incompletely erupted tooth.[1-6] Mandibular
third molars are the most frequently affected. However, mandibular second molars
may become involved when they are the most distal teeth in the arch. The most distal
maxillary molar may become involved with pericoronitis, but this is an infrequent
occurrence.

## Anatomic relationships

The occlusal surface of an involved tooth may be partly covered by a flap of tissue,
the operculum, which exists during the eruption of the tooth and may persist afterward
(Fig. 20-1). Various degrees of eruption, malposition, or impaction may further complicate the soft tissue architecture. In addition, pocket formation and bony deformities
are not uncommon in the molar region.

### SIGNS AND SYMPTOMS

The operculum is particularly vulnerable to irritation and is often directly traumatized when it is caught between the crown that it covers and the antagonist tooth
during closure. The cryptlike form of the pericoronal tissues favors the proliferation
of microorganisms, particularly since the performance of adequate oral hygiene in this
area is difficult. These factors predispose to acute infection, including acute necrotizing
ulcerative gingivitis (ANUG).[1]

A pericoronal flap may be asymptomatic, but it is a potential site for infection and
pocket formation. It thus provides for additional retention of bacteria and exudate.
Plaque accumulates on the exposed and operculum-covered surfaces of mandibular
third molars. Coccoid organisms are found interspersed between filamentous and rod-
shaped organisms. Spirochetes are also present. The numbers of spirochetes increase
apically in the plaque boundaries and on the plaque surface. Their position implies
that they may be at the vanguard in the development of pericoronitis. Since the spirochetes are superficial and in close contact with the epithelium of the pouch (oper-

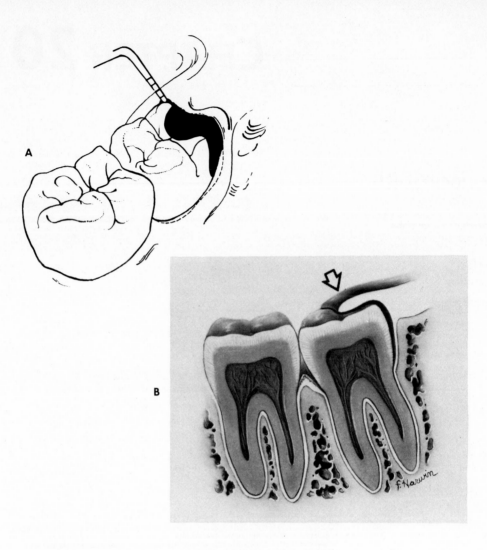

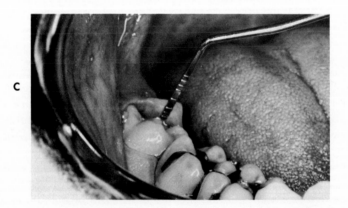

**Fig. 20-1.** Pericoronitis about a third molar. **A,** The tooth is partially enveloped by tissue, and, **B,** the operculum *(arrow)* covers the distal portion of the occlusal surface. **C,** Operculum retracted by a probe. Note ulceration below the operculum.

culum), their presence along with fusobacteria may be associated with the occurrence of NUG in these sites.[2] Streptococcal and staphylococcal infection may also occur.[1]

With accumulation and retention of bacterial plaque, acute exacerbation may ensue. Further enlargement of the tissue then inhibits drainage from the sulcus, inducing deeper spreading of the process beyond the gingival tissues. Often the enlarged tissues become traumatized during mastication, adding to the discomfort of the patient. Pus may issue from under the operculum. As the condition becomes more severe, swelling increases, mandibular movement is limited (trismus), and temperature is elevated. In addition, there may be leukocytosis, lymphadenopathy, foul breath (fetor oris), and referred pain to the ear. Pus may accumulate in the tissues subjacent to the buccal (vestibular) fornix.

## Treatment

In the treatment of pericoronitis, the following factors should be considered[5]:

1. Severity of the inflammatory process
2. Systemic complications
3. Advisability of retaining the involved tooth

Before undertaking treatment the dentist should review the medical history to determine if the patient has valvular heart disease, uveitis, or a cardiovascular or joint prosthesis. In these cases immediate coverage with ample doses of antibiotics is indicated because of the health risk.[7]

Steps in the treatment of pericoronitis are as follows:

1. Medicate with antibiotics as necessary. Antibiotics should be employed if fever, swelling, or lymphadenopathy is present.[8] If penicillin is contraindicated, erythromycin or metronidazole may be used as alternatives.[9] Tetracyclines and possibly chlorhexidine irrigation may be effective in some cases.
2. Cleanse the area by lavage and gentle curettage, and establish drainage. Remove all debris from below the operculum. Insert a single thickness of ¼-inch iodoform gauze below the operculum.
3. Instruct the patient to rinse frequently with warm solutions of saline (1 teaspoonful of salt to a pint of warm water).
4. At the second appointment (24 hours later) remove the drain. Insert a new drain for another 24 hours, if necessary. The patient should feel better.
5. Decide to either extract, or retain the offending tooth and remove the operculum. If NUG is an etiologic factor in the pericoronitis, appropriate treatment should be given (Chapter 18).
6. At times, selective grinding of the occlusal surface of the opposing molar may help to resolve the infection. At times, retention of the mandibular third molar and extraction of its opponent may be indicated.

Since the muscular floor of the oral cavity proper terminates mesial to the mandibular third molar, an infection lingual to the mandibular third molar could descend through the fascial planes of the neck and mediastinum. Because of this, pericoronitis should be carefully controlled.

## Prevention

Removal of third molar flaps (opercula) about the most distal, incompletely erupted teeth can prevent pericoronitis. Semi-impacted teeth should be removed carefully at an early time, taking care not to damage the bone on the distal surface of the adjacent tooth.

## Complications

Some cases of pericoronitis occurring in partly erupted, vital teeth give rise to cyst formation.[10] These are all reported to affect lower third molars, most frequently occurring on the buccal surface, possibly in association with an enamel projection in the buccal bifurcation. These cysts are generally unsuspected at the time of clinical and roentgenographic examination. Histologically, the cysts are lined by reduced enamel epithelium.

Pericoronal infections must be controlled before surgery. If the initial infection is not contained or is carried more deeply during surgical procedures, it may spread along fascial planes into the surgical spaces of the head and neck. Retropharyngeal, peritonsillar, masseter space, and temporal space abscesses, Ludwig angina, laryngeal edema, cavernous sinus thrombosis, and acute meningitis are relatively rare but can be serious consequences of pericoronitis.

### REFERENCES

1. Kay, H.L.W.: Investigation into the nature of pericoronitis, Br. J. Oral Surg. **4:**52, 1966.
2. Hurlen, B., and Olsen, I.: A scanning electron microscopic study on the microflora of chronic periodontitis of lower third molars. Oral Surg. **58:**522, 1984.
3. Leone, S., et al.: Correlation of acute pericoronitis and the position of the mandibular third molar, Oral Surg. **6:**245, 1986.
4. Nitzan, D.W., et al.: Pericoronitis: a reappraisal of its clinical and microbiologic aspects, J. Oral Maxillofac. Surg. **43:**510, 1985.
5. Kay, H.L.W.: The management of pericoronitis, Dent. Pract. **11:**80, 1960.
6. Bean, L.R., and King, D.P.: Pericoronitis; its nature and etiology, J. Am. Dent. Assoc. **83:**1074, 1971.
7. Kaplan, E.L., et al.: (Committee on Prevention of Rheumatic Fever and Bacterial Endocarditis of the American Heart Association): Prevention of bacterial endocarditis: a committee report of the American Heart Association, J. Am. Dent. Assoc. **95:**600, 1977.
8. Killey, H.C., and Kay, L.N.: The impacted wisdom tooth, ed. 2, Edinburgh, 1975, Churchill Livingstone, Inc.
9. McGowan, D.A., Murphy, K.J., and Sheiham, A.: Metronidazole in the treatment of severe acute pericoronitis: a clinical trial, Br. Dent. J. **142:**221, 1977.
10. Craig, G.T.: The paradental cyst: a specific inflammatory odontogenic cyst, Br. Dent. J. **141:**9, 1976.

### ADDITIONAL SUGGESTED READING

Andrews, A.G.: Pericoronitis, Appl. Ther. **8:**688, 1966.

Birn, H.: Spread of dental infections, Dent. Pract. **22:**347, 1972.

Crystal, D.K., et al.: Emergency treatment in Ludwig's angina, Surg. Gynecol. Obstet. **129:**755, 1969.

Wallace, J.R.: Pericoronitis and military dentistry, Oral Surg. **22:**543, 1966.

# CHAPTER 21

# Abscesses and cysts

**Abscesses**
Periodontal abscess
Gingival abscess
Periapical abscess
Differential diagnosis
Prognosis
Treatment

**Cysts**
Gingival cyst
Periodontal cyst
Incidence and origin

## Abscesses

A dental abscess is a circumscribed, acute, purulent infection of the soft tissues in **Definition**
or about the teeth. The area involved becomes swollen and painful. Pus may distend
the gingiva and extend into tissues subjacent to the vestibular fornix.

Bacteria are not normally present in the tissues. When they gain entrance a rapid **Pathogeneses**
migration of leukocytes occurs to contain the infection. The area is walled off by
thrombosis of the vessels and by a fibrinous blockade. The numbers of leukocytes and
microorganisms continue to increase. This is followed by necrosis and liquefaction of
the central area, with formation of pus. *Streptococcus viridans* has been reported as
the most common organism found when abscesses are cultured,[1,2] although staphylococci are being found increasingly.[3] Cultures taken of four patients with abscesses
showed that 90.2% of organisms in the exudate are obligate anaerobes. Gram-negative
anaerobic rods account for 59% of the flora and include *Bacteroides melaninogenicus*
ss. *asaccharolyticus, Capnocytophaga* species, *Vibrio corrodens,* and *Fusobacterium*
species. Gram-positive anaerobic cocci account for 13.7%. Streptococci are the most
frequent facultative isolate.[4,5]

### PERIODONTAL ABSCESS

The periodontal abscess can be an acute exacerbation of chronic periodontal disease.
It may occur when the infection passes into tissues through the pocket epithelium.
Such abscesses frequently result from the occlusion of the narrow mouths of tortuous
or deep intrabony pockets (Figs. 21-1 and 21-2). Since the virulence of the organisms
is an important factor, even shallow pockets may become involved. Occasionally, lateral
periodontal cysts (Fig. 21-3) may abscess.[6,7]

### GINGIVAL ABSCESS

The gingival abscess is a relative rarity that occurs when the bacteria invade through
a break in the gingival surface. Such abrasions may be the result of mastication, oral
hygiene procedures, or dental treatment (Fig. 21-4). Although the gingival sulcus is
not involved at the onset, the abscess may extend deep into the connective tissue,

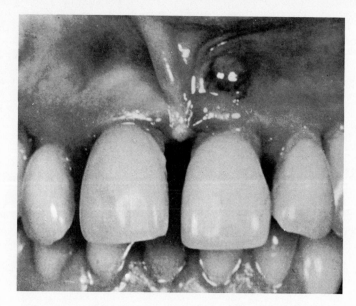

**Fig. 21-1.** Periodontal abscess in the region of the maxillary incisor.

involving the alveolar bone and communicating with the sulcus. The resistance of the patient is an important factor. The patient with an uncontrolled diabetes, for example, may be more susceptible to abscesses.

Histologically, gingival and periodontal abscesses are identical.[8]

## PERIAPICAL ABSCESS

The periapical (dentoalveolar) abscess is the result of pulpal infection that extends through the apical foramen to the periapical tissues. Such abscesses may develop fistulous tracts that communicate with the oral cavity. They may also develop a communication with the periodontal pocket or the gingival sulcus. It is possible for the pulpal infection to reach these periodontal tissues through an aberrant canal, root fracture, or a perforation. Of all the dental abscesses the periapical is the most common type.

The infective organisms include *Fusobacterium, Bacteroides, Streptococcus, Staphylococcus,* and *Peptostreptococcus.*[9,10]

**Cytologic characteristics**    The cytologic characteristics of the periapical abscess are typical. Polymorphonuclear leukocytes predominate at the apex and are massively congregated in the area of the abscess and in ulcerated areas. These cells migrate from dilated blood vessels in an attempt to protect the tissues from invading organisms by their phagocytic and enzymatic action. The more virulent the bacteria, the greater the leukocytic migration into the affected tissue area. The presence of pus exuding through a fistula is an indication of this leukocytic activity. Gingival and periodontal abscesses have similar cytologic characteristics, but the exudate may come from a pocket or stoma.

## DIFFERENTIAL DIAGNOSIS

The differential diagnosis of an abscess must distinguish periapical, periodontal, and gingival abscesses. Periodontal treatment is concerned primarily with periodontal and gingival abscesses. The periapical abscess is from pulpal infection, the periodontal abscess develops through the pocket, and the gingival abscess is an infection that occurs through a break in the gingival surface (Fig. 21-5). Although an abscess may

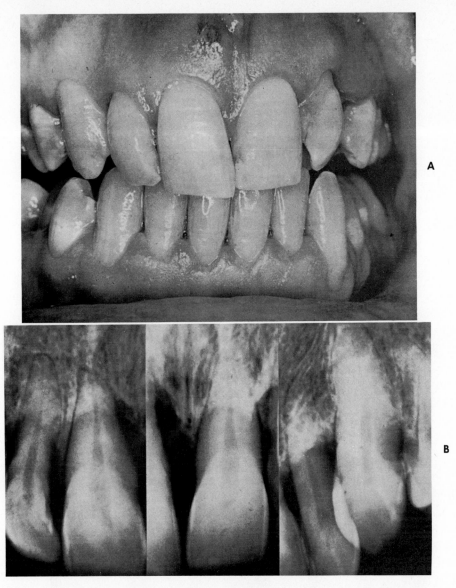

**Fig. 21-2.  A,** Periodontitis with a fistula mesial to the maxillary right central incisor, next to the frenum. **B,** Roentgenograms of the same patient, exhibiting considerable bone destruction in the region of the abscess.

originate in any one place, it can extend to involve other areas. For example, the periodontal abscess may cause pulpal necrosis and periapical abscesses and may ultimately lead to pocket formation.

The infective process and clinical symptoms of the various dental abscesses tend to resemble each other. The abscesses differ only in origin and avenue of infection.[8] Many periodontal abscesses are misdiagnosed as periapical abscesses, and teeth are extracted when the dentist is reluctant to treat this condition. Proper diagnosis, on the other hand, could lead to proper treatment and retention of many abscessed teeth. Diagnosis depends on clinical findings, roentgenographic examination, and pulp testing. Caries, pulpal involvement, and periapical pathosis are suggestive of periapical abscess, whereas pocket formation, alveolar bone loss, and periodontal pathologic con-

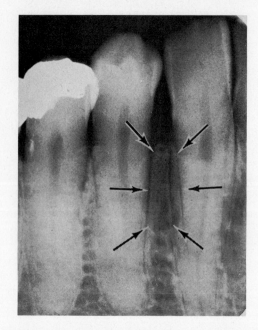

**Fig. 21-3.** Roentgenogram of a periodontal cyst. (Courtesy T. Gilmore, Portland, Oregon.)

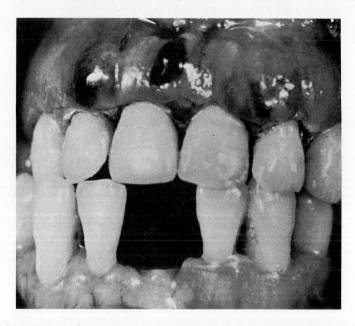

**Fig. 21-4.** Acute abscesses (gingival abscesses) produced by mechanical injury to the gingival tissues.

ditions are suggestive of periodontal abscess. When neither set of circumstances is obvious, a gingival abscess should be suspected. Periodontal abscesses can occur about nonvital teeth; conversely, periapical abscesses can occur in periodontally involved teeth. Moreover, the infection can spread from periodontium to pulp and vice versa so that an abscess may be both periodontal and periapical (Chapter 42). Fortunately, complications such as these are infrequent. Abscesses tend to have periods of exacerbation and remission. Repeated exacerbations are responsible for bizarre and extensive loss of bone.

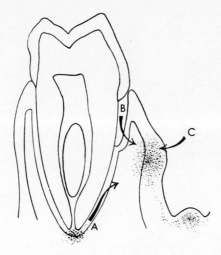

**Fig. 21-5.**  Portals of entry in abscess formation: *A,* periapical abscess; *B,* periodontal abscess; *C,* gingival abscess. A primary infection in any one area may travel to the other areas and involve them secondarily. In addition, extension to the vestibular fornix may occur.

## PROGNOSIS

The purpose of the diagnosis is to establish the type of abscess, the prognosis, and the choice of treatment. The prognosis of an abscessed tooth depends on the amenability of the infection to treatment. The gingival abscess is completely treatable and its prognosis favorable. The prognosis of the periapically abscessed tooth depends on whether root canal therapy is possible. The prognosis of the periodontally abscessed tooth depends on the amount and nature of the bone loss and the strategic position of the tooth. During the height of the abscess, mobility is increased and is an inconclusive symptom. The prognosis of a tooth with a periodontal abscess is generally promising, except in rare cases when a localized osteomyelitis follows.[11]

## TREATMENT

Treatment of the abscessed tooth varies with the decision to retain or to extract the tooth and with the type of abscess present. Treatment therefore has exodontic, periodontal, and endodontic aspects. The details of periodontal treatment are dealt with more fully in later chapters. The first step in treatment is the reduction of the abscess. The administration of antibiotics is indicated in the presence of fever and malaise.[2] Drainage should be established if it is not already present. This may involve curetting the pocket or incising the abscess ( Fig. 21-6). If the tooth is being traumatized, selective grinding procedures should be used to reduce the prematurity. When necessary, extraction of the tooth will serve to establish drainage. Reduction of the abscess should be followed by the appropriate treatment.

In some instances rinsing the mouth with hot water every 2 hours will help the abscess to point. If an incision is needed a horizontal cut over the center of the abscess is favored. Iodoform gauze may be inserted. Vertical incisions involving the gingival margin may lead to unsightly recessions and should be avoided. On occasion a flap may lead to unsightly recessions and should be avoided. On occasion a flap may be reflected[12,13] ( Figs. 21-6 and 21-7).

During the acute stages of the abscess, portions of the alveolar bone may become necrotic. Small sequestra may form. When a sequestrum forms the abscess will not resolve in the usual manner, and the sequestrum may have to be removed unless it is exfoliated. Observations of the presence of pus and necrotic bone associated with

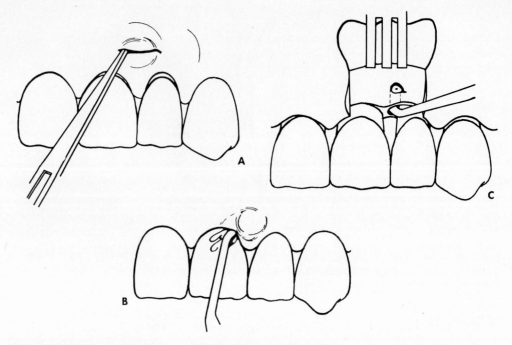

**Fig. 21-6.** Means of establishing drainage. **A,** Horizontal incision. **B,** Curettage through the gingival sulcus. **C,** Raising a small flap.

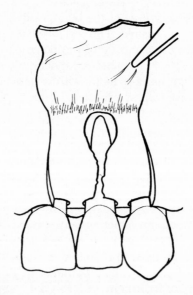

**Fig. 21-7.** Flap raised to give access to periapical and periodontal tissues. Apical resection and root curettage can be performed in instances requiring simultaneous endodontic and periodontal treatment. (Modified from Trott, J.R.: J. Can. Dent. Assoc. **25:**601, 1959.)

periodontal abscesses may have influenced the development of the early mistaken concept of periodontal disease as a flow of pus from the bone (pyorrhea alveolaris).

After the abscess is reduced, further treatment is determined by diagnosis and prognosis. If a tooth is hopelessly involved, it should be extracted. The gingival abscess will usually resolve completely after drainage. Periapical lesions are treated by endodontic procedures; the involved sulcus may subsequently heal.

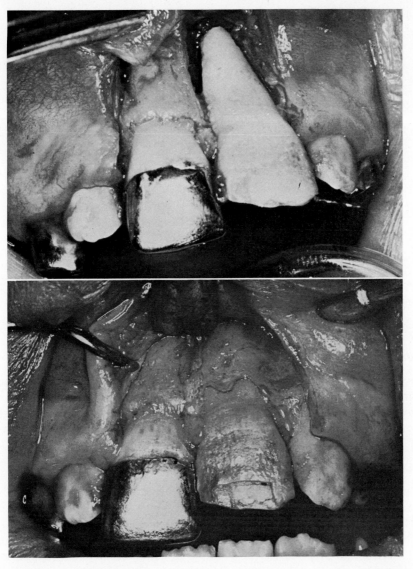

**Fig. 21-8.** **A,** A flap has been elevated to show the bone destruction caused by an abscess. The vestibular bone is completely destroyed, the apex of the tooth is involved, and the bone destruction extends orally to the palatal surface of the apical half of the tooth. (Courtesy W.H. Hiatt, Denver, Colorado.) **B,** Reoperation showing remarkable regeneration of vestibular bone after successful endodontic treatment. (Courtesy W.H. Hiatt, Denver, Colorado.)

Since the bone loss associated with periodontal abscesses may be extensive, osseous surgical procedures that might require further sacrifice of bone may be contraindicated. Reattachment or bone graft procedures are more conserving of bone and are therefore preferable.[14] Moreover, after periodontal abscesses are treated the potential for repair and attachment is enhanced.[12,13,15-17] Successful treatment is often followed by regeneration of bone.[17] Reattachment attempts depend on the location of the abscess and access to the area. In addition, adequate stabilization and minimization of occlusal traumatism may be called for.

If an abscess has involved both periapical and periodontal tissues, combined periodontal-endodontic treatment may be necessary (Chapter 42). This can be accomplished by exposing the area with a broad flap to gain access to the root surface and

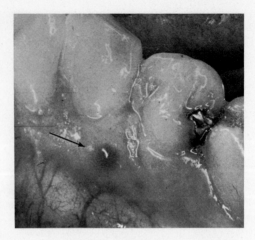

**Fig. 21-9.** Gingival cyst.

the apex (Figs. 21-7 and 21-8). In this way both curettage and apicoectomy can be performed in one operation.[13,17]

# Cysts

### GINGIVAL CYST

The gingival cyst occurs as a painless, bluish gray nodule in the gingiva (Fig. 21-9) and has the appearance and consistency of a mucocele.[18] Because such a cyst is located superficially it may not be apparent on the roentgenogram. The gingival cyst can provoke bone destruction by expanding. The destruction will occur from outside inward, whereas the periodontal cyst expands from the inside outward.

### PERIODONTAL CYST

A periodontal cyst (sometimes called a lateral periodontal cyst) may be seen on roentgenograms (see Fig. 21-3) as a well-defined radiolucent lesion adjacent to a root.[18,19] It occurs most frequently in the canine-bicuspid areas.[20] It lies mainly in the bone, sometimes breaking through the cortical plate and resulting in a swelling of the gingiva. Periodontal cysts have been reported in pericoronitis about mandibular third molars (Chapter 18).

### INCIDENCE AND ORIGIN

Gingival and periodontal cysts are infrequent. Their highest incidence is in the maxilla.[21,22] They may arise from remnants of odontogenic epithelium in the periodontal ligament or the gingiva.[23-28] Other mechanisms leading to the formation of such cysts undoubtedly operate occasionally and include cyst formation at an accessory pulp canal, dentigerous cysts assuming a lateral position, rests of Malassez, traumatic implantation of surface epithelium that later undergoes cystic degeneration, development from heterotopic glandular epithelium, or cystic development within a lateral periodontal abscess.[27] Solitary (extravasation) cysts may also occur in the alveolar region.[29] Some reports assert that most gingival and periodontal cysts occur in the region of the maxillary lateral incisor.[22] Others indicate the cuspid-bicuspid area.[18,20] Cysts can become infected and then form an abscess of puzzling origin in a vital tooth with no demonstrable pocket.

Attention should be directed to tooth vitality in periodontal diagnosis. Extensive and precipitous bone loss may have pulp disease as an associated cause. Proper diagnosis of such cases will promote success in treatment.

## REFERENCES

1. Ludwig, T.G.: An investigation of the oral flora of suppurative oral swelling, Aust. Dent. J. **2:**259, 1957.
2. Epstein, S., and Scopp, I.W.: Antibiotics and the intraoral abscess, J. Periodontol. **48:**236, 1977.
3. Goldberg, M.H.: The changing biologic nature of acute dental infection, J. Am. Dent. Assoc. **80:**1048, 1970.
4. Newman, M.G., and Sims, T.N.: The predominant cultivable microbiota of the periodontal abscess, J. Periodontol. **50:**350, 1979.
5. Moore, J.R., and Russell, C.: Bacteriologic investigation of dental abscesses, Dent. Pract. **22:**390, 1972.
6. Knolle, G.: Der Paradontalabscess, Dtsch. Zahnarztl. Z. **27:**290, 1972.
7. Miyasato, M.C.: The periodontal abscess, Periodont. Abstr. **23:**53, 1975.
8. O'Brien, T.J.: Diagnosis and treatment of periodontal and gingival abscesses, J. Ontario Dent. Assoc. **47:**16, 1970.
9. Williams, B.L., McCann, E.S., and Schoenknecht, F.D.: Bacteriology of dental abcesses of endodontic origin, J. Clin. Microbiol. **18:**770, 1983.
10. van Winkelhoff, A.J., et al.: *Bacteroides endodentalis* and other black-pigmented *Bacteroides* species in odontogenic abscesses, Infect. Immun. **49:**494, 1985.
11. Moskow, B.S., et al.: Repair of periodontal tissues following acute localized osteomyelitis, Periodontics **5:**29, 1967.
12. Prichard, J.F.: Management of the periodontal abscess, Oral Surg. **6:**474, 1953.
13. Trott, J.R.: The acute periodontal abscess, J. Can. Dent. Assoc. **25:**601, 1959.
14. Kareha, M.J., Rosenberg, E.S., and DeHaven, H.: Therapeutic considerations in the management of a periodontal abscess with an intrabony defect, J. Clin. Periodontol. **8:**375, 1981.
15. Nabers, J.M., et al.: Chronology, an important factor in the repair of osseous defects, Periodontics **2:**304, 1964.
16. Knewitz, K.W., Devine, K.D., and Waite, D.E.: Differential diagnosis of cervicofacial swellings, Oral Surg. **25:**43, 1968.
17. Hiatt, W.H.: Regeneration of the periodontium after endodontic therapy and flap operation, Oral Surg. **12:**1471, 1959.
18. Rickles, N.H., and Everett, F.G.: Gingival and lateral periodontal cysts, Parodontologie **14:**41, 1960.
19. Moskow, B.S., et al.: Gingival and lateral periodontal cysts, J. Periodontol. **41:**249, 1970.
20. Cohen, D.A., et al.: The lateral periodontal cyst: a report of 37 cases, J. Periodontol. **55:**230, 1984.
21. Stafne, E.C., and Milhon, J.A.: Periodontal cyst, J. Oral Surg. **3:**102, 1945.
22. Browne, W.G.: Periodontal cysts: an analysis of over 500 cysts, Oral Surg. **14:**1104, 1961.
23. Moskow, B.S., and Bloom, A.: Embryogenesis of the gingival cyst, J. Clin. Periodontol. **10:**119, 1983.
24. Gregg, T.A., and O'Brien, F.V.: A comparative study of the gingival and lateral periodontal cysts, Int. J. Oral Surg. **11:**316, 1982.
25. Neville, B.W., Mishkin, D.J., and Traynhom, R.T.: The laterally positioned odontogenic keratocyst: a case report, J. Periodontol. **55:**98, 1984.
26. Wysocki, G.P., et al.: Histogenesis of the lateral periodontal cyst and the gingival cyst of the adult, Oral Surg. **50:**327, 1980.
27. Fantasia, J.A.: Lateral periodontal cyst: an analysis of forty-six cases, Oral Surg. **48:**237, 1979.
28. Filipowicz, F.J., and Page, D.G.: The lateral periodontal cyst and isolated periodontal defects, J. Periodontol. **53:**145, 1982.
29. Peters, R.A., and Wussow, G.C.: Extravasation cyst of the maxilla: report of a case, Oral Surg. **26:**742, 1968.

## ADDITIONAL SUGGESTED READING

Lynch, D.P., and Madden, C.R.: The botryoid odontogenic cyst: report of a case and review of the literature, J. Periodontol. **56:**163, 1985.

Newman, M.G., and Goodman, A.D.: Guide to antibiotic use in dental practice, Chicago, 1984, Quintessence Publishing Co.

Oguntebi, B., et al.: Predominant microflora associated with human dental periapical abscesses, J. Clin. Microbiol. **15:**964, 1982.

Ritchey, B., and Orban, B.: Cysts of the gingiva, Oral Surg. **6:**765, 1953.

Shear, M., and Pindborg, J.J.: The periodontal cyst, Scand. J. Dent. Res. **83:**103, 1975.

Swan, R.H., Houston, G.D., and Moore, S.P.: Peripheral calcifying odontogenic cyst (Gorlin cyst), J. Periodontol. **56:**340, 1985.

Weine, F.S., and Silverglade, L.B.: Residual cysts masquerading as periapical lesions: three case reports, J. Am. Dent. Assoc. **106:**833, 1983.

# CHAPTER 22

# Vesicular and bullous diseases (desquamative gingivitis)

**Clinical appearance**

**Microscopic features**
Ultrastructure
Immunofluorescent study
Pemphigus vulgaris
Cicatricial pemphigoid and bullous pemphigoid
Lichen planus
Desquamative gingivitis
Allergic gingivostomatitis

**Treatment**
Systemic and topical therapy with steroids

**General periodontal management**
Multidisciplinary consultation
Periodontal therapy
Periodontal emergencies

---

**Definition**

There are a variety of intensely inflamed oral lesions characterized by clinical or subclinical vesiculation and red to magenta coloration of the affected area. These symptoms are found in a variety of conditions, including *benign mucous membrane pemphigoid (cicatricial pemphigoid), pemphigus vulgaris, bullous lichen planus (erosive lichen planus), bullous pemphigoid,* and *allergic gingivostomatitis*. All these diseases have been called *desquamative gingivitis*. Both cicatricial pemphigoid and pemphigus vulgaris have possible serious sequelae.[1] A precise and accurate diagnosis should be made. Histopathologic and immunologic tests must be made to determine the proper diagnosis. Desquamation should be regarded as a symptom. It is a reaction pattern common to several diseases. The detachment of the tissue is a result of vesiculation (blistering).

**Desquamation as a clinical sympathy**

**Blisters**

Blisters affecting the gingiva or other portions of the oral cavity are generally manifestations of systemic disease.[2-5] A vesicle is a small elevated lesion (less than 5 mm) containing fluid. Bullae are larger, ranging in size from 5 mm to a few centimeters. The vesiculobullous lesion may initially appear as an erythematous area and depending on pathologic stage may become a vesicle, ulcer, or healing lesion. The vesicular or bullous stage is infrequently observed since blisters burst easily following irritation or local trauma and are then seen as flaccid vesicles or bullae without fluid content (Fig. 22-1).

**Vesicles**

**Bullae**

## Clinical appearance

In desquamative oral lesions the gingival color may range from a diffuse rose to a fiery red. The gingival surface is smooth and shiny. The microscopic lesion (except for pemphigus) is at the basement membrane where blebs form. Stroking the gingiva with the finger or a probe may peel away the epithelium, exposing the raw surface of the connective tissue. Ulceration may occur after the chewing of some foods, or it may occur spontaneously and be accompanied by bleeding and pain.

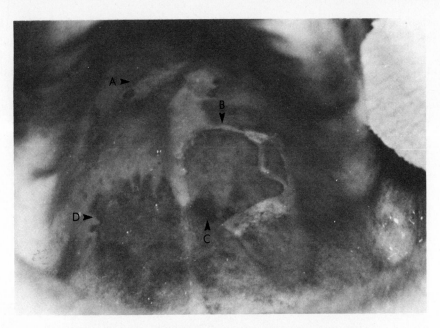

**Fig. 22-1.** Edentulous patient with a vesiculobullous disease, showing different clinical manifestations of the same entity. A, Flaccid bulla. B, Ruptured bulla. C, Ulcerated area. D, Healing lesion.

The lesions may involve the whole gingiva uniformly or may occur as single or multiple, discrete or irregular patches. They may be seen in the cheeks, hard and soft palate, tongue, vestibular surfaces of the lips, and floor of the mouth.[6-14]

Some patients may have lesions on other mucosal surfaces (conjunctiva, vagina, esophagus, larynx, pharynx, rectum) or on the skin. The oral lesions may be bullous erosions or the hyperkeratotic or parakeratotic striae of Wickham, which form a reticular or linear lichenoid pattern.

Although desquamative lesions most frequently affect young and middle-aged women, they are also seen in men.

Physical appearance of the lesion, its site, prevalence, chief complaint produced, and sex of the patient are often sufficient to make a presumptive diagnosis. Some other signs useful in differential diagnosis have been proposed.[15] These include (1) type of bulla (flaccid or tense), (2) rapid bursting of the bullae (pemphigus vulgaris blisters break faster), (3) reaction to pressure (pemphigus vulgaris lesions spread laterally), and (4) appearance (cicatricial pemphigoid and lichen planus tend to be more hemorrhagic; pemphigus vulgaris ulcers are shallow). The patient with a positive Nikolsky sign may facilitate the diagnosis of pemphigus vulgaris. A positive Nikolsky sign is observed when a blister is produced after minimal friction of mucosa or skin (a tongue blade can be used to perform the test). Atrophic or bullous lichen planus may be confirmed when typical lesions are found in other portions of the oral cavity.

Tissue should be taken from the site of the lesions and from adjacent healthy tissue, fixed in 10% neutral buffered formalin, and processed for routine histologic examination. Table 22-1 summarizes the main features associated with these diseases. The microscopic findings will depend, in part, on when the biopsy is taken in that the bullae may be at any stage of development, exacerbation, remission, or healing.

Early lesions may present a partial or inconclusive picture. Ulcers will show only nonspecific inflammatory infiltrate. The epithelium may lack keratinization; the epithelial–connective tissue interface may appear as a straight line without epithelial ridges or connective tissue papillae. The epithelium may be edematous, with widened

*Correlated lesions*

*Age and sex*

*Clinical diagnostic features*

*Histologic examination*

intercellular spaces. Basal cells may show lytic destruction. Spots or blebs may occur between epithelium and connective tissue. The basement membrane zone is not periodic acid–Schiff positive as it is in health[8,16,17] (Figs. 22-2 to 22-5) (Table 22-1).

**Inflammatory cells**

Inflammatory cells of all types are seen in the lamina propria and in the epithelium before the bullae form. The region of the basement membrane may be altered because of the presence of antibiodies to the basement membrane.[9-11] The inflammatory infiltrate is primarily chronic.[18] Plasma cells, lymphocytes, eosinophilic leukocytes, and macrophages are present. Mast cells can be detected with special stains[19] (Fig. 22-6).

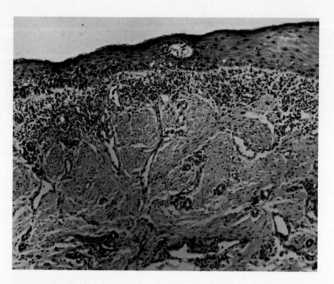

**Fig. 22-2.** Biopsy specimen of erosive lichen planus. The epithelium is atrophic. Connective tissue papillae are lacking, and there is severe subepithelial inflammation.

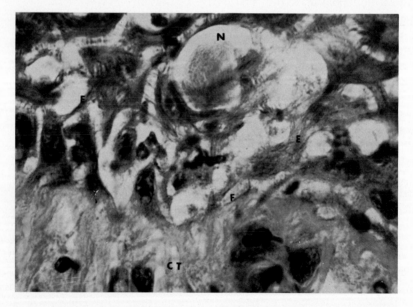

**Fig. 22-3.** Lytic destruction of basal cells in a desquamative gingival inflammation of the lichenoid type. The pattern of destruction is such that some of the tonofibrillar elements are preserved, as well as the connection of the epithelium to the connective tissue. *CT,* Connective tissue; *E,* epithelium; *N,* necrosis and lysis of cellular material; *F,* epithelial connective tissue junction. (Trichrome stain; ×600.) (Courtesy J.S. Bennett, Portland, Oregon.)

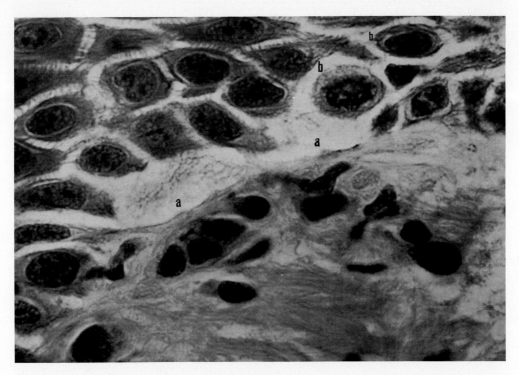

**Fig. 22-4.** Microscopic changes in early bullae formation in a clinical desquamative gingivitis. Note, *a,* the separation of the epithelial cells from the lamina propria and, *b,* widened intercellular spaces. (Trichrome stain; ×600.) (Courtesy J.S. Bennett, Portland, Oregon.)

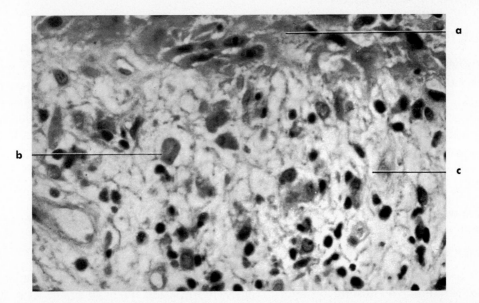

**Fig. 22-5.** Washed-out appearance of connective tissue. No basement membrane is apparent. *a,* Epithelium; *b,* macrophages; *c,* degenerated connective tissue.

**Table 22-1** Histologic features of oral lesions

| Disease or lesion | Gross picture | Epithelial changes | Fluid content | Inflammatory infiltrate |
|---|---|---|---|---|
| Pemphigus vulgaris (PV) | Separation of epithelial cell from the basal cell layer | Disappearance of intercellular bridges Acantholysis | Edema, polymorphonuclear leukocytes, lymphocytes, and Tzanck cells | Mild to moderate Scarce in early lesions |
| Cicatricial (benign mucous membrane) pemphigoid (CP or BMMP) | Epithelial separation from the underlying connective tissue | Basal layer may remain intact Atrophy as the lesion becomes older | Clear fluid with scattered inflammatory cells | Dense Plasma cells, lymphocytes, and eosinophils |
| Bullous pemphigoid (BP) | Epithelial separation from the underlying connective tissue | Minor degenerative alterations | Fibrinous exudate with inflammatory cells | Dense Plasma cells and lymphocytes |
| Lichen planus (LP) (bullous or erosive) | Subepithelial vesicle | Parakeratosis, atrophy, hydropic degeneration, shortening or disappearance of rete pegs, and colloid bodies | Edema with inflammatory cells | Dense Subepithelial T-lymphocytes |
| Desquamative gingivitis (DG) | Thin epithelium | Atrophy Disrupted basal layer and connective tissue boundary | Epithelial intercellular edema | Dense Bullous and lichenoid type Lymphocytes, plasma cells, and histiocytes |

Based on data from McCarthy, P.L. and Shklar, G.: Diseases of the oral mucosa, ed. 2, Philadelphia, 1980, Lea & Febiger; Shafer, W.G., Hine, M., and Levy, B.G.: A textbook of oral pathology, ed. 3, Philadelphia, 1974, W.B. Saunders Co.; and Andreasen, J.O.: Oral Surg. **25**:158, 1968.

## Microscopic features

### ULTRASTRUCTURE

Ultrastructure studies[9] of patients with desquamative lesions report that the collagen fibers may be slightly separated. There is a decreased number of anchoring fibrils. The basal lamina may be replicated.[8] The subepithelial connective tissue may be vacuolated and disorganized.[20] The basal lamina in the region of a bulla has been reported to be adherent to the basal cells,[20] the connective tissue,[21] or both.[9] Pseudopodia from the basal cells enter the bullae.[1,9,21] The bullae may contain fibrin, red blood cells, and cellular debris.

**Differential diagnosis**

Histologic studies may lead to the conclusion that the tissue appearance is consistent with the diagnosis of one of these diseases but may not provide confirmatory proof. Immune studies may then provide a differential diagnosis.

### IMMUNOFLUORESCENT STUDY

**Serum and biopsy**

Serum from 8 to 10 ml of blood collected without anticoagulants is sent at ambient temperature to the testing laboratory. Biopsies of the lesion and of an adjacent normal site should be obtained. The crevicular epithelium should be excluded. The tissue must be unfixed, quick frozen, and transported on dry ice. Quick freezing requires placing the tissue into liquid nitrogen or into a slush of dry ice mixed with acetone or ethanol. Alternatively, the biopsy may be placed in Michel's holding solution and transported at ambient temperature.[6]

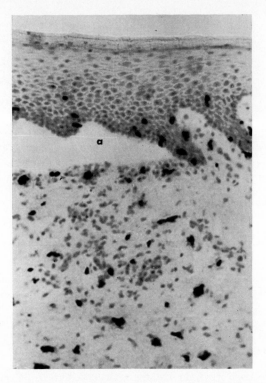

**Fig. 22-6.**   Bulla *(a)* in desquamative gingival inflammation showing mast cells stained dark with a specific mast cell stain. Mast cells are found in the connective tissue and the epithelium. (Courtesy W.B. Hall, San Francisco, California.)

Immunologic techniques with labelled (conjugated) antibodies can be used to perform a differential diagnosis. The most commonly used fluorescent marker is fluorescein isothiocyanate, which emits an apple-green color with a fluorescent light source. Conjugated antibodies are immunoglobulins prepared in swine, rabbits, and other animals against human IgG, IgM, IgA, complement fractions, fibrin, and fibrinogen.[22,23] They are commonly used in the differential diagnosis of the oral vesicular lesions.[24] There are two basic methods, direct immunofluorescence (DIF) and indirect immunofluorescence (IIF) (Fig. 22-7).

> **Diagnosis through immunologic techniques**

Direct immunofluorescence (DIF) uses host tissue and conjugated swine or rabbit antibodies against human immunoglobulins. In the indirect method (IIF) serum from the patient is used and tested against monkey mucosa. If there are sufficient circulating antibodies in the serum, these will cross-react with antigens in the monkey mucosa.

> **Direct (DIF) and indirect (IIF) immunofluorescence**

The immunoperoxidase technique[25-28] may be used in place of immunofluorescence. In immunoperoxidase techniques, horseradish peroxidase–conjugated antibodies are prepared. Visualization is obtained by adding diaminobenzidine with hydrogen peroxide, which results in dark brown precipitates in positive areas. There are both direct and indirect procedures, but the peroxidase-antiperoxidase immune complex method is most often used (Fig. 22-7).

> **Immunoperoxidase**

When pemphigus vulgaris is suspected, a cytologic smear can be taken instead of a biopsy, and a DIF can be performed on the acantholytic cells (Tzanck cells) of undisturbed bullae.[29-31] Typically what will be observed by immunofluorescence[24-32] will be an intercellular trace (Fig. 22-8, *A*) between suprabasal cells of immunoperoxidase.[33] Immunofluorescent findings are highly diagnostic in pemphigus vulgaris,[32] and DIF procedures are more sensitive than IIF procedures for pemphigus vulgaris confined to the oral cavity.[34,35]

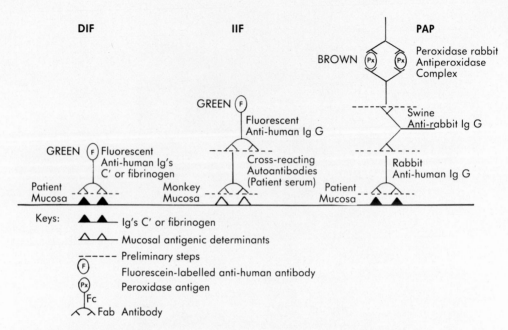

DIF                    IIF                         PAP

BROWN (Px) (Px) Peroxidase rabbit
                              Antiperoxidase
                              Complex

GREEN (F)
Fluorescent
Anti-human Ig G                Swine
                               Anti-rabbit Ig G

GREEN (F) Fluorescent
Anti-human Ig's
C' or fibrinogen        Cross-reacting          Rabbit
                        Autoantibodies          Anti-human Ig G
Patient                 (Patient serum)   Patient
Mucosa                  Monkey           Mucosa
                        Mucosa

Keys:        ▲▲ —— Ig's C' or fibrinogen

             △△ —— Mucosal antigenic determinants

             ------ Preliminary steps

             (F) Fluorescein-labelled anti-human antibody

             (Px) Peroxidase antigen

             Fc
             ∕\⟩ Fab Antibody

**Fig. 22-7.** Graphic representation of procedures for direct immunofluorescence *(DIF)*, indirect immunofluorescence *(IIF)*, and peroxidase-antiperoxidase *(PAP)* methods. (Based on data from Taylor, C.: Arch. Pathol. Lab. Med. **102:**113, 1978; Handlers, J., et al.: Oral Surg. **54:**207, 1982; and Nisengard, R.J., Alpert, A.M., and Krestow, V.: J. Periodontol. **49:**27, 1978.)

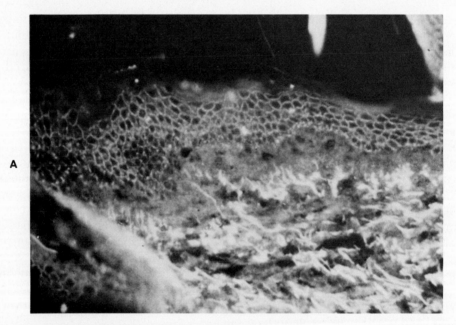

A

**Fig. 22-8.** Immunofluorescent assessment. **A,** Interepithelial pattern of staining in a skin lesion compatible with *pemphigus vulgaris;* antiserum against human IgG.

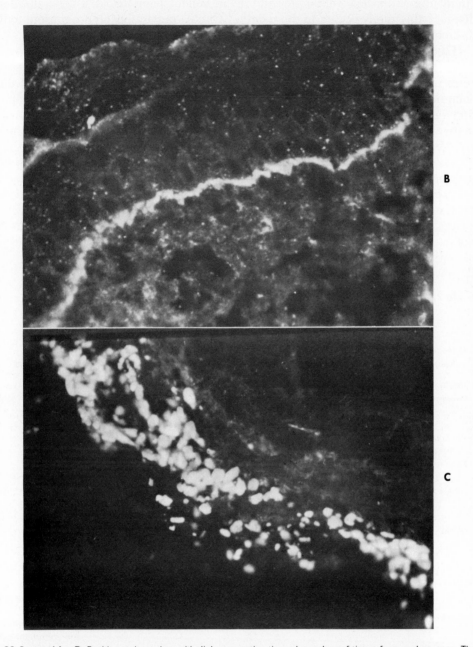

**Fig. 22-8, cont'd.   B,** Positive stain at the epithelial–connective tissue boundary of tissue from oral mucosa. The pattern of stain is similar for cicatricial and bullous pemphigoid; antiserum against human IgG. **C,** Globular staining pattern (Civatte bodies) from a desquamative lesion of the gingiva. Stain is suggestive of lichen planus; antiserum against IgM. (Courtesy Russell J. Nisengard, D.D.S., Ph.D., Buffalo, New York.)

Cicatricial pemphigoid and bullous pemphigoid cannot be distinguished by DIF studies.[36] Both techniques exhibit immunofluorescence at the epithelial basal cell layer[36-38] (Fig. 22-8, *B*). In this case IIF may be a complementary diagnostic aid, since circulating antibodies will be present only in bullous pemphigoid, a generalized skin disease[38] that rarely occurs in the mouth.[38] Circulating antibodies are present only in discrete amounts[18] or even absent in cicatricial pemphigoid.[39,40]

**Lichen planus**

Findings in lichen planus are indicative or suggestive but not diagnostic (Fig. 22-8, *C*). In lichen planus there may be visible plugs of fibrinogen[32] at the underlying connective tissue, perivascular deposits of immunoglobulins,[41] and globular deposits of immunoglobulins and complement (also known as cytoid or Civatte bodies).[42] Similar findings occur in lupus erythematosus and erythema multiforme. Table 22-2 summarizes immune responses observed in pemphigus vulgaris, cicatricial pemphigoid, bullous pemphigoid, lichen planus, and desquamative gingivitis.

The region of the basement membrane may be altered by antibodies to the basement membrane.[9-11] Immunofluorescence of the basement zone may be diagnostic for bullous pemphigoid, a dermatologic condition that rarely has oral involvement[11] and for benign mucous membrane pemphigoid.[37] Immunofluorescence of the intracellular spaces of the epithelium may be diagnostic for pemphigus. Erosive lichen planus does not have a linear immunofluorescence at the basement membrane. Cytoid bodies may be indicative of lichen planus but are found in other similar conditions.[7]

**Table 22-2**   Immunofluorescence features of oral lesions

| Disease or lesion | Pattern of staining | Positive reaction percentage* | | | Comments |
|---|---|---|---|---|---|
| | | Direct (DIF) | Indirect (IIF) | Reference number source | |
| Pemphigus vulgaris (PV) | Epithelial Intercellular | 98-100 | 86 | 32,34 | Positive reaction to immunoglobulins and complement[1] Diagnostic |
| Cicatricial (benign mucous membrane) pemphigoid (CP or BMMP) | Basal membrane zone | 97 | 36-50 | 35,36 | Positive reaction to immunoglobulins and complement Diagnostic |
| Bullous pemphoid (BP) | Basal membrane zone | 90 | 70-83 | 35,38 | Positive reaction to immunoglobulins and complement Diagnostic |
| Lichen planus (LP) | Coarse deposits in lamina propria and basal membrane zone Globular deposits in lamina propria (cytoid or Civatte bodies) | 99-100 | — | 32,42 | Positive reaction to: a. Fibrin and fibrinogen (coarse deposits) b. Immunoglobulins and complement (Civatte bodies) Suggestive Nondiagnostic |
| Desquamative gingivitis (DG) | Varies according to associated lesion | PV 100 CP 80-100 BP 100 LP 75-97 | 100 17 80 — | 24,89 | Positive reaction in 77% of DG lesions of different origin |

*Positive reaction to various combinations of antiglobulins, anticomplement fractions, and antifibrin or fibrinogen.

Most initial diagnoses of desquamative gingivitis progress to an ultimate diagnosis of erosive lichen planus or of benign mucous membrane pemphigoid (see Table 22-4). The latter diagnosis requires concomitant progressive involvement of other areas (conjunctiva, vagina, soft palate, perianal tissues, larynx, pharynx) accompanied by scarring. If neither progression nor scarring occurs, a diagnosis of desquamative gingivitis may be presumed. It has been suggested that these desquamative gingivitis cases are variants of benign mucous membrane pemphigoid that are nonprogressive.[4]

Desquamative gingivitis may be associated with other causes. It has been suggested that hormonal malfunction or menopause is related in some cases.[12] Similar clinical appearance may occur with some ordinary gingivitis, after certain medications, in acute monocytic leukemia, in plasmocytosis, and idiopathically.

**Hormonal interrelationship**

## PEMPHIGUS VULGARIS

Pemphigus vulgaris is a blistering disease of the mucous membrane and skin.[2,4,43] In the mouth it appears as flaccid vesicles that immediately rupture, leaving mucosal erosion or ulcers. Oral lesions may precede skin lesions and even be the only or main manifestation of pemphigus vulgaris.[34] The gingiva is frequently involved.[22] Gingival manifestations occur in approximately 25% of cases.[44] Pemphigus vulgaris onset is usually mild, appearing after the fifth decade. Women are more susceptible than men. The soft palate seems to be the oral tissue most frequently affected. Pemphigus vulgaris may be confined to mucous membranes in 45% of the patients.[45]

Statistical data suggest that Jewish people and Mediterranean ethnic groups have a greater susceptibility. Although the disease is one of old age, some cases have been reported in children.[45] Prognosis and sequelae depend on early diagnosis. Oral lesions usually heal without scarring, but severe skin involvement may lead to prostration, massive loss of fluid and protein, aggravated infection, and death. The potential of fatal consequences and the frequency of only oral manifestations makes the early diagnosis and treatment imperative. A gap of more than a year between the first symptoms and the diagnosis of oral lesions of pemphigus vulgaris has been reported.[44,46]

An immune pathogenesis has been suggested for pemphigus vulgaris.[47] Autoimmune phenomena can be firmly identified.[48] The appearance of immunoglobulins in the prickle-cell layer of oral epithelium may produce an intraepithelial vesicle by disrupting intercellular attachment apparatus. This is known as *acantholysis*. The intercellular separation is filled with an edematous fluid arising from the connective tissue, thus creating the clinical appearance of a blister. Lysed cells (acantholytic cells or Tzanck cells), which are diagnostic, remain floating in the vesicular fluid. The presence of immunoglobulins, specifically IgG, may induce the activation of the complement system and further increase acantholysis through an enhanced inflammatory response.[49] Histologically the pemphigus vulgaris lesion appears as an intraepithelial blister caused by acantholysis (Fig. 22-9).

**Pathogenesis**

Other lesions closely related to pemphigus vulgaris may occur in mucosa. Pemphigus vegetans is an exophytic variation of pemphigus vulgaris.[16] An untoward result of penicillamine therapy may be pemphigus-like mucosal lesions.[50] There is some question whether pyostomatitis vegetans, an oral manifestation of bowel disease[51] characterized by intraepithelial abscesses, might be a variant of pemphigus vegetans.[52,53]

## CICATRICIAL PEMPHIGOID AND BULLOUS PEMPHIGOID

Cicatricial (benign mucous membrane) and bullous pemphigoid share many pathologic and histologic features. Their ultimate distinction is established clinically, since even sophisticated direct immunofluorescent studies fail to distinguish them. They might be considered to be variants of the disease entity.[36] Cicatricial pemphigus is a

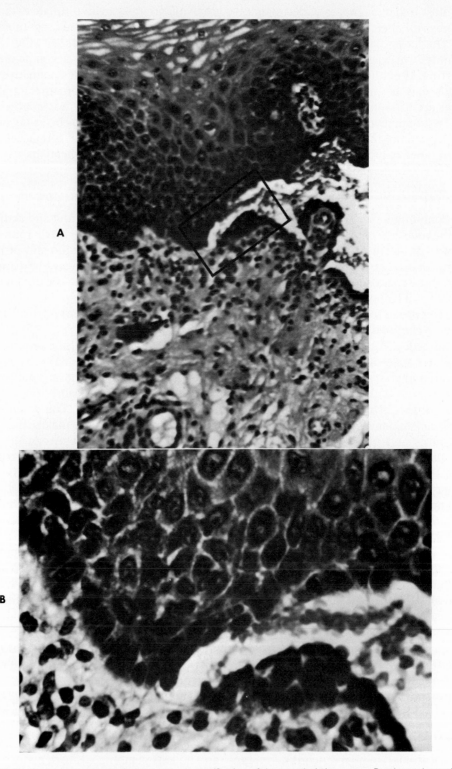

**Fig. 22-9.**   Pemphigus vulgaris. **A,** Low-power magnification of the acantholytic process. Basal membrane layer remains attached to the underlying connective tissue. Some acantholytic (Tzanck cells) and hemorrhagic cells can be observed in the space formed by acantholysis. Inflammation is rather scarce. **B,** High-power magnification of the region marked in **A.** (Hematoxylin and eosin stain; **A,** ×125 and **B,** ×400.)

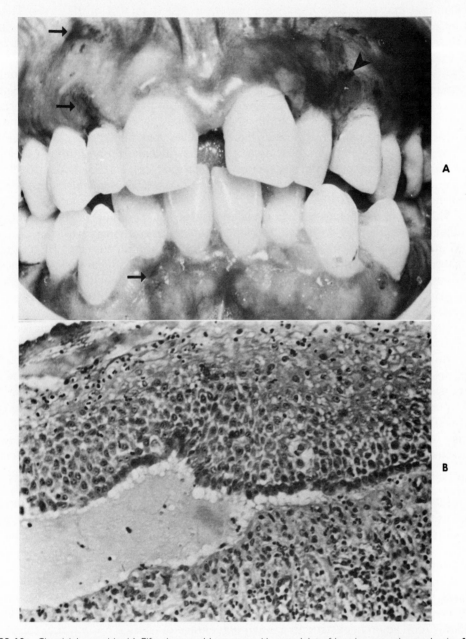

**Fig. 22-10.**   Cicatricial pemphigoid. Fifty-six-year-old woman with complaint of burning sensation and pain. **A,** Intraoral view shows atrophic *(arrows)* and hemorrhagic *(arrowhead)* changes. **B,** High-power magnification, Basal cell layer remains relatively intact and epithelium looks infiltrated subsequent to blister rupture. (Hematoxylin and eosin stain; **B,** ×125.)

vesicular or bullous disorder that may attack the oral cavity, eyes, vagina, rectum, urethra, pharynx, larynx, or nasal cavity. As in pemphigus vulgaris, unruptured vesicles and bullae are infrequent. The common finding is of a recently collapsed vesicle or bulla. The epithelial roof of the vesicle is easily removed leaving a bleeding, ulcerated lesion that may scar. Skin lesions are present in less than 10% of the cases. The oral mucosa is the anatomic area most frequently affected. Gingiva shows cicatricial pemphigoid changes in 64% of such cases, mainly as a desquamative lesion.[44] The incidence in women is greater (62%). The onset is after the sixth decade of life (ranging from age 50 to 80),[44] although early cases in children and adolescents have been reported.[54,55] Primary signs and symptoms, as well as the clinical course, are generally benign. Patients usually complain of an itching sensation and pain subsequent to ulceration. Patients may be free from symptoms for long periods. Scarring is not a common oral mucosal complication. On the other hand, the eyes may be seriously damaged even to the point of causing blindness as a result of symblepharon and ankyloblepharon, which lead to entropion, trichiasis, conjunctival erosion, and corneal damage by fibrous repair, all of which cause physical obstruction.[4] Oral clinical and histologic features are shown in Fig. 22-10.

Although clinical characteristics related to cicatricial pemphigoid suggest different etiologic possibilities,[56] an immune origin seems more consistent with the evidence. IgG and complement are bound to the basement membrane zone.[37,48] Histologically, cicatricial pemphigoid and bullous pemphigoid show subepithelial vesicles caused by the detachment of the epithelium from the underlying connective tissue, which is densely infiltrated by polymorphonuclear leukocytes and chronic inflammatory cells (Fig. 22-11). Collagen fibers may be slightly separated and a reduced number of anchoring fibrils can be observed. Bullae contain fibrin, mucoid material, red blood cells, and antibodies.[56]

Bullous pemphigoid (Fig. 22-11) differs clinically from cicatricial pemphigoid because it is a nonscarring blistering disease mainly affecting the skin,[38,44,57] and only occasionally involving the oral mucosa. When oral lesions are present, they occur most frequently on the buccal mucosa.[38,44] Gingival tissues are affected in 16% of the cases of oral bullous pemphigoid, whereas in cicatricial pemphigoid the incidence is greater than 60%.[44] Other dermatologic lesions may be found in the mouth, including lichen planus, dermatitis herpetiformis, erythema multiforme, and epidermolysis bullosa.[38]

## LICHEN PLANUS

Lichen planus is a rather common dermatitis that may also occur in the oral mucosa. It has different clinical manifestations including papular, reticular, ulcerative, erosive, and vesicular patterns.[58] The buccal mucosa and the tongue are most frequently affected. There is a higher incidence in women (1 : 1.7). Onset is generally between the fifth and sixth decades, with an earlier onset in men.[57-59]

Gingivae are affected by the erosive and reticular forms in 30% and 15% of the cases, respectively[60] (Fig. 22-12). Symptomatology is similar to benign mucous membrane pemphigoid.[59] The cause is unknown at this time. Stress is implicated.[61] Lichen planus may be preneoplastic in a small percentage of cases,[60,62-64] but this conclusion is disputed by other data.[65,66]

**Histologic appearance** Pathogenesis of lichen planus corresponds to a delayed immunopathologic response.[67] It is a cell-mediated immunologic disease dominated by T cells (thymus-dependent lymphocytes).[68,69] A humoral response with immunoglobulin and complement participation has not been demonstrated.[42,44,45,70] The typical histologic description of lichen planus corresponds to (1) hyper-, ortho-, or parakeratosis, (2) increase in thickness of stratum granulosum, (3) acanthosis in reticular patterns, (4) atrophy in

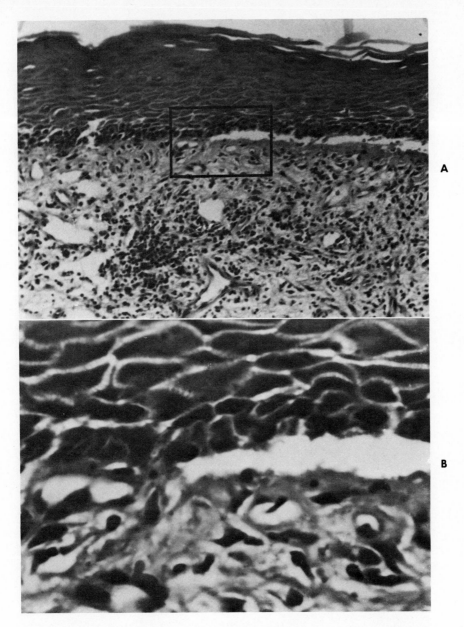

**Fig. 22-11.** Cicatricial pemphigoid. **A,** Atrophic keratinized epithelium separated from the underlying connective tissue, which shows a moderate and diffuse chronic infiltration. **B,** High-power magnification from **A.** Basal cell layer persists with some disturbance; it appears as a double layer. Infiltrate is mainly composed of mononuclear cells. (Hematoxylin and eosin stain; **A,** ×125 and **B,** ×600.)

erosive and ulcerative patterns, (5) detachment of the epithelial layer from connective tissue in vesiculobullous lichen planus lesions, (6) liquefactive degeneration of the epithelial basal cell layer, (7) colloid bodies, (8) characteristic degenerated epithelial cells, and (9) a subepithelial chronic lymphocytic band[16,71] (Fig. 22-13). Bullae develop as a result of extensive destruction and edema following degeneration of the stratum germinativum. A clear eosinophilic fluid containing scattered erythrocytes[72] can be obtained from unruptured blisters. A patient with oral lichen planus may develop a lowered rate of salivary secretion, since the disease may affect salivary glands.

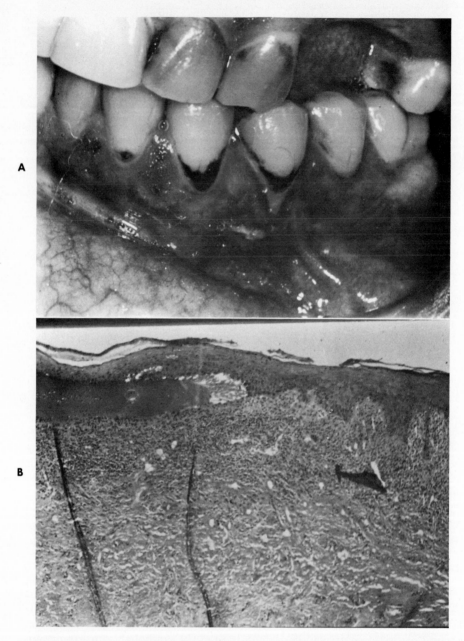

**Fig. 22-12.** Bullous lichen planus. **A,** Forty-six-year-old woman with chief complaint of an itching blister at the left mandibular bicuspid region. A ruptured vesicle between the canine and first bicuspid, with an erythematous change spreading over the second bicuspid, was observed. **B,** Biopsy taken from the gingiva, demonstrates an atrophic keratinized epithelium with an eosinophilic fluid-filled vesicle and typical subepithelial infiltrate. (Hematoxylin and eosin stain; ×40.)

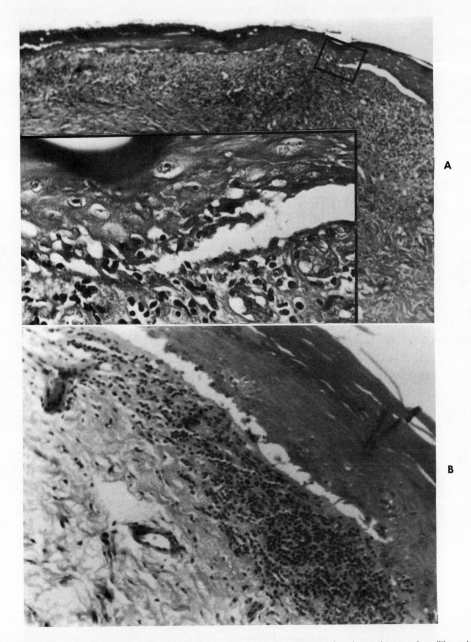

**Fig. 22-13.**   Bullous lichen planus. **A,** Keratinized atrophic epithelium; connective tissue shows a bandlike subepithelial lymphocytic infiltrate. A disturbed attachment from the connective tissue is observed along the epithelium; a frank vesicle has already formed on the right side. *Inset,* few epithelial rows remain because of severe atrophy and degeneration. No cells from the basal cell layer are detectable. A mononuclear infiltrate dominates the picture. **B,** Another example of bullous lichen planus, where bandlike subepithelial infiltrate can be clearly observed. (Hematoxylin and eosin stain; **A,** ×40. *Inset,* ×400. **B,** ×125.)

Other lesions such as discoid lupus erythematosus may have some characteristics resembling lichen planus.[72,73]Intraoral recurrent herpes simplex may show a blistering stage. Bullae are pathognomonic in genetic disorders such as epidermolysis bullosa.[74] Erythema multiforme, a vesiculobullous disease,[75] may affect the gums.[76] Additional clinical information; clinical patterns of the disease; and appropriate immune, serologic, and histologic studies may be useful in differential diagnosis (Fig. 22-14).

## DESQUAMATIVE GINGIVITIS

*Desquamative gingivitis* is a term frequently used to describe a variety of pathologic gingival alterations. It is a descriptive term representing a sign (desquamation) and not a disease. The desquamation is an important diagnostic sign that may be common to many of the lesions discussed in this chapter (Fig. 22-15). It is an atrophic change of the gingival epithelium that might be seen in dermatoses,[77] nutritional disturbance,[78] irritation and trauma,[79] hormonal influences,[80] hypersensitivity and intolerance,[81-84] acute and chronic infections,[85] and idiopathic causes.[86] It is possible to observe atrophic changes from psoriasis, vitamin deficiency, improper use of toothbrushes, abnormal habits, Turner syndrome, menopause, chewing gum, allergies, drug intake, herpesvirus infection, and so forth. The importance of this clinical sign, desquamative gingivitis, is that it may lead to early diagnosis of pemphigus vulgaris, cicatricial pemphigoid, and lichen planus.[87] Desquamative gingivitis is the most characteristic clinical sign of cicatricial pemphigoid.[88] The frequency of desquamative gingivitis in skin disease[89] is pemphigus vulgaris, 18%; bullous pemphigoid, 3%; cicatricial pemphigoid, 64%; and lichen planus, 25%.

Immunofluorescent studies[66,87,89,90] demonstrate the relationship of desquamative gingivitis and pemphigus vulgaris, bullous pemphigoid, cicatricial pemphigoid, and lichen planus and may distinguish those entities from each other. They are important planus and may distinguish those entities from each other. They are important because

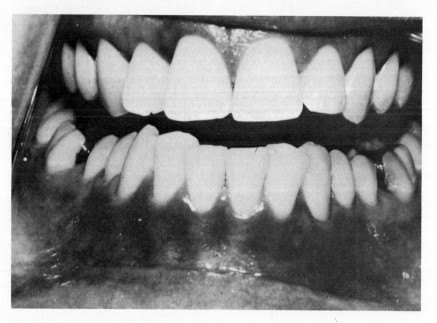

**Fig. 22-14.** Erythematous atrophic changes of the gums at the anterior mandibular region. The patient was a 24-year-old woman whose chief complaints were occasional burning and soreness sensations, which had developed over a period of more than 18 months. After consultation with several practitioners, the lesions were found to be consistent with lichen planus by immunofluorescence studies.

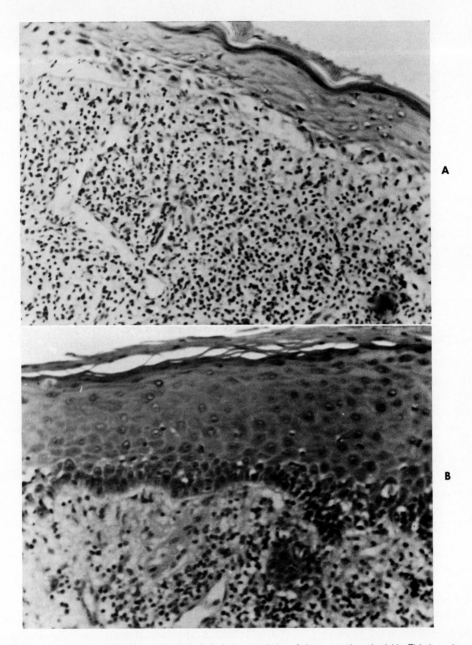

**Fig. 22-15.   A** to **C,** Views of lesions that had clinical characteristics of desquamative gingivitis. This is an inconclusive diagnosis as can be seen by the three different histologic pictures presented; the only factor they have in common is epithelial atrophy. **A** is suggestive of lichen planus, **B** and **C** are not indicative of a specific pathologic condition. (Hematoxylin and eosin stain; **A, B,** and **C,** × 125, × 400, and × 600, respectively.)          *Continued.*

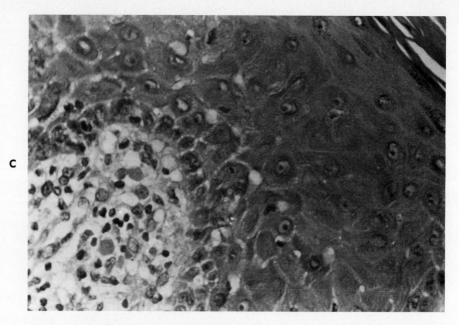

c

**Fig. 22-15, cont'd.** For legend see p. 451.

because they may predict which patients will go on to involvement of other mucosal tissues (Tables 22-3 and 22-4).

### ALLERGIC GINGIVOSTOMATITIS

An intensely red gingivitis accompanied by cheilitis and glossitis has been described in a number of patients.[81,91,92] The basement membrane is intact. There is neither acantholysis nor bullae formation. The epithelium is hyperplastic with deep rete "pegs" and connective tissue papillae that reach nearly to the surface. Leukocytes may be found in the epithelium. There is a heavy plasma cell infiltration. Many patients are heavy gum chewers. Types of chicle incorporated into the gum or into toothpaste have been incriminated. On discontinuation of the gum chewing or the use of their dentifrice or mouthwash, the lesion disappears. The condition is believed to be an allergic reaction to a constituent in these products.

## Treatment

Treatment depends on the diagnosis of the underlying condition. The more serious conditions, pemphigus and benign mucous membrane pemphigoid, may require systemic steroid therapy. Erosive lichen planus, the rare oral involvement of bullous pemphigoid, and the nonprogressive cases that show only desquamative gingivitis may be treated locally. Allergic gingivostomatitis requires the elimination of the offending allergen from food, chewing gum, toothpaste, and mouthwash.

### SYSTEMIC AND TOPICAL THERAPY WITH STEROIDS

In severe cases a combination of systemic and local steroids is appropriate. Oral prednisone, 40 to 50 mg/day in split doses,[93] plus local application of fluocinonide, 0.05%, may be adequate. The dosage of prednisone is decreased as the clinical condition subsides. Subsequently, local steroids may be sufficient. Topical therapy is adequate for mild cases[94] (Fig. 22-16).

Greater improvement has been obtained with topical application of corticoids. Cor-

**Table 22-3** Immunologic findings of importance in the diagnosis of desquamative gingivitis

| Underlying disease | Serum | | Biopsies | |
|---|---|---|---|---|
| | Types of antibodies | Findings | Pattern of immunofluorescence | Findings |
| Cicatricial (benign mucous membrane) pemphigoid | Basement membrane antibodies | − or +* | Basement membrane zone | + |
| Bullous pemphigoid | Basement membrane antibodies | + (80%) | Basement membrane zone | + (100%) |
| Pemphigus vulgaris | Epithelial intercellular spaces | + (over 95%) | Intercellular deposits | + (100%) |
| Lichen planus | | | Globular deposits in dermis and epidermis (cytoid bodies) | + (97%) |

From Nisengard, R.J., Alpert, A.M., and Krestow, V.: Desquamative gingivitis: immunologic findings, J. Periodontol. **49**:27, 1978.
*Most cases are negative for serum antibodies.

**Table 22-4** Clinical features of desquamative gingivitis in six women (postmenopausal) and one man

| Diagnosis* | Patient | Age/sex | Disease duration† (months) | Initial examination | Initial involvement | Latest examination | Latest involvement‡ |
|---|---|---|---|---|---|---|---|
| CP | 1 | 54/F | 36 | 2/74 | Gingiva | 5/76 | Gingiva, palate, buccal mucosa, nasal, tongue |
| CP | 2 | 69/F | 56 | 10/71 | Gingiva | 8/75 | Gingiva, palate, buccal mucosa, nasal, tongue |
| CP | 3 | 65/F | 44 | 10/72 | Gingiva | 5/76 | Gingiva, palate, buccal mucosa, nasopharynx, tongue |
| DG | 4 | 61/F | 69 | 9/71 | Gingiva | 10/74 | Gingiva |
| CP | 5 | 60/F | 30 | 12/73 | Gingiva | 5/76 | Gingiva, nasal mucosa, buccal mucosa, esophagus, tongue, rectum, palate |
| LP | 6 | 82/F | 42 | 4/73 | Gingiva | 2/76 | Gingiva, tongue, buccal mucosa, skin |
| CP | 7 | 74/M | 35 | 12/73 | Gingiva | 4/76 | Gingiva, nasal mucosa, buccal mucosa, conjunctiva, tongue |

From Rogers, R.S. III, Sheridan, P.J., and Jordon, R.E.: Desquamative gingivitis, Oral Surg. **42**:316, 1976.
*CP, Cicatricial pemphigoid (benign mucous membrane pemphigoid); DG, desquamative gingivitis; LP, lichen planus.
†Duration from onset to May 1976.
‡Patient 5, esophageal and rectal by history only.

ticoid ointment (0.1%) in an adhesive base (fluocinonide [Topsyn] or triamcinalone [Kenalog] in Orabase) is recommended.

In edentulous patients, the prosthesis can be used as a carrier. In dentate patients protective plastic devices covering the gingival tissues may be fabricated. These procedures may assist in reducing systemic steroid dosages, but some systemic uptake of the cortisone by mucosal absorption or swallowing will result even with topical application. Thus when topical and systemic therapy are combined, there may be an additive effect.

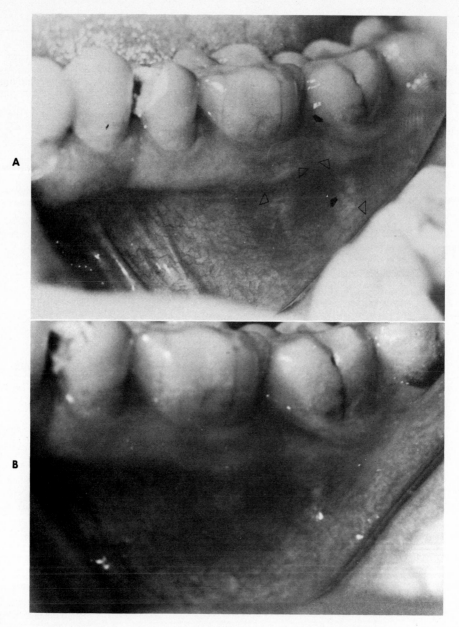

**Fig. 22-16.** Fifty-five-year-old woman with complaint of soreness on the buccal area between the left first and second mandibular molars. **A,** Atrophic *(arrowheads)* and hyperplastic *(open arrows)* lesions could be clinically identified in an area sensitive to palpation. Lesions were compatible with lichen planus. **B,** After 2 weeks of treatment with fluocinonide, 0.05% applied topically four times a day, signs had diminished and symptoms disappeared.

**Adjuvant therapy**

Systemic prescription of antiinflammatory steroids is not without complications,[95] and adverse effects appear in almost half the patients,[93] some extremely serious.[96] Adjuvant therapy may be advisable, and several compounds, such as immunosuppressive drugs, gold salts, dapsone, plasmapheresis, submucosal injection of corticosteroids,[97] and adrenocorticotropic hormone,[46] have been used. The combination of levamisole, an immunostimulant,[98] or azathioprine, an immunosuppressant,[99] with low doses of prednisone is reported to yield satisfactory results.

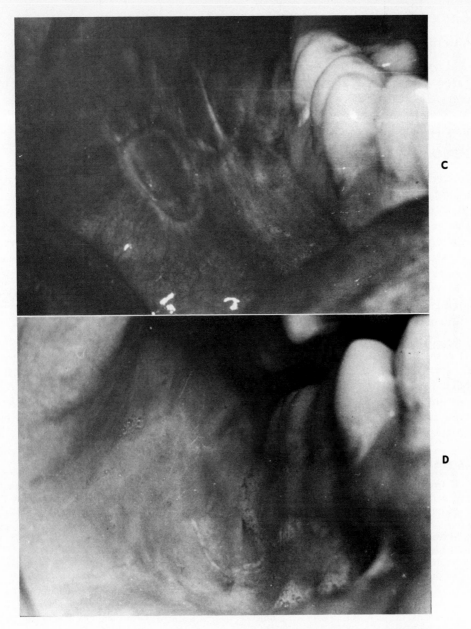

**Fig. 22-16, cont'd.    C,** Opposite side of the same patient. Typical asymptomatic lesions of lichen planus are present on the buccal mucosa and gingiva. No skin lesions were detected. **D,** Appearance of the lesions after 2 weeks. Therapy was continued for 8 additional weeks until lesions subsided completely.

In ulcerated and atrophic lesions oral surface anesthetics such as dyclone hydrochloride,[100] benzocaine, or diphenhydramine may relieve pain. Lichen planus steroid therapy combined with fungistatic agents such as amphotericin B, nystatin, and griseofulvin[61,101] may be helpful, although the mechanisms of action remain unclear. The topical application of estrogenic hormones in the form of ointment has brought inconsistent and temporary improvement in a few cases.[12]

In general, most pharmaceuticals offer only temporary or partial relief, but this may be sufficient to make the patient comfortable.

**Other therapeutic modalities**

# General periodontal management

## MULTIDISCIPLINARY CONSULTATION

Cooperation with a dermatologist and internist is advisable in the more serious cases. The biopsy is read by a pathologist, and the eyes should be examined by an ophthalmologist.

Scaling and oral hygiene measures should be initiated. The use of chlorhexidine may be helpful on occasion.

## PERIODONTAL THERAPY

Periodontal treatment may be undertaken during periods of remission or if the condition is not vesicular. The beneficial effect of some antimicrobials implies that there may be some relationship between plaque and lichen planus or other inflammatory conditions. Treatment of patients with vesiculobullous conditions must be cautious, since it is believed that they are autoimmune conditions. A conservative approach by scaling and root planing may be appropriate. Long-term systemic steroid therapy may impair healing, increase the susceptibility to infection, and suppress adrenal function. In such patients the doubling of systemic steroid dosage is recommended to avoid adrenal shock during stressful periodontal treatment.[102] Prophylactic antibiotics must be prescribed.

## PERIODONTAL EMERGENCIES

Infectious stomatitis, including gingival involvement, is rather common in hospitalized patients with pemphigus vulgaris. In these cases broad-spectrum antibiotics and antifungals are prescribed. Immediate microbial cultures for aerobic and anaerobic flora and bacterial antibiotic sensitivity testing should be ordered. As soon as results are available, scaling and oral hygiene measures should be undertaken.

**REFERENCES**

1. Greenberg, M.S.: Ulcerative vesicular and bullous lesions. In Lynch, M.A., et al., editors: Burket's oral medicine, ed. 8, Philadelphia, 1984, J.B. Lippincott Co.
2. Shklar, G., and McCarthy, P.L.: The oral manifestations of systemic disease, Boston, 1979, Butterworth Publishers.
3. Shklar, G., et al.: Oral lesions in bullous pemphigoid, Arch. Derm. **99:**663, 1970.
4. Dolby, A.E.: Oral ulcerations: immunological aspects. In Dolby, A.E., editor: Oral mucosa in health and disease, Oxford, 1975, Blackwell Scientific Publications.
5. McCarthy, P.L., and Shklar, G.: Diseases of the oral mucosa, ed. 2, Philadelphia, 1980, Lea & Febiger.
6. Nisengard, R.J., Alpert, A.M., and Krestow, V.: Desquamative gingivitis: immunologic findings, J. Periodontol. **49:**27, 1978.
7. Rogers, R.S., III, Sheridan, P.J., and Jordon, R.E.: Desquamative gingivitis, Oral Surg. **42:**316, 1976.
8. Forman, L., and Nally, F.F.: Oral nondystrophic bullous eruption mainly limited to the gingivae: a mechanical bullous response. A variant of cicatricial mucous membrane pemphigoid? Br. J. Dermatol. **96:**111, 1977.
9. Susi, F.R., and Shklar, G.: Histochemistry and fine structure of oral lesions of mucous membrane pemphigoid: preliminary observations, Arch. Dermatol **104:**244, 1971.
10. Jandinski, J.J., and Shklar, G.: Lichen planus of the gingiva, J. Periodontol. **47:**724, 1976.
11. Shklar, G., Meyer, I., and Zacarian, S.A.: Oral lesions in bullous pemphigoid, Arch. Dermatol. **99:**663, 1969.
12. Ziskin, D.E., and Zegarelli, E.V.: Chronic desquamative gingivitis; report of 12 cases, Am. J. Orthodont. (Oral Surg. Sect.) **31:**1, 1945.
13. Foss, C.L., Grupe, H.E., and Orban, B.: Gingivosis, J. Periodontol. **24:**207, 1953.
14. Sibulkin, D., and Cohen, H.J.: Oral mucosal erosions, Oral Surg. **34:**203, 1972.
15. Moore, D.S., and Nally, F.F.: A method of differential diagnosis of some bullous lesions, J. Oral Med. **29:**92, 1974.
16. Shafer, W.G., Hine, M., and Levy, B.G.: A textbook of oral pathology, ed. 3, Philadelphia, 1974, W.B. Saunders Co.
17. Andreasen, J.O.: Oral lichen planus. II. A histologic evaluation of ninety-seven cases, Oral Surg. **25:**158, 1968.
18. Glickman, I., and Smulow, J.B.: Histopathology and histochemistry of chronic des-

quamative gingivitis, Oral Surg. **21:**325, 1966.

19. Hall, W.B.: Staining mast cells in human gingiva, Arch. Oral Biol. **11:**1325, 1966.

20. Whitten, J.B.: The fine structure of desquamative gingivitis, J. Periodontol. **39:**75, 1968.

21. Brusati, R., and Bracchetti, A.: Electron microscopic study of chronic desquamative gingivitis, J. Periodontol. **40:**388, 1969.

22. Johnson, G.D., Holborow, E.J., and Dorling, J.: Immunofluorescence and immunoenzyme techniques. In Weir, D.M., editor: Handbook of experimental immunology, ed. 3, Oxford, 1978, Blackwell Scientific Publications.

23. Peters, J.H., and Coons, A.H.: Fluorescent antibody as specific cytochemical reagents: histochemical methods. In Williams, C.A., and Chase, M.W., editors: Methods in immunology and immunochemistry, vol. V, New York, 1976, Academic Press, Inc.

24. Nisengard, R.J., and Neiders, M.: Desquamative lesions of the gingiva, J. Periodontol. **52:**500, 1981.

25. Mesa-Tejada, R., Pascal, R.R., and Fenoglio, C.M.: Immunoperoxidase: a sensitive immunohistochemical technique as a "special stain" in the diagnostic pathology laboratory, Hum. Pathol. **8:**313, 1977.

26. De Lellis, R.A., et al.: Immunoperoxidase techniques in diagnostic pathology, Am J. Clin. Pathol. **71:**483, 1979.

27. Taylor, C.: Immunoperoxidase techniques, Arch. Pathol. Lab. Med. **102:**113, 1978.

28. Zanin, L.G., et al.: Immunofluorescence et immunoperoxidase: comparaison de la sensibilité en immunopathologie cutanée, Ann. Dermatol. Venereol. **105:**793, 1978.

29. Riva, R.D.: Exfoliative cytology: a review of literature and presentation of a fluorescent technique, J. Oral Med. **32:**98, 1977.

30. Acosta, A.E., Hietanen, J., and Ivanyi, L.: Direct immunofluorescence on cytological smears in oral pemphigus, J. Dermatol. **105:**645, 1981.

31. Laskaris, G., Papanicolaou, S., and Angelopoulos, A.: Immunofluorescent study of cytologic smears in oral pemphigus: a simple diagnostic technique, Oral Surg. **51:**531, 1981.

32. Daniels, T.E., and Quadra-White, C.: Direct immunofluorescence in oral mucosal disease: a diagnostic analysis of 130 cases, Oral Surg. **51:**38, 1981.

33. Handlers, J., et al.: Immunoperoxidase technique diagnosis of oral pemphigus vulgaris: an alternative method to immunofluorescence, Oral Surg. **54:**207, 1982.

34. Laskaris, G.: Oral pemphigus vulgaris: an immunofluorescent study of fifty-eight cases, Oral Surg. **51:**626, 1981.

35. Hodge, L., et al.: Indirect immunofluorescence in the immunopathological assessment of bullous pemphigoid cicatricial pemphigoid and herpes gestationalis, Clin. Exp. Dermatol. **3:**61, 1978.

36. Laskaris, G., and Angelopoulos, A.: Cicatricial pemphigoid: direct and indirect immunofluorescent studies, Oral Surg. **51:**48, 1981.

37. Dabelsteen E., et al.: Demonstration of basement membrane autoantibodies in patients with benign mucous membrane pemphigoid, Acta Derm. Venereol. **54:**189, 1974.

38. Laskaris, G., and Nicolis, G.: Immunopathology of oral mucosa in bullous pemphigoid, Oral Surg. **50:**340, 1980.

39. Bean, S.F., et al.: Cicatricial pemphigoid: immunofluorescent studies, Arch. Dermatol. **106:**195, 1972.

40. Griffith, M.R., et al.: Immunofluorescent studies in mucous membrane pemphigoid, Arch. Dermatol. **109:**195, 1974.

41. Holmstrup, E., Dabelsteen, E., and Ullman, S.: Deposits of immunoglobulins in oral lupus erythematosus, lichen planus and leukoplakia, Oral Surg. **51:**603, 1981.

42. Laskaris, G., Sklavounou, A., and Angelopoulos, A.: Direct immunofluorescence in oral lichen planus, Oral Surg. **53:**483, 1982.

43. Shklar, G., Frim, S., and Flynn, A.: Gingival lesions of pemphigus, J. Periodontol. **49:**428, 1978.

44. Lynde, C.W., Ongley, R.C., and Rigg, J.M.: Juvenile pemphigus vulgaris, Arch. Dermatol. **120:**1098, 1984.

45. Laskaris, G., Sklavounou, A., and Stratigos, J.: Bullous pemphigoid, cicatricial pemphigoid and pemphigus vulgaris, Oral Surg. **54:**656, 1982.

46. Markitziu, A., and Pisanty, S.: Gingival pemphigus vulgaris: report of a case, Oral Surg. **55:**250, 1983.

47. Talal, N., Fye, K.H., and Moutsopoulos, H.M.: Autoimmunity. In Fudenberg, H.H., et al., editor: Basic and clinical immunology, ed. 2, Los Altos, 1978, Lange Medical Publications.

48. Beutner, E., et al.: Autosensitization in pemphigus, bullous pemphigoid and other chronic bullous diseases. In Miescher, P.A., and Muller, H.J.: Textbook of immunopathology, ed. 2, New York, 1976, Grune & Stratton Inc.

49. Jordon, R.E., et al.: Classical and alternate pathway activation of complement in pemphigus vulgaris lesions, J. Invest. Dermatol. **63:**256, 1974.

50. Eisenberg, E., et al.: Pemphigus-like mucosal lesions: a side effect of penicillamine therapy, Oral Surg. **51:**409, 1981.

51. Van Hale, H., Rogers, R.S., and Zone, J.T.: Pyostomatitis vegetans: a reactive mucosal marker for inflammatory disease of the gut, Arch. Dermatol. **121:**94, 1985.

52. Cataldo, E., Covino, M.C., and Tesene, P.E.: Pyostomatitis vegetans, Oral Surg. **52:**172, 1981.

53. Hansen, L.S., Silverman, S., and Daniels, T.E.: The differential diagnosis of pyostomatitis vegetans and its relation to bowel disease, Oral Surg. **55:**363, 1983.

54. Moy, W., et al.: Cicatricial pemphigoid: a case of onset at age 5, J. Periodontol. **57:**39, 1986.

55. Barnett, M.L., Wittwer, J.W., and Miller, P.L.: Desquamative gingivitis in a 13-year-old male, J. Periodontol. **52:**270, 1981.

56. Pindborg, J.J.: Altas of diseases of the oral mucosa, ed. 3, Copenhagen, 1973, Munksgaard.

57. McCarthy, P.L.: Benign mucous membrane pemphigoid, Oral Surg. **33:**75, 1972.

58. Andreasen, J.O.: Oral lichen planus. I. A clinical evaluation of 115 cases, Oral Surg. **25:**31, 1968.

59. Cook, B.E.: The oral manifestations of lichen planus: 50 cases, Br. Dent. J. **96:**1, 1954.

60. Silverman, S., and Griffith, M.: Studies and oral lichen planus. II. Follow-up on 200 patients, clinical characteristics and associated malignancy, Oral Surg. **37:**705, 1974.

61. Lacy, M.F., Reade, P.C., and Hay, K.D.: Lichen planus: a theory of pathogenesis, Oral Surg. **56:**521, 1983.

62. Hyman, G. et al.: Autoradiographic studies of oral lichen planus, Oral Surg. **54:**172, 1982.

63. Mander, Z.M., and Deesen, K.C.: Transformation of oral lichen planus to squamous cell carcinoma: a literature review and report of a case, J. Am. Dent. Assoc. **105:**55, 1982.

64. Pogrel, M.A., and Weldon, L.L.: Carcinoma arising in erosive lichen planus in the midline of the dorsum of the tongue, Oral Surg. **55:**62, 1983.

65. Krutchkoff, D.J., Cutter, L., and Laskowski, S.: Oral lichen planus: the evidence regarding malignant transformation, J. Oral Pathol. **7:**1, 1978.

66. Fulling, H.S.: Cancer development in oral lichen planus, Arch. Dermatol. **108:**667, 1973.

67. Wells, J.V.: Immune mechanisms in tissue damage. In Fundenberg, H.H., et al., editor: Basic and clinical immunology, ed. 2, Los Altos, 1978, Lange Medical Publications.

68. Regezi, J.A., Deegan, M.J., and Hayward, J.R.: Lichen planus: immunologic and morphologic identification of the submucosal infiltrate, Oral Surg. **46:**44, 1978.

69. Walker, D.M.: Identification of subpopulation of lymphocytes and macrophages in the infiltrate of lichen planus lesion of skin and oral mucosa, Br. J. Dermatol. **94:**529, 1976.

70. Sklavounou, A.D, Laskaris, G., and Angelopoulos, A.P.: Serum immunoglobulins and complement (C3) in oral lichen planus, Oral Surg. **55:**47, 1983.

71. Ellis, F.A.: Histopathology of lichen planus: based on analysis of the one hundred biopsy specimens, J. Invest. Dermatol. **48:**143, 1967.

72. Schiött, M., and Pindborg, J.J.: Oral discoid lupus erythematosus. I. The validity of previous histopathologic diagnostic criteria, Oral Surg. **57:**46, 1984.

73. Buchner, A., Lozada, F., and Silverman, S.: Histopathologic spectrum of oral erythema multiforme, Oral Surg. **49:**221, 1980.

74. Wright, J.: Epidermolysis bullosa: dental and anesthetic management of two cases, Oral Surg. **57:**155, 1984.

75. Orfanos, C.E., Schaumburg-Lever, G., and Lever, W.F.: Dermal and epidermal types of erythema multiforme, Arch. Dermatol. **109:**682, 1974.

76. Bean, S.F., and Quezada, R.K.: Recurrent oral erythema multiforme: clinical experience with 11 patients, JAMA **249:**2810, 1983.

77. Jones, L.E., and Dolby, A.E.: Desquamative gingivitis associated with psoriasis, J. Periodontol. **43:**35, 1972.

78. Siegel, C., Barker, B., and Kunstadter, M.: Conditioned oral scurvy due to megavitamin C withdrawal, J. Periodontol. **53:**453, 1982.

79. Pattison, M.L.: Self-inflicted gingival injuries, J. Periodontol. **54:**299, 1983.

80. Michaelides, P.L.: Treatment of periodontal disease in a patient with Turner's syndrome, J. Periodontol. **52:**386, 1981.

81. Kerr, D.A., McClatchey, K.D., and Regezi, J.A.: Idiopathic gingivostomatitis, Oral Surg. **32:**402, 1971.

82. Lubow, R., et al.: Plasma-cell gingivitis: report of case, J. Periodontol. **55:**235, 1984.

83. Newcomb, G.M, Seymour, G.J., and Adkins, K.F.: An unusual form of chronic gingivitis: an ultrastructural, histochemical, and immunologic investigation, Oral Surg. **53:**488, 1982.

84. Murray, V.K., and De Feo, C.: Intraoral fixed drug eruption following tetracycline administration, J. Periodontol. **53:**267, 1982.

85. Scully, C.: Ulcerative stomatitis, gingivitis, and skin lesion, Oral Surg. **59:**261, 1985.

86. Jacobsen, P.L., et al.: Idiopathic gingival ulcerations: ten cases of a previously unreported entity, Oral Surg. **50:**517, 1980.

87. Roger, R., Sheridan, P.J., and Jordon, R.E.: Desquamative gingivitis: clinical, histopathologic and immunopathologic investigation, Oral Surg. **42:**316, 1976.

88. Shklar, G., and McCarthy, P.L.: Oral lesions of mucous membrane pemphigoid, Arch. Otolaryngol. **93:**354, 1971.

89. Sklavounou, A., and Laskaris, G.: Frequency of desquamative gingivitis in skin disease, Oral Surg. **56:**141, 1983.

90. Nisengard, R.J., Alpert, A.M., and Krestow, V.: Desquamative gingivitis: immunologic findings, J. Periodontol. **49:**27, 1978.

91. Kerr, D.A., McClatchey, K.D., and Regezi, J.A.: Allergic gingivostomatitis (due to gum chewing), J. Periodontol. **42:**709, 1971.
92. Perry, H.O., Deffner, N.F., and Sheridan, P.J.: Atypical gingivostomatitis, Arch. Dermatol. **107:**872, 1973.
93. Silverman, S., Lozada, F., and Migliorati, C.: Clinical efficacy of prednisone in the treatment of patient with oral inflammatory ulcerative diseases: a study of fifty-five patients, Oral Surg. **59:**360, 1985.
94. Orlowski, W.A., et al.: Chronic pemphigus vulgaris of the gingiva: a case report with a 6-year follow-up, J. Periodontol. **54:**685, 1983.
95. Harris, S.C.: The use of adrenal steroid in dental practice, Dent. Clin. North Am. **14:**845, 1970.
96. Negosanti, M., et al.: Severe herpetic gingivostomatitis associated with pemphigus vulgaris, Arch. Dermatol. **120:**540, 1984.
97. Bystryn, J.C.: Adjuvant therapy of pemphigus, Arch. Dermatol. **120:**941, 1984.
98. Lozada, F., Sylverman, S., and Cram, D.: Pemphigus vulgaris: a study of six cases treated with levamisole and prednisone, Oral Surg. **54:**161, 1982.
99. Lozada, F.: Prednisone and azathioprine in the treatment of patients with vesiculoerosive oral disease, Oral Surg. **52:**257, 1981.
100. Ship, I.I., Williams, A.F., and Osheroff, B.S.: Development and clinical investigations of a new oral surface anesthetic for acute and chronic oral lesions, Oral Surg. **13:**630. 1960.
101. Aufdemorte, T.B., De-Villez, R.L., and Gieseker, D.R.: Griseofulvin in the treatment of the three cases of oral erosive lichen planus, Oral Surg. **55:**459, 1983.
102. Kalkwarf, K.L., et al.: Management of the dental patient receiving corticosteroid medications, Oral Surg. **54:**396, 1982.

## ADDITIONAL SUGGESTED READING

Laufer, J., and Kuffer, R.: Le lichen plan buccal, Paris, 1970, Masson & Cie.
Nikai, H., Rose, G.G., and Cattoni, M.: Electron microscopic study of chronic desquamative gingivitis, J. Periodont. Res. Suppl. **6,** 1971.

# CHAPTER 23

## Gingival recession

**Anatomic factors**

**Etiologic factors**

**Prognosis**

**Therapeutic measures**

---

Recession of the gingiva with exposure of facial root surfaces and interdental embrasures may occur. This can occur on posterior teeth as well as anterior teeth. It can occur lingually as well as facially and interdentally. The patient, however, is most concerned esthetically with recession in the anterior part of the mouth.

Recession can be localized, about a single tooth or individual tooth units, or it may be generalized involving segments of teeth or arches.

Some generalized recession has been noted coincident with ageing.[1-4] Recession may also be related to periodontal disease,[1,2] developmental defects,[5] trauma,[6] and dental procedures.[7,8]

Gingival recession may occur in the presence or absence of visible inflammation. It may be accompanied by pocket depth or occur with shallow sulci (Fig. 23-1). When the sulci are shallow, the gingiva may be thin, finely textured, and pale pink in color. Papillary architecture may be normal or slightly receded. Although plaque may be minimal, it may still have influenced the recession.

Recession may also occur as a result of plaque-induced periodontal disease (periodontitis). When there is preexisting periodontal disease, plaque, and pockets, one may surmise that the recession is the result of inflammatory periodontal disease.

When there is no plaque, no apparent inflammation, and no pocket, the recession may have resulted from prior gingival disease or nonplaque-related causes. Nonplaque-related causes include ageing, developmental anatomic abnormalities such as tooth position, and dehiscences that relate to tooth eruption or to mechanical trauma (brushing, accidents, orthodontic movement, dental appliances, restorations, and procedures).

## Anatomic factors

Gingival recession may be related to certain predisposing anatomic factors. The position of gingival margins is partly determined by the height and thickness of the underlying bone, the thickness and texture of the gingiva, and tooth alignment. Teeth that are malposed (e.g., toward the labial or lingual surface) tend to have a thinner alveolar plate in the direction toward which they are malposed. They have a thicker

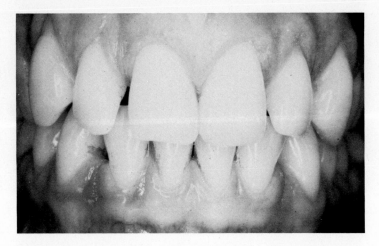

**Fig. 23-1.**    Gingival recession. Facial margins of the gingiva are receded. Papillae are long and fill the interdental embrasures. Sulcular depth is minimal. No inflammation can be discerned.

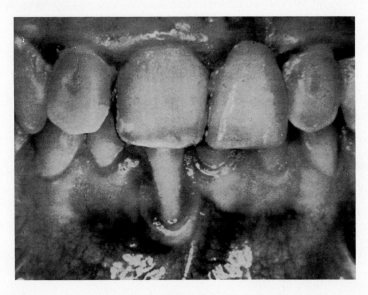

**Fig. 23-2.**    Localized recession of a vestibularly (labially) located mandibular central incisor.

alveolar plate on the side from which they are malposed.[9,10] Vestibularly malposed teeth (Fig. 23-2) usually have a thinner vestibular alveolar plate and some degree of root exposure. The gingival margins are thus positioned in accordance with tooth alignment and with bone thickness and height. Thin and delicately textured gingiva supported by a thin alveolar bone is more vulnerable to recession than thicker and more fibrous gingiva supported by a heavy alveolar plate. When the thinner and more delicate tissues are subjected to mechanical trauma and plaque, destruction of bone and gingiva may take place and result in recession.

Clefts of the gingiva (Fig. 23-3, *A*) apparently are caused by an uneven destruction of the marginal gingiva. They may develop on the lingual surface but are most often seen on the facial surface. Downgrowth and fusion of long epithelial ridges have been observed in the subepithelial connective tissue clefts. The fusion of such proliferated epithelial ridges with sulcular epithelium may be responsible for the formation of gingival clefts.[11,12] When there is no intervening alveolar bone, some clefts extend to

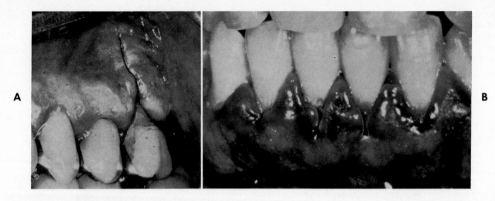

**Fig. 23-3. A,** Extensive cleft on the vestibular surface of a maxillary molar possibly associated with toothbrush injury. **B,** Pseudoclefts on the vestibular surfaces of the mandibular incisors primarily caused by hyperplastic overgrowth of the adjacent tissues.

the root surface. Occasionally clefts may result from faulty brushing (Fones' method) with a hard brush made of sharp bristles.[6] Some such clefts disappear spontaneously.[11] Pseudoclefts may be formed by overgrowth of adjacent tissue (Fig. 23-3, *B*). In such cases the alveolar bone may not be extensively affected.

## Etiologic factors

The cause of gingival recession, whether localized or generalized, is not always easy to determine.[13] The following factors have been incriminated[2,6,8,13-16]:

1. Inflammatory periodontal disease (considered to be the principal etiologic factor)[12]
2. Ageing
3. Developmental anatomic abnormalities (dehiscences, thin bony plates, high frenum attachments)
4. Faulty tooth alignment[14]
5. Toothbrush injury (Fig. 23-3, *A*)
6. Orthodontic forces (Fig. 23-4) that have moved a tooth through the alveolar plate
7. Pressure from such sources as bands, arch wires, and crowns[7,8]
8. Deleterious habits (pressure of foreign objects, fingernails, pencils, hairpins)
9. Clasps and mandibular oral (lingual) denture bars or aprons in partial dentures that have settled (pressure atrophy)
10. Surgical treatment of inflammatory periodontal disease

Repeated and prolonged toothbrush injury is often assumed to lead to recession.[6,11,13,14] Fig. 23-5 shows a recession associated with extensive abrasion at the cementoenamel junction. The patient reported brushing vigorously in a horizontal direction with a hard toothbrush. This type of recession is common on the left canines of right-handed persons.

Periodontal traumatism is another factor incriminated in gingival recession and cleft formation.[12] Available evidence tends to indicate that occlusal trauma does not produce recession.

The case of a young person shown in Fig. 23-6 demonstrates recession. Several primary teeth were missing. Two mandibular incisors were in crossbite to the maxillary incisors. The gingival margin on one tooth was receded compared with the gingiva of the other teeth. The gingival recession was brought about by the vestibular position of this tooth.

A seemingly similar occlusal situation without any recession of the gingiva, shown in Fig. 23-7, is of a 20-year-old adult. The incisor in Fig. 23-6, showing some recession,

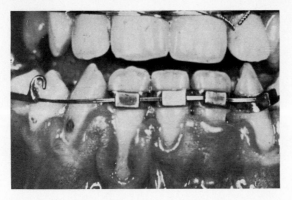

**Fig. 23-4.** Recession of the gingiva brought about during orthodontic therapy when a tooth was moved too rapidly or too far in a labial direction.

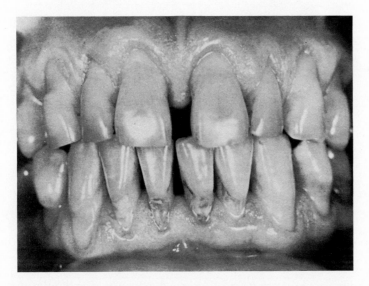

**Fig. 23-5.** Recession of the gingiva and abrasion of the teeth brought about by overly vigorous and incorrect brushing or the use of a brush with sharp, hard bristles.

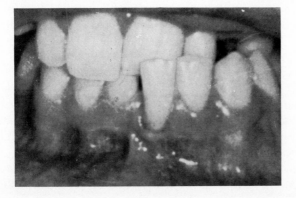

**Fig. 23-6.** Mandibular incisors in a crossbite relationship, allegedly producing periodontal traumatism and recession. In fact, the malposition of the central incisor labially produced the recession. (Courtesy J.R. Thompson, Chicago, Illinois.)

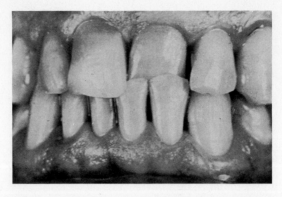

**Fig. 23-7.** Occlusal arrangement of teeth similar to that shown in Fig. 23-6 without recession. (Courtesy H.A. Brayshaw, Denver, Colorado.)

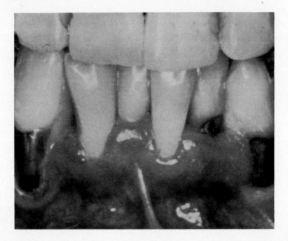

**Fig. 23-8.** Tooth position influences bony anatomy and the position of gingival margins. Teeth that are lingually positioned have higher gingival margins (on the vestibular surface) than do their more buccally positioned neighbors.

was considerably vestibular to its neighbors, whereas the mandibular incisors in Fig. 23-7 were not equally malpositioned. Obviously, the labioversion of the incisor in Fig. 23-6 resulted in a thinner labial alveolar plate. In the case in Fig. 23-7 an adequate thickness of vestibular bone was present, and, despite the similarity of the occlusal relationships, no gingival recession occurred. This point is illustrated further in Fig. 23-8. Six anterior teeth are present. The two canines are prominent labially, and the gingiva is receded. Two incisors are lingual and show no recession, whereas the labially positioned incisors show recession. The vestibular alveolar plate is thin in the incisor and canine regions. If a tooth becomes inclined vestibularly or orally, the thin alveolar covering bone can easily become resorbed. A relatively constant spatial relationship exists between the gingival attachment and the alveolar crest in health.[4,17,18] If the alveolar crest is resorbed, the gingival margin may follow, particularly when the overlying gingiva is thin and finely textured. Contributing factors might be injury from brushing or mastication.

Gingival recession may also result from mechanical irritation or pressure from dental appliances.[12,19] Some people respond to irritation by recession, some by overgrowth, and some by no change in the position of the gingival margin. Imperfect margins on dental restorations, clasps, and ill-fitting prostheses (Fig. 23-9) may traumatize the gingiva. Indicated therapy is removal of the mechanical irritants.

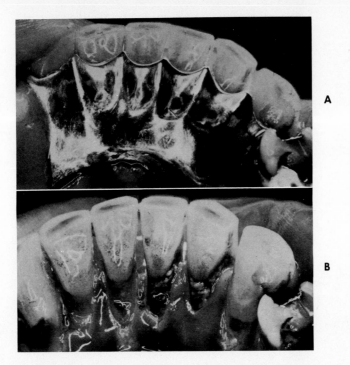

**Fig. 23-9.  A,** Lower partial denture with lingual apron from canine to canine. The apron presses against the linguogingival margins. **B,** Denture removed. The gingiva has been sheared away by the settling metal apron. Plaque is present.

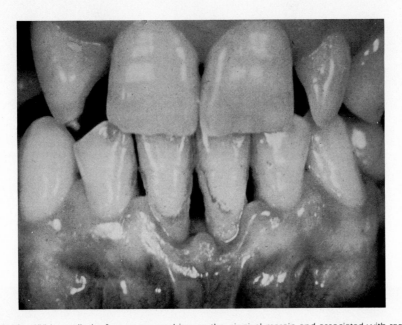

**Fig. 23-10.**  Wide vestibular frenum encroaching on the gingival margin and associated with recession.

The vestibular frenum, as seen in Fig. 23-8, is an anatomic structure that often is associated with recession of the gingiva on the mandibular central incisors. This factor was not contributory in the patient shown in the illustration. The influence of the frenum on gingival recession is controversial. A high vestibular frenum might play a part in recession shown in Fig. 23-10.

**Influence of frenum**

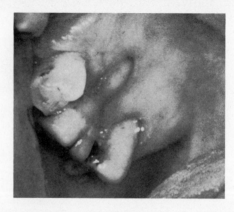

**Fig. 23-11.** Recession on the palatal root of a maxillary molar.

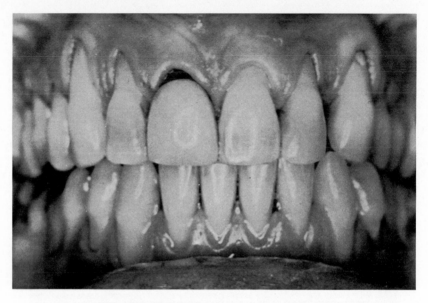

**Fig. 23-12.** Slowly progressive generalized recession.

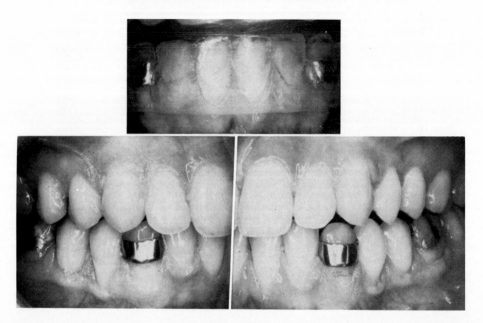

**Fig. 23-13.** Pressure atrophy by an orthodontic acrylic positioner has provoked recession of the mandibular gingiva.

In some instances isolated recession can occur on the palatal root of a maxillary molar (Fig. 23-11). Conceivably toothbrush friction or tongue pressure[20] can contribute to recession of the gingiva over a prominent root.

Gingival recession may also be an expression of a physiologic process. A gradual recession of the gingival margins has been noted with ageing.[17] This is apparent in older persons who have receded gingival margins, flattened papillae, and widened embrasures in a clinically healthy mouth. Whether ageing is the direct cause of the recession is unknown. Recession also occurs as an expression of passive eruption in young people.[21-23] These types of recession should be differentiated from the obvious pathologically induced recessions.

Physiologic gingival recession can be correlated with an apical migration of the junctional epithelium,[17,18] which occurs coincident with ageing and possibly with atrophy of alveolar bone. Physiologic bone atrophy may be postulated as an alteration in the delicate balance of continual bone replacement. Theoretically this would involve a decrease in bone replacement rather than an increase in bone destruction. Since the distance between the bottom of the junctional epithelium and the alveolar crest remains relatively constant in health,[4] the clinical expression of this process might be gingival recession.

## Prognosis

Some recessions can be arrested; others slowly progress with time despite all measures to arrest them. The patient shown in Fig. 23-12 had been under treatment for about 10 years. The mouth was reasonably clean. Brushing was fairly efficient, careful, and nontraumatic, yet slow progressive recession was evident with anatomic factors a likely contributing cause. In another case recession has been produced in a 16-year-old orthodontic patient by an acrylic positioner (Fig. 23-13). Removal of the appliance arrested the gingival recession.

Teeth are rarely lost because of gingival recession.[13-23] Recession may advance during some periods and then slow and remain stationary for years. In a few cases pocket formation might complicate the picture. Whether gingival recession requires surgical correction to prevent tooth loss is controversial.[22-28]

## Therapeutic measures

Therapeutic measures include the institution of proper oral hygiene (correct method of brushing; soft brush with polished, rounded bristle tips; nonabrasive dentifrice; and routine scaling to improve gingival contour.[22] There is some controversy as to how much gingiva is required for health. Some maintain that at least 2 mm of gingiva are needed to avoid inflammation[23]; this is denied by others who claim that less than 1 mm is maintainable.[24-26] Therefore in the absence of recession, a narrow gingival width may not be significant. Gingival grafts are sometimes used to correct localized defects or to create a new zone of gingiva for esthetic or prosthetic reasons.

**REFERENCES**

1. Akpata, E.F., and Jackson, B.: The prevalence and distribution of gingivitis and gingival recession in children and young adults in Lagos, Nigeria, J. Periodontol. **50:**79, 1980.
2. Woofter, C.: The prevalence and etiology of gingival recession, Periodontal Abstr. **17:**45, 1969.
3. Burch, T.R.J., et al.: Gingival recession ("getting long in the tooth"), colorectal cancer: degenerative and malignant changes as errors of growth control, Mech. Growth Dev. **2:**51, 1973.
4. Gargiulo, A.W., Wentz, F.M., and Orban, B.: Dimensions and relations of the dentogingival junction in humans, J. Periodontol. **32:**261, 1961.
5. Löst, C.: Depth of alveolar bone dehiscenses in relation to gingival recession, J. Clin. Periodontol. **11:**583, 1984.
6. Hirschfeld, I.: The toothbrush: its use and

abuse, Brooklyn, 1939, Dental Items of Interest Publishing Co.

7. Donaldson, D.: The etiology of gingival recession associated with temporary crowns, J. Periodontol. **45**:264, 1972.

8. Donaldson, D.: Gingival recession associated with temporary crowns, J. Periodontol. **44**:691, 1973.

9. Hirschfeld, L.: A study of skulls in the American Museum of Natural History in relation to periodontal disease, J. Dent. Res. **5**:241, 1923.

10. Morris, M.L.: The position of the margin of the gingiva, Oral. Surg. **11**:969, 1958.

11. Everett, F.G.: The case of the disappearing clefts, J. Periodontol. **39**:296, 1968.

12. Novaes, A.B., et al.: The development of the periodontal cleft: a clinical and histopathologic study, J. Periodontol. **46**:701, 1976.

13. Moskow, B.S., and Bressman, E.: Localized gingival recession, Dent. Radiogr. Photogr. **38**:3, 1965.

14. Gorman, W.J.: Prevalence and etiology of gingival recession, J. Periodontol. **38**:316, 1967.

15. O'Leary, T.J., et al.: The incidence of recession in young males: a further study, J. Periodontol. **42**:264, 1971.

16. Green, L.H., and Levin, M.P.: The treatment of an unusual case of incipient gingival recession exhibiting a familial tendency: a case report, J. Periodontol. **44**:519, 1972.

17. Gottlieb, B.: Der Epithelansatz am Zahn, Dtsch. Monatsschr. Zahnheilkd. **39**:142, 1921.

18. Orban, B., and Köhler, J.: Die physiologische Zahnfleischtasche, Epithelansatz und Epitheltiefenwucherung, Z. Stomatol. **22**:353, 1924.

19. Merritt, A.H.: Periodontal diseases, ed. 3, New York, 1945, The Macmillan Co.

20. Ray, H., and Santos, H.A.: Consideration of tongue-thrusting as a factor in periodontal disease, J. Periodontol. **25**:250, 1954.

21. Volchansky, A., Cleaton-Jones, P., and Fatti, L.P.: A three-year longitudinal study of the gingival margin in man, J. Clin. Periodontol. **6**:231, 1979.

22. Powell, R.N., and McEniery, T.M.: A longitudinal study of isolated gingival recession in the mandibular incisor region of children 6-8 years, J. Clin. Periodontol. **9**:357, 1982.

23. Lang, N.P., and Löe, H.: The relationship between width of keratinized gingiva and gingival health, J. Periodontol. **43**:623, 1972.

24. Bowers, C.: A study of the width of attached gingiva, J. Periodontol. **34**:201, 1963.

25. Miyasato, M., Crigger, M., and Egelberg, J.: Gingival conditions in areas of minimal and appreciable width of keratinized gingiva, J. Clin. Periodontol. **4**:200, 1977.

26. Tenenbaum, H.: A clinical study comparing the width of attached gingiva and the prevalence of gingival recession, J. Clin. Periodontol. **9**:86, 1982.

27. Ericsson, I., and Lindhe, J.: Recession in sites with inadequate width of the keratinized gingiva, J. Clin. Periodontol. **11**:95, 1984.

28. Wennström, J., and Lindhe, J.: Plaque-induced gingival inflammation in the absence of attached gingiva in dogs, J. Clin. Periodontol. **10**:266, 1983.

## ADDITIONAL SUGGESTED READING

Kalkwarf, K.L., and Krejci, R.F.: Effect of inflammation on periodontal attachment levels in miniature swine with mucogingival defects, J. Periodontol. **54**:361, 1983.

Mathur, R.M., et al.: Study of gingival recession as it relates to oral cleaning habits, J. Indian Dent. Assoc. **41**:159, 1969.

Moskow, B.S., and Baden, E.: Unusual gingival characteristics having a familial tendency: a case report, Periodontics **5**:259, 1967.

O'Leary, T.J.: The incidence of recession in young males, Periodontics **6**:109, 1968.

Orban, G.: Clinical and histologic study of the surface characteristics of the gingiva, Oral Surg. **1**:827, 1948.

Schoo, W.H., and van der Velden, U.: Marginal soft tissue recessions with and without attached gingiva: a five year longitudinal, J. Periodontol. **20**:209, 1985.

# CHAPTER 24

# Gingival enlargement: hyperplastic and inflammatory enlargement

**Gingival hyperplasia**
Localized hyperplasia
Generalized hyperplasia
Idiopathic gingival hyperplasia (fibromatosis)
Other enlargements
Phenytoin hyperplasia

**Treatment**

**Summary**

---

Enlargement of the gingiva may be caused by fibrous hyperplasia, inflammation, a combination of hyperplasia and inflammation, or bony growths such as thick alveolar processes, exostosis, and tori.

## Gingival hyperplasia

Gingival fibrous hyperplasia is an overgrowth caused by an increase in the fibrous tissue elements of the gingivae. It is not an inflammatory condition, although hyperplasia and inflammation of the gingiva most often occur together. Either can cause gingival enlargement.

### LOCALIZED HYPERPLASIA

Gingival hyperplasia may occur as a localized overgrowth, limited to a certain area[1-4] (Fig. 24-1). The cause of such localized fibromas is unknown. Local irritation may be responsible for their development. Microscopically such overgrowths are characterized by an increase in fibrous as well as cellular elements. Calcification and ossification may take place within them. Since irritation may induce localized overgrowths, they are also known as irritation fibromas.

Indicated therapy is the surgical removal of the overgrowth and elimination of the local irritating factor responsible for it. Excision is usually successful, although these lesions sometimes recur. Complete removal and elimination of the local irritating factor (cavities, open contacts) are probably the only ways to avoid recurrence.

### GENERALIZED HYPERPLASIA

Generalized gingival fibrous hyperplasia is a rare disease. It may develop in childhood and may be quite extensive.[5-11] A case occurring in a 24-year-old man is shown in Fig. 24-2, *A*. Microscopic examination revealed an increase in fibrous tissue elements (Fig. 24-2, *B*) with accompanying atrophic changes in the surface epithelium. No etiologic factor could be determined.

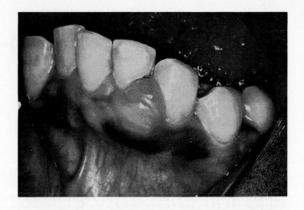

**Fig. 24-1.** Localized, gingival hyperplasia. (Courtesy F. Howell, San Diego, California.)

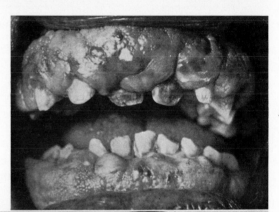

**Fig. 24-2. A,** Idiopathic gingival hyperplasia (fibromatosis). **B,** Microscopic specimen of gingival hyperplasia showing extensive overgrowth of the fiber bundles with little inflammation. (Courtesy O.J. Shaffer, El Paso, Texas.)

A

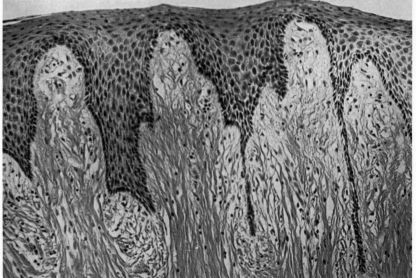

B

## IDIOPATHIC GINGIVAL HYPERPLASIA (FIBROMATOSIS)

Idiopathic gingival hyperplasia has a genetic background as indicated by multiple occurrences in a family.[5-10] Six of eight children in one family had fibrous hyperplasia. Fig. 24-3 shows the gingiva of one of the children, who still had some primary teeth. The father had a similar condition in childhood. A gingivectomy was performed at the

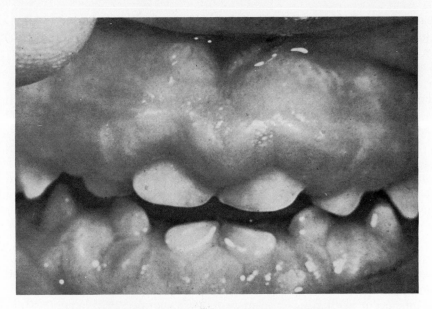

**Fig. 24-3.** Familial hereditary gingival hyperplasia.

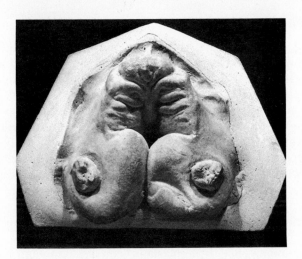

**Fig. 24-4.** Enormously enlarged tuberosities. (Courtesy H. Mathis, West Berlin, West Germany.)

age of 15, but the overgrowth recurred. Finally, all teeth were extracted and dentures were made. No systemic disease could be found in any member of this family.

Therapeutic judgment will govern the treatment for each specific case.[2,11] Gingival enlargement has a tendency to recur after excision but not after extraction of teeth. Gingival fibromatosis patients do not suffer from keloid formation. A few show hirsutism[9] and mental underdevelopment.[12]

## OTHER ENLARGEMENTS

Enlarged tuberosities may form that can extend almost to palatal midline and mesially to the premolar area (Fig. 24-4).[13] These enlargements usually consist of soft tissue.

Bony enlargements can also occur.[3] Tori and exostosis may provoke gingival enlargement consisting principally of fibrous tissue. At other times, the bony enlargements may be covered by a thin gingiva.

**Enlarged tuberosities**

**Bony enlargements**

**Inflammatory hyperplasia (hyperplastic gingivitis)**

Heavy alveolar ridges may be seen as gingival enlargement, occasionally causing teeth to seem "submerged." Inflammatory hyperplasia, an overgrowth in response to plaque, may occur in the course of periodontal disease. It may be localized or generalized and can be resolved with treatment.

**Localized inflammatory enlargements**

Localized inflammatory lesions are seen frequently and are not neoplastic. They are nonspecific inflammatory reactions. Circumscribed, localized overgrowths over one tooth or between two teeth have been called *epulis*. Today, they are classified as *pyogenic granuloma* (including *pregnancy tumor*), *ossifying fibroblastic granuloma, ossifying fibroma, fibrous hyperplasia,* or *fibrous epulis* and *peripheral giant cell granuloma.*[14] All have a tendency to recur and are classified as reactive lesions. The gingival enlargement, pyogenic granuloma, occurs at times in conjunction with periodontal abscesses and periodontal diseases.[15-17] A significant percentage of patients who exhibit pyogenic granulomas are pregnant. In these instances the tumor is referred to as a *pregnancy tumor*. Enlargements may occur with the use of contraceptive drugs.[18]

Other enlargements occur in the course of puberty, pregnancy, leukemia,[19] blood dyscrasias,[20] solid tumor neoplasia (including Kaposi sarcoma and carcinoma of the gingiva),[21] Wegener's granulomatosis,[22] and lymphangiomas.[23] Still other enlargements occur with drug therapy with cyclosporine,[24-26] nifedipine,[27] and phenytoin.

## PHENYTOIN HYPERPLASIA

Administration of phenytoin (Dilantin, Epanutin) in the treatment of epilepsy is frequently followed by a hyperplastic and inflammatory overgrowth of the gingiva,[28-43] usually within weeks to months following initiation of dosage. Gingival overgrowth has a tendency to reduce when another drug is substituted.[36,44,45] Not all patients receiving phenytoin develop gingival hyperplasia.[46] Different investigators have reported widely differing incidences of hyperplasia in patients with epilepsy treated with phenytoin. The average figure for hyperplasia is about 50%.[46,47] Sixty-six percent have some degree of hyperplasia, 26% moderate hyperplasia, and 6% severe enlargements.[32] The tendency toward hyperplasia varies considerably in amount and location. The hyperplasia is more pronounced about the anterior teeth and is more extensive on the vestibular than on the oral surfaces. It is also greater in the upper than in the lower jaw.[28] Oral hygiene may influence the amount and location of the enlargement.[46,47] Patients with better oral hygiene may have less hyperplasia.[42] Among hospitalized patients of normal intelligence, hyperplasia is seen less often and is less severe than among the severely retarded.[48]

It is unknown whether the effect on the gingiva is a result of the plasma level of the drug,[49,50] the salivary level,[49,51] or the sulcular fluid level[52] (phenytoin is excreted in crevicular fluid).[53] However, concentration of phenytoin in the tissue of patients with hyperplasia[49] is increased. The sulcular circulation may serve as a second source of phenytoin to the gingival tissue, or the hyperplastic effect of the drug may be through an intermediate metabolite.[37] The serum concentration of IgA may be decreased, thus influencing gingival inflammation.[37] Also there may be a genetic predisposition to this drug-induced IgA deficiency.[37] An increase in IgG levels has been reported.[43] There also may be decreased folate levels.[37]

The clinical picture of phenytoin-induced hyperplasia is different from that of idiopathic fibrous hyperplasia. The administration of phenytoin often leads to overgrowth of the papillae, leaving the margin unaffected or less affected (Fig. 24-5, *A*). Signs of inflammation are almost always present.

**Microscopic features**

The microscopic picture of phenytoin-induced hyperplasia also differs somewhat from that of idiopathic fibrous hyperplasia. In addition to an increase in the fibrous

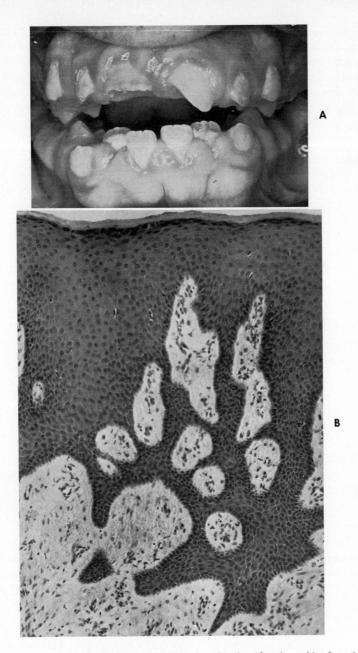

**Fig. 24-5.  A,** Phenytoin-induced hyperplasia in a child. Note the migration of teeth resulting from the proliferation of dense connective tissue. The gingiva has become so enlarged that the greater portion of the crowns has become submerged. **B,** Gingival biopsy of phenytoin-induced hyperplasia. The section is characterized by overgrowth of the epithelium with accompanying inflammatory reaction and fibrous overgrowth. (**A** courtesy J.M. Nabers, Wichita Falls, Texas.)

tissue elements,[41,54] there is a proliferative tendency in the epithelium (Fig. 24-5, *B*) and an increased accumulation of inflammatory cells.

The biologic mechanism for the gingival overgrowth in phenytoin therapy is not fully known. Local tissue chemistry is altered. Increased strength of scars in experimental animals receiving phenytoin has been demonstrated.[55] Phenytoin may be a stimulant of fibroblast protein synthesis or of mitosis,[39,41,56] although some reports do not support this. Phenytoin may interfere with collagenolysis, leading to a piling up of collagen, or there may be reduced prolylhydroxylation. Increased phenytoin content occurs in the saliva of patients on this therapy.[47,49,51] Saliva of patients with overgrowth has a reduced capacity to aggregate *Streptococcus sanguis*[35] and is altered in other parameters. However, examination of the oral flora of patients with and without overgrowth does not support a specific marginal plaque cause for the overgrowth.[40] The fact that overgrowth can be prevented or minimized in some cases by good oral hygiene may indicate that two elements interact to produce hyperplasia—a systemic factor and a local triggering stimulus.

## TREATMENT

**Supplemental therapy**

If phenytoin therapy is instituted, some gingival hyperplasia is likely to occur; however, with excellent oral hygiene the extent of overgrowth can be kept to a minimum or avoided.[58-60] This may reduce inflammation, but the microscopic features of hyperplasia may persist.[61] At times the physician may be able to substitute other drugs that can control convulsions and do not induce hyperplasia.

**Substitute drugs**

The drugs that may be substituted for phenytoin are phenobarbital, primidone-phenobarbital, carbamazepine mephenytoin, and valproic acid. Valproic acid may produce defective clotting and spontaneous hemorrhage. Consequently surgery should be avoided in these patients and they should be carefully monitored.[62,63] Carbamazepine appears to be without oral side effects.[36]

At other times the dosage of phenytoin can be reduced by using it in combination with other drugs.[44,54,64] Such substitution should be done only at the discretion of the attending neurologist. Phenytoin and phenobarbital are reported to induce hypocalcemia, rickets, and osteomalacia in some patients receiving long-term anticonvulsant therapy.[65-67] Close attention should be paid to calciferol intake.[65] The effect on bone may be a phenytoin inhibition of parathormone-induced inhibition of bone calcium mobilization.[66,68] Others feel the inactivity of some patients produces the bone changes, terming them a *disuse osteoporosis*.[69] Despite the occurrence of gingival hyperplasia, phenytoin remains the drug of choice for grand mal seizures. Although there is no effective drug therapy for the treatment of gingival enlargement in phenytoin therapy, a program of diligent oral hygiene should be instituted to prevent or minimize the development of hyperplasia. Where overgrowth is already present, the following measures may be taken:

1. Institution of rigid oral hygiene practices. With excellent oral hygiene, the extent of overgrowth can be minimized or avoided.[58-60] Oral hygiene may reduce inflammation, but the hyperplasia may persist.[61] Unfortunately some persons needing phenytoin therapy are not capable of following instructions for rigorous plaque control. Others may have a physical disability, and a few are mentally retarded.
2. Surgical treatment. Hyperplastic tissues are most often removed surgically. Unfortunately there is a tendency for recurrence that may begin immediately following surgery. Without effective plaque control measures, recurrence is assured. Sometimes reduction or alteration of the medication is effective. Substitution for phenytoin should be made immediately before surgery and for a variable period of weeks thereafter. Pressure devices may be used to prevent postsurgical gingival hyperplasia.[70]
3. Pressure devices to control tissue enlargement.[45,71] For patients taking phenytoin, the above plus the following is used.
4. Adequate zinc[53] and folic acid[72] should be maintained in the diet.
5. When short roots are present caused by early phenytoin therapy, the short roots may influence surgical and prosthetic measures.
6. Substitution of drugs or the reduction of dosage of phenytoin may be considered by the neurologist but not until the other controlling measures have been tried.[63]

Alginate impressions are taken presurgically (Fig. 24-6, *A*). Stone models are made and carved to the postsurgical gingival form. Alternatively the models may be made

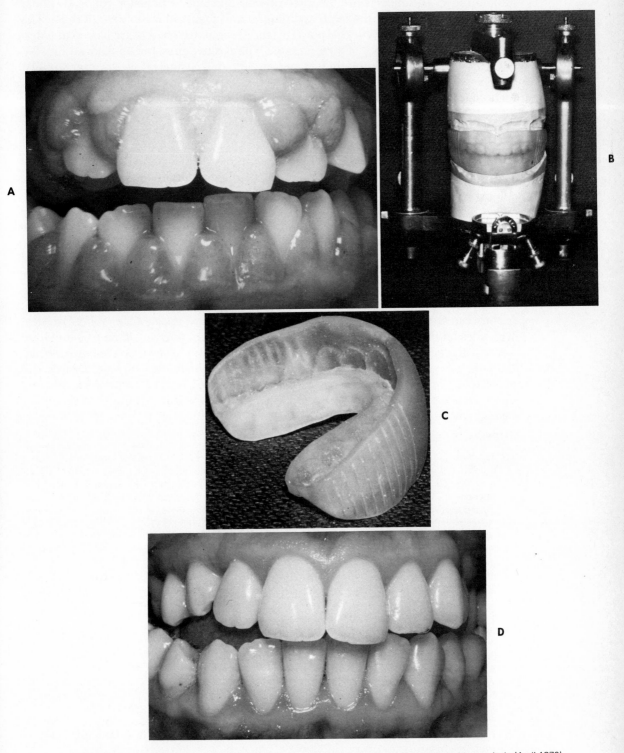

**Fig. 24-6.** **A,** An 18-year-old girl with caries, gross malocclusion, and phenytoin gingival hyperplasia (April 1970). A daily dose of 300 mg of phenytoin (Dilantin) was being taken to control grand mal seizures. Gingival surgery was performed, and a positive-pressure appliance fabricated (**B** and **C**). Carious teeth were restored. Phenytoin therapy was continued without recurrence of hyperplasia at 16 months postoperatively (**D**).

after surgery. The models are mounted on an adjustable articulator. Silicone rubber (hard) is packed around the teeth and gingiva and then trimmed (Fig. 24-6, *B*). The rubber surface is varnished with polyethylene. Articulated models are placed in a dry-heat oven at 350° F (176.7° C) for an hour. The positive-pressure appliance (Fig. 24-6, *C*) may be delivered at the time of dressing removal, usually 2 weeks after surgery.

The positive-pressure (Fig. 24-6, *D*) appliance is delivered following healing. This technique may provide better postsurgical results in some patients.

## Summary

Gingival enlargement may be viewed as a spectrum extending from idiopathic gingival hyperplasia (fibromatosis), in which inflammatory elements are absent, to phenytoin hyperplasia, in which inflammatory elements are present, to hyperplastic inflammation, seen in mouth breathers, to gingivitis in pregnancy, which is a hormonally conditioned increase in the inflammation and an overwhelming predominance of inflammatory elements.

The student may have difficulty understanding the difference between gingival fibrous hyperplasia and hyperplastic gingivitis. *Gingival hyperplasia* is caused mainly by an increase in the number of local cellular elements and intercellular fibers. The enlargement in *hyperplastic gingivitis* is primarily the result of inflammation. The lesions can frequently be differentiated by their clinical appearance. When we deal with a lesion that is primarily hyperplastic, the enlarged gingiva will be pale and hard because the enlargement is a result of the increase in fibrous connective tissue. When the gingival enlargement is primarily inflammatory, the gingiva will be inflamed. The consistency will be edematous because of the presence of inflammatory elements and blood vessels. The spectrum of hyperplastic gingivitis will range from a pale, rather firm gingiva to a boggy, soft, red tissue.

**REFERENCES**

1. Anneroth, G., and Sivurdson, Ä.: Hyperplastic lesions of the gingiva and alveolar mucosa, Acta Odontol. Scand. **41:**75, 1983.
2. Buchner, A., Caldron, S., and Ramon, Y.: Localized hyperplastic lesions on the gingiva: a clinico-pathologic study of 302 lesions, J. Periodontol. **48:**191, 1977.
3. Saito, I., et al.: Periosteal ossifying fibroma of the palate, J. Periodontol. **55:**704, 1984.
4. Bhaskar, S.N., and Jacoway, J.R.: Peripheral fibroma and peripheral fibroma with calcification, J. Am. Dent. Assoc. **73:**1312, 1966.
5. Savara, B.S., et al.: Hereditary gingival fibrosis; study of a family, J. Periodontol. **25:**12, 1954.
6. Winstock, D.: Hereditary gingivofibromatosis, Br. J. Oral Surg. **2:**59, 1964.
7. Zackin, S.J., and Weisberger, D.: Hereditary gingival fibromatosis, Oral Surg. **14:**828, 1961.
8. Jorgenson, R.J., and Cocker, M.E.: Variation in the inheritance and expression of gingival fibromatosis, J. Periodontol. **45:**472, 1974.
9. Horning, G.H., et al.: Gingival fibromatosis with hypertrichosis: a case report, J. Periodontol. **56:**344, 1985.
10. Redman, R.S., Ward, C.C., and Patterson, R.H.: Focus of epithelial dysplasia arising in hereditary gingival fibroma, J. Periodontol. **56:**158, 1985.
11. McIndoe, A., and Smith, B.O.: Congenital familial fibromatosis of the gums and teeth as a probable aetiological factor: report of an affected family, Br. J. Plast. Surg. **11:**62, 1958.
12. Willett, E.: Ein seltener Fall einer echten Fibromatosis gingivae, Oest. Z. Stomatol. **51:**663, 1954.
13. Mathis, H.: Zur Frage der Hyperplastic der Gingiva unter Dilantinbehandlung, Dtsch. Z. Zahnheilkd. **9:**1280, 1954.
14. Kfir, Y., Buchner, A., and Hansen, L.S.: Reactive lesions of the gingiva: a clinicopathologic study of 741 cases, J. Periodontol. **51:**655, 1980.
15. Bhaskar, S.N., and Jacoway, J.R.: Pyogenic granuloma—clinical feature, incidence, histology and result of treatment: report of 242 cases, J. Oral Surg. **24:**391, 1966.
16. Angelopolous, A.P.: Pyogenic granuloma of the oral cavity statistical analysis of clinical features, J. Oral Surg. **29:**840, 1971.
17. Leyden, J.J., and Master, G.H.: Oral cavity pyogenic granuloma, Arch. Dermatol. **108:**226, 1973.
18. Pearlman, B.A.: An oral contraceptive drug and gingival enlargement: the relationship between local and systemic facts, J. Clin. Periodontol. **1:**47, 1974.
19. Michaud, M., et al.: Oral manifestations of

acute leukemia in children, J. Am. Dent. Assoc. **95:**1145, 1972.

20. McKelvey, B., Satinover, F., and Sanders, B.: Idiopathic thrombocytopenic purpura manifesting as a gingival hypertrophy: case report, J. Periodontol. **47:**661, 1976.

21. Mathis, H.: Gingivitis chronica und Carcinomatosis, Stoma **20:**272, 1967.

22. Israelson, H., Binnie, W.H., and Hurt, W.C.: The hyperplastic gingivitis of Wegener's granulomatosis, J. Periodontol. **52:**81, 1981.

23. Josephson, P., and van Wyk, C.W.: Bilateral symmetrical lymphangiomas of the gingiva: a case report, J. Periodontol. **55:**47, 1984.

24. Daley, T.D., and Wysocki, G.P.: Cyclosporine therapy: its significance to the periodontist, J. Periodontol. **55:**708, 1984.

25. Adams, D., and Davies, G.: Gingival hyperplasia associated with cyclosporin A, Br. Dent. J. **157:**80, 1984.

26. Rateitschak-Plüss, E.M., et al.: Initial observation that cyclosporine-A induces gingival enlargement in man, J. Clin. Periodontol. **10:**237, 1983.

27. Lucas, R.M., Howell, L.P., and Wall, B.A.: Nifedipine-induced gingival hyperplasia: a histochemical and ultrastructural study, J. Periodontol. **56:**211, 1985.

28. Aas, E.: Hyperplasia gingivae diphenylhydantoinea: a clinical, histological, and biochemical study, Acta Odontol. Scand. **21:**(34), 1963.

29. Triadan, H.: Ueber die parodontale Nebenwirkung, der chronischen Hydantoinbehandlung, Heidelberg, 1968, Dr. Alfred Hüthig Verlag.

30. Church, L.F., Jr., and Brandt, S.K.: Phenytoin-induced gingival overgrowth resulting in delayed eruption of the primary dentition: a case report, J. Periodontol. **55:**19, 1984.

31. Hall, B.K., and Squier, C.A.: Ultrastructural quantitation of connective tissue changes in phenytoin-induced gingival overgrowth in the ferret, J. Dent. Res. **61:**942, 1982.

32. Sreedevi, B.T., and Narayana Rao, M.S.: Diphenylhydantoin gingival hyperplasia: an epidemiologic study, ISP Bull. **7:**3, 1983.

33. Hassell, T., et al.: Phenytoin induced gingival overgrowth in institutionalized epileptics, J. Clinical Periodontol. **11:**242, 1984.

34. Addy, V., et al.: Risk factors in phenytoin-induced gingival hyperplasia, J. Periodontol. **54:**373, 1983.

35. Smith, Q.T., and Hamilton, M.J.: Salivary composition, phenytoin ingestion and clinical overgrowth, J. Periodontol. **52:**673, 1981.

36. Lundström, A., Eeg-Olafsson, O., and Hamp, S.-E.: Effects of anti-epileptic drug treatment with cabazapine or phenytoin on the oral state of children and adolescents, J. Clin. Periodontol. **9:**482, 1982.

37. Hassell, T.M., et al.: Summary of an international symposium on phenytoin-induced teratology and gingival pathology, J. Am. Dent. Assoc. **99:**652, 1979.

38. Girgis, S.S., et al.: Dental root abnormalities and gingival overgrowth in epileptic patients receiving anticonvulsant therapy, J. Periodontol. **51:**474, 1980.

39. Al-Ubaidy, S.S., Al-Janabi, N.Y., and Al-Tai, S.A.: Effect of phenytoin on mitotic activity of gingival tissue and cultured fibroblasts, J. Periodontol. **52:**747, 1981.

40. Smith, Q.T., et al.: Microbial flora and clinical parameters in phenytoin associated gingival overgrowth, J. Periodontol. Res. **18:**56, 1983.

41. Hassell, T.M., et al.: Quantitative histopathologic assessment of developing phenytoin-induced gingival overgrowth in the cat, J. Clin. Periodontol. **9:**365, 1985.

42. Steinberg, S.C., and Steinberg, A.D.: Phenytoin-induced gingival overgrowth control in severely retarded children, J. Periodontol. **53:**429, 1982.

43. Setterstrom, J.A., et al.: Immunoglobulins in periodontal tissues. III. Concentration of immunoglobulins in Dilantin-induced and idiopathic gingival hyperplastic tissues, J. Periodontol. **51:**25, 1980.

44. Staple, P.H.: Regression of gingival hyperplasia following substitution of "Mysoline" for phenytoin sodium, Br. Dent. J. **9:**432, 1955.

45. Babcock, J.R.: The successful use of a new therapy in Dilantin gingival hyperplasia, Periodontics **3:**196, 1965.

46. Babcock, J.R.: Incidence of gingival hyperplasia associated with Dilantin therapy in a hospital population, J. Am. Dent. Assoc. **71:**1447, 1965.

47. Angelopoulos, A.P., and Goaz, P.W.: Incidence of diphenylhydantoin hyperplasia, Oral Surg. **34:**898, 1972.

48. Collins, J.M., and Fry, B.A.: Phenytoin gingival hyperplasia and chronic gingival irritation, Aust. Dent. J. **5:**165, 1960.

49. Conard, G.J., et al.: Levels of 5,5-diphenylhydantoin and its major metabolite in human serum, saliva, and hyperplastic gingiva, J. Dent. Res. **53:**1323, 1974.

50. Larmas, L.A., Mackinen, K.K., and Paunio, K.O.: A histochemical study of amylaminopeptidase in hydantoin-induced hyperplastic healthy and inflamed gingiva, J. Periodont. Res. **8:**21, 1973.

51. Little, T.M., Girgis, S.S., and Masotti, R.E.: Diphenylhydantoin induced gingival hyperplasia: its response to changes in drug dosage, Dev. Med. Child Neurol. **17:**421, 1975.

52. Steinberg, A.D., Jeffay, H., and Allen, P.: Transport of 14C-diphenylhydantoin and 14C-leucine through rabbit crevicular epithelium, J. Dent. Res. **53:**1387, 1974.

53. Joseph, C.E., et al.: Zinc deficiency changes in the permeability of rabbit periodontium to 14C-phenytoin and 14C-albumin, J. Periodontol. **53:**251, 1982.

54. Panuska, H.J., et al.: The effect of anticonvulsant drugs upon the gingiva, I.J. Periodontol. **31**:336, 1960; II, J. Periodontol. **32**:15, 1961.

55. Shafer, W.G., Beatty, R.E., and Davis, W.B.: Effect of Dilantin sodium on tensile strength of healing wounds, Proc. Soc. Exp. Biol. Med. **98**:348, 1958.

56. Shafer, W.G.: Response of radiated human fibroblast-like cells to Dilantin sodium in tissue culture, J. Dent. Res. **44**:671, 1965.

57. Babcock, J.R., and Nelson, G.H.: Gingival hyperplasia and Dilantin content of saliva, J. Am. Dent. Assoc. **68**:195, 1964.

58. Hall, W.B.: Dilantin hyperplasia; a preventable disease, J. Periodont. Res. Suppl. **4**:36, 1969.

59. Pihlstrom, B.A., et al.: Prevention of phenytoin associated gingival enlargement: a 15 month longitudinal study, J. Periodontol. **51**:311, 1980.

60. King, D.A., Hawes, R.R., and Bibby, B.G.: The effect of oral physiotherapy on Dilantin gingival hyperplasia, J. Oral Pathol. **5**:1, 1976.

61. Donnenfeld, O.W., Stanley, H.R., and Bagdonoff, L.: A nine month clinical and histologic study of patients of diphenylhydantoin following gingivectomy, J. Periodontol. **45**:547, 1974.

62. Hassell, T.M., et al.: Valproic acid: a new antiepileptic drug with potential side effects of dental concern, J. Am. Dent. Assoc. **99**:983, 1979.

63. Reynolds, N.C., Jr., and Kirkham, D.B.: Therapeutic alternatives in phenytoin-induced gingival hyperplasia, J. Periodontol. **51**:516, 1980.

64. Trott, J.R., and Neuman, K.: Improved gingival and mental condition following reduction of diphenylhydantoin medication for epilepsy, J. Can. Dent. Assoc. **30**:518, 1964.

65. Villareale, M., et al.: Diphenylhydantoin: effects on calcium metabolism in the chick, Science **183**:671, 1974.

66. Stamp, T.C.B.: Effects of long-term anticonvulsant therapy on calcium and vitamin D metabolism, Proc. R. Soc. Med. **67**:64, 1974.

67. Hahn, T.J., et al.: Serum 25-hydroxycalciferol levels and bone mass in children on chronic anticonvulsant therapy, N. Engl. J. Med. **229**:550, 1975.

68. Harris, M., and Goldhaber, P.: Root abnormalities in epileptics and the inhibition of parathyroid hormone induced bone resorption by diphenylhydantoin in tissue culture, Arch. Oral Biol. **19**:981, 1974.

69. Murchison, L.E., et al.: Effects of anticonvulsants and inactivity on bone disease in epileptics, Postgrad. Med. J. **51**:18, 1975.

70. Sheridan, P., and Reeve, C.M.: Effective treatment of Dilantin gingival hyperplasia, Oral Surg. **35**:42-46, 1973.

71. Davis, R.K., Baer, P.N., and Palmer, J.H.: A preliminary report on a new therapy for Dilantin gingival hyperplasia, J. Periodontol. **34**:17, 1963.

72. Mallek, H.M., and Nakamoto, T.: Dilantin and folic acid status: clinical implications for the periodontist, J. Periodontol. **52**:255, 1981.

**ADDITIONAL SUGGESTED READING**

Becker, W., et al.: Hereditary gingival fibromatosis, Oral Surg. **24**:313, 1967.

Falconer, M.A., and Davidson, S.: Coarse features in epilepsy as a consequence of anticonvulsant therapy: report of cases in two pairs of identical twins, Lancet **2**:112, 1973.

Forscher, B.K., and Cecil, H.C.: Biochemical studies on acute inflammation. II. The effect of Dilantin, J. Dent. Res. **36**:927, 1957.

Fritz, M.E.: Idiopathic gingival fibromatosis with extensive osseous involvement in a 12-year-old boy: report of a case, Oral Surg. **30**:755, 1970.

# CHAPTER 25

## Role of occlusion in periodontal disease

**Periodontium**
Mesial migration
Active eruption
Functional changes
Microscopic features

**Tissue changes in experimental occlusal traumatism**
Occlusal traumatism in animals

**Human autopsy findings**
Primary and secondary traumatism

**Tissue changes caused by periodontal traumatism**

**Combined periodontal disease**

---

It has been said that when the teeth, jaws, muscles of mastication, and temporomandibular joint (components of the stomatognathic system) are in a harmonious relationship, this balance will contribute to the health of the periodontium. Conversely, it has also been said that when the interrelationship is disturbed, periodontal disease may follow.

More has been written, but perhaps less known, about the precise role of occlusion in periodontal disease than about most other aspects of periodontology. The therapist is confronted with contradictory theories and methods. Therapy must depend on an understanding of the mechanisms of occlusion in both normal and pathologic physiology. The development of such an understanding is based on histologic observation of clinical material, clinical studies, and animal experimentation. From such a base one can more meaningfully employ the various methods of dealing with periodontal disease involving occlusion. Such disease is known as *periodontal trauma;* this term refers to changes produced in the periodontal tissues. Some students confuse malocclusion with occlusal traumatism. The two are most frequently unrelated. To fully understand the role of occlusion in periodontal disease, one must distinguish between malocclusion and occlusal traumatism.

*Periodontal trauma* is a morbid condition produced by repeated mechanical forces exerted on the periodontium exceeding the physiologic limits of tissue tolerance and contributing to a breakdown of the supporting tissues of the tooth. These forces produce local circulatory disturbances in the periodontal tissues. Other tissue changes, such as those of crushing and tearing, are produced when the tooth impinges on the alveolar bone. *Trauma* refers to the precise pathologic changes occurring in the tissues, whereas *traumatism* refers to the act or acts of producing the trauma. *Occlusal traumatism* implies that the forces are occlusal. **Definitions**

The muscles of the cheek, tongue, and lip can also be important in the causation of periodontal trauma. This is particularly noticeable in abnormal lip and tongue actions

479

and in abnormal swallowing patterns. In addition, habitual actions performed with the teeth, such as playing wind instruments, bobby pin opening, and pipestem biting, may contribute to traumatism.

## Periodontium

Each tooth is suspended in the alveolus by the periodontal ligament, which permits some movement of the teeth. Short-term tooth displacements are brought about by lip, tongue, and occlusal forces. When the application of the force is stopped, the tooth returns to position. There are long-term migratory movements in which growth and wear also play a role. Growth, wear, and lip-tongue-occlusal forces cause continuing changes in the position of the teeth. These movements require the supporting tissues to be constantly remodeled and adapted in response to the changing functional demands. Thus there is an ever-present functional interdependence between the teeth and the periodontium.

The periodontal ligament consists of the principal fiber bundles arranged in varying directions according to functional demands. Loose connective tissue that surrounds the blood vessels and nerve fibers is found between the bundles of the principal fibers. The cellular elements consist primarily of fibroblasts, but there are also epithelial cells (Malassez epithelial rests) that are remnants of Hertwig's epithelial sheath. The surface of the cementum of the functioning tooth has an uncalcified layer (cementoid) along which the cementoblasts are aligned. The periodontal surface of the alveolar bone may show a similar arrangement of osteoblasts. Osteoclasts may occasionally be seen within Howship's lacunae.

The osseous side of the periodontal space shows continuous change as in any other bone. The bone alongside different areas of the periodontal ligament varies in structure, depending on functional stimuli. This fact is of utmost importance for the proper understanding of periodontics and, in particular, for the proper appreciation of the role of the occlusal factor in periodontal diseases.

### MESIAL MIGRATION

The teeth move continually toward the midline. This is the so-called physiologic mesial migration of teeth.[1] Black[2,3] estimated that the ageing dental arch becomes shorter by about 1 cm. This shortening of the dental arch is caused by the attrition of contact points and contact planes. Despite this loss of tooth substance, the teeth remain in contact. It takes almost a lifetime for an entire dental arch to lose 0.5 to 1 cm in length. Therefore the physiologic mesial migration of teeth is an extremely slow process. Despite the slowness of this movement, we can distinguish the side *toward which* the teeth are moving (mesial) from the side *from which* they are moving (distal) by differences in microscopic specimens. A chronologic history of some of the changes may be seen in the alveolar bone.

The mesial and distal surfaces of a tooth are shown in Fig. 25-1. The bone and periodontal ligament of the two sides have a different structure. On the distal surface (A) the fiber bundles of the periodontal ligament appear stretched and under tension. On the mesial surface (B) they appear wavy, as though relaxed. This is not the only difference. On the distal (tension) side the alveolar bone is of bundle bone type, which signifies that coarse fiber bundles (Sharpey's fibers) are incorporated in the bone.

Loose connective tissue areas between the principal bundles of the periodontal ligament on the distal side appear oval in shape as the result of the tension of the fiber bundles. On the mesial side of the same tooth (in the direction of migration), the fiber

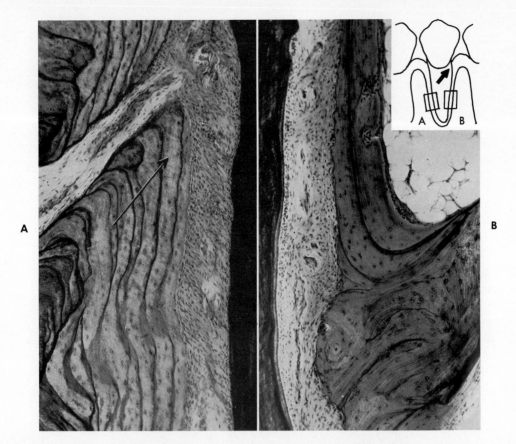

**Fig. 25-1.** Histologic sections showing the distal, **A,** and mesial, **B,** surfaces of a tooth. On the distal surface, **A,** the fibers are under tension. Some are embedded in bundle bone. The bundle bone is limited on the left by an irregular line known as a reversal line, which indicates that resorption has taken place up to that line from the marrow side. The resorption stopped, the process was reversed, and new lamellated bone was laid down in the form of haversian systems and parallel lamellae, replacing the bundle bone that had been resorbed. On the pressure side, **B,** the fiber bundles are relaxed. The surface of the bone has undergone resorption. (Arrow in inset shows the direction of movement of the tooth.) This bone is also lamellated, as can be seen by the tierlike arrangement, which indicates alternating periods of formation and rest. The lines between periods of bone formation are known as resting lines. (From the collection of J.P. Weinmann.)

bundles in the periodontal ligament are rather wavy and less stretched. The loose connective tissue areas are round. No differences are perceptible in the character of the cementum. Resorption of the lamellated alveolar bone by osteoclastic activity is in progress while new bone is being laid down from the endosteum in the marrow spaces (Figs. 25-1, *B,* and 25-2).

These histologic differences are a clear indication of different stimuli influencing the periodontium on the mesial and distal surfaces of the tooth as a result of this slow tooth migration. The extremely delicate mechanism of the interdependence of tissue structure and function in the periodontium is thus illustrated.

## ACTIVE ERUPTION

Mesial migration is not the only movement of teeth. There is also movement in an occlusal direction,[4,5] which leads to eruption of the teeth into the oral cavity and brings about occlusal contact. The period of active eruption is characterized by a rather rapid movement of the teeth and is manifested in the structural arrangement of the bone

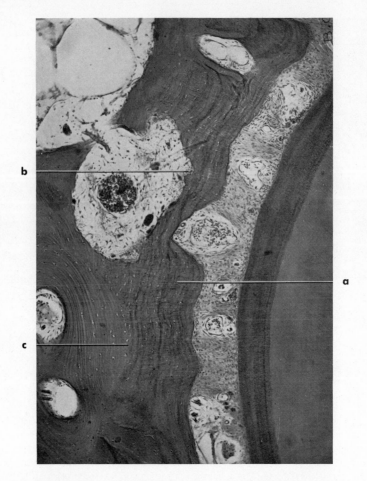

**Fig. 25-2.** *Internal remodeling of bone. Horizontal section of the distal surface of a tooth showing, a, formation of bundle bone on the side of tension and, b, resorption from the marrow spaces. Nonfunctioning parts of the bundle bone are thus eliminated, and the resorbed bone is replaced by newly formed haversian systems, c.*

trabeculae (Fig. 25-3), which are deposited in parallel layers at the fundus of the alveolus as well as at the alveolar crest. After the teeth come into occlusal contact, the active eruption process slows but never stops completely.[6] Eruption continues, and under ideal conditions, there is a correlation between occlusal attrition and active eruption.

A few illustrations will show how active eruption affects the surrounding structures. The bifurcation of a lower molar[7] is shown in Fig. 25-4. The interradicular bony septum shows layer-by-layer appositional growth in a mesio-occlusal direction. Resorption is taking place on the side of pressure. Thick cementum covers the root surface. The continuous formation of cementum is a necessary link in active eruption.

The buccal alveolar crest of a lower premolar is shown in Fig. 25-5, *A*. The bottom of the pocket is close to the cementoenamel junction, and the junctional epithelium extends about 2 mm apically along the cementum. The alveolar crest is about 1 mm apical to the deepest penetration of the epithelium and shows layer-by-layer apposition of bone in an occlusal direction. Higher magnification (Fig. 25-5, *B*) of the alveolar crest clearly shows the arrangement of the resting lines, which indicate a predomi-

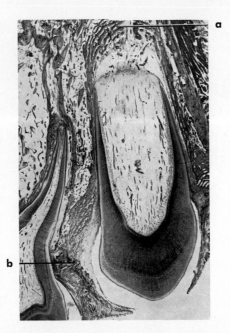

**Fig. 25-3.** During rapid active eruption of the tooth, bone is laid down, *a,* layer by layer at the fundus of the alveolus and, *b,* as a functional adaptation at the alveolar crest. (From Kronfeld, R.: N.Y.J. Dent. **6:**112, 1936.)

nantly occlusal growth of this alveolar crest. There is a reversal line on the buccal surface of the bone below the periosteum and close to the surface. The resorption was reversed; at the time of the patient's death, active bone formation was in progress on the periosteal side of this crest. Such functionally directed tissue changes not only occur in the immediate surroundings but also have their effect deep in the supporting alveolar bone (Fig. 25-2). The bony trabeculae are rebuilt constantly in response to functional influences by a process of resorption and formation. This takes place constantly in the jaws, showing the interdependence between function and structure.

Active occlusal eruption of the teeth has also been observed clinically. By way of illustration, a patient complained that a tooth was growing shorter.[8] On observation and examination the dentist noted that the seemingly shortened tooth was not actually getting shorter but was remaining fixed because of a pathologic process that stopped its eruptive movement, whereas the other teeth erupted normally. When such teeth are removed, extensive resorption of the roots and ankylosis with the bone may be noted.[9] These processes also can affect the primary teeth. If they remain in the jaw longer than is physiologically normal, they may appear shorter than adjacent permanent teeth. In fact, they may become totally or partially submerged, with bone and soft tissue slowly growing up around them.[10]

Other histologic findings indicate that teeth erupt even after they have reached the occlusal plane. Such a finding is supported by the presence of epithelial remnants far below the apex of a tooth in a nutrient canal[11] (Fig. 25-6). The epithelial rests are remnants of Hertwig's epithelial root sheath and are normally found in the periodontal ligament. If epithelial remnants remain below the apex (as in Fig. 25-6), it can be assumed that the apex was once at the place where the epithelial remnants are now

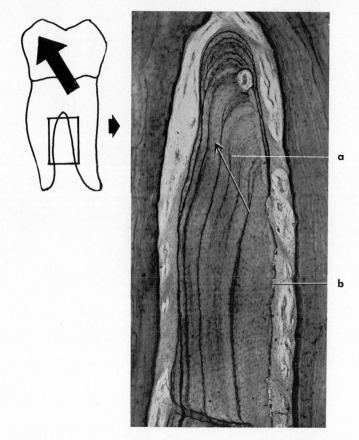

**Fig. 25-4.** Interradicular bone septum. Direction of tooth movement indicated by arrow. *a*, Layer-by-layer apposition of bone; *b*, bone resorption in pressure areas. (From Kronfeld, R.: N.Y.J. Dent. **6:**112, 1936.)

seen. These epithelial structures cannot actively change their position. They have been left behind by the eruption of the tooth. Deeper bony areas may contain isolated islands of bundle bone that were once alveolar bone but were left behind, unresorbed and unreplaced by lamellated bone.

Resorption and repair of alveolar bone take place as adaptive physiologic processes as long as the natural dentition remains, although these processes are slowed in old age.[12] The adaptive activities of the periodontal tissues may be upset whenever an endogenous or exogenous disturbance occurs. However, tissue breakdown also occurs as a physiologic process as cells and tissue elements are replaced. The form that the rebuilding takes depends primarily on functional demands.

The alveolus normally has an hourglass shape, being widest at the apex and at the alveolar crest. This is because there is movement in the physiologic range. The maximal displacement of a tooth depends on the shape of the bony housing. If, for example, a severe tipping displacement brings the cervical part of the tooth into contact with the alveolar margin, or the apex into contact with the alveolar bone, damage must occur. The bundles of the periodontal ligament are composed of collagen fibers that are essentially inelastic. Therefore they can scarcely stretch under tension. The major change in these fiber bundles is from a normal, wavy state to a straightened state. That these fibers do not significantly stretch beyond their normal length provides protection against total compression of the periodontal tissues under normal functional pressure. This is one of the most important functions of the periodontal ligament.

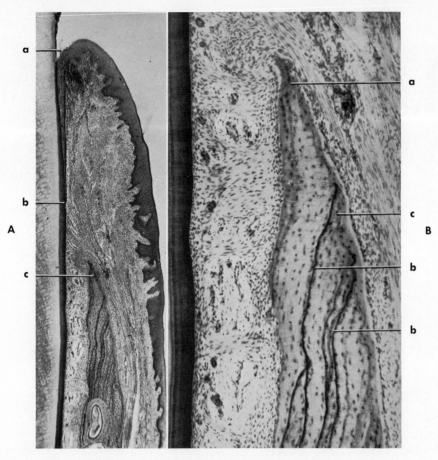

**Fig. 25-5. A,** As the result of active eruption of the tooth, bone apposition takes place at the alveolar crest. *a,* Bottom of the gingival sulcus; *b,* apical end of the epithelial attachment; *c,* tip of the alveolar crest. **B,** Higher magnification of, *a,* the tip of the alveolar crest showing, *b,* the layer-by-layer apposition of bone and, *c,* the increase in height of the alveolar crest. Bone formation is from the periosteal side, starting from a reversal line.

## FUNCTIONAL CHANGES

Function represents a range from nonfunction to hypofunction to physiologic function to hyperfunction to trauma. The tissues of the periodontium respond to these functional stimuli. Their form and structure reflect the effects of function.

Nonfunction and hypofunction may be expressed in disuse atrophy. The atrophy of disuse of the periodontal tissues is characterized by a rearrangement of the fibers of the periodontal ligament and of the trabeculation of the alveolar bone without gingival recession.

**Disuse atrophy**

The connective tissue elements of the periodontium—the periodontal ligament, cementum, and alveolar bone—are also arranged functionally. The trabeculation of cancellous bone is arranged in response to the load placed on the bone.[13] The alveolar process of the mandible and the maxilla (Fig. 25-7) shows a trabecular arrangement radiating toward the roots as if to form bracing scaffolds or girders. These trabecular patterns also vary from individual to individual[14] partly because of the size and shape of the mandible and the maxilla, their interrelationship, the arrangement and function of the teeth, and the strength of the musculature. There is a difference in bone density when normal function is present and when function is reduced or absent. The side of a mandible that is not in occlusal function (Fig. 25-8, *A*) appears porous as compared with a side that is in function (Fig. 25-8, *B*). The trabeculae are thin and sparse. The

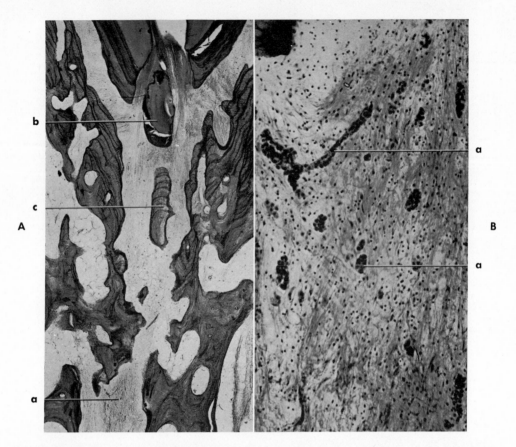

**Fig. 25-6. A,** Epithelial rests, *a,* far below the apex of the tooth, *b,* suggest that the apex once was at the level of these epithelial remnants and then actively erupted. This is also manifested by bundle bone, *c,* around the apex. **B,** Higher magnification showing the epithelial remnants, *a.*

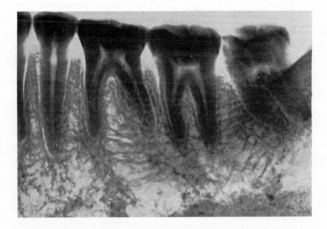

**Fig. 25-7.** Functional arrangement of the bone trabeculae in the cancellous bone of the mandible.

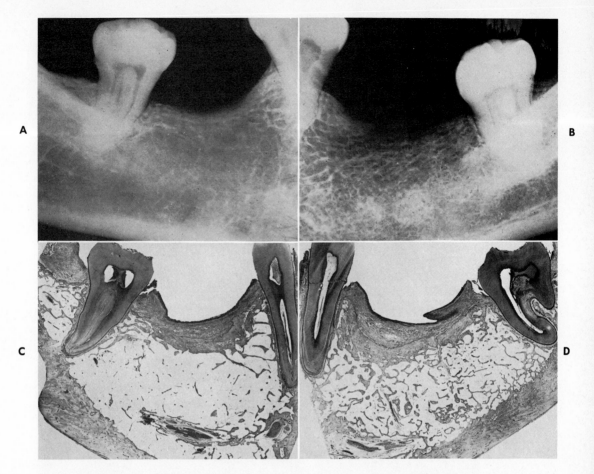

**Fig. 25-8.** Differing density of trabecular arrangement of bone tissue in the mandible as seen in roentgenograms and accompanying microscopic sections. On **A** and **C,** the side without occlusal function, the bone trabeculae are thin and less densely arranged than those on **B** and **D,** the side with function. (From the collection of J.P. Weinmann.)

marrow spaces are wide. The functional side has more and heavier trabeculae. The marrow spaces are smaller.[15]

## MICROSCOPIC FEATURES

Microscopically disuse atrophy and hypofunction appear as an enlargement of the bone marrow spaces with a corresponding decrease in trabeculae. Two maxillary molars are shown in Fig. 25-9: *A* represents a tooth out of function for years, and *B* a tooth in function. The most striking difference is the sparse amount of cancellous bone around one and the heavy trabeculation of bone around the other. A lamina dura is present around both teeth.

When osteoporosis develops in disuse atrophy, it takes place by osteoclastic resorption of bone trabeculae in areas of functional inactivity. Localized osteoporotic areas in the jaw caused by lack of function cannot be treated by medication. Proper therapy would be to restore function.

**Osteoporosis of disuse atrophy**

On closer examination of the photographs shown in Fig. 25-9, in higher power, several other differences can be detected between the functioning and the nonfunctioning tooth. The functioning tooth has a wider periodontal ligament and a thinner cementum than does the nonfunctioning tooth[15] (Fig. 25-10). In addition, the periodontal ligament is well organized in the functioning tooth *(A)*. The principal fibers

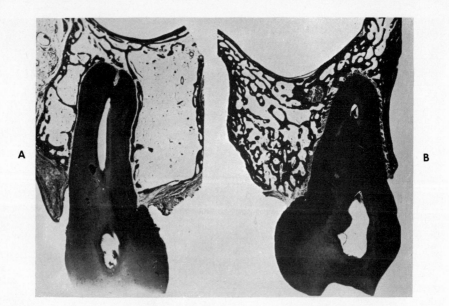

**Fig. 25-9.** Histologic sections of the periodontium of a nonfunctioning, **A,** and functioning, **B,** tooth showing differences in bone trabeculation and width of the periodontal ligament.

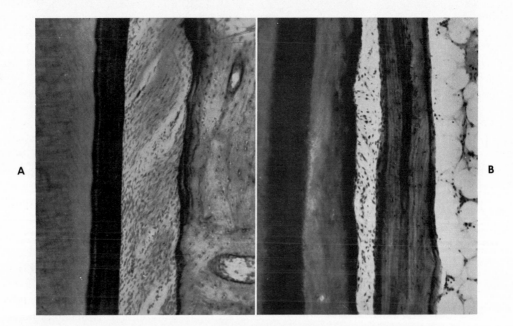

**Fig. 25-10.** Higher magnification of the functioning, **A,** and nonfunctioning, **B,** periodontal ligament. **A,** The periodontal space is wider, the cementum thinner, and the periodontal ligament well organized on the side of function. **B,** On the side of disuse, the periodontal space is narrow, cementum is thick, and the periodontal ligament has been replaced by a loose connective tissue. The bone also shows changes caused by the functional influences.

are extended between bone and cementum and enter the hard structures as Sharpey's fibers. In the thin periodontal ligament of the nonfunctioning tooth *(B)*, no principal fibers are demonstrable. Only loosely organized connective tissue without functional orientation is present. A thick layer of cementum is deposited on the old cementum. The bone is laid down parallel to the surface incrementally. The periodontal surface of the alveolar plate appears as a thick, dark line—a so-called resting line.

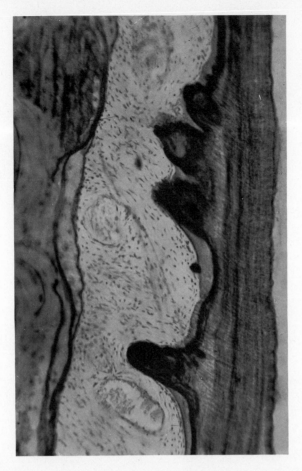

**Fig. 25-11.** Spikelike cemental overgrowth caused by increased function of a tooth (hypertrophy).

These changes in the bone, periodontal ligament, and cementum are all expressions of a lack of functional stimuli.

Hyperfunction in the presence of health (absence of inflammatory periodontal disease) provokes a functional adaptation in which additional structural elements are formed on cementum and in bone to withstand the added force. These are expressed clinically and microscopically as a thickened lamina dura, buttressing bone formation, osteosclerosis, and cemental spurs (Figs. 25-11 and 25-12). Periodontal ligament fiber bundles become thicker and are functionally oriented. **Hyperfunction**

## Tissue changes in experimental occlusal traumatism

### OCCLUSAL TRAUMATISM IN ANIMALS

Extensive investigations in occlusal traumatism have been conducted on dogs.[16] In an attempt to establish what damage is done by occlusal traumatism, high crowns were cemented on opposing maxillary and mandibular teeth. This caused the two teeth to strike each time the animal closed its jaws (premature contact). The tissue changes induced in the periodontium were observed from a few hours to more than a year later. A tooth exposed to such traumatic forces is shown at 36 hours (Fig. 25-13). The tooth was tipped around an axis close to the center of the root, as indicated in Fig. 25-7. Small hemorrhages were noted, but no gross tears occurred at either the alveolar crest or the apex. In other experiments on monkeys, thrombosis of blood vessels was noted **Premature contact**

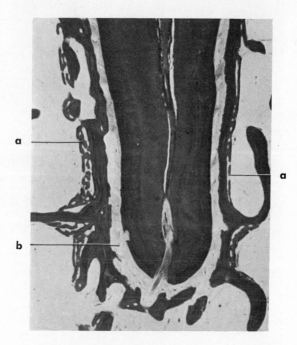

**Fig. 25-12.** Microscopic specimen showing formation of new bone, *a,* around the alveolar bone proper, increasing bone thickness in response to increased functional demands. Widening of the apical periodontal ligament, *b,* has occurred by bone resorption in response to increased functional influences.

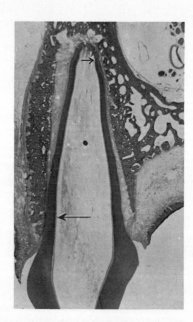

**Fig. 25-13.** Histologic section of a dog's tooth exposed to occlusal traumatism for 36 hours. The tooth was rotated around an axis in the center of the root *(dot).* The periodontal ligament is compressed at the alveolar margin on the buccal side and at the apex on the palatal side *(arrows).* The periodontal ligament is widened on the corresponding areas on the opposite sides.

on the tension side[17] (Fig. 25-14, *A*), leading to resorptions on the surface of the adjacent alveolar bone. Gross tears were not observed in these experiments either. Six months later the bone resorption was repaired, and the periodontal ligament had regenerated (Fig. 25-14, *B*).

The precursors of the collagen molecules are formed in adjacent fiber-forming cells and pass into the extracellular space. The precursors then combine to form new collagen fibrils.[18-20] This repair is a result of the activity of fibroblasts, cementoblasts, and osteoblasts. The collagen fibers of the periodontal ligament have a much more rapid turnover than was previously believed possible.[21-24] Collagen synthesis occurs anywhere in the ligament, and additional collagen molecules can be fabricated and joined to preexisting fibrils. Thus changes in the width of the periodontal ligament (Fig. 25-14) can take place.

**Rapid collagen turnover**

The response to this type of traumatic injury and the process of repair make a fascinating study. Fig. 25-15, *A*, shows an incisor that was ligated firmly to a labial arch wire for 48 hours. The tooth was tipped so far labially that it touched the alveolar crest. This caused a complete compression and necrosis of the periodontal ligament at the area of contact between tooth and bone (*B*). There was also a contact between tooth and bone close to the apex on the lingual side. During the 48 hours in which this intensive pressure was applied, the only tissue reaction seen in the area was in the bone marrow spaces adjacent to the pressure area where osteoclastic bone re-

**Increased fibroblastic activity**

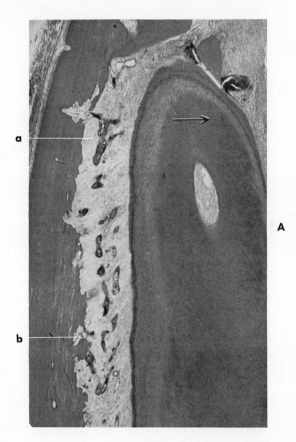

**Fig. 25-14.** Experimental occlusal traumatism in a monkey. **A,** Thrombosed blood vessels in the periodontal ligament caused by extensive tension, *a,* with resorption of bone, *b.* Movement of the apex is indicated by the arrow.                                         *Continued.*

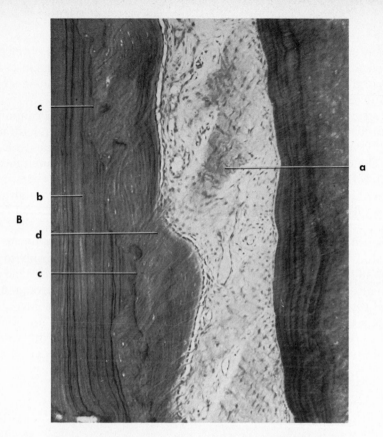

**Fig. 25-14, cont'd.** **B,** Higher magnification of a tension area corresponding to that shown in **A,** 6 months later. In **B,** the periodontal ligament, *a,* is completely regenerated, and the alveolar bone repaired. Between the old bone, *b,* and new bone, *d,* a resorbed surface, *c,* (reversal line), is evident. The new bone is of bundle bone character, forming the periodontal surface of the alveolar bone.

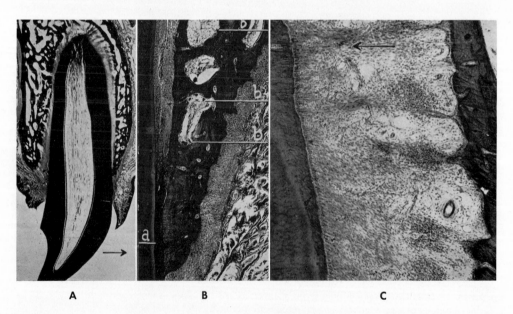

A                              B                              C

**Fig. 25-15.** Trauma in a dog; (*arrow,* direction of tooth movement). **A,** The tooth was ligated to an orthodontic arch wire for 48 hours. Pressure areas occurred on the labial marginal and lingual apical aspects. Tension areas occurred in the opposite regions. **B,** Higher magnification showing, *a,* necrotic compressed periodontal ligament between the tooth and the alveolar crest and, *b,* beginning osteoclastic bone resorption in the marrow spaces. **C,** Tension side at the apex shows formation of new bone spicules and increased cellular activity to repair the damage done by the overextension; (*arrow,* direction of tooth movement).

sorption was apparent. There was considerably more activity in the tension zone—at the alveolar margin on the palatal side and at the apex on the labial side; the periodontal space was double its normal width. Higher magnification (C) showed that the periodontal ligament was wider and more cellular than normal. Dense masses of cells had accumulated in certain areas. Osteoblasts lined the bony spicules being formed in the direction of tension. These extended toward the fiber bundles in a growth pattern. Obviously the cellular elements are of as much significance as the fibers of the periodontal ligament. Moreover, they are of prime importance in the processes of repair and healing. In observing the adaptive process in the pressure and the tension areas, the sequence in which repair takes place can be seen.

The necrotic mass that is so characteristic of damage inflicted by excessive pressure is slowly eliminated by resorption of the bone adjacent to the area of pressure necrosis. This type of bone resorption of the bone adjacent to the area of pressure necrosis has been called *undermining resorption*. The necrotic area is resorbed from the rear, where the tissue is vital. The process of bone resorption must proceed from the periphery since no osteoclasts or macrophages can develop in the area of maximal pressure, which has become necrotic (Fig. 25-16). The time necessary to eliminate the necrotic tissue will largely depend on the extent of the involved area. Fig. 25-17 shows an alveolar crest with a small necrotic area 14 days after application of excessive pressure. Here the necrotic area was almost entirely eliminated. Complete regeneration would have taken place in 2 or 3 more days.

**Undermining resorption**

Fig. 25-18 shows the alveolar margin of a tooth 15 days after cementation of a high crown. Resorption proceeded considerably more slowly than in the previous case because of the size of the necrotic area. Resorption was forced to progress along the boundaries of the bone marrow spaces. These appeared widened so that only a thin plate of bone lined the necrotic periodontal ligament. This specimen shows an interesting and important feature: new formation of bone on the periosteal side of the alveolar crest. This is a functional adaptation. The progress of functional adaptation

**Functional adaptation**

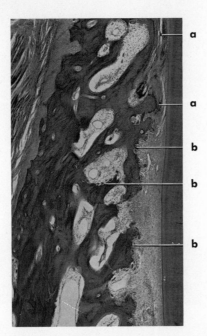

**Fig. 25-16.** Undermining bone resorption in progress 60 hours after beginning of the traumatic influence. *a*, Necrotic area without bone resorption; *b*, undermining bone resorption in progress.

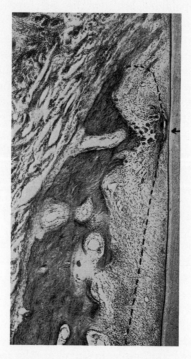

**Fig. 25-17.** Alveolar crest with necrotic pressure area (arrow) 14 days after beginning of the trauma. The necrotic area is almost completely eliminated. The probable former shape of the alveolar bone is sketched with a dotted line.

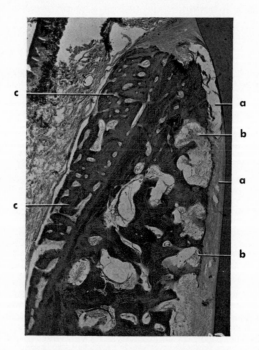

**Fig. 25-18.** Alveolar margin 15 days after beginning of the trauma. a, Extensive area of necrosis; b, undermining resorption in progress; c, new formation of bone on the periosteal side of the alveolar crest.

on both the pressure and the tension sides can be seen at the apex of a tooth (Fig. 25-19) exposed to traumatism for 3 weeks. The apex was moved in the direction of the arrow. Two areas of necrosis can be seen. Both were almost completely undermined and eliminated. The width of the periodontal ligament was once again almost normal.

New bundle bone had been formed on the tension side, reestablishing the normal functional width of the periodontal ligament. The extent to which the apex was moved can be seen by the amount of newly formed bone. Where the two necrotic spots are present, there must originally have been bone. Cementum is present in the area formerly occupied by the periodontal ligament. On the tension side the surface of the old alveolar bone is shown by a dark resting line, indicating the amount of bone that was produced.

If traumatism is maintained for a long time, the process of necrosis, resorption, and repair is repeated or continues as long as the trauma occurs. Eventually the periodontium, as well as the entire jaw, will adapt to the new functional demands. *No changes in the gingiva or the junctional epithelium were evident in any of these experiments; neither did occlusal traumatism cause pocket formation.*

The longest experiment conducted on a dog was for 13 months. The result can be seen in Fig. 25-20. Compare the right side, *A* (traumatic side), with the left side, *B* (control side). The experimental tooth was displaced apically and lingually. The apex almost perforated the cortical plate of the mandible. No acute traumatic changes were detectable on the pressure side of the periodontal ligament. No pocket formation or migration of the epithelial attachment occurred on the pressure side. On the buccal side, which was the side of tension, the development of an infrabony pocket could be seen. This was the only pocket that was observed in the entire series of experiments on 34 dogs. One explanation for the development of this pocket is that the tooth tipped so far buccally that the crown on the antagonist tooth wedged food into the gingival

**Infrabony pocket**

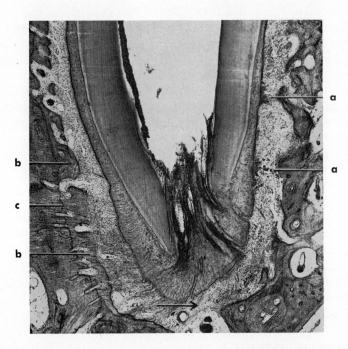

**Fig. 25-19.** Apex of a tooth exposed to trauma for 3 weeks. *a,* Necrotic areas and osteoclasts indicating the former location of the periodontal ligament and alveolar bone; *b,* newly formed bone on the tension side indicative of the amount of tooth movement; *c,* resting line showing the surface of the alveolar bone before trauma; (*arrow,* direction of tooth movement).

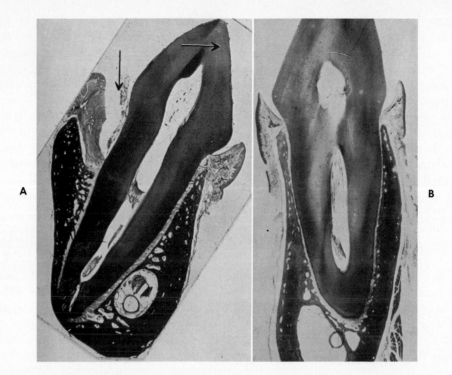

**Fig. 25-20. A,** Tooth exposed to trauma for 13 months. No traumatic tissue changes were evident in the periodontium. Intra-alveolar pocket formation on the vestibular side probably caused by food impaction is the result of extensive tipping of the tooth. **B,** Control tooth.

sulcus. Another explanation is that the combined effects of plaque-induced periodontal disease and trauma combined to give a heightened emphasis to the destructive potential of inflammation. This pocket was not caused by occlusal traumatism per se but may have resulted from the combination of trauma and plaque-induced inflammation.

Other investigators have confirmed these findings.[25] Excessive occlusal forces were reported to have altered the pathway of the inflammatory infiltrate. In the absence of occlusal traumatism, the inflammatory infiltrate is said to follow a perivascular course.[26] When occlusal traumatism is superimposed, the inflammatory infiltrate is purported to be deflected directly into the periodontal ligament.[27]

In an effort to duplicate the combined effects of inflammation and traumatism, high crowns with extensive overhangs were placed on second premolars.[28,29] Mesial and distal contacts were opened to permit the mobile tooth to move mesiodistally as well as buccolingually. The animals were killed at 3 days, 3 weeks, 3 months, and 6 months. The teeth had become mobile and extensively depressed. Cemental and dentinal resorption had occurred. The periodontal ligament space had widened. The direction of transseptal and principal fibers had become almost vertical. The fibers were tensely stretched (Fig. 25-21). *There was neither pocket formation nor gingivitis or apical proliferation of the epithelial attachment. No alteration occurred in the pathway of the inflammatory infiltrate up to 3 months.* However, at 6 months gingivitis was apparent with some apical proliferation of the junctional epithelium.

## Human autopsy findings

The tissue responses to occlusal traumatism in humans duplicate those observed in experimental animals.

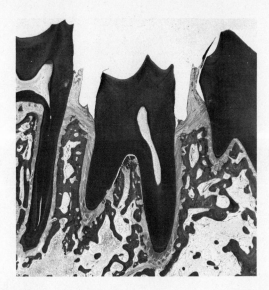

**Fig. 25-21.**    Premolar of a monkey with high crown and overhang. Proximal contacts were opened. At 3 weeks the tooth was depressed, and the direction of periodontal fibers changed. The periodontal ligament was widened, and the tooth was loose. Some acute traumatic changes were still present in the bifurcation. By 3 months an adaptation had taken place. No pockets or apical proliferation of the junctional epithelium had occurred. (Courtesy A. Gargiulo, Chicago, Illinois.)

The first observation of traumatic tissue changes in a human dentition was made on an autopsy specimen of a 24-year-old man who had died of tuberculosis.[30] The pertinent area of interest is shown in Fig. 25-22. The mandibular first molar was missing, and the second molar had tipped mesially. In the maxilla the second premolar and second molar were missing (*A*). The first molar was present and had been restored with a gold crown. The occlusal relation was such that, on closure, the mesiobuccal cusp of the mandibular molar came into contact with the distobuccal cusp of the maxillary molar. Microscopic examination (*B*) revealed pressure areas, with necrosis and its sequelae in the three areas outlined.

Necrosis was present at the mesial alveolar margin of the molar (Fig. 25-23), with undermining resorption advancing from the adjacent marrow spaces. Necrosis was also seen in the bifurcation (Fig. 25-24) and on the distal sides of both apices (Fig. 25-25). The location of pressure areas could be explained by the presence of a rotational fulcrum in the interradicular area. The characteristic features of necrosis, undermining resorption, and endosteal bone formation were present. New bone formation had taken place as a repair process.

Further information was gained from the study of an autopsy specimen of two mandibular premolars in a 64-year-old man. The two teeth exhibited extensive occlusal wear[31,32] (Fig. 25-26, *A*). The roentgenogram showed that the second premolar was tipped mesially and the occlusal surface abraded obliquely. The periodontal ligament of the second premolar was considerably wider than normal. Judging from this evidence alone, one might suspect that an infrabony pocket was present. The microscopic picture showed no pocket. In fact, the bottom of the sulcus was still located on enamel. Only a mild gingivitis was present. The periodontal ligament on the distal surface of the first premolar was of normal width. The fiber bundles were functionally arranged. A few cementum spicules were seen, probably caused by increased function.[33] The periodontal ligament of the second premolar showed a funnel-shaped widening coronally. It was bordered by numerous open marrow spaces, causing the radiolucency in the x-ray film. A higher magnification of the periodontal ligament revealed necrosis in a

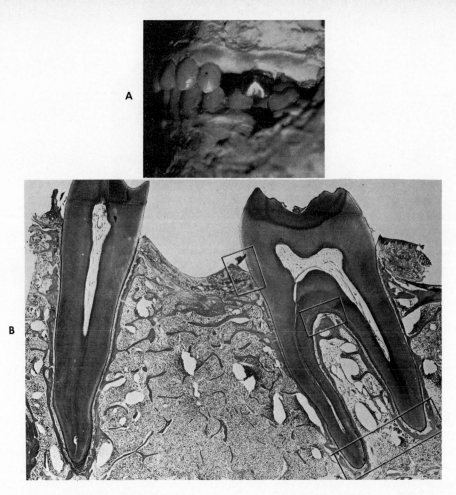

**Fig. 25-22.** Autopsy specimen of a human jaw (24-year-old man). Note the occlusal relation of the maxillary first molar, mandibular second premolar, and mandibular second molar. **B,** Gross microscopic specimen of the mandibular second molar and second premolar shown in **A.** The outlined areas indicate the pressure areas produced by occlusal traumatism.

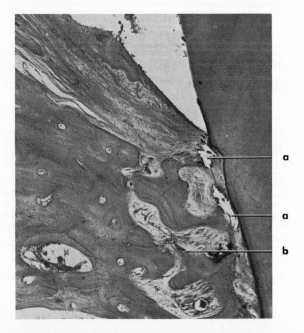

**Fig. 25-23.** Mesial alveolar marginal area of the molar shown in Fig. 25-22, *B.* Necrotic areas in the periodontal ligament are indicated by *a;* resorption of bone by *b.*

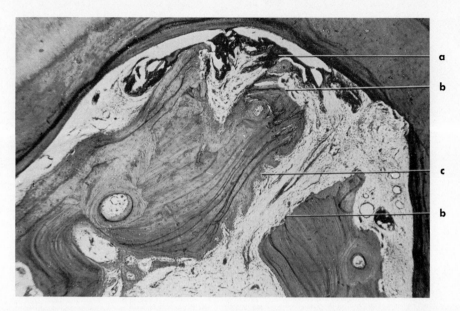

**Fig. 25-24.** Bifurcation area of molar shown in Fig. 25-22. Necrosis, *a*, and undermining bone resorption, *b*, are evident. The new formation of bone, *c*, is occurring on the endosteal side of the bone trabeculum.

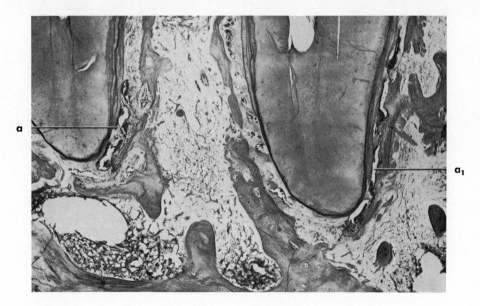

**Fig. 25-25.** Apices of the roots of the molar shown in Fig. 25-22. Necrotic areas are present on the distal aspect of both apices (*a* and *a_1*). Undermining resorption and endosteal bone formation are also taking place.

circumscribed area ( Fig. 25-26, *B*) and an irregular pattern of root resorption extending into the dentin. The periodontal ligament did not show a regular arrangement of the principal fibers. It was rather loose and poorly organized and showed signs of compression.

This case is of special interest because of the roentgenographic suggestion of an infrabony defect. There must have been occlusal traumatism of considerable duration, as indicated by the occlusal wear and the accompanying obliteration of the pulp chamber by irregular dentin. There was no sign of injury to the gingival tissue, even though the occlusal surface was abraded and the tooth was tilted mesially.

Tissue changes indicative of trauma are frequently found in autopsy material.[34,35]

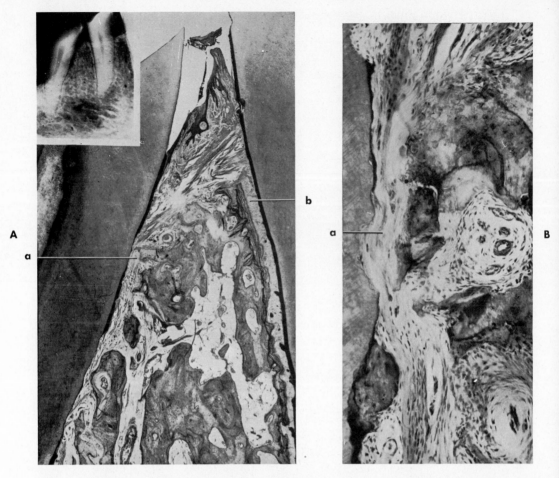

**Fig. 25-26. A,** Human autopsy specimen. Two mandibular premolars show extensive occlusal wear. The second premolar is tipped mesially. The roentgenogram *(inset)* shows considerable widening of the periodontal ligament space on the mesio-occlusal aspect. The microscopic specimen shows disarrangement of the lamina dura (cribriform plate) in this area, *a,* as compared with the regular outline of the lamina dura of the distal surface of the first premolar, *b.* **B,** Higher magnification of the mesial surface. Cementum resorption and the necrotic area *(a)* are indications of repeated trauma. (**A** from Kronfeld, R.: N.Y.J. Dent. **6:**112, 1936.)

In one study in which fifty human jaws were examined, moderate to extensive traumatic tissue changes were found in all specimens. Such findings may include a necrotic area of the pressure side. A case with early bone resorption can be seen in Fig. 25-27. This specimen had many empty lacunae, indicating the presence of necrosis. Similar findings are also made in orthodontically moved teeth.[36]

Sensitivity of teeth and pulp necrosis sometimes are related to occlusal traumatism. Such disturbances can occur whenever the anatomic relation of the apical foramen is such that the circulation of the pulp is disturbed (Fig. 25-28).

There is no reason to believe that widening of the periodontal space affects the depth of the gingival sulcus. The epithelial attachment is some distance from the alveolar crest (1 to 2 mm).[37] The blood supply to the marginal gingiva is derived primarily from superficial periosteal vessels. Since occlusal forces do not cause thrombosis of these vessels, the gingiva apparently is not adversely affected.

## PRIMARY AND SECONDARY TRAUMATISM

Most cases discussed have demonstrated traumatic tissue changes in otherwise healthy periodontal structures. Under such conditions these tissue changes are called

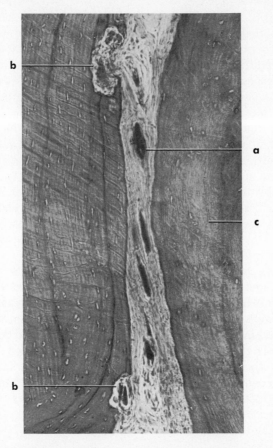

**Fig. 25-27.** Histologic section of traumatized area near the apex of a human tooth. *a,* Necrotic tissue with thrombosed blood vessels evident in the periodontal ligament; *b,* bone resorption bay; *c,* cementum.

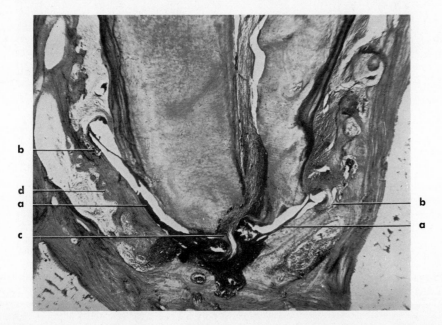

**Fig. 25-28.** Apical area of a human tooth that has been severely traumatized. *a,* Necrosis; *b,* undermining bone resorption; *c,* severe necrosis at the apical foramen; *d,* endosteal bone formation.

*primary traumatism,* that is, an excessive force exerted on a tooth with normal bone support. If prior periodontal disease has caused bone loss and weakening of the supporting tissue and normal occlusal forces are causing periodontal damage, the condition is known as *secondary traumatism.* In other words, secondary traumatism occurs when the force is excessive for diminished bone support. If a tooth has lost a significant amount of its periodontal support, even normal masticatory forces can become excessive.

A condition of this type is illustrated in Fig. 25-29, *A,* which shows a maxillary lateral incisor with about half its cemental surface exposed. There are heavy calcified deposits on this surface. The severely inflamed gingiva, with pocket formation and exudation, is typical of periodontitis. The periodontal ligament is considerably widened at the crest, probably because of mobility. At higher magnification of the labial alveolar margin (Fig. 25-29, *B*), active resorption can be observed. There are osteoclasts in lacunae of the thin alveolar plate. The periodontal ligament consists of loosely organized connective tissue. On close inspection a few small bone spicules are evident, remnants of the former alveolar bone proper.

Another human autopsy specimen with similar findings is shown in Fig. 25-30. The age of this patient is unknown, but he was apparently over 40. The occlusion had been mutilated by extractions. The second and third mandibular molars were tipped anteriorly. Microscopic examination *(B)* revealed a deep infrabony pocket on the mesial aspect of the second molar. Below the pocket a dark body could be seen in the widened periodontal space. Higher magnification of the area *(C)* revealed a cemental tear. Such cemental tears are the result of trauma, most often a blow. A sudden forceful closure might also have caused this. A necrotic tissue mass lined with macrophages could be seen distal to the root *(D).* This necrotic area presumably was once the periodontal ligament, destroyed by pressure from the tipping tooth. The adjacent bone showed

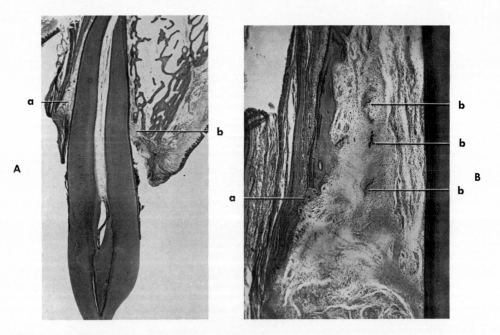

**Fig. 25-29.** Histologic section of a maxillary lateral incisor with severe periodontitis and gingival recession exposing the root surfaces. The periodontal ligament is funnel shaped on both the labial, *a,* and the palatal, *b,* surfaces. **B,** Higher magnification of the marginal alveolus on the labial surface. The periodontal ligament space is wide and without principal fibers. *a,* Osteoclastic activity; *b,* several bone spicules in the periodontal ligament, indicating the former position of the alveolus.

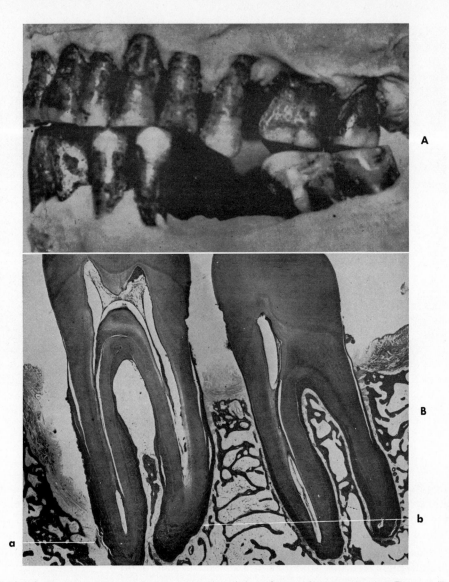

**Fig. 25-30.** **A,** Human autopsy specimen showing the relation of the molars to each other. The mandibular molars are tipped mesially. The second premolar and first molar are missing. **B,** Microscopic section of the two molars. A deep infrabony pocket is present on the mesial surface of the second molar. The bifurcation is involved. The lamina dura of the alveolar bone at the distal aspect of the apical areas of both molars (pressure areas) appears more discontinuous than elsewhere. *a,* Cemental tear; *b,* pressure area.                    *Continued.*

osteoclastic activity. Such tissue changes are possible only if adjacent teeth are not in firm contact. If arch contact exists, traumatic changes of this type are not likely, since teeth brace one another.

These cases are typical of secondary traumatism. The reduced or weakened periodontium cannot withstand occlusal forces that previously were normal and nontraumatic.

*It should be reemphasized that occlusal traumatism per se does not cause gingivitis, periodontitis, or pocket formation.*[17] *The pathologic features of traumatism are different from those of inflammation.*[16,17] Traumatic tissue damage heals by formation of granulation tissue, proliferation of capillaries and fibroblasts, and activity of macrophages. This healing process need not be considered an inflammatory process. It will

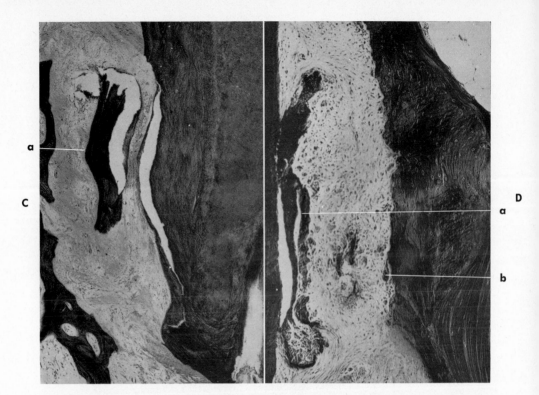

**Fig. 25-30, cont'd.** **C,** Higher magnification of the mesial aspect of the second molar. *a,* Cemental fragment torn loose by trauma. **D,** Necrotic area on the distal surface of the second molar; *a,* resorption of the necrotic ligament and, *b,* bone in progress.

be helpful at this point to review Chapter 11. Inflammation always includes cellular infiltration. In traumatism, circulatory disturbance is present, created by the obstruction of blood flow. Although circulatory disturbance leads ultimately to necrosis, it does not show the cellular infiltrate. *There are no leukocytes, lymphocytes, or plasma cells in or around these necrotic areas.* Elimination of such lesions starts from the periphery, where circulation is not impaired. Repair and regeneration are initiated without the classical signs of inflammation.

## Tissue changes caused by periodontal traumatism

The following changes caused by occlusal trauma may occur in periodontal structures.

**Periodontal ligament**  In the *acute* phase of trauma, there is compression on the pressure side of the periodontal ligament. Crushing, hemorrhage, thrombosis, and necrosis may occur. Stretching takes place on the tension side; sometimes this may cause thrombosis of the vessels and tearing of the ligament. In the *chronic* phase the periodontal ligament becomes wider; this may be reflected in clinical mobility.[38] There may be hyalinization and a subsequent formation of fibrocartilage.[12,39] Ankylosis may occur.[12]

**Cementum**  In the *acute* phase there may be cemental tears[12] and fractures. Cemental and dentinal resorption may follow. In the *chronic* phase reparative changes such as cemental hyperplasia and formation of cementum spurs may occur. Resorbed areas may be repaired by cemental apposition.

**Alveolar bone**  The physiologic reaction of alveolar bone to moderate pressure is resorption; to moderate tension, it is apposition. During the *acute* phase, necrosis of bone may occur in areas of total compression of the periodontal ligament. This is followed by resorption. These mechanisms work to reestablish a functional width of the periodontal ligament. If, however, the traumatism is continued, excessive widening of the periodontal ligament may result. This may be seen roentgenographically as a wider or funnel-shaped periodontal ligament. Occasionally the widening appears as a rarefaction in the apical and furcation areas.

No evidence exists that either gingival changes (festooned gingival margins, recession, or clefts) or pocket formation occurs as a consequence of occlusal traumatism per se. An early explanation given for exaggerated marginal festooning of the gingiva and gingival clefts was that occlusal traumatism caused an impingement on the blood supply reaching the gingiva through the periodontal ligament. It has been shown, however, that the supply to the buccal and lingual gingivae is mainly through periosteal vessels coursing along the buccal and lingual surfaces of the alveolar process. Compression of the periodontal ligament will not occlude these vessels. Blanching of the gingiva can occur, however, if loose teeth are luxated. In this case there will be direct impingement of the tooth against the soft tissues, and the alveolar crest must have previously been resorbed to much lower levels because of periodontitis.

*Gingiva*

Odontoblastic activity may be stimulated, and secondary dentin may be formed. The pulp chamber and canal may become narrower and even obliterated. Pulp stones may be formed. In some cases pulpitis and loss of pulpal vitality may occur.

*Pulp*

## Combined periodontal disease

*Occlusal trauma cannot initiate inflammatory periodontal disease.* Whether occlusal trauma in the presence of preexisting inflammatory disease can cause the formation of pockets is controversial.[27,40-43] There is evidence that occlusal trauma in the presence of periodontitis can influence the progression and course of the disease.[27,39-58]

Morphologic changes in bone and in the periodontal ligament are caused by occlusal trauma.[*] The changes are adaptive as the periodontal ligament assumes a greater width in accord with the increased function. If the force is discontinued, the changes are reversible.[16,17,50]

Although the conversion of a gingivitis into periodontitis by the addition of occlusal trauma has not been demonstrated, Tilt[58] reported an apical proliferation of junctional epithelium in marmosets with naturally occurring gingivitis when occlusal trauma was superimposed.

It has been proposed that inflammation and trauma are codestructive factors leading to a widened periodontal ligament and horizontal and angular bone loss at the alveolar crest[35,40,43,45-47] and that periodontitis is accelerated by trauma.[43,45,46] A periodontitis with a superimposed traumatism produces more extensive bone loss than does periodontitis alone.[48,49] Bone alteration produced by trauma alone is reversible when the trauma is removed[16,17,29,50] However, when bone loss is the result of periodontitis in the presence of traumatism, removal of the traumatism does not result in any regeneration.[50]

*Combined periodontitis and occlusal trauma*

Institution of plaque removal in the presence of continued trauma results in some repair and no further loss of connective tissue attachment.[59] When both trauma and inflammation are controlled, there is a remarkable but not complete regeneration of bone.[49] This regeneration involves some restoration of alveolar crestal height and an increase in the volume of trabeculae in proportion to marrow spaces.[51] Combined periodontitis-traumatism results in an enlargement of the marrow spaces so that the volume of bone surrounding the marrow spaces becomes approximately 35% less than

*Effect of trauma*

*Effect of plaque and inflammation*

---

*See references 16, 17, 28-30, 32, 35, 38, 42, 45, 46, 48, and 57.

that present in similar areas of normal specimens.[51] There is loss of crestal height as well. The regeneration that follows control of trauma and inflammation would have been complete if the bone had regenerated to the level of loss produced by periodontitis alone. This did not occur. The crestal bone level was significantly lower.[60]

**Experimental trauma super-imposed on periodontitis**

If experimental traumatism is induced in teeth with lessened bone support but that are otherwise in good health, the results are similar to those found in healthy teeth. Widened periodontal ligaments and angular bone deformities may result with[58] or without[53,54] further apical displacement of the junctional epithelium. Plaque must be present for pocket formation.[55,56] Trauma superimposed on periodontitis in which angular bone loss and infrabony pockets are present results in more pronounced apical migration of the junctional epithelium than in periodontitis alone.[56-60] It also results in additional bone loss.[61]

These findings again reinforce the necessity of dealing with the plaque-induced periodontal disease and restoring the tissues to a noninflamed state before treating traumatism.[57] One may conclude that traumatism in the presence of an established inflammatory periodontal disease plays a role in the progression of the existing periodontal disease, even though it has no role in the genesis of inflammatory periodontal disease.[59,62-64]

Another type of interrelationship exists when advanced inflammatory periodontal disease causes so much bone loss that secondary traumatism results. Then the advanced inflammatory disease is complicated by the presence of traumatism. When the forces become tantamount to "extraction forces" in their dimension, the tooth may be naturally avulsed or have so hopeless a prognosis as to require extraction.[57] Another possibility is that a fulminating abscess may result as a consequence of periodontal infection. When mobility is extreme and only one third or less of the alveolar bone remains,[65] such abscesses may result in avulsion or extraction.

**Summary**

Several important results are apparent from these investigations:

1. Periodontitis with superimposed trauma produces more bone loss than periodontitis alone.[48,49] Endosteal bone loss produces an enlargement of marrow spaces, so that the volume of coronal bone surrounding these spaces was 35% less than that in control specimens. However, periodontitis and traumatism may or may not produce loss of connective tissue attachment.
2. Bone alterations resulting from trauma are reversible when the trauma is removed.[16,17,29,50] When the trauma is permitted to persist in the absence of inflammation, a functional adaptaton occurs that results in a mobile tooth without pocket formation.
3. When bone loss is the result of periodontitis in the presence of trauma, the removal of traumatism does not result in regeneration of lost crestal bone.[50]
4. When bone loss is the result of combined periodontitis-traumatism, eliminating the inflammation may result in some repair but not further loss of connective tissue attachment.[65]
5. When bone loss is the result of periodontitis and traumatism, the elimination of both results in a remarkable, but not complete, regeneration of bone.[49] Some but not all crestal bone is restored, and there is significant endosteal bone formation, increasing the volume of trabeculae in proportion to marrow spaces.[51]

**REFERENCES**

1. Stein, G., And Weinmann, J.P.: Die physiologische Wanderung der Zähne, Z. Stomatol. **23:**733, 1925.
2. Black, G.V.: Special dental pathology, Chicago, 1915, Medico-Dental Publishing Co.
3. Black, G.V.: Operative dentistry, vol. 1, ed. 6, revised by A.D. Black, Chicago, 1924, Medico-Dental Publishing Co.
4. Sicher, H.: Tooth eruption: the axial movement of teeth with limited growth, J. Dent Res. **21:**395, 1942.
5. Weinmann, J.P.: Bone changes related to eruption of the teeth, Angle Orthod. **11:**83, 1941.
6. Weinmann, J.P., and Sicher, H.: Correlation of active and passive eruption. Burd. **46:**128, 1946.
7. Kronfeld, R.: Structure, function and pathol-

ogy of the human periodontal membrane, N.Y.J. Dent. **6:**112, 1936.

8. Gottlieb, B.: Ein Fall von scheinbarer Verkürzung eines oberen Schneidezahnes, Z. Stomatol. **22:**501, 1924.

9. Kotanyi, E.: Ein weiterer klinishcer Beweis des kontinuierlichen Zahndurchbruches, Z. Stomatol. **28:**1055, 1930.

10. Noyes, F.B.: Submerging deciduous molars, Angle Orthodont. **2:**77, 1932.

11. Orban, B.: Ist das Paradentium eine organische Einheit? Z. Stomatol. **24:**515, 1932.

12. Grant, D.A., and Bernick, S.: The periodontium of ageing humans, J. Periodontol. **43:**660, 1972.

13. Wolff's law of transformation. Quoted in Weinmann, J.P., and Sicher, H.: Bone and bones, ed.2, St. Louis, 1955, The C.V. Mosby Co.

14. Brescia, N.: Applied dental anatomy, St. Louis, 1961, The C.V. Mosby Co.

15. Kellner, E.: Histologische Befunde an antagonistenlosen Zähnen, Z. Stomatol. **26:**271, 1928.

16. Gottlieb, B., and Orban, B.: Die Veränderungen der Gewebe bei übermässiger Beanspruchung der Zähne, Leipzig, 1931, Georg Thieme Verlag.

17. Bhaskar, S.N., and Orban, B.: Experimental occlusal trauma, J. Periodontol. **26:**270, 1955.

18. Stern, I.B.: An electron microscopic study of cementum, Sharpey's fibers and periodontal ligament in the rat incisor, Am. J. Anat. **115:**377, 1964.

19. Stallard, R.E.: The utlization of H³-proline by the connective tissue elements of the periodontium, Periodontics **1:**185, 1963.

20. Crumley, P.J.: Collagen formation in the normal and stressed periodontium, Periodontics **2:**53, 1964.

21. Carneiro, J., and Fava de Moraes, F.: Radioautographic visualization of collagen metabolism in the periodontal tissues of the mouse, Arch. Oral Biol. **10:**833, 1965.

22. Guis, M.B., Slootweg, R.N., and Tonino, G.J.: A biochemical study of collagen in the periodontal ligament from erupting and non-erupting bovine incisors, Arch. Oral Biol. **18:**253, 1973.

23. Rippin, J.W.: Collagen turnover in the periodontal ligament under normal and altered functional forces. I. Young rat molars, J. Periodont. Res. **11:**101, 1976.

24. Rippin, J.W.: Collagen turnover in the periodontal ligament under normal and altered functional forces. II. Adult rat molars, J. Periodont. Res. **13:**149, 1978.

25. Waerhaug, J., and Hansen, E.R.: Periodontal changes incident to prolonged occlusal overload in monkeys, Acta Odontol. Scand. **24:**91, 1966.

26. Weinmann, J.P.: Progress of gingival inflammation into the supporting structures of the teeth, J. Periodontol. **12:**71, 1941.

27. Macapanpan, L.C., and Weinmann, J.P.: The influence of injury to the periodontal membrane on the spread of gingival inflammation, J. Dent. Res. **33:**263, 1954.

28. Comar, M., Kollar, J., and Gargiulo, A.: Local irritation and occlusal trauma as co-factors in the periodontal disease process, J. Periodontol. **40:**193, 1969.

29. Wentz, F.M., Jarabek, J., and Orban, B.: Experimental trauma imitating cuspal interferences, J. Periodontol. **29:**117, 1958.

30. Orban, B.: Tissue changes in traumatic occlusion, J. Am. Dent. Assoc. **15:**2090, 1928.

31. Kronfeld, R.: Histologic study of the influence of function on the human periodontal membrane, J. Am. Dent. Assoc. **18:**1242, 1931.

32. Kronfeld, R.: Physiology of the human periodontal tissue under normal and abnormal occlusal conditions, Ill. Dent. J. **8:**13, 1939.

33. Bödecker, C.F.: Critical review of Gottlieb and Orban's "Die Veränderungen der Gewebe bei übermässiger Beanspruchung der Zähne," Orthod. Oral Surg. Rad. Int. J. **18:**895, 1932.

34. Orban, B., and Weinmann, J.: Signs of traumatic occlusion in average human jaws, J. Dent. Res. **13:**216, 1933.

35. Glickman, I., and Smulow, J.B.: Further observations on the effects of trauma from occlusion in humans, J. Periodontol. **38:**280, 1967.

36. Oppenheim, A.: Human tissue response to orthodontic intervention, Am. J. Orthod. **28:**263, 1942.

37. Gargiulo, A., Wentz, F.M., and Orban, B.: Dimensions and relations of the dentogingival junction in humans J. Periodontol. **32:**261, 1961.

38. Picton, D.C.A., and Slatter, J.M.: The effect on horizontal tooth mobility of experimental trauma to the periodontal membrane in regions of tension and compression in monkeys, J. Periodont. Res. **7:**35, 1972.

39. Everett, F.G., and Bruckner, R.J.: Cartilage in the periodontal ligament space, J. Periodontol. **41:**165, 1970.

40. Glickman, I.: Role of occlusion in the etiology and treatment of periodontal disease, J. Dent. Res. **50:**199, 1971.

41. Drum, W.: Parafunktionen und Autodestruktionsprozesse, Berlin, 1969, Quintessenz.

42. Stahl, S.S.: The responses of the periodontium to combined gingival inflammation and occluso-functional stresses in four human specimens, Periodontics **6:**14, 1968.

43. Glickman, I., and Smulow, J.B.: Alteration in the pathway of gingival inflammation into the underlying tissues induced by excessive occlusal forces, J. Periodontol. **33:**7, 1962.

44. Orban, B.: Traumatic occlusion and gum inflammation, J. Periodontol. **10:**39, 1939.

45. Glickman, I.: Inflammation and trauma from occlusion; co-destructive factors in chronic periodontal disease, J. Periodontol. **34:**5, 1963.

46. Glickman, I.: Occlusion and the peridontium, J. Dent. Res. **46:**53, 1967.

47. Glickman, I., and Smulow, J.B.: Adaptive alteration in the periodontium of the rhesus monkey in chronic trauma from occlusion, J. Periodontol. **39:**101, 1968.

48. Meitner, S.W.: Co-destructive factors of marginal periodontitis and repetitive mechanical injury, J. Dent. Res. **54:**C78, 1975.

49. Kantor, M., Polson, A.M., and Zander, H.A.: Alveolar bone regeneration after removal of inflammatory and traumatic factors, J. Periodontol. **47:**687, 1976.

50. Polson, A.M., Meitner, S.W., and Zander, H.A.: Trauma and progression of marginal periodontitis in squirrel monkeys. IV. Reversibility of bone loss due to trauma alone and trauma superimposed upon periodontitis, J. Periodont. Res. **11:**290, 1976.

51. Polson, A.M., Meitner, S.W., and Zander, H.A.: Trauma and progression of marginal periodontitis in squirrel monkeys. III. Adaptation of interproximal alveolar bone to repetitive injury, J. Periodont. Res. **11:**279, 1976.

52. Zander, H.A., and Polson, A.M.: Present status of occlusion and occlusal therapy in periodontics, J. Periodontol. **48:**540, 1977.

53. Lindhe, J., and Ericsson, I.: The influence of trauma from occlusion on reduced but healthy periodontal tissues in dogs, J. Clin. Periodontol. **3:**110, 1976.

54. Ericcson, I.: Thilander, B., and Lindhe, J.: Influence of tipping movements on experimental periodontitis in dogs, J. Dent. Res. **56:**A144, 1977.

55. Svanberg, G.: Influence of trauma from occlusion on the periodontium of dogs with normal or inflamed gingivae, Odontol. Rev. **25:**165, 1974.

56. Lindhe, J.A.: Influence of trauma from occlusion on the progression of experimental periodontitis in the beagle dog. J. Clin. Periodontol. **1:**3, 1974.

57. Lindhe, J.A., and Nyman, S.: The role of occlusion in periodontal disease and the biologic rationale for splinting in the treatment of periodontitis. Oral Sci. Rev. **10:**11, 1977.

58. Tilt, L.: Occlusal trauma and naturally occurring gingivitis in marmosets, Master's thesis, Chicago, 1977, Loyola University.

59. Polson, A.M., Kantor, M.A., and Zander, H.A.: Periodontal repair after reduction of inflammation, J. Periodontol. **14:**520, 1979.

60. Polson, A.M.: Interrelationship of inflammation and tooth mobility (trauma) in pathogenesis of periodontal disease, J. Clin. Periodontol. **7:**351, 1980.

61. Polson, A.M., and Zander, H.A.: Effect of periodontal trauma upon intrabony pockets, J. Periodontol. **54:**586, 1983.

62. Lindhe, J., and Ericsson, I.: The effect of jiggling forces on periodontally exposed teeth in the dog, J. Periodontol. **53:**562, 1982.

63. Ericsson, I., and Lindhe, J.: Effect of long-standing jiggling on experimental marginal periodontitis in the beagle dog, J. Clin Periodontol. **9:**497, 1982.

64. Nyman, S., Karring, T., and Bergenholz, G. Bone regeneration in alveolar bone dehiscences produced by jiggling forces, J. Periodontol. **17:**316, 1964.

65. Frank, R.M., and Voegel, J.C.: Bacterial bone resorption in advanced cases of human periodontitis, J. Periodont. Res. **13:**251, 1978.

## ADDITIONAL SUGGESTED READING

Dotto, C.A., et al.: Vascular changes in experimental trauma from occlusion. J. Periodontol. **38:**183, 1967.

Gaengler, P., and Merte, K.: Effects of force application on periodontal blood circulation: a vital microscopic study in rats, J. Periodont. Res. **18:**86, 1983.

Glickman, I.: Occlusion—a factor in periodontal health and disease in the circumpubertal and adolescent periods, J. Periodontol. **42:**513, 1971.

Gottlieb, B., and Orban, B.: Biology and pathology of the teeth and its supporting mechanism, New York, 1983, The Macmillan Co.

Grant, D.A., Chase, J., and Bernick, S.: Biology of the periodontium in primates of the *Galago* speicies, J. Periodontol. **44:**540, 1973.

Itoiz, M.E., Carranza, F.A., Jr., and Cabrini, R.I.: Histologic and histometric study of experimental occlusal trauma in rats, J. Periodontol. **34:**305, 1963.

Mailland, M.: Effets d'une surcharge occlusale experimentale sure le parodonte du rat, J. Bio. Buccale **2:**327, 1974.

Mailland, M., and Baron, R.: Etude quantitative des éffets d'une surcharge occlusale sure las densité osseuse interradiculaire chez le rat, J. Biol. Buccale **3:**41, 1975.

Mühlemann, H.R., and Herzog, H.: Tooth mobility and microscopic tissue changes produced by experimental occlusal trauma, Helv. Odontol. Acta **5:**33, 1961.

Palcanis, K.: Effect of occlusal trauma on interstitial pressure in the periodontal ligament, J. Dent. Res. **52:**903, 1973.

Rateitschak, K.H., and Herzog-Specht, F.A.: Reaktion und Regeneration des Parodonts auf orthodontische Behandlung mit festsitzenden Apparaten, Schweiz. Monatsschr. Zahnheilkd. **75:**741, 1965.

Reitan, K.: Tissue behavior during orthodontic tooth movement, Am. J. Orthod. **46:**881, 1960.

Shefter, G.J., and McFall, W.T., Jr.: Occlusal relations and periodontal status in human adults, J. Periodontol. **55:**368, 1984.

Stallard, R.E.: The effect of occlusal alterations on

collagen formation within the periodontium, Periodontics **2:**49, 1964.

Svanberg, G., And Lindhe, J.: Experimental tooth hypermobility in the dog, Odontol. Rev. **24:**269, 1973.

Svanberg, G., and Lindhe, J.: Vascular reactions in the periodontal ligament incident ot trauma from occlusion. J. Clin Periodontol. **1:**58, 1974.

Weinmann, J.P.: The adaptation of the periodontal membrane to physiologic and pathologic changes, Oral Surg. **8:**977, 1955.

Wentz, F.M., Jarabek, J., and Orban, B.: Experimental trauma imitating cuspal interferences, J. Periodontol. **29:**117, 1958.

Wingard, C.E., and Bowers, G.M.: The effects on facial bone from facial tipping of incisors in monkeys, J. Periodontol. **47:**450,l 1976.

# PART FOUR

## Elements of
## Therapeutic Judgment

# CHAPTER 26

# Psychologic aspects of periodontics

Although it is apparent that psychologic insight is required for the proper management of a dental practice, other relationships between psychology and dentistry are far less obvious but no less important. Psychoanalytic theory places great importance on the relationship of the oral cavity to the psyche. Other data also support the hypothesis that psychologic and social factors are involved in diseases of the oral cavity.

## Psychosomatic factors

Is periodontal disease related to psychogenic causes? A study of a hospitalized, emotionally ill population showed acutely disturbed patients had a higher incidence of periodontal disease than did apathetic patients. Other reports have indicated a correlation between periodontal disease and neurotic tendency, measured anxiety (a symptom of neurosis), and factors such as strained family relationships, hysteria, and hypochondriasis.[1,2]

These studies support the existence of an association between periodontal disease and psychologic factors; that is, certain measurable factors of periodontal disease and psychologic status vary proportionately.[3-5] Causality is not involved in these measurements, yet such a presumption is tempting to make. Bruxism, NUG, poor oral hygiene, depressed immune responses, and poor diet may in fact be manifestations of psychologic states. To the extent that this is so, periodontal disease may have psychologic roots. Although a case can be made for this argument, it is not yet proved. On the other hand, case histories indicate that psychoanalysis sometimes permits the elimination of neurosis-induced periodontal symptoms.[3]

### BRUXISM AND CLENCHING

The muscular force produced during bruxism and clenching may result in occlusal traumatism (Chapter 25). Therefore a fuller understanding of how these muscle actions may have a psychologic origin could prove valuable.

The psychologic explanation for bruxism is a construction.* All persons have drives that are associated with life goals. When these drives are blocked, the resultant frustration produces rage. Rage must have an outlet; for instance, an enraged child will not hesitate to bite. When the child learns that such biting behavior is socially unacceptable, the biting is repressed. Since the rage cannot be suppressed, new outlets for its dissipation must be found. Substitute satisfactions (sublimation) may be employed. When substitution is inadequate, one may still resort to biting to gain satisfaction. This satisfaction may be gained surreptitiously and symbolically on an unconscious level by bruxing or clenching. These activities occur during the waking hours, but they are especially prevalent during sleep, when the unconscious is most emergent (night grinding). The patient may be completely unaware of these repeated and sustained forced contacts of the teeth that seem to have no functional significance in humans (parafunction). However, there is evidence that bruxism in some primates is also a tooth-honing mechanism.[6]

The following evidence tends to support the psychologic correlation between bruxism and anxiety: In a word-association test given to a student with electrodes placed on the temporal muscles, spikes (muscle contractions) appeared with emotional words and disappeared with neutral words. Electromyographic recordings were made of the temporal and masseter muscles of eight dental students. During the recording, stress was provided by having the dean "unexpectedly" arrive on the scene and engage the student in a conversation that somehow turned to the subject of forthcoming examinations and the student's prospects. Action potentials increased with the stress.[7]

The electrical activity of the masseter and temporal muscles increases when a human experimental subject performs a task.[8] Increases in amplitude of electromyograms occur when the subject makes a mistake in the performance of the task.[9] In a study of 103 patients with bruxism who were compared with a control group, the bruxing patients had a significantly higher degree of depression and anxiety symptoms. They also had symptoms of muscular tension and latent or manifest aggressiveness.[10] A striking enlargement of the masseter muscles has been observed in some mental patients, which could be a form of work hypertrophy related to clenching and oral-aggressive energy.[11,12]

Bruxism and circulatory phenomena may be interrelated in a psychophysiologic manner.[13] Tooth contacts lasting up to 17 seconds have been reported concomitant with alterations in pulse rate and stroke. These periods of bruxing contact were directly related to periods of emotional reaction (stress and/or anxiety).[14] Although an emotional basis for bruxism may exist, the assumption that bruxism is diagnostic of emotional disturbance or psychopathology is not warranted. It appears that bruxism is universal.

## SALIVA

Just as "gnashing the teeth" and "shutting up like a clam" demonstrate emotional overtones, phrases like "spitting mad," "frothing at the mouth," and "drooling in anticipation" show that salivation has psychiatric implications. Although the relationship of emotionally controlled salivation to periodontal disease may not be so obvious as in the case of bruxism, it may be equally or more important. Psychologic factors are known to influence the rate of secretion and composition of saliva.[15] Saliva, in turn, relates to plaque formation, calculus deposition, and antibacterial and proteolytic activities, all of which may have a bearing on periodontal disease.

---

*A construction in geometry is an assumption that leads to the derivation of a proof. In psychiatry and in periodontics, there are many constructions (working hypotheses) that facilitate treatment. These constructions need not be true for treatment based on them to work. It is possible for both treatment and construction to be related to other true but as yet unknown foundations.

A transient reduction of salivary flow and changes in salivary enzyme content can be produced by mental activity, stress, muscular effort, or emotional disturbance.[16-18] Level of pH has also been observed to go up as salivation increases.[19]

These relationships between salivary physiology and psychologic status do not necessarily demonstrate causation of periodontal disease, but they show a pathway in which periodontal health is influenced by salivary changes.

## CIRCULATION

The tonus of the smooth muscle of blood vessels may be altered by the emotions[13] by way of the autonomic nervous system. For example, dilatation and contraction are related to blushing and blanching and well as to facial expression.[13] Prolonged contraction could alter the supply of oxygen and nutrients to the tissues. There is little evidence to support such a relationship with periodontal disease however. Metabolic studies indicate that the oxygen consumption of gingival tissues varies in health and disease, but this may relate to altered tissue activity.[19-23]

Rats caged in crowded conditions in which movement is inhibited demonstrate a lowered oxygen utilization by their oral tissues. This observation is related to the social stress provoked by the crowding.[23] Mice similarly treated have been observed to develop systolic hypertension.[24] Physical and psychologic stimuli (e.g., mental arithmetic) reduce the amplitude of the volume pulse of the gingiva as well as that of the finger. The gingival and cutaneous vascular responses occur simultaneously with other variables and are relatable to both the anticipation of stress and the actual cold pressor stimulation.[25,26]

## DIET AND APPETITE

Psychologic factors affect the choice of foods, the physical consistency of the diet, and the quantities of food eaten. These factors may have a direct on indirect influence on the periodontium.

## ORAL HYGIENE

It is obvious that proper oral hygiene is partially dependent on the mental health status of the patient. Some patients may be so disturbed or distracted psychologically that personal hygiene is neglected. Other patients may intentionally ignore oral hygiene to fulfill deep neurotic needs. Moulton, Ewen, and Thieman[27] suggest that oral hygiene may be neglected during depression, deep anxiety, and rebellion against authority. Dependent individuals may exhibit chronic neglect as if they were expecting such care to be the responsibility of others. The dentist's instructions concerning oral hygiene may be ignored as a form of "parental defiance."[28]

Techniques are available to the dentist for developing desired patient behavior with regard to oral hygiene. These techniques depend on psychologic approaches to reinforce desirable behavior and to extinguish undesirable behavior.[29,30]

## ORAL HABITS

Neurotic needs find oral expression. The mouth may be used to obtain satisfaction, to express dependency or hostility, and to inflict or receive pain. Sucking, biting, sensing, and feeling may become habitual, as in thumb sucking, tongue thrusting, infantile swallowing, and biting of tongue, lip, cheek, or fingernail. These actions also figure in bruxing, clenching, tooth doodling, and smoking. Such habits may lead to tooth migration, occlusal traumatism, and occlusal wear.

Other potentially harmful habits may act by affecting tissue moisture or temperature. Perhaps the most insidious of these is smoking, which according to some studies is related to NUG and possibly to other oral diseases as well.[31,32] Smoking is also

**Smoking**

inversely related to many psychosocial variables associated with mental health.[33] What is not known, however, is whether the smoking is in itself of direct etiologic significance or merely a symptom of some underlying psychologic disturbance that has a more important role in the pathogenesis of these diseases. This qualification would not minimize the direct local irritating effect of nicotine and tars on the tissue, nor would it probably influence the role of these irritants in the formation of calculus.[26] The rate of plaque formation is not increased in smokers, but smoking and periodontal disease are correlated.[34-37] Consequently other factors, possibly psychologic, may be present.

**Coffee drinking**

Coffee drinking is another habit that may act extrinsically (through thermal or chemical properties) and intrinsically (through caffeine content). Coffee drinking is more frequent among smokers[33] and has also been shown to be greater among patients with NUG than among those with healthy gingivae.[26]

## PERIODONTAL DISEASES

**Necrotizing ulcerative gingivitis**

Necrotizing ulcerative gingivitis (NUG) is a disease of special interest because it may have an emotional basis (Chapter 18). Some evidence exists to indicate that the suggested relationship between emotional stress and NUG is more than conjecture. Of the hospitalized patients examined by Mellars and Herms,[38] the acutely mentally ill were more prone to NUG than were the chronically mentally ill. The disease among military personnel may be related to fatigue, nervousness, and unusual dependence.[39] A group of patients with this disease examined by Moulton and co-workers[27] exhibited a pattern of oral dependence as a central life problem. The attacks of NUG among this group were brought on by acute anxiety. Case histories indicate that attacks of acute anxiety are often the precipitating factor.[40-42]

Patients with NUG have a tendency to cutaneous vasodilatation in response to irritation and, in addition, show a longer latency period for flare reaction.[43,44]

**Atypical gingivo-stomatitis**

An unusual gingivitis extending from the gingival margin to the mucogingival junction and limited almost entirely to the labial and buccal surfaces has been reported.[45,46] Evidence of an excessively dependent yet hostile relationship with either spouse or parent was found in the 7 patients studied.[45]

**Excoriative gingivitis**

Self-inflicted gingival excoriations that have a neurotic or unconscious habitual basis are periodically reported.[47-49] These may be so extensive as to involve self-extraction of teeth.

## OTHER FACTORS

**Denial**

The psyche may influence therapy in other areas. Patients may have unrealistic attitudes or protective mechanisms that lead them to deny their dental ills.[50]

**Somatic delusions**

Some patients seeking cosmetic surgery or dentistry because of somatic delusions may displace their dissatisfaction on the therapist.[51] Some middle-aged women go to periodontists, reassured that, if they can keep their teeth, they can hold back the ravages of age.[52]

Treatment may influence the psychiatric status of the patients.[52] In selected cases, patients may need psychiatric assistance and preparation to avoid posttreatment illness.[53] The acceptance of treatment and its course and success for some patients depends on the therapist's interaction with and management of their psychologic status.[54,55]

**Stress**

Selye has proposed the general adaptation syndrome, a set of nonspecific physiologic reactions to stress,[56] and now stress and psychosomatic influences are considered to be separate but parallel factors in the causation of diseases.[14] However, life events, in terms of stress, have not been shown to be predictors of the probability of future illness.[57] The pituitary and adrenal hormones play a role in regulating the response to stress,[58] involving a feedback mechanism. When the hydrocortisone level in blood is elevated, the central nervous system shuts off the secretion of adrenocorticotropic hormone (ACTH) and conversely increases production when the level of hydrocortisone is low. The levels of either of these two hormones have effects on the brain and play a role in learning behavior.[58]

In turn, psychologic factors can influence disease processes.[59] Now evidence is beginning to accumulate that psychosocial factors and the central nervous system (specifically the hypothalamus) may influence the humoral immune response[60-62] and, in this way, susceptibility to some infections and some neoplastic processes.

**Immune response**

## Summary

The conclusion that psychologic factors may alter tissue physiology and contribute to periodontal disease seems inescapable. Precise knowledge concerning definitive pathways and specific mechanisms is lacking or incomplete. Future studies should bring this area into sharper focus.

### REFERENCES

1. Ewen, S.J.: The dental interview, N.Y. J. Dent. **21:**392, 1951.
2. Witkin, G.J.: Management of the patient with periodontal disease, J. Am. Dent. Assoc. **55:**625, 1957.
3. Saul, L.J.: A note on the psychogenesis of organic symptoms, Psychoanal. Q. **4:**476, 1935.
4. Belting, C.M., and Gupta, O.P.: Incidence of periodontal diseases among persons with neuropsychiatric disorders, J. Dent. Res. **39:**744, 1960.
5. Manhold, J.H.: Report of a study on the relationship of personality variables to periodontal conditions, J. Periodontol. **24:**248, 1953.
6. Zingeser, M.R.: Canine tooth honing mechanism, Am. J. Phys. Anthropol. **31:**205, 1969.
7. Perry, H.T., et al.: Occlusion in a stress situation, J. Am. Dent. Assoc. **60:**626, 1960.
8. Yemm, R.: Variations in the electrical activity of the human masseter muscle occurring in association with emotional stress, Arch. Oral Biol. **14:**873, 1969.
9. Yemm, R.: A comparison of the electrical activity of masseter and temporal muscles of human subjects during experimental stress, Arch. Oral Biol. **16:**269, 1971.
10. Molin,C., and Levi, L.: A psycho-odontologic investigation of patients with bruxism, Acta Odontol. Scand. **24:**373, 1966.
11. Guggenheim, P., and Cohen, L.B.: The histopathology of masseteric hypertrophy, Arch. Otolaryngol. **71:**906, 1960.
12. Guggenheim, P., and Cohen, L.B.: External hyperostosis of the mandible angle associated with masseteric hypertrophy, Arch. Otolaryngol. **70:**674, 1959.
13. Zajonc, R.B.: Emotion and facial efference: a theory reclaimed, Science **228:**15, 1985.
14. Butler, J.H., and Stallard, R.E.: Physiologic stress and tooth contact, J. Periodont. Res. **4:**152, 1969.
15. Gottlieb, G., and Paulson, G.: Salivation in depressed patients, Arch. Gen. Psychiatry **5:**468, 1961.
16. Winsor, A.L.: Effects of mental effort on parotid secretion, Am. J. Psychol. **43:**434, 1931.
17. Brothers, J.D., and Warden, C.J.: Analysis of the enzyme activity of the conditioned salivary response in human subjects, Science **112:**751, 1950.
18. Bates, J.F., and Adams, D.: The influence of mental stress on the flow of saliva in man, Arch. Oral Biol. **13:**593, 1968.
19. Starr, H.E.: Hydrogen-ion concentration of mixed saliva considered as index of fatigue and emotional excitation, Am. J. Psychol. **33:**394, 1922.
20. Glickman, I., Turesky, S., and Hill, R.: Determinations of oxygen consumption in normal and inflamed gingival tissue using the Warburg manometric technique, J. Dent. Res. **28:**83, 1949.
21. Glickman, I., Turesky, S., and Manhold, J.H.: The oxygen consumption of healing gingiva, J. Dent. Res. **29:**429, 1950.
22. Manhold, J.H.: Introductory psychosomatic dentistry, New York, 1956, Appleton-Century-Crofts.
23. Manhold, J.H., Doyle, J.L., and Weisinger, E.H.: Effects of social stress on oral and other bodily tissues. II. Results offering substance to a hypothesis for the mechanism of formation of periodontal pathology, J. Periodontol. **42:**109, 1971.
24. Henry, J.P., Meehan, J.P., and Stephens, P.M.: The use of psychosocial stimuli to induce prolonged systolic hypertension in mice, Psychosom. Med. **29:**408, 1967.
25. Giddon, D.B., Cline, C.J., and Gustafson, L.A.: Studies of in vivo vascular reactions of normal human gingiva to cold pressor stimulation, J. Dent. Res. **43:**908, 1964.
26. Giddon, D.B.: Psychophysiology of the oral cavity, J. Dent. Res. Suppl. **45:**1627, 1966.
27. Moulton, R., Ewen, S., and Thieman, W.:

Emotional factors in periodontal disease, Oral Surg. **5:**833, 1952.

28. Sword, R.O.: Oral neglect—why, J. Am. Dent. Assoc. **80:**1327, 1970.

29. Winslow, E.K., and Ferris, R.T.: Developing desired patient behavior, Dent. Clin. North Am. **14:**269, 1970.

30. Ferris, R.T., and Winslow, E.K.: Reinforcing desired behavior with periodontal patients, Dent. Clin. North Am. **14:**279, 1970.

31. Goldhaber, P., and Giddon, D.B.: Present concepts concerning the etiology and treatment of acute necrotizing ulcerative gingivitis, Int. Dent. J. **14:**468, 1964.

32. Everett, F.G.: Necrotizing ulcerative gingivitis. II. Treatment plan, Oregon Dent. J. **26:**2, 1957.

33. Matarazzo, J.D., and Saslow, G.: Psychological and related characteristics of smokers and nonsmokers, Psychol. Bull. **57:**493, 1960.

34. Sheiham, A.: Periodontal disease and cleanliness in tobacco smokers, J. Periodontol. **42:**259, 1971.

35. Arno, A., et al.: Alveolar bone loss as a function of tobacco consumption, Acta Odontol. Scand. **17:**3, 1959.

36. Marrkanen, H., et al.: Smoking and periodontal disease in a Finnish population aged 30 years and over, J. Dent. Res. **64:**932, 1985.

37. Macgregor, I., Edgar, W.M., and Greenwood, A.R.: Effects of cigarette smoking on the rate of plaque formation, J. Clin. Periodontol. **2:**35, 1985.

38. Mellars, N.W., and Herms, F.W.: Investigation of neuropathologic manifestations of oral tissues, Am. J. Orthod. **32:**30, 1946; **33:**812, 1947.

39. Carter, W.J., and Ball, D.M.: Results of a three year study of Vincent's infection at the Great Lakes Naval Dental Dept., J. Periodontol. **24:**187, 1953.

40. Baker, E.G., Crook, G.H., and Schwabacher, E.D.: Personality correlates of periodontal disease, J. Dent. Res. **40:**396, 1961.

41. Davis, R.K., and Baer, P.N.: Necrotizing ulcerative gingivitis in drug addict patients being withdrawn from drugs: report of two cases, Oral Surg. **31:**200, 1971.

42. Formicola, A.J., Witte, E.T., and Curran, P.M.: A study of the personality traits and acute necrotizing ulcerative gingivitis, J. Periodontol. **41:**36, 1970.

43. Sekine, M., and Kakuday, Y.: Resistance or permeability of capillaries in gingiva. Abstracts of papers of oral physiological studies, Department of Physiology, Osaka Dental College, Kyoto, Japan: Rinsko-Shika-Sha, 1962, pp. 145-147. Cited in Giddon, D.B.: Psychophysiology of the oral cavity, J. Dent. Res. **45:**1627, 1966.

44. Giddon, D.B., Clark, R.E., and Vann, J.G.: Apparent vasomotor hypotonicity in the remission stage of acute necrotizing ulcerative gingivitis, J. Dent. Res. **48:**431, 1969.

45. Epstein, R.S., et al.: Psychiatric and histologic findings in an unusual type of chronic gingivitis: report of seven cases, J. Periodontol. **43:**110, 1972.

46. Owings, J.R.: An atypical gingivostomatitis: a report of four cases, J. Periodontol. **40:**538, 1969.

47. Stewart, D.J., and Kernohan, D.C.: Self-inflicted gingival injuries: gingivitis artefacta, factitial gingivitis, Dent. Pract. **22:**418, 1972.

48. Fisher, B.K.: Neurotic excoriations, Can. Med. Assoc. J. **105:**937, 1971.

49. Blanton, P.L., Hurt, W.C., and Largent, M.D.: Oral factitious injuries, J. Periodontol. **48:**33, 1977.

50. Golden, L.M.: Denial of dental problems by patients: a theoretical approach to this question as involved with early development, Ann. Dent. **23:**103, 1961.

51. Druss, R.G., Symonds, F.C., and Crikelair, G.F.: The problem of somatic delusions in patients seeking cosmetic surgery, Plast. Reconstr. Surg. **48:**246, 1971.

52. Lefer, L.: Psychic stress and the oral cavity, Postgrad. Med. **49:**171, 1971.

53. Cleary, M.F.: Postoperative psychiatric disturbance, Penn. Dent. J. **33:**269, 1966.

54. Lefer, L.: Failures in motivation of home care, Dent. Clin. North Am. **16:**3, 1972.

55. Weisenberg, M.: Behavioral motivation, J. Periodontol. **44:**489, 1973.

56. Selye, H.: The stress of life, New York, 1956, McGraw-Hill Book Co.

57. Rabkin, J.G., and Struening, E.L.: Life events, stress, and illness, Science **194:**1013, 1976.

58. Levine, S.: Stress and behavior, Sci. Am. **224:**26, 1971.

59. Weiss, J.M.: Psychologic factors in stress and disease, Sci. Am. **226:**104, 1972.

60. Stein, M., Schiavi, R.C., and Camerino, M.: Influence of brain and behavior on the immune system, Science **191:**435, 1976.

61. Adler, R., editor: Psychoneurobiology, 1981, New York, Academic Press, Inc.

62. Rogers, M.P., Dubey, D., and Reich, P.: The influence of the psyche and the brain on immunity and disease susceptibility: a critical review, Psychosomatic Med. **41:**147, 1979.

## ADDITIONAL SUGGESTED READING

Borland, L.R., and others: Psychology in dentistry: selected references and abstracts, Public Health Service Publication no. 929, Washington, D.C., 1962, U.S. Government Printing Office.

Boyens, P.J.: Value of autosuggestion in the therapy of "bruxism" and other biting habits, J. Am. Dent. Assoc. **27:**1773, 1940.

Cleary, M.F.: Postoperative psychiatric disturbance, Penn. Dent. J. **33:**269, 1966.

Dworkin, S.F.: Psychosomatic concepts and dentistry: some perspectives, J. Periodontol. **40:**647, 1969.

Frenkel, R.E.: Clinical management and treatment of rage, N.Y. State J. Med. **71:**1740, 1971.

Land, M.: Management of emotional illness in dental practice, J. Am. Dent. Assoc. **73:**631, 1966.

Miller, A.A.: Psychologic considerations in dentistry, J. Am. Dent. Assoc. **81:**941, 1970.

Miller, S.C., Thaller, J.L., and Soberman, A.: Use of the Minnesota Multiphasic Personality Inventory as a diagnostic aid in periodontal disease— a preliminary report, J. Periodontol. **27:**44, 1956.

Redman, R.S., et al.: A psychological component in the etiology of geographic tongue, Am. J. Psychiatry **121:**805, 1965.

Ross, M.G.: The contributions of social and behavioral sciences to the health sciences, J. Dent. Res. Suppl. **44:**1104, 1965.

Walsh, J.: Psychologic defense mechanisms in dentistry, Aust. Dent. J. **9:**455, 1964.

Winer, R.A., et al.: Composition of human saliva, parotid gland secretory rate, and electrolyte concentration in mentally subnormal persons, J. Dent. Res. Suppl. **44:**632, 1965.

# CHAPTER 27

# Doctor-patient relationship

## Interview

**Rapport**

The doctor-patient relationship begins to form when the patient first meets the dentist. It crystallizes during the interview. The interview gives the dentist an opportunity to establish rapport,[1] to introduce patient education, and to acquaint the patient with the way in which the practice is conducted. During the interview the chief complaint, the medical history, and the dental history are obtained. Simultaneously the patient is observed for the purpose of making a preliminary evaluation of the individual. The successful observer combines the skills of a clinician with those of the lawyer, psychiatrist, and detective.[2]

In the earlier days of medicine and dentistry, observation was the only tool available to the clinician. Today observation is still employed to evaluate the type of individual who has come for treatment. Moreover, it enables one to know whether there is any relationship between the patient's general health and mental health and his/her dental disease.[3] Such information can be gleaned by astute questioning, examining, recording, and observing.

**Observation**

A good share of observation consists of being attentive to the patient's manner of response. Much is revealed by the patient's choice of words, tone of voice, facial expression, and movements during the time of answering questions. These reactions tend to be heightened in the dental office, since dentistry represents a stress situation to many patients.[4]

While the dentist is observing the patient, most likely the patient will be appraising the dentist. Therefore the interview should be conducted in a relaxed, self-assured manner. A professional bearing is appropriate but be attentive and sympathetic rather than aloof and cool. Let the patient do the talking. Should the patient ask questions, limit answers to the shortest and simplest possible. Above all, do not lecture the patient on the subject of dentistry.[5]

**Questioning**

Sometimes, when the patient asks questions concerning dentistry, he/she may be expressing anxiety rather than an interest in dentistry. The more experienced practitioner will sense this anxiety and reassure the patient, thus dealing with what is at the root of the question. In addition to words, the dentist's manner of approach will convey a competence to the patient that will be reassuring. The less experienced practitioner will often deliver a long discourse on dentistry that does not satisfy the patient's need, leaving the patient with a feeling of frustration.

On occasion the patient will ask a question that in reality reflects a doubt not expressed in words. If this is sensed, attempt to make the patient verbalize the doubt so that it can be brought into the open and then dealt with. A question should be regarded as a clue. Unresolved doubts of the patient may interfere with the course of treatment at a later time.

## Psychologic factors

An awareness of the patient's emotional structure can be significant, since the patient relates with emotional overtones to the disease, its treatment, and to the dentist also. Since periodontal disease may have psychosomatic facets (Chapter 26), it is important for the dentist to be alert to such a likelihood in the patient. It is possible for the dentist to have psychologic awareness without specific training. Although a capacity for warmth and feeling for people may occur naturally, it can also be developed if one learns to relax and to listen to what the patient is really saying. Qualities of sensitivity, perception, and insight can be nurtured by devoting adequate time to the interview. Some knowledge of these qualities is as important to the dentist as it is to the physician.

Without being aware of it, patients exhibit clues to their emotional makeup and to what they are really thinking. The dentist who detects and interprets these clues correctly is in a position to help the patient so that a minimum of stress and a maximum of benefit are received from treatment.[6-9] Such an insight into the patient's behavior requires patience and diagnostic acumen. Everything the patient says or does usually has a reason. No reaction or response, not even a jest, is meaningless. Responses are clues to the unconscious. The unconscious is generally well hidden, and the patient is unaware of its influence on his/her behavior, but the observer can detect the behavior and through it interpret the unconscious.

**Parent-child relationship**

The dentist, in a sense, symbolizes a parent; a parent-child relationship may develop with many patients. With it, such childhood attitudes as dependence, rebelliousness, and affection may be reenacted during the course of treatment. Since dentistry may be threatening or painful, ingrained attitudes toward sickness, pain, and death may be displayed. The patient may come to the dentist with many preconceived notions. These tend to set the stage for the actual relationship and color the technical aspects of treatment.

The mouth provides satisfactions and is used in eating, talking, fighting, sensing, and loving. Many neurotic conflicts are centered about the mouth. The dentist must deal with the patient's psychologic structure and the mouth as a center for emotional manifestations. Unfortunately the dentist is not a neuter in treatment; his/her psyche enters into treatment through the patient-dentist relationship in a manner that is reflected in the attitude toward and treatment of the patient.[10]

### PSYCHIATRIC MANIFESTATIONS DURING THERAPY

**Occlusal dis-harmony**

Several relatively common situations occur during treatment that are laden with emotional significance. For example, some patients with mental distress may complain of an imbalance of occlusion, unconsciously hoping that a balancing of the occlusion will result in a "balancing" of the mind. Other patients, detesting some phase of their emotional structure and unconsciously wishing to have it removed, may repeatedly seek surgery of other structures (polysurgical addiction), including peri-

**Polysurgical addiction**

**Rigidity**

**Omnipotence**

**Value judgments**

**Referral**

odontal surgery. Naturally the dental treatment cannot eliminate the mental symptoms.

Some situations involve the patient who, because of deep anxiety and rigidity, attempts to ensure the success of treatment by choosing a therapist who will serve in an omnipotent, godlike capacity. This distortion of the role of the therapist supports the neurotic dentist who feels endowed with such godlike abilities. Such an interaction results in an unhealthy dentist-patient relationship. Treatment is not regarded as a joint venture. The patient cannot tolerate untoward or unexpected developments. The situations can be traumatic to both neurotic personalities.

The degree to which behavior is logical, purposeful, and free of anxiety is a measure of mental health in both dentist and patient; the reverse is a measure of neurosis. All people have neuroses. Neuroses should not indicate disgrace or stigma since they are matters of personal health. The neurosis represents some carefully self-selected adjustment to inner conflict. Although people are not consciously aware of the roots of their neuroses, they nurture and hold these neuroses dear on an unconscious level. Essentially we approve of our own neuroses, but we are critical of the neuroses of other people.

The dentist should treat the patient with friendliness and respect, not with criticism or condemnation. He/she should not develop "holier-than-thou" feelings, make snide remarks, or render value judgments. The patient should be treated with tact and courtesy. The dentist must be sincerely concerned with the welfare of the patients and this should take precedence over dentistry as a business. He/she should try to understand the patient as well as the patient's dental illness. The dentist is often not sufficiently well prepared to meet the psychologic demands of the patient or guide the development of new attitudes in patients concerning treatment and health; yet all facets of treatment, in particular those involving reeducation of the patient, require such training. Although the dentist should conduct a practice in a psychologically sensitive manner, he/she should not attempt psychotherapy per se.

Some dentists state that they have patients in their practice whom they regard as "a pain in the neck." After a particularly bad session with such a patient, the dentist may feel ready to give up dentistry. These feelings are indicative of the fact that not every dentist can treat every patient; neither can the dentist truly understand what role the patient is acting out during the dental visit. If the dentist perceives a rising level of nervousness or anger, he/she would be best advised to try to determine what he/she or the patient may be doing to precipitate this state of events and if possible deal with its basic cause. When the situation appears to be unmanageable, the patient should be referred to another dentist or physician. The dentist feels less angry when there is no compulsion to comply with impossible demands. This can be done by setting limits for the patient's behavior. The dentist should not view the patient as a threat to himself/herself or his/her competence.

The patient should be reassured, not threatened. By developing a therapeutically appropriate relationship with the patient, the dentist is capable of providing the utmost of comfort and benefit to the patient.

## Patient compliance in health care

No other area in health care has more psychological overtones than patient compliance with prescriptions for medication, exercise, diet, smoking, drinking, and plaque control. Measures to increase patient compliance with home care instructions are needed and are being studied with increasing frequency. Self-care motivation is a necessary basis for successful preventive dentistry. The following example of a student-patient interaction during a period of plaque-control instruction is illustrative of the importance of psychologic sensitivity in patient motivation.

**July 17** This was Leo H.'s first plaque-control visit. He is a very pleasant man and seems eager to learn. I used disclosing solution and pointed out all the plaque to him. There was plaque everywhere; his plaque-free score was 1.1%.* Leo told me he had not brushed after lunch, but I told him that the amount of plaque in his mouth was not solely the result of failing to brush after lunch. He had brought his toothbrush with him, so I asked him to show me how he brushed. Basically, he is doing it correctly. He gets the bristles in at a 45-degree angle and vibrates, following with a sweep down the tooth. He is a bit awkward with the lingual surfaces, but at least he can control the brush. I suggested a couple of ways to make holding the brush easier, and he was receptive. I asked him if he used floss, and he said yes. I gave him some, and he showed me how he flossed. Again, he *knows* how to do it. I just reminded him how important it is to draw the floss tightly around the line angles of each tooth. I then went over the basics of plaque control and its relation to periodontal disease. Leo knew all about it and promised a drastic improvement on the next visit.

**July 20** Leo was true to his word. After disclosing, I was encouraged to see a great reduction in the amount of plaque. His score was 56.6%. Most of the plaque was in the maxillary lingual and mandibular interproximal areas. He forgot his brush, so we went over flossing and inter-proximal areas. Leo was happy with the improvement and told me how much better his mouth feels. He seemed gung ho, and I really believe he will continue the good work.

**July 24** Bad day. Leo was full of excuses, ranging from "I was so busy this weekend, I just couldn't find enough time" to the old "I didn't brush after lunch." His score was 20.7%. I was disappointed and let him know it. Again, no brush. He is flossing correctly. The basic problem here is laziness and just not enough concern. Even though his mouth *feels* better when he takes care of it, and even though he has paid a lot of money and had surgery, he does not seem to care about maintaining oral health. More promises.

**July 28** Leo forgot his appointment because it was a Friday instead of Thursday. He was very sorry when I called him but couldn't leave his office. We arranged another appointment for Monday.

**July 31** Again, no Leo. It turned out he was on his way to the clinic and suddenly became violently ill. *Very* sorry. I was worried about him but am getting to the point where I didn't quite believe everything he tells me. Next appointment for tomorrow.

**August 1** Leo made it to this one. Today he had an additional line: "I haven't been feeling well, so. . . ." Plaque-free score was 7.7%. I can't believe it. He had a gingivoplasty done recently and says his mandibular centrals are much too tender to touch. I told him he could *not* ignore the area any more and to brush and floss, but gently at first. I explained how the tissues need the stimulation to heal. This made sense, but whether he will do it remains to be seen. He is really beginning to make me angry, and I will probably start screaming the next time I see him. How angry can I get? How much can I lecture him? Why won't he do what he says he will? Why won't he do what he says he *does*? Why should I care if he has a lot of plaque in his mouth if he doesn't even care? This is a *very frustrating* business!

## Summary

Psychologic factors may affect tissue physiology and contribute to periodontal disease. Knowledge concerning the definitive mechanisms of such alteration is lacking or incomplete. Nevertheless, understanding of periodontal disease and its treatment requires some awareness of the patient and his/her particular psychologic makeup. Although specific steps in treatment may be performed on a symptomatic basis, it is well to keep in mind that symptoms occur in people. Some dentists prefer to think of teeth, jaws, and mouth in an isolated sense. What in a living organism is really isolated?

---

*Score ranges from 0% to 100%, with scores of 85% or higher indicating good plaque control.

The patient of today readily accepts that psychologic stress affects other body organs, so why not the oral structure? Even in the most technical manipulation, the dentist is required to treat the whole patient[11]; only by doing so does he/she fulfill his/her professional responsibility.

## REFERENCES

1. Cinotti, W.R., and Grieder, A.: Applied psychology in dentistry, St. Louis, 1964, The C.V. Mosby Co.
2. Stern, I.B.: Case history and examination: University of Washington periodontics syllabus, Seattle, 1959, University of Washington Press.
3. Beck, F.M., Kaul, T.J., and Weaver, J.N. II: Recognition and management of the depressed dental patient, J. Am. Dent. Assoc. **99:**967, 1979.
4. Dember, W.N.: The psychology of perception, New York, 1960, Holt, Rinehart & Winston, Inc.
5. Gale, E.N., et al.: Effects of dentists' behavior on patient's attitudes, J. Am. Dent. Assoc. **109:**444, 1984.
6. Raper, H.R.: The art of consultation with the dental patient, N.Y. J. Dent. **33:**176, 1963.
7. Beldoch, M.: Sensitivity to the communication of feelings, Trans. N.Y. Acad. Sci. **24:**317, 1962.
8. Weckstein, M.S.: Practical applications of basic psychiatry to dentistry, Dent. Clin. North Am. **14:**397, 1970.
9. Cowen, J., and Friedman, W.F.: Psychologic considerations in long-term dental care, Dent. Surveys, p. 34, 1971.
10. Rankin, J.A. and Harris, M.B.: Patients' preferences for dentists' behaviors, J. Am. Dent. Assoc. **110:**323, 1985.
11. Corah, N.L., O'Shea, R.M., and Skeels, D.K.: Dentists' perceptions of problem behaviors in patients, J. Am. Dent. Assoc. **104:**829, 1982.

## ADDITIONAL SELECTED READING

Baume, P.: The doctor in the doctor-patient relationship, Med. J. Aust. **2:**323, 1974.

Ewen, S.: Dynamics of the dental interview—a guided psychological process, N.Y. J. Dent. **37:**139, 1967.

Fusco, M.A.: Munchausen's syndrome: report of a case, J. Am. Dent. Assoc. **112:**210, 1986.

Garfield, E.: Treating the whole person: the use of social sciences information in medical libraries, Curr. Contents **22:**5, 1977.

Glavind, L.: The result of periodontal treatment in relationship to various background factors, J. Clin. Periodontol. **13:**789, 1986.

Korsch, B.M., and Negrete, V.F.: Doctor-patient communication, Sci. Am. **227:**66, 1972.

Morrow, R.G.: Communication with patients in a general practice, Dent. Clin. North Am. **14:**241, 1970.

Newberger, H.M.: Psychologic factors influencing the dentist patient relationship, J. Dent. Med. **11:**16, 1956.

Shour, E.: Interpersonal relationships in dental practice, Alpha Omegan **58:**123, 1965.

Sword, R.O.: Psychologic aspects of the doctor-patient relationship, Dent. Surv., p. 64, Nov. 1965.

Ward, N.G., and Stein, L.: Reducing emotional distance: a new method to teach interviewing skills, J. Med. Educ. **50:**605, 1975.

# CHAPTER 28

# Examination and diagnosis: classification

**Examination**
Interview
Medical history
Medical laboratory tests
Dental history
Dental laboratory tests
Oral examination
Periodontal examination
Roentgenographic examination
Occlusal analysis

**Integration of data**

**Diagnosis**

**Classification**

**Reexaminations**

---

Before dental diseases can be treated, they must be recognized and diagnosed. Adequate dental care demands that all patients receive an acceptable clinical examination. This examination should include a medical and dental history as well as a clinical and roentgenographic examination. The purpose of the history, clinical examination, and diagnosis is to arrive at a logical plan of treatment to eliminate or alleviate the patient's signs and symptoms of dental disease and to prevent further destructive changes.[1]

## Examination

The procedures of examination lend themselves to a systematic routine. All the information obtained should be charted. This is a simple means of documentation, which helps in the development of a diagnosis and treatment plan. The findings of the examination, the diagnosis, the prognosis, and the treatment plan, all of which relate directly to each other, may be determined with a greater degree of accuracy on the basis of measured observations. A flow sheet, such as that on p. 526, is helpful. The individual steps can be followed sequentially.

In addition to the disease process, another threat to longevity of the natural dentition is lack of awareness on the part of the patient. The patient may not know about periodontal disease or may not be motivated toward treatment. The responsibility then falls on the dentist to educate and motivate the patient. This is possible when an appropriate dentist-patient relationship has been established. This step occurs during the interview and examination.

**EXAMINATION AND DIAGNOSIS FLOW SHEET**

☐ Interview (case history)        ☐ Occlusal examination        ☐ Etiologic factors
☐ Clinical examination            ☐ Listing of findings          ☐ Prognosis
☐ Roentgenographic examination    ☐ Diagnosis                    ☐ Treatment plan

The examination must contain the following elements noted in the chart:
1. Chief complaint
2. Medical history
3. Soft tissue examination
4. Periodontal charting
    a. Pocket depths
    b. Outline of margins, particularly if recession is present or the gingiva is narrow
    c. Mobilities
5. Occlusal analysis, if mobility or roentgenographic signs of periodontal traumatism are present
6. Synopsis of past dental treatment

The report should relate the above findings condensed to narrative form and should list the following in table form:
1. Diagnosis
2. Etiology
3. Prognosis
4. Treatment plan

The report should defend each step in the reasoning process involved in establishing (1) the diagnosis, (2) the etiology, (3) the prognosis, and (4) the treatment plan.

The treatment plan is divided into three phases as follows (recharting of pocket depths and gingival response should follow each phase of treatment before proceeding to the next phase):

Phase I     Plaque control instruction, root planing, occlusal adjustment, gingival and subgingival curettage

Phase II    Reconstructive surgery (grafting, mucogingival surgery, osseous surgery) and excisional surgery (gingivectomy, open curettage, Widman flap, ostectomy)

Phase III   Final occlusal adjustment, tooth polishing, scaling and root planing, plaque control instruction, treatment of tooth sensitivity, gingivoplasty

## INTERVIEW

The first step in an examination is the patient interview. It should be used with all new patients. It may be dispensed with for old patients if the objectives of the interview have been reached previously. The interview gives the dentist an opportunity to establish rapport.

Preliminary information pertaining to the interview may be obtained through printed forms. These are not intended to supplant but rather to supplement and expedite the interview.

During the interview the following information should be elicited[2]: (1) vital statistics, (2) chief complaint, (3) medical history, and (4) dental history.

**Vital statistics**      The vital statistics include the patient's name, home and business addresses and phone numbers, age, sex, marital and family status, and occupation. These are all significant. They give information about the patient and his/her background. By the mode of response, the dentist may be able to gauge the patient's intelligence and estimate the degree of patient cooperation. The source of referral is important too. If the patient was referred by another patient who had periodontal treatment, chances are that he/she is partly informed about periodontal disease and therefore requires less time for patient education. The patient can be tested with a comment such as, "I guess that Mrs. _____ has told you all about periodontal disease." If the answer is negative, proceed as usual. If the answer is positive, the patient should be rewarded with some remark about how unusual it is to have such a well-informed patient.

What is the reason for the patient's visit? Does the patient have pain, discomfort, or any other complaint? Often the patient will come for a routine checkup. However, there will be times when he/she arrives in an emergency, with pain, bleeding, or swelling. In these instances, attend to the emergency as soon as its location and cause have been determined. When there are no medical contraindications or precautions to be taken, the remainder of the interview may be postponed. In any event the dentist may want to know when the condition started and whether it has ever occurred previously.

**Chief complaint**

## MEDICAL HISTORY

To assess the medical status of a new patient, a questionnaire may be filled out by the patient before the actual interview. A typical questionnaire (pp. 528-529) provides a guide to obtaining a complete medical history but does not replace the interview. Some practitioners prefer a questionnaire; others work without such printed guides.

The patient should be asked, "How is your health?" Some patients will respond by giving a detailed answer. Most patients, however, will answer, "Fine." Test this answer by asking some of the following questions: "Have you ever been seriously ill?" "When were you last examined by a physician?" "Who is your physician?" "What was the reason for your last visit to the physician?" "What were the findings?" "Are you under treatment now?" "Have you taken out insurance in the last few years?" "Did you have any difficulty with the insurance examination?" "Did you serve in the armed forces?" "Were you discharged for any medical reason?" "Have you ever been hospitalized? When and for what reason?" "Have you had any operations?" "Do you take any medication or drug regularly?" "Have you had an adverse reaction to any medication?"

When the patient denies a history of diseases of the various organ systems, the negative answers need not be recorded.[3,4] Generally, specific inquiries should be made concerning the heart and circulatory system, respiratory system, genitourinary system, allergies, endocrinopathies, and blood dyscrasias. If all the answers are negative, the notation should read, "Medical history noncontributory." Certain negative answers, however, must be recorded. These are the answers to questions such as: "Have you ever had rheumatic fever?" "Have you had hepatitis?" "Have you ever taken antibiotics?" "Are you allergic to any antibiotics?" "Are you sensitive to aspirin, or have you ever experienced any unusual reactions from local anesthetics or codeine?" "Do you take aspirin regularly?" All information of medical significance should be recorded. List briefly the essential factors in the patient's medical history that might be of significance to his/her periodontal disease (e.g., pregnancy, diabetes, dysfunction of ovaries, thyroid, or other endocrine gland) or that might affect the course of the treatment or require certain precautions (history of rheumatic or valvular heart disease, joint replacements, high blood pressure, use of anticoagulants or regular use of aspirin, blood dyscrasia, hepatitis, syphilis, kidney disease, AIDS). If the patient is receiving anticoagulants or aspirin, the dentist must confer with the patient's physician as to the feasibility of surgery; the use of anticoagulants or drugs containing aspirin should be discontinued before surgery. Inquiry should be made regarding the adequacy of the patient's diet, disturbances of the digestive tract, diseases of the lungs, and allergic

## MEDICAL HISTORY

Name _____ Home address _____

Physician's name _____ Address _____

How old are you? _____ Circle if you are: single, married, widowed, separated, divorced

Circle the highest year you reached in school:

| 1 2 3 4 5 6 7 8 | 1 2 3 4 |
|---|---|
| Elementary | High |

| 1 2 3 4 5 6 7 8 |
|---|
| College |

What is your occupation? _____

_____

**Directions:** If your answer is yes to the question asked, put a circle around "Yes." If your answer is no, put a circle around "No." Answer all the questions. Answers to these questions are for our records only, and they will be considered confidential.

| | | |
|---|---|---|
| 1. Are you being treated for any condition by a physician now? | No | Yes |
| 2. Are you taking any medicines now? | No | Yes |
| 3. Have you been examined by your physician within the last year? | No | Yes |
| 4. Has there been any change in your general health in the last year? | No | Yes |
| 5. Have you ever been seriously ill? | No | Yes |
| 6. Have you ever been hospitalized? | No | Yes |
| 7. Have you ever had a major operation? | No | Yes |
| 8. Have you ever had a blood transfusion? | No | Yes |
| 9. Have you ever had any of the following diseases? | | |
|     Rheumatic fever | No | Yes |
|     Inflammatory rheumatism | No | Yes |
|     Jaundice (yellow skin and eyes) | No | Yes |
|     Tuberculosis | No | Yes |
|     Venereal disease | No | Yes |
|     Heart attack or stroke | No | Yes |
|     AIDS | No | Yes |
| 10. Have you ever been told by a physician that you have a heart murmur? | No | Yes |
| 11. Do you ever have asthma or hay fever? | No | Yes |
| 12. Do you ever have hives or skin rash? | No | Yes |
| 13. Have you ever experienced an unusual reaction to any of the following drugs? | | |
|     Aspirin | No | Yes |
|     Penicillin | No | Yes |
|     Iodine | No | Yes |
|     Sulfonamides (sulfa) | No | Yes |
|     Barbiturates (sleeping pills) | No | Yes |
|     Other medicines | No | Yes |
| 14. Have you ever experienced an unusual reaction to a dental anesthetic? | No | Yes |
| 15. Do you have diabetes (sugar disease)? | No | Yes |
| 16. Do you have high blood pressure? | No | Yes |
| 17. Do you bleed for a long time when you cut yourself? | No | Yes |
| 18. Have you ever had an injury to your face or jaws? | No | Yes |
| 19. Have you ever had surgery or x-ray treatment for a tumor, growth, or other condition in your mouth or on your lips? | No | Yes |

## MEDICAL HISTORY—cont'd

**Systems review**

20. Do you have frequent severe headaches?    No    Yes
21. Do you have any complaints regarding your eyes?    No    Yes
22. Do you have any ear trouble?    No    Yes
23. Do you have frequent colds?    No    Yes
24. Do you have sinus trouble?    No    Yes
25. Do you have nosebleeds?    No    Yes
26. Do you have frequent sore throats?    No    Yes
27. Do you have any sensitive teeth?    No    Yes
28. Have you ever had a toothache?    No    Yes
29. Do you have bleeding gums?    No    Yes
30. Do you have frequent canker sores or cold sores?    No    Yes
31. Have you ever had a severely sore mouth?    No    Yes
32. Is it difficult for you to open your mouth as wide as you would like?    No    Yes
33. Does your jaw click when you chew?    No    Yes

**Cardiorespiratory**

34. Do you have any chest pain on exertion?    No    Yes
35. Are you ever short of breath on mild exertion?    No    Yes
36. Do your ankles swell?    No    Yes
37. Do you have a persistent cough?    No    Yes
38. Do you ever cough blood?    No    Yes

**Gastrointestinal**

39. Has your appetite changed recently?    No    Yes
40. Are there any foods you cannot eat?    No    Yes
41. Do you have any difficulty swallowing?    No    Yes
42. Do you have frequent indigestion?    No    Yes
43. Do you vomit frequently?    No    Yes

**Genitourinary**

44. Do you have kidney trouble?    No    Yes
45. Do you urinate more than six times a day?    No    Yes
46. Are you thirsty much of the time?    No    Yes

**Bones and joints**

47. Have you ever had painful and swollen joints?    No    Yes

**Neuromuscular**

48. Do you have any numb or prickling areas on your skin?    No    Yes
49. Do you ever have fits or convulsions?    No    Yes
50. Do you have a tendency to faint?    No    Yes

**Hematology**

51. Do you bruise easily?    No    Yes
52. Do you have any blood disorder such as anemia (thin blood)?    No    Yes

**Endocrines and metabolism**

53. Does hot weather bother you more than it does other people you know?    No    Yes
54. Are you excessively nervous?    No    Yes
55. Do you get tired easily?    No    Yes

**Women**

56. Are you pregnant at the present time?    No    Yes
57. Have you passed the menopause (change of life)?    No    Yes
58. Are your menstrual periods irregular?    No    Yes

Courtesy A.E. Fry, University of Oregon Dental School.

reactions.* Note should be made of the date and any type of general surgery that has been performed. Whether the patient has ever been uprated or rejected by an insurance company as an impaired risk should also be noted.[1-3]

During this portion of the examination, the dentist-patient relationship tends to crystallize. Rapport is established, which can be significant in all future relationships. Throughout the questioning period the examiner should be conscious of cancer and alert to any leads such as weight loss, swellings, and ulcers. Most patients are cancer conscious, too, so the examiner must be careful never by word or action to arouse a patient's anxiety and then leave his/her fears unanswered. Even a chance remark such as "hmm" will frighten some people. Observations of nervous habits and any abnormal condition of the skin, hair, and fingernails should be noted. Also any tic, ptosis, unusual expression, or unusual posture or gait should be recorded.

There are separate questions to ask women relating to childbearing, menarche, and menopause. If the patient is or has been married, ask her whether she has any children and how many. "Did you have any unusual trouble at the time of their births?" "Did you have trouble with your gums or teeth during pregnancy?" "Is your menstrual cycle regular?" Where appropriate, determine whether the patient has reached menopause.

An attempt should also be made to determine the patient's nervous state. "Do you get up tired?" may elicit a laugh and the answer "I'm always tired." Then the examiner must determine whether this is a joke or the patient is indeed serious. "Do you sleep well at night?" "Is your heartbeat regular?" "How is your appetite?" While asking these questions, reach out and gently take the patient's hand to examine the palm. Is it wet? Does the patient consider himself/herself nervous? Any affirmative answers may be suggestive of neurosis. Develop the habit of watching the patient's upper lip and brow for perspiration, which may be a sign of tension. The patient who yawns during the interview may be tense not bored.[1-3]

Careful interrogation of the patient may yield significant information concerning present physical status or may provide clues to undetected disease. Medical inventory questionnaires are available, but these have shortcomings if used routinely. They do not constitute an interview. Also an interview does not constitute an examination; rather the patient relates his/her history and symptoms, which may not be completely accurate. However, the manner in which the patient expresses himself/herself may be significant. The medical inventory questionnaire cannot detect nuances in the patient's response.

The dentist is handicapped in the total evaluation of the patient's health insofar as he/she does not do and interpret physical examinations at the present time. Dental education is currently preparing dentists to make physical examinations. There is no reason, however, why the dentist cannot call for competent medical consultation when he/she believes it necessary. On the other hand, routine medical examination may fail to supply additional information. When specific positive findings are present, there may be a relationship to the patient's dental status.

When both medical and oral signs of disease are present, important relationships

---

*Colored tags may be affixed to the patient's chart to alert the dentist to some systemic or local condition that must be considered. A red tag indicates the presence of a systemic condition that should be noted on the tag (cardiovascular disease, history of rheumatic fever, diabetes, ulcers, allergies, or that the patient is taking medication such as cortisone or anticoagulants). A yellow tag may be used to indicate that the patient is apprehensive and that some premedication such as a tranquilizer should be given or prescribed. A green tag may indicate tooth or gingival sensitivity to probing or to other instrumentation such as root planing. The condition may then be entered in a prominent place on the outside of the chart entitled "Alert."

may be demonstrable. Protein-calorie nutritional deficiency has been related to periodontal disease and to a depressed immune response. Gingival bleeding and bruisability may be related. Tooth mobility can be related to ascorbic acid metabolism or carbohydrate metabolism. Clinical experience may indicate that changes in tissue form, color, and consistency may be suggestive of intrinsic disturbance even if the examiner cannot demonstrate the specific deficiency.

## MEDICAL LABORATORY TESTS

Sometimes after the interview the dentist may believe that laboratory tests should be performed or that medical consultation might be desirable. Blood smears, biopsies, blood tests, and urine tests may at times be indicated to identify systemic factors that might affect or modify periodontal treatment.

**Medical laboratory tests and consultation**

Although the routine use of medical laboratory tests is rarely productive for the periodontist, such tests are of undisputed value when the examiner is suspicious of specific intrinsic pathologic conditions. No startling results have been forthcoming when routine clinical tests were made on patients with periodontal disease. This fact may indicate that patients with periodontal disease can be intrinsically well, which would be an oddity, since studies indicate that 92% of presumably healthy patients are actually afflicted with disease. Finally, one would presume that when specific intrinsic factors are present and are related to periodontal disease, intrinsic medication would cure the disease. This has not been the case. However, when a related intrinsic deficiency has been adequately altered, local treatment appeared to be more effective. Beyond this, except for gingival changes in intrinsic diseases, such as leukemia, nutritional deficiencies, diabetes, and bone changes in osteodystrophies, little is known about the precise relationship between intrinsic factors and periodontal disease.

## DENTAL HISTORY

When the chief complaint is of a nonemergency nature, obtain in the patient's own words the history of the present oral illness from its inception until the present time. "Have you ever had any treatment for this condition?" "What was it as you recall?" "Did you complete your treatment?" "Did you carry out your part of the treatment?" On occasion, the fact that the patient is stoic and has minimized an emergency situation will become evident. Conversely, occasionally an anxious patient may appear as an emergency case with what is actually a minor complaint. Whatever information the patient volunteers should be followed by questions in logical order so that as much as possible can be learned. Some particularly astute examiners pose the same question in two different ways to check the accuracy of the answers.

The dental history should include all dental treatments rendered in the past (orthodontics, prosthetic appliances, removal of impacted teeth). Additionally the history should include such items as the following: approximate dates of previous periodontal treatment (root planing, curettage, gingival surgery, osseous surgery, occlusal adjustment, splinting, plaque control instruction). Note the history of previous complaints (gingival bleeding, periodontal abscesses, pain, burning, bad taste, bad breath, pathologic tooth migration). Question the patient with regard to rapidity of new formation of plaque, stain, and calcified deposits. The patient's periodontal complaint should be recorded in his/her own words. Entries such as the following should be made: "gums bleed on brushing," "gums hurt," "certain teeth loose," "some teeth moved," "teeth extremely sensitive to cold," "bad breath or bad taste."

Many patients will present a preconceived idea of dentistry that does not include periodontal treatment. Such patients must be educated as to why the examination is conducted as it is. They will have to be made aware of the existence of periodontal disease. Their education is best accomplished with casual sentences during the interview and the examination.

If the interview has progressed smoothly, a 1-minute introduction to periodontal treatment (such as the following) may be in order, which will lead directly to the examination.

"At one time patients came to the dentist only in emergency situations, when they had a toothache or needed an extraction. Of course, each diseased tooth once had a very small cavity or beginning periodontal disease that could have been treated simply. It is now seldom necessary to extract a tooth unless caries or periodontal disease are far advanced. I am now going to make a careful examination to detect decay and periodontal disease. Is that all right?"

Most patients will consent to this examination. Some may ask what periodontal disease is. An explanation that this condition was once called "pyorrhea" should be sufficient. Then give a brief, simple description of periodontal disease and mention that the word "pyorrhea" was used when the disease was considered hopeless. The disease can now be treated successfully, so the name is no longer used.

Some patients will ask more detailed questions at this point; these represent clues to deeper-lying doubts. The examiner's objective is then to unmask the basic reason for the question and to properly educate the patient. Do not become hostile and argumentative. Responses should consist of a repetition of the preceding explanation and of gaining the patient's acceptance of the principle that it is important to find dental defects when they are just beginning. Elicit why the patient questions the need for the examination. Once the patient has indicated the source from which doubts may stem, the examiner may effectively deal with the doubt in a way that reassures the patient.

## DENTAL LABORATORY TESTS

**Identification of microbial populations in pockets**

At the present time, laboratory tests are not used regularly in the periodontal examination. These may, however, become a part of the periodontal examination in the future. Specific laboratory tests for the sampling and identification of bacteria are available. Routine sampling is complex and time-consuming; recently, however, simplified techniques have been and continue to be developed. These include the use of selective media, immunofluorescence antibody tests, gas-liquid chromatography, sulcular fluid analysis, dark-field and phase-contrast microscopy to assay types of flora.[5-13]

**Gingival sulcular fluid**

The examination of gingival fluid holds particular promise, especially in the monitoring of specific constituents.[14-16]

The flow of gingival fluid may be used to monitor gingival inflammation.[17-22] The clinician may examine subclinical gingival inflammation by measuring sulcular fluid flow and then analyzing the fluid sample for immunologic, chemical, or other constituents (e.g., anaphosphatase, myeloperoxidase, lysozyme, lactoferrin, endotoxin).[15,23-25] The degree of activity can thus be gauged. For example, collagenolytic activity may be measured, or complement components may be identified.[11,20-22]

**OMR**

Orogranulocytic migratory rate (OMR),[26-30] that is, the rate of entry of leukocytes into saliva or gingival fluid, may become a clinical tool if there is improvement and simplification of harvesting techniques.[31] A positive correlation has been demonstrated between OMR and the gingival index.[32-34] There is an increased concentration of endotoxins obtained from gingival washings in gingivitis.[35]

**Gingivitis fluorescein test**

Sodium fluorescein swallowed in a capsule for the gingivitis test enters the saliva through the gingival fluid. The amount recovered correlates with the clinical severity of gingivitis.[36,37]

Advances in immunology have suggested that rapid diagnostic tests may soon be available on a routine basis. These include tests designed to measure polymorphonuclear (PMN) leukocyte chemotaxis and phagocytosis. Tests involving chemotaxis of PMNs include the following: **Immune function tests**

1. Adherence assay
2. Leukotaxis assay of both cells and serum
3. Stimulated nitroblue tetrazolium reduction
4. Phagocytosis and killing of *Staphylococcus aureus*
5. Levels of immunoglobulins in saliva or serum[38-40]

## ORAL EXAMINATION

The intraoral examination consists of an inspection of the soft tissues (including the gingiva), the teeth, the occlusion, and the temporomandibular joint. Full-mouth roentgenograms should be taken. In addition, study models and Kodachrome photographs of the dentition may be helpful. It may be necessary to test the vitality of the teeth. The date of the examination should be noted. All data should be carefully charted because they become a part of the patient's record. **Intraoral examination**

A proper dental examination pays attention to the soft tissues as well as the teeth. The condition of the following should be observed: tongue, buccal mucosa, floor of the mouth, palate, frena, throat, and oral mucosa. Do the amount and consistency of saliva appear normal? Are there variations in the color, contour, or firmness of the gingiva (see Chapter 15, Plate 6)? Is the form of the gingiva physiologic: (Plate 7, p. 534, and Fig. 28-1)? Is the gingiva firm or is it retractable and does it bleed easily (Fig. 28-2)? Is the vestibule shallow or deep? Is the zone of gingiva narrow or broad (Fig. 28-3)? Does the patient have pain? Are there areas of food impaction? Are any other possible local causes evident? Does the patient relate a history of trench mouth or pyorrhea, recurrent cold sores, cankers or mouth blisters, dental abscesses, sinus trouble, swellings, or pain? Is there evidence of these in the mouth? **Soft tissues**

The clinical gingival findings can be classified according to the following:

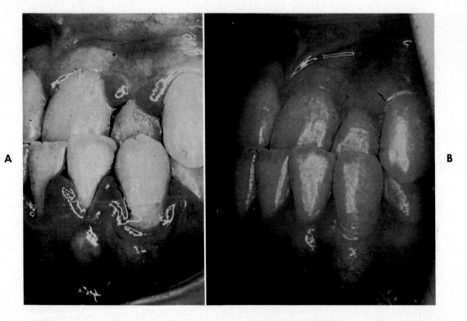

**Fig. 28-1.** *Compare the nonphysiologic,* **A,** *and physiologic,* **B,** *forms of the gingivae in the same patient before and after treatment.*

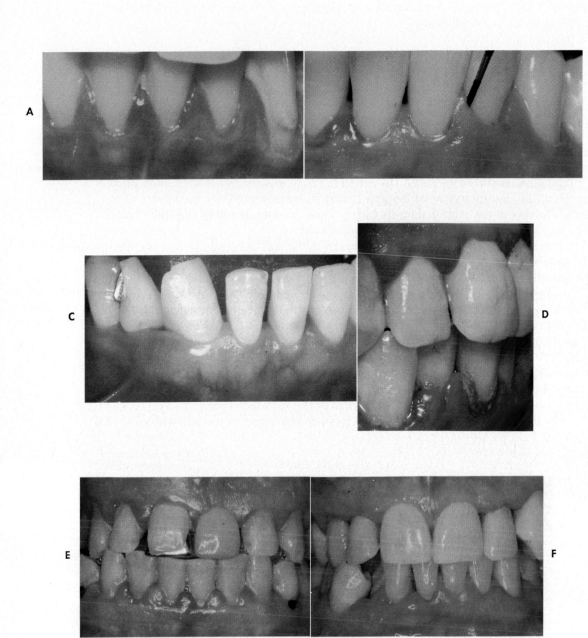

**Plate 7.** Variations in gingival inflammatory responses to plaque. **A,** Edematous papilla, recession under canine. **B,** Papillary and marginal inflammation, pocket formation. **C,** Crater formation between malpositioned lateral incisor and canine. **D,** Enlarged, swollen papillae and heavy calculus deposits. **E,** Fibrotic enlarged papillae. **F,** Combination of cratering and gingival enlargement. (Color courtesy Hu Freidy Dental Manufacturing Co.)

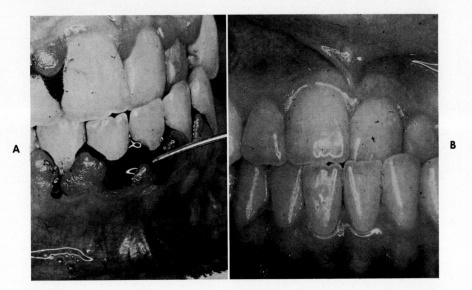

**Fig. 28-2.** Compare the edematous, bleeding gingivae before **(A)** and the firm, noninflamed gingivae after **(B)** treatment.

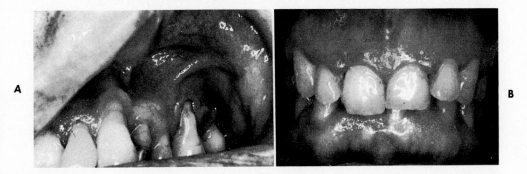

**Fig. 28-3.** **A,** Note the narrow gingiva associated with recession at canine and first molar. Pockets extend beyond the mucogingival junction. **B,** Wide gingiva. Pockets are present but do not extend beyond the mucogingival junction.

1. *Distribution of lesions.* Localized or generalized
2. *Extent of lesions.* Papillary, marginal, or gingival
3. *State of inflammation.* Acute or chronic
4. *Clinical factors.* Gingival color changes, hyperplasia, ulceration, necrosis, formation of pseudomembranes, depth of pockets, exudation, bleeding on probing, abnormal muscle attachments or frena, recession or cleft, width of gingiva, relation of pockets to mucogingival junction, furcation involvements.

In examining the gingiva, the clinician must keep the picture of the "normal" gingiva in mind. With this as a guide, he/she can more readily observe the extent and state of inflammation and the distribution of the lesions.

The size of the teeth should be noted, and the degree of caries susceptibility should **Teeth** be gauged by the number of restorations and cavities. The type and quality of restorations should be evaluated. In addition, erosions should be noted. The biting surfaces should be examined for excessive occlusal wear. When this is evident, the patient should be questioned as to whether he/she grinds the teeth or chews on one side only.

| Tooth no. | 3 | | 9 | | 12 | | |
|---|---|---|---|---|---|---|---|
| Facial and lingual scores | F M G D | L | F M G D | L | F M G D | L | Record in circle the score on all 6 teeth. |
| Total | | | | | | | |
| Facial and lingual scores | F M G D | L | F M G D | L | F M G D | L | |
| Total | | | | | | | |
| Tooth no. | 28 | | 25 | | 19 | | |

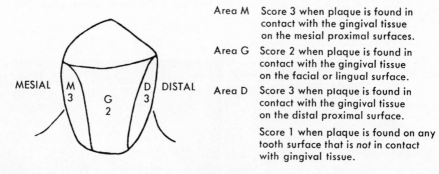

MESIAL  M 3  G 2  D 3  DISTAL

Area M  Score 3 when plaque is found in contact with the gingival tissue on the mesial proximal surfaces.

Area G  Score 2 when plaque is found in contact with the gingival tissue on the facial or lingual surface.

Area D  Score 3 when plaque is found in contact with the gingival tissue on the distal proximal surface.

Score 1 when plaque is found on any tooth surface that is *not* in contact with gingival tissue.

**Fig. 28-4.** Plaque Index survey form useful for screening and for patient education. (Modified from F. Grossman, United States Navy.)

Does he/she chew tobacco? Is he/she unhappy with the appearance of the mouth? Diastemata should be noted, and proximal contacts tested with dental floss. Conditions such as toothbrush abrasion, tooth mobility, tooth malpositions, hypoplastic enamel, supernumerary teeth, nonvital teeth, and tooth sensitivity should be recorded. For tooth sensitivity, questions may be asked concerning the effects of temperature extremes and sweets. The teeth may be percussed.

**Oral hygiene**
The general status of oral hygiene should be ascertained. Note the presence of plaque, stain, and calculus. A disclosing solution may be used to show the patient the presence of plaque. In addition, the patient may be questioned concerning the date of the last prophylaxis, the method and frequency of toothbrushing, and cleaning aids used in an attempts to gauge the rate of calculus deposition.

**Plaque survey**
At this time some practitioners take a plaque survey. The score indicates the status of the patient's oral hygiene as shown by the stained plaque. During treatment complete indices can be taken and compared with earlier indices to note improvement or lack of improvement in plaque control.

A typical survey index is shown in Fig. 28-4. Originally such indices were designed for epidemiologic studies. These studies have shown that a direct relationship exists between plaque and gingivitis. The oral hygiene index has been extended to office use for preventive periodontics and screening examinations.

**Disclosing solutions and tablets**
Disclosing solutions and tablets may be used to make plaque visible. Disclosing solutions impart a bright red color to the plaque, stains, and calcified deposits. Two-

toned disclosing solutions may be applied to distinguish between old and new plaque. The solutions also stain the imperfect margins of plastic fillings and the mucosa of the lips, cheeks, tongue, and floor of the mouth. Because these stains tend to last on mucosal surfaces for several hours, some patients object to the regular use of disclosing solutions. The stain of disclosing tablets, on the other hand, does not last as long nor is it as intense.

When disclosing tablets are used, the patient is instructed to chew the wafer thoroughly, working it into the saliva, and then to swish the fluid vigorously about the mouth for a minute. Care must be taken that the solution reaches all parts of the mouth. If it does not, surfaces of some teeth may not be stained, even when plaque is present. Proper staining can be attained by a vigorous pumping action of the cheeks to force the solution between the teeth. After about a minute the mouth may be emptied and rinsed gently with water. Examination should be made immediately. The patient should observe the procedure with a mirror.

Obviously the use of stains such as basic fuchsin, Bismark brown, or erythrosin can facilitate the patient's efforts at plaque removal. Stains facilitate the patient's objective: the complete removal of plaque from the tooth surfaces. They provide an effective means of determining whether this objective has been reached by the absence of a stain on exposed tooth surfaces.

The following data should be recorded on the periodontal chart (p. 540):

1. Plaque (plaque-free score)
2. Subgingival calculus
3. Supragingival calculus
4. Food impaction or retention
5. Location of dental caries
6. Erosion
7. Abrasion
8. Inadequate restorations
9. Diastemata
10. Rotated teeth
11. Intruded or extruded teeth

**Temporomandibular joint**

The patient should be questioned as to temporomandibular joint symptoms (e.g., pain, subluxation, clicking, popping). The joint should be palpated in both protrusive and lateral excursions. In addition, the pathway of the chin point should be observed during mandibular movements. Deviation to the right or left may be indicative of joint or muscular dysfunction. In the majority of cases, however, the joints will be found to be functioning normally.

## PERIODONTAL EXAMINATION

**Screening**

The student, the dental hygienist, or the practitioner inexperienced in charting often finds it to be a time-consuming exercise. To improve efficiency, a periodontal screening form (p. 538) may be used to quickly differentiate the healthy patient from the patient who needs a more detailed periodontal workup. Such screening differs from the screening used by epidemiologists. It is used to quickly identify the periodontally ill patient early in the course of the disease so that curative and preventive treatment can be undertaken at the earliest possible time.[41]

The oral and roentgenographic examinations are performed first. Any tooth showing inflammation, mobility, pocket depths of 4 mm or greater, furcation involvement, widened periodontal ligament spaces, horizontal bone loss, or angular or vertical bone loss is circled in red. If no circle appears on the screening sheet, the patient does not need a detailed examination. The patient may be periodontally healthy or have class I periodontal disease. This screening form can reduce examination time significantly. As soon as the examiner has accumulated 4 or 5 red circles, he/she may conclude that the patient has periodontal disease and may proceed to definitive periodontal charting. This conclusion may be reached in as little as 5 minutes. If the screening indicates a disease of class II to IV, the examiner proceed to a full periodontal examination and charting. A work sheet to assist the student in the steps of periodontal examination will facilitate the routine (p. 539).

# PERIODONTAL SCREENING FORM

| Name | Patient's name |
|---|---|

| Date | Record number |
|---|---|

Circle involved tooth numbers in *red*.

**Oral examination**

Occlusal checklist

Inflammation

| 1 | 2 | 3 | 4 | 5 | 6 | 7 | 8 | 9 | 10 | 11 | 12 | 13 | 14 | 15 | 16 |
|---|---|---|---|---|---|---|---|---|----|----|----|----|----|----|----|
| 32 | 31 | 30 | 29 | 28 | 27 | 26 | 25 | 24 | 23 | 22 | 21 | 20 | 19 | 18 | 17 |

Mobile teeth*

| 1 | 2 | 3 | 4 | 5 | 6 | 7 | 8 | 9 | 10 | 11 | 12 | 13 | 14 | 15 | 16 |
|---|---|---|---|---|---|---|---|---|----|----|----|----|----|----|----|
| 32 | 31 | 30 | 29 | 28 | 27 | 26 | 25 | 24 | 23 | 22 | 21 | 20 | 19 | 18 | 17 |

☐

Pocket depths 4 mm or more

| 1 | 2 | 3 | 4 | 5 | 6 | 7 | 8 | 9 | 10 | 11 | 12 | 13 | 14 | 15 | 16 |
|---|---|---|---|---|---|---|---|---|----|----|----|----|----|----|----|
| 32 | 31 | 30 | 29 | 28 | 27 | 26 | 25 | 24 | 23 | 22 | 21 | 20 | 19 | 18 | 17 |

Oliver index (probe mesials only)

Furcation involvements

| 1 | 2 | 3 | 4 | 5 | 6 | 7 | 8 | 9 | 10 | 11 | 12 | 13 | 14 | 15 | 16 |
|---|---|---|---|---|---|---|---|---|----|----|----|----|----|----|----|
| 32 | 31 | 30 | 29 | 28 | 27 | 26 | 25 | 24 | 23 | 22 | 21 | 20 | 19 | 18 | 17 |

☐

Other

| 1 | 2 | 3 | 4 | 5 | 6 | 7 | 8 | 9 | 10 | 11 | 12 | 13 | 14 | 15 | 16 |
|---|---|---|---|---|---|---|---|---|----|----|----|----|----|----|----|
| 32 | 31 | 30 | 29 | 28 | 27 | 26 | 25 | 24 | 23 | 22 | 21 | 20 | 19 | 18 | 17 |

Describe (i.e., hyperplasia, lack of zone of attached gingiva)

**Radiographic examination**

Angular bone loss

| 1 | 2 | 3 | 4 | 5 | 6 | 7 | 8 | 9 | 10 | 11 | 12 | 13 | 14 | 15 | 16 |
|---|---|---|---|---|---|---|---|---|----|----|----|----|----|----|----|
| 32 | 31 | 30 | 29 | 28 | 27 | 26 | 25 | 24 | 23 | 22 | 21 | 20 | 19 | 18 | 17 |

☐

Significant horizontal bone loss

| 1 | 2 | 3 | 4 | 5 | 6 | 7 | 8 | 9 | 10 | 11 | 12 | 13 | 14 | 15 | 16 |
|---|---|---|---|---|---|---|---|---|----|----|----|----|----|----|----|
| 32 | 31 | 30 | 29 | 28 | 27 | 26 | 25 | 24 | 23 | 22 | 21 | 20 | 19 | 18 | 17 |

Widened periodontal ligament

| 1 | 2 | 3 | 4 | 5 | 6 | 7 | 8 | 9 | 10 | 11 | 12 | 13 | 14 | 15 | 16 |
|---|---|---|---|---|---|---|---|---|----|----|----|----|----|----|----|
| 32 | 31 | 30 | 29 | 28 | 27 | 26 | 25 | 24 | 23 | 22 | 21 | 20 | 19 | 18 | 17 |

☐

Check one   ☐ Normal   ☐ Class I periodontal disease   ☐ Class II to IV periodontal disease

*Occlusal examination: Are any teeth mobile? Mobility is defined as anything beyond the least perceptible mobility that the eye can detect, which is noted as 1. The scale of mobility ranges from 0 (ankylosed) to—(between 0 and 1), to 1 (defined above), to 1− (twice the mobility of 1), to 2 (twice the mobility of 1−), etc. If you have any checks in the occlusal checklist boxes, the patient will require an occlusal examination. The examination should be performed on an occlusal analysis and diagnosis form after scaling and curettage have been completed and immediately preceding the occlusal adjustment.

---

**WORK SHEET FOR PERIODONTAL EXAMINATION**

Name _____

A. Interview examination
  1. Medical history

   Age _____ Birth date _____ Marital status _____

   Children (number and ages) _____

   Date of last physical examination _____ Military service _____
   History
     a. Serious illnesses
     b. Hospitalizations
     c. Diabetes, high blood pressure, cardiac disease, infectious hepatitis, rheumatic fever
   Current medications
   Sensitivity to any medications
   Synopsis
  2. Dental history
B. Clinical examination (periodontal aspects to be performed if screening indicates that the patient
  has periodontal disease)
  Head-neck-regional lymph nodes
  Oral mucosa, tongue, cheeks, lips, tonsillar region
  Gingiva: color, size, consistency
  Charting (note the following on the clinical chart):
    Missing teeth
    Recession (gingival margin)
    Mucogingival junction
    Zone of gingiva: narrow or lacking
    Pain on percussion
    Diastemata
    Mobility
    Pocket depths
    Furcation involvements
    Whether the patient has wear facets
C. Roentgenographic examination
  Level of bone (percent)
  Horizontal or vertical loss
  Angular bone loss
  Furcation involvements
  Widening of periodontal ligament space
  Crown-root ratio
D. Is traumatism present?   Yes _____ No _____ Why? _____
  If yes, after scaling and curettage have been completed, take study models and complete occlusal
  analysis.

---

As one proceeds with the examination, the findings should be recorded on a suitable chart. A pictorial diagrammatic chart is helpful since the patient can also read it (Figs. 28-5 and 28-6). Missing teeth, impactions, anomalies, periapical pathology, caries, pain on percussion, poor contacts, food impactions, premature contacts, recessions, and rotations all have been entered by this time. If some notations have been overlooked, go back and enter them. Notations require more time in the beginning when one is unaccustomed to using them. Ultimately, when skill and accuracy are attained, they take only a short time. Standardized symbols should be used so that notations are universally understood and the charts may be readable in the future and by others (Fig. 28-7). Auxiliary personnel may assist in recording data, which may be dictated.

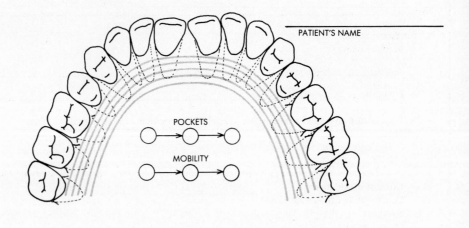

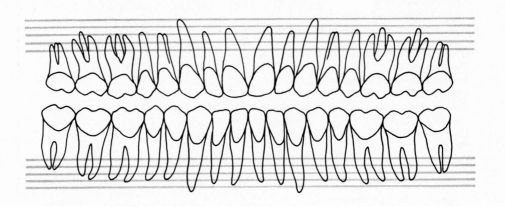

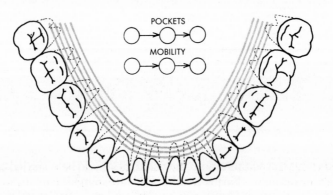

**Fig. 28-5.**    Diagrammatic chart for recording examination findings (Stern Examination Chart).

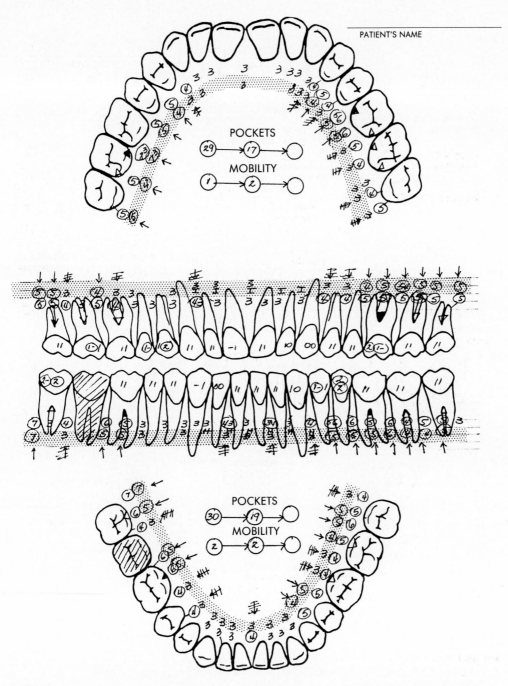

PATIENT'S NAME

**Fig. 28-6.** There are two chartings on this chart—one is the initial examination and one is the examination after initial therapy. In this diagram the stippled numbers represent the second examination. In practice, a black pen is used for the initial examination and a red pen for the second examination. Each buccal, lingual and pair of interproximal readings are circled if they are 4 mm or more, and they are indicated by an arrow. Pockets reduced to 3 mm at the time of the second examination have the arrow struck. In this case the maxillary pockets are reduced from 29 to 17; the mandibular from 30 to 19. (Stern Examination Chart.)

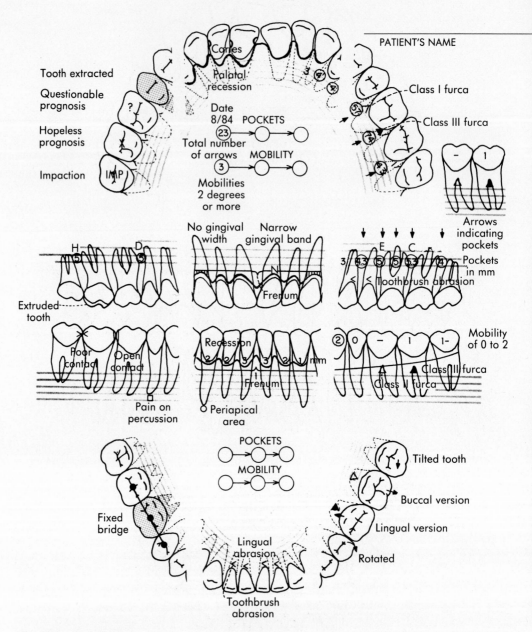

**Fig. 28-7.** Symbols used in charting. Letters over pocket depths are used to indicate: C = crater, B = bleeding, D = deposits, E = exudate, H = hyperplasia, and I = inflammation. (Stern Examination Chart.)

Hygienists may chart during treatment and on maintenance (recall) visits.

At this point the all-important charting of mobility and pocket depth still remains. The patient should be told that some discomfort may be experienced during the measurement of the pockets, particularly when inflammation is present. A topical anesthetic can usually minimize any pain. If the patient has reported a history of rheumatic fever with permanent valvular impairment or orthopedic joint replacement an adequate dose of antibiotics must be given before probing. When the case is to be documented with photographs or when study models are to be taken, it is best to obtain these before probing since the gingiva may bleed. Bleeding tends to mar the photographs and the models. The armamentarium used in the examination is shown in Figs. 28-8 and 28-9.

Probing may measure from the gingival margin[42] or from a fixed reference point, such as the cementoenamel junction, a filling margin, or a plastic stent. Probing from the gingival margin records pocket depth. Probing from a fixed reference point (such as the cementoenamel junction or a restoration) records attachment level.[42,43]

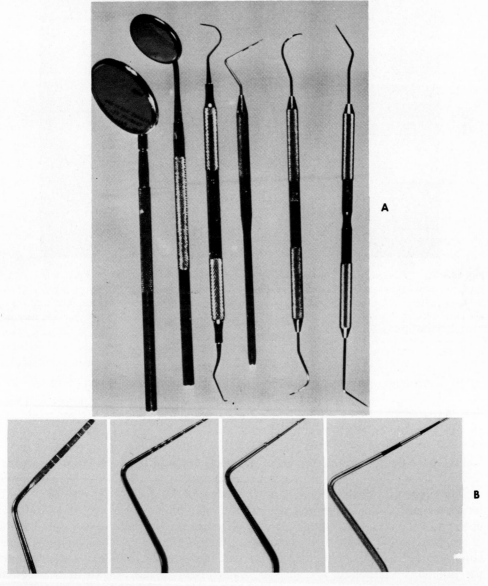

**Fig. 28-8.** **A,** Armamentarium for examination: mouth mirrors, explorers, and probe. **B,** Calibrated periodontal probes used in charting pocket depth: Goldman-Fox probe; Williams probe; University of Michigan "O" probe; color-coded 3-6-9-12-mm probe (from *left* to *right*).

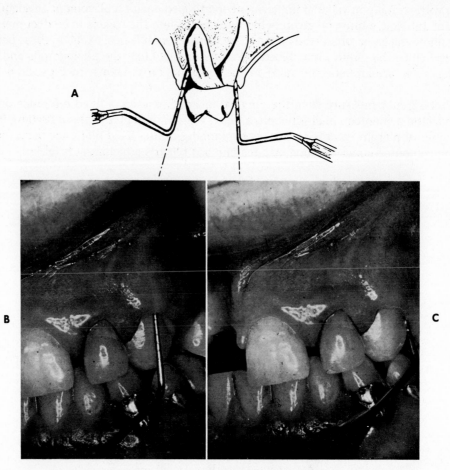

**Fig. 28-9. A,** *Circumferential probing method. The probe is drawn along the base of the pocket from proximal contact to proximal contact. Positioning of the probe for pocket measurement.* **B,** *The sulcular depth is 4 mm on the labial surface of the canine.* **C,** *On the distal surface of the same tooth, an 8-mm pocket is present. The sulci and pockets should be probed carefully since readings on different surfaces of the same tooth may vary extensively. (Courtesy of G. Tussing, Lincoln, Nebraska.)*

In determining pocket depth, one should use a periodontal probe (Figs. 28-8 and 28-9). The periodontal probe is useful because it is calibrated. The probe should be passed under the gingiva along the circumference of the tooth. Three measurements should be made on the buccal aspect and three on the lingual aspect of each tooth (Fig. 28-10). The probe should be manipulated so that it does not stop at calculus. In addition, the entire circumferences of the pocket should be inspected in a sweeping traverse so as not to miss a narrow pocket entrance.

The probe may or may not stop at the bottom of the pocket[43-47] (Fig. 28-11). How far it reaches will depend on the size of the probe, the force exerted, the dimensions of the pocket, access to it, the angle of application, the presence of deposits, the state of gingival health,[46,48-50] and the accuracy of the examiner in reading the probed measurement.[49-53] In the presence of inflammation, however, the probe may extend through the junctional epithelium and give a greater (1 to 1.5 mm) depth than is actually present.[49,50] Probe penetration varies with the degree of health and disease at the probing site.[45] For example:

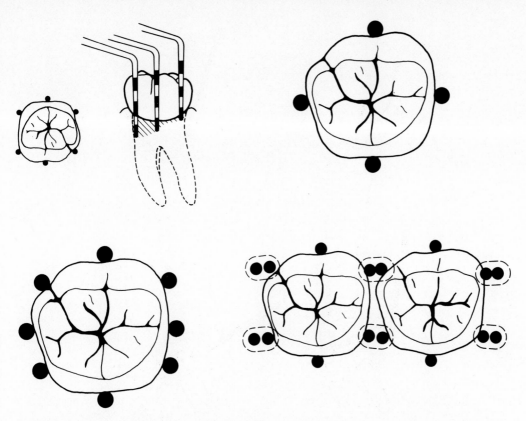

**Fig. 28-10.** Probing positions used by different schools of therapists. Four to eight points are measured and recorded. Picture *(lower right)* illustrates the coupling of the two interproximal notations, which are then counted as one unit (as shown in Fig. 28-6).

1. In healthy specimens, the probe tends to fall short of the apical termination of the epithelial attachment by an average of 0.4 mm.
2. In experimental gingivitis specimens, the probe tends to fall short of the apical termination of the epithelial attachment by an average of 0.2 mm.
3. In periodontitis specimens, the probe tends to go past the apical termination of the epithelial attachment by an average of 0.2 mm.

Following treatment, the pocket wall may become tighter and prevent the probe from reaching the bottom of the pocket.[54-56] However, changes in probing depths obtained at different examinations may accurately reflect changes in health or disease (Fig. 28-12). In general, probing is performed with a very light pressure of not more than one or two ounces of force.

Calculus deposits often cause errors in probing by either preventing the probe from entering the sulcus at the proper angulation or impeding insertion to the depth of the pocket. In these instances the probe should be manipulated in several directions so as to pass by the calculus. It may be held horizontally when the shape of the interdental pocket is being explored (see Fig. 28-11, *C* and *D*), but, in general, it is held with a slight inclination to the long axis of the tooth with the shank of the probe close to the contact point. If the angle is too large, an error in the reading will result (see Fig. 28-11, *A* and *B*). In tortuous pockets, when the probe is held absolutely parallel

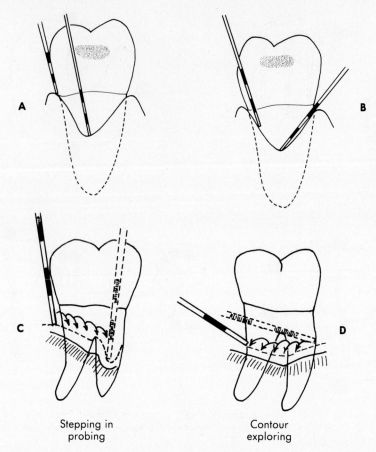

Stepping in
probing

Contour
exploring

**Fig. 28-11. A,** Proper angulation for buccal/lingual and interproximal measurements. Note probe shaft position close to contact point. **B,** When improper angulation is used, the probe may not extend to the base of the pocket and at times even when it does extend to the pocket base the reading may be larger than it should be since the probe is measuring the diagonal dimension. If the probe shaft is brought to the contact point (as in **A**), the reading will be more accurate. **C,** Stepping is performed to explore the pocket, looking for the narrow entrances of precipitous pockets. **D,** Contour exploring is done to determine the outline of a pocket or of the attachment.

to the long axis of the tooth and is used for measuring but not exploring, the deepest portions of the pocket may be completely missed (Fig. 28-13).

Probing is particularly important because roentgenograms do not offer a sufficiently accurate picture of pocket depth. Bone levels may be high, yet pockets may be deep.[57] Extensive bone loss may exist and yet be unaccompanied by pockets if the gingiva has receded. Measurements of bone height by transgingival probing can be quite accurate.[58] One objective of periodontal therapy is the reduction of probing depth. This cannot be achieved unless one realizes to what extent pockets are present and if they are suprabony or infrabony. The patient's periodontal condition may often be prejudged on the basis of the excellent clinical appearance of the gingiva (Fig. 28-14). The dentist may then decide that the patient is not a "periodontal case." Such patients frequently have pockets that go undetected at a time when proper diagnosis and treatment could have rectified the condition more easily.

Once a surgical flap has been retracted, measurement of pocket depth can no longer be made. Defects of alveolar bone are often referred to as "pockets." This is inaccurate. Although pockets are related to bony lesions, the terms are not synonymous. When one desires to document relationships for purposes of research, roentgenograms may be taken with calibrated silver points[59] or gutta-percha points inserted in the pocket. Dental floss may be tied to the neck of the point to prevent aspiration or loss.

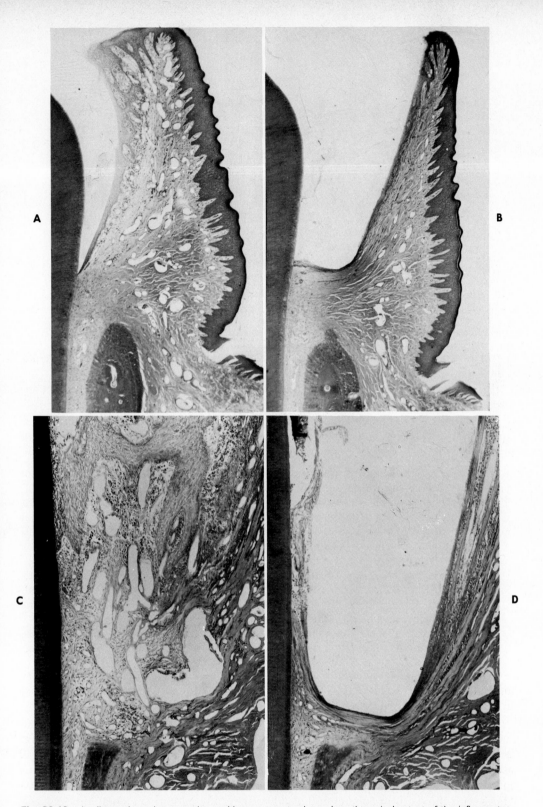

**Fig. 28-12.** In diseased specimens probe position appears to depend on the apical extent of the inflammatory infiltrate. In the healthy specimens (little or no infiltrate) it has not been possible to establish what determines final probe position. **A,** Buccal gingiva of lower premolar of beagle dog in 60-day experimental gingivitis; no apical migration of junctional epithelium. **B,** Same premolar as in **A** (in a different plane of section). Plastic probe with a terminal diameter of ~ 0.35 mm inserted. **C,** Buccal gingiva or lower premolar of beagle dog; periodontium with substantial apical migration of the epithelial attachment. **D,** Same premolar as in **C** (different plane of section). Plastic probe with a terminal diameter of ~ 0.35 mm inserted on facial aspect less than 1 mm mesial to the site shown in **C.** The probe goes apical to the apical termination of the epithelial attachment. Probes in **B** and **D** were inserted with the same force. (Courtesy G. Armitage, San Francisco, California.)

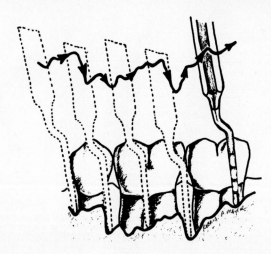

**Fig. 28-13.** Sounding (transgingival probing) after anesthesia reveals irregular character of bone loss in periodontitis. Bone loss is shown along vestibular tooth surfaces. (Bone height can be recorded by transgingival probing.) (Courtesy G. Tussing, Lincoln, Nebraska.)

A grid incorporated on the roentgenogram has proved valuable in documenting alveolar crest and tooth relationships[59] (Fig. 28-15).

**Furcation involvements**

Furcation involvements may be detected in roentgenograms. Early furcation invasions may not be recognized on roentgenograms, and bone may be lost in the furcation without pocket involvement. Therefore detection and accurate classification of furcation involvements requires probing. Furcation involvements have been classified into three groups based upon *horizontal* probing characteristics.

1. *Class I, incipient.* This may not be detectable in an x-ray series. Such a furcation cannot be entered by an explorer primarily because it is an indentation.
2. *Class II, moderate.* This is an incomplete furcation involvement. Bone loss may be present on only one surface of the furcation. An explorer or curette can be inserted but cannot pass completely through from buccal to lingual or from mesial to distal surfaces. Roentgenographic evidence of bone loss may not always be obvious.
3. *Class III, advanced.* This is a through-and-through involvement. A radiolucency is apparent in roentgenograms. The furcation may be entered from buccal and lingual surfaces of mandibular molars or from two or three surfaces on maxillary molars—buccal, mesial, and distal. Involvements also occur on maxillary first premolars. Other classifications involve the horizontal and vertical depths of furcation involvements.

    Subclassification measures probeable *vertical* depth from the roof of the furcation. Class A is a probing depth of 1 to 3 mm. Class B is 4 to 6 mm and Class C is 7 mm or more.

**Tooth mobility**

The prognosis of periodontally involved teeth depends often on the initial mobility and whether it can be altered by treatment. The measurement of mobility is essential in determining the therapy required and in evaluating the results of such treatment.[60,61]

**Clinical measurement**

Mobility can be determined by luxating a tooth with a light force and observing its movement. The tooth may be moved between the handles of two instruments (Fig. 28-16) or between the finger and instrument handle. The degree of movement is ascertained by comparison with adjacent teeth that are not being moved. Further information may be gained by having the patient move through lateral and protrusive glides with the teeth in contact and also by asking the patient to clench and rock the teeth. The occlusal contacts will cause the mobile teeth to move; this can be seen by observing highlights of reflected light on the tooth surface or by holding the fingertips partly on the teeth and partly on the gingivae. Visual perception may be enhanced by placing a piece of blue articulating paper between the teeth during the glide movements. The movement of the teeth is more obvious against this dark background.

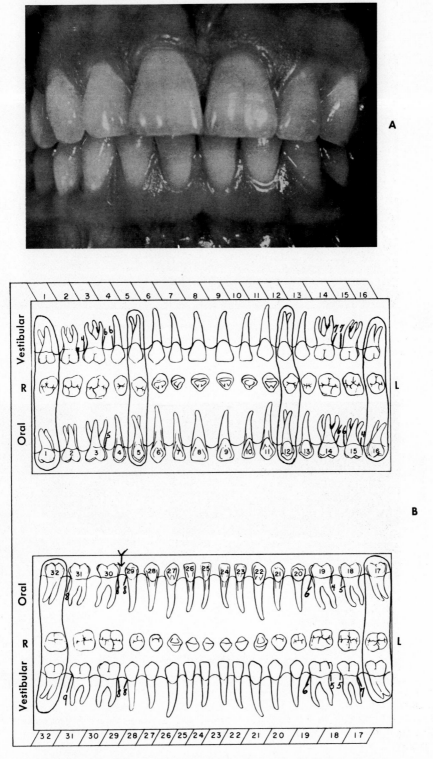

**Fig. 28-14. A,** Periodontitis in a case that appears fairly normal clinically. Despite the excellent appearance, extensive periodontal disease is present around some posterior teeth (see charting). **B,** Recorded findings of patient. Chart is one of several types in use.

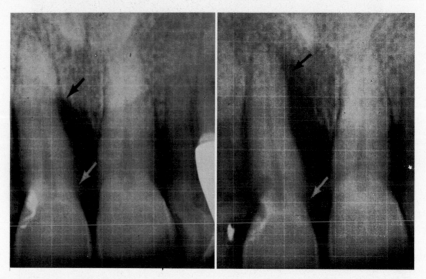

**Fig. 28-15.** A grid incorporated on the roentgenogram can be used to document and compare bone levels. The sequence is of an untreated case of periodontosis. Roentgenograms were taken a year apart and show rapid alveolar bone loss.

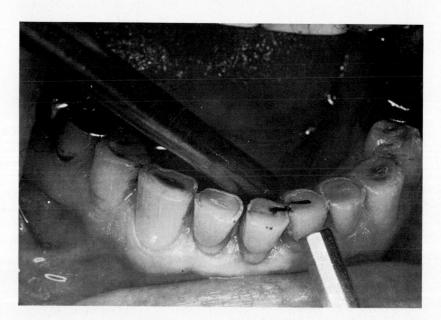

**Fig. 28-16.** Method of measuring mobility with handles of two instruments. Fix the jaw in place by hand and forearm. In this instance a line was drawn with indelible pencil to indicate the proximal relationship of the central incisors before movement. The lingual displacement of the mandibular left central incisor indicates a mobility of 2½ degrees.

The degree of movement is indicated on an arbitrary scale of 0 to 3. A reading of 0 indicates no perceptible movement; 1 refers to the least perceptible movement of a healthy lower incisor; 1½ to 2½ are increasing degrees that end at 3, a degree of mobility indicating a hopeless prognosis. Teeth that can be depressed have a mobility of 3. The readings of trained observers correspond closely. The use of these numbers is not precisely equated to movement in millimeters; such measurements are possible in experiments that make use of mobility-measuring devices (see box, p. 538).

**Degree of movement**

Normal teeth may have a range of mobility that is barely perceptible.[62-65] Beyond this range, mobility is a symptom that occurs early in periodontal traumatism but late in periodontitis. The causes of mobility may be intrinsic, involving morphology or condition of the tissue, or extrinsic, involving the loading of these tissues. Thus the length and shape of the clinical root and crown, the height of the alveolar bone, and the width of the periodontal ligament may determine the firmness of a tooth. Firmness also depends on the biologic status of the supporting tissues. Teeth tend to loosen during acute inflammation, as may occur in infection or after surgery. Teeth may also loosen during pregnancy and in diabetes and severe nutritional deficiency. The alteration of tooth mobility in these instances may be mediated on a biochemical level.

**Causes of mobility**

Physical forces are exerted on the periodontium, superimposing their influence on whatever local and intrinsic factors are present. Habits, dental appliances, dental procedures, and traumatic impact may produce such forces. Stresses are also applied during mastication, swallowing, bruxism, and clenching. Primary traumatism is the production of mobility in a tooth with normal support subjected to a force in excess of physiologic limits. Secondary traumatism is the production of mobility by normal forces in a tooth with weakened support. When local and intrinsic factors such as inflammation and metabolic disturbance are present, normal forces may produce mobility in a tooth with a full osseous support.

**Primary and secondary traumatism**

Much knowledge concerning tooth mobility rests on subjective clinical observation. It would be desirable if laboratory techniques could be applied to the study of mobility. Mechanical, optical, and electronic devices for the quantitative measurement of tooth mobility have been developed for this reason.[60,62-67] Generally these may be either mechanical devices or electrical conductivity-sensing devices (transducers or strain gauges), through which tooth movement can be measured and recorded. A known load is applied to the tooth, and a measurement of movement is obtained. The findings in these instances are experimental, but they may have clinical significance. Studies on healthy teeth indicate that the application of small loads to the tooth will produce a considerable initial displacement. When increasing loads are applied, further displacement occurs but of lesser magnitude. The range of movement varies up to 0.2 mm horizontally and 0.02 mm vertically. In pathologic states this movement may be increased tenfold.

**Mobility-measuring devices**

**Experimental findings in tooth mobility**

Mobility has been found to vary between individuals of the same age and between teeth in the same person. It is greater in children, young adults, and in some women. It decreases after completion of active tooth eruption. Anterior teeth are looser than posterior teeth. There are fluctuations during the day; a tooth is twice as mobile in the morning as it is in the evening. Lying down for a few moments will increase mobility. After a tooth is traumatically loosened, it slowly recovers in a matter of weeks. In some instances mobility may be increased during pregnancy or menstruation. Drugs that alter blood pressure may also alter mobility. The range of these experimental mobility measurements is enormously increased in the presence of periodontal disease.[65,68]

The opportunity to make objective measurements of tooth mobility and of force applied to the tooth will ultimately permit a better clinical evaluation of the factors that affect mobility. This is important since mobility is a basic symptom of periodontal disease.[69-71]

**Bleeding indices**

Bleeding (Sulcus and Papillary Bleeding Indices and Gingival Bleeding Time Index) are regarded as measures of disease activity. They correlate well with amount of sulcus fluid and with gingival index.[72-76] These indices correlate weakly with pocket depth.[72,75-77] Bleeding on probing may represent an earlier sign of inflammation than various tissue color changes.[73,75] Bleeding may be used to assess healing.[84] Bleeding may be recorded by coloring the central circle (Fig. 28-17) in red.

**Halitosis**

Halitosis (fetor ex ore) is important to the patient[77-83] and many times is the symptom that brings the patient to the dentist. It may be caused by periodontal disease. Halitosis may originate in areas in which retention of food particles occurs. Decomposing soft deposits may cause it. Another cause is acute necrotizing gingivitis. Deep carious lesions may also cause it. Halitosis is often seen in patients suffering from febrile diseases and from psychiatric depression. If, after the elimination of dental and periodontal causes and the exclusion of offensive foods and drink, bad breath persists, competent medical specialists should examine the nose, nasopharynx, tonsils and lungs, since diseases of these organs may on occasion cause halitosis.[85]

## ROENTGENOGRAPHIC EXAMINATION

Roentgenograms are of greatest diagnostic value in periodontics when the angulation of projection and the density of the films show trabecular patterns and discrete changes in bone density and bone levels. Roentgenograms can give some of the following information:[84,86,87]

1. Interdental bone height and presence of a lamina dura
2. Trabecular patterns
3. Areas of bone destruction that can be confirmed by probing (teeth with angular or horizontal bone loss greater than one tenth root length)
4. Bone loss in furcations
5. Width of periodontal ligament space (Is there a noticeable widening?)
6. Crown-to-root ratio
7. Root shape and length
8. Caries, general quality of restorations, heavy calculus deposits
9. Location of antrum relative to alveolar crest
10. Missing teeth, supernumerary teeth, impactions

Roentgenograms give a two-dimensional representation of three-dimensional structures. They are most useful as a diagnostic tool when they are correlated with visual oral examination, clinical probing, and pocket charting.

Surveys employing the long cone–paralleling technique of projection are desirable. A minimum of sixteen films should be used; this results in each area being exposed at more than one angulation. Technical errors that produce elongation, foreshortening, and/or overlapping severely impair the diagnostic usefulness of the roentgenograms. Panoramic roentgenographic surveys have limited use. The bisecting technique should be used to discern periapical disease about individual teeth.

The place of the roentgenogram in periodontal diagnosis is important, on the one hand, and much misunderstood, on the other. Too often the diagnosis of periodontal disease is made only from inspection of bone loss that becomes evident in roentgenograms when the disease is advanced.

**Inspection before probing**

Before making a systematic oral examination, the clinician should study the roentgenograms in a sequential manner for gross oral pathologic conditions (cysts, granulomas, cementomas, foreign bodies, impactions, unerupted or supernumerary teeth, neoplasms). Next the clinician should view the patterns of alveolar bone trabeculation. Several types of trabecular patterns have been described. Deviations from normal trabeculation, such as disuse atrophy, and rare general involvements, such as hyper-

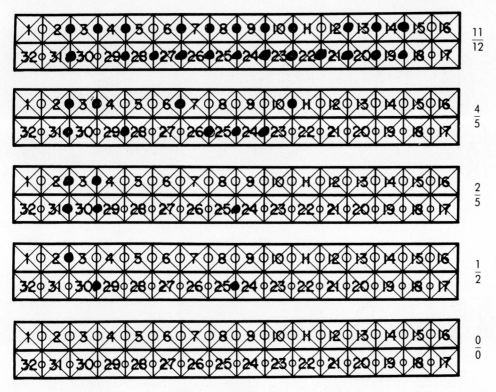

**Fig. 28-17.**  Bleeding points (darkened circles) are noted and totaled before treatment. Weekly readings were made after treatment and home care were instituted; they show gradual improvement.

parathyroidism and Paget's disease, should be noted. The loss of trabeculation caused by disuse atrophy will be readily apparent around teeth long out of occlusion and around extraction sites.

Roentgenograms should be inspected for calculus, caries in the crown or root surfaces, and overhanging or defective restorations. Are there open contact points? Are these defects related to areas of bone loss? Is any immediate treatment necessary to prevent or cope with pulpal involvement? The roentgenograms should further be examined for height of septal bone, continuity of lamina dura, and width of periodontal ligament.[86-91]

**Etiologic factors**

Normal, healthy alveolar bone has characteristic appearances on radiographs. The alveolar crests are situated approximately 2 to 3 mm apical to the cementoenamel junctions of the teeth. The shape of the alveolar crests may vary from rounded to flat. The interdental septa may be wide or thin. The angulation of the crests may be horizontal, or they may be angulated mesiodistally (Fig. 28-18, *A* and *B*).

**Normal radiographic appearance**

The shape of the alveolar crest is influenced by crown form, tooth position, and tooth angulation, the distance between roots, and root form. Where roots are close together, the interdental septum is narrow and usually rounded at the crest; where roots are more widely separated (because of convexity of crown form or diastemata), the septum is broad and flat (Fig. 28-18, *A*).

Where the cementoenamel junctions are at the same level, the crests will be horizontal; where teeth are tilted or inclined, the alveolar crests will be inclined. The height of the "normal" crest will be maintained at 2 to 3 mm apical to the cementoenamel junctions (Fig. 28-18, *B*).

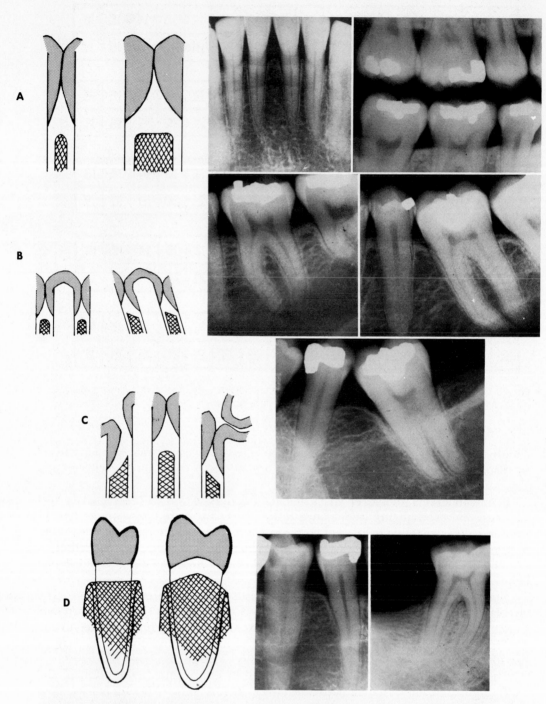

**Fig. 28-18. A,** Where teeth are closely approximated and crowns are relatively flat, a narrow rounded septum is seen. Where teeth are more widely separated, by convexity of crowns or diastemata, the alveolar crest will appear flat. **B,** Diagrammatic illustration of the influence of tooth inclination on the alveolar crests. *Left,* Crests are horizontal when teeth are placed vertically; *right,* crests are oblique whenever teeth present a deviation from the vertical in their long axes, an effect produced by the relative positions of the cementoenamel junctions. **C,** Configuration of the alveolar crest as it is governed by the state of eruption. *Left,* Undereruption; *center,* normal eruption; *right,* overeruption. **D,** The thickness of the bone as influenced by the width of the roots will influence roentgenopacity. *Left,* A thinner root with bone loss, therefore less roentgenopacity; *right,* a thicker root with less bone loss, therefore thicker bone and greater roentgenopacity. At the crest, however, the rounded form may give a lesser density than the flat form at the left. Roentgenopacity is also influenced by thickness of cortical bone and by trabecular patterns and density.

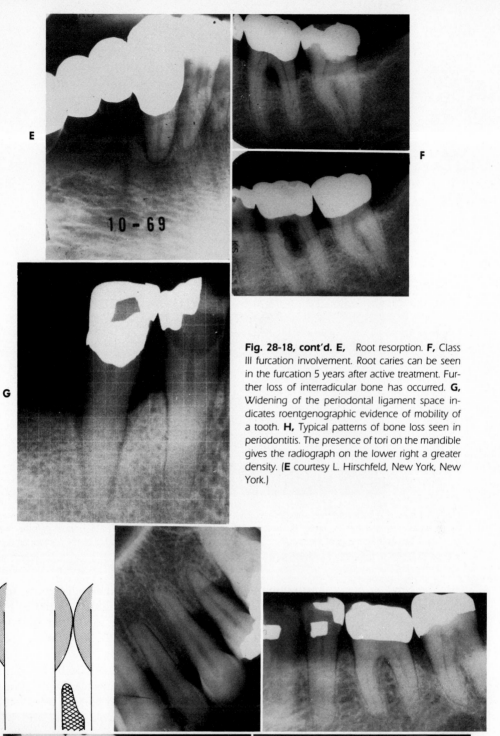

**Fig. 28-18, cont'd. E,** Root resorption. **F,** Class III furcation involvement. Root caries can be seen in the furcation 5 years after active treatment. Further loss of interradicular bone has occurred. **G,** Widening of the periodontal ligament space indicates roentgenographic evidence of mobility of a tooth. **H,** Typical patterns of bone loss seen in periodontitis. The presence of tori on the mandible gives the radiograph on the lower right a greater density. (**E** courtesy L. Hirschfeld, New York, New York.)

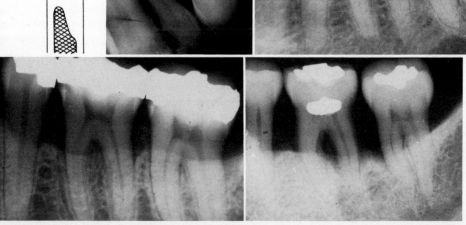

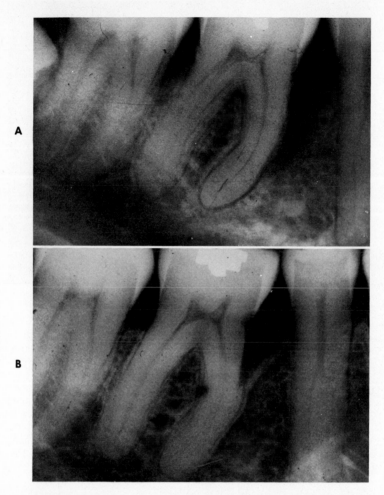

**Fig. 28-19. A,** Vertical bone destruction and thickening of the periodontal ligament around the mesial root of the mandibular molar has occurred. **B,** Posttreatment results reveal restoration of lost bone and the removal of tooth structure on the mesial of the molar incident to root planing, a carious lesion at the cementoenamel junction, and open contacts. (Courtesy H. Meador, San Antonio, Texas.)

The stage or state of eruption of approximating teeth will also influence the form of the alveolar crests. Where cementoenamel junctions of neighboring teeth are at the same level, the crest will be flat or rounded; where teeth are incompletely erupted or are overerupted, the crest will be angulated and will follow the levels of the adjacent cementoenamel junctions (Fig. 28-18, *C*).

The opacity or density of the roentgenogram will be influenced by the density of bone trabeculation, the thickness of the bone, and the thickness of cortical bone. Thus in areas of wide roots, dense trabeculation, and thick cortical bone, a relatively *dense* radiographic bone is seen. Where roots are narrower buccolingually and where a narrower alveolus, thinly trabeculated, or thin cortical plate is present, a radiolucent roentgenogram is seen (Fig. 28-18, *D*).

Root resorption (Fig. 28-18, *E*), caries of the crown (*H*) or of the root (*F*), and widening of the periodontal ligament area (*G*) may be seen on the x-ray films and the clinical examination.

**Periodontal bone loss**

Osseous defects resulting from periodontal disease may become evident in roentgenograms (Fig. 28-18, *H*) and must be confirmed and correlated with the data derived from probing and clinical examination. The patterns of bone loss may be horizontal

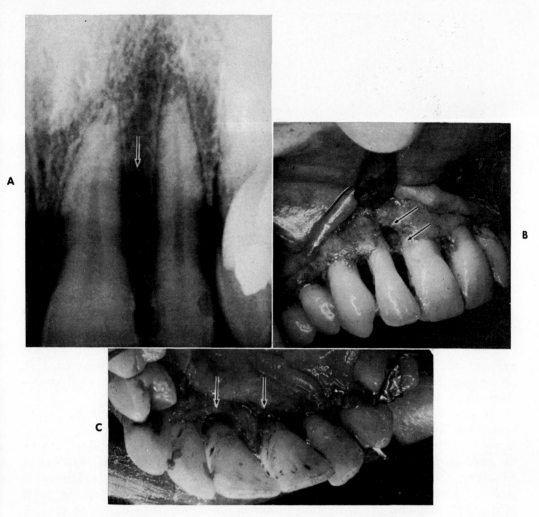

**Fig. 28-20. A,** Roentgenogram of the maxillary right central and lateral incisors shows an area of radiolucency interproximally bordering the central incisor. The bizarre bone configuration caused by the destruction was seen when a flap was retracted, **B.** An isthmus of bone is all that remains of the alveolar crest. A large area of bone destruction is apical to this and extends palatally. **C,** Troughlike, infrabony destruction can be seen on the palatal surface around the central incisor. The defect communicates with the bony defect on the interproximal and labial surfaces of the teeth.

or vertical. Bony craters or troughs may be distinguishable. There may be furcation involvements (classes I to III). The maxillary antrum may be close to the alveolar crest in areas of bone loss.

After studying the roentgenograms, the therapist should make a clinical examination. When this is completed, he/she should peruse the roentgenograms once more to determine whether the findings agree or disagree with the prior clinical findings. If there are any obvious differences, they should be accounted for. Spot reprobing may be necessary. Roentgenograms taken at predetermined angles may be needed to visualize bony defects. The use of calibrated silver points or grids may be helpful.[59,90,91]

Roentgenograms may reveal information about the occlusion. There may be evidence of periodontal traumatism.[60] Roots may be long or they may be short and tapering. Root resorption may be present, and the crown-to-root ratio may be poor. There may be thickening of the periodontal ligament (Fig. 28-18, *G*); only part of the root

**Occlusion**

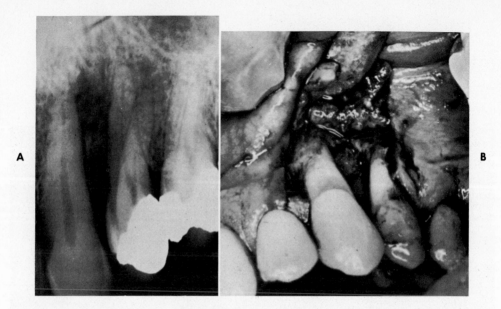

**Fig. 28-21.** Degree of density in a roentgenogram can mask pathologic conditions. The bone loss shown in **B** is greater than the roentgenogram, **A,** would indicate.

**Limitations**

may actually be covered by bone. Teeth may be malaligned, tilted, overerupted, or submerged. There may be sclerotic areas related to overfunction, medication, or disease.

The value of roentgenograms is readily appreciated. However, their limitations should also be understood. Roentgenograms cannot give an accurate picture of pocket depth; this can be judged only by probing. When attachment levels are assessed by probing and roentgenographic interproximal bone height (by the method of Björn and associates[58]), there is a good correlation in longitudinal records of the same patient. Roentgenograms do not show the earliest disease changes. Roentgenographic evidence of bone changes in treatment must be confirmed by clinical probing (Fig. 28-19).

Investigators have been unable to correlate roentgenographic findings and gingivitis (as measured by the gingival index).[92,93] Roentgenograms rarely are indisputable indicators of successful treatment. They may not depict bony deformities accurately or show bone changes on oral (lingual) and vestibular (buccal) aspects of teeth (Fig. 28-20). Roentgenograms show few soft-to-hard tissue relationships. Changes in angulation, direction of the roentgen rays, and factors such as inflammation that affect the radiographic density of alveolar bone will all affect the x-ray image[92-94] (Fig. 28-21). Moreover, there may be wide variation between classical roentgenographic measurements of bone loss and those based on clinical probing,[34,95,96] when the bone levels are checked with measurements made after reflecting a surgical flap.[97,98]

Despite these limitations, a periodontal examination is incomplete without good roentgenograms. Good roentgenograms, viewed under good diffused light with a magnifying lens or loupe, can reveal most bone lesions in periodontal disease. Roentgenograms are an essential part of the examination even though the sensitivity of roentgenograms to accurately measure bone loss in periodontal disease is only fair (see Fig. 28-20). The use of roentgenograms alone can result in serious underestimation of bone loss.[97,98]

## OCCLUSAL ANALYSIS

The dentition should be rated as complete or mutilated by extractions. When there are missing teeth, it should be noted whether or not they have been replaced. Has the dentition then maintained itself, or is the arch collapsing and the teeth drifting? When the dentition is complete (or if the status can otherwise be ascertained), what is the orthodontic classification? Has the patient ever had orthodontic treatment? Has malocclusion or tooth malposition contributed to the patient's present disease status? Has perfect occlusion, when present, preserved good oral health? These factors are not always correlated. Does the patient have centric prematurities? Note their location. Does the patient have interferences in excursions (lateral and protrusive)? Are there balancing side contacts or prematurities? Are the teeth mobile to testing? Do they exhibit fremitus in function? Does the patient complain that fillings squeak when he/she chews? Do the restorations contribute to pathologic changes or do they promote oral health? Does the patient swallow with the mouth open or closed? Does he/she thrust the tongue between the teeth during swallowing? Does the patient have oral compulsions such as lip, tongue, or cheek biting? Does he/she bite or chew on objects such as eyeglasses, pencils, or fingernails? Does he/she lick the lips? Is the patient a mouth breather? Does he/she clench the masseter muscles? The patient should be questioned concerning whether he/she grinds or clenches the teeth or sets the jaw in determination. The teeth should be checked for corroborative wear facets or mobility. Occlusal analysis is assisted by the use of charts to record the pertinent information (see pp. 560-561.)

## Integration of data

Having studied the components of a diagnosis, the student will be required to integrate these in the examination of a patient. The work sheets on pp. 526 and 539 will make this easier. The examination includes (1) an interview examination, (2) a clinical examination, and (3) a roentgenographic examination. The data may be entered in pencil and then rewritten on the patient's chart. The case report required by some schools may be included as part of the patient's chart. Item D asks, "Is traumatism present?" If the answer is positive, study models may be made after root planing and curettage. At this time a thorough occlusal examination can be performed (pp. 560-561). However, the order of examination is flexible.

## Diagnosis

The documented observations made in charting enable the clinician to make a diagnosis. Although the diagnostic statement is brief, it represents the information gathered from detailed, systematic observations. Treatment is planned from the observation and the diagnosis and a prognosis is made.

The diagnosis of the patient's condition should be stated. For example, the dentist might indicate a condition such as necrotizing ulcerative gingivitis (NUG); marginal papillary hyperplastic gingivitis; periodontitis (mild, moderate, advanced, rapidly progressive, localized, or generalized); or primary or secondary periodontal traumatism. The salient findings that lead to this diagnosis should be enumerated. Furthermore the most likely primary and contributory etiologic factors should be summarized. As pointed out earlier, we reason from the findings to their causes and from the causes to the required treatment, all on a biologic basis. When the etiologic factors are unknown, we must treat on a symptomatic basis.

After the examination, a concise listing of pertinent findings of the interview and

# OCCLUSAL ANALYSIS AND DIAGNOSIS

Patient's name _____     Record number _____

**A. Pertinent items abstracted from medical and dental history**

1. Chief complaint (related to occlusion) _____
2. History of orthodontic treatment or previous occlusal adjustment:

   ☐ No    ☐ Yes    Date _____

3. Mobile teeth

| 1 | 2 | 3 | 4 | 5 | 6 | 7 | 8 | 9 | 10 | 11 | 12 | 13 | 14 | 15 | 16 |
|---|---|---|---|---|---|---|---|---|----|----|----|----|----|----|----|
| 32 | 31 | 30 | 29 | 28 | 27 | 26 | 25 | 24 | 23 | 22 | 21 | 20 | 19 | 18 | 17 |

4. Furcations

| 1 | 2 | 3 | 4 | 5 | 6 | 7 | 8 | 9 | 10 | 11 | 12 | 13 | 14 | 15 | 16 |
|---|---|---|---|---|---|---|---|---|----|----|----|----|----|----|----|
| 32 | 31 | 30 | 29 | 28 | 27 | 26 | 25 | 24 | 23 | 22 | 21 | 20 | 19 | 18 | 17 |

**B. General appraisal**

1. Facial form:    Normal ☐    Asymmetric ☐    Hypertrophy right ☐    or left ☐
2. Habits (describe) _____
3. Tension _____

**C. Radiographic findings**

1. Angular bone loss

| 1 | 2 | 3 | 4 | 5 | 6 | 7 | 8 | 9 | 10 | 11 | 12 | 13 | 14 | 15 | 16 |
|---|---|---|---|---|---|---|---|---|----|----|----|----|----|----|----|
| 32 | 31 | 30 | 29 | 28 | 27 | 26 | 25 | 24 | 23 | 22 | 21 | 20 | 19 | 18 | 17 |

2. Significant horizontal bone loss

| 1 | 2 | 3 | 4 | 5 | 6 | 7 | 8 | 9 | 10 | 11 | 12 | 13 | 14 | 15 | 16 |
|---|---|---|---|---|---|---|---|---|----|----|----|----|----|----|----|
| 32 | 31 | 30 | 29 | 28 | 27 | 26 | 25 | 24 | 23 | 22 | 21 | 20 | 19 | 18 | 17 |

3. Widened PDL or funneling

| 1 | 2 | 3 | 4 | 5 | 6 | 7 | 8 | 9 | 10 | 11 | 12 | 13 | 14 | 15 | 16 |
|---|---|---|---|---|---|---|---|---|----|----|----|----|----|----|----|
| 32 | 31 | 30 | 29 | 28 | 27 | 26 | 25 | 24 | 23 | 22 | 21 | 20 | 19 | 18 | 17 |

4. Changes in alveolar bone density
   a. Overall trabeculation: Increased ☐    Decreased ☐
   b. Lamina dura thickening ___|___    Crestal lamina dura indistinct ___|___
5. Evaluation of teeth
   a. Root form: conical, clubbed, divergent (specify) _____
   b. Crown-root ratio: Adequate ☐    Disproportional (specify) _____

**D. Parafunctional tooth contacts**

1. Habits: Bruxism ☐    Clenching ☐    Tapping ☐    Tongue thrusting ☐
   Mouth breathing ☐    Lip, tongue, or cheek biting ☐
   Other (explain) _____
2. Patient awareness of habits
   a. Bruxism:   None ☐   In sleep ☐   On awakening ☐   Daytime ☐   Under tension ☐
   b. Clenching: None ☐   In sleep ☐   On awakening ☐   Daytime ☐   Under tension ☐

3. Wear facets

| 1 | 2 | 3 | 4 | 5 | 6 | 7 | 8 | 9 | 10 | 11 | 12 | 13 | 14 | 15 | 16 |
|---|---|---|---|---|---|---|---|---|----|----|----|----|----|----|----|
| 32 | 31 | 30 | 29 | 28 | 27 | 26 | 25 | 24 | 23 | 22 | 21 | 20 | 19 | 18 | 17 |

**E. Static analysis from study casts**

1. Angle's classification (circle):    I    II    II, Div. 1    II, Div. 2    III
2. Midline position (mandibulary to maxillary central incisors):
   Normal ☐    Mandibular teeth displaced to right ☐    or left ☐    _____ mm

3. Arch form
   a. Symmetric ☐     Asymmetric ☐     Describe _____
   b. Occlusal plane configuration (curve of Spee):
      Normal ☐     Exaggerated ☐     Flat (horizontal) ☐     Reverse ☐
4. Missing teeth: Distribution _____|_____
5. Positions of groups of teeth
   a. Open bite (indicate opposing teeth not in contact) _____
   b. Anterior overbite (vertical overlap):
      Normal to slight (incisal one third) ☐
      Moderate (middle one third) ☐
      Severe (cervical one third) ☐
      Very severe (mandibular incisors occlude with maxillary palatal gingiva) ☐
      Edge-to-edge _____
   c. Anterior overjet (horizontal overlap) _____ mm (measure with probe)     ☐ (1 to 2 mm)
   d. Teeth in crossbite _____|_____ Crowding _____|_____
6. Position of individual teeth (note on patient's clinical charting)
   a. Rotation
   b. Inclinations
   c. Extrusion
   d. Drifting
   e. Pathologic migration
7. Morphology of teeth
   a. General morphology: Cusps  Steep ☐     Shallow ☐
   b. Marginal ridge relations (note uneven ridges with arrow)
      Relation to restorations _____|_____
   c. Occlusal and/or incisal wear
      (1) General:  Slight ☐     Moderate ☐     Severe ☐
      (2) Facets _____|_____ (Correlate
          with parafunctional.) (See section E.)
8. Observe lingual surfaces of teeth with casts in occlusion
   a. Severe anterior overbite with contact of mandibular incisor with palatal surface of maxillary
      gingiva?
      _____|_____
   b. Cusp points that may wedge into proximal areas of opposing teeth?
      _____|_____

**F. Musculature**
1. Function
   a. Maximum opening _____ mm (incisal edge to incisal edge at midline)
   b. Restrictions on opening? Yes ☐     No ☐     Describe _____
   c. Jaw manipulation: Easy ☐     Difficult ☐
      (1) Inhibited voluntary movement: To right lateral ☐     To left lateral ☐
          Protrusive ☐
      (2) Deflections on opening or closing (right, left, S, etc.: specify)
      _____
2. Spasm and/or pain (circle):  None     On palpation: R L     Temporal area: R L
   Masseter area: R L     Pterygoid: R L
3. Freeway space _____ mm
4. Occlusion/disocclusion ratio (in laterals) _____

**G. Summary of evidence for occlusal adjustment**
Based on the interpretation of the accumulated data:
1. Is an occlusal adjustment indicated? Yes ☐     No ☐
2. Defend your answer: _____

If your answer is yes, proceed with the face-bow transfer and mounting of study casts.

the clinical, roentgenographic, and occlusal examinations should be correlated. From such correlation, the diagnosis, the etiology, the prognosis, and the treatment plan are derived.

From Chapter 1, it can be seen that there are many periodontal diseases. However, the bacterially induced diseases—gingivitis and periodontitis—are the most frequently encountered. From the data obtained during the examination, the patient may be categorized in one of the ADA case types (see box, below).

## Classification

No generally accepted classification for periodontal diseases exists at the present time. Nevertheless a classification is needed. A classification should not be rigid, but it must be adaptable, responding to changing knowledge. Its function is the logical and systematic separation and organization of knowledge about diseases, so that one may reason from the signs and symptoms seen in the patient to a presumed etiologic history, from the presumed etiologic history to the identification of the condition, and

---

### PERIODONTAL DIAGNOSIS BY CASE TYPE

| American Dental Association Code Number | Case Type | Description |
|---|---|---|
| 04500 | I | Gingivitis (shallow pockets, no bone loss) |
| | IA | Gingivitis with complicating factors (systemic disease, physical disabilities) |
| 04600 | II | Early periodontitis (moderate pockets, minor-to-moderate bone loss, satisfactory topography, usually no tooth mobility) |
| | IIA | Early periodontitis with complicating factors |
| 04700 | III | Moderate periodontitis (moderate-to-deep pockets, moderate-to-severe bone loss, unsatisfactory topography, usually slight mobility of teeth) |
| | IIIA | Moderate periodontitis with complicating factors |
| 04800 | IV | Advanced periodontitis (deep pockets, severe bone loss, advanced mobility patterns, usually missing teeth; may become prosthetic reconstruction case) |
| | IVA | Advanced periodontitis with complicating factors |

I    II    III    IV

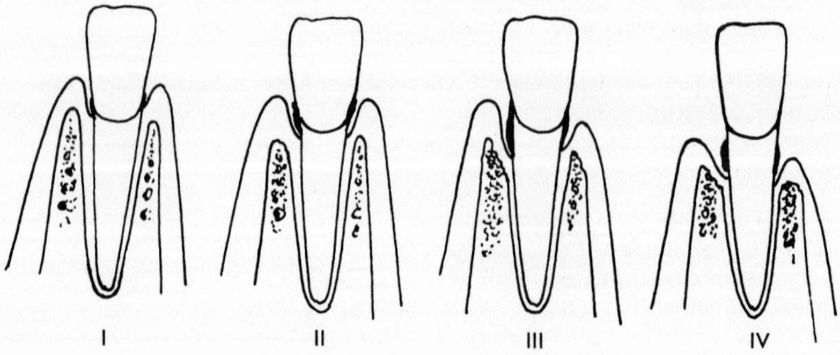

from there to the prescribed course of treatment. With a classification, facts can be filed for future reference. There is no reason for not adding to a classification or changing its sequence to simplify it if the changes are based on new findings[98-107] (see box, p. 565).

A system of classifying or grouping the pathologic processes affecting the periodontium serves to identify the etiologyy and to facilitate communication among clinicians, researchers, educators, students, epidemiologists, and public health workers.

Dentists commonly use the singular term *periodontal disease,* but a plurality of diverse conditions afflict the periodontium. The periodontium, being an organ made of several basic tissues, is subject to infectious, metabolic, developmental, neoplastic, nutritional, hormonal, dystrophic, and traumatic maladies. Inflammation is the most common pathologic process affecting the periodontium and is what the dentist has in mind when speaking of periodontal disease(s).

Classification systems use the term *gingivitis* to mean inflammation of the superficial investing layer of the periodontium and reserve *periodontitis* for the extension of the inflammatory process to the underlying supporting structures. The idea that gingivitis and periodontitis are a continuum has prevailed in the past and is expressed in concepts such as, "while not all gingivitis proceeds to periodontitis, all periodontitis originates as gingivitis." Probably neither of these concepts is correct.

The problems in distinguishing between gingivitis and periodontitis are magnified when classifications are expanded to include other disorders. The difficulties inherent in classification are obvious when some examples are reviewed. In many instances, the disease process may be influenced by a past response of the periodontium or an etiologic factor no longer present.

Since we are still delineating the precise pathogenesis of periodontal diseases, names that indicate these pathogenetic pathways are not yet in use. Instead, the presently used names depict the signs, symptoms, and, at times, the histopathologic characteristics of the disease—e.g., gingivitis and periodontitis.

Periodontal disease entities can frequently be classified in more than one category. The diseases may be multifactorial and in their advanced stages may be combined with other disease entities; for example, a patient with juvenile periodontitis may have a typical flora for the disease and also have tooth mobility and defective immunologic responses. Thus this disease may appear in more than one classification category, depending upon the basis for the classification.

One useful property of a good classification is consistency. For instance, Orban, 1949, (see box, p. 565) established a classification based upon tissue response, dividing reactions into inflammatory, dystrophic, and neoplastic.[98] When later developments proved this classification to be inadequate, the value of the consistency remained.

Another classification by Weatherford can be seen in the box on p. 565. It uses elements from the classifications of Pritchard[114] and Page and Schroeder[117] and combines rate of destruction with age of the patient. This classification differentiates gingivitis, gingival enlargement, NUG, periodontitis, and so on, and is useful in teaching students. Another classification used for insurance purposes emphasizes *case type* (of complexity) (see box, opposite), which in turn relates to extent and complexity of treatment. The interplay of infection, inflammatory response, metabolic status of the cells are all part of the disease process. Some of the factors that influence the disease process can be outlined as follows:

   I. Inflammatory response to bacterially induced disease
  II. Immunological response

III. Metabolic influences
   A. Genetic
   B. Nongenetic
      1. Hormonally induced
      2. Nutritionally induced
      3. Drug induced
IV. Neoplastic
 V. Other factors

A classification based solely on etiologic agents would be desirable. It may not be realized, however, since many factors influence the manifestations of the disease and no single agent or cluster of agents can be proven to cause the disorder. The current evidence concerning microbial specificity in the causation of periodontal disease is presented and discussed in Chapter 8. However, the diagnosis of a "bacteroidal periodontitis" or an "actinomycetal periodontitis" or an "actinobacillary/capnocytophagal periodontitis" is premature. While there are many types of periodontal diseases, some of which may be noninflammatory, inflammatory disorders are the predominant forms of the disease. Thus a utilitarian classification should emphasize the inflammatory conditions.

No infection (defined as a disease caused by bacteria) is likely to exist without a concomitant immune response. The immune response has been shown to play a role in all infections and is likely to do so in gingivitis and periodontitis. Any suppression of the immune response can result in bacterial overgrowth. Genetic factors may predispose or even trigger periodontal diseases. Systemic diseases such as diabetes mellitus are positively related to increased incidence and severity of periodontitis. Factors governing leukocyte migration and chemotaxis influence host response and susceptibility to infection. Thus systemic/genetic/immunologic factors exert important pathogenetic influences.[117-119]

Any alteration in salivary composition or flow—be it the result of immune disease (Sjögren's syndrome, and so on), x-irradiation, medication, or mouthbreathing—will affect the bacterial population of the mouth. Even though our concern may be primarily with bacterially induced inflammation of the periodontal tissues, we must give consideration to the interrelationships that influence the pathogenesis of the disease.

A single clinical entity such as hyperplasia could be fitted into the several classifications shown in Tables 28-1 and 28-2. Thus the classification system may be useful in differential diagnosis.

Periodontitis may not be a homogenous disease but rather a family of *several different, yet related, diseases* (Table 28-1). The clinical features of inflammation are similar, but distinct differences may exist in the etiology, progression, natural history, and in responses to treatment. Genetic, hematologic, and immunologic influences have been reported for several types of periodontitis, lending validity to the inclusion of a class reflecting these modifying factors (see box opposite, classification of Grant, Stern, and Everett, 1979[113]).

Juvenile periodontitis has been described in two forms; a localized one in which the incisors and first molars are the areas of predominant involvement and in another, more generalized, form. These may be the result of age of onset and degree of immune response rather than the manifestations of two distinct disease entities. In fitting periodontitis and gingivitis into the proposed classification, several considerations may be pertinent. There is accumulating evidence that even in inflammatory states that appear to be slowly and continuously progressive, the process is more likely periodic with episodes in which tissue destruction occurs, interspersed with periods of remission during which time some repair may occur. These cyclic occurrences may go undetected in screening

# CLASSIFICATIONS OF PERIODONTAL DISEASE

**Gottlieb, 1928[108]**

*Inflammatory*
Schmutz pyorrhea (poor oral hygiene)
*Degenerative or atrophic*
Diffuse alveolar atrophy (systemic or metabolic causes)
Paradental pyorrhea

**Box, 1940[109]**

*Gingivitis*
Acute
Chronic
*Periodontitis*
Acute
Chronic
Periodontitis simplex (exogenous factors)
Periodontitis complex or rarefying pericementitis fibrosa (endogenous factors)

**Bernier, 1957[110]**

*Inflammation*
Gingivitis
Periodontitis
Primary (simplex)
Secondary (complex)
*Dystrophy*
Occlusal traumatism
Periodontal disuse atrophy
Gingivitis
Periodontosis

**Orban, 1949[111]**

*Inflammatory conditions*
*Gingivitis*
Acute or chronic according to duration
Ulcerative, purulent, etc., according to symptoms
Local or systemic according to etiology
Local (extrinsic)
Infectious
Physical
Chemical
Systemic (intrinsic)
Dietary deficiency
Endocrine disturbance
*Periodontitis*
Simplex—following gingivitis
Complex—following periodontosis
*Degenerative conditions*
*Gingivosis*—systemic etiology
Degeneration of connective tissue
*Periodontosis*
Early—no inflammation
Late—deep pockets with periodontitis
*Atrophic conditions*
Periodontal atrophy—bone recession
*Periodontal traumatism*
Primary—overstress, bruxism, etc.
Secondary—loss of supporting tissue

**Orban—cont'd**

*Gingival hyperplasia*
Infectious—pyogenic granuloma
Endocrine dysfunction—pregnancy
Drugs—Dilantin
Idiopathic

**Goldman and Cohen, 1972[112]**

*Inflammation*
*Gingivitis*—with or without gingival enlargement (acute and chronic)
*Periodontitis*
Secondary to long-standing gingivitis
Initial lesion
May occur in conjunction with occlusal traumatism
Secondary to periodontosis
*Dystrophy*
Occlusal traumatism
Degenerative disease of attachment apparatus: periodontosis

**Grant, Stern, and Everett, 1979[113]**

*Inflammatory*
Gingivitis
Periodontitis
Juvenile periodontitis
*Traumatic/degenerative*
Periodontal trauma
Gingival recession
Alveolar atrophy
*Systemic/genetic/immunologic*
Hereditary gingival fibromatosis
Chédiak-Higashi syndrome
Down syndrome
Hypophosphotasla
Cyclic neutropenia
Lazy leukocyte syndrome
Diabetes mellitus
Juvenile periodontitis
Hyperkeratosis palmaris et plantaris

**Prichard, 1972[114]**

*Inflammation with surface destruction*
Necrotizing ulcerative gingivitis
Herpetic gingivostomatitis
Desquamative gingivitis
Oral ulcers
*Diseases affecting the surface or gingiva*
Inflammation without surface destruction
Marginal gingivitis
Generalized diffuse gingivitis
Gingival enlargement
*Disease that affect the deeper structures*
Chronic destructive periodontal disease or periodontitis
Periodontal abscess
Periodontal traumatism
Primary traumatism
Secondary traumatism

**Schluger, Yuodelis, and Page, 1977[115]**

*Gingivitis*
Plaque-associated gingivitis
Acute ulcerative necrotizing gingivitis
Hormonal gingivitis
Drug-induced gingivitis
*Marginal periodontitis*
Adult type
Juvenile type

**Ramfjord and Ash, 1979[116]**

*Gingivitis*
Simplex
Complex
Gingival hyperplasia
Necrotizing lesions
Traumatic
*Gingival atrophy or recession*
Systemic factors
Local causes
*Trauma from occlusion*
*Periodontitis*
Simple
Complex
Juvenile, etc.

**Page and Schroeder, 1982[117]**

*Periodontitis*
Prepubertal
Generalized
Localized
Juvenile
Rapidly progressing periodontitis
"Adult" type periodontitis

**Weatherford, 1987**

*Diseases affecting the surface of gingiva*
Inflammation without surface destruction
Marginal gingivitis
Generalized diffuse gingivitis
Gingival enlargement
Inflammation with surface destruction
Necrotizing ulcerative gingivitis
Herpetic gingivostomatitis
Desquamative gingivitis
Oral ulcers
*Diseases affecting deeper structures*
Early onset periodontitis
Prepubertal periodontitis
Generalized
Localized
Juvenile periodontitis
Rapidly progressing periodontitis
Postpubertal periodontitis
"Adult" type periodontitis
Rapidly progressing periodontitis
Periodontal traumatism
Primary traumatism
Secondary traumatism
Periodontal abscess

**Table 28-1** Etiologies in the classification of periodontal disease (Grant, Stern, Listgarten)

| Etiology | Disease |
| --- | --- |
| **BACTERIALLY INDUCED DISEASES** | |
| Gingivitis | |
| Periodontitis | Adult type (slow and intermittently progressive) |
| | Post-juvenile periodontitis (slow and intermittently progressive) |
| | Early onset periodontitis |
| |    Juvenile type (molar-incisor) |
| |    Juvenile type (generalized) |
| |    Prepubertal (mixed dentition) |
| | Adult type (rapidly progressive) |
| Acute necrotizing ulcerative gingivitis | |
| Acute abscess | |
| Pericoronitis | |
| **FUNCTIONALLY INDUCED DISEASES** | |
| Traumatic occlusion | Bone resorption |
| Disuse atrophy | Alveolar atrophy (resorption of supporting bone) |
| **TRAUMA** | |
| Habits, accident | Gingival recession, bone resorption |

**Table 28-2** Modifying factors in gingivitis and periodontitis

| Etiology | Disease |
| --- | --- |
| Genetic influence | Down syndrome |
| | Hypophosphatasia |
| | Familial gingival enlargement (fibromatosis) |
| Neutrophil dysfunction | Cyclic neutropenia |
| | Chédiak-Higashi syndrome |
| | Lazy leukocyte syndrome |
| | Juvenile periodontitis (familial) |
| | Hyperkeratosis palmar-plantaris |
| | Infantile hereditary agranulocytosis |
| | Congenital neutropenia |
| | Agranulocytosis |
| Dermatologic | Benign mucous membrane pemphigoid |
| | Erosive lichen planus |
| Autoimmune | Sjögren's syndrome |
| Immune deficiency | AIDS |
| | Immunosuppressive cancer |
| Metabolic influences | |
|   Hormonal | Gingivitis related to androgens, estrogens, oral contraceptives |
|   Nutritional | Scurvy |
| | Protein-calorie malnutrition |
|   Drug induced | Dilantin-induced hyperplasia |
| | Nifedipine-induced hyperplasia |
| | Cyclosporin A-induced hyperplasia |
| | Immunosuppressive chemotherapy |
|   Neoplastic | Leukemias |
| | Metastatic tumors to periodontium |

**Table 28-3**  Characteristics of various forms of periodontitis

|  | AP | RP-A | RP-B | JP | Post-JP | PP |
|---|---|---|---|---|---|---|
| Age | 35 yrs or over | 14-26 yrs | 26-35 yrs | 12-26 yrs | 26-35 yrs | <12 yrs |
| Sex ratio F:M | 1:1 | 2-3:1 | ? | 3:1 | 3:1 | 1:1 |
| Lesions | Variable | Generalized | Generalized | First molar incisor | First molar incisor | General or localized mixed dentition |
| Tooth-associated materials | Yes | Yes/no | Yes/no | No/yes | Yes | Minimal |
| Caries rate | Variable | Variable | Variable | Low | Variable | Low |
| Immune factors | | | | | | |
| PMN | Normal | Depressed | Depressed or normal | Depressed | ? | Depressed |
| Lymphocytes, AMLR | Normal | Depressed | Normal | Increased | Increased (not significant) | ? |
| Genetic | ? | Yes | ? | Yes | Yes | Yes |

From Suzuki, J.B.: Current diagnosis and classification of periodontal diseases, Dent. Clin. N. Am. In press, 1988.
 AP—Adult periodontitis.
 RP-A—Rapidly progressive periodontitis, type A.
 RP-B—Rapidly progressive periodontitis, type B.
  JP—Juvenile periodontitis.
Post-JP—Post-juvenile periodontitis.
  PP—Prepubertal periodontitis.
 AMLR—Autologous mixed lymphocyte reaction.
 PMN—Polymorphonuclear leukocytes.

studies in which all data is pooled and there are few active sites. Not all sites are equally affected and some sites are not affected at all. The periods of exacerbation may be short and therefore may be missed. Fitting patients into inflexible classes is difficult because of the possibility that the disease might change, or more than one class of disease may be present in the same patient at the same time. Some characteristics of the adult, rapidly progressing, juvenile, postjuvenile, and prepubertal forms of periodontitis are listed in Table 28-3.

## REEXAMINATIONS

Only by repeated measurement (of bone level,[120,121] of bacterial types present,[10,11,13] of number of bacteria, of the constituents in crevicular gingival fluid,[22,23,30,31] of tooth mobility, of degree of imflammation,[12,13,29-31,90] and of probing depth and attachment level) can we make comparisons of the health or disease of the patient through periods of time. Such monitoring helps us decide if the patient has improved or worsened, if the disease is quiescent or active, and if the therapy has been effective. Ultimately, probing and charting must be correlated with microbiologic data, sulcular fluid examination, bone density and other test results.[120,121] Some progress has been made in this regard. Keyes and associates[124] have proposed a microbiologic monitoring of spirochetes, motile rods, and polymorphonuclear leukocytes in subgingival plaque samples as a means of assessing the presence of active, ongoing disease. Together with evaluation of the anatomic and morphologic features of cases, evaluations of the efficacy of treatment are possible[122-124] under specific conditions. On the other hand, since the particular species of bacteria responsible for the active episodes of periodontal breakdown and the mode of action involved are unknown, such monitoring may yield only limited information in adult periodontitis[125] (see Chapter 8). Moreover, dark-field examination of plaque samples from active sites of breakdown and inactive sites as determined by changes in attachment level or stability do not support this hypothesis.[126] Some populations of periodontitis-resistant people exhibit a high proportion of spirochetes and intermediate percentages of motile rods.[127]

Charting is the major recording tool in common use at the present time. If periodic chartings are compared, retrospective analysis becomes possible. The form used for such comparisons is shown in Fig. 28-22. In quiescent periods, examinations are made annually. In active periods the examinations must be performed more frequently. The changes in the patients' health-disease status are more easily followed. Both numbers and depths of pockets are compared. Such awareness leads to more effective delivery of therapeutic interventions during times of breakdown, and a more careful analysis of the effectiveness of therapy during and following treatment. However, precise identification of beginning and end of disease activity remains an elusive goal. Treatment without careful moinitoring cannot be proven to be necessary or effective. Monitoring a patient during a period of disease activity without providing treatment constitutes negligence.

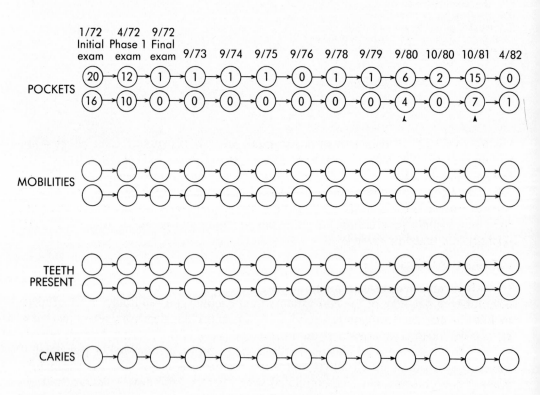

**Fig. 28-22.** Examination synopsis form permits the entry and comparison of periodic recordings. Pockets, mobilities, number of teeth present, and new carious lesions are tallied at the outset of treatment, after initial and surgical therapy, and during periodontal maintenance therapy or at reevaluation examinations. When an increase in number occurs (see *arrowheads*), either surgical or conservative or other therapeutic steps are taken. Measurements are then made at short intervals (monthly or in 6-week periods) until the number returns to normal. Any increase in the number of pockets, mobility, or caries signifies a recurrence and a need for further treatment.

## REFERENCES

1. Guidelines for the clinical assessment of periodontal therapy, The California Society of Periodontists.
2. Cohen, H.: The nature, methods and purpose of diagnosis, Lancet **1**:23, 1943.
3. O'Leary, T.J., Shannon, I.L., and Prigmore, J.R.: Clinical and systemic findings in periodontal disease, J. Periodontol. **33**:243, 1962.
4. Maguire, G.P., and Rutter, D.R.: History-taking for medical students, I. Deficiencies in performance, Lancet **2**:556, 1976.
5. Wolff, L.F., Bakdash, M.B., and Bandt, C.L.: Microbial interpretation of plaque relative to the diagnosis and treatment of periodontal disease, J. Periodontol. **56**:281, 1985.
6. Listgarten, M.A., and Schifter, C.: Differential dark-field microscopy of subgingival bacteria as an aid in selecting recall intervals: results after 18 months, J. Clin. Periodontol. **9**:305, 1982.
7. Leggott, P.J., et al.: Phase contrast microscopy of microbial aggregates in the gingival sulcus of *Macaca mulatta:* subgingival plaque bacteria in *Macaca mulatta,* J. Clin. Periodontol. **10**:412, 1983.
8. Greenwell, H. III, and Bissada, N.F.: Variations in subgingival microflora from healthy and intervention sites using probing depth and bacteriologic identification criteria, J. Periodontol. **55**:391, 1984.
9. Wolff, L.F., et al.: Distinct categories of microbial forms associated with periodontal disease, J. Periodont. Res. **20**:497, 1985.
10. Zambon, J.J., et al.: Rapid identification of periodontal pathogens in subgingival dental plaque: comparison of indirect immunofluorescence microscopy with bacterial culture for detection of *Bacteroides gingivalis,* J. Periodontol. Suppl. **56**:32, 1985.
11. Genco, R.J., Zambon, J.J., and Murray, P.A.: Serum and gingival fluid antibodies as adjuncts in the diagnosis of *Actinobacillus actinomycetemcomitans*–associated periodontal disease, J. Periodontol. Suppl. **56**:41, 1985.
12. Ebersole, J.L., Taubman, M.A., and Smith, D.J.: Local antibody responses in periodontal disease, J. Periodontol. Suppl. **56**:51, 1985.
13. Greenstein, G., and Polson, A.: Microscopic monitoring of pathogens associated with periodontal diseases: a review, J. Periodontol. **56**:740, 1985.
14. Golub, L.M., and Kleinberg, I.: Gingival crevicular fluid, a new diagnostic aid in managing the periodontal patient, Oral Sci. Rev. **8**:49, 1976.
15. Löe, H., and Holm-Pedersen, P.: Absence and presence of fluid from normal and inflamed gingivae, Periodontics **3**:171, 1965.
16. Alfano, M.C., et al.: Passively generated increase in gingival crevicular fluid flow from human gingiva, J. Dent. Res. **55**:1132, 1976.
17. Egelberg, J., and Attström, R.: Comparison between orifice and intracrevicular methods of sampling gingival fluid, J. Periodont. Res. **8**:384, 1973.
18. Tsuchida, K., and Hara, K.: Clinical significance of gingival fluid measurement by "Periotron," J. Periodontol. **52**:697, 1981.
19. Friedman, S.A., Mandel, I.D., and Herrera, M.S.: Lysozyme and lactoferrin quantitation in the crevicular fluid, J. Periodontol. **54**:347, 1983.
20. Golub, L.M., et al.: Collagenolytic activity of crevicular fluid from pericoronal gingival flaps, J. Dent. Res. **55**:177, 1976.
21. Winer, R.A., et al.: Enzyme activity in periodontal disease, J. Periodontol. **41**:449, 1970.
22. Schenkein, H.A., and Genco, R.J.: Gingival fluid and serum in periodontal diseases. I. Quantitative study of immunoglobulins, complement components, and other plasma proteins, J. Periodontol. **48**:772, 1977.
23. Schenkein, H.A., and Genco, R.J.: Gingival fluid and serum in periodontal diseases. II. Evidence for cleavage of complement components C3, C3 proactivator (factor B) and C4 in gingival fluid, J. Periodontol. **48**:778, 1977.
24. Botta, G.A., et al.: Gas-liquid chromatography of the gingival fluid as an aid in periodontal diagnosis, J. Periodont. Res. **20**:450, 1985.
25. Klinkhamer, J.M., and Mitchell, M.D.: Orogranulocyte peroxidase activity as a measure of inflammatory periodontal disease, J. Dent. Res. **58**:531, 1979.
26. Hase, M.P., and Reade, P.C.: The oral leukocyte migration rate index as a method of assessing periodontal disease in an individual, J. Periodont. Res. **14**:153, 1979.
27. Klinkhamer, J.M.: Quantitative evaluation of gingivitis and periodontal disease. I. The orogranulocytic migratory rate, Periodontics **6**:207, 1968.
28. Skougaard, M.R., Bay, I., and Klinkhamer, J.M.: Correlation between gingivitis and orogranulocytic migratory rate, J. Dent. Res. Suppl. **48**:717, 1969.
29. Iacono, V.J., et al.: *In vivo* essay of crevicular leukocyte migration: its development and potential applications, J. Periodontol. Suppl. **56**:56, 1985.
30. Lamster, I.B., Hartley, L.J., and Vogel, R.I.: Development of a biological profile for gingival crevicular fluid: methodical considerations and evaluation of collagen-degrading and ground substance-degrading enzyme activity during experimental gingivitis, Periodontol. Suppl. **56**:13, 1985.
31. Mukherjee, S.: The role of crevicular fluid iron in periodontal disease, J. Periodontol. Suppl. **56**:22, 1985.
32. Woolweaver, D.A., et al.: Relation of the orogranulocytic migratory rate to periodontal disease and blood leukocyte count, J. Dent. Res. **51**:929, 1972.

33. Löe, H., and Silness, J.: Periodontal disease in pregnancy. I. Prevalence and severity, Acta Odontol. Scand. **21**:533, 1963.

34. Suomi, J.D., Palumbo, J., and Barbano, J.P.: Comparative study of radiographs and pocket measurements in periodontal disease evaluation, J. Periodontol. **39**:311, 1968.

35. Tzamouranis, A., et al.: Increase of endotoxin concentration in gingival washings during experimental gingivitis in man, J. Periodontol. **50**:175, 1979.

36. Mörmann, W., Regolati, B., and Mühlemann, H.R.: The gingivitis fluorescein test, Helv. Odontol. Acta **18**:1, 1974.

37. Mörmann, W., et al.: Gingivitis fluorescein test in recruits, Helv. Odontol. Acta **19**:27, 1975.

38. Reiff, R.L.: Serum and salivary IgG and IgA response to initial preparation therapy, J. Periodontol. **55**:299, 1984.

39. Tolo, K., and Schenck, K.: Activity of serum immunoglobulins G, A, and M to six anaerobic, oral bacteria in diagnosis of periodontitis, J. Periodont. Res. **20**:113, 1985.

40. Polson, A.M., and Goodson, J.M.: Periodontal diagnosis: current status and future needs, J. Periodontol. **56**:25, 1985.

41. Sheiham, A.: Screening for periodontal disease, J. Clin. Periodontol. **5**:237, 1978.

42. Sibertson, J.F., and Burgett, F.G.: Probing of pockets related to attachment level, J. Periodontol. **48**:148, 1978.

43. Everett, F.G.: Grenzen der Behandlung parodontotischer Zähne, Dtsch. Zahnaerztl. Z. 1972.

44. Armitage, G.C., Svanberg, G.K., Löe, H.: Microscopic evaluation of clinical measurements of connective tissue attachment levels, J. Clin. Periodontol. **4**:173, 1977.

45. Robinson, P.J., and Vitek, R.M.: The relationship between gingival inflammation and resistance to probe penetration, J. Periodont. Res. **14**:239, 1979.

46. Polson, A.M., et al.: Histological determination of probe tip penetration into gingival sulcus of humans using electronic pressure sensitive probe, J. Clin. Periodontol. **7**:479, 1980.

47. Listgarten, M.A.: Periodontal probing: what does it mean? J. Clin. Periodontol. **7**:165, 1980.

48. Freed, H.K., Gapper, R.L., and Kalkwarf, K.L.: Evaluation of probing forces, J. Periodontol. **54**:488, 1983.

49. Listgarten, M.A., Mao, R., and Robinson, P.J.: Periodontal probing and the relationship of the probe tip to periodontal tissues, J. Periodontol. **47**:511, 1976.

50. Spray, J.R., et al.: Microscopic demonstration of the position of periodontal probes, J. Periodontol. **49**:148, 1980.

51. Hassell, T.M., Germann, M.A., and Saxer, U.P.: Periodontal probing: interinvestigator discrepancies and correlations between probing force and recorded depth, Helv. Odontol. Acta **17**:38, 1973.

52. Flemming, I., Karring, T., and Attström, R.: Reproducibility of pocket depth and attachment level measurements when using a flexible splint, J. Clin. Periodontol. **11**:662, 1984.

53. Durwin, A., et al.: Significance of probing force for evaluation of healing following periodontal therapy, J. Clin. Periodontol. **12**:306, 1985.

54. Stambaugh, R., et al.: The limits of subgingival scaling, Int. J. Periodont. Restor. Dent. **5**:31, 1981.

55. Aeppli, D.M., Boen, J.R., and Bandt, C.L.: Measuring and interpreting increases in probing depth and attachment loss, J. Periodontol. **56**:262, 1985.

56. Magnusson, I., and Listgarten, M.A.: Histologic evaluation of probing depth following periodontal treatment, J. Clin. Periodontol. **7**:26, 1980.

57. Björn, H., Halling, A., and Thyberg, H.: Radiographic assessment of marginal bone loss, Odontol. Rev. **20**:165, 1969.

58. Greenberg, J., Laster, L.L., and Listgarten, M.A.: Transgingival probing as a potential estimator of alveolar bone level, J. Periodontol. **47**:514, 1976.

59. Everett, F.G., and Fixott, H.C.: Use of an incorporated grid in the interpretation of dental roentgenograms, Oral Surg. **16**:1061, 1963.

60. O'Leary, T.J., Rudd, K.D., and Nabers, C.L.: Factors influencing horizontal tooth mobility, Periodontics **4**:308, 1966.

61. Adriaens, P.A.: Summary of the Sixth Belgian Congress of Dentistry: tooth mobility and tooth movement, J. Am. Dent. Assoc. **103**:897, 1981.

62. Körber, K.H., and Körber, E.: Untersuchungen zur Biophysik des Parodontiums, Dtsch. Zahnaerztl. Z. **17**:1585, 1962.

63. Körber, K.H., and Körber, E.: Untersuchungen über die kaufunktionelle Beanspruchung des Zahnes, Dtsch. Zahnaerztl. Z. **18**:576, 1963.

64. Picton, D.C.A.: A study of normal tooth mobility and the changes with periodontal disease, Dent. Pract. **12**:167, 1962.

65. Mühlemann, H.R.: Tooth mobility: a review of clinical aspects and research findings, J. Periodontol. **38**:686, 1967.

66. Persson, R., and Svensson, A.: Assessment of tooth mobility using small loads. I. Technical devices and calculations of tooth mobility in health and disease, J. Clin. Periodontol. **7**:259, 1980.

67. Rydén, H., Bjelkhagen, H., and Sandström, U.: A laser instrument for measuring tooth movements, J. Periodontol. **50**:265, 1979.

68. Laster, L., Laudenbach, K.W., and Stoller,

N.H.: An evaluation of clinical tooth mobility measurements, J. Periodontol. **46:**603, 1975.

69. O'Leary, T.J.: Indices for measurement of tooth mobility in clinical studies, J. Periodont. Res. Suppl. **14:**94, 1974.

70. Wasserman, B.H., Geiger, A.M., and Turgeon, L.R.: Relationship of occlusion and periodontal disease. VII. Mobility, J. Periodontol. **44:**572, 1973.

71. O'Leary, T.J., Shanley, D.B., and Drake, R.B.: Tooth mobility in cuspid-protected and group-function occlusions, J. Prosthet. Dent. **27:**21, 1972.

72. Caton, J., Greenstein, G., and Polson, A.M.: Depth of periodontal probe penetration related to clinical and histologic signs of gingival inflammation, J. Periodontol. **52:**626, 1981.

73. Engelberger, T., et al.: Correlations among Papilla Bleeding Index, other clinical indices and histologically determined inflammation of the gingival papilla, J. Clin. Periodontol. **10:**579, 1983.

74. Nowicki, D., et al.: The gingival bleeding time index, J. Periodontol. **52:**260, 1981.

75. Greenstein, G.: The role of bleeding on probing in the diagnosis of periodontal disease: a literature review, J. Periodontol. **55:**684, 1984.

76. Löe, H.: The gingival index, the plaque index and the retention index systems, J. Periodontol. **38:**610, 1967.

77. Polson, A.M., and Caton, J.G.: Current status of bleeding in the diagnosis of periodontal diseases, J. Periodontol. Suppl. **56:**1, 1985.

78. Massler, M., Emslie, R.D., and Bolden, T.F.: Fetor ex ore, Oral Surg. **4:**110, 1951.

79. Hine, M.K.: Halitosis, J. Am. Dent. Assoc. **55:**37, 1957.

80. Burnette, E.W.: Limitations of roentgenograms in periodontal diagnosis, J. Periodontol. **42:**293, 1971.

81. Convery, L.: Halitosis, Irish Dent. Rev. **9:**44, 1963.

82. Spouge, J.D.: Halitosis, Dent. Pract. **14:**307, 1964.

83. Wright, W.H.: Local factors in periodontal disease, J. Periodontol. **1:**163, 1963.

84. Hurt, W.C.: Periodontal diagnosis—1977: a status report, J. Periodontol. **48:**533, 1977.

85. Everett, F.G.: Halitosis, Oregon Dent. J. **41:**13, 1971.

86. Rosling, B., et al.: A radiographic method for assessing changes in alveolar bone height following periodontal therapy, J. Clin. Periodontol. **2:**211, 1975.

87. Baumhammers, A., and Ceravolo, F.J.: An improved diagnostic point to aid in radiographic interpretation, J. Periodontol. **48:**52, 1977.

88. Bassiouny, M.A., and Grant, A.A.: Radiographic assessment of proximal infrabony pocket topography, J. Periodontol. **47:**440, 1976.

89. Snyder, M.B., et al.: The advantages of xeroradiography for panoramic examination of the jaws and teeth, J. Periodontol. **48:**467, 1977.

90. Hirschfeld, L.: A calibrated silver point for periodontal diagnosis and recording, J. Periodontol. **24:**94, 1953.

91. Biggerstaff, R.H., and Phillips, J.R.: Equantative comparison of paralleling long cone and bisection of angle periapical radiography, Oral Surg. **41:**673, 1976.

92. Hollender, L., Lindhe, J., and Koch, G.: A roentgenographic study of clinically healthy and inflamed periodontal tissues in children, J. Periodont. Res. **1:**146, 1966.

93. Ainamo, J., and Tammisalo, E.H.: Comparison of radiographic and clinical signs of early periodontal disease, Scand. J. Dent. Res. **81:**548, 1973.

94. Patur, B: Roentgenographic evaluation of alveolar bone changes in periodontal disease, Dent. Clin. North Am., vol. 47, 1960.

95. Grondahl, H.-G., Johnson, E., and Lindahl, B.: Diagnosis of marginal bone destruction with orthopantomography and intraoral full mouth radiography, Sven. Tandläk. Tidskr. **64:**439, 1971.

96. Kelly, G.P., et al.: Radiographs in clinical periodontal trials, J. Periodontol. **46:**381, 1975.

97. Theilade, J.: An evaluation of the reliability of the radiographs in the measurement of bone loss in periodontal disease, J. Periodontol. **31:**143, 1960.

98. Stern, I.B.: Comparisons of periodontal techniques and philosophies as taught by different schools. I. The periodontal examination, Nihon Dent. Rev. **500:**177, 1984.

99. Lyons, H., Bernier, H., and Goldman, H.M.: Report of the Nomenclature and Classification Committee, J. Periodontol. **30:**74, 1959.

100. Fish, E.W.: Parodontal disease, ed. 2, London, 1952, Eyre & Spottiswoode Ltd.

101. Hine, M.K., and Hine, C.L.: Classification and etiology of periodontal disturbances, J. Am. Dent. Assoc. **31:**1297, 1944.

102. Hulin, C.: Nomenclature and classification, Parodontologie **3:**82, 1949.

103. Held, A.J., and Chaput, A.: Les parodontolyses, Paris, 1959, Prélat.

104. Orban, B.: Classification and nomenclature of periodontal diseases, J. Periodontol. **13:**88, 1942.

105. Box, H.K.: Periodontal studies, Dent. Items Interest **62:**915, 1940.

106. Kantorowicz, A.: Klinische Zahnheilkunde, Berlin, 1924, Hermann Meusser.

107. Weski, O.: Parodontopathien und Parodontosis, Berichte des 9ten internationalen Zahnärzte Kongresses der F.D.I., Vienna, 1936, Urban & Schwarzenberg.

108. Gottlieb, B.: Parodontal pyorrhea and alveolar atrophy, J. Am. Dent. Assoc. **15:**2196, 1928.

109. Box, H.K.: Periodontal studies, Dent. Items Interest **62:**915, 1940.

110. Bernier, J.L.: Report of the Committee on Classification and Nomenclature, J. Periodontol. **28:**56, 1957.

111. Orban, B.: Classification of periodontal disease, Paradontologie **3:**159, 1949.

112. Goldman, H.M., and Cohen, D.W.: Periodontal therapy, ed. 5, St. Louis, 1972, The C.V. Mosby Co.

113. Grant, D.A., Stern, J., and Everett, F.: Periodontics, ed. 5, St. Louis, 1979, The C.V. Mosby Co.

114. Prichard, J.F.: Advanced periodontal disease, ed. 2, Philadelphia, 1972, W.B. Saunders Co.

115. Schluger, S., Yuodelis, R., and Page, R.: Periodontal disease, Philadelphia, 1977, Lea & Febiger.

116. Ramfjord, S.P., and Ash, M.M.: Periodontology and periodontics, Philadelphia, 1979, W.B. Saunders Co.

117. Page, R.C., and Schroeder, H.E.: Periodontitis in man and other animals, Basel, 1982, S. Karger.

118. Brady, W.F., and Martinoff, J.T.: A simplified examination, diagnosis, and treatment classification of periodontal disease, J. Am. Dent. Assoc. **104:**313, 1982.

119. Cianciola, L.J., et al.: Defective polymorphonuclear leukocyte functions in a human periodontal disease, Nature **265:**445, 1977.

120. Hausmann, E., et al.: Usefulness of subtraction radiography in the evaluation of periodontal therapy, J. Periodontol. Suppl. **56:**4, 1985.

121. Jeffcoat, M.K., et al.: Nuclear medicine: an indication of "active" alveolar bone loss in beagle dogs treated with a non-steroidal anti-inflammatory drug, J. Periodontol. Suppl. **56:**8, 1985.

122. Rams, T.E., et al.: Long-term effects of microbiologically modulated periodontal therapy on advanced adult periodontitis, J. Am. Dent. Assoc. **111:**429, 1985.

123. Keyes, P.H., and Rams, T.E.: A rationale for the management of periodontal diseases: rapid identification of microbial therapeutic targets with phase-contrast microscopy, J. Am. Dent. Assoc. **106:**803, 1983.

124. Keyes, P.H.: Microbiologically monitored and modulated periodontal therapy, Gen. Dent. **33:**105, 1985.

125. Greenwell, H., and Bissada, N.F.: A dispassionate scientific analysis of Keyes' technique, Int. J. Periodont. Restor. Dent. **5:**65, 1985.

126. Haffajee, A.D., Socransky, S.S., and Goodson, J.M.: Clinical parameters as predictors of destructive periodontal disease activity, J. Clin. Periodontol. **10:**257, 1983.

127. Africa, C.W., Parker, J.R., and Reddy, J.: Bacterial studies of subgingival plaque in a periodontitis-resistant population. I. Darkfield microscopic studies, J. Periodont. Res. **20:**1, 1985.

## ADDITIONAL SUGGESTED READING

Brady, W.F., and Martinoff, J.T.: Validity of health history data collected from dental patients and patient perceptions of health status, J. Am. Dent. Assoc. **101:**642, 1980.

Burstone, C.J., Pryputniewicz, R.J., and Bowley, W.W.: Holographic measurement of tooth mobility in three dimensions, J. Periodont. Res. **13:**283, 1978.

Chilton, N., et al.: Proceedings of the Workshop on Quantitative Evaluation of Periodontal Disease by Physical Measurement Techniques, J. Dent. Res. **58:**547, 1979.

Dombrowski, J.C., et al.: A rapid chairside test for the severity of periodontal disease using gingival fluid, J. Periodontol. **49:**391, 1978.

Green, E., Clayton, J.A., and Schork, M.A.: Longitudinal periodontometry, J. Periodont. Res. **6:**301, 1971.

Oliver, R.C., Holm-Pedersen, P., and Löe, H.: The correlation between clinical scoring, exudate measurements and microscopic evaluation of inflammation in the gingiva, J. Periodontol. **40:**201, 1969.

Orban, B.J., and Orban, T.R.: Three-dimensional roentgenographic interpretation in periodontal diagnosis, J. Periodontol. **31:**275, 1960.

Orban, J.E., and Stallard, R.E.: Gingival crevicular fluid: a reliable predictor of gingival health? J. Periodontol. **40:**231, 1969.

van der Velden, U., and de Vries, J.H.: Introduction of a new periodontal probe: the pressure probe, J. Clin. Periodontol. **5:**188, 1978.

Vitek, R.M., Robinson, P.J., and Lautenschlager, E.P.: Development of a force-controlled periodontal probing instrument, J. Periodont. Res. **14:**93, 1979.

# CHAPTER 29

# Prognosis

**Definitions**

**Prognostic judgment and treatment planning**
Past history (rate of destruction)
Other considerations in establishing prognosis
Preserving the dentition

**Objectives of treatment**

---

## Definitions

Prognosis is a forecast. It developed as a prediction of the probable course of a disease and of the chances of the patient's recovery or death. In ancient times this forecast involved superstitious auguries and practices. Medicine was primitive and could not deal with infections and tumors. The death rate was high, the life span short. *Prognosis* was and is a word of urgency and importance to the patient, to whom the significance of the diagnosis lies in the prognosis.

Prognosis has different connotations and nuances. After diagnosis and before treatment the patient may ask, "Is my disease fatal?" "Will I lose my teeth?" The treatment prognosis is involved: "Will your treatment help me?" "What can you do to help me?" The estimation of the value of prosthetic dentistry and its relative effectiveness differs between a patient who is essentially well and another who has suffered from advanced periodontal disease. What are the therapeutic "odds"? What are the financial risks? What are the chances that the treatment will be of benefit? The patient has every right to know the answers to these questions. The patient can then be said to have accepted **Informed** treatment after being fully informed (i.e., informed consent). **consent**

Prognosis has three meanings in dentistry.

1. *Diagnostic prognosis.* An evaluation of the course of the disease without treatment. **Diagnostic** What is the status of the teeth now, and what is the anticipated future of these **prognosis** teeth?
2. *Therapeutic prognosis.* Given the state of the art and science of periodontics and the **Therapeutic** knowledge and skill of the practitioner, what effect will periodontal treatment have on **prognosis** the course of the disease?
3. *Prosthetic prognosis.* Given the anticipated result of periodontal treatment and the peri- **Prosthetic** odontal health status obtained for the patient, what is the forecast for the success of the **prognosis** prosthetic restoration? Will the prosthesis be therapeutic or detrimental? What specific needs dictate that it be prescribed? One must also take the state of the art and science of prosthetic and reconstructive dentistry and the skill and knowledge of the practitioner into consideration.

When a dentist performs an examination and presents the findings and diagnosis to the patient, evaluation of the health status of the teeth carries an implied prognosis of the first definition (diagnostic prognosis). A periodontal treatment plan is presented with a verbalized or implied prognosis of the second definition (therapeutic prognosis). A prosthetic treatment plan involves the third definition (prosthetic prognosis).

The prognosis can be hopeless for the dentition of a patient exhibiting extremely advanced rampant caries or extremely advanced periodontal disease. Similarly, the prognosis of a patient who is caries-immune and has no inflammatory periodontal disease is excellent.

**Range of diagnostic prognosis**

Between the extremes of hopeless and excellent is an entire range of gradations:

1. Excellent
2. Good
3. Fair
4. Guarded
5. Poor
6. Hopeless

## Prognostic judgment and treatment planning

Treatment can alter prognosis. If a patient has a mild gingivitis and some simple carious lesions, proper treatment and maintenance implies excellent health for decades. The patient may well ask, "I want to keep my teeth. How will your treatment alter the disease status of my teeth?" This depends on the diagnostic findings and the diagnostic prognosis (first definition). The severity and distribution of the lesions, the ADA classification type, and complicating factors of the disease must all be assessed to determine the effect of therapy.

**Severity and distribution of inflammatory and traumatic factors**

The severity of the disease might be slight, moderate, or severe (i.e., mildly, moderately, strongly, or extremely advanced periodontal disease). Severity depends on pocket depth, degree of bone loss, tooth mobility, and crown-root ratio. The distribution of disease may be generalized or localized. Inflammatory factors may have a generalized or a localized distribution. Traumatic factors may have a generalized or a localized distribution. The precise combination of both inflammatory and traumatic factors must be considered and may produce a variation in prognosis for individual teeth. There is an overall prognosis that may differ from that of an individual tooth.

**Individual tooth therapeutic prognosis**

Individual tooth therapeutic prognosis includes such factors as the following:

1. Percentage of bone loss
2. Probing depth
3. Distribution and type of bone loss
4. Presence and severity of furcation involvements
5. Mobility
6. Crown-root ratio
7. Pulpal involvement
8. Tooth position and occlusal relationship
9. Strategic value

**Overall therapeutic prognosis**

Following are factors included in overall prognosis:

1. Age
2. Medical status
3. Individual tooth prognoses (distribution and severity)
4. Degree of involvement, duration, and history of the disease (rate of progression)
5. Patient cooperation
6. Economic considerations
7. Knowledge and ability of the dentist
8. Etiologic factors

Only when all these factors are considered can a judgment be developed as to whether periodontal therapy could influence the etiologic factors inherent in the patient's disease and correct the sequelae of the disease process.

The development of a realistic therapeutic prognosis depends on the accuracy and completeness of the information gathered at the examination. It represents a considered judgment of the future course of the disease and a prediction of the response to treatment.

In general the therapeutic prognosis depends on the dentist's ability to recognize and eliminate or control the factors causing the disease, the ability to correct any damage that may have been caused by the disease, and the patient's ability and determination in maintaining the health of the periodontium and teeth.

The overall prognosis depends on the prognoses of the individual teeth. Periodontal disease often is very selective. Much destruction may occur about some teeth and little or none about others. Therefore the treatment plan prognosis must be weighed on two scales, one for the individual teeth and the other for the dentition as a whole.

## PAST HISTORY (RATE OF DESTRUCTION)

Probably the most important factor in forecasting the future health status of a dentition is knowledge of its past health status. The dentition that had a great breakdown many years ago but has remained unchanged since would have a better future than one which has more bone at present but which is going downhill rapidly. This forecast applies regardless of how few or many teeth remain. Comparisons of present records with older chartings, examinations, and roentgenograms that contain data concerning pocket depth, mobility, and bone level are of great value in determining rate of disease progression. Steady progression implies a poorer prognosis than does arrested disease, even at an advanced stage. Rapid progression about many teeth, simultaneously or sequentially, carries a poorer prognosis than does a rapid destruction of the periodontal tissues of a single tooth. Let us consider pocket formation, tooth mobility, and bone loss as elements of the natural history of the disease in the patient.

Shallower pockets have a better prognosis than do deep pockets. Deep pockets of 8 mm or more have a poor prognosis generally. Deep pockets can have a favorable prognosis if bone levels are high. Pockets around single-rooted teeth are usually easier to eliminate. Pockets around multirooted teeth present a special problem if furcations are involved. In general, the more amenable the pocket is to treatment, the better the prognosis.[1] *Pocket formation*

*Extent*

The location of the pocket is important. Some deep infrabony pockets on the proximal surfaces respond by fill and reattachment (Fig. 29-1, *A* to *E*). Others do not: a deep infrabony proximal pocket that does not respond will result in reverse architecture and will have a poor prognosis. Deep circumferential bony defects also carry a poor prognosis. Shallow defects can be treated by either fill or elimination. Pockets made deeper by inflammatory hyperplasia (pseudopockets) have a good prognosis. At times treatment may result in the clinical closure of a pocket by means of a long junctional epithelium (Fig. 29-1, *A* and *B*). *Location*

Formation of a long epithelial attachment is quite predictable in specific situations. Long narrow palatal pockets and deep labial pockets not involving the proximal surface will often close completely after thorough subgingival curettage even when they extend below the mucogingival junction.

Some pockets are more amenable than are others to surgical elimination by virtue of their depth, shape, and distribution. The morphologic characteristics of some retromolar regions, shallow vaults, or shallow mylohyoid attachments can complicate the potential for surgical pocket reduction. Although some teeth with pockets can be maintained for many years, it is generally true that successful pocket elimination results in a better prognosis than if residual pockets are left or reform after surgery. *Depth and complexity*

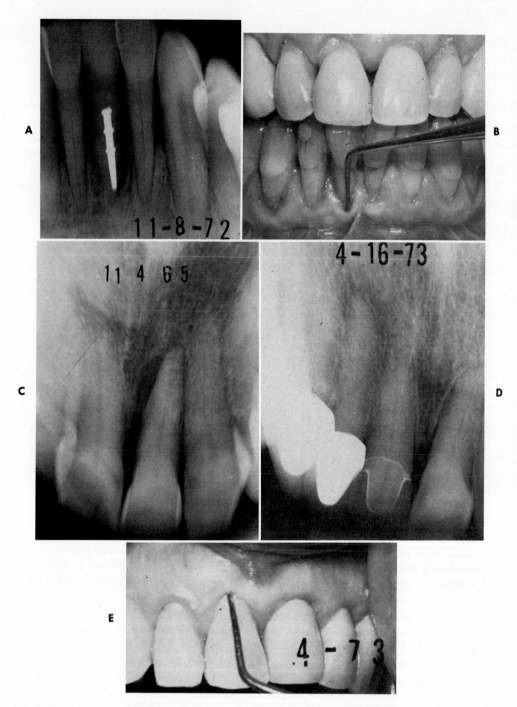

**Fig. 29-1.** **A,** Very deep labial pocket indicated by calibrated silver points to apex. **B,** After treatment, probe does not penetrate pocket to same extent. **C,** Roentgenogram showing bone destruction on mesial surface of the left central incisor. **D** and **E,** After treatment by curettage via flap bone has regenerated, and probe does not penetrate pocket. (Courtesy L. Hirschfeld, New York, New York.)

Teeth with pocket depth and bone loss have a more favorable prognosis when the teeth are firm rather than loose. With extensive bone loss, tooth mobility becomes increasingly important. Teeth with only 4 or 5 mm of remaining bone or with a mobility degree of 2 to 3 have a doubtful, if not hopeless prognosis. If the cause of tooth mobility can be eliminated, and if the mobility can be controlled or eliminated, the prognosis is better.[2] When traumatism produces forces of extraction dimension, the prognosis becomes hopeless.[3] This can occur particularly when the bone loss is extensive or when too few teeth remain.

The term *firm* is an oversimplification, since all teeth, unless they are ankylosed, have a range of mobility. In general, however, a direct association exists between increasing mobility and worsening prognosis. Prognosis is poor in the presence of advanced bone loss and uncontrolled systemic factors. A tooth that can be rotated or depressed is much more seriously involved than a tooth that has horizontal mobility. Mobility that relates to a widened periodontal ligament (primary occlusal trauma) rather than to loss of alveolar support has a more favorable prognosis. Occlusal adjustment and stabilization through splinting are procedures intended to reduce tooth mobility. Successful application of these procedures will also alter prognosis.

Mobility must be correlated with other clinical and roentgenographic findings in determining prognosis. Unless its cause is understood, mobility cannot be properly evaluated. Tooth mobility directly reflects disturbance; its measurement is useful in planning treatment and evaluating results. Mobility need not be progressive; some mobile teeth remain equally mobile for years.

The greater the bone loss, the poorer the prognosis. As bone loss exceeds 50%, the prognosis worsens rapidly. The more irregular the bone loss, the poorer the prognosis. When the pattern of bone loss is horizontal, pocket elimination is usually easier. When irregular, vertical, or troughlike bone defects are present, the feasibility of osteoplasty, new attachment attempts, or bone grafting must be considered. As a rule, vertical bone losses with one- and two-walled infrabony defects or interproximal bony craters have a worse prognosis than a more generally horizontal type of destruction. The architecture of these infrabony defects influences their prognosis considerably. Three-walled infrabony defects, for instance, which provide a scaffold for repair and good regenerative potential offer predictable regeneration of new ligament and bone. Two-walled craters have a poorer, and one-walled the poorest, prognosis for bone regeneration.

Other factors related to the rate of progression of the disease are the age of the patient and the etiologic factors involved in the patient's disease.

Treatment prognosis is also related to the extent, nature, and duration of the involvement. When extensive involvement occurs in an older patient, there is more likelihood of stretching the serviceability of the dentition to match the patient's life expectancy than there is when a young patient exhibits an advanced condition. Of two patients with equally advanced bone loss, one of whom is 30 and the other 70 years old, the younger will have the poorer prognosis. The rate of progression was more rapid in the younger patient, and the length of the needed lifetime of the dentition is greater. These factors result in poor odds. However, it should be noted that, although some younger patients have dentitions which deteriorate steadily in repeated episodes, other respond to treatment with few repeated episodes.

When the causative factors of the disease are easily recognized, such as poor oral hygiene or the presence of plaque and deposits, the correction can be more easily accomplished. When teeth have tilted, drifted, or rotated, hygiene may be more difficult and elimination of pockets impaired, in which case the prognosis is poorer. In general, the more obvious the etiology, the easier the treatment.[4] The patient who shows a severe response to minimal amounts of plaque has a poorer prognosis than does the patient who exhibits a resistant response in the presence of a considerable amount of plaque.[5]

Systemic involvement

A patient with a systemic involvement presents more of a problem than does a patient who is in excellent health. A patient's health and associated capacity for repair are important factors to consider in developing the treatment plan prognosis. When periodontal disease is complicated by active systemic factors such as uncontrolled diabetes and other diseases with altered leukocyte chemotaxis, the progression often is continuous even in the face of periodontal and prosthetic treatment (Fig. 29-2). When periodontal disease is complicated by traumatism, the prognosis is worse than when it is not.

Traumatism

Other factors influencing treatment prognosis are essentially morphologic in nature and include the number and distribution of teeth, tooth morphology, and furcation involvement.

**Number and distribution of teeth**

The number of teeth present is important. If there are relatively few, they must bear all the forces of mastication and parafunctional stress. They must also support bridges or dentures, which may further overload them. On the other hand, when more teeth are present, forces can be distributed through many more ligaments and their alveolar housings. In addition, prostheses may be unnecessary or may involve only short spans that would not overload abutment teeth. If the contact relationships are

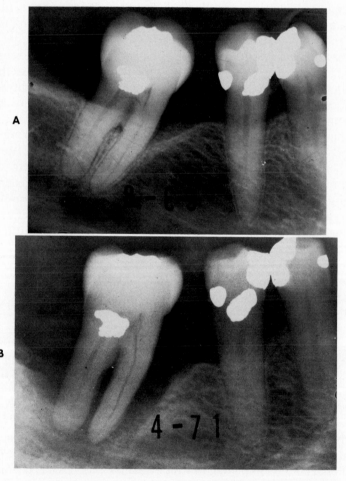

**Fig. 29-2.** Rapid breakdown in an uncontrolled diabetic. **A,** Radiographs before breakdown. **B,** Radiographs 2 years later. (Courtesy L. Hirschfeld, New York, New York.)

good, valuable support is obtained against trauma in a mesial and distal direction.

When a considerable number of teeth are missing, the distribution of the remaining ones will influence prognosis. If there are only ten teeth left, for instance, it is better to have them all in the lower arch, opposing a full upper denture, than vice versa. It is certainly better than having five teeth in each arch. If the number of remaining teeth is reduced, it is better to have molars, bicuspids, and cuspids than incisors. Bilateral is better than unilateral distribution. The worst arrangement is to have unilateral distributions in each arch that do not contact (Fig. 29-3).

The prognosis is better if the remaining teeth are distributed alternately rather than grouped. Then the arch might extend from molar to molar rather than from first bicuspid to first bicuspid. In the latter situation the interseptal bone is narrower, interproximal hygiene is more difficult, and a distal extension partial would be needed. When only anterior teeth are present, it is better that they be arranged in a curve rather than in a straight line.

The more favorable the crown-root ratio, the better the prognosis. Teeth with short, slender or tapering roots have a poorer prognosis than do those with long and broad roots. Multirooted teeth usually resist traumatic forces better than do single-rooted teeth. Flared molar roots give better support than do fused, conical roots. Broad occlusal tables and large crowns can contribute to increased mobility. **Tooth morphology**

The support of the tooth is determined by the height of the alveolar crest and the length and shape of the root. Cuspids can withstand loss of support better than lateral incisors by virtue of their longer roots and root concavities. Maxillary first premolars show early mobility because of the tapered roots. Some patients have teeth with short roots. Others have root resorption, which is sometimes the result of orthodontic therapy (Fig. 29-4). Such teeth are less resistant to excessive occlusal forces.

In general teeth with furcation involvements have a poor prognosis. They do not make satisfactory abutments. They are more difficult to scale and may abscess more frequently. Some furcation-involved teeth can be treated by endodontics followed by root resection; others can be maintained. **Furcation involvements**

The following factors should be considered in projecting a prognosis for teeth with furcation involvements:

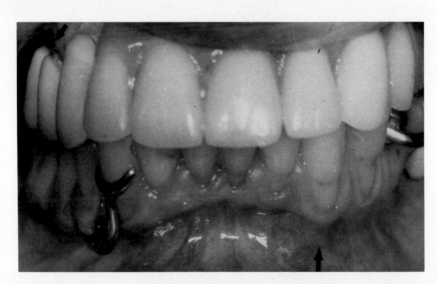

**Fig. 29-3.**    Patient with unfavorable distribution of teeth. The maxillary teeth are all on the left side *(arrow)* and the mandibular on the right *(arrow)*. (Courtesy L. Hirschfeld, New York, New York.)

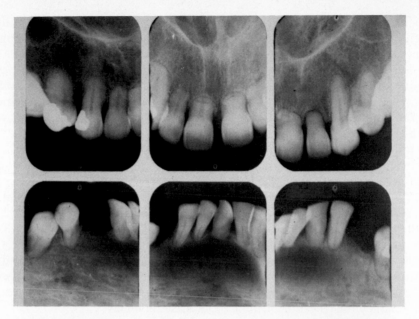

**Fig. 29-4.** Extensive resorption after orthodontic therapy. Although the crown-root ratio is highly unfavorable, the teeth have been retained for the past 18 years. (Courtesy L. Hirschfeld, New York, New York.)

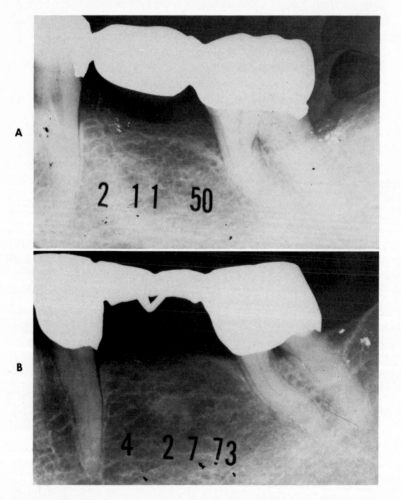

**Fig. 29-5.** Furcation involvements do not always enlarge significantly with time. **A,** Radiograph at time of treatment by curettage. **B,** Radiograph 20 years later, showing minimal change. (Courtesy L. Hirschfeld, New York, New York.)

1. *Extent of involvement*. Is the furcation partially or totally involved?
2. *Status of bone support*. If the bone levels are relatively sound, the effort to save the tooth may be justifiable. Root length and crown-root ratio must be considered since these factors are measures of the amount of bone support present.
3. *Angulation of root spread*. If a furcation-involved tooth is to be retained as is, the furcation is more accessible for home care if the roots are widely spread and root concavities are shallow. If root resection is planned, the roots to be retained must be aligned with the crown. If they are not, the roots may not be able to withstand occlusal forces. Proximal furcation or a deep furcation on one surface is difficult to maintain.
4. *Health of neighboring teeth*. When good abutment teeth are present mesial as well as distal to the involved tooth, extraction should be considered. At one time furcation-involved teeth were considered to have a hopeless prognosis and were extracted almost routinely. At the present time many prosthodontists will not make use of a furcation-involved tooth unless it is treated by root resection. Nevertheless, some furcations do not become larger after treatment (Fig. 29-5). Of 499 well-maintained periodontal patients with 387 mandibular first and second molars having furcation involvements, 61 (15.5%) were extracted over a period of 22 years (see Chart 1, Table 29-1, below). Of 101 patients who were not as well maintained, the loss of such molars was greater.[6]

A furcation-involved tooth is hopeless if the entire interradicular septum has been resorbed. Gutta-percha or silver points can be used to determine the extent of loss. If the roots converge and fuse at the apices, root resection is difficult and the prognosis

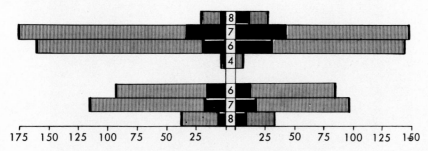

**Chart 1.** Histograph of presence of posterior teeth with furcation involvements and relative loss over 22-year average period. These figures describe loss in 499 well-maintained patients in a group of 600 surveyed. Striped areas indicate the total number of teeth with furcation involvement. Black areas indicate the number of teeth lost. (From Hirschfeld, L., and Wasserman, B.: J. Periodontol. **49:**226, 1978.)

**Table 29-1**   Furcation-involved teeth lost, by response group*

| Tooth number | WM (499) Lost/present | Percent | D (76) Lost/present | Percent | ED (25) Lost/present | Percent | Total group Lost/present | Percent |
|---|---|---|---|---|---|---|---|---|
| 1,16 | 15/48 | 31.2 | 17/20 | 85.0 | 3/4 | 75.0 | 35/72 | 48.6 |
| 2,15 | 76/322 | 23.6 | 46/60 | 76.7 | 19/20 | 95.0 | 141/402 | 35.1 |
| 3,14 | 50/304 | 16.5 | 42/64 | 65.6 | 15/16 | 93.7 | 107/384 | 27.9 |
| 4,13 | 1/8 | 12.5 | 0/1 | 00.0 | 0.0 | 00.0 | 1/9 | 11.1 |
| 18,30 | 27/176 | 15.3 | 16/27 | 59.2 | 16/19 | 84.2 | 59/222 | 26.5 |
| 17,31 | 34/211 | 16.1 | 27/43 | 62.9 | 16/23 | 69.5 | 77/277 | 27.8 |
| 16,32 | 17/71 | 23.9 | 17/21 | 80.9 | 6/6 | 100.0 | 40/98 | 40.8 |
| TOTAL | 220/1140 | 19.3 | 165/236 | 69.9 | 75/88 | 84.4 | 460/1464 | 31.4 |

From Hirschfeld, L., and Wasserman, B.: A long-term survey of tooth loss in 600 treated periodontal patients, J. Periodontol. **49:**225, 1978.
*WM, Well maintained; D, downhill; ED, extreme downhill.

is poor. When adequate root spread is present, hemisection is often possible (Fig. 29-6). Radiographs should be taken at different angles. Sometimes an additional root may be detected. When the defect is caused by a nonvital pulp, regeneration of an involved septum is possible after endodontic therapy (Fig. 29-7).

When a partial furcation is present on a mandibular molar, further opening by osseous surgery or closure by bone grafting should be considered as alternatives to root resection. These alternatives are less successful for the maxillary molars. Bifurcated maxillary premolars are difficult to treat except if hemisection is possible.

The treatment of furcation is discussed in Chapter 42.

Other factors involved in establishing a treatment prognosis are related to personal psychologic, sociologic, and financial considerations.

## OTHER CONSIDERATIONS IN ESTABLISHING PROGNOSIS

**Plaque control**

When the performance of home care is acceptable and the caries incidence is low, the prognosis is better than when home care is not acceptable and the caries rate is high. The patient who does not have the motivation, dexterity, and discipline to keep the plaque score down has a poorer prognosis. Some patients have a more viscous saliva than others, which provides for a more rapid plaque accumulation. Others ac-

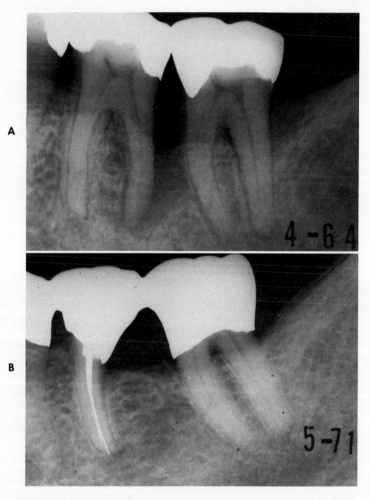

**Fig. 29-6.** Hemisection of the distal root of a mandibular first molar. Before **(A)** and after **(B)** hemisection and bridge, showing bone regeneration. (Courtesy L. Hirschfeld, New York, New York.)

cumulate plaque slowly and in scanty amounts; they have a better prognosis. Persons with high caries rates will exhibit decay in furcations and under crowns (Fig. 29-8) resulting in a poor prognosis.

The dentist must be able to realize treatment objectives of creating a healthy gingiva, of eliminating pockets, and of establishing conditions whereby the patient can maintain the health of his/her mouth. If these objectives can be reached, the prognosis will be better than when they cannot be reached. For instance, a patient who is not a good surgical candidate because of health or emotional reasons has a poorer prognosis than would be the case if he/she were a surgical candidate. If the patient lacks the time, patience, or wherewithal to undertake treatment, the prognosis is worsened. If the patient resists treatment or abdicates responsibility, the prognosis is worsened. Alternative treatment plans can be considered, but often the effort is frustrating and success is limited. The patient must be interested in retaining the teeth. If he/she is not, chances are that the therapy will be less effective.[7,8]

**Feasibility of treatment objectives**

When complex and extensive prostheses are involved, the prognosis tends to be more guarded than when the integrity of the dentition can be maintained with less involved prostheses or when no prosthesis is needed.

**Complexity and extent of prosthesis**

The value of the tooth must be considered. It is not worth putting the patient

Value of tooth

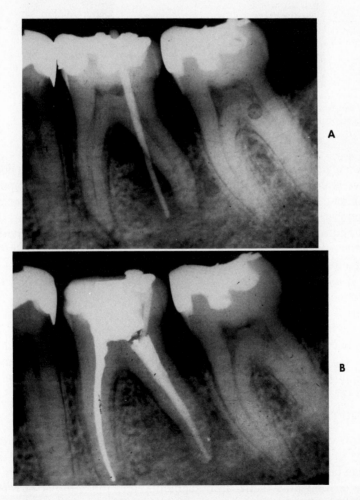

**Fig. 29-7.** Combined periodontal-endodontic lesion. **A,** Destruction to apex, involving interradicular bone. **B,** Regeneration of periodontium 1 year after endodontic therapy. (Courtesy L. Hirschfeld, New York, New York.)

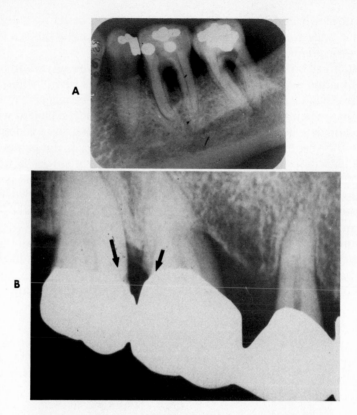

**Fig. 29-8.** Caries susceptibility will influence prognosis. **A,** Caries in furcation. **B,** Caries under a splint. (Courtesy L. Hirschfeld, New York, New York.)

through heroic procedures for a tooth of questionable value. It is often better to extract it or to leave it alone until it causes trouble. A carious extruded, unopposed maxillary third molar might be indicated for extraction ordinarily, but, if the second molar has a poor prognosis, the third molar may be retained as an abutment. A questionable tooth should not be included in a splint unless its presence is a necessity. Statistics indicate that a relatively large number of upper second molars with furcation involvement are lost during a long maintenance period (see Table 29-1). This fact might influence the use of such a tooth as a bridge abutment. On the other hand, lower molars with furcation involvements might be used with more assurance.

Malaligned teeth may be made serviceable through orthodontic therapy, but the potential benefit must be weighed against the effort and expense.

The complexity and extent of any necessary associated prosthesis should be carefully evaluated. If extensive restoration of the dentition, fixed splinting, and orthodontic movement and other procedures are necessary, the patient's ability to have all associated procedures performed must be considered.

### PRESERVING THE DENTITION

The prime consideration is the preservation of the dentition as a functioning unit. This means that the loss of individual components can be tolerated if the remaining dentition can be retained and restored to function and esthetics. Therefore the strategic importance of individual teeth, arch segments, and the number of remaining teeth and their distribution cannot be overemphasized. Often extracting one tooth will improve the chances of a neighboring tooth, particularly where buckling or bone loss is present. Teeth with untreatable caries or endodontic problems should be eliminated. Extruded teeth may traumatize opposing teeth in excursive movements. When this cannot be corrected, the tooth extruded should be extracted.

Unfortunately dental treatment is often conceived of in terms of absolutes. Good and poor prognoses are viewed as black and white. In actuality, a zone of gray exists between the black and white in periodontal prognosis. Some confusion exists because of our inability to perceive all the factors involved in a prognosis. The inexperienced diagnostician will often recognize and treat only the most overt periodontal conditions. These become more obvious with the severity of the situation. Moreover, such conditions are often treated inadequately. Naturally, then, the rate of failure is high. Disillusionment with the effectiveness of periodontal treatment may follow. The pendulum may swing to the other extreme, and further attempts at periodontal therapy may be abandoned in a retreat to the forceps. Neither approach is rational. Sometimes extractions are indicated; at other times periodontal treatment is indicated. It is important to be able to differentiate between the two.

Judgments should be made on a tooth-to-tooth basis with the entire dentition in mind. In some instances the extraction of a single tooth will make the whole situation untenable. In other situations isolated extractions will simplify the problem.

Each practitioner should define what is considered to be a hopeless tooth. This will make treatment planning simpler. Criteria vary; no list is completely applicable. However, use may be made of the following list of characteristics of hopeless or relatively hopeless periodontally involved teeth:

**Hopeless tooth**

1. Associated with intractable pain relieved by extraction
2. Associated with massive infection reduced by extraction
3. Mobility beyond 3 degrees
4. Furcation involvement with little or no interradicular bone
5. Bone loss beyond the apex
6. Bone loss to the apex on one side of the tooth
7. Generalized circumferential bone loss to within 3 mm of the apex
8. Pocket depth to the apex without pulpal involvement
9. Vertical cracks or fractures
10. Inaccessible perforations or accessory canals
11. Number and position of remaining teeth precluding prosthetic restoration
12. Extreme caries susceptibility

In general, a tooth with a hopeless prognosis should be extracted. Yet a tooth may have a hopeless prognosis and still be retained. Some remarkable long-term results have been achieved with such teeth, particularly when it has been possible to avoid involving them in splinting (Fig. 29-9). However, one cannot rely on the chance of obtaining such a result in formulating a treatment plan prognosis. The predictability of a successful result is low. Whereas prognosis is a qualitative term, predictability is quantitative. It may be defined as the success/failure ratio or the number of successful results in the total number of similar situations. The predictability goes up if all judgments concerning diagnosis and etiologic factors are correct and if the skill of the clinician is adequate to the task.

**Predictability**

Let us consider a tooth with roentgenographic evidence of extensive bone loss. Bone may be lost about a tooth for a variety of reasons, some of which follow. The likelihood of regeneration of bone decreases as the list descends:

**Bone loss**

1. *Endodontic involvement.* When the pocket is a narrow fistula exiting through the sulcus, regrowth of bone usually follows successful endodontic therapy.
2. *Localized acute osteomyelitis.* In this relatively rare condition, pocket formation and bone loss occur rapidly and are associated with severe pain. Temporary stabilization, gentle drainage, and antibiotic therapy result in bone regeneration.

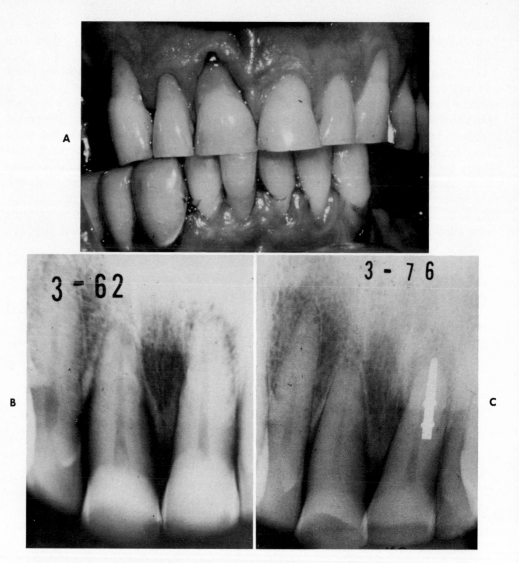

**Fig. 29-9.** Pocket extending to apex of maxillary central incisor. Treatment did not produce closure or regeneration, yet the tooth was maintained for more than 14 years. (Courtesy L. Hirschfeld, New York, New York.)

3. *Loss from a lesion on an adjacent tooth or root.* If the lamina dura and periodontal ligament are present when alveolar bone loss results from a periodontal lesion about an adjacent tooth, there is a good likelihood of regeneration after extraction of the offending tooth. The same regeneration may be observed after root amputation.

4. *Proliferation of granulation tissue.* Proliferative granulation tissue (Fig. 29-10) is often associated with rapid bone loss. Complete removal of the granulation tissue by a localized flap procedure often results in the regeneration of the lost periodontium (Fig. 29-11). Removal of granulation tissue may also be done by subgingival curettage. Regeneration rarely occurs in furcations.

5. *Periodontal abscess.* When rapid bone loss is associated with a periodontal abscess, prompt treatment and healing will usually be followed by regrowth of bone (Fig. 29-12). One must distinguish between a periodontal abscess and a proliferation of granulation tissue (Fig. 29-13). In addition, periodontal abscesses are sometimes mistakenly diagnosed as periapical (pulpal) lesions. The distinction is made by pulp testing.

6. *Cysts.* Cysts tend to have a more chronic course than abscesses. The potential for bone regeneration is good.

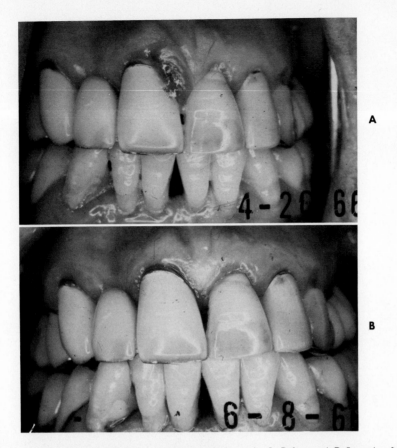

**Fig. 29-10.** Rapid proliferation of granulation tissue at gingival margin. **A,** Before and, **B,** 3 weeks after removal with curette. (Courtesy L. Hirschfeld, New York, New York.)

7. *Periodontitis.* Regeneration is not a frequent sequel to treatment of inflammatory peri-odontal disease unless three-walled infrabony defects are present. Bone grafting or ortho-dontic movement can be of value.
8. *Combined periodontal-endodontic involvement.* When a pocket extends to the apex of a tooth or to an accessory canal and pulp death ensues, the prognosis is not nearly as good as in the endodontic-periodontic lesion, which is initiated by the pulpal problem. To differentiate between the two is sometimes difficult although the history of the symptoms and the rapidity of bone destruction may be indicative.

A similar scale may be constructed for tooth mobility. Although a mobility of 3 degrees or greater may be hopeless, a tooth may have a transient mobility of 3 when it is in trauma, when it is abscessing, or during pregnancy. The clinician must employ an element of perceptivity and thought in scrutinizing all clinical findings.

**Tooth mobility**

## Objectives of treatment

Treatment goals should be evaluated in every case. Can treatment objectives of a firm nonretractable gingiva that does not bleed be reached? Can the pocket be elim-inated?[1] Will the bone regenerate? Can the tooth be stabilized? Can the tooth be restored? Can the patient tolerate the treatment? If you believe the answers to these questions to be "yes," then plan and proceed with the treatment. If "no," alternative treatment, compromise, or extraction is advisable.

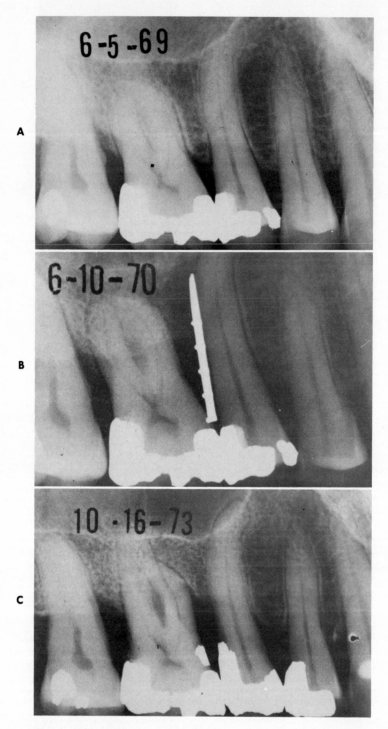

**Fig. 29-11.** Regrowth of bone after flap procedure to remove rapidly growing granulation tissue. **A,** One year before rapid bone loss. **B,** Just before flap procedure. **C,** Forty months later, showing considerable regeneration. (Courtesy L. Hirschfeld, New York, New York.)

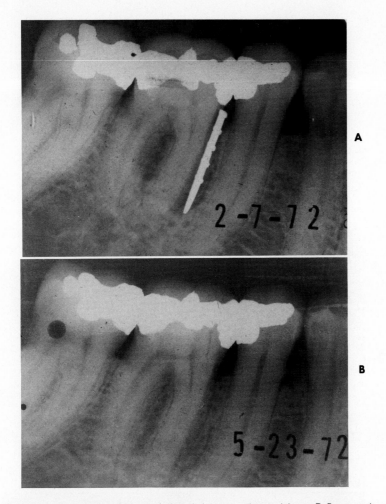

**Fig. 29-12.**    **A,** Bone destruction produced by a periodontal abscess on the mesial root. **B,** Regeneration following treatment. (Courtesy L. Hirschfeld, New York, New York.)

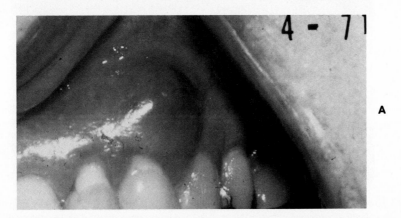

**Fig. 29-13.**    Subgingival mass of granulation tissue simulating a periodontal abscess. **A,** Firm rather than fluctuant.

*Continued.*

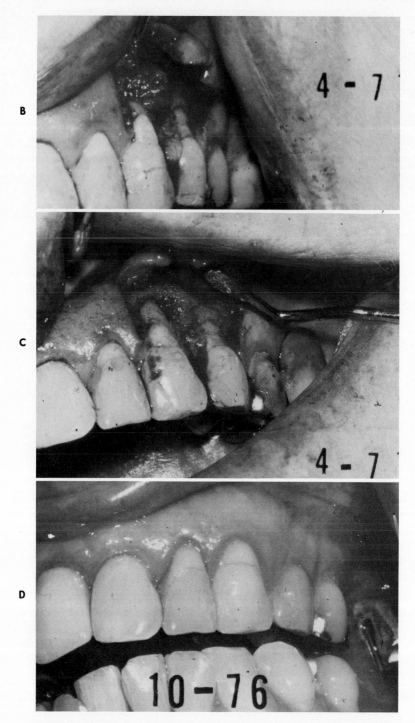

**Fig. 29-13, cont'd.   B,** Granulation tissue revealed by reflection of a flap. **C,** Granulation tissue removed. **D,** Five and a half years later, showing return to normal gingival form and contour. (Courtesy L. Hirschfeld, New York, New York.)

You may arrive at a periodontal or prosthetic treatment plan that you believe has a poor or guarded prognosis. Then treatment would carry a high risk, and the case would be designated as a high-risk case. The patient should be advised of the risk factor of the treatment plan. There are also moderate- and low-risk cases, and some with a good, very good, or excellent prognosis.

**Low-, moderate-, and high-risk treatment plans**

As definitive laboratory tests are developed to make diagnosis more accurate, and as further knowledge concerning the etiology and pathogenesis of periodontal diseases is developed, prognosis will change from a qualitative to a quantitative judgment. In addition, information is becoming available from clinical[9] and retrospective studies of treated cases observed over periods of time. These data should be considered in the diagnosis and prognosis and on the effectiveness of therapeutic procedures (Chapter 49).

### REFERENCES

1. Williams, C.H.M.: Rationalization of periodontal pocket therapy, J. Periodontol. **14:**67, 1943.
2. Everett, F.G., and Stern, I.B.: When is tooth mobility an indication for extraction? Dent. Clin. North Am. **13:**791, 1969.
3. Lindhe, J.A., and Nyman, S.: The role of occlusion in periodontal disease and the biologic rationale for splinting in the treatment of periodontitis, Oral Sci. Rev. **10:**11, 1977.
4. Wade, A.B.: Causes in failure of treatment of localized pocketing, Dent. Health **4:**9, 1965.
5. Homan, B.T.: A prescription for periodontal therapy: curettage, Aust. Dent. J. **9:**515, 1964.
6. Hirschfeld, L., and Wasserman, B.: A long-term survey of tooth loss in 600 treated periodontal patients, J. Periodontol. **49:**225, 1978.
7. Awwa, I., and Stallard, R.E.: Periodontal prognosis: educational and psychological implications, J. Periodontol. **41:**183, 1970.
8. Derbyshire, J.C.: Patient motivation in periodontics, J. Periodontol. **41:**630, 1970.
9. Lindhe, J., et al.: Long-term effect of surgical–non-surgical treatment of periodontal disease, J. Clin. Periodontol. **11:**448, 1984.

### ADDITIONAL SUGGESTED READING

Fleszar, T.J., et al.: Tooth mobility and periodontal therapy, J. Clin. Periodontol. **7:**495, 1980.

Forsberg, A., and Hägglund, G.: Mobility of teeth as a check of periodontal therapy, Acta Odontol. Scand. **15:**305, 1957.

Haffajee, A.D., Socransky, S.S., and Goodson, J.M.: Clinical parameters as predictors of destructive periodontal disease, J. Clin. Periodontol. **10:**257, 1983.

Lindhe, J., et al.: Critical probing depths in periodontal therapy, J. Clin. Periodontol. **9:**323, 1982.

Lindhe, J., Haffajee, A.D., and Socransky, S.S.: Progression of periodontal disease in adult subjects in the absence of periodontal therapy, J. Clin. Periodontol. **10:**433, 1983.

Toersky, A., and Kahneman, D.: The framing of decisions and the psychology of choice, Science **211:**453, 1981.

# Treatment plan

**Definition**  The treatment plan is the scheduled sequence of therapeutic measures used to cure or arrest the patient's periodontal disease. It is developed to meet the patient's specific needs as revealed during the examination and diagnosis. The plan includes a judgment of the presumed etiology, as well as of the prognosis. It is as individualistic as are the patient and the disease. It is best to remember that the disease is an interaction between the causative factors and the patient and that the result differs in every patient. Dentists do not treat diseases per se; they treat people.

## Presentation

The treatment plan presentation, of necessity, must be preceded by a presentation of the findings of the examination and by an explanation of the nature of periodontal disease processes. The patient should have the charting explained and should be taught to read it. For this reason, a diagrammatic chart is preferred (see Fig. 28-5). In addition, it is useful to sketch and explain on patient educational diagrams how plaque accumulates, (Figs. 30-1 and 30-2) how pockets form and progress, how alveolar bone is lost, and how teeth loosen. A patient who does not understand the pathogenesis of the disease will be ill-prepared to accept an explanation of treatment. A full explanation, in a layperson's terminology, given in a short period of time is necessary before informed consent can be obtained. In addition, it is necessary to discuss the length of treatment[1] and the costs involved. A planned, cooperative effort between patient and dentist is required; this is based on a full presentation of the facts to the patient. The patient should be encouraged to ask questions. Informed consent requires that the patient has understood the presentation. It may be advisable to have the patient sign consent forms.[1,2] Informed consent requires that the patient understand the advantages and disadvantages of treatment—the expected and probable as well as the unexpected but possible sequelae. If informed consent is not obtained, the patient may involve the dentist in legal action even if the expected goals are obtained but the result comes as

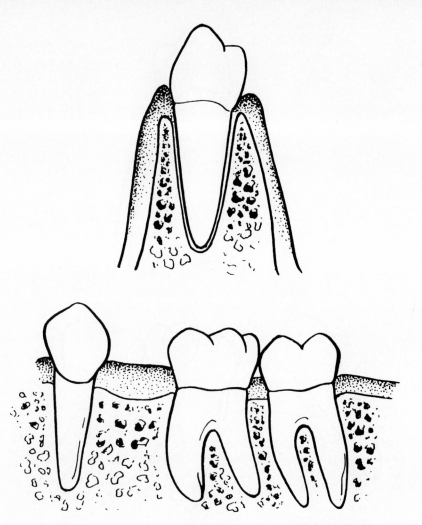

**Fig. 30-1.** *Diagram of the normal periodontium, useful in sketching during patient education.*

a surprise to the patient. If the patient was not forewarned of the possible but unlikely sequelae, legal action is more of a certainty.[2-5]

**Rationale**

The goal of periodontal treatment is to arrest the process of breakdown, which may otherwise lead to ultimate loss of teeth, and to establish oral conditions conducive to periodontal health.[6] Within limits one should be able to use therapeutic measures on a predictable basis. In general, treatment should be limited to direct measures necessary to achieve the result.[7]

Insofar as possible, therapy should be definitive. Treatment should not generally resort to trial and error. Treatment should not be a sequence of alternatives to be used when the earlier steps fail. Therapy should consist of various clinical approaches that are the armamentarium of periodontics[8] and which are described in the following chapters.

**Examination**

The examination visits consist of the steps in the checklist on p. 595, the first five of which are facets of data collection.[9]

After completion of the examination, the findings, diagnosis, and prognosis should be presented to the patient and explained. These items are the result of the examination and must be understood by the patient before a treatment plan is presented. The

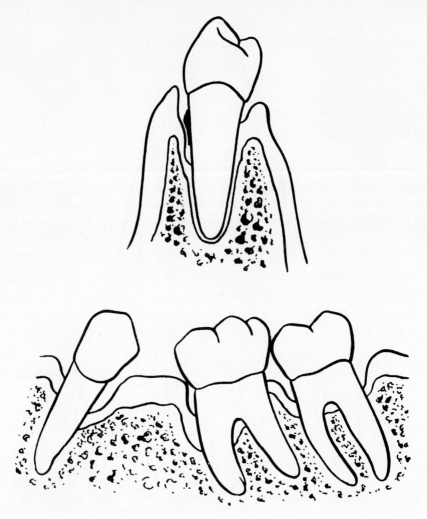

**Fig. 30-2.** Diagram of a diseased periodontium, useful in sketching during patient education.

treatment plan (opposite and pp. 596-597) is presented only to patients who understand their condition and who are properly motivated. This is basic to obtaining an informed consent. Such patients frequently ask what can be done for them. At this point, the case presentation should be made. Attempt to be objective with the patient. Never do an "off-the-cuff" presentation. All the needed facts should be known, fully digested, and a written plan prepared before a presentation is made. Do not make rash promises, great pronouncements, or profound judgments. The expectations of the patient stem in part from the case presentation. Do your best to ensure that the expectations are realistic and that the patient understands them.

The evaluator of the periodontal patient is not obligated to perform therapy, but he/she is obligated to make a diagnosis and to inform the patient if periodontal disease is present. Treatment planning is not accomplished by a rigid set of rules. Many factors will influence the sequence and selection of therapy; they are numerous and varied. The choice of methods is available in rich array, and their sequencing is a matter of many combinations and permutations. However, time and effort may be wasted if an orderly, systematic approach is not used. A well-devised treatment plan avoids these pitfalls and also allows the patient, dentist, and consulting specialists to

---

### EXAMINATION CHECKLIST

1. Interview (case history)
   a. Vital statistics
   b. Medical history
   c. Dental history
   d. Chief complaint
2. Clinical examination
3. Occlusal examination
4. Radiographic examination
5. Listing of findings
6. Diagnosis and prognosis (evaluation of health status)
7. Etiology
8. Treatment plan and therapeutic prognosis

---

### TREATMENT PLAN

**Steps**        **Specific reasons for treatment**

_____     _____

_____     _____

_____     _____

_____     _____

### ALTERNATIVES

**Steps**        **Specific reasons for treatment**

_____     _____

_____     _____

_____     _____

---

be aware of what the treatment will consist of, how long it will take, and what the anticipated results may be.

It is useful for a student to list the steps of the treatment plan and the specific reasons for the treatment he proposes to perform. He/she may do the same for an alternative treatment plan. The practitioner may communicate the steps and reasons verbally by reading from the entries made in the list (above).

The treatment sequence is divided into three phases. Phase I (initial therapy) includes all steps involved in reducing inflammation, bringing plaque accumulation and bacterial infection under control, removing accretions, controlling bruxism, stabilizing loose teeth, and adjusting the occlusion. Phase I may include steps involving surgical access to eliminate accretions, depending on the philosophy of the dental school or of the practitioner. Scaling and root planing may be done in several visits: sequential full-mouth, half-mouth, or quadrant visits. Similarly, gingival curettage, subgingival curettage, and the modified Widman flap may be employed here. A checklist for the different pathways in initial therapy is shown on p. 596.

At the end of this phase of treatment, an all-important reevaluation will be made to gauge the degree of improvement obtained. The results of initial treatment will be

**Phase I checklist (initial therapy)**

---

**PHASE I TREATMENT**

☐ Extractions

☐ Mouth preparation: A, B, or C—one to four visits (depending on whether full mouth, half mouth, or single quadrants are treated each visit)

| **A** | **B** | **C** |
|---|---|---|
| 1 { ☐ Initial scaling (full mouth) / ☐ Plaque control 1 | 1 { ☐ Initial scaling (full mouth) / ☐ Plaque control 1 | 1 { ☐ Initial scaling (full mouth) / ☐ Plaque control 1 |
| 2 { ☐ Definitive scaling and root planing* / ☐ Plaque control 2 | 2 ☐ Perform A, 2 | 2 { ☐ Gingivectomy, subgingival curettage, or modified Widman flap and scaling and root planing†‡ (half mouth)§ / ☐ Plaque control 2 |
| 3 { ☐ Definitive scaling and root planing* / ☐ Plaque control 3 | 3 ☐ Perform A, 3 | 3 { ☐ Gingivectomy, subgingival curettage, or modified Widman flap and scaling and planing†‡ (half mouth) / ☐ Plaque control 3 |
| | 4 ☐ Gingival (soft tissue) curettage (half mouth)†‡ | |
| | 5 ☐ Gingival (soft tissue) curettage (half mouth)†‡ | |

☐ Occlusal adjustment (one or two visits)
  ☐ Indirect intraoral approach
    ☐ Study casts
    ☐ Face-bow transfer and mounting
  ☐ Direct intraoral approach
    ☐ Study casts

{ ☐ Centric
  ☐ Protrusive
  ☐ Laterals
  ☐ Balancing

☐ Night guards (one or two visits)
  ☐ Study casts                    ☐ Prescription                    ☐ Insertion

☐ Splinting
  ☐ Acid-etch technique                    ☐ Wire ligation
  ☐ Others _____

☐ Periodontal orthodontics

☐ Reexamination (charting and consultation)

---

*Two visits if full-mouth rounds or half mouth is done in one visit; four visits if one quadrant is done in one visit.
†One visit if done as a full-mouth procedure and four visits if done by the quadrant.
‡Will require surgical dressing(s) to be placed. These will be removed at a subsequent visit(s).
§May also be performed after sequence A.

---

checked against the charting. Residual inflammation and its presumptive causes will be noted, and changes in pocket depth and tooth mobility will be assessed. The treatment plan will be reevaluated and changed as needed. If no further treatment is necessary, the case will be considered completed and will be placed into recall and maintenance; otherwise, restorative and prosthetic treatment will be started, after which the patient will be listed in recall and maintenance. In general, only provisional restorative dentistry is performed before the completion of phase I treatment.

**Phase II checklist (surgical therapy)**

The phase II treatment plan consists of reconstructive surgical steps, as opposed to surgery performed in phase I, which is performed to gain access to accretions and plaque. Surgery in phase II has the primary goal of adding to the alveolar bone and gingival tissues and the secondary goal of correcting osseous and gingival form. It basically includes osseous surgery, bone grafting, and mucogingival surgery but under

---

### PHASE II TREATMENT

☐ Surgery*          **Procedure**

 ☐ First quadrant _____

 ☐ Second quadrant _____

 ☐ Third quadrant _____

 ☐ Fourth quadrant _____

☐ Postsurgical examination (charting and evaluation)

*Surgery may be performed in one, two, or four visits (full mouth, half mouth, or quadrants). Each surgery visit will require one or more postsurgical visits.

---

### PHASE III TREATMENT

**Phase III checklist (finishing steps)**

☐ Occlusal adjustment
☐ Scaling
☐ Plaque-control efficacy evaluation
☐ Gingivoplasty (surgical corrections)
☐ Postoperative x-ray films (for class III or IV patients in treatment for more than 12 months and to check teeth with bone grafting, root resection, or a questionable prognosis)
☐ Final examination
☐ Prosthetic and restorative prescription
☐ Consultation visit

### MAINTENANCE TREATMENT

**Maintenance**

☐ Patient to be placed into recall and maintenance program (to include periodic reevaluation)

---

certain circumstances may include gingivectomy and reattachment procedures when these aim primarily at improvement of tissue level and tissue form. Phase II surgery generally has more complicated goals, is more involved, and calls for a greater degree of skill and effort than surgery performed in phase I. Phase I surgery may be performed as a prerequisite for phase II surgery; however, even where it is intended to be definitive, the goals of phase II surgery may be unmet, and the need for phase II surgery may remain. In either of these events phase II surgery will be required. If phase II treatment has been performed, the treatment plan will involve phase III therapy (refer to phase III checklist above).

At this point the patient, having been informed of the sequence of treatment, should be advised of the duration of treatment, the number of visits, and the approximate length of each visit. The course of treatment may be outlined by placing check marks in the squares provided in the checklists for phases I and II treatment. Practitioners can develop similar treatment plan outlines for themselves. After an explanation of time involved,[9,10] the approximate cost should be developed. A similar type of checklist (p. 598) may be employed to calculate and present the fee.

**Length and timing of treatment**

**FEE CHECKLIST**

| | Cost |
|---|---|
| Examination and consultation | _____ |
| Full-mouth x-ray films | _____ |
| Extractions | _____ |
| Scale and root planing | _____ |
| Plaque control | _____ |
| Gingival curettage | _____ |
| Phase I surgery ____|____* ____† | _____ |
| Occlusal adjustment | _____ |
| Night guards | _____ |
| Splint | _____ |
| Minor tooth movement (MTM) | _____ |
| Phase I examination | _____ |
| Surgery | _____ |
| Phase II examination | _____ |
| Final occlusal adjustment | _____ |
| Final scale—full-mouth x-ray films | _____ |
| Miscellaneous | _____ |
| Prophylaxis during treatment | _____ |
| TOTAL | _____ |

*Quadrant involved.
†Type of surgery.

## Patient consent

After hearing the presentation, the patient must decide whether to undergo treatment. This decision is based on the patient's understanding of his/her health status, the treatment plan, and of his/her perception and confidence in the therapist. Liability may result if treatment proceeds without full disclosure, without referral when indicated, and without informed consent. Some practitioners use informed consent forms[2-5] (Figs. 30-3 and 30-4). These may be prepared to parallel the three phases of therapy and be presented for signature before each phase. Some consent forms are written defensively and may prove frightening to the patients. Some are too general and obscure. A good rule to apply is to inform the patient if the likelihood of an occurrence is, in general, 1 in 150 or more and not to inform the patient if the occurrence is more rare. However, given the examination findings of a specific patient, when a postoperative sequela is common in similar cases, then the patient must be informed. Some dentists may prefer to use the informed consent checklist (Fig. 30-3). These practitioners verbalize the risks of not having treatment. They tell the patient about the temporary treatment sequelae of swelling, bleeding, pain, thermal sensitivity, infection, trismus, and the more permanent possibilities of recession, tooth mobility, and food impaction. Some dentists include this information in a letter to the patient.

## Order of treatment

### PHASE I

Phase I treatment consists of a number of steps. The initial effort should be directed toward the elimination of inflammation and the institution of a program of plaque control. This may require a number of visits to remove all deposits and to establish

## CONSENT TO PERIODONTAL (GUM) TREATMENT

I hereby authorize Doctor _____ (herein after called "Doctor"), and whomever he/she may designate as his/her assistant(s) to perform following treatment and/or surgery upon _____ .

### DIAGNOSIS

I have been informed that I have periodontal (gum) disease and/or deformities that could lead to the loss of certain of my teeth. I have been advised that the proposed therapy is intended to extend the life expectancy of my teeth. This consent form outlines that treatment program, its expected consequences, and limitations.

### TREATMENT PLAN

- Oral hygiene/disease prevention
- Root planing and curettage (tooth and/or gum scraping)
- Bite adjustment
- Tooth-straightening procedures with fixed and/or removable appliance(s)
- Semipermanent splints (stabilization)
- Biteguard

- Mucogingival surgery with/without bone recontouring
- Gingivectomy
- Curettage
- Tissue grafts
- Extraction of teeth as determined during surgery
- Periodontal maintenance therapy (professional recall care)

### ALTERNATIVES

Further, I have been informed that possible alternatives to the above treatment include:

- Maintenance therapy only
- Curettage and maintenance therapy only
- Root planing and maintenance therapy only

- Presurgical and maintenance therapy only
- Extraction(s)
- Other _____

### NONTREATMENT RISKS

I further understand that if no treatment is rendered the risks to my dental health include, but are not limited to, the following:

- Premature loss of teeth
- Gum recession
- Halitosis
- Loosening of teeth

- Abscesses (gum boils)
- Tooth drifting, flaring, or other tooth movement
- Further deepening of periodontal and/or pus pockets

### TREATMENT RISKS

Risks of the treatment include, but are not limited to:

- Swelling
- Pain
- Thermal sensitivity
- Exposure of margins of crowns (caps)
- Phonetic interferences
- Infection

- Tooth mobility
- Food impaction between teeth
- Temporary restricted mouth opening
- Numbness of jaw or gum nerves
- Other _____

### UNFORESEEN CONDITIONS DURING SURGERY

If any unforeseen condition should arise in the course of the operation, calling for the Doctor's judgement for procedures in addition to or different from those now contemplated, I further request and authorize the Doctor to do whatever he/she may deem advisable.

### NO WARRANTY

No guarantee, warranty, or assurance has been given to me that the proposed treatment will be curative and/or successful to my complete satisfaction. Due to individual patient differences, a risk of failure, or relapse, or worsening of my present periodontal condition may result despite treatment and may require retreatment and/or extraction of teeth. However, it is Doctor's opinion that therapy will be helpful and that any further loss of supporting tissues or bone would occur soon without the recommended treatment.

It has been explained to me that the long-term success of treatment requires my cooperation and performance of daily removal of bacterial deposits (plaque) from my teeth, as well as periodic periodontal maintenance therapy after the proposed treatment at a dental office.

I certify that I have read fully and have had all of my questions answered so that I understand the above consent to treatment, the explanation therein referred to or made, and that all blanks or statements requiring insertion or completion were filled in and in applicable sections, if any, were stricken before I signed.

DATE _____ SIGNED _____
Patient or legal guardian

WITNESS _____

**Fig. 30-3.** *Suggested authorization and informed consent to periodontal surgery. (Courtesy Department of Periodontology, University of Southern California School of Dentistry.)*

---

GENERAL CONSENT FORM*

I hereby consent to the performance of treatment upon _____

myself/name of patient

by Dr. _____.

Such treatment will consist of: _____

_____

(description in general terms)

The nature and purpose of the treatment rendered, possible hazards, and alternative methods of treatment have been fully explained to me. No guarantee, warranty, or assurance has been given to me that the treatment will be successful or to my complete satisfaction.

Dated: _____    _____

(Name of Patient or Legal Guardian)

WITNESS:

_____

---

*Unspecific and of questionable legal value

**Fig. 30-4.** *Sample general consent form. (From Zinman, E.J.: J. West. Soc. Periodontol./Periodont. Abstr.* **24**:101, 1976.)

effective plaque control. During this phase chemical control of plaque by rinses, irrigations, antibiotics, and so on may be employed. The patient's level of oral hygiene performance should be evaluated at each visit with the aid of a plaque score, and further coaching in plaque control given as necessary. The patient should achieve a plaque-free score of 85% or better.

**Reduction of pocket depth**

In addition, phase I therapy is intended to reduce pocket depth wherever possible. Scaling and root planing are accompanied by inadvertent soft tissue curettage and produce some degree of pocket reduction. Gingival curettage, subgingival (closed) curettage, gingivectomy, and the Widman (open curettage) procedure will also produce a degree of pocket reduction and possibly reattachment.

**Reduction of traumatism**

Phase I therapy also attempts to minimize periodontal traumatism by means of occlusal adjustment, night guards, and negative feedback training (operant conditioning). If the teeth are extremely malposed or if the arch is collapsed (see Fig. 30-2), periodontal orthodontics may be indicated. The succeeding steps are generally performed in phase I.

### Occlusal adjustment

Occlusal adjustment should follow scaling and root planing. If a tooth is extremely mobile, gross occlusal adjustment may be done before scaling to reduce mobility. Generally, occlusal adjustment is performed as a step of phase I therapy. However, some correction is usually needed in phase III since there is some accommodation and movement of teeth during surgical therapy.

### Orthodontics

Orthodontic tooth movement may precede or follow any surgical interventions. When orthodontic tooth movement is performed to help eliminate inflammation resulting from tooth position or bony deformities resulting from tooth malalignment, tilting, or drifting, it should precede surgery. When orthodontic tooth movement is done for purposes of reconstruction or esthetics, it may follow surgery. A schedule should be devised for frequent, regular scaling during orthodontic interventions and for appraisal of plaque control. If the case is complex or if the practitioner is not skilled in tooth movement, the patient should be referred to an orthodontist.

### Extractions

Teeth with hopeless prognoses should be extracted early in treatment unless they are being retained temporarily for esthetics or for space maintenance.[6,7] The failure to remove such teeth early in treatment may lead to abscess formation. Hopeless teeth can interfere with treatment and make it more complex. The patient may forget the hopeless prognosis of a tooth and become upset when extraction is ordered later in treatment. The surgical situation may involve impactions, cysts, and complex extractions. If the requirements for the surgery transcend the skill and training of the practitioner, he/she should refer the patient to an oral surgeon.

### Restorations

Usually periodontal therapy should precede restorative interventions. At times, however, caries may be so extensive as to require immediate attention. Depending on the patient's needs, these restorations should be temporary, since the completion of periodontal treatment may be followed by reconstruction. The necessity of provisional splinting during the treatment period should be evaluated. Scheduling of restorative treatment should be done according to the following general rules (this is particularly true for students who may feel pressured to seek shortcuts in order to reach restorative requirements):

1. Normal patients. (Restorative treatment starts immediately.)
2. Class I (ADA periodontal disease classification)
   a. Without occlusal treatment need. (Caries control and scaling and root planing, including plaque control, may be simultaneous. Definitive restorative treatment should follow completion of scaling and plaque control.)
   b. With occlusal treatment need. (Definitive restorative treatment may immediately follow completion of scaling, plaque control, and occlusal adjustment.)
   c. With surgical treatment need. (Definitive restorative treatment should not be instituted for at least 4 to 6 weeks after the patient has healed.)

Caries control (temporary fillings) can be performed at any time in the course of periodontal treatment if it is used to prevent pulp exposure. In addition, measures to maintain occlusal relationships may be taken on a provisional basis. Amalgam and composite restorations may be performed to close contacts, to correct food impaction, and to remove overhangs. Restorative dentistry is performed by the generalist and is not in the province of the periodontist. Appropriate referrals should be made if the patient does not have a dentist.

### Splinting

Wire ligation and composite acid-etch splinting are generally performed during phase I therapy. Provisional or conditional splinting[10] may be done in phase I or in phase III therapy. Permanent splinting should be instituted at the end of a waiting period of 6 to 8 weeks after healing at the earliest. Whereas the periodontist may perform the wire ligation or composite acid-etch splinting, the provisional splinting and permanent splinting are to be performed by the generalist or by a prosthodontist. If the patient does not have a dentist, or if the case is complex, appropriate referrals should be made. In addition, it is necessary, when one expects that extensive restorative dentistry will follow periodontal treatment, that the nature of treatment, time, and cost be established in advance as part of full disclosure and informed consent.[11] This relaying of information requires that the patient have a consultation visit with the generalist or prosthodontist who will do the reconstruction. It may also require consultation(s) between the restorative and periodontal therapists. The periodontal and dental status of the patient will dictate restorative needs and will be modified by the patient's desires and financial considerations.

### Emergency

When the patient has an emergency involving pain, swelling, infection, and discomfort, the emergency condition must be resolved after the history and examination of the area involved in the chief complaint. Occasionally, an emergency condition will arise in the course of therapy. Then, too, the treatment plan must be suspended until the emergency is resolved. Generally, emergency visits may involve the treatment of such conditions as abscesses, necrotizing gingivitis, endodontic problems, hopeless teeth, various oral ulcerations, and temporomandibular joint problems. At other times, the patient may present with acute anxiety because of an oral lesion or an occlusal problem. These emergencies all take priority over other treatment scheduling.

### Medical status

When the history and examination finds that the patient has a systemic condition that would complicate treatment, a medical consultation is necessary. If the patient has not been to a physician in a number of years, a medical examination should be required before proceeding with treatment. Blood pressure readings and blood tests are in the province of the dentist. When positive findings are made, the patient should be referred to a physician.

## PHASES II AND III

When the patient has ADA class II, III, or IV periodontal disease, treatment phases I through III must be instituted and completed. Phase II surgery permits pocket elimination or reduction when infrabony pockets are present. The restoration of normal osseous form by ostectomy-osteoplasty procedures is possible if the deformities are not more than 3 or 4 mm deep and the bone loss generally is slight. Otherwise the therapist must resort to osseous surgery combined with grafting procedures in an attempt to restore lost bone.[12] At the same time root resections and mucogingival and gingivectomy procedures may be blended in an attempt to produce the best result possible.

Restorative treatment performed at this stage may be related to the periodontal-endodontic cases, to odontoplasty, and to provisional splinting.

## MAINTENANCE THERAPY

If the patient has been referred to a periodontist by another dentist, the patient should be returned to the referring dentist when the patient's periodontal disease is completely reversed (e.g., gingivitis, frenectomy, gingival clefts). In many instances, this also applies to patients of ADA types I and II periodontal disease. However, some type II and all types III and IV patients should be seen alternately by the periodontist and the generalist: one responsible for periodontal health, the other for the dental status of the patient. The specialist may see the patient once a year or every other year for the less involved cases, whereas the generalist maintains the patient in the recall system. On the other hand, advanced cases may be seen alternately at 2- to 4-month intervals or, with the consent of the generalist, may be seen primarily by the periodontist and yearly by the generalist.

## PROSTHETIC PRESCRIPTION

Reconstructive treatment should follow periodontal surgery after a waiting period of at least 2 months. When bone loss is very advanced and the status of the teeth guarded, it is best to consider partial dentures. If the teeth can support a fixed prosthesis and be helped by it, then splinting is advisable.

## ALTERNATIVE TREATMENT PLANS

Alternative treatment plans should be prepared for the patient who elects to forego splinting and surgery when these are indicated. In this case the patient may be treated through phase I therapy and be placed on a maintenance schedule. The patient who chooses neither to be treated, nor to accept an alternative treatment plan must be prepared to accept "crisis care"[10] and to go on to full dentures at a future time. Sometimes treatment planning may provide for a divided prescription spanning several years. This is done particularly where the patient cannot afford the complete sequence at once. Divided prescription may also be done, however, where the longevity of the teeth is very doubtful. At times patients elect alternative treatment because of anxiety. When they perceive that treatment is not threatening, these patients may change their minds and continue with phases II and III.

The establishment of an alternative plan generally calls for a rigorous maintenance schedule with scaling and planing performed more frequently than is otherwise usual.

# Treatment criteria

## QUALITY OF CARE

The quality of care that the patient receives is a matter of knowledge and technical skill. It maximizes the benefits of treatment and minimizes its risks, taking into account, on one hand, the preferences of the patient[13]; on the other, it reflects a precise adjustment of the care to the requirements of the case. Categorical criteria exist that list procedures that must or must not be performed in every case in a class. There are contingent criteria also that list procedures that should be performed or may be performed, depending on the nature and circumstances of the case.[13] These criteria permit varying the strategies of care as judged by their benefits, risks, and costs.[13] Given the possibility of varying the strategy of treatment, the essence of quality is gauged by relative success in treatment as shown by retrospective studies and reflects *clinical judgment*, which is the choice of the most appropriate strategy in the management of a given patient.[13]

**Strategy of care and clinical judgment**

In general, periodontal care seeks the following (Fig. 30-5):

**Concept of cure**

1. Removal of known etiologic factors
2. Reduction of all pockets to a minimal depth to facilitate maintenance by the patient *and* the dental hygienist
3. Creation of a maintainable gingival and osseous architecture
4. Restoration of a functional and esthetic dentition
5. Maintenance of the resulting health by the patient, doctor, and hygienist

Any periodontal treatment plan, to be fully successful, should be directed at satisfying these five details of therapy. The well-designed treatment plan should strive to accomplish the best result, with a minimal procedure, in maximum comfort.[1] Above all, the result should remove all subjective symptoms and create a state of oral health suitable for maintenance, with comfort such that the patient feels a complete oral unawareness—a negative oral sense. To accomplish this, each case may be assayed as to its individual demands, and a plan of treatment devised that will reach a successful conclusion.

## PHILOSOPHY OF TREATMENT

It is well recognized that periodontal diseases can be treated successfully and that the health of the diseased periodontium can be restored and the teeth maintained. The

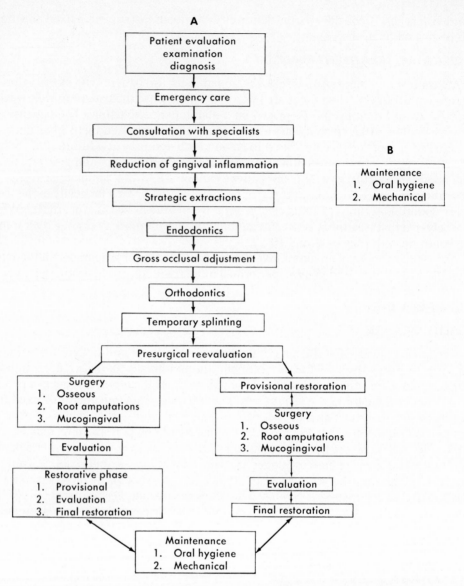

**Fig. 30-5.** *Sequence of therapy for the periodontal patient.* **A,** *This sequence of therapy is usually the most practical but is not to be considered inviolate (see text).* **B,** *At any stage of therapy the patient will be in maintenance and may be held there.*

therapeutic regimen selected will reflect the "concept of cure" embraced by the therapist.

All therapists agree that the elimination of inflammation is a primary objective of therapy. However, some difference of opinion exists as to how this is best accomplished. All forms of therapy have indications and contraindications; none is sacrosanct or inviolate. The therapeutic concept of today includes all forms of therapy, conservative and complex, selected and blended for the successful management of the *individual patient*. Therapy must be tailored to the needs, both physical and psychologic, of the patient. The treatment plan is a strategy to develop dental health. There are various possible goals. Decisions must be made as to whether a "long initial preparation" phase will be attempted or full treatment followed by maintenance. The role of the patient in oral hygiene must be understood. The patient's commitment to final restorative procedures, the possibility of losing teeth that do not respond to treatment or are jeopardizing adjacent teeth, possible changes in treatment plan, and provisional steps in therapy must be considered by the therapist and discussed with and understood by the patient. It may not always be practical or possible to follow "ideal" treatment sequence in every patient; these situations must be recognized and considered in the development of the treatment plan. For example, in a patient with very deep pockets and advanced bone loss, flap curettage after initial scaling may be the therapy of choice. In this type of case one must consider that a prolonged initial preparation may not achieve total débridement, whereas the surgical approach to scaling would. On the other hand, the patient may respond well to an extended initial preparation and may, in time, avoid surgical intervention. It is possible, given time, effort, skill, and patience on the part of the therapist, to maintain some periodontal patients with a curette and oral hygiene. But it is not practical to consider this approach to be applicable to all patients. The clinical judgment of the dentist should decide which treatment plan would be best for each patient. Although differences in philosophy will alter each doctor's choices, dentistry is committed to technical and intellectual excellence. One cannot hide a choice based on lack of technical skill or knowledge behind the argument that the choice was based on a different philosophic approach. The patient's needs are too important for such a rationalization.

## RECORD KEEPING

The treatment performed should be recorded carefully at each visit. An exact record of every step that has been taken is essential. As each step is completed, it should be checked off against the treatment plan checklist. Charting must be repeated at the phase I, II, and III reevaluations and compared with the initial charting. In this way one can gauge the success of therapy. Recall reevaluations and roentgenograms make up the history of the disease in a given patient and of the effectiveness of treatment. Such data are of immense value in retrospective studies. When sufficient data are accumulated, the validity of various approaches for different categories of patients will become firmly established.

# Referral

There are three basic reasons for referral: (1) professional, (2) moral and ethical, and (3) legal.

1. *Professional:* Professional referrals are classified as follows:
   a. *Medical:* Referral/consultation is indicated when a patient's medical history discloses significant information that may contribute to or influence the course and outcome of the treatment or when the dentist suspects illness.
   b. *Dental:* Referral/consultation is indicated when the dentist cannot provide the entire dental therapy the patient needs. When the examination reveals periodontal disease that the generalist cannot or does not wish to treat, referral to a periodontist is in order. Equally the periodontist is obligated to refer patients for treatment to the general practitioner or other specialists.
2. *Moral and ethical:* The American Dental Association (ADA) code of professional conduct regarding consultation and referral states: "Dentists shall be obligated to seek consultation, if possible, whenever the welfare of patients will be safeguarded or advanced by utilizing those who have special skills, knowledge, and experience. When patients visit or are referred to specialists or consulting dentists for consultation:
   a. The specialists or consulting dentists upon completion of their care shall return the patient, unless the patient expressly reveals a different preference, to the referring dentist, or if none, to the dentist of record for future care.
   b. The specialists shall be obligated when there is no referring dentist and upon a completion of their treatment to inform patients when there is a need for further dental care."[14]

3. *Legal:* Dentists are obligated by law to keep their diagnostic and treatment capabilities up to the standards imposed by other members of the profession in good standing. Furthermore, dentists must exercise reasonable judgment in deciding whether to treat or refer their patients. Even though the dentist is not required to consult with a specialist on every conceivable complication that may arise in his/her practice, he/she has the duty to seek consultation/referral with a specialist when he/she knows, or in the exercise of reasonable care should know, that the services of a specialist are indicated. Legally, when expert testimony supports that a reasonably careful and prudent dentist would have sought consultation/referral under similar circumstances, the dentist may be held negligent for failing to do so.[15]

Other reasons for referral include: patient relocation, dentist-patient personality conflict, and dentist's preference.

Some dentists do not use specialty service because of the following reasons.[16]

1. *Patients' limited dental budget.* The dentist may fear that using specialty service will necessarily mean loss of patient's fees. On the contrary, the specialist is interested in promoting good dentistry and will, by the nature of his/her specialty position, educate and inform the patient of the necessity of complete oral health care; thus supporting the dentist's position in the health care team.
2. *Dentist's "loss of face" with patients.* The dentist should never view patients as a threat to himself/herself or his/her competence. Today most patients are aware of the complexity of dental treatment. Furthermore, with the scientific advancement in dentistry, it is now possible for the public to receive the benefits of the increased knowledge and skill with specialty utilization. The specialist can communicate this point directly to the patient and confirm that the dentist's decision to refer was made with the patient's welfare being of utmost importance.
3. *Dentist's fear of possible loss of patients because of referral.* It is a source of embarrassment to the dentist and the specialist alike, if at the conclusion of specialty treatment the patient decides to seek another dentist. The establishment of confidence and rapport between the dentist and his/her patients will minimize the likelihood of this occurrence. Patients who decide to seek another dentist after specialty treatment usually are motivated by some dissatisfaction with the services of the referring dentist or his/her staff. Often "lost" patients are referred too late for successful dental treatment even by the specialist. Examples of potential patient dissatisfaction in these cases occurs when a patient is referred to a specialist as a "last resort." Periodontal breakdown that is simply "observed" or even undiagnosed for years and not referred by the dentist often can become so advanced that successful treatment is not possible.[17]

## Elements of referral

### Communication

Once the decision to refer has been made, effective communication among the dentist, the patient, and the specialist becomes an essential function. This communication triad must exist in order to enhance the patient management process.

Informing the patient about the disease condition is the first step in the dentist-patient communication process. This discussion must be honest and presented in readily understood terms. The need and reasons for referral to a specialist are discussed. All patient questions should be encouraged and answered with sensitivity and empathy. The dentist should transmit to the specialist a brief summary of his/her findings, appropriate records and tentative restorative treatment plan. In return, the specialist should provide the dentist with a timely and concise report of his/her findings, including specific suggestions and recommendations for treatment. When treatment is completed, the specialist should provide a posttreatment report, stating achieved results, prognosis, and recommendations for maintenance therapy.

The specialist-patient communication begins with the interview and examination process as discussed earlier in Chapter 28. Following treatment, the need for restorative care and other measures should be explained to the patient, who is then returned to the dentist of record. If the patient's first contact is with the specialist and no dentist of record is noted, the specialist is obliged to inform/refer the patient to a dentist for further dental care. In addition, a recall-maintenance schedule should be made.

## Documentation

All communication, written or verbal, must be properly documented on the patient's chart. Accurate communication and documentation between the dentist and the specialist allows for continuity of patient care and treatment as well as more efficient patient management.

Patients have the right of access to their records and may acquire copies of the original documents. However, the patient should never be allowed to handle the original documents.[18]

## Summary

It is difficult for the dentist or specialist to possess expert knowledge and skill in all areas of dentistry because of the ever-expanding scope and complexity of dental therapy. Today's dentist is confronted with a wide range of treatment procedures and available alternatives. Knowing his/her treatment capabilities and limitations, the dentist must exercise reasonable and prudent judgment in deciding whether to treat patients or refer them. At all times during the course of treatment, the primary focus is the patient's welfare. Effective communication and interaction among the dentist, the patient, and the specialist are vital elements of proper treatment.

**REFERENCES**

1. Bellini, J., and Johansen, J.: Average time required for scaling and surgery in periodontal therapy, Acta Odontol. Scand. **31:**283, 1973.
2. Morgenstein, W.M.: Informed consent—the doctrine evolves, J. Am. Dent. Assoc. **93:**637, 1976.
3. Zinman, E.J.: Informed consent to periodontal surgery—advise before you incise, J. West. Soc. Periodontol./Periodont. Abstr. **24:**101, 1976.
4. Zinman, E.J.: Common dental malpractice errors and preventive measures, J. West. Soc. Periodontol./Periodont. Abstr. **23:**149, 1976.
5. Morris, W.O.: Recent developments in dental litigation, J. Am. Dent. Assoc. **92:**766, 1976.
6. Everett, F.G., and Stern, I.B.: When is tooth mobility an indication for extraction? Dent. Clin. North Am. **13:**791, 1969.
7. Corn, H., and Marks, M.H.: Strategic extractions in periodontal therapy, Dent. Clin. North Am. **13:**817, 1969.
8. Cohen, D.W.: Principles and concepts of treatment derived from these studies, and their application to dentistry, J. Clin. Periodontol. **10:**542, 1983.
9. Despeignes, J.: Synthesis of current periodontal therapy: on the need for a system in treatment planning, Bull. Acad. Dent. **10:**9, 1966.
10. Stern, I.B.: The status of temporary fixed-splinting procedures in the treatment of periodontally involved teeth, J. Periodontol. **31:**217, 1960.
11. Ingelfinger,F.J.: Medicine: meritorious or meritricious, Science **200:**942, 1978.
12. Zander, H.A., Polson, A.M., and Heijl, L.C.: Goals of periodontal therapy, J. Periodontol. **47:**261, 1976.
13. Donabedian, A.: The quality of medical care, Science **200:**356, 1978.
14. American Dental Association: Principles of Ethics and Code of Professional Conduct, J. Am. Dent. Assoc. **102:**680, 1981.
15. Zinman, E.J.: Usual and customary vs. prudent practice, Dent. Student, Jan. 1981.
16. Chace, R.: Place of the specialist in dentistry, J. Am. Dent. Assoc. **69:**181, 1964.
17. Johnson, R.L.: In Prichard, J,: The diagnosis and treatment of periodontal disease in general dental practice, Philadelphia, 1979, W.B. Saunders Co.
18. Sheppard, G.A.: Medical-legal considerations. In Malamed, S.F.: Handbook of medical emergencies in the dental office; St. Louis, 1982, The C.V. Mosby Co.

## ADDITIONAL SUGGESTED READING

Chasens, A.I.: Periodontal disease: a major responsibility in the general practice of dentistry, N.Y. J. Dent. **30:**87, 1960.

Deasy, M.J., et al.: Periodontal therapy: principles of pocket elimination, J. Am. Dent. Assoc. **92:**1173, 1976.

Dixon, R.A., and Henry, J.L.: Overall philosophy of treatment of periodontal disease and case analysis, J. Periodontol. **26:**21, 1955.

Ekanayaka, A.N.I., and Sheiham, A.: Estimating the time and personnel required to treat periodontal disease, J. Clin. Periodontol. **5:**85, 1978.

Howells, J., et al.: A logical approach to periodontal pocket therapy, J. Periodontol. **29:**128, 1958.

Thomas, B.O.A., et al.: What is periodontal maintenance care and whose responsibility is it? J. West. Soc. Periodontol. **8:**11, 1963.

# PART FIVE
## Initial Nonsurgical Therapy

# CHAPTER 31

# Plaque control (oral hygiene, chemical plaque control), root sensitivity, and halitosis

## Plaque control (oral hygiene)

Plaque control refers to procedures that are intended to remove bacterial plaque from teeth. This may be accomplished via professional plaque removal, patient-performed oral hygiene, or chemical plaque control. Plaque control is the most effective means of preventing accumulation of microbial dental deposits, thereby interfering with the initiation, development, or progression of periodontal disease.[1]

## Objectives

The objective of oral hygiene is to reduce the number of microorganisms on the teeth.[2] All accessible dental plaque and debris should be removed from the gingival margins, proximal tooth surfaces, and, where possible, gingival sulci. Doing this reduces the factors that produce irritation and inflammation.[3] One of the causes of halitosis is also removed by these measures. Gingival stimulation (massage) may play a role in increasing gingival tone, surface keratinization, gingival vascularity, and gingival circulation; however, conclusions in this area are not well documented.

## Requirements

Requirements for care will vary from patient to patient and even in different areas of the same mouth.

## CLINICAL EXAMINATION

**Anatomic considerations and patient interview**

Clinical examination will enable the dentist to evaluate the needs of each patient. This evaluation should include an appraisal of the anatomy and alignment of the teeth, the relationship of the teeth to the gingiva, and the type and amount of deposits present. The patient should be questioned as to current oral hygiene practices. During the discussion the dentist should note the responses of the patient to both oral hygiene questions and suggestions regarding the home dental care program. Some patients may be free of gingival disease or resistant to it. Oral hygiene will not be a therapeutic necessity for these people.

**Saliva**

**Diet**

The plaque-reducing effect of hard fibrous foods has been shown in dogs.[4] Diet, however, apparently plays a small part in removal of plaque in humans.[5,6] This difference may be explained by variations in tooth anatomy in human and canine dentitions. Diet composition may influence plaque formation because diet along with saliva provides nutrients for plaque microorganisms. Refined carbohydrates may increase plaque formation by providing additional energy supply for microorganisms.[7] In a study comparing carbohydrate-free diet and supplementation with sucrose-, xylitol-, or sorbital-containing sweets, more plaque formed during periods of dieting with sucrose supplements.[8] Studies have investigated whether sucrose may influence bacterial composition of dental plaque.[9,10] Quantitative proportions of some bacteria may be altered by diet. In conclusion, the clinical impact of sugar consumption is complex, with research indicating that intake of refined carbohydrates is instrumental in development and maintenance of plaque.

## PATIENT EVALUATION AND EDUCATION

In teaching plaque control, first evaluate the patient. Note the quality of oral hygiene and try to determine attitudes toward home dental care. Discuss the patient's daily schedule. Individuals may have differing social attitudes toward oral hygiene. This does not mean that such attitudes cannot be altered; what it means is that the dentist may perceive a basis from which to proceed in educational efforts.[11,12]

One should create an environment (and develop rapport) that enhances communication. Present small units of information to the patient. Add information and alternate techniques in increments at subsequent visits, thus varying the rate of instruction to each patient's needs. Demonstrate techniques in the patient's mouth, then follow up with patient participation and immediate feedback. Constant positive reinforcement is an important part of all dental therapy.

**Disclosing solutions and plaque index**

Show the patient the plaque on the teeth. It may not be readily visible. Use an explorer or other instrument to collect a small amount of this material. When a phase microscope is available, take a smear from the interdental tooth surfaces, place it on a slide, add a drop of water and a coverslip, and demonstrate to the patient the motile bacteria.[13] This can be dramatic. Now ask the patient to rinse with a disclosing solution or to chew a disclosing tablet (Red-Cote).[14,15] Using a hand mirror and good light, show the patient the stained areas on the teeth.

**Disclosing solutions and tablets**

The use of disclosing agents provide a measure of plaque accumulation that the patient can see. It is an objective criterion for adequate oral hygiene. Disclosing solutions also stain mucosa of lips, tongue, cheeks, and gingiva. However, some of the tissue discoloration can be removed by rinsing. Fluorescent disclosing solutions that are invisible may be used in place of stains.[16] The *location of bacterial plaque in proximity to the gingiva and the consequences* of its presence should be explained to the patient. Record specific areas of plaque in a diagram and develop a plaque index. Plaque index may be expressed as percentage of tooth surfaces with plaque:

$$\left( \frac{\text{Number of surfaces with plaque}}{\text{Total number of tooth surfaces}} \times 100 \right)$$

or as percentage of plaque-free surfaces:

$$\left\{ \left( \frac{\text{Number of surfaces with plaque}}{\text{Total number of tooth surfaces}} \times 100 \right) = X \right\} 100 - X$$

The plaque-free score has an important motivational role in the prevention of disease by stressing clean surfaces; it encourages the patient. **Plaque-free score**

A rubber stamp (Fig. 31-1) may be imprinted on the patient's record at each visit and at the time of completion of phase I treatment. Apply disclosing solution to all teeth. Instruct the patient to rinse. Note in red on the chart and count all surfaces with remaining plaque. Strike out missing teeth with a single line. Then complete the plaque index score (plaque-free score or plaque-infected score). Reinforcement of oral hygiene techniques should continue until a patient maintains a plaque-free score of better than 85% or a plaque-infected score of 15% or less.

The little circles between tooth numbers in Fig. 31-1 represent the interdental papillae. When the interdental papillae bleed easily the circles should be filled in to score bleeding on this form. Each papilla is provoked with a probe and scored if it bleeds. Improvement in health would be indicated by repeated charting showing progressively fewer papillae filled in. In this way a record of bleeding papillae can be kept.

This method of scoring plaque index and bleeding assesses both oral hygiene status and gingival inflammation. Repeated scores at the beginning of subsequent office visits may be compared to previous scores and specific sites, providing patient participation and patient visualization. Patients are encouraged when the therapist stresses success in plaque removal (clean surfaces). Then the therapist should assess the technique used in the plaque-infected areas, and new or alternate techniques for their care may be introduced.

Keep in mind, however, that the generalized (nonspecific) plaque hypothesis has been replaced by the specific plaque hypothesis, and therefore the relationship between disease and plaque quantity may not be linear. All plaque, per se, may not be pathogenic in all patients.

In Plate 8, *A* to *C*, p. 614, a gingivitis around the mandibular right lateral incisor can be seen in a 25-year-old woman who did not brush for 2 weeks. In *D* to *F* of this plate a 26-year-old woman formed extensive plaque that literally covered the crowns; however, no clinical gingival inflammation could be detected.

## HOME CARE DENTAL CLEANSING AIDS

There are a number of aids that can be used in home care dental cleansing:

I. Toothbrush (manual or electric) (Butler, Roto-Dent, Interplak, Broxodont)
II. Interdental aids
    A. Dental floss (unbonded unwaxed or waxed)
    B. Triangular toothpicks
        1. Hand-held triangular toothpicks
        2. Proxapic
    C. Brushes
        1. Proxabrush system

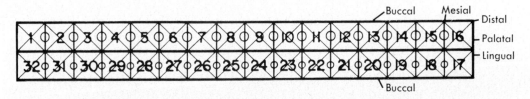

**Fig. 31-1.** Form for recording plaque-free score and bleeding papillae.

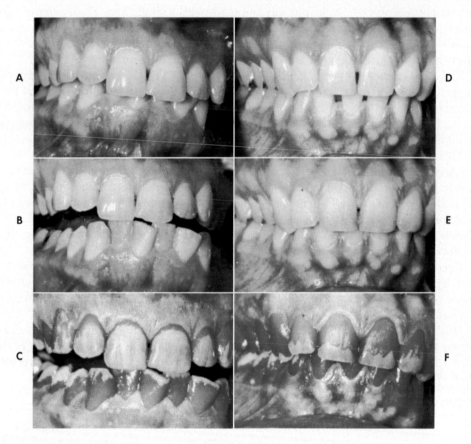

**Plate 8.** **A,** Gingival inflammation in a 25-year-old woman at the start of a study on the relationship of oral hygiene and gingival inflammation. **B,** After 2 weeks of no oral hygiene, plaque is visible even without disclosing solution. A mild, marginal, papillary gingivitis is present. **C,** Use of a disclosing solution vividly illustrates abundant plaque. **D,** Plaque in a 26-year-old dental assistant at the start of a plaque experiment. **E,** After 14 days without oral hygiene, plaque may be seen on teeth and gingiva. Very little inflammation could be detected. **F,** Rinsing with 0.2% basic fuchsin solution reveals the extent of plaque collected. (Color page donated as a service to the profession by The John Butler Toothbrush Co., Chicago, Illinois.)

2. Bottle brushes
3. Single-tufted brushes (flat or tapered)
  D. Yarn
  E. Variable-diameter floss
  F. Perio-Aid (round toothpick holders)
III. Others
  A. Gauze strips
  B. Pipe cleaners
  C. Rubber-tip stimulator
  D. Water irrigation device
  E. Floss holders

## INSTRUCTION IN TOOTHBRUSHING

Before any instruction in brushing begins, make the patient aware of several concepts:

1. *Frequency of brushing.* The necessity of brushing once or twice daily to remove all plaque and debris and to stimulate the surrounding tissue should be emphasized.
2. *Nature and composition of debris.* The location of plaque and the consequences of its presence should be explained. Diagrams are helpful, if not indispensable, teaching aids. The patient should be made aware of what the dentist is attempting to accomplish and what favorable results can be obtained.
3. *Type of toothbrush to be used.* Toothbrush recommendations should be based on the patient's individual needs.

**Frequency of brushing**

The frequency of toothbrushing and cleansing should be timed with the aim of preventing gingival disease and caries. Only daily cleansing may be necessary to prevent gingivitis.[17] It has also been established that, for maintenance of periodontal health, *complete* plaque control has to be performed only every 24 to 48 hours.[18,19] However, the requirements for control of caries or control of breath odors are more demanding. Acidogenic microorganisms can, in the presence of a proper substrate, lower the pH on the tooth surface in an incredibly short time. Breath odors are found immediately after ingestion of foods. Moreover, the feeling of personal comfort that clean teeth can give requires frequent brushing. On the basis of these factors consider twice-daily brushing to be empirically necessary. If two daily brushings are recommended two brushes are to be used at alternate sessions. They should be rinsed thoroughly and air dried.

Once the patient is aware of the reasons for brushing, begin the technical instruction. Visual aids will help to convey the message. The recommended sequence for instruction is as follows:

1. Designate which brush or brushes to use.[20-24]
2. Demonstrate the maxillary and mandibular anterior areas in the patient's mouth. The patient should observe with a mirror.
3. Have the patient brush his/her own teeth with a moistened brush.
4. Point out any errors in technique, including placement of the brush and position of hand and arm.
5. Correct these efforts in subsequent demonstrations until the desired technique is perfected in the anterior area.
6. Repeat the sequence of instruction for other areas of the mouth.

**Toothbrushes**

The following should be taken into consideration when recommending a toothbrush (Fig. 31-2):

1. *Type.* Decide which type or types of toothbrush should be used.[20] There are manual and mechanical brushes. In the majority of cases the manual brush is the instrument of choice. In some instances, however, the mechanically operated brush should be recommended.[25]

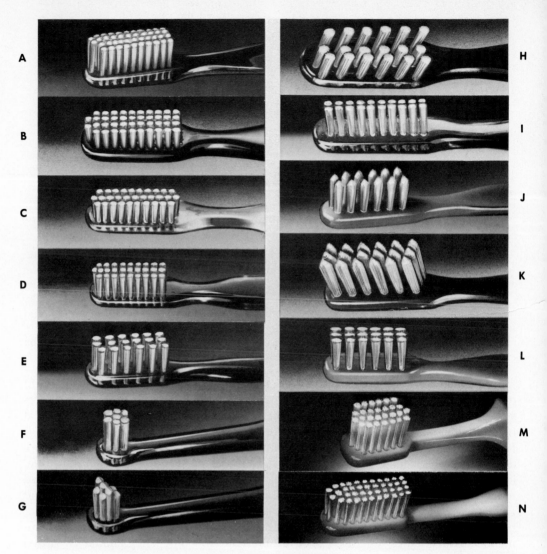

**Fig. 31-2.**  Toothbrushes in varying shapes, sizes, bristle lengths, and firmness. Brushes should be prescribed according to individual patient needs. **A,** Four-row, multitufted, soft nylon with dome-top trim and rounded bristle ends; Butler No. 411 Adult, G-U-M (0.008). **B,** Four-row, multitufted, soft natural bristle; Butler No. 511 Adult, G-U-M. **C,** Three-row, multitufted, soft nylon, rounded bristle; Butler No. 311 Adult, G-U-M (0.008). **D,** Three-row, multitufted, soft nylon; Butler No. 111 Junior, G-U-M (0.008). **E,** Three-row, soft nylon; Butler Adult/Bass Brush (0.007). **F,** Soft nylon; Butler No. 307 End-Tuft (0.008). **G,** Soft nylon; Butler No. 308 Tapered End-Tuft (0.008). **H,** Orthodontic brush with depressed center row; Butler No. 123 (0.009). **I,** Two-row, sulcular, soft nylon; Butler No. 210 Sulcular, G-U-M (0.008). **J,** Two-row, multitufted, medium nylon; Butler Adult (0.012). **K,** Three-row, multitufted, hard nylon; Butler Adult (0.014). **L,** Three-row, soft nylon; Lactona Adult. **M,** Four-row; Reach. **N,** Four-row, soft nylon; INAVA Adult, France. (Courtesy John O. Butler Co., Chicago, Illinois.)

2. *Size.* The handle should be shaped for a firm, comfortable grip. The brush should be small enough for easy insertion into all areas of the mouth, yet large enough to cover several teeth.

3. *Bristles.* The bristles may be of equal length. If they are soft they should be closely set. If they are hard they should be more widely spaced. They may be of either synthetic or natural boar fibers. The synthetic variety has been improved in resiliency. The ends are rounded, with a diameter of 0.007 to 0.011 inch, so that the bristles can be used to advantage in either the soft[22] (Fig. 31-3, *A* and *B*) or the hard type of brush.[23] Synthetic bristles are more easily cleansed and are more durable, and their stiffness is not so easily affected by water.[20] Brushes are available with supersoft synthetic bristles arranged in

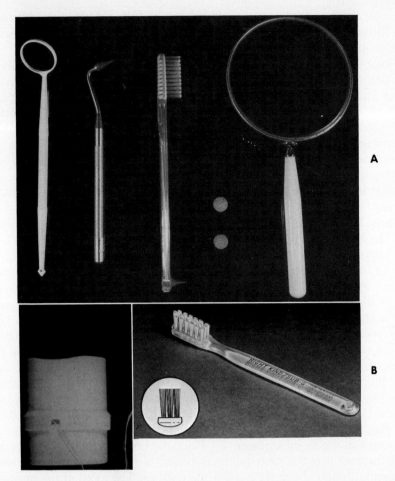

**Fig. 31-3.** **A,** Basic armamentarium *(top)* for oral hygiene. *Left to right,* Mouth mirror, interdental stimulator, toothbrush, disclosing tablets, and hand mirror. **B,** Dental floss and soft-bristled brush with rounded ends for sulcular brushing.

two or three rows. These types are generally employed for only a short time, usually during the healing period after periodontal surgery.

Instruct the patient to brush systematically, starting posteriorly and moving progressively toward the anterior and then returning to the posterior region on the opposite side of the same arch.

**Sequence of brushing**

The length of time required for mouth cleansing will vary for each patient, depending in part on the frequency of brushing. Suggest a prescribed time, emphasizing the fact that initially more time (10 to 20 minutes) will be required until the patient becomes adept. Later, 3 to 5 minutes may suffice.

**Length of brushing time**

Brushing should be performed before a mirror with a good light so that the patient can check the placement of the brush and bristles. Patients who wear glasses for reading should wear them for brushing. Some patients who claim to brush often may not accomplish as thorough a debridement as others who may brush conscientiously once a day.[26] The patient should brush at night before going to bed. Thus during the hours of sleep, the mouth will be as clean as possible, and plaque will not be left in situ for 12 or more hours.

At successive appointments examine the patient's mouth to evaluate the plaque accumulation. If plaque remains in some areas examine the patient's technique and correct any errors. In many cases several weeks may elapse before the patient is able to carry out a home dental care regimen successfully. Monitor the efficacy of oral hygiene throughout treatment and suggest changes as necessary in home dental care methods or in the treatment plan based on this evaluation.

**Intrasulcular method**

No single method of toothbrushing has been demonstrated to be totally adequate for all patients.[27] The intrasulcular method advocated by Talbot[28] in 1899 and by Bass[21] in 1944 is currently popular. This method is efficient in removing dental plaque from the exposed gingival margin of the tooth and approximately a half millimeter or so into the sulcus.[29] The interdental sulci are better cleansed with floss when there are no concavities. The occlusal surface must be cleansed by a vibrating motion of the bristle ends over the occlusal surfaces. In mouths where periodontal disease has created large interproximal spaces, the Charters method of toothbrushing may be used after the intrasulcular method, to be followed by use of interdental brushes, dental floss, or cotton yarn.

**Modified intrasulcular method**

In the modified intrasulcular method a brush with soft, multitufted synthetic bristles is used. The bristles have rounded, polished ends (0.007 inch in diameter). Place the brush so that the sides of the bristles are flat against the facial, palatal, or lingual surfaces of the teeth, the inside bristles are next to the teeth, and the ends of the bristles are at the gingival margin of these teeth (Fig. 31-4, *A*). Rotate the handle of the brush slightly so that the outer two or three rows of bristles overlap both the gingival margin and the attached gingiva adjacent to that margin (*B*). Perform a vibrating (reciprocating) motion in an anteroposterior direction, forcing the fine bristles next to the tooth into the gingival sulcus. At the same time the vibrating motion by the outer two or three rows of bristles will cleanse the plaque from the part of the attached gingiva under the bristle ends and stimulate the gingiva. This vibrating motion should be applied for about 10 seconds in any area. The sides of the bristles help loosen the plaque. After the vibrating motion is applied roll the brush toward the occlusal surface. Begin the sequence of brushing in the posterior part of the mouth on the maxillary arch at the facial surfaces (*C*). Place the brush as described to complete the cycle. Then move it to the next segment toward the mesial surface (*D*), overlapping the segments slightly (*E*). Repeat the cycle until the last tooth of the opposite side of the arch is cleansed. Brush the distal surface of the last tooth in the arch by placing the ends of the bristles against this surface and vibrating the brush. Repeat the procedure on the palatal surface (*F*). Next, place the bristle ends on the occlusal surfaces, vibrating them into the fissures and moving around the arch.

When the maxillary arch is completed, brush the mandibular teeth in the same manner.

**Modified Stillman method**

The modified Stillman brushing method[30] enjoys widespread popularity since it permits good cleansing and excellent massage. Because of the stimulation that it provides it is sometimes recommended in managing problems of gingival hyperplasia. It is a forerunner of the intrasulcular method.

In this technique place the bristles first on the attached gingiva just coronal to the mucogingival junction (Fig. 31-5, *A*). Direct the tips of the bristles apically at a 45-degree angle. With the sides of the bristles pressed firmly against the gingiva, introduce a slight mesiodistal vibratory motion simultaneously with the gradual movement of the brush toward the occlusal plane. This slight yet firm mesiodistal massage is believed to clean the teeth effectively, especially since the vibratory movement forces the bristles into interproximal spaces and adjoining tooth areas (the so-called unclean area of the tooth). The gingiva is also massaged simultaneously. The ill effects of improper placement of bristles should be shown so that injury to the soft tissues is avoided (Fig. 31-5, *E*). Be sure that the patient knows how easy it is to miss the gingiva (*B*) and the cervical areas of the teeth, thus leaving plaque (*C*). Apply sufficient pressure to produce a blanching of the tissues (*D*). In brushing the vestibular areas of the maxillary molars,

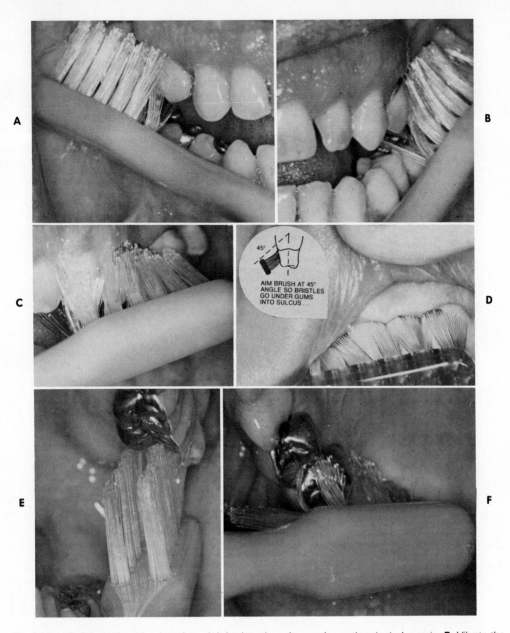

**Fig. 31-4.   A,** Sulcular brushing introduces bristles into the sulcus and over the gingival margin. **B,** Vibrate the bristles in place. **C,** Brush each segment in turn, overlapping the segments. Start on the upper right. **D,** Apply even pressure. **E,** Brush the distal surface of the last tooth *(upper left)*. **F,** Palatal brushing is difficult for some persons. Bristles should be placed carefully against the margin and in the sulcus. (Courtesy E. Moser, San Francisco, California.)

show how cheek clearance for the brush can be obtained by moving the mandible toward the side being brushed. Show how to brush the distal surfaces of the last molars, working the bristles up and around these areas.

Demonstrate the placement of brush to teeth and gingiva on the palatal and lingual surfaces. The technique can be shown first in the mandibular anterior region. Patients with a narrow arch should use only part of the bristles (split-brush technique). In some cases the patient can effectively cleanse the mandibular incisors by biting on a finely textured brush. Another effective way to brush the lingual surfaces of mandibular

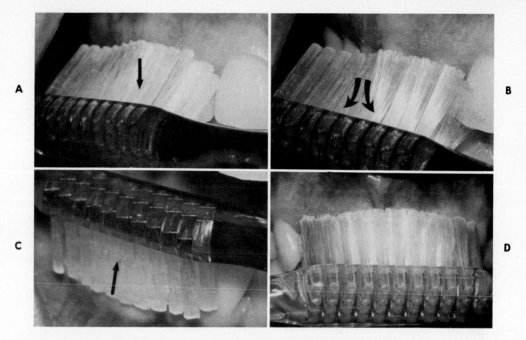

**Fig. 31-5. A,** Placement of the toothbrush at a 45-degree angle on the attached gingiva. Press the brush against the tissues until blanching is achieved. Then shimmy or pump the brush with a reciprocal motion of the handle, and, **B,** carry the brush coronally without turning or twisting the brush head in the direction of the arrows (modified Stillman technique). **C,** Brush with the bristle tips toward the gingiva and into the sulci to cleanse the interdental spaces and the sulci (modified Stillman technique). **D,** The massaging action is shown in the blanching of the gingiva.

incisors is as follows: Hold the brush at the end, and, bending over the basin, bring the full force of the arm to bear in the downward stroke. Since the lingual surfaces of the mandibular incisor teeth often are difficult areas to clean, many types of brushes can be employed (stiff, one-row bristled brushes for cases of crowding or buckling or during orthodontic treatment; lingual brushes with bristles inserted on a curved head; brushes with a small head that can be turned on an adjustable swivel to various positions).

Emphasize to the patient that the entire lingual surface of mandibular molars must be reached. Show how the last molar may be missed completely if the brush is not carried down on the gingiva and far enough back. In situations where the incisal edges of anterior teeth engage the toothbrush handle and interfere with proper placement of the bristles at the gingival margin, a toothbrush with a handle that is easily bent without heating (i.e., Butler Co.) by the dental therapist or patient may be recommended (Fig. 31-6).

When a patient is troubled by a gag reflex or by difficulty of access, instruct the patient to place the bristles on the occlusal surfaces, retaining half the bristles in this position and carrying the remaining bristles toward the gingiva. A brush with a narrow head (two rows or three rows) will also benefit patients who have a gag reflex. The use of a minimal amount of toothpaste and brushing the lingual aspect of lower molar first also benefits these patients.

On the palatal surfaces of the maxillary premolars and molars, hold the brush so that it is parallel to the median line of the maxilla. In this manner the bristles reach all areas evenly. If the handle is held to one side some bristles will miss the teeth.

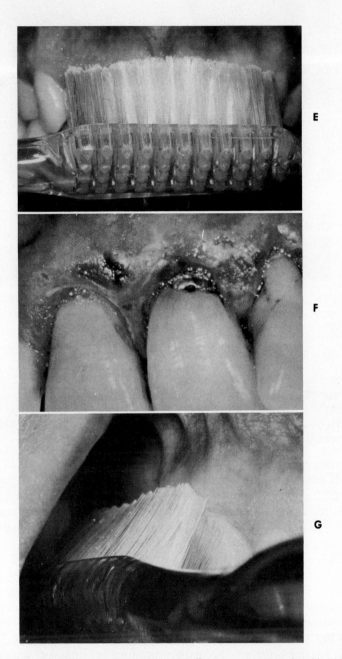

**Fig. 31-5, cont'd.   E,** Press the brush against the gingiva with sufficient pressure to produce blanching. **F,** Improper brushing may cause tissue injury. **G,** To brush the vestibular surfaces of maxillary molars, do not open the mouth too wide. Instead, shift the mandible laterally to the side that is to be brushed to create more space.

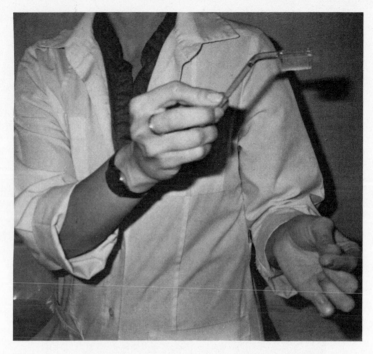

**Fig. 31-6.** Bending the toothbrush handle can facilitate access to lingual surfaces. Toothbrush handles made of a "memory" plastic may be easily bent and may resume or be bent back to the original shape.

The benefits of the modified Stillman method are as follows:

1. The gingiva is mechanically stimulated.
2. The gingival third of the tooth is contacted with a short vibratory motion over the surface, and plaque is removed between the gingival margin and the height of contour.
3. The tips of the bristles tend to reach the interproximal areas and to clean and stimulate the interdental papillae without injury.

The preceding is a description of the *modified* Stillman method. In the original (unmodified) method there is no brush movement toward the occlusal plane.[30] The bristles are placed on the gingival margin and the cervical portion of the tooth, and the mesiodistal vibratory pressure is applied without any movement of the bristle tips from their original placement. A hard brush may be prescribed for the management of gingival hyperplasia by the modified Stillman method.

**Charters technique (interdental brushing)**

When the interdental papillae are receded, leaving interdental areas open, the Charters method may be used. Work the bristles between the teeth, and point them incisally or occlusally at a 45-degree angle. After the bristles are engaged interproximally use a firm but gentle shimmying motion for 10 to 15 seconds in each area.[31] The proper placement of the brush for the labial area of the maxillary anterior teeth is shown in Fig. 31-7, *A,* and that for the buccal area of the mandibular teeth in Fig. 31-7, *B.* For lingual brushing the same procedure is employed, except that only the tip of the brush may be used effectively. On the lingual and palatal areas of the maxillary posterior teeth, advise the patient to place the brush head against the palate to permit the bristles to work between the teeth. If the proper angle is not maintained, some bristles may impinge on the gingiva and prevent the patient from working the rest of the bristles interdentally.

The Charters, Stillman, and intrasulcular methods are difficult for many patients to master. Just as important, no method is particularly efficient in removing debris

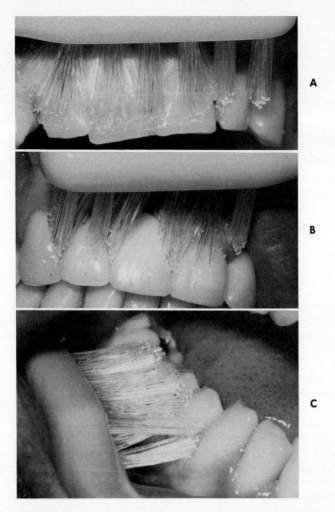

**Fig. 31-7.** **A,** Place the bristles firmly at a 45-degree angle toward the incisal or occlusal edges of the teeth. **B,** Brush the interdental spaces by a gentle shimmying motion. **C,** Position the brush for interdental brushing as shown on the mandible (Charters technique).

once it has been loosened. Therefore a thorough and vigorous rinsing should follow each brushing procedure.

The roll technique is easily performed and is used by many people. It is most **Roll technique** appropriate when the patient is in normal health. In this technique the bristles are placed well up on the gingiva at a 45-degree angle. Press the sides of the bristles against the tissue and simultaneously roll them incisally or occlusally against the gingiva and teeth, similar to the turning of a latchkey.

The electric toothbrush is both efficient and surprisingly appealing to patients. For **Electric tooth-** these reasons it has a definite use for some patients,[24,32,33] especially the handicapped **brush** and those who lack digital dexterity. Currently available electric toothbrushes have various types of actions or movements. Most brushes have small removable heads of synthetic fibers. The bristles are of a soft texture; damage to the tissues is rare because the brush action tends to stop on application of excessive pressure.

In the arc oscillating brushes, the bristles rotate vigorously in an arc of approximately 60 degrees. In using this instrument hold the brush lightly against the teeth so that the bristles move in a gently sweeping arc from the incisal edge to the attached gingiva and back again.

Another type provides a reciprocating horizontal movement. The action of this brush is somewhat similar to that used in the Charters, Stillman, and intrasulcular methods. When a reciprocating type of brush is used in a Bass-like stroke, the bristles are believed to enter into the sulci better and to cleanse them better. In any of the three types of brushes the action can be modified by a mere turning of the handle.

A third type (elliptic) combines the oscillating with the reciprocating, and a fourth type uses a rotary motion of the bristles.

## INTERDENTAL AIDS

**Instructions in use of dental floss**

In most mouths plaque will be found primarily on the interdental tooth surfaces and secondarily at the gingival margins. Toothbrushing may clean only the facial and lingual aspects of the teeth, so interdental cleaning is necessary where gingivitis is present. There is no clear evidence that any particular oral hygiene routine is better than any other for all patients.[33] What is extremely important is thoroughness of plaque removal. Show the patient how to remove plaque. Because interdental areas are rarely cleansed as thoroughly as other areas, they tend to have the deepest pockets.

1. Give the patient a hand mirror and have him/her observe.[15]
2. Start with unwaxed floss (many authorities prefer unwaxed floss, but no significant differences have been found in cleansing ability of waxed and unwaxed floss).[34-36]
3. Demonstrate the use of floss in the patient's mouth. Floss all proximal tooth surfaces, starting at the most posterior tooth in the maxillary right quadrant, completing all maxillary teeth, and progressing from the mandibular left quadrant to end on the mandibular right.
4. When dental floss is used, discuss the composition of plaque, the role plaque plays in producing inflammation, the relative invisibility of plaque, and therefore the need for the use of disclosing tablets or solution to make plaque readily visible. Emphasize that daily plaque removal can eliminate inflammation and that after cure this care can prevent or minimize future periodontal disease.
5. Emphasize that the floss can remove plaque in areas where the toothbrush cannot or where the toothbrush is inefficient.[37-39] Tell the patient that plaque is adherent and that firm pressure is necessary to remove it.
6. Avoid value judgments concerning the patient's oral hygiene. Establish a visual objective that can be reached, such as removal of all the disclosant stain on the tooth surfaces. Where tooth stains such as those from tobacco are found or where calculus is present, explain that you will remove these by scaling.

A procedure for the use of floss is as follows (Fig. 31-8):

1. Draw an 18- to 24-inch length of dental floss from the container, using the small sharp device on the container for cutting the desired length.
2. Twist the floss three times around the middle finger of the right hand and three times around the middle finger of the left hand, leaving a space of 1 to 4 inches between the hands. The thumbs and forefingers should be left free. Use them to guide the floss (Fig. 31-8, *A*).
3. Work the floss gently through the contact points to avoid damaging the gingiva (Fig. 31-8, *B* and *C*).
4. Make the floss firm by stretching it. Press the floss against the tooth and carry it carefully under the free gingival margin of the papilla (Fig. 31-8, *D*).
5. Once the floss is in the sulcus wrap it firmly against the mesial tooth surface by applying pressure with both hands (toward the distal). Carry the floss apically until resistance is met (Fig. 31-8, *E*). Then, engaging any plaque, move it incisally or occlusally toward the contact point. You do not have to pass through the contact point at this time. Repeat the procedure for the adjacent proximal tooth surface.

Thumbs and forefingers are appropriate for all teeth (Fig. 31-8, *F*). For additional cleansing efficiency apply a dentifrice or stain remover to the tooth before using the

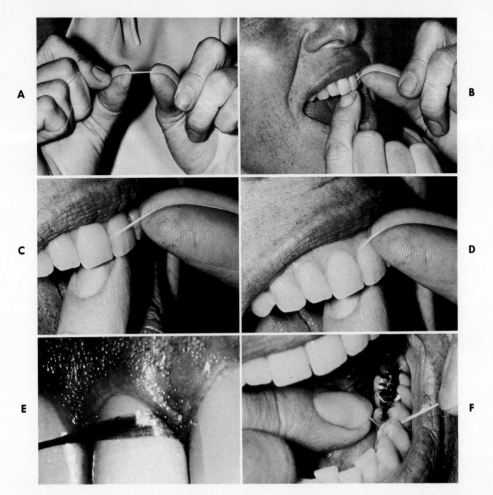

**Fig. 31-8.** **A,** Wrap most of the floss on the middle finger of the right hand and the rest around the middle finger of the left hand. As you are flossing, take up the floss on the other finger like a scroll to provide fresh floss. Use index fingers and thumbs as guides for flossing the upper teeth and index fingers for the lower teeth. **B,** Hold the floss tightly and work it gently between the teeth. Be very careful not to snap the floss between teeth and under gums because this can harm the delicate tissue. **C,** Curve the floss around the tooth and carefully work it apically. **D,** Work the floss into the sulcus. **E,** Holding the floss tightly against the tooth, scrape toward the point where the tooth touches its neighbor. Repeat this step on the adjacent tooth. **F,** Set a pattern for flossing, and follow the same pattern every time so that all the teeth are flossed.

floss. Incorrect use of floss may damage the gingiva.[37-39] Some patients may maneuver floss better if it is tied into a 6- to 8-inch diameter loop. Individuals who lack dexterity or who have large fingers or long fingernails may require a floss carrier (Fig. 31-9) to effectively remove proximal plaque without damaging soft tissue.

## Training routine

To establish an educational procedure that will train the patient, a program of regular, closely spaced visits is advised. Programs of daily visits (or visits every other day) encourage learning retention and permit patient feedback. They also permit the dentist to reinforce learning and to help establish new habit patterns by the patient.[26,40]

Such repeated instruction is valuable, since the patient is actively involved in the treatment procedure. The patient is shown what to do and then allowed to do it himself.

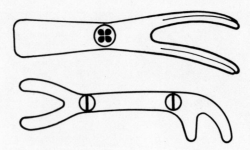

**Fig. 31-9.** Two types of floss carriers that are particularly useful for patients with poor digital dexterity.

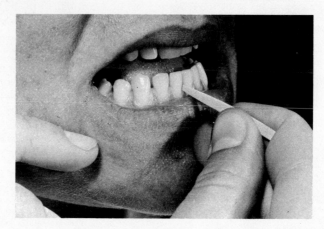

**Fig. 31-10.** Use Stim-U-Dents for interproximal cleansing and gingival stimulation. A to-and-fro motion works best.

The daily visits or every other day should be followed by several weekly visits to further establish habit patterns.[27]

At one visit have the patient rinse with a disclosing solution or use a disclosing tablet, and take another plaque index. Point out areas of successful efforts and areas of deficiency.

Then have the patient demonstrate flossing. If the patient is found to injure himself/herself with floss, the use of flat dental tape may be indicated in place of the floss.[23] Praise accomplishments and correct errors.

**Triangular toothpicks**    Interproximal areas with gingival recession and loss of interdenta papilla accumulate more plaque than normal interproximal areas. Therefore alternative aids are often necessary for periodontal patients. Specifically, triangular toothpicks may be recommended in areas with open interdental spaces, and interdental brushes may be recommended for cleansing concave interproximal tooth surfaces (Figs. 31-10 and 31-11). Floss generally removes plaque better than triangular toothpicks,[41] but interdental brushes (Proxabrush) are even more effective.

**Perio-Aid**    A device that is useful in reducing dental plaque at gingival margins and interproximally is called Perio-Aid (Fig. 31-11). This instrument consists of a plastic handle that will receive round, polished toothpicks and that permits the patient to cleanse the teeth at gingival margins, where accessible, and in areas of difficult access. The tip can be dipped into the sulcus.

**Interproximal brushes**    Interproximal brushes (Fig. 31-12) are useful in cleansing interdental areas.[42] Some patients prefer these brushes to floss, since less dexterity is required. Some interproximal brushes are constructed like "test-tube" brushes in various sizes. Other types

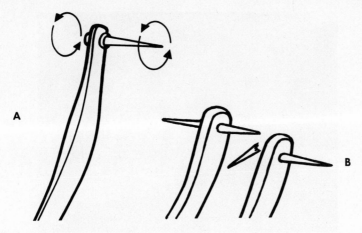

**Fig. 31-11.** **A,** Proxapic Butler triangular toothpick holder allowing 360-degree rotation of the triangular toothpick to facilitate interdental placement. **B,** Perio-Aid round toothpick holder used for cleansing at the gingival margin and interdentally. A tapered, round toothpick is inserted into the hole in the carrier and is then broken off; the tip is left and is used in a tracing motion along the gingival margins.

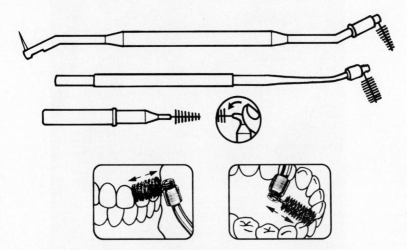

**Fig. 31-12.** Interdental brush (Proxabrush), useful for interdental cleansing when the interdental space is wide. The brushes are replaceable (three different sizes of replaceable bristles).

consist of replaceable brushes that insert into handles (Fig. 31-12). They are made in a variety of shapes and sizes (test tube, pine tree) to facilitate cleansing in posterior areas of the dentition. The interproximal brushes should be chosen to fit specific areas.[43]

Areas not easily reached with other oral hygiene aids (i.e., distal aspect of posterior molars, furcation areas, areas of root amputation) may be cleansed with flat or tapered, single-tufted brushes (Fig. 31-12) or with the Roto-Dent or Interplak.[44]

When larger interproximal spaces are present or near posterior pontics, four-ply **Yarn** cotton yarn may be helpful. When necessary the yarn can be reduced in width by unraveling. Attach the yarn to the floss by knotting, and introduce it into the interproximal areas by drawing the floss through the contact followed by the yarn through the embrasure (Fig. 31-13). The yarn can remove plaque in such areas. Its size and surface are effective where floss is sometimes inefficient because of tooth anatomy (e.g., fluting of the root) or embrasure form. Variable-diameter floss can also be effective in wider interdental spaces (Fig. 31-14).[45]

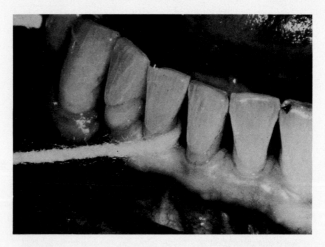

**Fig. 31-13.** Use yarn for interdental cleansing and stimulation.

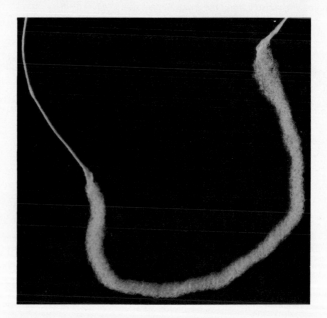

**Fig. 31-14.** Variable-width floss useful in widened embrasures and around flat roots.

## Other aids

**Gauze strips**

Teeth bordering edentulous areas may be cleansed with the brush turned so that the bristles strike the proximal surfaces. Four-ply cotton yarn or gauze strips may be used when the tooth surfaces are not readily accessible to a brush (Fig. 31-15, *A*). The gauze material for this technique may be 1-inch gauze bandage cut into strips 6 inches in length and folded down the center. Place the fold on the tooth, and carry the gauze as far gingivally as possible, even under the margin. Move the gauze, in a shoeshine motion, several times across the area.[38]

**Floss threaders**

Floss or tape can be threaded through the embrasures, and pontics and abutment teeth can be cleansed (Fig. 31-15, *B*).

**Pipe cleaners**

Pipe cleaners (without metal bristles) are sometimes effective in cleansing inaccessible interproximal areas and exposed bifurcations and trifurcations. The cleaners

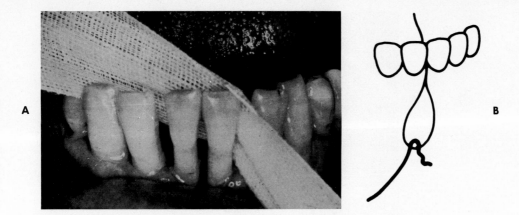

**Fig. 31-15.** **A,** Use gauze strips to cleanse proximal areas of widely spaced teeth. **B,** Thread dental tape or floss between abutment teeth or pontics with the help of a plastic needle (Butler).

are carefully teased between the exposed roots of the furcations and pulled through (tooth abrasion in the furcation is common with this technique).

**Interdental stimulator**

The interdental stimulator consists of a rubber tip of smooth or ribbed conical shape attached to a handle or to the end of a toothbrush. Its action massages and stimulates circulation of the interdental gingiva and may increase the tone of the tissue. It may also aid in cleansing debris from interproximal areas where papillary height is reduced and embrasures are open. An interdental stimulator is not recommended for areas in which the papillae are normal and fill the interproximal spaces. It may cause injury to the gingival tissue.

This physiotherapy is useful in areas in which the interdental tissue has been destroyed by disease or removed by surgery. Instruct the patient to use the interdental stimulator once a day. The tip of the stimulator is placed interdentally and slightly coronally. Pressure is exerted on the gingiva in a rotary motion from both the buccal and lingual aspects (Fig. 31-16). The pressure is useful in causing deliberate tissue recession.

**Water irrigation devices**

Water irrigation devices may be useful. There are several types. One uses faucet water to irrigate between and around the teeth. The water pressure is steady and is controlled by turning the faucet handle. Others use an intermittent water jet[46,47]; water placed in a receptacle is propelled by a motor-driven pump to the teeth and gingiva.

When complicated bridgework and fixed orthodontic appliances are present in the mouth, they tend to accumulate debris. The rinsing device helps to keep the mouth clean. For some patients it is useful to add an irrigation device to the oral hygiene regimen for more effective removal of debris. *The impression prevails that water pressure helps remove food debris and even some plaque, but it does not remove all dental plaque.*[48]

Such devices may be used to deliver plaque-inhibiting medicaments by adapting a blunt syringe needle to the device. Pocket irrigation is thus feasible.[49] They may also be useful in the immediate postsurgical cleansing of tender gingiva.

The patient would be overwhelmed if instruction in the use of all the oral hygiene aids were given at once. Therefore one technique should be presented at a time. When the patient shows reasonable progress in mastering the use of the first (i.e., floss) begin education in the use of toothbrush and other aids.

Manuals, visual aids, filmstrips, and group instruction have all been advocated in attempts to establish or improve plaque control efforts by patients.[50-52]

Correct cleansing is of inestimable value in the treatment of periodontal disease

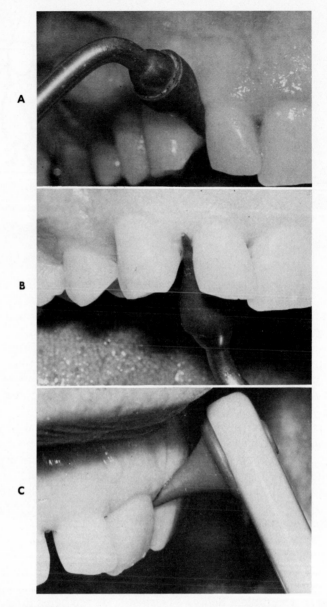

**Fig. 31-16.** **A,** Use the rubber-tipped stimulator in a rotary motion, exerting pressure on the gingiva—vestibular (labial) application. **B,** Rubber-tipped stimulator—oral (palatal) application. **C,** Some stimulators are attached to the toothbrush handle. If they are of proper dimension and shape, they are useful.

and in the maintenance of health. Instituting a program of plaque control will improve gingival health. Strict attention should be given to the needs of each patient. The topography of the teeth and tissues, digital dexterity, and patient idiosyncrasies may create problems in individual cases.

## POSTSURGICAL PLAQUE CONTROL

The postsurgical removal of plaque is vital to successful treatment.[53,54] Directly after sutures and/or dressings are removed, institute a plaque control schedule for the patient. Some patients are reluctant to floss and brush because the gingivae are tender and bleeding is easily provoked. Prescription of topical anesthetics for use before brushing is usually indicated. Special soft toothbrushes may be prescribed. Medicaments for control of tooth sensitivity are also applied at this time.

When no dressing is placed, institute home plaque control with an extrasoft brush as soon as practical after surgery. Interproximal cleansing with floss, triangular toothpicks, or interdental brushes (depending on postsurgical interdental space size) should be introduced as soon as epithelialization of interdental wounds has occurred.

After sutures and/or dressings are removed, polish the teeth with fine pumice, apply any medicaments for desensitization, caries control, and the like, and then start the patient on flossing and brushing. When healing is complete and the tissues are firm and not sensitive, the patient should resume regular plaque removal.

## CHEMICAL PLAQUE CONTROL

Given the well-known inability or lack of desire of many individuals to remove plaque daily from the tooth surfaces, research has been directed toward drugs administered in mouthwashes, dentifrices, and chewing gums, and other vehicles or by syringes for pocket irrigation, in an effort to control dental plaque. Theoretically it is possible to interfere with dental plaque by chemical plaque control.[55] Such control does the following:

1. Inhibition of plaque development
2. Elimination of existing plaque
3. Inhibition of calcification of plaque
4. Inhibition of microbial colonization on tooth surfaces
5. Converting pathogenic bacterial plaque into a nonpathogenic plaque

The agents that can be used for these purposes include tensioactive agents, antibiotics, antiseptics, enzymes, fluorides, and dietary substances.

**Tensioactive agents**

Dental deposits have been described as less common in people living in areas with a high fluoride content in the drinking water.[56] Fluoride reduces the ability of hydroxyapatite powders to adsorb protein and diminishes the surface energy[57,58] of enamel surfaces and the formation of plaque. Laboratory and animal investigations have shown fluorides to inhibit bacterial multiplication[59] and, topically applied, to reduce plaque formation.[60-65]

**Fluorides**

Stannous fluorides have recently been shown to partially inhibit plaque formation.[61-64] Specifically, subgingival irrigation with 1.64% $SnF$[63] or other antimicrobial agents[65] may be important in eliminating bacteria in areas that are inaccessible to mechanical plaque control. They may also delay reinfection of pockets.

**Silicones**

Application of silicones seems to reduce calculus formation in vitro,[66] but further studies indicate that the application of various kinds of films involves technical difficulties, must be frequently repeated, and has only a limited effect on plaque formation. Such methods have proved of little practical value to date.[67-69]

**Antibiotics**

Several antibiotics can depress oral microorganisms (penicillin,[70-72] tetracyclines,[73] vancomycin,[74,75] actinobolin,[76] cc 10232,[77-79] kanamycin,[80] spiramycin,[81,82] and metronidazole[83,84]). Even though penicillin may inhibit plaque formation, this antibiotic should be reserved for the treatment of life-threatening infections because of the dangers of sensitization.

Systemic administration of tetracycline has no long-term advantage when compared to local débridement alone.[85] Tetracycline is excreted in the gingival sulcus in a higher concentration[86] and is effective against *Actinobacillus actinomycetemcomitans*.[87] Recent studies suggest a beneficial effect of tetracycline in conjunction with local débridement and surgery in juvenile periodontitis.[88,89] When tetracycline is applied locally by hollow fiber delivery systems, dosage can be reduced 1500 times and local concentration will be increased 100-fold.[90,91] Local delivery of tetracycline is being investigated. Ongoing research should determine any long-term clinical benefits of this mode of therapy.

Three daily rinses with an aqueous solution of vancomycin do not successfully inhibit plaque formation.[92]

Topical application of 5% kanamycin paste reduced plaque accumulation in mentally retarded children (who did not perform oral hygiene), although this antibiotic was not successful in treating existing gingivitis.[80]

Proponents of the use of spiramycin in the treatment and prevention of dental plaque infections cite its ability to be stored in salivary glands and released slowly in saliva.[93] Further controlled clinical studies are needed to assess the potential of spiramycin for use in routine periodontal therapy.

A drug that is highly effective against gram-negative anaerobes and spirochetes is metronidazole, which suggests it may be successful in treating rapidly progressive periodontitis, juvenile periodontitis, and necrotizing ulcerative gingivitis.[83,94] Possible side effects of metronidazole include blood dyscrasias, cancer in rats,[95] and a disulfiram (Antabuse) effect.

It is difficult to make direct comparisons of the benefits of the antibiotics mentioned. Variations are present in the mode of antibiotic administration and in the experimental models tested. In addition, the lack of uniformity and the criteria by which the clinical and bacteriologic effects were evaluated prohibit direct comparison. Although results of animal experiments with drugs directed against gram-positive microorganisms have proved promising, clinical trials in humans have generally been unsuccessful.[96,97]

**Enzymes**

Enzymes are theoretically capable of degrading the intermicrobial cementing matrix of plaque and thereby the framework for bacterial colonization.

It has been shown in vitro that established plaque is dissolved by dextranases[98] and that the addition of dextranase to animal diets containing sucrose inhibits plaque formation.[99,100] Dextranase preparations tested in humans, however, have had little[61,101,102] or no [103,104] effect on the microbial plaque. Apart from dextranase, enzyme preparations such as trypsin, chymotrypsin, pancreatin, amylase, lipase, and elastase have been tested for their ability to degrade dental plaque. At this time it seems justified to state that clinical trials with enzymes have not been encouraging.

Enzymes have been included in toothpastes to interfere with phosphorylation and calcification of plaque. The problem in the use of enzymes for chemical plaque control is the mode of application. Enzymes in mouthwashes, dentifrices, or chewing gums may not act long enough to be effective against plaque formation.

**Antiseptics**

Plaque inhibition in vivo has been demonstrated with sodium ricinoleate,[69] mercurials (e.g., sodium parahydroxymercuribenzoate[105]), and substances such as chloramine T, cetylpyridinium chloride, benzalkonium chloride,[74,103-105] chlorhexidine salts,[106,107] and alexidine.[108] These substances have attracted great attention. The chlorhexidine effect is the result of a local antibacterial action of the antiseptic bound to organic or inorganic components of the tooth surface.[109,110] Dental use of chlorhexidine as an antibacterial agent is based on the absorption of the drug by oral surfaces. This concept is referred to as *substantivity* and may be defined as a prolonged contact time between a substance and the substrate.

Some undesirable side effects are present. Discoloration of the teeth, silicate fillings, and the tongue is clearly seen in chlorhexidine rinsers. Some persons have complained of a bitter taste and an interference with their sense of taste.[106,111,112]

However, chlorhexidine has been the most widely used agent in periodontal therapy.[113] This agent is used throughout the world. The major objection to its use has been the brown stain that forms on the teeth with prolonged use. The stain is easily removed with common prophylaxis techniques. When this agent was used at a concentration of 0.2% twice daily as a mouthwash, bacterial colonization of the teeth was prevented in patients refraining from all oral hygiene measures. In addition, use of chlorhexidine has resulted in dissolution of plaque and elimination of gingivitis in humans and of dental caries in laboratory animals.[103] The performance of chlorhexidine warrants continued clinical and laboratory research on this and other chemical antimicrobial agents.[106,110]

New methods for subgingival delivery of chlorhexidine include subgingival irrigation via syringe[114] and cellulose dialysis tubes loaded with 20% chlorhexidine placed into periodontal pockets.[115]

Laboratories all over the world are working on problems related to chemical plaque control, and the day is approaching when topical application of antibacterial substances will facilitate achievement of a dentition with minimal amounts of microbial plaque.

**Topical antibacterial agents**

Considering the wealth of circumstantial evidence implicating local bacterial residents in the etiology of periodontal diseases, treatment by topical application of antibacterial agents would seem obvious. Why this approach has not been more universally advocated provides a basis for evaluating the relative merits of advocated procedures.

Treatment of periodontal disease by antibacterial therapy has several potential advantages: It is relatively inexpensive and relatively painless, and it gets to the heart of the disease problem. However, the pivotal issue is effectiveness, which in many instances remains to be demonstrated.

Effective use of antibacterial drugs in periodontal therapy depends on a clear understanding of the limitations associated with treatment by drug therapy. For any drug to be effective, the following must be true:

1. The agent must be intrinsically capable of exerting the drug action at an attainable concentration.
2. The agent must reach the site of action.
3. The concentration at the site of action must be sufficient to elicit the drug effect.
4. The duration over which an effective concentration is maintained must be sufficient to allow the drug to act.

The importance of these factors can be appreciated by realizing that failure in any one of these criteria can result in therapeutic failure. Most of the failings of antibacterial agents in periodontal therapy can be ascribed to failure to meet one or more of these criteria, and most of the successes can be related to conditions under which all of these criteria have been met.

**Plaque control by mouthrinses**

The area in which antibacterial agents have been most thoroughly tested is in the reduction of supragingival plaque by mouthrinses (see box below). There is little doubt that the amount of supragingival plaque can be reduced by this means. A review[116] evaluated data on clinical efficacy related to mouthrinses and classified agents broadly as "clearly effective" and "possibly effective" by one of the following four criteria:

1. Prevented most clinically detectable plaque
2. Prevented most clinically detectable gingivitis
3. Prevented development of white spot lesions during a sucrose change
4. Prevented development of bacterial shifts, which have been associated with caries or gingivitis

---

### REQUIREMENTS OF ANTIMICROBIAL AGENTS FOR MOUTH RINSING

1. Lack of oral or systemic toxicity
2. Poor absorption from alimentary tract
3. Substantivity
4. Broad antimicrobial spectrum?
5. Low induced drug resistance

From Newbrun, E.: Chemical and mechanical removal of plaque, Compend. Contin. Educ. Dent. Suppl. **6:**110, 1985.

Based on these criteria only the biguanides such as chlorhexidine were considered "clearly effective," whereas quaternary ammonium compounds, essential oils, sanguinarine, and stannous fluoride were considered as "possibly effective." Unfortunately this assessment must be considered as somewhat arbitrary because there are few comparative trials testing multiple agents under the same protocol.

Of the antibacterial mouthrinses, chlorhexidine (CH) (tested clinically in concentrations of 0.1% to 0.5%) has been studied most extensively (in more than 300 papers). It is an effective antibacterial agent in concentrations of 100 μg/ml (bactericidal) to 0.1 μg/ml (bacteriostatic) and capable of completely inhibiting plaque formation.[117] It is generally more effective for gram-positive than for gram-negative organisms. The ability of CH to bind to anionic groups on the tooth surface and on bacterial surfaces (intrinsic substantivity) is generally considered to contribute to its effectiveness by producing a sustained presence in the oral cavity. The principal side effects from prolonged use include objectionable taste and staining of the teeth, tongue, and restorations in some, but not all, individuals. In addition, the alteration of taste perception and oral desquamation have been reported.[118] Although they have been less extensively tested, alexidine and octenidine are chemically similar to CH and may be expected to produce similar effects.

Quaternary ammonium compounds such as cetylpyridinium chloride (CPC) and benzethonium chloride are widely marketed in over-the-counter mouthrinse preparations. However, their efficacy at concentrations of 0.05% to 0.1% has been generally lower than that of CH. These agents have little substantivity. At commercial available concentrations CPC does not completely inhibit the growth of *Streptococcus mutans* or *Actinomyces viscosus*, and in the presence of saliva, the antibacterial activity of CPC is reduced.[119]

Phenolic compounds have been used since 1867 as germicides. Their use as mouthrinses produces a moderate reduction in plaque mass with no reported side effects.[120] Thymol, the principal antibacterial component of commercial preparations, appears intrinsically incapable of completely inhibiting the growth of *A. viscosus*, *A. naeslundii*, or *S. mutans* at any attainable concentration.[121] Sanguinarine has been recently introduced as a mouthrinse. Preliminary results[122] indicate that sanguinarine inhibits growth of periodontal microorganisms at 16 μg/ml and is capable of reducing plaque mass and gingivitis.[123] However, because of the relatively small number of clinical tests reported, it is difficult to evaluate its comparative efficacy. Fluoride preparations in concentrations greater than 0.3% have been investigated for their ability to reduce plaque and gingivitis[124] and appear to be comparable to 0.1% CH. In addition, fluoride appears to produce specific reductions in supragingival plaque by reducing the proportions of *S. mutans*.

Several unanswered issues confuse the evaluation of antibacterial agents used as mouthrinses. First, it is not clear that reductions in supragingival plaque mass can be interpreted as being therapeutically beneficial. Several reports of population groups with large amounts of supragingival plaque and little associated periodontal disease have appeared.[125-127] Clearly, dental plaques differ greatly in pathogenicity. Second, since agents applied by mouthrinse do not penetrate beyond the orifice of the periodontal pocket,[65,128] effects on periodontal microbiota may be limited. Third, there is no information on the preventative effects of mouthrinses. Antibacterial mouthrinses can reduce supragingival plaque mass and decrease some signs of gingivitis. The therapeutic significance of these observations, however, remains to be clarified.

**Periodontal therapy by irrigation**

The treatment of periodontal pockets by professional administration and/or self-administration of antibacterial agents theoretically provides the basic means for delivering the drug to the site of action. Agents that have been most extensively tested for this purpose include CH, fluoride, and inorganic salts with hydrogen peroxide.

CH solutions administered by pump-driven irrigators have been tested and found effective as an adjunct in plaque control. Subsequent to demonstration that larger volumes of dilute solutions were effective and caused less staining,[129] it was found that one daily irrigator application of 400 ml of a 0.02% CH solution was the lowest concentration for complete inhibition of supragingival plaque.[117] It is generally reported that application by a pump-driven irrigator is more effective in the control of supragingival plaque than rinsing.[130]

Studies in which 0.2% CH has been used for subgingival irrigation[114,131,132] indicate that signs of gingivitis and periodontal inflammation can be reduced by this procedure. However, it is generally recognized by those conducting clinical studies that the result was to reduce the needed frequency of maintenance visits rather than to substitute for conventional therapy.

Sodium fluoride is an antibacterial agent with somewhat low potency in the order of 128 to 2048 $\mu$g/ml.[133] Subgingival irrigation with 1.65% $SnF_2$ produced a decrease in motile bacteria and spirochetes and a reduction in bleeding index scores[134] that persisted for 6 weeks. However, the use of this procedure as an adjunct for periodontal therapy has not been adequately explored.

Considerable interest has been focused on patient self-treatment with a paste made of hydrogen peroxide and sodium chloride, sodium bicarbonate, or magnesium sulfate.[135] Although attractive as a therapeutic method, owing to the low expense of agents employed, clinical testing of the procedure indicates that it is no more effective than conventional oral hygiene in controlling subgingival microflora.[136] Concentrated solutions of salt unquestionably have antibacterial activity. This is the basis for preservation by the pickling process. However, they have extremely low potency as compared to other antibacterial agents and no substantivity and therefore are limited in their ability to establish and maintain an antibacterial environment.

A fundamental problem related to patient self-treatment by application of antibacterial agents is the ability to effectively deliver the agent to areas where it is needed. When one considers the difficulty a practitioner may experience even with excellent light, positioning, specially designed instruments, and direct visualization, it is difficult to believe that patients can master the dexterity needed to control their periodontal disease by self-application of medicaments in all but the most accessible regions of the mouth. Clearly, if the product is not delivered in the site of action it will be not be effective.

**Intrapocket drug delivery devices**

The periodontal pocket is a logical site for controlled drug delivery directed toward the treatment of periodontal diseases. Devices with a drug reservoir of 1 to 5 mg that is released at the rate of a few released at the rate of a few micrograms per hour are sufficient to raise the gingival fluid level of a therapeutic agent to effective levels.[137,138]

A single-blind study was designed to test the efficacy of periodontal disease therapy by local drug delivery.[139] The clinical and microbiologic effects of this form of therapy were compared with effects of periodontal scaling. In periodontal sites treated by local drug delivery, tetracycline-loaded ethylene vinyl acetate fibers were gently pressed into the periodontal pocket to completely fill irregular defects. They were then circumferentially wound to fill the remainder of the pocket. To increase the effectiveness of the delivery system and reduce the likelihood of displacement, the treated area was covered by a periodontal dressing. By this procedure a tetracycline concentration of approximately 600 $\mu$g/ml (0.06%) was maintained throughout the 10-day therapeutic period. The average tetracycline dose used was 2.4 mg per tooth treated.

After the fiber delivery system was removed, bacterial counts from the periodontal pocket were extremely low.[91] After fiber therapy treated sites improved clinically,[140] as evidenced by decreased probing depths from a fixed referenced point. New lesion formation at fiber-treated sites decreased from a pretreatment rate of 26.5% of sites per year to a posttreatment rate of 4.8% of sites per year.

Principal ways in which clinical response with local drug delivery differed from that with scaling were in early (3 to 6 months) attachment gain and in the degree of reduction of new lesion formation. Effects on bacterial population by scaling were much smaller than by local drug delivery and failed to achieve statistical significance.[91] Treatment of refractory forms of periodontal disease constitutes an important potential use for this form of therapy. A case study illustrating this application has been reported.[138]

In addition to fiber devices, drug-containing slabs and films have been tested for intrapocket delivery. CH was incorporated into ethyl cellulose polymer films (30% loading), which were placed into periodontal pockets for clinical testing. Devices of this design, in which 80% of the CH was released over a 3-day period, were found to reduce the numbers of periodontal organisms as revealed by dark-field microscopy.[141]

Cast films of ethyl cellulose with propylene glycol[142] have been tested for delivery of CH[143,144] and metronidazole.[145] Two devices were constructed: One released 80% of the drug load in 3 days, and another released 50% in 6 days. Placement of these devices into periodontal pockets resulted in marked alteration of the periodontal flora that persisted for up to 10 days. Strips of polyethyl methacrylate containing CH and metronidazole have also been prepared.[146] Preliminary tests of these devices indicate potential utility in periodontal therapy.

Clinical investigation to date indicates that small devices may be placed within the periodontal pocket as a relatively painless procedure that does not produce visible signs of irritation. Also, in all studies in which antibacterial agents have been tested, effects have been produced that appear beneficial. No harmful side effects from this form of treatment have been reported.

Certain advantages relative to conventional therapy have been shown, including the following:

1. Higher concentrations of agents than are otherwise possible can be established and maintained at a local site.
2. Effective concentrations can be maintained for longer periods of time than possible by irrigation or rinse procedures.
3. Effective levels can be established at sites that are difficult to reach by other means, such as the base of a periodontal pocket.
4. Effective local levels of an agent can be achieved with little systemic load.

Drug delivery within the oral cavity represents an application of controlled-release technology with exceptional potential. The localized nature of dental diseases and the ease of accessibility for placing delivery devices suggests applications of greater diversity and sophistication than are possible elsewhere in the body.

Treatment of periodontal diseases by local application of antibacterial agents shows promise but will require more extensive evaluation before its full utility can be appreciated. Procedures employed can be evaluated on the basis of their mode of delivery and on the basis of the particular agents used. Table 31-1 can be useful in evaluating modes of delivery.

Clearly, mouthrinses fail to reach the pocket microbiota, and pocket irrigation may fail to maintain adequate duration of contact. Only local delivery devices can dependably achieve all pharmacodynamic criteria.

Concerning the agents used for local application (Table 31-2), several comparisons can be made as follows: with the exception of CH, sanguinarine, and tetracycline, most antibacterial agents require concentrations exceeding 100 µg/ml (0.01%) to be

**Table 31-1** Mode of delivery for antibacterial agents

| Results | Mouthrinses | Pocket irrigation | Local delivery devices |
|---|---|---|---|
| Reach the site of action | Poor | Good | Good |
| Attain adequate concentration | Good | Good | Good |
| Retained for adequate duration | Poor | Poor | Good |

effective and are therefore intrinsically lacking in antibacterial potency. The need to establish and maintain high concentrations can limit their utility. The ability to bind tissue or teeth (substantivity) and thereby prolong activity appears to be a useful attribute. Of the agents discussed, only CH, fluoride, tetracycline, and sanguinarine possess substantivity, and the side effects from the use of these agents are generally inconsequential. The most notable exception is taste and tooth staining with CH. In addition, water retention from sodium salts can be a problem, especially with hypertensive patients.

Treatment of periodontal disease by locally applied antibacterial agents is a procedure still in its infancy. However, with a clearer understanding of potential benefits and limitations, the use of these techniques as adjuncts to conventional therapy can be expected to provide substantial benefits (Tables 31-2 and 31-3).

**Table 31-2** Agents for local application

| Agents | Intrinsic activity | Substantivity | Side effects |
|---|---|---|---|
| Chlorhexidine | Good | Good | Tooth stain, taste |
| Quaternary ammonium compounds | Fair | Poor | Few if any, mild tooth stain |
| Fluoride | Fair | Good | Few if any |
| Phenols | Fair | Poor | Few if any |
| Inorganic salts | Poor | Poor | Water retention (sodium salts only) |
| Tetracycline | Good | Good | Few if any |
| Sanguinarine | Good | Good | Few if any |

**Table 31-3** Antibacterial agents tested for plaque prevention or reduction

| Antibiotics | | Other antibacterial agents | |
|---|---|---|---|
| Agent | Spectrum | Agent | Spectrum |
| Actinobolin | Broad | Bis-biguanides* | Broad |
| Chlortetracycline | | Alexidine | |
| Tetracycline | | Chlorhexidine | |
| Streptomycin† | | Bispyridines | Broad |
| Kanamycin† | | Octenidine | |
| Neomycin† | | Phenolic compounds | Broad |
| Niddamycin† | | Phenol | |
| Bacitracin† | Gram-positive | Betanaphthol | |
| Erythromycin | | Hexylresorcinol | |
| Penicillin | | Halogens | Broad |
| Vancomycin* | | Iodine and iodophors | |
| Gramicidin* | | Chloride | |
| Spiramycin† | | Oxychlorosene | |
| Polymyxin B* | Gram-negative | Chloramine T | |
| | | Fluoride | |
| | | Oxygenating agent‡ | Broad |
| | | Peroxide | |
| | | Perborate | |
| | | Metronidazole | Broad (only anaerobes) |
| | | Quaternary ammonium Compounds | |
| | | Cetylpyridinium chloride | Mostly gram-positive |
| | | Benzethonium chloride | |
| | | Domiphen bromide | |

From Newbrun, E.: Chemical and mechanical removal of plaque, Compend. Contin. Educ. Dent. Suppl. **6**:110, 1985.
*Not absorbed, or poorly absorbed, across gastrointestinal tract.
†Some gram-negative also.
‡Antiseptic action limited or questionable.

## Root sensitivity

Sensitivity of an exposed root surface is a vexing problem for the patient and is a not infrequent and distressing sequel to scaling, root planing, and surgical procedures. Such sensitivity is a result of stimulation of dentinal tubules. This discussion excludes sensitivity from occlusal trauma and pulpal changes caused by caries and restorative procedures.

Even though they may not have been especially sensitive originally, surgically exposed root surfaces often become hypersensitive. Routine, thorough brushing and use of adjunctive aids, such as toothpicks, stimulators, and dental tape, help to desensitize root surfaces. Plaque and food debris that are allowed to remain on exposed root surfaces often lead to increasing sensitivity. A vicious cycle[147] may be created. Exposed root surfaces are not kept clean and become hypersensitive. Because of the discomfort involved in brushing, the patient tends to avoid these areas, and the hypersensitivity is aggravated. In such cases root surfaces must be desensitized, and an adequate oral physiotherapy regimen instituted. Without effective home care, however, even the improvement that follows desensitization is likely to be short lived.

The stimuli responsible for hypersensitivity reactions to mechanical, chemical, or thermal stimuli include the following:

### Mechanical stimuli

1. Periodontal instrumentation (surgical and root planing)
2. Toothbrushing

### Chemical stimuli

1. Sweet or sour foods and drink
2. Plaque allowed to remain on the tooth surface

### Thermal stimuli

1. Hot and cold liquids or foods
2. Dental procedures (use of hot or cold fluids, compounds, hydrocolloid)

### THEORIES OF SENSITIVITY

Theories of sensitivity propose the following as likely explanations for root discomfort:

1. There is direct stimulation of sensory nerve endings in dentin.[148]
2. Odontoblasts and their processes in dentinal tubules are sensory cells that receive stimuli.[148]
3. Nerve impulses are modulated by the release of certain polypeptides during pulp injury.[149]
4. Pulp nerves are stimulated by hydrodynamic mechanism.[150,151]

Evidence for the stimulation of pulp nerve fibers by a hydrodynamic mechanism appears to be the most likely mechanism.[152]

The rationale of desensitization procedures is not fully understood. Some techniques may depend on denaturation of the superficial ends of Tomes fibers or of nerve endings in dentin. Other procedures are designed to deposit an insoluble substance on the ends of the fibers or nerves to act as a barrier to stimuli. Still others are designed to stimulate secondary dentin formation, thus insulating the pulp from external stimuli. The anti-inflammatory and antihyperemic properties of corticoids may prevent or relieve hypersensitivity by reducing hyperemia in the pulp.

Grossman[153] has suggested the following requirements for a satisfactory method of treating hypersensitivity: The method should be nonirritating to the pulp, painless on application, easily applied, and rapid acting; it should be consistently effective for long periods of time; and it must not discolor the teeth. No method meets all these requirements.

Some procedures for treatment may be carried out in the office. Others are done by the patient at home. A combination of both is sometimes indicated. Various desensitizing agents are discussed in Table 31-4.

## DESENSITIZATION

In all patients in whom office treatment is used, the root surfaces must be clean, dry, and carefully isolated.

**Office treatment**

Silver nitrate has been a traditional "nostrum" in dental offices. This treatment is obsolete, since it produces unsightly discoloration. In its stead Gottlieb's impregnation has been used.[154] Cleanse and dry the tooth with a solution of benzene (U.S.P.). Apply a 40% aqueous solution of zinc chloride for 1 minute. (Care should be taken to protect adjacent soft tissues.) Follow this by the application of a 20% aqueous solution of potassium ferrocyanide to the root surface still moist from the zinc chloride. Rub the potassium ferrocyanide into the root surface with a cotton pellet or porte-polisher for 1 minute. A whitish, curdy, insoluble precipitate forms, which reduces hypersensitivity.

Sodium fluoride* may be used for office treatment of hypersensitive root surfaces.[155] It is in the form of a paste, consisting of equal parts of sodium fluoride, kaolin, and glycerin.[156] After the hypersensitive areas are cleaned, rub the paste into the exposed root surfaces with a porte-polisher and orangewood stick or a rubber cup for 1 to 5 minutes. Satisfactory results are usually obtained. No caustic effects on gingiva or mucosa result from contact with the paste; however, it is toxic if accidentally ingested.

A modification of the fluoride treatment for hypersensitive teeth is the use of sodium silicofluoride.[157] A saturated watery solution (0.7% to 0.9%†) is applied for 5 minutes to the cervical areas and rubbed into the surface for 5 minutes. The patient may also use the solution at home. Results are said to be better than those with the sodium fluoride paste.

Stannous fluoride prophylactic paste containing 8.9% stannous fluoride in the mixture has been introduced for use in the dental office and seems to have desensitizing properties when used in prophylaxis.[158] Such preparations are available commercially.

Iontophoresis has also been used in the obtunding of hypersensitive exposed root surfaces.[158-161] Sodium fluoride solutions (1% to 2%) are the electrolytes used. Acidulated phosphofluoride solutions have also been employed. Low-voltage batteries creating a galvanic current of fractions of 1 mA are employed. The appliances are so used that a sable brush serves as the cathode, which is wetted with the fluoride solution and brought into contact with the sensitive root surface. The desensitization achieved by iontophoresis is the result of stimulation of secondary dentin formation by the current.[161,162]

Corticoids have been used with some success for the desensitization of exposed root surfaces.[152]

After 30 or 60 days' use of a toothpaste containing formaldehyde, response to thermal and mechanical stimuli was assessed, with no significant alteration of hypersensitivity noted.[163] Other desensitizing toothpastes contain strontium chloride,[163] potassium nitrate,[164,165] sodium citrate pluronic gel,[166] monofluorophosphate,[167] and formalin–sodium monofluorophosphate combined formula[168]; positive results for all these agents have been cited in the literature.

Office treatments and home treatment often must be combined for best results.

---

*Fluoride solutions should be stored in plastic bottles to avoid reactions with the glass, which would cause deterioration of the solutions.

†Sodium silicofluoride is soluble in cold water up to 0.7% and in boiling water up to 0.9%.

**Table 31-4**  Desensitizing medicaments

| Agent | Summary of results | Mode of action |
|---|---|---|
| Fluoride | Claimed effective for 1 to 2 years | Replaces calcium carbonate complex and forms hard, insoluble calcium fluoride structure; dentinal tubules decrease in diameter as it creates a physiologic zone of hypercalcification |
| Glycerin | Extreme pain, relieved after 10 treatments | Lipid solvent |
| Silver nitrate | Conflicting results: some good, some poor and even not as effective as controls; yields a very black stain | Dentinal tubule obliteration |
| Strontium chloride | Conflicting reports: moderately effective or ineffective; however, most showed good relief | Bicolloidal binding and blocking action with or in organic material of tooth structure; strontium ion–stimulated secondary dentin formation; modification of transmission of neural impulses or stimulation of recalcification |
| Formalin | Conflicting: range of results from no relief to 74% relief | Protein precipitator |
| Sodium monofluorophosphate | All found more relief than controls: up to 58.5% relief obtained | Occlusion of exposed dentinal tubules |
| Sodium silicofluoride | In treatment of periodontal cases this found superior to sodium fluoride, formalin, zinc chloride, and silver nitrate | Hypercalcification of dentinal tubules |
| Calcium hypophosphate | 86% showed significant improvement | Dentinal surfaces closed |
| Corticosteroids | Consensus was very favorable | Sedative action; anti-inflammatory action on pulp; action on vascular tone of endothelium |
| Glucorticoid | 87.4% had excellent and/or good results vs. 0% of control group | Not understood |
| Calcium hydroxide | Positive results up to 6 months after treatment | Promotes hypermineralized cementum or brings about occlusion of exposed dentin tubules; also thought to promote increase in dentinal hardness |
| Sodium fluoride and iontophoresis | Good relief in some patients | Ionization increases fluoride uptake |
| Sodium citrate pluronic gel | | Forms a nonionized calcium complex in dentinal tubules; pluronic gel precipitates proteins out of solution; both mechanisms act to occlude dentinal tubules |
| Potassium nitrate | Significant relief | Oxidizing effect or blocking of dentinal tubules |
| Stannous fluoride | Fair to good relief | Replaces calcium carbonate and decreases diameter of dentinal tubules |
| Tresiolan | Good relief report in experimental group | Forms organosiloxane resinous skin |

Modified from Peden, J.: J. West. Soc. Periodontol. **25:**75, 1977.

Office treatment may have to be repeated. Home treatment alone may produce desensitization after several weeks, but usually several methods must be tried before satisfactory results are obtained. Diligent oral hygiene alone often solves the problem.

Prevention and treatment of dentinal hypersensitivity require a greater understanding of the etiology and mechanisms of action of the different treatments. If sensitivity is caused by hydrodynamic fluid movement, then therapeutic agents that decrease dentin permeability should be recommended. In vitro studies of experimental dentifrices containing oxalate as the active agent signifiant decrease in hydraulic conductance of dentin compared to that of marketed dentifrices.[169]

## Halitosis

Fear of offending by bad breath is a powerful motivating force driving people to seek dental attention, perhaps third in importance after cosmetic considerations and pain. If a person has any doubts one need only watch television to see the number of commercials recommending mouthwashes that purport to prevent or cure this condition.

Two terms appear in the literature—*halitosis* and *fetor ex ore* (fetor oris). Some authors make a distinction between the two: Bad mouth odor not arising in the mouth is halitosis, whereas odors that are caused orally are fetor ex ore.[170] This distinction does not seem to be important, and the term *halitosis* is used for any kind of bad breath.

An important clinical feature of halitosis is that the offending person may be unaware of the condition. Howe[171] stated in 1874 that "few of the afflicted persons detect the cause of their isolation."

Attempts have been made to measure the intensity of bad breath by means of an instrument called an osmoscope[172,173] and lately by spectrometer analysis and a titrilog,[174] which is an instrument capable of measuring volatile oxidizable sulfur components (hydrogen sulfide, methylmercaptan, methyl disulfide), thought to be responsible for oral bad breath. A number of other instruments have also been employed for objective measurement of halitosis.

Breath comes from the lungs and is exhaled through bronchi, trachea, larynx, and nose or mouth. Therefore bad breath may arise in any of these areas: the lungs, the breathing passages, the nose, or the mouth. Among breath odors originating in the lungs are the smell of garlic and of alcohol. These odors are caused by the excretion into the lungs of the volatile oils flavoring these foods. Similarly, there may be acetone on the breath of uncontrolled diabetics. In addition, bronchiectasis, advanced malignancy, and some other diseases in the respiratory tract may impart bad odor to the breath. Furthermore, a certain number of cases of bad breath exist as a result of conditions of the nose and the nasopharynx, for instance, chronic atrophic rhinitis (ozena), purulent sinusitis, and adenoids (see box on p. 642).

In the older writings diseases of the stomach and the gastrointestinal tract were also mentioned as possible causes.[171] However, such conditions are no longer considered to be etiologic factors for halitosis.

In the majority of cases bad breath originates in the oral cavity; it may be a result of one of the following forms of tissue destruction: acute necrotizing ulcerative gingivitis, bad oral hygiene, advanced chronic periodontal disease, Vincent's angina, open gangrenous pulps, and large unfilled cavities containing decomposing food remnants. Smoking imparts characteristic odors offensive to many. Bad mouth odors are also found in the leukemias and the terminal stages of cirrhosis of the liver; these are caused by decomposition of blood oozing from the hemorrhagic gingiva.[175]

## CAUSES OF HALITOSIS

Physiologic
  Lack of flow of saliva during sleep
  Food
  Smoking
  Menstruation
Pathologic
  Disorders of the oral cavity
    Poor oral hygiene
    Dental plaque
    Dental caries
    Gingivitis
    Stomatitis
    Periodontitis
    Hairy tongue
    Oral carcinoma
  Disorders of upper respiratory tract
    Breathing through the mouth
    Chronic sinusitis
    Foreign bodies
    Atrophic rhinitis (ozena)
    Wegener granulomatosis (midline granuloma)
    Tuberculosis
    Syphilis
    Rhinoscleroma

Adenoiditis
Nasopharyngeal abscess
Carcinoma of the larynx
Laryngoscleroma
Disorders of lower respiratory tract
  Pulmonary abscess
  Carcinoma of the lung
  Other
    Bronchiectasis
    Necrotizing pneumonitis
    Empyema
Gastrointestinal conditions
  Salivary gland dysfunction
    Dehydration
    Anticholinergic drugs
    Radiotherapy
    Sjögren syndrome
  Peritonsillar abscess
  Retropharyngeal abscess
  Cryptic tonsillopathy
  Vincent's angina
  Carcinoma of the tonsil or pharynx
  Pharyngitis sicca
  Gangrenous angina
  Zenker's diverticulum
  Postcricoid carcinoma

Congenital bronchoesophageal fistula
Disorders of lower gastrointestinal tract
  Gastric carcinoma
  Hiatus hernia
  Pyloric stenosis
  Enteric infections
Neurologic disorders
  Dysosmia
  Dysgeusia
  Zinc deficiency
Systemic diseases
  Leukemia
  Agranulocytosis
  Febrile illness with dehydration
  Ketoacidosis
  Hepatic failure
  Azotemia
Drugs
  Lithium salts
  Penicillamine
  Griseofulvin
  Thiocarbamide
  Dimethyl sulfoxide
Functional
  Psychoses
  Depression

From Attia, E.L.: Halitosis, originally published in *Canadian Medical Association Journal*, vol. 126, June 1, 1982.

A rather common cause for halitosis is mouth breathing[175,176]; this habit prevents the mucosa and teeth from being washed and flushed with saliva and thereby interferes with the removal of cells, bacteria,[177] and their products. A specific microorganism responsible for bad breath has not been determined, however. A coated tongue may sometimes be the source of halitosis; reduction of salivary flow in febrile diseases and old age often contributes heavily to bad breath. Other situations in which bad breath is often observed include morning breath and hunger breath. The latter condition is more strongly manifested the longer the time passed since the last meal. Some women have a characteristic bad breath during menstruation.[175]

The drug dimethyl sulfoxide[178] gives the breath a characteristic unpleasant odor of not-quite-fresh oysters.

A congenital esophagobronchial fistula had been reported as the cause of halitosis in a 38-year-old man.[179] Another unexpected cause of halitosis was foreign body ingestion (a plywood well) in the pharynx, almost obliterating openings to the larynx and esophagus.[180]

## TREATMENT

In view of the many factors causing or contributing to bad breath, the taking of good medical and dental history is essential. Keep in mind the possible systemic ramifications of this problem; however, the majority of cases will be seen to be caused by local oral factors.

Early extraction of broken-down root stumps is recommended as well as the restoration of carious teeth. Strive for sufficiently wide embrasure spaces, well-contoured and well-polished restorations, removal of overhangs, and well-placed contact points. These measures will prevent food retention and the attending bad odors and irritation of the underlying gingiva. Furthermore, be sure to institute a regimen of good oral hygiene with toothpaste. Brushing of teeth, gingivae, and tongue produces a sizable reduction of bad odor for 2 hours.[181] Several years ago claims were made touting chlorophyll toothpastes for use in halitosis; these claims have not been fully proved.

The use of mouthwashes may have a temporary effect in reducing halitosis. The Food and Drug Administration, however, citing a study of the National Academy of Sciences–National Research Council Drug Efficacy Group,[182] has advised manufacturers of nine brands of mouthwashes to stop using such advertising claims as "effectively destroys bacteria that cause bad breath in the mouth." The study concluded that there is a lack of substantial evidence for such claims. These mouthwashes may be advertised as "aromatic mouth fresheners," "an aid to the daily care of the mouth," and "causing the mouth to feel clean."[183]

Antiseptic mouthwashes may help to reduce halitosis for as long as 2 to 3 hours.[173] Clinical research indicates the antiodor properties of mouthwash are related to its antimicrobial activity.[184,185] Another mouthrinse with the active agent of sanguinarine has demonstrated decrease in volatile sulfur compounds (responsible for malodor). The results demonstrated that sanguinarine in combination with zinc ion is more effective in controlling volatile sulfur compounds than zinc alone or the strictly antimicrobial action of conventional mouthrinses.[186] However, the effect of proper personal periodontal care is in only small part the result of a masking effect. To a much greater degree it is the result of the friction of brushing, the removing of squames and their bacterial colonies, and the increased salivary flow caused by flavoring agents. Prolonged use of so-called deodorants, such as a sodium perborate or hydrogen peroxide, is discouraged because of the attending undesirable side effects, which include the possible production of black, hairy tongue. Mouth breathing and lack of lip seal should be treated whenever possible. To do this first establish whether an obstacle to normal respiration exists (e.g., deviated nasal septum or large adenoids). To combat the accompanying halitosis suggest that the patient brush the teeth, gums, and tongue vigorously three times a day with a mild dentifrice and a mildly aromatic mouthwash. In older patients sometimes the use of sour lozenges not containing sugar may be suggested in the interval between brushing to increase salivary flow.

In conclusion, halitosis is, for objective as well as subjective reasons, most important to the patient. It may interfere with married life, dating, and business and social contacts. The dentist himself may offend patients.[182,183] More importantly, bad breath may indicate the presence of an underlying systemic condition. Therefore, whenever local measures prove ineffective, the consultation of a competent internist is indicated.

## Conclusion

The rationale for periodontal treatment is to arrest the process of breakdown, which may otherwise lead to ultimate loss of teeth, and to establish oral conditions conducive to periodontal health. Microbial plaque is the main factor of clinical importance in the etiology of gingivitis. It has been stated that an undisturbed plaque around the tooth will eventually cause a breakdown of the attachment apparatus. In spite of the argument that the *rate* of progression of periodontal breakdown may be influenced by factors such as the type of bacteria in the plaque and host susceptibility, the therapist must keep in mind that treatment must be primarily directed toward elimination of microbial plaque and the prevention of its recurrent formation. Studies have shown that it is possible to successfully treat periodontal disease by instituting a proper plaque control regimen and regular maintenance recall.

## REFERENCES

1. Hirschfeld, I.: The toothbrush; its use and abuse, Brooklyn, 1939, Dental Items of Interest Publishing Co.
2. Arnim, S.S.: Microcosms of the human mouth, J. Tenn. Dent. Assoc. **39:**3, 1959.
3. Schultz-Haudt, S.D., Bruce, M.A., and Bibby, B.G.: Tissue destructive products of gingival bacteria from non-specific gingivitis, J. Dent. Res. **33:**624, 1954.
4. Egelberg, J.: Local effect of diet on plaque formation and development of gingivitis in dogs, Odontol. Rev. **16:**50, 1965.
5. Lindhe, J., and Wicen, P.O.: The effect of the gingivae of chewing fibrous food, J. Periodont. Res. **4:**193, 1969.
6. Wade, A.B.: Effect on dental plaque of chewing apples, Dent. Pract. **21:**194, 1971.
7. Gugenheim, B.: Extracellular polysaccharides and microbial plaque, Int. Dent. J. **20:**675, 1970.
8. Rateitschak-Plüss, E.M., and Guggenheim, B.: Effects of a carbohydrate-free diet and sugar substitutes on dental plaque accumulation, J. Clin. Periodontol. **9:**239, 1982.
9. Gehring, F., et al.: Turku sugar studies. IV. An intermediate report on the differentiation of polysaccharide-forming streptococci, Acta Odontol. Scand. **32:**435, 1974.
10. De Stoppelaar, J.D., van Houte, J., and Dirks, D.B.: The effect of carbohydrate restriction on the presence of *Streptococcus mutans, Streptococcus sanguis* and iodophilic polysaccharide-producing bacteria in human dental plaque, Caries Res. **4:**114, 1970.
11. Stewart, R.T.: What is the most effective means of changing patients' plaque control behavior? Periodont. Abstr. **21:**63, 1973.
12. Wentz, F.M.: Patient motivation: a new challenge to the dental profession for effective control of plaque, J. Am. Dent. Assoc. **85:**887, 1972.
13. Shulman, J.: Clinical evaluation of the phase contrast microscope as a motivational aid in oral hygiene, J. Am. Dent. Assoc. **92:**759, 1976.
14. Arnim, S.S.: The use of disclosing agents for measuring tooth cleanliness, J. Periodontol. **34:**227, 1963.
15. Everett, F.G., and Passmore, D.J.: Mirror as an aid to toothbrushing and oral physiotherapy, J. West. Soc. Periodontol. **6:**104, 1958.
16. Lang, N.P., Ostergaard, E., and Löe, H.: A fluorescent plaque disclosing agent, J. Periodont. Res. **7:**59, 1972.
17. Löe, H., et al.: How frequently must patients carry out effective oral hygiene procedures in order to maintain gingival health? J. Periodontol. **42:**309, 1971.
18. Lang, N.P., Cummings, B.R., and Löe, H.: Toothbrushing frequency as it relates to plaque development and gingival health, J. Periodontol. **44:**396, 1973.
19. Lang, N.P., et al.: Longitudinal therapeutic effect on the periodontal attachment level and pocket depth in beagle dogs. I. Clinical findings, J. Periodont. Res. **14:**418, 1979.
20. Hine, Jr., M.K., Wachtl, C., and Fosdick, L.S.: Some observations on the cleansing effect of nylon and bristle toothbrushes, J. Periodontol. **25:**183, 1954.
21. Bass, C.C.: The optimum characteristics of toothbrushes for personal oral hygiene, Dent. Items Interest **70:**696, 1948.
22. Gilson, C.M., Charbeneau, G.T., and Hill, H.C.: A comparison of physical properties of several soft toothbrushes, J. Mich. Dent. Assoc. **51:**347, 1969.
23. Puckett, J.B.: Bristles in hand-manipulated toothbrushes, J. Periodontol. **41:**398, 1970.
24. Bechlem, D.N., Saxe, S.R., and Stern, I.B.: A histologic study of the effect upon the gingivae of using an electric toothbrush in the presence of marginal periodontitis, Periodontics **3:**90, 1965.
25. McAllan, L.H., et al.: Oral hygiene instruction in children using manual and electric toothbrushes, Br. Dent. J. **140:**51, 1976.
26. Goldman, H.M.: Effect of single and multiple toothbrushing in the cleansing of the normal and periodontally involved dentition, Oral Surg. **9:**203, 1956.
27. Kimmelman, B.J.: Teaching two toothbrushing techniques: observations and comparisons, J. Periodontol. **39:**36, 1968.
28. Talbot, E.S.: Interstitial gingivitis, Philadelphia, 1899, S. S. White Dental Mfg. Co.
29. Gibson, J.A., and Wade, A.B.: Plaque removal by the Bass and roll brushing techniques, J. Periodontol. **48:**456, 1977.
30. Stillman, P.R., and McCall, J.O.: A textbook of clinical periodontia, ed. 2, New York, 1937, The Macmillan Co.
31. Charters, W.J.: Proper home care of the mouth, J. Periodontol. **19:**136, 1948.
32. Aronovitz, R., and Conroy, C.W.: Effectiveness of the automatic toothbrush for handicapped persons, Am. J. Phys. Med. **48:**193, 1969.
33. Strahn, J.D., Bashaart, A., and Greenslade,

R.N.: Control of plaque by non-chemical means, J. Clin. Periodontol. **4**:13, 1977.

34. Hill, C.H., Levi, P.A., and Glickman, I.: The effects of waxed and unwaxed floss on interdental plaque accumulation and interdental gingival health, J. Periodontol. **44**:411, 1974.

35. Lamberts, D.M., Wunderlich, R.C., and Caffesse, R.G.: The effect of waxed and unwaxed dental floss on gingival health. I. Plaque removal and gingival response, J. Periodontol. **53**:393, 1982.

36. Wunderlich, R.C., Lamberts, D.M., and Caffesse, R.G.: The effect of waxed and unwaxed dental floss on gingival health. II. Crevicular fluid flow and gingival bleeding, J. Periodontol. **53**:397, 1982.

37. Parfitt, G.J.: Cleansing the subgingival space, J. Periodontol. **34**:133, 1963.

38. Smith, J.H., O'Connor, T.W., and Radentz, W.: Oral hygiene of the interdental area, Periodontics **1**:204, 1963.

39. Everett, F.G., and Kunkel, Sr., P.W.: Abrasion through the abuse of dental floss, J. Periodontol. **24**:186, 1953.

40. Stanmeyer, W.R.: Measure of tissue response to frequency of toothbrushing, J. Periodontol. **28**:17, 1957.

41. Gjermo, P., and Flötra, L.: The effect of different methods of interdental cleaning, J. Periodontol. Res. **5**:230, 1970.

42. Nabak, R.P., and Wade, A.B.: The relative effectiveness of plaque removal by Proxabrush and rubber oral stimulator, J. Clin. Periodontol. **4**:128, 1977.

43. Waerhaug, J.: The interdental brush and its place in operative and crown and bridge dentistry, J. Oral Rehabil. **3**:107, 1976.

44. Glavind, L., and Zeuner, E.: The effectiveness of a rotary electric toothbrush on oral cleanliness in adults, J. Clin. Periodontol. **13**:135, 1986.

45. Stevens, A.W., Jr.: A comparison of the effectiveness of variable diameter vs. unwaxed floss, J. Periodontol. **51**:666, 1980.

46. Crumley, P.J., and Sumner, C.F.: Effectiveness of a water pressure cleansing device, Periodontics **3**:193, 1965.

47. Krajewski, J.J., Robach, W.C., and Higgenbotham, T.L.: Current status of water pressure cleansing in oral hygiene, J. Calif. Dent. Assoc. **42**:433, 1966.

48. Fine, D.H., and Baumhammers, A.: Effect of water pressure irrigation on stainable material on teeth, J. Periodontol. **41**:468, 1970.

49. Bhaskar, S.N.: Clinical use of toothpaste and oral rinse containing sanguinarine, Compend. Contin. Educ. Dent. Suppl. **5**:87, 1984.

50. Friedman, L.A., et al.: Bacterial plaque disclosure surgery, J. Periodontol. **45**:439, 1974.

51. Radentz, W.H., et al.: Teaching dental flossing to patients via television reinforced by individual instructions, J. Periodontol. **46**:426, 1975.

52. Zaki, H.A., and Bandt, C.L.: The effective use of a self-teaching oral hygiene manual, J. Periodontol. **45**:491, 1974.

53. Lindhe, J., and Nyman, S.: The effect of plaque control and surgical pocket elimination on the establishment and maintenance of periodontal health: a longitudinal study of periodontal therapy in cases of advanced disease, J Clin. Periodonol. **2**:67, 1975.

54. Nyman, S., Lindhe, J., and Lundgren, D.: The role of occlusion for the stability of fixed bridges in patients with reduced periodontal tissue support, J. Clin. Periodontol. **2**:53, 1975.

55. Gjermo, P.: Chemical cleaning of teeth. In Frandsen, A., editor: Oral hygiene, Copenhagen, 1972, Munksgaard.

56. Möller, I.J.: Dental fluorose og caries, Copenhagen, 1965, Rhodos, International Science & Art Publishers.

57. Glantz, P.-O.: On wettability and adhesiveness, Odontol. Rev. **20**(suppl. 17), 1969.

58. Bibby, B.G., and Van Kestern, M.: The effect of fluorine on mouth bacteria, J. Dent. Res. **19**:391, 1940.

59. Ericsson, T., and Ericsson, Y.: Effect of partial fluorine substitution on the phosphate exchange and protein absorption of hydroxyapatite, Helv. Odontol. Acta **11**:10, 1967.

60. Weiss, E., Gedalia, I., and Zilberman, Y.: The effect of topical application with an organic and inorganic fluoride compound on the inhibition of dental plaque in humans, J. Dent. Res. **56**:1345, 1977.

61. Keyes, P.H., et al.: Bio-assays of medicaments for the control of dentobacterial plaque, dental caries and periodontal lesions in Syrian hamsters, J. Oral Ther. **3**:157, 1966.

62. Shern, R., Swing, K.W., and Crawford, J.J.: Prevention of plaque formation by organic fluorides, J. Oral Med. **25**:93, 1970.

63. Schmid, E., Kornman, K.S., and Tinanoff, N.: Changes of subgingival total colony forming units and black pigmented bacteroides after a single irrigation of periodontol pockets with 1.64% $SnF_2$, J. Periodontol. **56**:330, 1985.

64. Tinanoff, N., and Weeks, D.B.: Current status of $SnF_2$ as an antiplaque agent, Pediatr. Dent. **1**:199, 1979.

65. Hardy, J.H., Newman, H.H., and Strahn, J.D.: Direct irrigation and subgingival plaque, J. Clin. Periodontol. **9**:57, 1982.

66. Draus, F.J., Leung, S.W., and Miklos, F.: Towards a chemical inhibition of calculus, Dent. Prog. **3**:79, 1963.

67. Schaffer, E.W., Schindler, C.H., and McHugh, R.B.: The effects of two ion exchange resins on the inhibition of calculus-like deposits in vitro, J. Periodontol. **35**:296, 1964.

68. Bowen, W.H.: The prevention or control of dental plaque. In McHugh, W.D., editor: Dental plaque, Edinburgh, 1970, E & S Livingstone, Ltd.

69. Stookey, G.K., Hudson, J.R., and Muhler, J.C.: Polishing properties of zirconium silicate on enamel, J. Periodontol. **37**:200, 1966.

70. Littleton, N.W., and White, C.L.: Dental findings from a preliminary study of children receiving extended antibiotic therapy, J. Am. Dent. Assoc. **68**:520, 1964.

71. Mühlemann, H.R., et al.: The cariostatic effect of some antibacterial compounds in animal experimentation, Helv. Odontol. Acta **5**:18, 1961.

72. Dossenbach, W.F., and Mühlemann, H.R.: Effect of penicillin and ricinoleate on early calculus formation, Helv. Odontol. Acta **5**:25, 1961.

73. Löe, H., et al.: Experimental gingivitis in man, J. Periodont. Res. **2**:282, 1967.

74. McCormick, M.H., et al.: Vancomycin, a new antibiotic. I. Chemical and biologic properties, Antibiot. Ann., p. 606, 1956.

75. Jordan, D.C., and Mallory, H.D.C.: Site of action of vancomycin and *Staphylococcus aureus,* Antimicrob. Agents Chemother. **4**:489, 1964.

76. Armstrong, P.J., and Hunt, D.E.: In vitro evaluation of actinobolin as an antibiotic for the treatment of periodontal disease, I.A.D.R. Abstr. no. 142, 1971.

77. Volpe, A.R., et al.: The long term effect of an antimicrobial formulation on dental calculus formation, J. Periodontol. **41**:463, 1970.

78. Stallard, R.E., et al.: The effect of an antimicrobial mouthrinse on dental plaque, calculus and gingivitis, J. Periodontol. **40**:683, 1969.

79. Hazen, S.P., Rokita, J., and Volpe, A.R.: Histologic study of a potential plaque inhibiting agent, I.A.D.R. Abstr. no. 285, 1971.

80. Loesche, W.J., and Wafe, D.: Reduction of supragingival plaque accumulations in institutionalized Down's syndrome patients by periodic treatment with topical kanamycin, Arch. Oral Biol. **18**:1131, 1973.

81. Harvey, R.F.: Clinical impressions of a new antibiotic in periodontics, spiramycin, J. Can. Dent. Assoc. **27**:576, 1961.

82. Mills, W.H., Thompson, G.W., and Beagrie, G.S.: Clinical evaluation of spiramycin and erythromycin in control of periodontal disease, J. Clin. Periodontol. **6**:308, 1979.

83. Lozdan, J., et al.: The use of nitrimidazine in the treatment of acute ulcerative gingivitis: a double blind controlled trial, Br. Dent. J. **130**:294, 1971.

84. Heijl, L., and Lindhe, J.: The effect of metronidazole on the development of plaque and gingivitis in the beagle dog, J. Clin. Periodontol. **6**:222, 1979.

85. Listgarten, M.A., Lindhe, J., and Helldén, L.: Effect of tetracycline and/or scaling on human periodontal disease: clinical, microbiological and histological observations, J. Clin. Periodontol. **5**:246, 1978.

86. Gordon, J.M., et al.: Tetracycline: levels achievable in the gingival crevice fluid and in vitro effect on subgingival organisms. I. Concentrations in crevicular fluid after repeated doses, J. Periodontol. **52**:609, 1981.

87. Slots, J., et al.: In vitro antimicrobial susceptibility of *Actinobacillus actinomycetemcomitans,* Antimicrob. Agents Chemother. **18**:9, 1980.

88. Slots, J., and Rosling, B.G.: Suppression of the periodontopathic microflora in localized juvenile periodontitis by systemic tetracycline, J. Clin. Periodontol. **10**:465, 1983.

89. Kornman, K.S., and Robertson, P.B.: Clinical and microbiological evaluation of therapy for juvenile periodontitis, J. Periodontol. **56**:443, 1985.

90. Goodson, J.M., Haffajee, A., and Socransky, S.S.: Periodontal therapy by local delivery of tetracycline, J. Clin. Periodontol. **6**:83, 1979.

91. Goodson, J.M., et al.: Periodontal disease treatment by local drug delivery, J. Periodontol. **56**:265, 1985.

92. Jensen, S.B., et al.: Experimental gingivitis in man. IV. Vancomycin induced changes in bacterial plaque composition as related to development of gingival inflammation, J. Periodont. Res. **3**:284, 1968.

93. Yankell, S.L., et al.: Spiramycin excretion in animals, J. Dent. Res. **50**:1359, 1971.

94. Lindhe, J., et al.: The effect of metronidazole therapy on human periodontal disease, J. Periodont. Res. **17**:534, 1983.

95. Roe, F.J.: Metronidazole: review of uses and toxicity, J. Antimicrob. Chemother. **3**:206, 1977.

96. McFall, W.T., Shoulars, H.W., and Carnevale, R.A.: Effect of vancomycin in the inhibition of bacterial plaque formation, I.A.D.R. Abstr. no. 46, 1968.

97. Jensen, S.B., et al.: Experimental gingivitis in man. IV. Vancomycin induced changes in bacterial plaque, J. Periodont. Res. **3**:284, 1968.

98. Fitzgerald, R.J., Spinell, D.M., and Stoudt, T.H.: Enzymatic removal of artificial plaques, Arch. Oral Biol. **13**:125, 1968.

99. Fitzgerald, R.J., et al.: The effects of a dextranase preparation on plaque and caries in hamsters: a preliminary report, J. Am. Dent. Assoc. **76**:301, 1968.

100. König, K.G., and Guggenheim, B.: In vivo effects of dextranase on plaque and caries, Helv. Odontol. Acta. **12**:48, 1968.

101. Jensen, S.B., and Löe, H.: The effect of dextranase on plaque and gingivitis in man. In The prevention of periodontal disease, proceedings of a European symposium, London, 1971, Henry Kimpton.

102. Lobene, R.R.: A clinical study on the effect of dextranase on human dental plaque, J. Am. Dent. Assoc. **82**:132, 1971.

103. Caldwell, R.C., et al.: The effect of a dex-

tranase mouthwash on dental plaque in young adults and children, J. Am. Dent. Assoc. **82:**124, 1971.

104. Nyman, S., Lindhe, J., and Janson, J.C.: The effect of a bacterial dextranase on human dental plaque formation and gingivitis development, Odontol. Rev. **23:**243, 1972.

105. Hanke, M.T.: Studies on the local factor in dental caries. I. Destruction of plaques and retardation of bacterial growth in the oral cavity, J. Am. Dent. Assoc. **27:**1379, 1940.

106. Löe, H., and Schiött, C.R.: The effect of mouthrinses and topical application of chlorhexidine on the development of dental plaque and gingivitis in man, J. Periodont. Res. **5:**79, 1970.

107. Davies, R.M., et al.: The effect of topical application of chlorhexidine on the bacterial colonization of the teeth and gingiva, J. Periodont. Res. **5:**69, 1970.

108. Spolsky, V.W., and Forsythe, A.: Effects of alexidine 2HCl mouthwash on plaque and gingivitis after six months, J. Dent. Res. **56:**1349, 1977.

109. Rölla, G., Löe, H., and Schiött, C.R.: The affinity of chlorhexidine for hydroxyapatite and salivary mucins, J. Periodont. Res. **5:**90, 1970.

110. Lindhe, J., et al.: Influence of topical application of chlorhexidine on chronic gingivitis and gingival wound healing in the dog, Scand. J. Dent. Res. **78:**471, 1970.

111. Schroeder, H.E.: Formation and inhibition of dental calculus, Berne, 1969, Hans Huber Medical Publisher.

112. Löe, H., and Schiött, C.R.: In International conference on periodontal research, J. Periodont. Res. **4**(suppl.):38, 1969.

113. Bayer, I., Gedalia, I., and Gover, A.: Chlorhexidine and fluoride in prevention of plaque and caries in hamsters, J. Dent. Res. **56:**1365, 1977.

114. Soh, L.L., Newman, H.N., and Strahan, J.D.: Effects of subgingival chlorhexidine irrigation on periodontal inflammation, J. Clin. Periodontol. **9:**66, 1982.

115. Coventry, J., and Newman, H.N.: Experimental use of a slow release device employing chlorhexidine gluconate in areas of acute periodontal inflammation, J. Clin. Periodontol. **9:**129, 1982.

116. Kornman, K.S.: The role of supragingival plaque in the prevention and treatment of periodontal diseases: a review of current concepts, J. Periodontol. Res. **51**(suppl. 16):5, 1986.

117. Lang, N.P., and Ramseier-Grossman, K.: Optimal dosage of chlorhexidine digluconate in chemical plaque control when applied by the oral irrigator, J. Clin. Periodontol. **8:**189, 1981.

118. Flotra, L., et al.: Side effects of chlorhexidine mouthwashes, Scand. J. Dent. Res. **79:**119, 1971.

119. Baker, P.J., et al.: The *in vitro* inhibition of microbial growth and plaque formation by surfactant drugs, J. Periodont. Res. **13:**474, 1978.

120. Fine, D.H., Letizia, J., and Mandel, I.D.: The effect of listerine antiseptic mouthrinse on the biomass of developing dental plaque, J. Clin. Periodontol. **12:**660, 1985.

121. Evans, R.T., et al.: *In vitro* antiplaque effects of antiseptic phenols, J. Periodontol. **48:**156, 1977.

122. Lindhe, J.: Clinical assessment of antiplaque agents, Compend. Contin. Educ. Dent. Suppl. **5:**78, 1984.

123. Socransky, S.S.: Microbiology of plaque, Compend. Contin. Educ. Dent. Suppl. **5:**53, 1984.

124. Svantun, B., et al.: A comparison of the plaque-inhibiting effect of stannous fluoride and chlorhexidine, Acta Odontol. Scand. **35:**247, 1970.

125. Reddy, J., et al.: Prevalence and severity of periodontitis in a high fluoride area in South Africa, Community Dent. Oral Epidemiol. **13:**108, 1985.

126. Johannson, L., Oster, B., and Hamp, S.: Evaluation of cause-related periodontal therapy and compliance with maintenance care recommendations, J. Clin. Periodontol. **11:**1689, 1984.

127. Löe, H., et al.: Natural history of periodontal disease in man: rapid, moderate and no loss of attachment in Sri Lankan laborers 15 to 45 years of age, J. Clin. Periodontol. **13:**431, 1986.

128. Newman, H.N.: The apical border of plaque in chronic inflammatory periodontal disease, Br. Dent. J. **141:**105, 1976.

129. Cumming, B.R., and Löe, H.: Optimal dosage and method of delivering chlorhexidine solutions for the inhibition of dental plaque, J. Periodont. Res. **8:**57, 1973.

130. Lang, N.P., and Raber, K.: Use of oral irrigators as vehicle for the application of antimicrobial agents in chemical plaque control, J. Clin. Periodontol. **8:**177, 1981.

131. Wieder, S.G., Newman, H.N., and Strahan, J.D.: Stannous fluoride and subgingival chlorhexidine irrigation in the control of plaque and chronic periodontitis, J. Clin. Periodontol. **10:**172, 1983.

132. Yeung, F.I.S., Newman, H.N., and Addy, M.: Subgingival metronidazole in acrylic resin vs. chlorhexidine irrigation in the control of chronic peridontitis, J. Periodontol. **10:**651, 1983.

133. Mandell, R.L.: Sodium fluoride susceptibilities of suspected periodontopathic bacteria, J. Dent. Res. **62:**706, 1983.

134. Mazza, J.E., Newman, M.G., and Sims, T.H.: Clinical and antimicrobial effect of stannous fluoride on periodontitis, J. Clin. Periodontol. **8:**203, 1981.

135. Rams, T.E., and Keyes, P.H.: A rationale for the management of periodontal diseases: effects of tetracycline on subgingival bacteria, J. Am. Dent. Assoc. **107:**37, 1983.

136. Greenwell, H., et al.: Clinical and microbiologic effectiveness of Keye's method of oral hygiene on human periodontitis treated with and without surgery, J. Am. Dent. Assoc. **106:**457, 1983.

137. Goodson, J.M.: Dental applications. In Langer, R.S., and Wise, D.L., editors: Medical applications of controlled release technology, Vol. II, Boca Raton, Fla., 1984, CRC Press.

138. Goodson, J.M.: Controlled drug delivery: a new means for treatment of dental diseases, Compend. Contin. Educ. Dent. **6:**27, 1985.

139. Goodson, J.M., Hogan, P., and Dunham, S.: Clinical responses in a four-quadrant study of periodontal therapy, J. Dent. Res. **63:**268, 1984. (Abstr. no. 874.)

140. Goodson, J.M., Dunham, S., and Hogan, P.: Darkfield microbiologic responses in a four-quadrant study of periodontal therapy, J. Dent. Res. **63:**268, 1984. (Abstr. no. 875.)

141. Soskolne, A., et al.: Sustained release reservoirs of chlorhexidine in periodontal pockets, J. Dent. Res. **61:**273, 1982.

142. Samuelov, Y., Donbrow, M., and Friedman, M.: Sustained release of drugs from ethyl-cellulose-polyethylene glycol films and kinetics of drug release, J. Pharm. Sci. **68:**325, 1979.

143. Friedman, M., and Golomb, G.: New sustained release dosage form of chlorhexidine for dental use. I. Development and kinetics of release, J. Periodont. Res. **17:**323, 1982.

144. Soskolne, A., et al.: New sustained release dosage form of chlorhexidine for dental use. II. Use in periodontal therapy, J. Periodont. Res. **18:**330, 1983.

145. Golomb, G., et al.: Sustained release device containing metronidazole for periodontal use. (In press.)

146. Addy, M., et al.: The development and *in vitro* evaluation of acrylic strips and dialysis tubing for local drug delivery, J. Periodontol. **53:**693, 1982.

147. Everett, F.G., Hall, W.B., and Phatak, N.M.: Treatment of hypersensitive dentin, J. Oral Ther. **2:**300, 1966.

148. Fearnhead, R.W.: Innervation of dental tissues. In Miles, A.E.W., editor: Structural and chemical organization of teeth, vol. 1, New York, 1967, Academic Press, Inc., p. 249.

149. Rapp, R., Avery, J.K., and Strachan, D.S.: Possible role of acetylcholinesterase in neural conduction within the dental pulp. In Finn, S.B., editor: Biology of the dental pulp organ, a symposium, Birmingham, 1968, University of Alabama Press, p. 309.

150. Brännström, M.: Sensitivity of dentine, Oral Surg. **21:**517, 1966.

151. Greenhill, J.D., and Pashley, D.H.: The effects of desensitizing agents on hydraulic conduction of human dentin in vitro, J. Dent. Res. **60:**686, 1981.

152. Gangarosa, L.P.: Iontophoretic application of fluoride by tray techniques for desensitization of multiple teeth, J. Am. Dent. Assoc. **102:**50, 1981.

153. Grossman, L.E.: The treatment of hypersensitive dentin, J. Am. Dent. Assoc. **22:**592, 1935.

154. Gottlieb, B.: Technique of impregnation for caries prophylaxis, J. Mo. Dent. Assoc. **28:** 366, 1948.

155. Lukomsky, E.H.: Fluorine therapy for exposed dentin and alveolar atrophy, J. Dent. Res. **20:**649, 1941.

156. Hoyt, W.H., and Bibby, B.G.: Use of sodium fluoride for desensitizing dentin, J. Am. Dent. Assoc. **30:**1372, 1943.

157. Bhatia, H.L.: Use of sodium silicofluoride as a desensitizing agent for exposed sensitive cementum and cervical dentin, Burd. **54:**4, 1953.

158. Bixler, D., and Muhler, J.C.: Effect of dental caries in children in a nonfluoride area: combined use of three agents containing stannous fluoride: a prophylactic paste, a solution, and a dentifrice, J. Am. Dent. Assoc. **68:**792, 1964.

159. Schlegel, P.L., Stowell, E.C., and Emmerson, C.C.: The influence of an electrical potential on topically applied fluorides, J. South. Calif. Dent. Assoc. **30:**321, 1962.

160. Jensen, A.L.: Hypersensitivity controlled by iontophoresis, J. Am. Dent. Assoc. **68:**216, 1964.

161. Lefkowitz, W., Burdick, H.C., and Moore, D.L.: Desensitization of dentin by bioelectric induction of secondary dentin, J. Prosthet. Dent. **13:**940, 1963.

162. Bowers, G.M., and Elliott, J.R.: Topical use of prednisolone in periodontics, J. Periodontol. **35:**486, 1964.

163. Ross, M.R.: Hypersensitive teeth: effect of strontium chloride in a compatible dentifrice, J. Periodontol. **32:**49, 1961.

164. Tarbet, W.J., et al.: Home treatment for dentinal hypersensitivity: a comparative study, J. Am. Dent. Assoc. **105:**227, 1982.

165. Hodosh, M.: A superior desensitizer potassium nitrate, J. Am. Dent. Assoc. **88:**831, 1974.

166. Zinner, D.D., Duany, L.P., and Lutz, H.J.: A new desensitizing dentifrice, J. Am. Dent. Assoc. **95:**982, 1977.

167. Addy, M., and Morgan, T.: Scanning electron microscope and electrical resistance changes in dentine treated with toothpastes, J. Dent. Res. **61:**547, 1982. (I.A.D.R. Abstr. no. 102.)

168. McFall, W.T., and Morgan, W.C.: Effectiveness of a dentifrice containing formalin and sodium monofluorophosphate on dental hypersensitivity, J. Periodontol. **56:**288, 1985.

169. Pashley, D.H., et al.: Dentin permeability: effects of desensitizing dentifrices in vitro, J. Periodontol. **55:**522, 1984.

170. Crohn, B.B., and Drosd, R.: Halitosis, JAMA **117:**2242, 1941.

171. Howe, J.W.: The breath and diseases which give it a fetid odor, New York, 1874, Appleton-Century.

172. Brening, R.H., Sulser, G.F., and Fosdick, J.S.: Determination of halitosis by use of osmoscope and cryoscopic methods, J. Dent. Res. **18:**127, 1939.

173. Morris, P.P., and Read, R.R.: Halitosis, J. Dent. Res. **28:**324, 1949.

174. Richter, V.J., and Tonzetich, J.: The application of instrumental technique for the evaluation of odoriferous volatiles from saliva and breath, Arch. Oral Biol. **9:**47, 1964.

175. Massler, M., Emslie, R.D., and Bolden, T.E.: Fetor ex ore, Oral Surg. **4:**110, 1951.

176. Fox, N., and Kesel, R.G.: Hyperplastic sinopharyngitis, Arch. Otolaryngol. **42:**368, 1945.

177. Berg, M., and Fosdick, L.S.: Studies in periodontal disease. II. Putrefactive organisms in the mouth, J. Dent. Res. **25:**73, 1946.

178. Kutscher, A.H., Zegarelli, E.V., and Everett, F.G.: DMSO in stomatologic research, Ann. N.Y. Acad. Sci. **141:**465, 1967.

179. Lawson, R.A.M., and Carrol, K.: Delayed halitosis—a rare cause, Postgrad. Med. J. **58:**52, 1982.

180. Harma, N.K.: An unexpected cause of halitosis, Br. Dent. J. **157:**281, 1984.

181. Sulser, R.H., Lesney, T.A., and Fosdick, L.S.: Reduction of breath and mouth odors by means of brushing teeth, J. Dent. Res. **19:**193, 1940.

182. Everett, F.G.: Halitosis, Ore. Dent. J. **41:**13, 1971.

183. Morgenroth, J.: Ueber den Foetor ex ore, Dtsch. Zahnarztl. Z. **20:**67, 1966.

184. Pitts, G., et al.: The in vivo effects of an antiseptic mouthwash on odor-producing microorganisms, J. Dent. Res. **60:**1891, 1981.

185. Pitts, G., et al.: Mechanism of action of an antiseptic, anti-odor mouthwash, J. Dent. Res. **62:**738, 1983.

186. Boulware, R.T., and Southard, G.L.: Sanguinarine, in the control of volatile sulphur compounds in the mouth: a comparative study, Compend. Contin. Educ. Dent. **5:**S62, 1984.

## ADDITIONAL SUGGESTED READING

Aziz-Gandour, I.A., and Newman, H.N.: The effects of a simplified oral hygiene regimen plus supragingival irrigation with chlorhexidine or metronidazole on chronic inflammatory periodontal disease, J. Clin. Periodontol. **13:**228, 1986.

Löe, H., and Kornman, K.: Strategies in the use of antibacterial agents in periodontal disease in host-parasite interactions. In Genco, R.J., and Mergenhagen, S.E., editors: Periodontal diseases, Washington, D.C., 1982, American Society for Microbiology, p. 376.

Mandell, R.L., et al.: The effect of treatment of *Actinobacillus actinomycetemcomitans* in localized juvenile periodontitis, J. Periodontol. **57:**94, 1986.

Wennström, J., and Lindhe, J.: The effect of mouthrinses on parameters characterizing human periodontal disease, J. Clin. Periodontol. **13:**86, 1986.

# CHAPTER 32

# Scaling and root planing

---

Current periodontal therapy is directed toward establishing a periodontium that can be maintained free of disease. The goal of treatment is to establish a healthful situation in which the dentition can be maintained by recall maintenance and home care measures. Scaling and root planing are the basic procedures used by the dentist and the hygienist in this effort.

Definition

Scaling and root planing are techniques of instrumentation applied to the root surface to remove plaque, calculus, and altered or roughened cementum. When thoroughly performed, these techniques leave a smooth, clean, hard, and polished root surface. Scaling/root planing is a primary treatment for periodontal inflammation. In simple cases it may be the only treatment necessary. In severely advanced periodontal disease, scaling/root planing may be the only treatment feasible. Since the removal of plaque and deposits is basic to the control of periodontal inflammation, root planing and scaling are more frequently used than any other types of therapies. Root instrumentation is one of the most difficult procedures in dentistry. It requires dexterity, tactile acuity, and judgment, which is only gained through experience. Root instrumentation must be meticulously performed to achieve success.

## Goals

Goals

The purpose of scaling and root planing is to eliminate the etiologic agents causing inflammation, bacterial plaque, and its products on and in the tooth, and calculus.[1-7] Other factors, such as overhanging and marginally deficient restorations that are associated with plaque retention are often corrected during scaling and root planing. Together with plaque control, débridement is vital in the prevention of inflammatory periodontal disease. In an epidemiologic study Russell[8] noted, "The conclusion seems inescapable that much of the current high tooth mortality from periodontal disease could have been prevented by early and adequate scaling."

The pocket is a haven for bacterial activity. It contains concealed spicules of calculus covered by plaque, which initiates the inflammatory process and promotes the deepening of the pocket. Obviously elimination of these deposits is basic to therapy. Scaling and root planing, together with plaque control, constitute the major means by which the disease is prevented.

When plaque and calcified deposits are removed,[1-7,9] the diseased gingival tissues can heal. The chronic inflammatory tissue in the lamina propria can be replaced by healthy connective tissue organized to form a healthy lamina propria. The ulcerated sulcular epithelium can heal, and a diseased pocket can be converted into a healthy sulcus.

Scaling and root planing coupled with plaque control[4,5] is a part of every treatment plan for inflammatory periodontal disease.

When the gingivae are edematous, the edema may be reduced or eliminated by scaling and root planing.[4,9-23] The resolution of inflammation may eliminate some of the shallower pockets. When the gingivae are fibrotic, less shrinkage may occur, but some reduction in pocket depth is possible. Even in advanced disease, scaling and root planing coupled with improved plaque removal will commonly bring about a resolution of inflammation and produce reduced probing depth. This reduced probing depth may occur because of receded gingival margins, gain in attachment levels, or the inability to probe a pocket because of close adaptation of the gingiva to the tooth.[12-21] Clinical health, however, may not be reflected histologically in specimens of clinically healthy gingiva.[13]

**Edematous and fibrotic gingivae**

All periodontal therapy is based on the successful performance of initial or phase I therapy. Since phase I therapy includes all measures used before surgical therapy, this stage of treatment has been frequently referred to as *conservative therapy*.

**Phase I therapy**

Root instrumentation and plaque control should precede surgical procedures, except in the event of emergency. In many cases, surgery may become unnecessary as inflammation is eliminated and probing depths are reduced. When surgery is needed, prior root instrumentation creates a cleaner environment, which assists the surgeon. Tissues cut smoothly when inflammation with attendant hyperemia and edema are reduced. The surgical field is not as bloody and the potential for uneventful healing is improved.[14,15] Scaling and root planing may be repeated during and after surgical procedures and after healing.[4,14-17,19-21] They should also be continued as a routine part of periodontal maintenance therapy.[4,14,16] Scaling and root planing done at regular intervals minimizes the reaccumulation of plaque and calculus, alters the microbial flora in sulci, and aids in maintaining gingival health.[10,15-18]

**Maintenance therapy**

The rationale for planing root surfaces is to remove calculus and cementum containing endotoxin and to smooth the root surfaces.[19-29] Although a rough surface will enhance bacterial plaque retention and make oral hygiene more difficult,[10] persons with effective oral hygiene can keep rough as well as smooth tooth surfaces clean supragingivally. Subgingivally, however, it appears that increased roughness will favor plaque retention.[26,29] Rough root surfaces should be deliberately planed to decrease potential for plaque retention subgingivally.[10] Since residual calculus cannot be easily distinguished from a rough surface, root planing ensures calculus is removed. In addition, the presence of cementum-bound lipopolysaccharide endotoxins has been demonstrated within root surfaces.[27,28,30] Root planing has been advocated for the re-

**Rationale for root planing**

moval of root cementum contaminated by endotoxin.[29,30] It is known how deeply endotoxin penetrates the root and therefore how much of the root surface needs to be removed.[22,27-29] Total removal of cementum by instrumentation does not appear to be practical.[20] In addition to endotoxin, residual calculus is often encountered following scaling. This residual calculus is usually located in root irregularities and is covered by plaque.[29,31] In areas where the roots have been planed completely, there is less likelihood of residual calculus.[12,32] Thus root planing will help ensure a more complete elimination of calcified deposits and root-associated endotoxins and may assist in reducing subgingival plaque retention.

Calculus on the root surface is covered with bacterial plaque and degenerated epithelial cells and is associated with epithelial proliferation into the lamina propria and the apical migration of junctional epithelium. The removal of calculus and plaque promotes healing.[3,14-17,19,20,33-35]

## Periodontal prophylaxis

Oral prophylaxis is a scaling and polishing procedure performed on dental patients in normal or good periodontal health to remove coronal plaque, stain, and deposits thus preventing caries and periodontal disease. Since pockets and recessions are absent in a completely normal periodontium, scaling and polishing are performed on the anatomic crown and into very shallow, healthy sulci (less than 3 mm deep). Consequently, prophylactic scaling may be performed with instruments called *scalers*. Such instruments have straight-line, angular cutting edges. Polishing may be performed with polishing agents applied by handpiece-mounted rubber cups.[36,37] Another instrument, the Prophy-Jet, polishes with a polishing mixture applied by air pressure.[36,37]

Generally prophylactic scaling procedures may be sufficient to deal with patients with normal periodontal health and some with mild disease (AAP type 1), but they are not adequate in dealing with the subgingival deposits in patients with more severe periodontal disease (AAP types II to IV). In mild instances of type 1 periodontal disease, inflammation may be reversed by scaling, and good health may be maintained by daily home care and periodic prophylaxis. Patients with the more advanced (AAP types II to IV) periodontal disease will require periodontal (therapeutic) scaling and root planing, possibly in conjunction with other forms of periodontal therapy. Maintenance scaling is performed thereafter for the lifetime of their dentitions.

## Scaling

Gingival inflammation and pocket depth are cardinal signs of periodontal disease. Except in type I cases, the junctional epithelium will have migrated onto the cemental surface. Whereas the inflammatory aspect is reversible, the positional defect (i.e., recession) generally is not. Thus major differences occur when a patient develops periodontitis. First, the junctional epithelium migrates onto the cementum. Second, pocket formation results in deeper and less accessible areas into which plaque and calculus extend and are thus more difficult to remove. Finally, both the "exposed" cementum and the inflamed sulcular tissues are submarginal and must be instrumented to restore the periodontium to a healthy state. This instrumentation is referred to as scaling and root planing.

**Scaling**  Root instrumentation can be divided arbitrarily into two separate procedures: scaling and root planing. *Scaling* consists of the removal of calculus, bacteria, and their products from the root surfaces of the teeth without special effort to making the root smooth. Scaling is accomplished by powerful, short working strokes. Depending on the location of the calculus, scaling is divided into either supragingival or subgingival instrumentation. The objective of supragingival scaling is the removal of deposits from the clinical crowns of the teeth. Subgingival scaling is the removal of deposits below the gingival margin. Subgingival scaling and root planing are performed as either closed or open procedures. The closed procedure implies subgingival instrumentation without surgical (incisional) displacement of the gingiva. The root surface is not accessible for direct visual inspection. The open procedure calls for exposure of the affected root surface by surgery. The gingivae are incised and a flap is reflected to facilitate access and visibility for the operator.

## Root planing

The objectives of *root planing* include the systematic smoothing of roughened root surfaces and the removal of contaminated surface cementum or dentin. Root planing is often performed using local anesthesia. Clinically, root planing is an extension and refinement of scaling and is generally not a separate procedure. Often the only difference between these procedures is one of intent.[14] Some clinicians refer to root planing as *root curettage*.[6,38] Root planing is performed with fine curettes using a pull stroke. After exploration with a periodontal explorer to sense the character of the root surface, fine, flexible curettes are applied to the tooth with a light but firm touch for root planing. The angle of these curette blades to the tooth surface is approximately 45 to 90 degrees. Strokes are made in various directions, completely smoothing the root surface and leaving it with a glasslike, hard finish. The operator confines the instrument to the root surface and tries to avoid wounding soft tissues, although this may occur inadvertently. It should be stressed that some removal of cementum occurs in the root planing procedure.

**Objectives**

### PREMEDICATION

When a history of rheumatic fever, mitral valve prolapse, or aortic or orthopedic implants is elicited, premedication with antibiotics is indicated. Two gm of penicillin V should be taken 30 to 60 min before the appointment, followed by 1.0 gm 6 hours later. When penicillin allergy is present, 1 gm of erythromycin should be substituted and taken 1½ to 2 hours before the procedure followed by 500 mg 6 hours later (see box, below).

For more extensive discussion of patients requiring antibiotic protection see box, p. 722.

### ANESTHESIA

It is useful for the student to use anesthesia (block or infiltration) and/or analgesia in periodontal cases requiring scaling and root planing. In maintenance cases, it may

---

- The new standard recommendation is to prescribe 2 gm of penicillin V 1 hour before treatment and a single 1 gm dose 6 hours later.
- Parenteral regimens for use in cases requiring maximal protection: ampicillin, 1 to 2 gm intramuscularly or intravenously, plus gentamicin, 1.5 mg/kg intramuscularly or intravenously, 30 minutes before the procedure, followed by 1 gm oral penicillin V 6 hours later. Instead of oral penicillin V, the parenteral regimen may also be repeated once 8 hours later.
- The oral regimen for patients allergic to penicillin is vancomycin, 1 gm intravenously, administered slowly for 1 hour before treatment. No repeat dose is necessary.
- Erythromycin, 1 gm orally, 1½ hours before the appointment then 1 dose, 500 mg, 6 hours later may be given in the event of penicillin allergy.

not be essential to use anesthesia unless tooth sensitivity is present. Topical anesthesia may suffice in some cases.

## Basic armamentarium

**Designs for specific needs**

Since root instrumentation is the basic method of treatment and of all techniques has been in use the longest, it is not surprising that many instruments have been introduced.[39] The purpose of an instrument should be well understood. Some instruments are more effective in removing bulky, calcified deposits but are not designed to reach to the bottom of the pocket. Others are made so that their blades can be carried below the apical end of the calculus at the bottom of the pocket without causing undue damage to the attachment tissues.

The names given to the instruments usually describe the shape and design of the blades or the mode of action of the instruments. There are chisels, hoes, sickles, files, and curettes. Each of the five types of instruments is designed for a specific use and sometimes for access to a specific tooth surface.[39] The chisel, hoe, and sickle are designed for the removal of heavy calculus, whereas curettes and files are intended to remove finer or residual deposits and to smooth the root surface. Only curettes and scalers have universal application in root instrumentation procedures. Hoes, files, and chisels have a more limited application, and they have a greater potential to damage periodontal tissues when used by an inexperienced practitioner. In addition, a sharp cutting edge is difficult to maintain in this group of instruments. With the advent of ultrasonics, hoes and chisels are used less frequently.

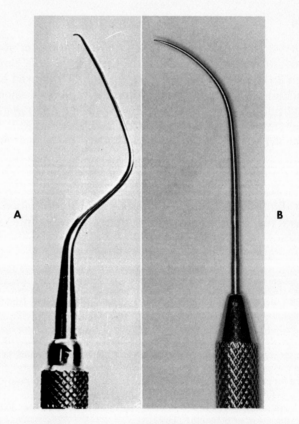

A          B

**Fig. 32-1.** **A** and **B,** Pocket explorers, an indispensable instrument in periodontal diagnosis.

## PERIODONTAL EXPLORER

The periodontal explorer (Fig. 32-1) has a long and more flexible working end (tyne) than does the common explorer. It is used to explore the depth and shape of the pocket and the amount and configuration of calculus in the pocket.

This instrument is also used to feel the texture of the root surface. When the tip of the instrument is placed with its side to the surface of the tooth and guided into the pocket (Fig. 32-2), it transmits a feeling of the character of the root surface to the operator's fingers; this is referred to as *tactile sensitivity*. Accretions, indentations, furcations, or ledges can be determined more easily than they can with a straight explorer.

The pocket explorer can also indicate the hardness and smoothness of the root after planing.[39]

## CURETTES

The curette is the most versatile of all subgingival instruments and is the most commonly used instrument for scaling, root planing, and the removal of the soft tissue lining of the periodontal pocket. The shape of the instrument allows for easy entry

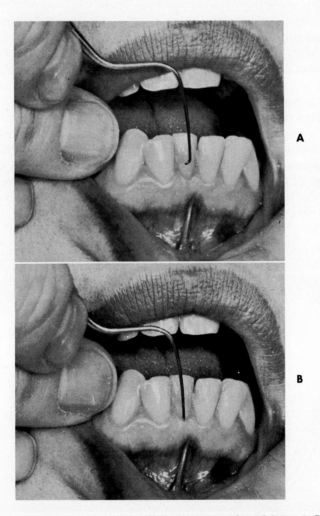

**Fig. 32-2. A,** Place the pocket explorer with the side of the tip on the surface of the tooth. **B,** Guide the tip of the explorer gently to the bottom of the pocket. Surface irregularities will be transmitted to the fingers.

into a pocket because its shank design enables it to conform to the curvatures of the root more readily and with more safety than any other instrument. The curette facilitates greater tactile sensitivity than any other subgingival instrument with the possible exception of the explorer. Curettes are primarily pull-type instruments. "Pull type" refers to the working stroke direction. Curette pull strokes may be lateral, circumferential, or coronal in direction on any tooth surface in any area of the arch. Unquestionably, the use of the curette will produce the smoothest subgingival root surface when compared with any other instruments.[32,40,41]

Curettes may be single or double ended. Double-ended instruments have two working ends (blades), one at either end of the instrument handle. The blades are mirror images of each other. Single-ended instruments have only one working end. Thus two instruments are needed in this case to obtain a matched set. Curettes are usually identified by the name of the designer and are numbered in sets. For example, the Gracey 5/6 curette was designed by Dr. Gracey. It is also a double-ended instrument. The blades (5/6) are mirror images.

Curette blades usually have two cutting edges that are formed by the two lateral borders of the back of the blade converging with the face of the blade (Fig. 32-3). Only one cutting edge is used against the tooth in scaling and root planing procedures. The toe of the blade is the rounded tip of the blade.

Curette handles vary in size and shape. Usually a larger and textured handle is best for a secure and comfortable grasp. A hollow handle will enhance tactile sensitivity (Fig. 32-4).

Curette shank designs differ greatly depending on the area of use and the instrument purpose. Generally, a well-designed instrument is balanced so that the shank and blade are in line with the handle[42] (Fig. 32-5).

Curettes have two cutting edges: an outside edge and an inside edge (Fig. 32-6). The outside cutting edge is used on facial, lingual, and mesial surfaces of posterior teeth and on all surfaces of anterior teeth. The inside cutting edge is used on distal surfaces of posterior teeth. When using the outside cutting edge, the handle of the instrument should be parallel to the tooth surface being scaled. When using the inside cutting edge, the handle of the instrument should approach a perpendicular angle to the tooth surface being instrumented (Fig. 32-7).

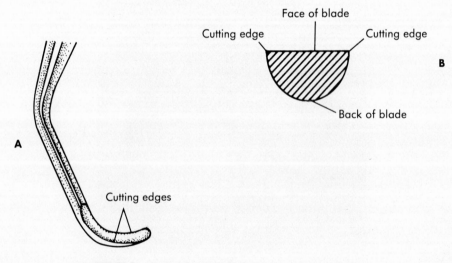

**Fig. 32-3.  A,** Curette blade. **B,** Curette blade in cross section.

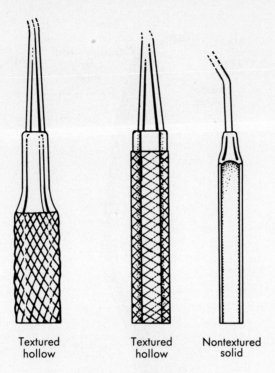

Textured      Textured      Nontextured
hollow        hollow        solid

**Fig. 32-4.**   Handle types.

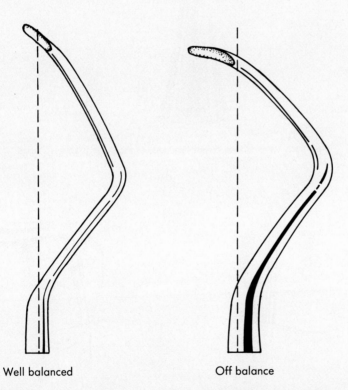

Well balanced              Off balance

**Fig. 32-5.**   Instrument balance. Curette with blade in line with the handle is well balanced. Curette with blade and handle in different planes is off balance.

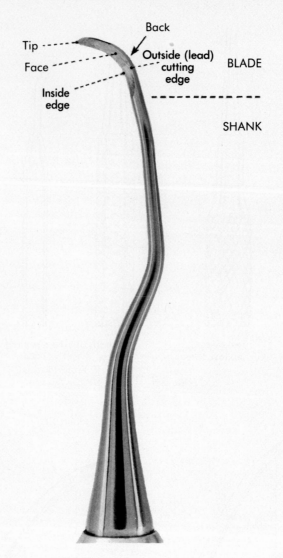

**Fig. 32-6.** Periodontal curette. The face of the blade is spoon shaped.

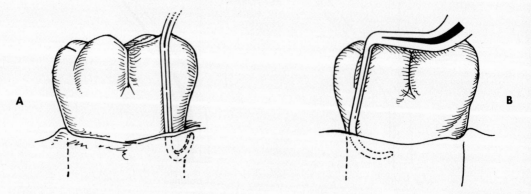

**Fig. 32-7.** Inside blade being used. The handle is parallel to the tooth surface. The curette tip is guided into the sulcus with the back of the blade used to displace the gingiva without impinging and with the cutting edge used against the tooth surface to detect calculus. **A,** On the proximal surface. **B,** On the vestibular surface.

There are two types of curettes: universal curettes and area-specific curettes. Universal curettes may be used throughout the mouth on any surface (Table 32-1). Blade size and shank length may vary, but the cutting edges are straight, rounded at the tip. The face of the blade is always at a 90-degree angle to the lower shank of the instrument. Universal curettes are especially good for removing ledges of supragingival calculus and in shallow sulci. They may be used on healthy mouths where there is no evidence of pocket depth, recession, or furcation involvement. Common universal curettes are the Barnhart 1/2 and 5/6 and the Columbia-McCall 13/14 and 4R/4L (Fig. 32-8).

**Universal and area-specific curettes**

## Gracey curettes

Gracey curettes are referred to as *area-specific curettes,* meaning that each blade and shank was designed for access to a specific area of the mouth (Fig. 32-9 and Table 32-2). Although they are designed to be used on specific tooth surfaces, they can be adapted to several different areas by altering hand and patient positions.

Gracey curette design differs from that of universal curettes in several ways:

**Gracey vs. universal curettes**

1. Unlike the universal curette whose blade is angled at 90 degrees to the lower shank of the instrument, the Gracey curette blade is angled at 70 degrees to the lower shank of the instrument. This is referred to as an *offset blade* (see Fig. 32-6).
2. To engage the working blade of the Gracey curette, the angle of the *lower shank* of the instrument must be parallel to the tooth surface being instrumented. The working blade of a universal curette is engaged when the *handle* is parallel to the tooth surface. For distal surfaces of posterior teeth, the handle is positioned almost perpendicular to the tooth surface.
3. The blade of the Gracey curette is curved rather than straight. This curvature is particularly important in terms of sharpening and in terms of adapting the blade to the tooth surface. Generally speaking, only the toe third of the Gracey curette blade can be adapted effectively.
4. Although the Gracey curette has two cutting edges, only the outside (cutting) edge is used (see Fig. 32-6).

**Table 32-1.** Universal curettes

| Curettes | Purpose |
|---|---|
| Barnhart 1/2 | Good for heavy calculus ledges, particularly in the posterior areas |
| Barnhart 5/6 | Good for routine oral prophylaxis maintenance cases with light to moderate subgingival calculus |
| | Supragingival calculus and limited to sulcus areas with no evidence of loss of attachment |
| Columbia-McCall 4R/4L | Can be used universally throughout the mouth, good for the same uses as the Barnhart 1/2 |
| Columbia-McCall 13/14 | Especially useful in the anterior areas for supragingival and subgingival calculus in sulcus areas |

**Table 32-2.** Gracey curettes*

| Curettes | Purpose |
|---|---|
| Gracey 1/2, 3/4, and 5/6 | For anterior teeth; have long, straight shanks |
| Gracey 7/8 and 9/10 | For facial and lingual surfaces of posterior teeth |
| Gracey 11/12 | For mesial surfaces of posterior teeth |
| Gracey 13/14 | For distal surfaces of posterior teeth |

*Gracey curettes come in sets of several instruments. Each blade and shank is designed to adapt to a specific area or tooth surface.

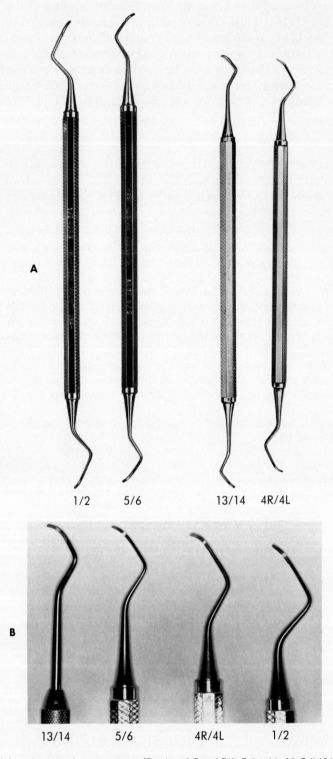

**Fig. 32-8.** **A,** Universal curettes in common use (Barnhart 1/2 and 5/6, Columbia-McCall 13/14, Columbia 4R/RL). **B,** The curette blades of the Columbia-McCall 13/14, Barnhart 5/6, Columbia 4R/4L, and Barnhart 1/2.

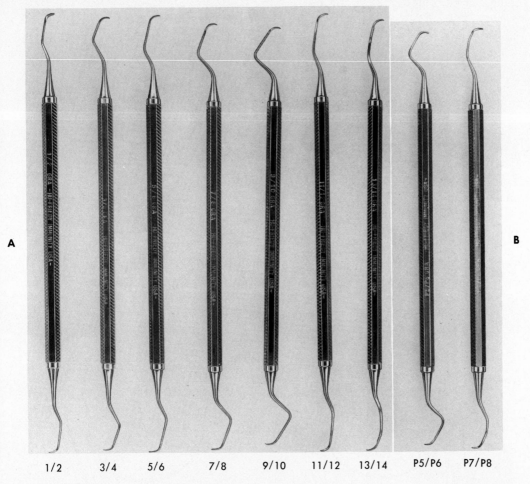

A                                                                                    B

| 1/2 | 3/4 | 5/6 | 7/8 | 9/10 | 11/12 | 13/14 | P5/P6 | P7/P8 |

**Fig. 32-9.** **A,** Gracey periodontal finishing curettes. Following are descriptions and uses of the instruments: *1* and *2* (short) for incisors and cuspids; *3* and *4* (short contra-angle) for incisors and cuspids; *5* and *6* (medium) for bicuspids and molars; this right and left pair features the shank and blade at a slight contra-angle for use under normal conditions for anteriors as well; *7* and *8* (medium contra-angle) for bicuspids and molars, buccal locations; *9* and *10* (long contra-angle) for molars, featuring the shank and blade at a more acute angle for less accessible root surfaces; *11* and *12* for mesiolingual and mesiobuccal locations; designed to work, from the lingual direction, on the mesial surfaces of bicuspids and molars; may be used in so many areas and on so many root surfaces that they might correctly be called "universal"; *13* and *14* for distoposterior locations; a right and left pair designed to reach distal surfaces of all posterior teeth with minimal cheek tissue distention (in such inaccessible areas, each instrument may be used to cross-check the work of its opposite by varying slightly the degree of blade surface placement). **B,** Gracey prophylactic instruments differ from the finishing curette in shank construction. The blades are of the same delicate size, but the shank of the prophylactic instrument is shorter and slightly heavier. This slightly more rigid design feature has proven most efficient to the practitioner of dental hygiene. These instruments carry the prefix "P."

## Sickles

Sickle scalers are instruments designed to remove gross supragingival calculus. The blades of sickle scalers are triangular in cross section with a pointed tip (Fig. 32-10). The cutting edges may be straight or rounded. The back of the blade comes to a point and is formed by the junction of two flat lateral sides. The sickle scaler is too bulky for adequate subgingival scaling or root planing. Subgingival use leads to tissue distention and laceration. Also its design limits the sickle's ability to adapt to root contours, leading to root gouging, missed calculus, and laceration of the gingiva at times (Fig. 32-11).

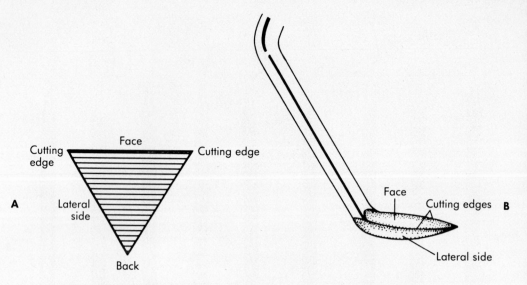

**Fig. 32-10.** Sickle scalers. **A,** Blade in cross section. **B,** Sickle blade.

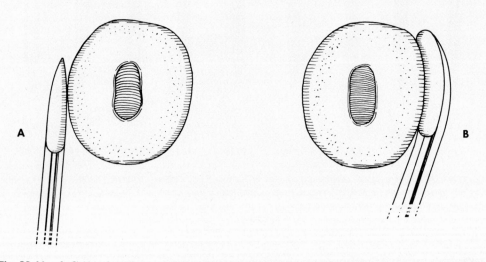

**Fig. 32-11.** **A,** Sickle adaptation is limited, and the tip of the blade may lacerate the gingiva. **B,** Curette adapts to the tooth surface when held in the closed position because the curvatures tend to match.

There are two types of sickles: anterior sickle scalers and posterior or modified sickle scalers. Anterior sickle scalers may be straight or hooked (Fig. 32-12). The blade and shank of anterior sickles are in a straight line with the handle. The blades are at 90 degrees to the shank and have two cutting edges that adapt to the tooth surface like curettes (45- to 90-degree angle). Sickle scalers are used with pull strokes. Both straight and hooked sickles are good for removing supragingival calculus on mandibular anterior teeth. The hooked sickle is helpful on the lingual surfaces of lingually averted teeth. Posterior sickles (contra-angled) have the same blade design as anterior sickles, but they have a modified shank, designed to adapt interproximally in premolar and molar areas (Fig. 32-13).

The blades of some sickle scalers are rectangular and extremely thin, sometimes as fine as 0.2 to 0.4 mm. These may be used with a push or a pull stroke.

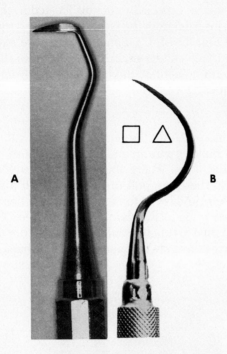

**Fig. 32-12.** Sickle scalers. The blades may be square or triangular (**A** and **B**).

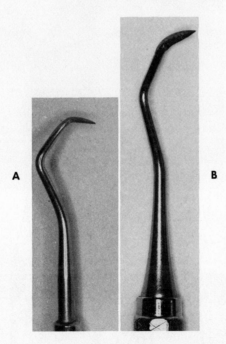

**Fig. 32-13.** **A** and **B,** Sickle scalers with biangled shanks that make for easier access to the posterior interproximal surfaces.

### Chisels

Like the sickle scaler, the chisel (Fig. 32-14, *A* and *B*) is designed for gross and supragingival calculus removal, especially calculus located in the mandibular anterior region. The instrument is inserted from the facial surface, and a push stroke is engaged to dislodge the deposits (Fig. 32-14, *C*). Some chisels have extremely sharp corners that may nick the tooth surface and traumatize tissue. These corners may be rounded by the operator. With the refinement of curettes and the advent of ultrasonic devices, chisels are used less frequently.

### Hoes

Hoes are instruments intended for the removal of heavy subgingival and supragingival calculus. They are bulky instruments with limited use. Hoes tend to distend tissue in deep pockets and areas where the gingiva tightly conforms to the tooth. Shaped like a garden hoe, these are pull instruments with a single straight cutting edge (Fig. 32-15). The cutting edge is formed by the junction of the blade face and the beveled toe. The blade angle to the shank is 100 degrees. Hoes may be single or double ended and are designed to function either in the anterior or the posterior regions of the mouth. Anterior hoes have shorter and straighter shanks, posterior hoes have

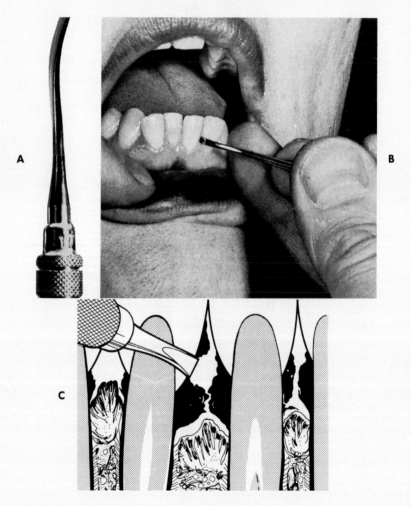

**A**  **B**

**C**

**Fig. 32-14.** **A,** Periodontal chisel. **B** and **C,** Proper application. **C,** Diagrammatic view of calculus removal.

longer and angled shanks. All hoes are best suited for facial and lingual surfaces and for proximal surfaces adjacent to edentulous areas. Hoes are best used when tissue is easily displaced. The straight cutting edge limits the hoe's ability to access root contours. Like the chisel, ultrasonics and rigid curettes have replaced the hoe in today's armamentarium.

### Files

Files may be considered to be a series of small hoes.[42,43] Like hoes, most files are designed for removing supragingival and subgingival deposits where the gingiva is easily displaced. The file blade consists of multiple cutting edges that crush or fracture heavy and/or tenacious deposits. The shank design is like that of the hoe and therefore limits the file's ability to adapt to root form. The file is used like a hoe on facial and lingual surfaces, with a pull stroke. The file is difficult to sharpen, and when used improperly, it can nick the root surface. Like the hoe, files are used less frequently since the advent of ultrasonics and rigid Gracey curettes (Fig. 32-16). There are very fine files, however, that are useful in narrow, deep pockets.

### ULTRASONIC UNITS

Ultrasonic units are a useful adjunct to (but not a substitute for) hand scaling and instrumentation. There are two common types of ultrasonic units, the piezoelectric and the magnetostrictive.[44-46] Both types of units are composed of the following:

1. An electric power generator that delivers energy in the form of high-frequency vibrations to a handpiece
2. A handpiece
3. Electrical and water outlets
4. A foot control

Both types of units have handpieces that have interchangeable tips. Piezoelectric ultrasonic units are less common than magnetostrictive ultrasonic units but tend to provide safety for use on patients with cardiac pacemaker devices. With a magnetostrictor handpiece, energy is carried from the power generator through strips that

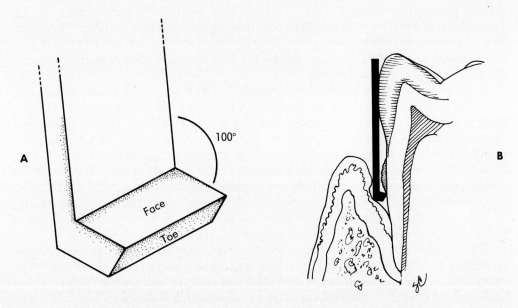

**Fig. 32-15.** **A,** Working end of a hoe. **B,** Cross section of a hoe in use.

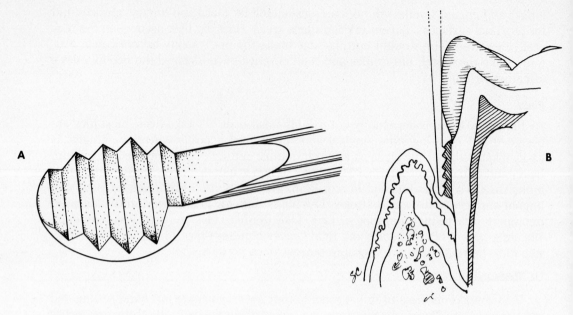

**Fig. 32-16.**   Use of file to remove deposits in deep, narrow pocket. **A,** Working end of file. **B,** Cross section of file in use.

encircle the handpiece (Fig. 32-17). The insert is composed of many magnetostrips that convert the electrical energy in the handpiece to mechanical energy in the form of rapid vibrations. The vibrations may vary from 20,000 to 29,000 cycles per second. These cycles cause the tip of the insert to alternatingly increase or decrease, thus the tip moves approximately 1/1000 of an inch in a back-and-forth, circular, or figure-eight motion. It is the tip motion that disrupts the calculus deposits.

Ultrasonic instruments are mainly employed for the gross removal of calculus supragingivally and in shallow, accessible pockets. Although ultrasonic units can plane the root surface,[47-56] hand curettes have proven more effective. Access in periodontal pockets deeper than 4 mm is easier with hand instruments. The water spray (Fig. 32-18), helpful in some ways in the ultrasonic unit, tends to impede visibility. The bluntness of the instrument tip also tends to limit tactile sensitivity, and the vibrations have been shown to disrupt tissue by lifting off epithelium and dismembering collagen bundles in young, growing tissue.

**Clinical application**   In general, the lowest power setting consistent with effectiveness should be used. After the instrument has been prepared for use, the tip should be run between the fingers to guard against excessive vibration and heat production.[56] The handpiece and tip should be applied with very light but firm pressure—a feather touch and brush stroke.[57] The time of application should be kept as short as is practical. The tip should be kept in motion at all times as the instrument is being used. A periodontal explorer should be used during ultrasonic instrumentation to check the root surface. The water spray should be ample (Fig. 32-18), particularly in areas where the flow at the tip may be blocked (subgingivally). It is important not to use tips that have rough surfaces or spurs as they would scratch the tooth surface.

**Influence on hard and soft tissues**   The effect of ultrasonic instruments on the tooth surface may range from little or no change to a characteristic, fine, stippled or granular pattern of varying depth.[58] The main effect on the soft tissue is a fragmenting and washing away of the sulcular lining and adjacent tissue[59,60] (gingival curettage). Coagulation has also been reported.[46] The depth and degree of these tissue effects are governed by the quantity of ultrasonic

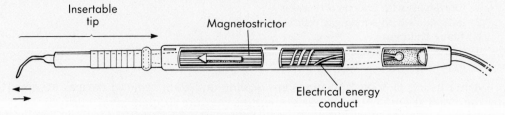

**Fig. 32-17.** Diagram of a magnetostrictor (ultrasonic) scaler.

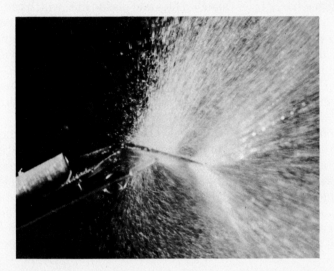

**Fig. 32-18.** Ultrasonic tip showing the direction of the water spray (cavitation). The water spray is used primarily as a cooling device for the tip, which would otherwise become too warm. The water, however, is also useful for lavage and the removal of debris.

energy applied[46]; this quantity is determined by the following factors[57]: (1) power setting (amplitude of tip motion), (2) applied pressure, (3) relative sharpness of the tip, (4) angle of application, and (5) time of exposure per unit area. The healing of wounds produced by ultrasonic instrumentation appears to be similar to that of wounds produced by hand instrumentation.[61] Both the time required for epithelization and the reappearance of an inflammatory infiltrate in the adjacent connective tissue during healing have been studied and are reported to be similar to that for hand scaling.[47,62-64]

Ultrasonic curettage is particularly useful in the early phases of treatment and when tissues are hemorrhagic. The washed field also makes the instruments convenient for calculus removal during periodontal surgery. In addition, the instrumentation with lavage is helpful in the treatment of acute necrotizing ulcerative gingivitis; it enhances resolution of the acute phase of this disease. Gingival healing is reported to occur more rapidly after ultrasonic planing and curettage. This may be a result of the lavage.[48-50] The instrumentation is also useful in patients with heavy supragingival calculus. Many patients experience less pain during instrumentation. Contraindications for the use of ultrasonic instruments have not been clearly defined. Some patients have experienced pain; others have reported tooth sensitivity after repeated use. Caution is called for in the presence of baked porcelain inlays or jacket crowns. Root surfaces treated with an ultrasonic scaler should be finished with curettes.[51] Curettes produce surfaces with least roughness,[52,53] although the reverse has also been reported.[47,54]

Ultrasonic units have been contraindicated in the following instances:

**Indications and contraindications**

1. Individuals with infectious diseases
2. Individuals with strong gag reflexes
3. Young children
4. Individuals who experience pain on use
5. Individuals with cardiac pacemakers[65]

A full listing of sonic and ultrasonic scaling and stain removal devices accepted by the Council on Dental Materials, Instruments, and Equipment is given in Table 32-3.[66]

**EVA system**

The EVA system[67] is an instrument consisting of a contra-angle that attaches to a straight slow-speed handpiece. Diamond files and plastic tips, which can hold polishing materials, are inserted into the contra-angle (Fig. 32-19). The tip vibrates along its long axis. This instrument is useful for interproximal root planing and polishing but should not be used on subgingival tooth surfaces unless these surfaces have been exposed. Polishing should always follow the use of the diamond files. This device is most useful for correcting overhanging or overcontoured interproximal restorations and for removing hard deposits that are inaccessible to hand and ultrasonic instruments.

**Chemotherapy**

The question might be asked to what extent should chemical or chemotherapy be combined with scaling and root planing? Locally applied germicide used in combination with instrumentation appears to offer no enhanced effect,[13] although chlorhexidine rinses are reported to eliminate gingivitis.[68] Germicides have been employed to reduce postinstrumentation bacteremias.[69] Orally administered systemic tetracycline is reported to influence the colonization of the pocket by nonpathogenic flora for up to 6 months.[70,71] However, concurrent treatment with antibiotics or chlorhexidine appears to yield clinical improvement that may not be mirrored microscopically.[13]

## Reexamination

Areas once scaled should be carefully reexamined on subsequent visits when other quadrants are scaled. Probably with even the most meticulous instrumentation some fragments of calculus may remain and cause inflammation. The reddish or bluish color of the gingiva may contrast with the pink color of areas where the root has been

**Table 32-3.** Professional scaling and stain-removal devices classified by the Council on Dental Materials, Instruments, and Equipment

| Acceptable | Provisionally acceptable |
| --- | --- |
| Ultrasonic-magnetostrictive | Ultrasonic-magnetostrictive type and Hydraulic |
|   Dentsply-Cavitron Model 2001, Dentsply International, Inc. |   (air-powered) |
|   Dentsply-Cavitron Model 2002, Dentsply International, Inc. |   A-dec Ultrasonic Scaler, A-dec, Inc. |
|   LT-200, California Technics |   Odontoson 3, Teledyne Densco |
|   Midwest XGT, Ritter-Midwest |   Son-Au-Tec, Macan Engineering and Manufacturing Co. |
|   Tec-Son II, California Technics | Ultrasonic-piezoelectric |
|   Ultrason 770, California Technics |   Piezo-Electric, Spartan USA, Inc. |
|   Ultrason 990, California Technics | Sonic |
| Hydraulic (air-powered) |   Orbison, Columbus Dental |
|   Prophyjet, CooperCare, Inc. |   Titan-S, Star Dental |
| Ultrasonic-magnetostrictive type and Hydraulic (air-powered) | |
|   Cavijet, CooperCare, Inc. | |

From Council on Dental Materials, Instruments, and Equipment: Status report on professional scaling and stain-removal devices, J. Am. Dent. Assoc. **111:**801, 1985; copyright by the American Dental Association. Reprinted by permission.

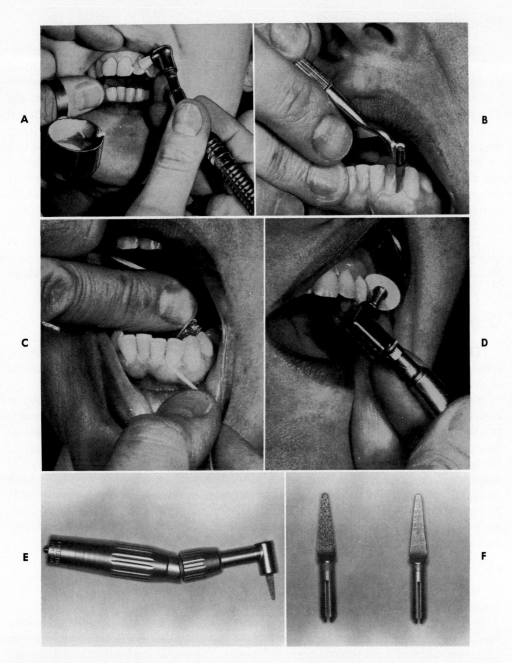

**Fig. 32-19.** **A,** Polishing tooth surfaces with a rubber cup. The polishing agent is retained in the thumb cup. **B,** Use of porte-polisher. **C,** Use of waxed dental tape for interproximal polishing. **D,** Use of cuttlefish disks for polishing. **E,** EVA contra-angle handpiece. **F,** EVA tips.

completely divested of deposits, making such areas obvious. With the resolution of inflammation, remaining fragments of subgingival deposits sometimes become supra-gingival.

## Polishing

After root planing has been completed, the teeth should be polished thoroughly with fine polishing agents.[14,15] Polishing can be done adequately with the motor-driven rubber cup (see Fig. 32-19, *A*) on accessible areas of the tooth. The use of the rubber cup rather than the brush for the buccal and lingual areas allows surfaces below the gingival margins to be polished simultaneously. Interproximal areas should be polished with shaped balsa wood sticks; a porte-polisher; wide, waxed dental tape; or fine linen strips. In polishing with a porte-polisher, use soft orangewood points (*B*). These can be shaped with a knife to fit any area. The fine polishing agent should be carried to the area, and the tape applied in a shoeshine fashion (*C*). Fine cuttlefish disks may be used on surfaces that need more than pumice polishing (*D*). A special contra-angle handpiece for cleansing and polishing interproximal surfaces is also available (Eva handpiece, Dentatus, Sweden) (Fig. 32-19, *E* and *F*).

The most widely used polishing agent is a paste consisting of flour of pumice and glycerine with flavoring and color additives. Sodium fluoride or stannous fluoride may be added to this mixture for a desensitizing effect. Other polishing agents such as zirconium oxide or kaolinite pastes have been suggested.

## Sharpening instruments

**Dull instru-ments**

The objective of sharpening instruments is to restore the sharpness of the cutting edge of the blade and to maintain the original design and shape (and thus function) of the instrument.

Keeping instruments sharp (well honed) is important because dull instruments limit efficiency and effectiveness in calculus removal. With sharp instruments, calculus is severed from the tooth surface; dull blades tend to crush calculus, leaving residual fragments. With dull instruments, more pressure must be exerted to remove calculus, decreasing the control and precision of instrumentation and increasing the danger of instrument slippage. Dull instruments limit the operator's effectiveness by decreasing tactile sensitivity and are less efficient because more strokes are needed to débride and plane the root. Dull instruments tend to increase the time expended in treating each patient. Finally they are more likely to leave calculus with a burnished or smoothed surface, making it difficult to detect clinically.

### HOW TO SHARPEN

Instruments are sharpened in different ways.[72-75] Any method is acceptable if it results in a sharp blade edge without destroying the blade form.

A sharpening stone is used to restore the cutting edge to a dull periodontal instru-ment. There are several types of sharpening stones. Some stones are synthetic whereas others are quarried from natural mineral deposits. The stones are harder than the metal of the instrument. This allows the stone to shave metal away in the sharpening process.

Sharpening stones come in a variety of coarseness grades, types, and shapes. Coarseness grades are designated as fine, medium, and coarse. Coarse grades are used on very dull instruments and for instrument recontouring. Medium and fine grades are used for rehoning blade edges when they are only slightly dulled. Sharpening stones may be mounted or unmounted. Mounted stones are used on a handpiece and are employed to sharpen the face of the instrument blade (Fig. 32-20, *A*). Mounted

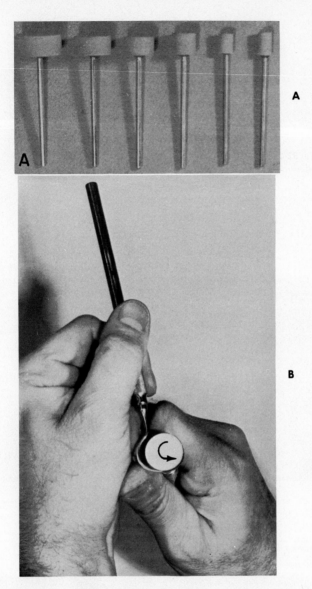

**Fig. 32-20.  A,** Mounted Arkansas stones used mainly to sharpen the face of the blade. **B,** Use of stone rotating toward tip of sickle.

stones have limitations. It is difficult to control the uniformity of metal removal, which may ruin the contour of the instrument. Also even light applications of pressure remove large and needless amounts of metal. The unmounted or hand-held sharpening stones are the most popular and most efficient (Fig. 32-21). Hand-held stones come in a variety of shapes. They may be flat and rectangular or they may be cylindric or conical in shape. The cylindric and conical stones are generally used to sharpen the face of the blade (Fig. 32-22). Flat, rectangular stones are probably the most popular and are used to sharpen the cutting edge by recontouring the back and sides of the instrument blade.

There are basically three types of sharpening stones; Arkansas, India, and carborundum stones. Arkansas stones are a fine grade. India stones are a fine or medium grade and are the most universally used. Both the Arkansas and India stones should be lubricated with mineral oil. The mineral oil reduces heat produced by the friction

**Fig. 32-21.** **A,** Arkansas unmounted stone. **B,** Fine-grade India stones.

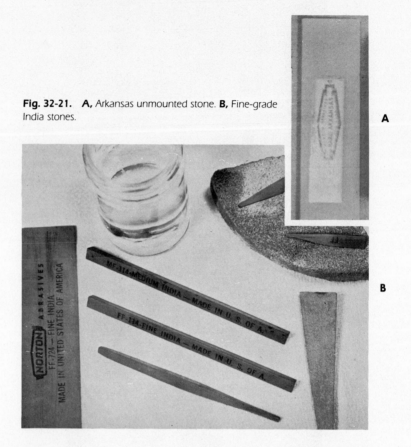

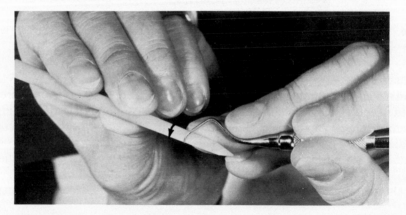

**Fig. 32-22.** Sharpening the face of a curette on a conical Arkansas stone.

of sharpening, thus preserving the temper of the metal. The oil also prevents metal filings from becoming embedded in the stone, thus ruining the effectiveness of the stone. Carborundum stones are very coarse and are ideal for recontouring instrument blades and rehoning very dull instruments; they are used with water as the lubricant.

Methods of sharpening may vary. A simple and systematic method employs an unmounted India stone. In this method the instrument is stabilized and the sharpening stone is moved along the cutting edge. The following steps should be followed to effectively sharpen a periodontal instrument:

1. Set up a clean sharpening area that has suitable illumination, a magnifying glass, and a hard countertop approximately elbow height.
2. Choose a stone grade appropriate to the amount of sharpening and/or recontouring needed. The stone should be sterilized if sharpening is done before patient treatment.
3. Properly lubricate the stone with a few drops of oil.
4. Hold the instrument to be sharpened in a firm palm grasp and stabilize the hand against the countertop. Grasp the sharpening stone between the thumb and fingers of the opposing hand.
5. Hold the instrument so that the face of the blade is parallel to the floor.
6. Place the stone against the lateral surface of the blade edge to be sharpened. Establish an angle between the face of the blade and the stone that is 100 degrees to 110 degrees. This ensures an angle of 70 to 80 degrees between the face and the lateral surface of the blade.
7. Gracey instruments and some sickle scalers have rounded blades. Preserving the shape of these blades is essential. Therefore, sharpen the Gracey curette in three parts beginning with the back third of the blade and working toward the toe third (see Fig. 32-33). Move the stone in short, consistent, firm, up-and-down strokes with emphasis on the down stroke. Sharpening of each third of the blade should end with a down stroke. If the edges of these rounded blades are flattened, the tip will be weakened and may break during use. Universal curettes and some sickle scalers have blades that are straight. These blades may be sharpened along the total length of the blade.
8. A sludge of oil and metal filings will appear on the face of the blade. Remove the sludge with a 2 × 2 gauze square. Check the instrument for sharpness with an acrylic stick and/or visual inspection.
9. Periodically sharpen the toe of the blade to keep the contour rounded. If the toe becomes pointed, it is weakened and may become susceptible to breakage. Also a pointed toe tends to gouge tissue and is uncomfortable to the patient. With continued sharpening the instruments become proportionally smaller. Such instruments are useful in areas of narrow access.

## WHEN TO SHARPEN

Instruments may be sharpened before, during, or after an appointment. How often an operator needs to sharpen an instrument depends on the amount and tenacity of calculus present and the extent of root planing necessary. Extensive root planing and/ or heavy deposits may require the instruments to be sharpened several times during an appointment. Lighter deposits may require the instruments be sharpened only before or just after the appointment. The most effective sharpening is before the instrument becomes too dull because at this time it is easier to rehone, takes less time, and ultimately conserves metal.

A good idea in the sharpening process is to keep a separate stone for each set of instruments. By having separate stones for each instrument setup, the stone can be used before patient appointments to prepare the instruments and during patient appointments. Also, the stone can be sterilized with the instruments.

## TESTING FOR SHARPNESS

The most direct method for determining the sharpness of an instrument is how the instrument works during scaling and root planing. A sharp instrument will grab or "bite" into the calculus/tooth surface during the working stroke. A sharp instrument will transmit the sense of root morphology and calculus to the operator. With a sharp instrument, calculus will be removed with an adequate but not excessive amount of pressure.

Sharpness may also be assessed tactilely with an acrylic stick. Adapt the blade in the working position to an acrylic stick. Evaluate how well the blade edge "bites" into the stick. If the blade does not firmly "bite" into the stick, the instrument needs sharpening.

The sharpness of an instrument may be determined by a visual inspection. The cutting edge can be easily discerned by holding the instrument under good illumination and magnification. An almost invisible even-looking edge indicates that the blade edge is sharp. If light is reflected off of the edge, the instrument is dull. A visual inspection should also include an assessment of the shape of the blade to ensure maintenance of the original form.

## Primer on instrumentation

The removal of calculus by scaling and root planing is complex and the result of the mastery of many subskills. Identifying and developing these subskills (often referred to as process skills) is difficult. It requires diligence and persistence. Proper development of these subskills leads to a clinically rewarding experience.

### GRASP

How an instrument is held influences the effectiveness of instrumentation. A proper grasp permits better tactile sensitivity, precise control of movements, instrument stability, and flexibility in movement. It reduces fatigue of the fingers, hands, and arms. With a proper grasp, less trauma is inflicted on hard and soft tissues, providing comfort to the patient during and after treatment.

### Modified pen grasp

The modified pen grasp is the most effective and stable grasp (Figs. 32-23 and 32-24). This grasp differs from the common pen grasp mainly by the position of the middle

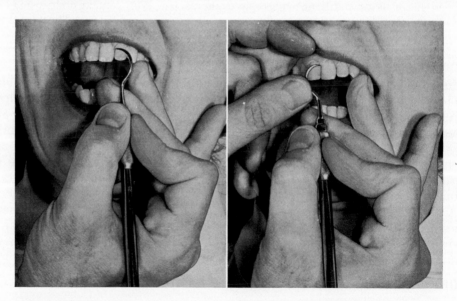

**Fig. 32-23.** The pen grasp with fourth finger rest commonly used for scaling and root planing.

finger on the handle of the instrument. The grasp is a three-point contact of the thumb, index, and middle fingers. The instrument is held by the thumb and index finger near the junction of the handle and shank. The thumb opposes the index and middle fingers on the handle. The index finger is bent at the second joint from the fingertip. The middle finger is positioned so that the lateral surface of the pad is resting on the instrument. The middle finger is also held snugly against the fourth finger. On the opposite side of the handle, the pad of the thumb rests between the middle and index fingers, creating a tripod effect. The instrument handle rests somewhere between the second knuckle and the V formed by the thumb and index finger.

The tripod effect of the modified pen grasp enhances control and allows the operator to rotate the instrument between the index and middle fingers. This precise rotation is essential in adapting the instrument blade to the continuously changing tooth contours as one moves along the root.

### Palm grasp

In the palm grasp the instrument is held by cupping all the fingers (except the thumb) around the handle (Fig. 32-25). The thumb serves as a fulcrum and simultaneously applies pressure against the instrument. Although used by some clinicians, the palm grasp has limitations in scaling and root planing because it offers limited maneuverability and reduced tactile sensitivity. These limitations render the palm grasp impractical for any precise and controlled movements. The palm grasp is good, however, for stabilizing instruments during sharpening.

### FULCRUMS

A fulcrum is a pivotal point from which work (scaling and root planing) is done (Fig. 32-26). The fourth (or ring) finger is the fulcrum preferred. The fulcrum may act as a finger rest or stabilizing point for light, exploratory strokes, or it may act as a pivotal point when power is needed. Although it is possible to use the third or middle finger, this is not recommended because it restricts movement during the activation of strokes and limits instrument control and tactile sensitivity.

An adequate fulcrum is essential for instrument control. It prevents laceration of the gingiva and injury to surrounding tissues and thus enhances patient comfort and protection. It also enhances patient confidence.

Maximal instrument control is achieved when the middle finger is kept next to the

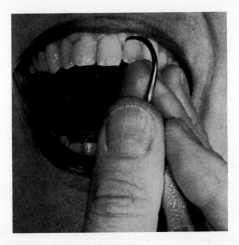

**Fig. 32-24.** The modified pen grasp with fourth finger rest helps to minimize fatigue from cramped fingers and enhances tactile sensitivity. Fatigue reduces tactile sensitivity.

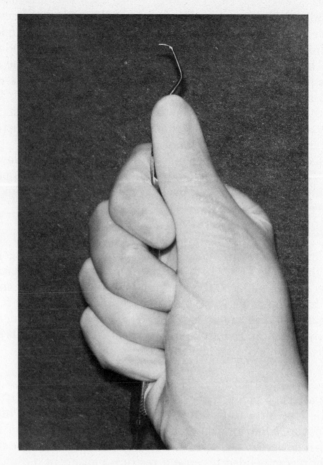

**Fig. 32-25.** Palm and thumb grasp in root planing.

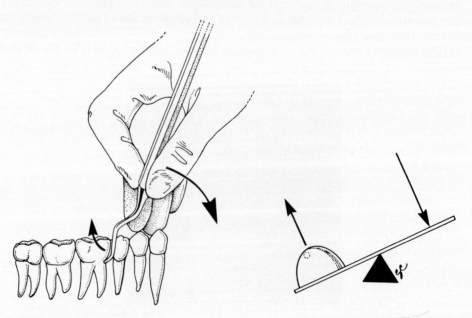

**Fig. 32-26.** The fulcrum is the stabilizing and pivotal point from which the working stroke used in scaling and root planing can occur.

ring finger while still maintaining its position on the shank of the instrument. This proximity of the third and fourth fingers is referred to as a *built-up fulcrum* (Fig. 32-27). Separation of the third and fourth fingers is termed a *split fulcrum* and results in a loss of power but no lessening of control (Fig. 32-28).

Proper finger rest is important in preventing injury to the patient's teeth and periodontal tissues and also for the patient's comfort. The operator who uses no finger rest or maintains an insecure rest may slip and cut the patient. The practitioner who applies excessive pressure during instrumentation will remove excessive tooth structure and

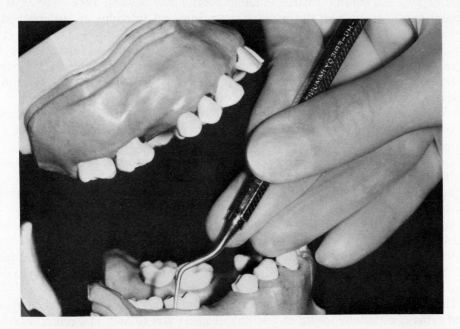

**Fig. 32-27.** Built-up fulcrum.

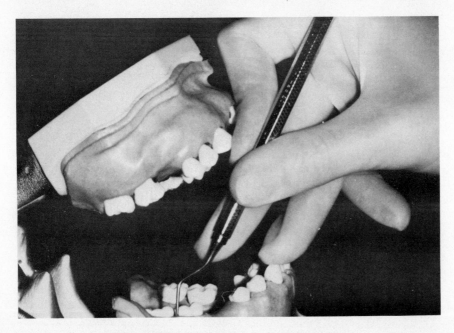

**Fig. 32-28.** Split fulcrum with fourth finger rest.

cause root sensitivity. Patients will be dissatisfied and will, in addition, characterize the dentist as having a heavy hand.

Touch perception is a necessity in finishing procedures and less important in scaling/planing. Remember that as tactile sensitivity goes down and more force is applied, it becomes easier to remove excess tooth structure, which will result in sensitivity.

Positions of fulcrums/finger rests tend to be area-specific in the mouth and may be approached in a variety of ways. Fulcrums may be classified as being either intraoral or extraoral. Intraoral fulcrums are ideally established near the working area and facilitate maximal control. Instrumentation control may become more difficult as the fulcrum moves away from the working area. Intraoral fulcrums are established by placing the pad of the ring finger on an occlusal surface near or adjacent to the working area. The whole hand may then pivot about the fulcrum. Intraoral fulcrums are universal and may be used on both the maxillary and mandibular arches. The fulcrum of choice is on the mandible; access may be restricted with an intraoral fulcrum on maxillary molars.

When the teeth, tongue, or facial muscles impede instrument access, variations of the basic fulcrums may be used. The following are some alternate fulcrums that may be used:

A *cross-arch fulcrum* is a finger rest placed on the occlusal surfaces of the teeth on the other side of the same arch. For example, for access to the distal and lingual surfaces of mandibular right molars, the fulcrum is on the biting surfaces of the left side of the arch (Fig. 32-29).

An *opposite-arch fulcrum* is a fulcrum placed on the occlusal surfaces of the arch opposite the working area. For example, for access to maxillary right posterior teeth, a fulcrum is placed on the mandibular right occlusal surfaces (Fig. 32-30). An equally effective fulcrum accesses the mesial surfaces of mandibular molars from the maxillary arch.

The *finger-on-finger fulcrum* is established on the index or thumb of the opposite hand. This is especially useful in edentulous areas and to help in gaining access to the palatal surfaces of posterior teeth on the operator's side (Fig. 32-31).

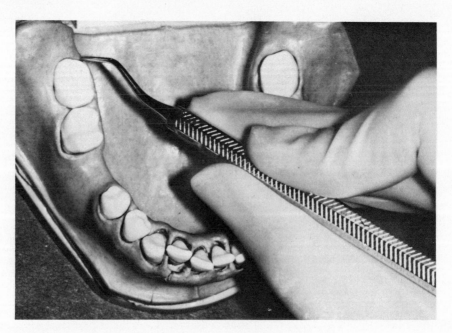

**Fig. 32-29.** Cross-arch fulcrum.

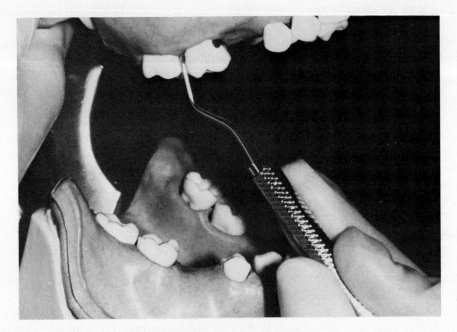

**Fig. 32-30.** Opposite-arch fulcrum.

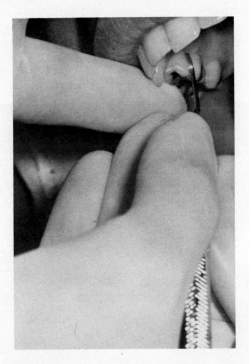

**Fig. 32-31.** Finger-on-finger fulcrum.

*Extraoral fulcrums* are often helpful for effective instrumentation of maxillary posterior teeth. The fingers rest on the lower border of the mandible, which facilitates optimal access and power (Fig. 32-32).

If control seems to be compromised, the fulcrum should be reinforced to stabilize the instrument. A *reinforced fulcrum* is accomplished by placing the index finger or thumb of the opposite hand on the shank of the instrument. Reinforced fulcrums are most commonly used with extraoral or opposite arch fulcrums (see Fig. 32-42).

## WORKING STROKE

The working stroke, or the way the instrument is activated and used against the tooth surface, is important for efficient and effective endotoxin, plaque, and calculus removal. Several components are important to the successful preparation, initiation, activation, and completion of working and exploring instrument strokes. These are: blade adaptation, instrument angulation, blade insertion, and lateral pressure, and the activation, direction, and nature of the working stroke itself.

*Blade adaptation* is the way in which the blade of the instrument is placed against the tooth surface. The primary goal of proper blade adaptation is to prevent tooth gouging, tissue mutilation, or patient discomfort. The instrument blade face is placed facing and conforming to the contour of the tooth surface without lacerating the gingiva or digging into the tooth structure.

The blade of a curette may be divided into three parts, the back third, the middle third, and the toe third (Fig. 32-33). The toe third of the blade must contact the tooth surface at all times. On the broad, flat buccal and lingual tooth surfaces of mandibular and maxillary molars, approximately half of the blade may be adapted. The most difficult areas for proper blade placement are the line angles, depressions, and concavities, narrow root surfaces, cervical areas, and furcations; there less of the blade surface can make proper contact. The toe third of the blade is used and the instrument is rotated slightly between the fingers as the instrument is advanced along the tooth surface (Fig. 32-34).

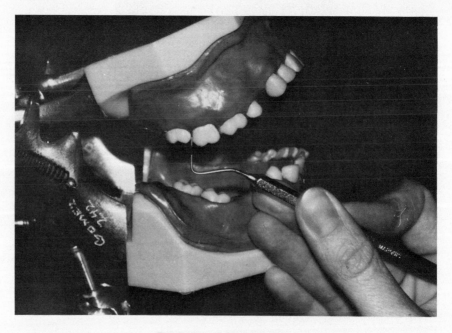

**Fig. 32-32.** Extraoral fulcrum.

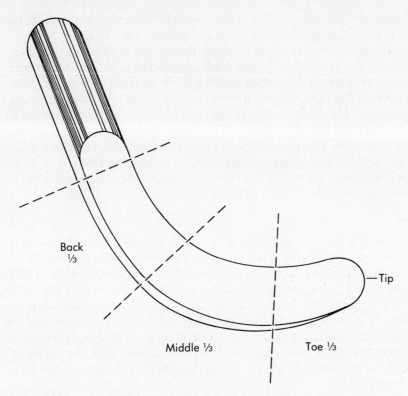

**Fig. 32-33.** The curette blade. The back third is that part nearest the shank of the instrument. The toe third extends from the rounded tip of the blade to approximately one-third the distance of the length of the blade.

Back
⅓

—Tip

Middle ⅓        Toe ⅓

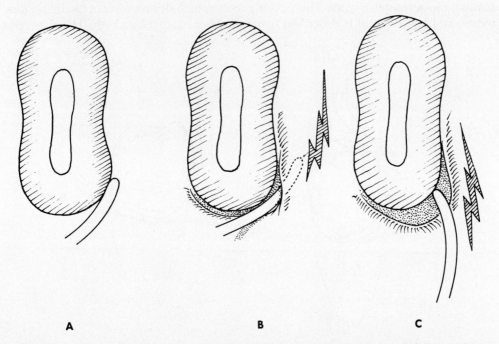

**A**                              **B**                              **C**

**Fig. 32-34.** Blade adaptation. **A,** Blade in proper contact. The toe third of the blade is used. **B,** Improper contact of back third of blade with tooth, leading to tissue laceration by toe of blade. **C,** Figure of the tip of the blade adapted to the tooth surface, leading to tissue distention and tooth gouging.

It is important that the toe third of the blade should be directed apically rather than coronally to ensure access to the base of the sulcus (Fig. 32-35).

*Blade angulation* is the angle or plane formed by the face of the blade and the tooth surface. The purpose of proper blade angulation is to form a cutting edge that is in contact with the tooth surface. For the work stroke the proper angulation is 70 to 90 degrees. If the blade is open more than 90 degrees, the blade angulation is said to be "too open." The blade no longer contacts the tooth surface, resulting in the loss of a cutting edge or tissue laceration. (The open blade may be used intentionally in soft tissue curettage. This procedure should not be confused with unintentional tissue laceration.) A blade angulation of less than 45 degrees is referred to as being "too closed" and will drag over rather than remove calculus. This leads to burnishing rather than removing calculus (Fig. 32-36).

### Insertion

Scaling begins with the insertion of the blade subgingivally. The blade is inserted closed face in an exploratory stroke. During insertion, the blade-to-tooth angulation approaches zero degrees or a parallel relationship with the tooth surface. This facilitates instrument access to the base of the sulcus or periodontal pocket (Fig. 32-36).

*Lateral pressure* is the force applied to the tooth surface by the cutting edge of the instrument. It is controlled by fulcrum force and grasp. This force may be altered depending on the amount and tenacity of deposits present. Hard pressure is exerted to chip ledges or rings of tenacious calculus. In most cases, firm but moderate pressure is required. As the amount and/or tenacity of calculus decreases, the force exerted may be diminished.

If too little pressure is applied in calculus removal, the calculus will be incompletely removed and burnished. If the pressure is not controlled (uneven pressure), the pressure will result in rippled root surfaces or root gouging.

*Instrument activation* (working stroke) refers to the movement made by the instrument to accomplish work. The working motion includes movement by the fingers, wrists, and forearm and is described by its direction, activity, or both. There are two

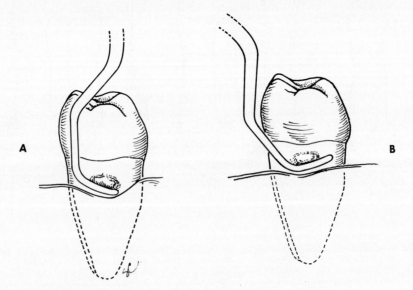

**Fig. 32-35.**  Insertion and blade adaptation. **A,** Proper insertion with toe third of blade on the tooth surface, tip of blade pointing apically. **B,** Improper positioning, tip of blade is pointing coronally and will be caught by the contact point. Back third of blade is adapted to the tooth surface.

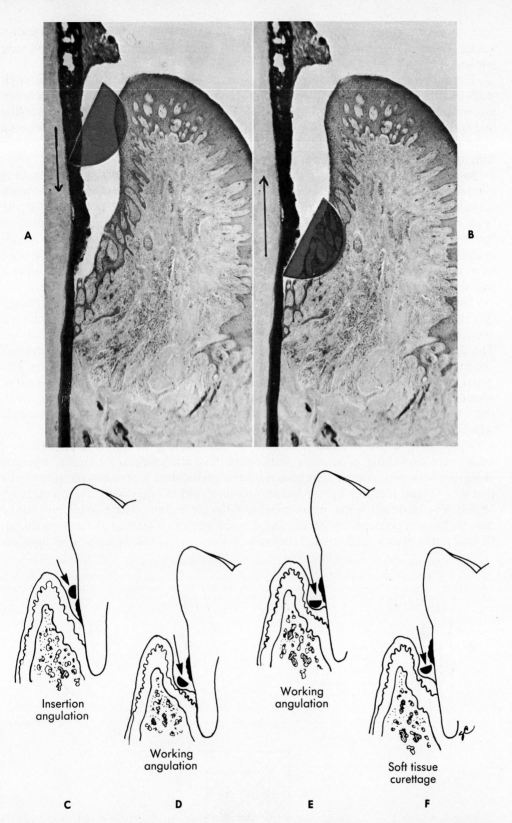

**Fig. 32-36.** **A,** Curette in exploratory stroke in closed-face position. **B,** The blade is manipulated past all concretions until the back of the blade comes to rest on the junctional epithelium. **C** to **E,** The sequential positions of the curette blade from insertion to positioning for engaging and removing calculus. All three illustrations imply that the working (lead) cutting edge is in contact with the tooth. **F,** Intentional soft tissue curettage. (Note the distention of the pocket wall in **E** and **F** and unintentional curettage.)

basic strokes used in root instrumentation: the exploratory stroke and the working stroke. The working stroke may be further divided into the scaling and the root planing stroke.

The purpose of the exploratory stroke is to determine the topography of the tooth surface subgingivally. The exploratory stroke is also used to evaluate the location, amount, and texture of calculus deposits. The exploratory stroke must be well controlled and deliberate in its execution. To accomplish an effective exploratory stroke, the grasp is firm, the fulcrum is stable, and lateral pressure against the tooth surface is light yet firm and controlled. The stroke is initiated as a feeling stroke.

In general, the direction, length, and pressure of the scaling/root planing stroke is determined by the amount of calculus, the shape of the sulcus or pocket, the tooth surface anatomy, and the tone of the gingival tissue. The typical stroke used is the "pull stroke" in a coronal direction. The Gracey curettes were originally designed as "push stroke" instruments. The "push stroke" was accomplished by moving the curette apically to dislodge calculus. The Gracey curette has since been redesigned to be used as a "pull stroke" instrument. Thus the "push stroke" is infrequently used because it might force calculus and debris into the soft tissues.

The scaling stroke is a short, powerful pull stroke designed to split or dislodge calculus from tooth surfaces. Movement for the power stroke is initiated by the finger, wrist, and forearm muscles, with the fingers locked on the fulcrum and the curette. The fulcrum acts as a pivot from which force can be applied at the blade. Power is obtained from the fulcrum by applying increased pressure to the fulcrum finger. The grasp should be controlled with the handle of the instrument locked between the second knuckle and the V of the hand. The stroke is initiated as a rocking motion with the wrist and forearm. This rocking may produce an undulation in the root surface, which is made smooth by the root planing strokes.

The scaling stroke is usually followed by root planing strokes. The root planing stroke is a smoothing or shaving stroke that, like the exploratory stroke, requires absolute instrument control. The root planing stroke differs from the scaling stroke in that it is longer, requires lighter lateral pressure, and is often multidirectional (Fig. 32-37). The blade angle may be reduced to 40 to 60 degrees. The root planing stroke may be likened conceptually to planing a wood surface. The root planing stroke, although initiated as a "pull stroke" (coronal direction), may also be vertical, oblique, or

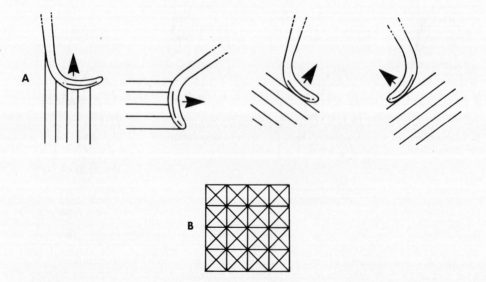

**Fig. 32-37. A,** Root planing strokes are multidirectional. **B,** Root planing strokes are cumulative.

horizontal. The vertical and oblique strokes are the most common. The vertical stroke is directed in the same plane as the long axis of the tooth and is most commonly used on the anterior teeth and the interproximal surfaces of posterior teeth. The oblique stroke is diagonal to the long axis of the tooth and is useful in approaching line angles and posterior facial and lingual surfaces where vertical strokes are difficult to achieve because of facial musculature. Both the vertical and oblique strokes help protect the epithelial attachment. Horizontal strokes are often employed at the cementoenamel junctions and line angles and are used to augment the vertical and oblique strokes.

Many clinicians use a separate set of curettes for final root planing. These instruments have fine blades and flexible shanks.[75] Regardless of technique used, remember the root surface should be explored repeatedly while planing, using the root explorer to determine if a smooth, hard finish has been produced.

**Finishing strokes**

The attachment of calculus in spaces formerly occupied by Sharpey's fibers and in cemental irregularities makes the removal of cementum necessary. However, the deliberate removal of extensive amounts of tooth structure cannot be justified. Clinical and histologic investigations have shown that more than half the cementum is removed during root planing. Dentin is exposed, and any remaining cementum is very thin when the root surface feels clinically hard and smooth. Clinicians have not been able to determine by touch whether cementum or dentin is being instrumented.[42] Overinstrumentation should be avoided; it is unnecessary and can lead to root sensitivity.

In summary, the steps involved in instrument activation are as follows:

1. Adapt the blade to the tooth surface
2. Close the blade
3. Insert the blade to the base of the sulcus or periodontal pocket
4. Open the blade to establish a cutting edge
5. Lock the fingers on the curette and the fulcrum
6. Apply fulcrum pressure
7. Apply lateral pressure against the tooth
8. Begin a wrist and arm motion, moving the instrument in a coronal direction (pull stroke); as the instrument is pulled coronally, finger flexion will accompany the wrist and forearm action

## HAND POSITION

Hand position is important for proper instrumentation, blade angulation, working stroke activation, and access. On the mandibular arch, for example, the hand must be high enough to activate the working stroke. The hand position changes for every surface of every tooth and is therefore explained in detail in the section "Atlas of instrumentation procedures," pp. 687-711.

## PATIENT/OPERATOR POSITION

Patient/operator positioning is commonly identified by the position of the small hand on a clock in relation to the face of the clock. The patient is represented by the face of the clock. The operator is represented by the small hand of the clock (Fig. 32-38).

For the maxillary arch, the patient position is usually supine with feet level or slightly elevated (Fig. 32-39). For the mandibular arch, the back of the chair is raised approximately 30 to 40 degrees from the supine position (Fig. 32-40).

The height of the chair should be about elbow height of the operator who should be in a relaxed and sitting position. For a right-handed operator, the field of positioning is within the 8 and 1 o'clock positions. For the left-handed operator, the field of positioning is within the 11 and 4 o'clock positions (see Fig. 32-38). To be comfortable for long periods of time the operator should work with feet flat on the floor and with back straight.

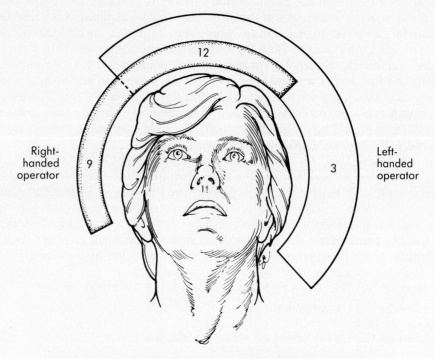

**Fig. 32-38.** Patient-operator positioning.

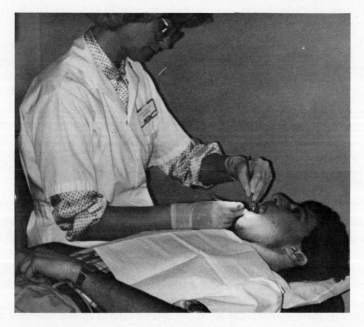

**Fig. 32-39.** The patient is supine for access to the maxillary arch.

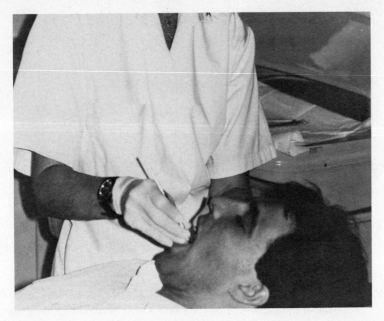

**Fig. 32-40.** The back of the patient's chair is raised to a 30- to 40-degree angle to the floor to access the mandibular arch.

## EXTENT AND PLAN OF INSTRUMENTATION

Teeth should be planed in a systematic order and sequence. Several approaches are possible. Treatment should be limited to specific areas so that tooth/root surfaces can be completely debrided and polished in the allotted time. In cases of early periodontitis, teeth may be scaled in quadrants. Often as much as half the mouth may be completed in a 1-hour appointment. In moderate or advanced cases the number of teeth scaled may be limited to one quadrant or even to one sextant (4 to 5 teeth). Although scaling/root planing may take multiple appointments, it is an efficient method of operation. Haphazard or spot scaling is time consuming, inefficient, and fails to remove all deposits.

The extent of root instrumentation depends on the condition of the tissues, the amount of calculus, and the time reserved for the patient. In very severe cases, it may not be possible to plane more than a few teeth. Whatever is done should be done thoroughly before proceeding to the next area. Local anesthesia or nitrous oxide analgesia may be required for patient comfort. If two quadrants are scaled in one visit, it is advisable to instrument both quadrants on one side of the mouth. This will permit the patient to chew comfortably on the uninstrumented side. Except in severe cases, the patient should not experience more than mild discomfort.

Surgical dressings may be used in selected cases after root planing, particularly if considerable inadvertent gingival curettage has been performed. This tends to reduce any bleeding and postoperative pain and makes the patient more comfortable. Saline rinses may be prescribed postoperatively as needed.

## Atlas of instrumentation procedures

This section deals in detail with the proper instrumentation by sextant for scaling and root planing (Figs. 32-41 to 32-52).

## Maxillary right posterior sextant (facial) Nos. 1-5 (Fig. 32-41).

**GRASP**
- Use a modified pen grasp (**C**).
- The fingers form a tripod near the junction between the instrument shank and the handle of the instrument. The instrument may be extended for extraoral fulcrums.
- The handle of the instrument rests in the V of the hand.

**FULCRUMS**
**A,** Extraoral with the palm up. The palm is facing toward the patient's ear. The back of the hand rests on the lower border of the mandible at about the first joint.
**B,** The fulcrum may be intraoral on the maxillary arch with the palm down and facing toward the chin. This fulcrum has limitations posterior to the premolars. (In general, intraoral fulcrums are used for control and extraoral fulcrums for strength.)
**D,** The fulcrum may be intraoral on the mandibular arch (opposite-arch fulcrum) with the palm down. In this instance, fulcrum on the anterior teeth.
**E,** The fulcrum may be extraoral and reinforced with the thumb of the opposite hand. The reinforcement will increase control.

**INSTRUMENTS**
- Gracey 7/8 for direct facial surfaces. Use vertical or oblique strokes from the distobuccal line angle to the mesiobuccal line angle.
- Gracey 11/12 for mesial surfaces, vertical strokes. (Lower shank of the instrument should be parallel to the tooth surface.)
- Gracey 13/14 for distal surfaces, vertical strokes. (Lower shank of the instrument should be parallel to the tooth surface.)

**BLADE**
- Adapt the toe third of the blade at line angles and interproximally.
- The shank should be parallel to allow the toe third to be apically positioned so that the back of the blade abuts the tissue.
- The toe half of the blade can be adapted on the facial surface.

**PATIENT POSITIONING**
Supine.

**OPERATOR POSITIONING**
9 to 10 o'clock position.

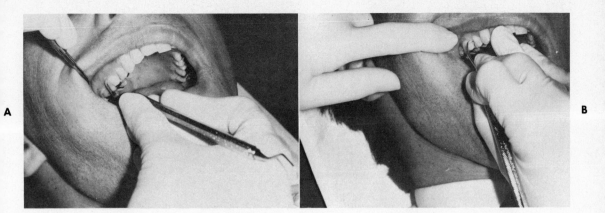

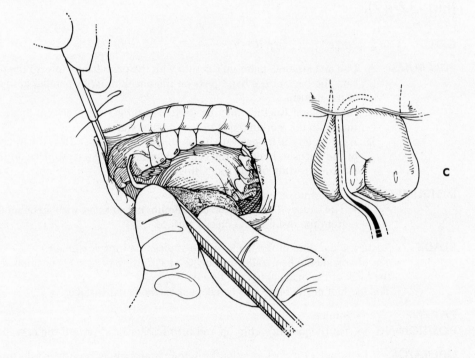

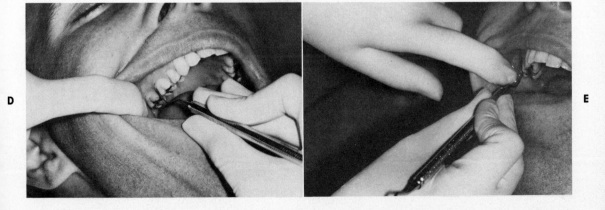

## Maxillary right posterior sextant (palatal) Nos. 1-5 (Fig. 32-42).

**GRASP**   Use a modified pen grasp **(C)**.

**FULCRUMS**   **A,** Use an extraoral, palm-up fulcrum with the palm facing toward the patient's ear. The back of the hand rests on the cheek muscles parallel to the corner of the mouth.

**B,** An intraoral fulcrum may be used. The finger rests on the tooth surface mesial to the working area in the maxillary arch.

**D,** A finger on the finger rest affords stability and facility. Rest the index finger of the opposite hand on the occlusal surfaces of the teeth. Use an intraoral fulcrum, resting on the index finger.

**INSTRUMENTS**   • The same as for the facial surfaces.
• The Gracey 13/14 may be used for lingual surfaces with an oblique stroke from the distal to the mesial surface.

**BLADE**   • Adapt the toe third of the blade at line angles and interproximally.
• The shank should be parallel to allow the toe third to be apically positioned so that the back of the blade abuts the tissue.
• The toe half of the blade can be adapted on the facial surface.

**PATIENT POSITIONING**   • Supine.
• Tilt the patient's chin up and turn his/her head toward the operator.

**OPERATOR POSITIONING**   • About 11 o'clock position for intraoral and finger-on-finger fulcrums.
• About 9 to 10 o'clock position if the extraoral fulcrum is used and as the hand rest moves toward the chin.

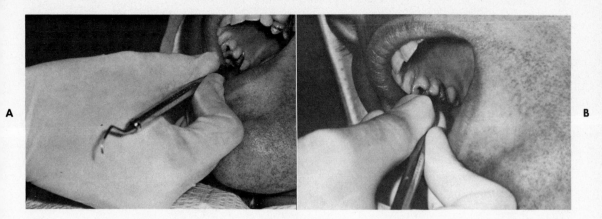

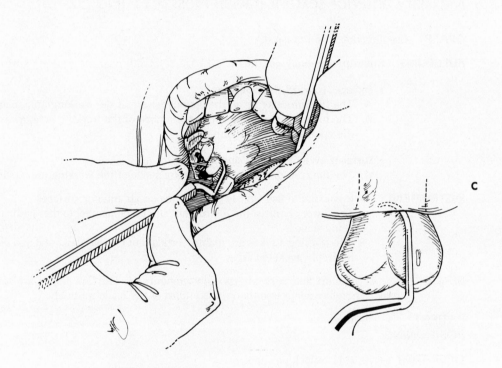

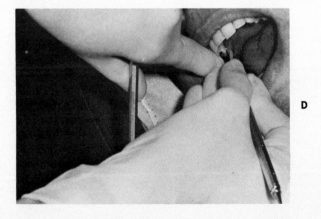

## Maxillary anterior sextant (facial) Nos. 6-11 (Fig. 32-43).

**GRASP**   Use a modified pen grasp (**C**).

**FULCRUMS**   Fulcrum intraorally on the incisal edge of a tooth near the working surface.

- **Surfaces toward the operator**
  **A,** The fulcrum may be on the operator's side of the working area, palm up.
  **B,** The fulcrum may be on the opposite side of the working area, away from the operator with the palm down.

- **Surfaces away from the operator**
  **D,** The fulcrum may be on the operator's side of the working area, palm up.

**INSTRUMENTS**   • It is usual to use Gracey 5/6 curettes on all anterior surfaces.
   • The lower shank of the instrument should be parallel to the tooth surface being scaled.
   • The working strokes are mainly vertical but can be horizontal and oblique in deeply pocketed areas.

**BLADE**   The root anatomy and curvature is quite pronounced. The line angles are severely curved. Therefore adapt less than the toe third of the blade routinely.

**PATIENT POSITIONING**   Supine.

**OPERATOR POSITIONING**   9 to 11 o'clock position.

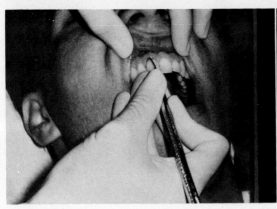
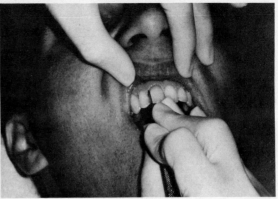

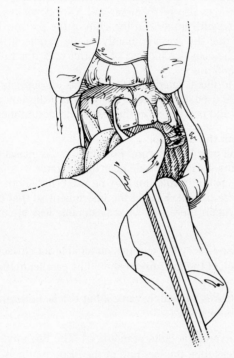
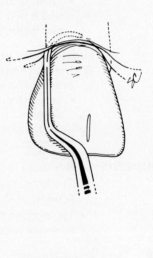

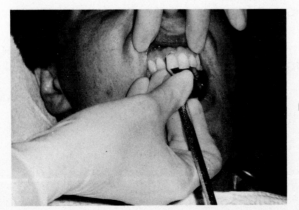

## Maxillary anterior sextant (palatal) Nos. 6-11 (Fig. 32-44).

**GRASP**    Use a modified pen grasp (**C**).

**FULCRUMS**
- **Surfaces toward the operator**

  **A,** Fulcrum on the incisal edge of the tooth adjacent to the working area on the side away from the operator. The fulcrum is intraoral and palm down.
  - The fulcrum may also be extraoral and palm down (not shown). Rest the fourth and fifth fingers on the chin of the patient. Extend the instrument so that the grasp is mainly on the handle of the instrument. (There may be considerable loss of control with this fulcrum, but it is useful for exploring.)
  - There is an intraoral fulcrum referred to as an opposite-arch fulcrum, which may be used occasionally (not shown). Fulcrum on the mandibular incisors and proceed as in the extraoral fulcrum mentioned above.

- **Surfaces away from the operator**

  **B,** Use an intraoral palm-up fulcrum. Fulcrum on the incisal edge of a tooth near the working area on the side near the operator.
  - An extraoral, palm-up fulcrum may be used (not shown). Fulcrum on the chin of the patient. Extend the instrument so that the grasp is on the handle. Again there may be considerable loss of control with this fulcrum.

**INSTRUMENTS**
- It is usual to use Gracey 5/6 curettes on all anterior surfaces.
- The lower shank of the instrument should be parallel to the tooth surface being scaled.
- The working strokes are mainly vertical but can be horizontal and oblique in deeply pocketed areas.

**BLADE**    The root anatomy and curvature is quite pronounced. The line angles are severely curved. Therefore adapt less than the toe third of the blade routinely.

**PATIENT POSITIONING**
- Supine.
- Lift the patient's chin.
- In many instances indirect vision is advised.

**OPERATOR POSITIONING**
- For surfaces toward the operator, an 8 to 9 o'clock position is advised.
- For surfaces away from the operator and an intraoral fulcrum, an 11 to 12 o'clock position is recommended.
- For surfaces away from the operator and an extraoral fulcrum, a 10 to 11 o'clock position is advised.

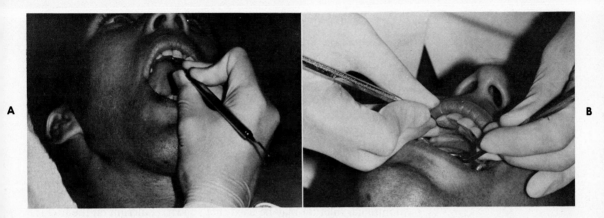

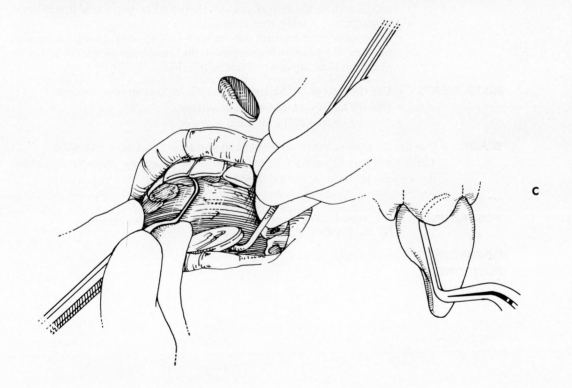

# Maxillary left posterior sextant (facial) Nos. 12-16 (Fig. 32-45).

**GRASP**  Use a modified pen grasp **(B)**.

**FULCRUMS**  **A,** An extraoral fulcrum is quite acceptable. The fourth and fifth fingers rest on the lower border of the mandible. The palm is facing toward the operator and cups the chin. This fulcrum affords the operator with both power and control.

- An intraoral fulcrum may be used (not shown). Fulcrum on the occlusal edge of the maxillary teeth near the working area. The fulcrum finger should rest on the buccal cusp(s). (It should be noted that this fulcrum, although quite stable, may limit power.)
- An opposite-arch fulcrum may be used (not shown). This is an intraoral fulcrum. The fulcrum finger rests on the mandibular incisors or bicuspids. The palm is facing down, cupping the chin.

**INSTRUMENTS**
- Use the Gracey 7/8 for the facial surfaces. Use an oblique stroke.
- Use the Gracey 11/12 for mesial surfaces.
- Use the Gracey 13/14 for distal surfaces.

**BLADE**
- Use the toe third of the instrument at all line angles and interproximally.
- The toe half may be used on the facial surface of the molars; however, if furcation depressions are present, the toe third is best.

**PATIENT POSITIONING**
- Supine.
- The patient's face should be turned toward the operator.
- Tilt the patient's chin up.

**OPERATOR POSITIONING**  9 to 10 o'clock position.

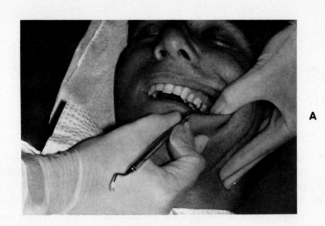

A

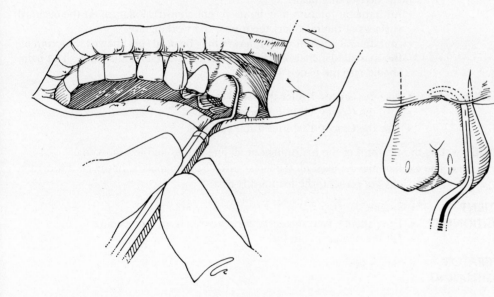

B

## Maxillary left posterior sextant (palatal) Nos. 12-16 (Fig. 32-46).

**GRASP**   Use a modified pen grasp **(C)**.

**FULCRUMS**   **A,** An extraoral fulcrum may be used. The fourth and fifth fingers should rest on the lower border of the mandible. The palm will cup the chin. This is the preferred fulcrum.

**B,** The extraoral and opposite-arch fulcrums may be reinforced by using the index finger of the opposite hand. This is a good way to increase control and still maintain strength. Place the index finger on the shank of the instrument near the working blade.

- An intraoral fulcrum may be used (not shown). Fulcrum on the occlusal surfaces of the maxillary teeth near the working area.
- An intraoral opposite-arch fulcrum may be used (not shown). Fulcrum on the mandibular incisors or bicuspids on the mandibular arch. The palm should cup the patient's chin.

**INSTRUMENTS**
- Use the Gracey 7/8 for the facial surfaces. Use an oblique stroke.
- Use the Gracey 11/12 for mesial surfaces.
- Use the Gracey 13/14 for distal surfaces.

**BLADE**
- Use the toe third of the instrument at all line angles and interproximally.
- The toe half may be used on the facial surface of the molars; however, if furcation depressions are present, the toe third is best.

**PATIENT POSITIONING**
- Supine.
- The patient's face should be turned away from the operator.
- Tilt the patient's chin up.

**OPERATOR POSITIONING**   9 o'clock position.

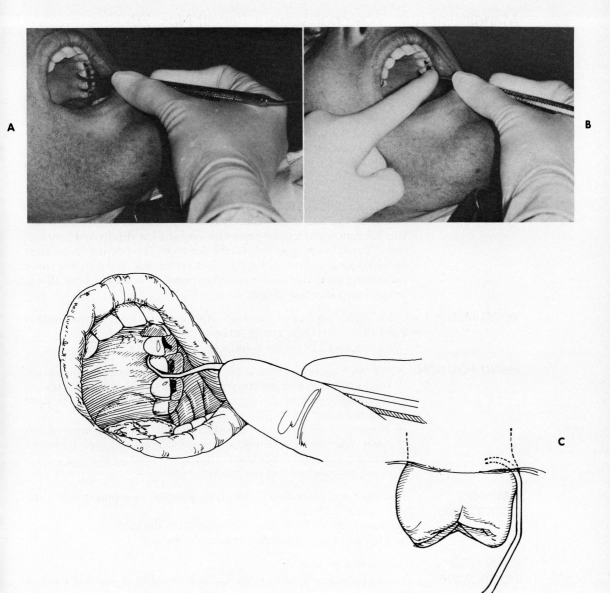

## Mandibular right posterior sextant (facial) Nos. 28-32 (Fig. 32-47).

**GRASP**   Use a modified pen grasp (**C**).

**FULCRUMS**   **A,** The basic fulcrum for all mandibular teeth is the built-up fulcrum. The fulcrum is intraoral with the fourth finger resting on the occlusal/incisal surfaces of the bicuspids and/or incisors. The palm is facing down.

**B,** For mesial surfaces, an opposite-arch fulcrum may be used. This fulcrum is especially good for removal of heavy calculus deposits or access to deep pockets. The fulcrum is intraoral on the maxillary incisors or bicuspids. The instrument is extended into the mesial surfaces of the mandibular teeth. Lateral pressure is exerted with the first and middle fingers.

- For mesial surfaces, a cross-arch fulcrum may also be used (not shown). This fulcrum is particularly suited for very shallow depths and light calculus. The fulcrum is on the mandibular arch. The fulcrum finger rests on the occlusal surfaces of the bicuspids on the side of the arch opposite the working area. This fulcrum sacrifices strength and control but affords better blade adaptation in tight areas.

**INSTRUMENTS**
- Use a Gracey 7/8 for facial surfaces. An oblique stroke is recommended.
- Use a Gracey 11/12 for mesial surfaces.
- Use a Gracey 13/14 for distal surfaces.

**HAND POSITION**
- For the traditional intraoral fulcrum and on the mesial surfaces, the hand must be raised and turned so that the thumb is pointing toward the mandibular teeth and is pushing against the instrument. The palm is facing down.
- There is an alternative hand position for the traditional intraoral fulcrum. Again for mesial surfaces, the second finger may apply the lateral pressure against the instrument. Rotate the hand so that the palm is facing toward the ear of the patient.

**PATIENT POSITIONING**
- Raise the back of the dental chair from a supine to approximately a 45-degree angle to the floor.
- The patient should be at about elbow height to the operator.
- Turn the patient's head slightly toward the operator.

**OPERATOR POSITIONING**
- 8 to 9 o'clock position.
- For the opposite arch fulcrum, the operator should be at the 12 to 1 o'clock position.

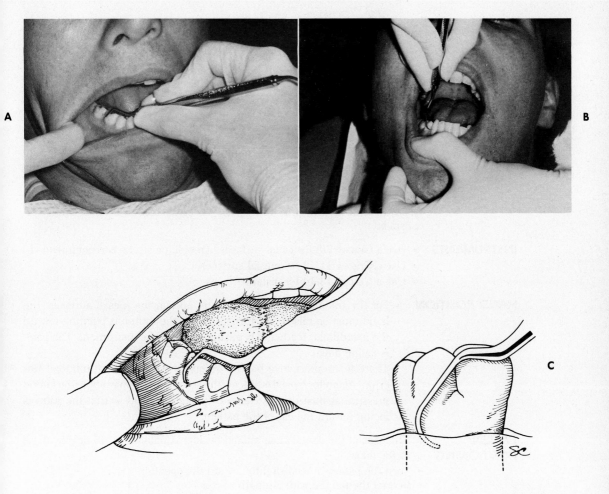

# Mandibular right posterior sextant (lingual) Nos. 28-32 (Fig. 32-48).

**GRASP**  Use a modified pen grasp (**C**).

**FULCRUMS**
**A,** An intraoral built-up fulcrum is best used. The ring finger rests on the incisal edge of the anterior teeth. The palm may be down or facing toward the patient's ear.

**B,** An intraoral maxillary fulcrum (opposite-arch fulcrum) may be used for mesial surfaces. The ring finger rests on the maxillary incisors and/or bicuspids.

**INSTRUMENTS**
- Use a Gracey 7/8 for facial surfaces. An oblique stroke is recommended.
- Use a Gracey 11/12 for mesial surfaces.
- Use a Gracey 13/14 for distal surfaces.

**HAND POSITION**
- For the traditional intraoral fulcrum and on the mesial surfaces, the hand must be raised and turned so that the thumb is pointing toward the mandibular teeth and is pushing against the instrument. The palm is facing down.
- There is an alternative hand position for the traditional intraoral fulcrum. Again for mesial surfaces, the second finger may apply the lateral pressure against the instrument. Rotate the hand so that the palm is facing toward the ear of the patient.

**PATIENT POSITIONING**
- The back of the dental chair should be approximately at a 45-degree angle to the floor.
- Turn the patient's head slightly toward the operator.
- Retract the tongue with a mouth mirror.

**OPERATOR POSITIONING**
- 9 to 10 o'clock position.
- For mesial surfaces and an opposite arch fulcrum, the operator needs to be at a 12 to 1 o'clock position.

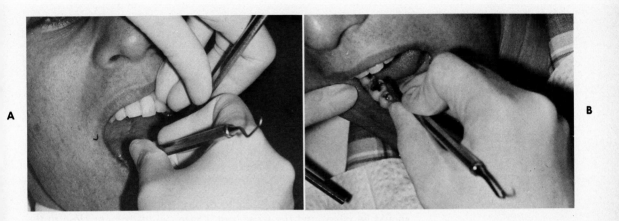

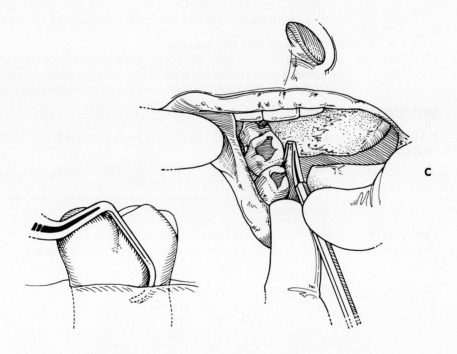

## Mandibular anterior sextant (facial) Nos. 22-27 (Fig. 32-49).

**GRASP**    Use a modified pen grasp (**C**). It is important to use fingers to rotate the blade around the sharp line angles of lower anterior teeth.

**FULCRUMS**
- **Surfaces toward the operator**
  **A,** Fulcrum on the incisal edge of a tooth near the working area. The hand should be raised and the wrist bent. Grasp the instrument close to the shank with the middle finger on the shank of the instrument. The thumb should point down toward the incisal edge and should press laterally against the instrument that will be pressing laterally against the tooth.

- **Surfaces away from the operator**
  **B,** Fulcrum on the incisal edge of the tooth, with the palm facing toward the patient's nose. Grasp the instrument, with the surfaces, toward the operator. The first finger and the thumb supply the lateral pressure.

**INSTRUMENT**    Gracey 5/6.

**PATIENT POSITIONING**
- The back of the dental chair should be approximately at a 45-degree angle to the floor
- Turn the patient's head slightly toward the operator.
- Retract the tongue with a mouth mirror.
- For surfaces toward the operator, turn the patient's head slightly toward the operator.

**OPERATOR POSITIONING**
- For surfaces toward the operator, 9 o'clock position.
- For surfaces away from the operator, 12 o'clock position.

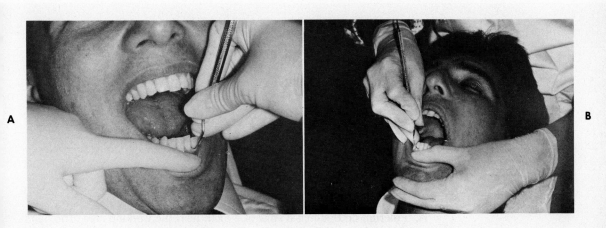

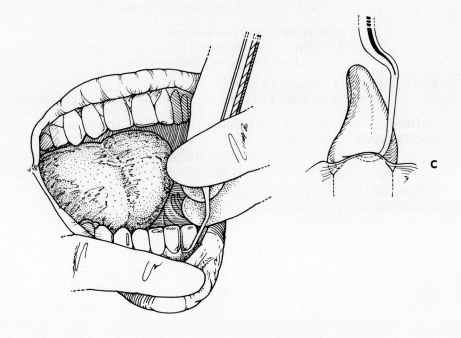

## Mandibular anterior sextant (lingual) Nos. 22-27 (Fig. 32-50).

**GRASP**   Use a modified pen grasp (**C**).

**FULCRUMS**   • **Surfaces toward the operator**
**A,** Fulcrum on the incisal edge of a tooth near the working area. The hand should be high with the wrist bent. Grasp the instrument close to the shank with the middle finger on the shank. The first finger and the thumb should press laterally against the instrument.

• **Surfaces away from the operator**
**B,** Fulcrum should be toward the operator except the thumb alone exerts the lateral pressure against the instrument.

**INSTRUMENTS**   • Use the Gracey 5/6.
• A Gracey 13/14 may be used on the direct lingual surfaces.

**PATIENT POSITIONING**   • The back of the dental chair should be approximately at a 45-degree angle to the floor.
• Turn the patient's head slightly toward the operator.
• Retract the tongue with a mouth mirror.

**OPERATOR POSITIONING**   • For surfaces toward the operator, 9 o'clock position.
• For surfaces away from the operator, 12 o'clock position.

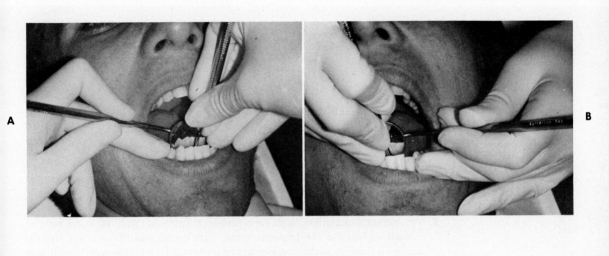

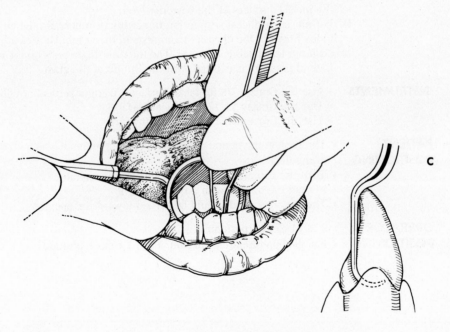

## Mandibular left posterior sextant (facial) Nos. 17-21 (Fig. 32-51).

**GRASP**   Use a modified pen grasp (**C**).

**FULCRUMS**  **A,** Use an intraoral, built-up fulcrum. Fulcrum on the incisal/occlusal surfaces of the lateral incisors, cuspids, or bicuspids.

**B,** An intraoral maxillary arch (opposite-arch fulcrum) may be used for the mesial surfaces of the posterior teeth. The fourth and fifth fingers rest on the incisal edges of the anterior maxillary teeth. Extend the instrument into the mesial surfaces of the posterior teeth.

**D,** For mesial surfaces, a finger-on-finger fulcrum may also be employed. The index finger of the opposite hand rests in the vestibular area adjacent to the posterior teeth being accessed. The fulcrum finger rests on the index finger. Lateral pressure is exerted with the thumb of the grasp.

**INSTRUMENTS**
- Use the Gracey 7/8 for facial surfaces, using a vertical or oblique stroke.
- Use the Gracey 11/12 for mesial surfaces.
- Use the Gracey 13/14 for distal surfaces.

**PATIENT POSITIONING**
- The back of the dental chair should be approximately at a 45-degree angle to the floor.
- Turn the patient's head slightly toward the operator.
- Retract the tongue with a mouth mirror.
- The patient's head should be turned toward the operator.

**OPERATOR POSITIONING**
- 9 to 11 o'clock position.
- For the opposite arch fulcrum, 12 to 1 o'clock position.

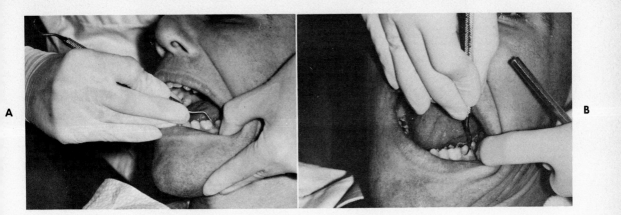

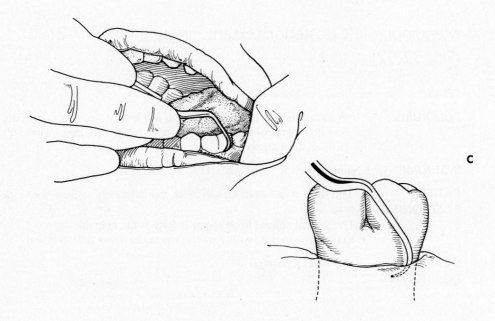

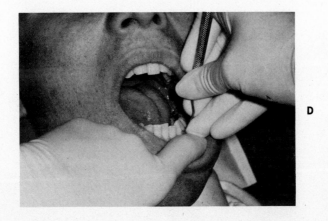

## Mandibular left posterior sextant (lingual) Nos. 17-21 (Fig. 32-52).

**GRASP**  Use a modified pen grasp **(B)**.

**FULCRUMS  A,**  Use an intraoral, built-up fulcrum on the incisal surfaces of anterior teeth.
- An intraoral maxillary arch (opposite-arch fulcrum) may be used for mesial surfaces (not shown).

**INSTRUMENTS**  Same as for the facial surfaces.

**PATIENT POSITIONING**
- The back of the chair should be at approximately a 45-degree angle to the floor.
- The patient should be at elbow height to the operator.
- Retract the tongue with a mouth mirror to better access vision.

**OPERATOR POSITIONING**  8 to 9 o'clock position.

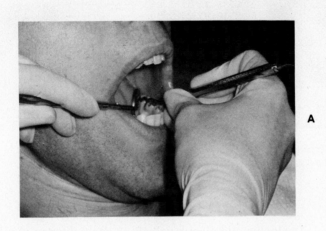

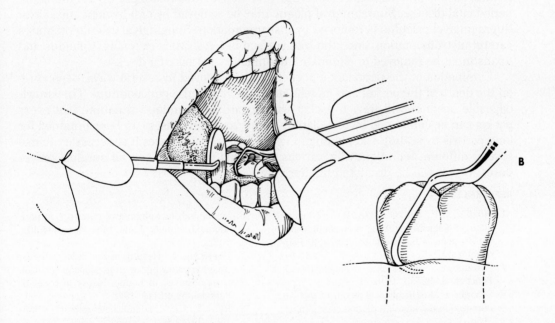

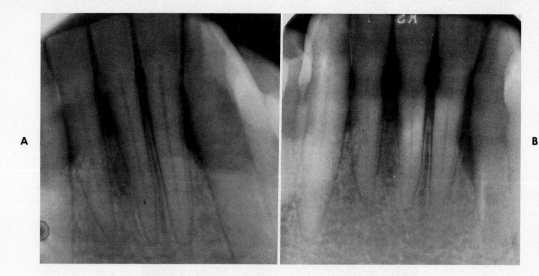

**Fig. 32-53.** **A,** Preoperative roentgenogram showing calculus and bone loss. **B,** A total of 15 years of maintenance scaling has removed a significant amount of tooth structure cervically. Bone levels are essentially unaltered.

## Summary

The removal of calculus and plaque will aid in the reduction of inflammation and reduce pocket probing depth. It is the first step in the treatment of inflammatory periodontal disease. Supragingival plaque may be removed by oral hygiene measures. Supragingival calculus is removed by instrumentation. Subgingival calculus requires careful instrumentation since the root surface is a reservoir for toxins. Calculus and toxins must be removed to eliminate inflammatory periodontal disease.

Elimination of the periodontal pocket can be achieved in several ways, depending on the depth of the pocket and its relation to the rest of the periodontium. The knowledgeable operator will treat a pocket with regard to its unique situation. Not every pocket can be eliminated by root planing. However, many cases can be maintained for long periods by scaling and planing (Fig. 32-53). In many cases it is necessary to use several different techniques for various situations, including special surgical procedures, which will be discussed in later chapters.

**REFERENCES**

1. Hughes, T.P., and Caffesse, R.G.: Gingival changes following scaling, root planing and oral hygiene: a biometric evaluation, J. Periodontol. **49:**245, 1978.
2. Garrett, J.S.: Root planing: a perspective, J. Periodontol. **49:**553, 1978.
3. Schaffer, E.M.: Histological results of root curettage of human teeth, J. Periodontol. **27:**296, 1956.
4. Morrison, E.C., et al.: Effects of repeated scaling and root planing and/or controlled oral hygiene on the periodontal attachment level and pocket depth in beagle dogs. I. Clinical findings, J. Periodontol. Res. **14:**428, 1979.
5. O'Leary, T.J.: The inflammation reduction phase of periodontal therapy: oral hygiene and root planing procedures, Alpha Omegan **76:**32, 1983.
6. Hirschfeld, I.: Subgingival curettage in periodontal treatment, J. Am. Dent. Assoc. **44:**301, 1952.
7. Waerhaug, J.: Healing of the dentoepithelial junction following subgingival plaque control. I. As observed in human biopsy material, J. Periodontol. **48:**119, 1978.
8. Russell, A.J.: Epidemiologic research 1960-1963, JAMA **68:**820, 1964.
9. Slavkin, H., et al.: Subgingival curettage, Periodontol. Abst. **27:**126, 1979.
10. Graham, C.J.: Home care effectiveness upon planed teeth and scaled teeth following surgery, J. Periodontol. **37:**43, 1966.
11. Caton, J.G., and Zander, H.A.: The attachment between tooth and gingival tissues after periodic root planing and soft tissue curettage, J. Periodontol. **50:**462, 1979.

12. Stambaugh, R., et al.: The limits of subgingival scaling, Int. J. Periodontics Rest. Dent. **5**:31, 1981.

13. Dragoo, M., et al.: Experimental periodontal treatment in humans. I. Root planing with and without chlorhexidine rinses, Int. J. Periodontics Rest. Dent. **3**:9, 1984.

14. Armitage, G.C.: Biologic basis of periodontal maintenance therapy, Berkeley, Calif., 1980, Praxis Publishing Co.

15. Ambrose, J.A., and Detamore, R.J.: Correlation of histologic and clinical findings in periodontal treatment: effect of scaling on reduction in gingival inflammation prior to surgery, J. Periodontol. **31**:238, 1960.

16. Jones, W.A., and O'Leary, T.J.: The effectiveness of in vivo root planing in removing bacterial endotoxin from the roots of periodontally involved teeth, J. Periodontol. **49**:337, 1978.

17. Ramfjord, S.P., et al.: Results following three modalities of periodontal therapy, J. Periodontol. **46**:522, 1975.

18. Mousques, T., Listgarten, M.A., and Phillips, R.W.: Effect of scaling and root planing on the composition of the human subgingival microbial flora, J. Periodontol. Res. **15**:144, 1980.

19. Tagge, D.L., O'Leary, R.J., and El-Kafrawy, A.H.: The clinical and histological response of periodontal pockets to root planing and oral hygiene, J. Periodontol. **46**:527, 1975.

20. O'Leary, T.J., and El-Kafrawy, A.H.: Total cementum removal: a realistic objective, J. Periodontol. **54**:221, 1983.

21. Proye, M., Caton, J., and Polson, A.: Initial healing of periodontal pockets after a single episode of root planing monitored by controlled probing forces, J. Periodontol. **53**:295, 1982.

22. Aleo, J.J., et al.: The presence and biologic activity of cementum-bound endotoxins, J. Periodontol. **45**:672, 1974.

23. Syed, S.A., Morrison, E.C., and Lang, N.P.: Effects of repeated scaling and root planing and/or controlled oral hygiene on the attachment level and pocket depth in beagle dogs. II. Bacteriological findings, J. Periodontol. Res. **17**:219, 1982.

24. Lie, T., and Meyer, K.: Tooth surface roughness in response to different periodontal instruments: a scanning electron microscope study, J. Clin. Periodontol. **4**:250, 1977.

25. Greene, E., and Ramfjord, S.P.: Tooth roughness after subgingival root planing, J. Periodontol. **37**:396, 1966.

26. Waerhaug, J.: Effect of rough surfaces upon gingival tissue, J. Dent. Res. **35**:323, 1956.

27. Aleo, J.J., De Renzis, F.A., and Farber, P.A.: In vitro attachment of human gingival fibroblasts to root surfaces, J. Periodontol. **46**:639, 1975.

28. Bravman, R.J., Everhart, D.L., and Stahl, S.S.: A cementum-bound antigen: its reaction with serum antibody and localization, *in situ*, J. Periodontol. **50**:656, 1979.

29. Baumhammers, A., and Rohrbaugh, F.A.: Permeability of human and rat dental calculus, J. Periodontol. **41**:279, 1970.

30. Nishimini, D., and O'Leary, T.J.: Hand instrumentation versus ultrasonics in the removal of endotoxins from root surfaces, J. Periodontol. **50**:345, 1979.

31. Rabbani, G.M., Ash, M.M., and Caffesse, R.G.: The effectiveness of subgingival scaling and root planing in calculus removal, J. Periodontol. **52**:119, 1981.

32. Walker, S.L., and Ash, M.M.: A study of root planing by scanning electron microscopy, Dent. Hyg. **50**:109, 1976.

33. Alexander, A.G.: Dental calculus and bacterial plaque and their relationship to gingival disease in 400 individuals, Br. Dent. J. **29**:116, 1970.

34. Rateitschak, K.H.: The therapeutic effect of local treatment on periodontal disease assessed upon evaluation of different diagnostic criteria. I. Changes in gingival inflammation, J. Periodontol. **35**:155, 1964.

35. Waerhaug, J.: Microscopic demonstration of tissue reaction incident to removal of subgingival calculus, J. Periodontol. **26**:26, 1955.

36. Muhler, J.C., Dudding, N.J., and Stookey, G.K.: Clinical effectiveness of a particular particle size distribution of zirconium silicate for use as a cleaning and polishing agent for oral hard tissues, J. Periodontol. **35**:481, 1964.

37. Stoll, F.A., and Werner, A.R.: New polishing agent for dental prophylaxis, J. Am. Dent. Hygien. Assoc. **37**:79, 1963.

38. Schluger, S., Yuodelis, R.A., and Page, R.C.: Periodontal disease, Philadelphia, 1977, Lea & Febiger.

39. Orban, B., and Manella, V.B.: A macroscopic and microscopic study of instruments designed for root planing, J. Periodontol. **27**:120, 1956.

40. Jones, S.J., Lozdan, J., and Boyde, A.: Tooth surface in situ with periodontal instruments: scanning electron microscopic studies, Br. Dent. J. **132**:57, 1972.

41. D'Silva, I.V., et al.: An evaluation of root topography following periodontal instrumentation: a scanning electron microscopic study, J. Periodontol. **50**:283, 1979.

42. Everett, F.G., Foss, C.L., and Orban, B.: Study of instruments for scaling (root planing), Parodontologie **16**:61, 1962.

43. Willman, D.E., Norling, B.K., and Johnson, W.N.: A new prophylaxis instrument: effect on enamel alterations, J. Am. Dent. Assoc. **101**:923, 1980.

44. Atkinson, D.R., Cobb, C.M., and Killoy, W.J.: The effect of an air-powder abrasive system on an *in vitro* surface, J. Periodontol. **55**:13, 1984.

45. Burke, S.W., and Green, E.: Effectiveness of periodontal files, J. Periodontol. **41**:39, 1970.

46. Ewen, S., and Glickstein, C.: Ultrasonic ther-

apy in periodontics, Springfield, Ill., 1968, Charles C Thomas, Publisher.

47. Breininger, D.R., O'Leary, T.J., and Blumenshine, R.V.H.: Comparative effectiveness of ultrasonic and hand scaling for the removal of subgingival plaque and calculus, J. Periodontol. **58:**9, 1987.

48. Woodruff, J.M., Levin, M.P., and Brady, J.M.: The effects of two ultrasonic instruments on root surfaces, J. Periodontol. **46:**119, 1975.

49. Suppipat, N.: Ultrasonics in periodontics, J. Clin. Periodontol. **1:**206, 1974.

50. Bhaskar, S.N., Grower, M.F., and Cutright, D.E.: Gingival healing after hand and ultrasonic scaling—biochemical and histologic analysis, J. Periodontol. **43:**31, 1972.

51. Stende, G., and Schaffer, E.M.: A comparison of ultrasonic and hand scaling, J. Periodontol. **32:**312, 1961.

52. Van Volkinburg, J.W., Green, E., and Armitage, G.C.: The nature of root surfaces after curette, cavitron and alpha-sonic instrumentation, J. Periodont. Res. **11:**374, 1976.

53. Pameijer, C.H., Stallard, R.E., and Hiep, H.: Surface characteristics of teeth following periodontal instrumentation: a scanning electron microscopic study, J. Periodontol. **43:**628, 1972.

54. Ewen, S., and Gwinnett, A.J.: A scanning electron microscopic study of teeth following periodontal instrumentation, J. Periodontol. **48:**92, 1977.

55. Antonini, C.J., et al.: Scanning electron microscope study of scalers, J. Periodontol. **48:**45, 1977.

56. Clark, S.M., Grupe, H.E., and Mahler, D.B.: Effect of ultrasonic instrumentation on root surfaces, J. Periodontol. **39:**135, 1968.

57. Clark, S.M.: The ultrasonic dental unit: a guide for the clinical application of ultrasonics in dentistry and in dental hygiene, J. Periodontol. **40:**621, 1969.

58. Thornton, S., and Garnick, J.: Comparison of ultrasonic to hand instruments in the removal of subgingival plaque, J. Periodontol. **53:**35, 1982.

59. Torfason, T., et al.: Clinical improvement of gingival conditions following ultrasonic versus hand instrumentation of periodontal pockets, J. Clin. Periodontol. **6:**165, 1979.

60. Frisch, J., Bhaskar, S.N., and Shell, D.: Effect of ultrasonic instrumentation on human gingival connective tissue, Periodontics **5:**123, 1967.

61. Ewen, S.J., et al.: A comparative study of ultrasonic generators and hand instruments, J. Periodontol. **47:**82, 1976.

62. Schaffer, E.M., Stende, G., and King, D.: Healing of periodontal pocket tissues following ultrasonic scaling and hand planing, J. Periodontol. **35:**140, 1964.

63. Goldman, H.M.: Histologic assay of healing following ultrasonic curettage versus handinstrument curettage, Oral Surg. **14:**925, 1961.

64. Sanderson, A.D.: Gingival curettage by hand and ultrasonic instruments: a histologic comparison, J. Periodontol. **37:**279, 1966.

65. Adams, D., et al.: The cardiac pacemaker and ultrasonic scalers, Br. Dent. J. **152:**171, 1982.

66. Council on Dental Materials, Instruments, and Equipment: Status report on professional scaling and stain-removal devices, J. Am. Dent. Assoc. **111:**801, 1985.

67. Axelsson, P.: Eva-systemet: Ett nytt hjälpmedel för approximal rengöring, puts och polering, Sveriges Tandläk Tidn. **61:**1086, 1969.

68. Löe, H., and Schiott, C.R.: The effect of mouth rinses and topical application of chlorhexidine on the development of dental plaque and gingivitis in man, J. Periodontol. Res. **5:**79, 1970.

69. Witzenberger, T., O'Leary, T.J., and Gillette, W.B.: Effect of a local germicide on the occurrence of bacteremia during subgingival scaling, J. Periodontol. **53:**172, 1982.

70. Listgarten, M.A., Lindhe, J., and Helldén, L.: Effect of tetracycline and/or scaling on human periodontal disease: clinical, microbiological and histological observations, J. Clin. Periodontol. **5:**245, 1978.

71. Slots, J., et al.: Periodontal therapy in humans. I. Microbiological and clinical effects of a single course of periodontal scaling and root planing, J. Periodontol. **50:**495, 1979.

72. Paquette, O.E., and Levin, M.P.: The sharpening of scaling instruments. I. An examination of principles, J. Periodontol. **48:**163, 1977.

73. Paquette, O.E., and Levin, M.P.: The sharpening of scaling instruments. II. A preferred technique, J. Periodontol. **48:**169, 1977.

74. Foss, C.L., and Orban, T.R.: Sharpening periodontal instruments, J. Periodontol. **27:**135, 1956.

75. Grant, D.A., Stern, I.B., and Everett, F.G.: Periodontics, ed. 5, St. Louis, 1979, The C.V. Mosby Co.

**ADDITIONAL SELECTED READING**

Deidrich, P., Vahl, J., and Bomfleur, W.: Rasterelektronenmikroskopische Untersuchungen der Wurzeloberfläche nach Anwendung verscheidener Hand- und Ultraschallinstrumente, Dtsch. Zahnaertzl. Z. **30:**396, 1975.

Ekanayaka, A.N.I., and Sheiham, A.: Estimating the time and personnel required to treat periodontal disease, J. Clin. Periodontol. **5:**85, 1978.

Kopczyk, R.A., and Conroy, C.W.: Attachment of calculus to root planed surfaces, Periodontics **6:**78, 1968.

O'Leary, T.J.: The impact of research on scaling and root planing, J. Periodontol. **57:**69, 1986.

Oshrain, H.I., Salkind, A., and Mandel, I.D.: Bacteriologic studies of periodontal pockets ten minutes after curettage, J. Periodontol. **43:**685, 1972.

Reinhardt, R.A., Bolton, R.W., and Hlava, G.: Effect of nonsterile versus sterile water irrigation with ultrasonic scaling on postoperative bacteremias, J. Periodontol. **53:**96, 1982.

Saglie, R.: A scanning electron microscopic study of the relationship between the most apically located subgingival plaque and the epithelial attachment, J. Periodontol. **48:**105, 1977.

Stone, S., Ramfjord, S.P., and Waldron, J.: Scaling and gingival curettage; a radioautographic study, J. Periodontol. **37:**415, 1966.

Stookey, G.K.: In vitro estimates of enamel and dentin abrasion associated with a prophylaxis, J. Dent. Res. **57:**36, 1978.

Winslow, M.B., and Kobernick, S.D.: Bacteremia after prophylaxis, J. Am. Dent. Assoc. **61:**69, 1960.

# PART SIX

## Surgery

# CHAPTER 33

# Preparations for periodontal surgery

**Preoperative evaluation**
Examination
Planning

**Surgical assistant**
Lighting of surgical field
Retraction for surgery
Aspiration
Control of bleeding
Suturing
Postoperative appointment

**Periodontal dressings**

**Postoperative period**
Instructions
Medication
Cleaning and sterilizing
Records

**Cooperative periodontal surgery (surgical training)**
Preoperative evaluation
Surgical design and planning
Sequence of cooperative surgery
Postoperative examinations

## Preoperative evaluation

Surgical steps are performed after débridement and plaque control are instituted, except for emergencies. Before undertaking surgery, the dentist should rechart findings on the patient. Medical and dental history should be reviewed. The charting should be reviewed and assessed. The patient's ability to remove plaque should be evaluated. Tooth sensitivity should be noted and measures taken to control it. From this evaluation the decision to proceed with surgery will be made.

### EXAMINATION

Presurgical examination includes recharting to evaluate changes in pocket depth and to note the form, contour, color, and texture of the gingiva.

The general indications for surgery are the presence of pockets and unphysiologic gingival form. Specific indications are discussed in appropriate chapters on surgical procedures. *General indications for surgery*

Surgery may be contraindicated in patients with certain organic or metabolic diseases (Addison disease, poorly controlled diabetes, severe cardiac disease, clotting problems) and in patients who have responded poorly to previous surgery. In addition, patients with a high caries index may be poor risks when root areas are exposed after surgery. When systemic or bleeding problems are present or anticoagulant therapy is being administered, consultation with a physician and appropriate laboratory tests are mandatory. *General contraindications*

In selecting the best treatment for the patient, the dentist should also consider the patient's emotional status. When the patient feels threatened by proposed surgery, alternative nonsurgical treatment may be indicated. *Emotional status of patient*

Any surgery should be approached cautiously when the patient is wary of esthetic *Esthetics* deformity that may be caused by the apical displacement of the gingival margins.

**Poor home dental care**

Finally, the patient who is unwilling or unable to perform proper plaque control is a poor candidate for surgery. The seeds for recurrence of the disease are present in this situation.

## PLANNING

If surgery is indicated, presurgical evaluation should be made. The area to be operated on, pocket depth, bony deformities, the type and extent of surgery, and the steps common for the procedure should be carefully planned. All this should be noted on an appropriate surgical chart for mandibular (Fig. 33-1, A) and maxillary arches (Fig. 33-1, B). The patient should be advised of the surgery and its steps and informed of its advantages and disadvantages. Any anxiety should be dealt with. The appointment should be made to accommodate the patient's social or business schedule.

**Premedication**

Premedication should be given when indicated and may include the administration of antibiotics to patients with valvular heart disease or other conditions requiring antibiotics. In such cases the medication should be started 1 hour before surgery to provide adequate levels and minimize bacterial resistance. Antibiotic medication should be adequate in amount and should be continued for several days after surgery[1-7] (Table 33-1 and box on p. 722).

Patients on anticoagulant therapy or aspirin should stop such medications 7 to 14 days before surgery and 3 or 4 days afterward with their physician's approval.

**Apprehension**

Anxiety or apprehension is present in most patients who are facing surgery.[2] At times verbal reassurance is all that is needed to allay anxiety. At other times premedication with a tranquilizer, barbiturate, or antihistamine may be indicated. Premedication may be given at the time of surgery. Intramuscular or intravenous[2,8,9-13] administration of scopolamine or meperidine-antihistamine and meperidine-diazepam combinations are widely used. Some practitioners use nitrous oxide analgesia.[14] If premedication for sedation is used in the office,[15] it should be administered 30 to 45 minutes before local anesthetic injections. Premedication, anesthesia, or postmedication may affect the patient's ability to drive or to take care of himself/herself properly. Preparations should be made for the patient to have adequate transportation and care.

At the time of surgery, the surgeon should reinspect the operative site to plan the design and extent of the incisions.

Before the anesthetic is given, the surgeon and assistant must scrub. The patient's partial dentures, eyeglasses, earrings, or other items that may interfere with surgery should be removed to a safe and convenient place. The patient should be suitably draped. Sterile technique, including rubber gloves and face mask, is necessary.[16-19]

**Instruments**

Surgical trays (Figs. 33-2, A and B, and 33-3) containing instruments for an indicated procedure are recommended. The tray should be placed in a position that is readily accessible to the dentist and assistant. The tray may be placed above and in front of the patient or behind the patient out of the patient's view. In addition to the surgical instruments, suction tips, mirrors, retractors, and gauze sponges should be at hand. Other instruments that might be needed for special procedures should be kept readily accessible in sterile packs (Figs. 33-4 and 33-5).

A basic list of instruments for periodontal surgery follows. Specific preferences in many schools cause such lists to differ. More instruments are listed than would be used, and individual preferences would determine selection.

| | |
|---|---|
| Mouth mirror | Periosteal elevators (Hirschfeld, Goldman-Fox) |
| Calibrated probe | Molt curette |
| Explorer | Burs |
| Anesthetic syringe (aspirating) | Carbide burs F6 |

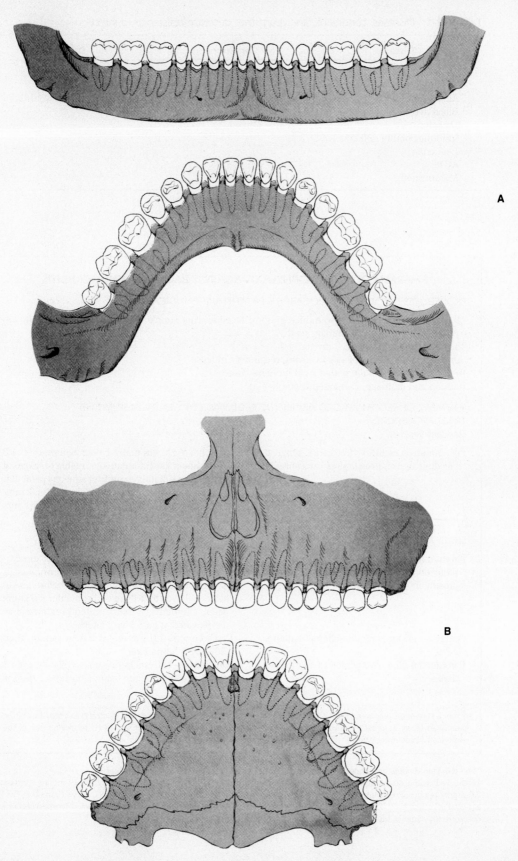

**Fig. 33-1.** Charts for delineating surgical steps (Stern).

**Table 33-1** Diseases, conditions, and drugs that decrease resistance to infection

| Diseases | Conditions | Drugs |
|---|---|---|
| Addison disease | Orthopedic implants | Adrenal corticosteroids |
| Agranulocytosis | Heart valve | Cytotoxic drugs |
| Alcoholism | prostheses | Immunosuppressive drugs |
| Blood dyscrasias | Aortic prostheses | |
| Diabetes | | |
| Immunoglobulin deficiency | | |
| Leukemia | | |
| AIDS | | |
| Malnutrition | | |

---

### PHARMACOLOGIC PROPHYLAXIS AGAINST BACTERIAL ENDOCARDITIS

#### PROCEDURES FOR WHICH ENDOCARDITIS PROPHYLAXIS IS INDICATED

All dental procedures likely to induce gingival bleeding (not simple adjustment of orthodontic appliances or shedding of primary teeth)
Tonsillectomy or adenoidectomy (or both)
Surgical procedures or biopsy involving respiratory mucosa
Bronchoscopy, especially with a rigid bronchoscope*
Incision and drainage of infected tissue

#### SUMMARY OF RECOMMENDED ANTIBIOTIC REGIMENS FOR DENTAL RESPIRATORY TRACT PROCEDURES†
##### Standard Regimen

| | |
|---|---|
| For dental procedures that cause gingival bleeding, and oral/respiratory tract surgery | Penicillin V 2.0 gm orally 1 hour before, then 1.0 gm 6 hours later; for patients unable to take oral medications, 2 million units of aqueous penicillin G intravenously or intramuscularly 30-60 minutes before procedure and 1 million units 6 hours later may be substituted |

##### Special Regimens

| | |
|---|---|
| Parenteral regimen for use when maximal protection desired (e.g., for patients with prosthetic valves) | Ampicillin 1.0-2.0 gm intramuscularly or intravenously, plus gentamicin 1.5 mg/kg intramuscularly or intravenously, 30 minutes before procedure, followed by 1.0 gm oral penicillin V 6 hours later; alternatively, the parenteral regimen may be repeated once 8 hours later |
| Oral regimen for penicillin-allergic patients | Erythromycin 1.0 gm orally 1 hour before, then 500 mg 6 hours later |
| Parenteral regimen for penicillin-allergic patients | Vancomycin 1.0 gm intravenously slowly over 1 hour, starting 1 hour before; no repeat dose is necessary |

From a statement prepared by the Committee on Prevention of Rheumatic Fever and Bacterial Endocarditis of the American Heart Association: Shulman, S.T., et al.: Circulation **70:**1123a, December, 1984; by permission of the American Heart Association.

*The risk with flexible bronchoscopy is low, but the necessity for prophylaxis is not yet defined.
†Note: Pediatric doses: Ampicillin 50 mg/kg per dose; erythromycin 20 mg/kg for first dose, then 10 mg/kg; gentamicin 2.0 mg/kg per dose; penicillin V full adult dose if greater than 60 lb (27 kg), one-half adult dose if less than 60 lb (27 kg); aqueous penicillin G 50,000 units/kg (25,000 units/kg for follow-up); vancomycin 20 mg/kg per dose. The intervals between doses are the same as for adults. Total doses should not exceed adult doses.

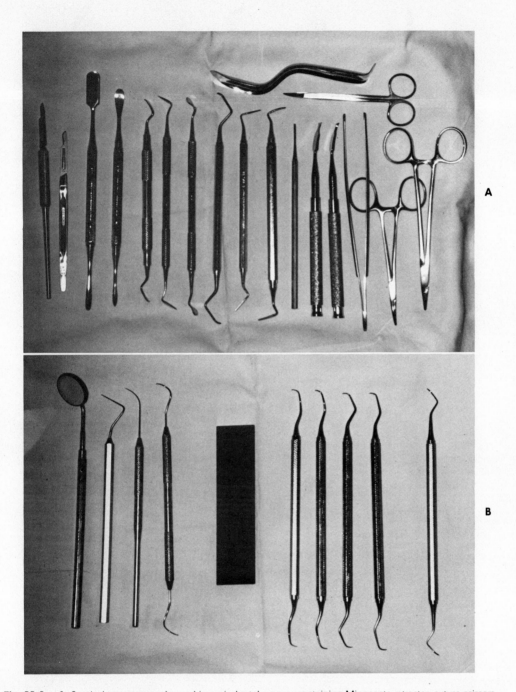

**Fig. 33-2.** **A,** Surgical tray commonly used in periodontal surgery containing Minnesota retractor, suture scissors, needle holder, curved needle holder, tissue forceps, Ochsenbein chisels, straight (Wedlestadt) chisel, curved and straight files, large curette (Prichard), kidney-shaped knife (Kirkland), back knife or Orban knives, back-action chisel, periostome, Prichard periostome, flat and rounded scalpels with 15 and 15C blades. (Not shown: calibrated periodontal probe, mirrors, cotton forceps, USC interdental knife, Gracey finishing curettes, cotton swabs, sponges, anesthetic syringe, sutures.) **B,** Surgical tray containing mirror, periodontal pocket probe, explorer, Nabors furcation probe, sharpening stone, and Gracey curettes. (**A,** courtesy of J. Corrigan, San Jose, California.)

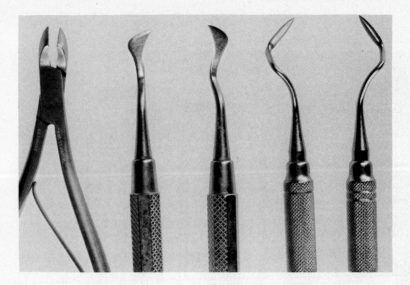

**Fig. 33-3.** Periodontal scalpels (knives) and soft tissue rongeurs.

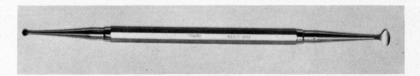

**Fig. 33-4.** Double-ended Molt curette for flap reflection, osteoplasty, and for obtaining cortical bone for grafts and transplants.

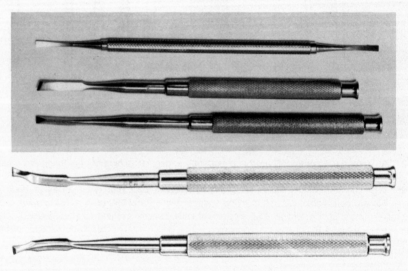

**Fig. 33-5.** Bone chisels used in osseous surgery and in separating secondary flaps from bone (Ochsenbein).

Aspirator
Cotton pliers
Tissue forceps
Curettes (as preferred)
    Gracey 1/2
    Gracey 3/4
    Gracey 5/6R
    Gracey 7/8R
    Gracey 11/12R
    Gracey 13/14R
    Goldman-Fox no. 2
    Goldman-Fox no. 3
    Goldman-Fox no. 4
    McCall 13/14
    McCall 17/18
   Surgical curettes
    Universal
    Kramer
    Prichard 1/2
    Ball
    Crane-Kaplan no. 6
   Interdental knives
    Orban knives
    Sanders knife
    Goldman-Fox no. 7
    Goldman-Fox no. 8
    Goldman-Fox no. 11
    USC DE knife

Surgical round burs nos. 6 and 8
Carbide surgical burs
Kidney-shaped knives
   Kirkland 15/16 knife
   Goldman-Fox no. 7
   Buck knife 5/6
Needle holder, carbide jaws
Soft tissue rongeurs
   Sugarman
   Goldman-Fox
Mosquito forceps
Suture scissors
   Goldman-Fox no. 16
   Orban scissors
Bone chisels
   Ochsenbein chisels
   TG chisel
   Back-action chisel 13K and 13KL
Minnesota mouth retractor
No. 3 Bard-Parker handle
Bard-Parker blades: nos. 11, 12, 12B, 15, and 15C
Files
   Schluger
   Buck
   Miller
   Sugarman
Dappen dish
Cavitron tips

**Local anesthetic**

Local infiltration and block anesthesia are the methods of choice. Standard techniques of dosage and administration should be used. After the initial administration, it may be desirable to inject a drop of anesthetic directly into the interdental papilla. This is particularly useful in gingivectomy. It makes the gingiva firmer and easier to incise and has a hemostatic effect because of the vasoconstrictor in the anesthetic solution.

Once premedication and a local anesthetic have been given, the patient should not be left alone. The assistant or the dentist should be present.

**Communications**

During the operation verbal instructions to the assistant should be worded to avoid creating anxiety. Requests for instruments and other materials should be made in a professional manner or by signals to maintain a calm atmosphere. Careless orders, remarks, angry glances, or unnecessarily rapid movements are alarming to the patient and may result in a tense and unsatisfactory atmosphere. The patient may interpret such events to mean the operation is progressing poorly. Thus a poor postoperative course of events can be anticipated.[20]

## Surgical assistant

The assistant is an active participant in all surgical procedures, serving as a second pair of hands. The assistant aspirates, retracts, passes, and retrieves instruments, and cleanses the surgical surface with water spray. The assistant should explain to the patient in brief, simple, and nonalarming terms the use of the aspirator so that the patient will not be apprehensive when it is used. The assistant should also inform the patient that, if the muscles tire or become painful from holding the mouth open, he/she will be given the opportunity to close the mouth and rest. A bite block may then be useful. Adroit explanation will properly prepare the patient for surgery and permit the operation to progress smoothly. Characteristics and duties of the surgical assistant are listed in this section.

**Instructions**

The following guide for surgical assistance presumes that periodontal disease progression and treatment are understood. The surgical assistant is a member of a team performing periodontal surgery. The team consists of a surgeon and a surgical assistant. The surgical assistant is responsible to the surgeon for the complete setup of the surgery, handling of instruments, photography, and patient management.

**Role**

The role of an assistant to a periodontal surgeon is to make it easier for the surgeon to administer treatment smoothly and efficiently. Without the assistant there can be no surgery. The better the assistant performs the job, the better the surgeon performs the surgery. The combined efforts will result in better treatment of the patient.

**Characteristics**

Following are characteristics of an excellent surgical assistant:

1. Is professional and efficient, yet relaxed. The assistant's good nature will help relax the patient at a time when the patient may be nervous and insecure. An excellent assistant inspires confidence in the physician and the office.
2. Has a genuine interest in the health care of the patient and a genuine desire to help.
3. Keeps patient records neat and orderly and sets the x-ray films on the view box before surgery.
4. Sharpens surgical instruments to perfection before each surgery, sterilizes all instruments, and prepares the tray of surgical instruments before surgery.
5. Prepares and stores the periodontal pack (when used) before or after the surgery as needed.
6. Protects the patient's lips by applying petroleum jelly before surgery.
7. Scrubs hands clean before surgery. Wears surgical rubber gloves and a face mask. Wears a cap to restrain the hair.
8. Knows both how to position mirrors and how to take photographs.
9. Knows all the surgical instruments by name and appearance.
10. Is aware of each stage of the operation and the sequence of operating.
11. Adjusts the intraoral light to provide access and vision for the surgeon.
12. Hands the instruments to the surgeon in proper sequence and replaces them to precise position on the surgical tray.
13. Is responsible for keeping the patient's face clean and for keeping instruments clean and in order during surgery.
14. Communicates with the surgeon without speaking, if at all possible, and certainly without alarming the patient.

Before surgery, the surgical assistant will perform the following:

1. Seat the patient
2. Drape the patient
3. Set the x-ray studies on the view box
4. Set up the surgical tray, including sterile gauze pads and anesthetic
5. Receive briefing by the surgeon and examine the surgical chart
6. Set the surgical chart on the cabinet

The surgical assistant is responsible for these measures:

1. Retracting the lips, tongue, and cheeks
2. Aspirating
3. Adjusting the lighting
4. Positioning flaps for stability and access while the surgeon operates and then sutures

After the surgery the surgical assistant will make sure that the patient understands the instructions given by the surgeon and will supply the patient with an instruction sheet, gauze, and a temporary ice pack. The assistant delivers and explains prescriptions and postsurgical care.

## LIGHTING OF SURGICAL FIELD

It should be the function of the assistant to control the lighting so that the operative field is adequately illuminated at all times. The dental spotlight must be properly positioned for visibility and illumination. In certain cases a small intraoral spotlight or headlamp may be necessary to provide additional lighting. A high-speed contra-angle handpiece with fiber-optic illumination is an asset.

## RETRACTION FOR SURGERY

It is the duty of the assistant to retract the lips, cheeks, and tongue to permit adequate access for the surgeon and to facilitate surgical procedures. Retraction is accomplished with a Minnesota retractor. It may also be accomlished with a no. 4 mouth mirror, which can be used to retract the tongue ( Fig. 33-6) or to distend the cheek ( Fig. 33-7). A finger placed in the vestibule may also be used to retract the cheek. The aspirator tip, in addition to keeping the field clear of blood and saliva, may occasionally be used to keep the tongue from the field of surgery ( Fig. 33-8). The assistant is responsible for retracting flaps while osseous surgery is being performed. Various instruments are used to retract flaps, including the periostome and tissue retractors ( Figs. 33-9 to 33-11). Protection of cheek, lips, and tongue is especially

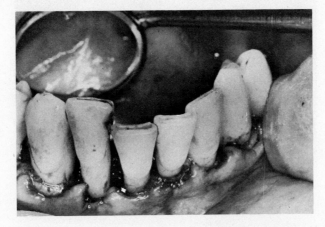

**Fig. 33-6.** Use of the no. 4 mouth mirror to retract the tongue.

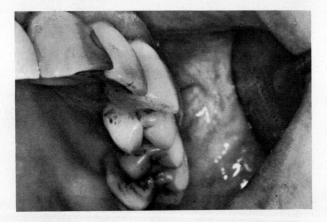

**Fig. 33-7.** Use of the no. 4 mouth mirror to retract the cheek.

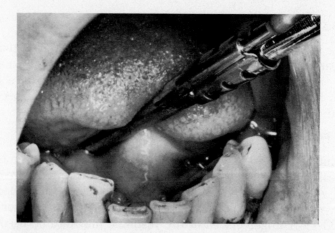

**Fig. 33-8.** Use of the aspirator tip to retract the tongue from the surgical field.

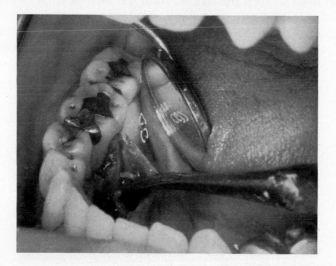

**Fig. 33-9.** Use of the mirror to retract the tongue and reflect light. The aspirator tip may aspirate, retract the flap, and protect the tongue and sublingual tissues during instrumentation.

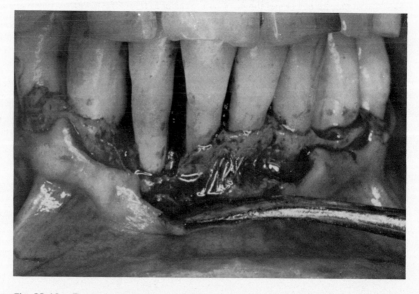

**Fig. 33-10.** The assistant retracts a full-thickness modified flap with a periosteal elevator.

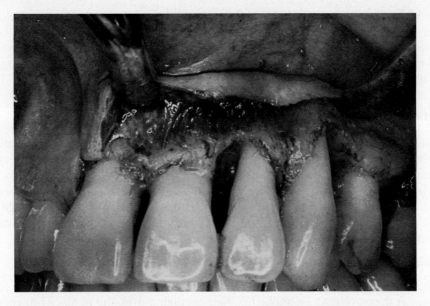

**Fig. 33-11.** The surgeon uses a periosteal elevator to retract a flap while the assistant uses the tip of the aspirator to retract and aspirate.

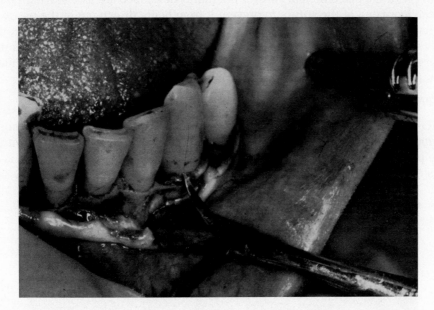

**Fig. 33-12.** Use of the aspirator tip to distend the cheek to provide better access for instrumentation during surgery.

important when surgical burs, stones, or chisels are used (Fig. 33-12). A mirror, a periostome, cheek retractors, or a surgical aspirator tip should be kept between the cheek or tongue and the revolving bur or other surgical instrument.

## ASPIRATION

The assistant will use an aspirator to remove blood, oral secretions, and water or saline solution spray. The size and shape of the aspirator tip used will depend on the type of aspirator (high volume or high pressure) and on the specific requirements of the surgical intervention. In general, it is desirable to have both a small and a larger tip available. The assistant may control the device by a foot pedal. The spray cleanses the surgical field of blood and removes small pieces of tissue loosened by the curette or scalpel. Flakes of calculus are also removed. Small bits of excised tissue, blood, and debris may be lifted from the end of surgical instruments by touching with the aspirator tip (Fig. 33-13). A saliva ejector occupies space and may be inconvenient. Proper surgical aspiration can adequately remove fluids and debris from the mouth.

## CONTROL OF BLEEDING

Bleeding must be controlled during surgery and at its completion, before suturing or applying the dressing. Bleeding may be controlled by sponges (Fig. 33-14). Capillary bleeding can be controlled by pressure; arterial bleeding requires suturing. Bleeding on incision may be more profuse and may diminish as the operation progresses. The dentist may at times apply cotton pellets under pressure to control hemorrhage (Fig. 33-14). Usually a wait of 3 to 5 minutes will permit the surgery to proceed without excessive bleeding.

## SUTURING

Flaps are sutured following surgery. This procedure alone usually achieves hemostasis. A dressing may be applied. When needed, a dressing is placed to cover the wound surface. During suturing the efforts of the assistant are extremely important. Assisting with the placement of sutures is a highly developed art. The assistant usually holds the loose end of the suture to prevent it from being drawn out of the tissue. The other hand is used to retract the cheek or lip. Flaps may be supported with a tissue forceps so that the needle can be more easily passed through. After the tie is made, the surgeon retracts the lips, cheek, or tongue and extends the suture while the assistant cuts it. (See discussion on suturing in Chapter 35.)

## POSTOPERATIVE APPOINTMENT

After the operation the assistant or the dentist gives postoperative instructions and prescriptions. Care should be taken in what is said to the patient. The patient often can be programmed for an easy or difficult postoperative experience by what is said. Postoperative complications and pain are often minimal; they are moderate or severe

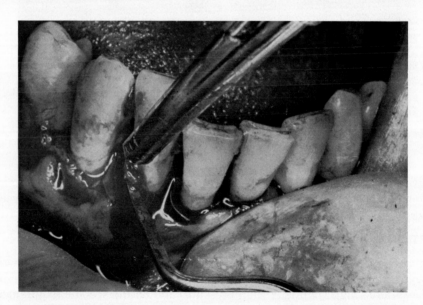

**Fig. 33-13.** Lifting of bits of tissue from the curette blade with the aspirator during surgery.

in only 5.5% of cases.[21] The assistant should take the patient to the desk and give instructions to the secretary for the date and time of the postoperative appointment.

## Periodontal dressings

Periodontal dressings are used to cover and protect wound surfaces after surgery. They shield the incised tissues from irritation by such factors as foods, air, and tongue or cheek movements.

Several types of dressings are available:

1. Zinc oxide—eugenol base dressings
2. Ready-mix dressings (These do not contain eugenol. The ingredients are calcium sulfate, zinc oxide, acrylate, and corrigents for taste and color.)
3. Rosins
4. Combinations of water-soluble metallic oxides and nonionizing carboxylic acids (COE-Pak) (These do not contain eugenol.)
5. Fat-base dressings (Baer)

Commercially available periodontal dressings[22]:

1. COE-Pak, Coe Laboratories, Inc.
2. Kirkland Periodontal Pack, Pulpdent Corp. of America
3. Peridres, Premier Dental Products Co.
4. Perio-Care Periodontal Dressing, Pulpdent Corp. of America
5. Periodontal Pack, Pulpdent Corp. of America
6. Perio Putty, Cadco Dental Products
7. Zone Periodontal Pak, Cadco Dental Products

Most dressings require the mixing of two pastes or powder and liquid to a paste-like consistency that is manageable. When the paste becomes manageable the dressing may be applied (Fig. 33-15). Some dressings can be stored by refrigeration. To apply the dressing, form it into strips and place on buccal and lingual wound surfaces, forcing it interproximally. If sutures are present, it sometimes helps to cover the cut ends with Gelfoam. Apply the strips to the wound surface and gently knead them into inter-

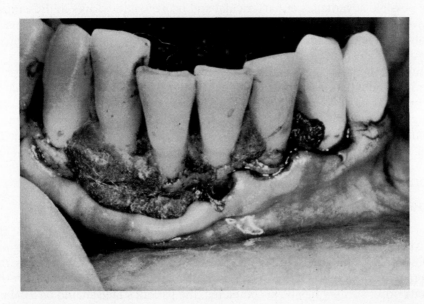

**Fig. 33-14.** Use of sponges and cotton pellets to control bleeding before osseous corrections.

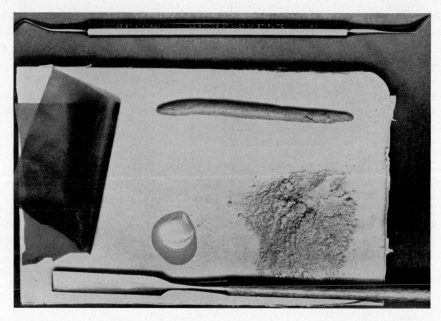

**Fig. 33-15.** Waxed-paper pad and instruments for mixing and applying surgical dressing when needed.

proximal spaces to connect the buccal and lingual segments. A moistened cotton swab may be used to shape the mass after application. The dressing should cover the wound but should not interfere with occlusion. Impingement on motile tissues may cause painful ulcerations, and the dressing should be muscle trimmed.

**Other types**   Noneugenol formulas[23,24] are believed to be less irritating to bone, although this belief has been challenged.[25] A noneugenol formula[26] contains the following: powder (rosin, 0.52 gm; zinc oxide, 0.41 gm; bacitracin, 3000 units) and liquid (Zinc oxide, 5%; hydrogenated fat, 95%).

Thermoplastic materials and oral adhesives are also marketed.[27] Cyanoacrylate dressing is reported to be advantageous in healing.[28,29]

The possible advantages of bactericidal and bacteriostatic drugs in dressings have been investigated.[30-32] The pack itself may exert a transient antibacterial effect,[33] and generally is not harmful to healing.[34-36] Sensitization, allergy, and candidiasis produced by dressings may occur.[37]

Stents may be used to retain dressings and to prevent displacement or loss.[38,39]

Many periodontists use no dressing when flaps are coapted and sutured. When reattachment operations and bone grafts are attempted, tinfoil, Telfa, Adaptic, or Surgicel may be placed over the site and the sutures before dressing placement. Some periodontists cover bone grafts with free gingival grafts or with freeze-dried skin, sutured to place, in order to slow epithelial cell migration on the root.

## Postoperative period

### INSTRUCTIONS

After the completion of suturing and the possible placement of dressings, the assistant should give the patient both verbal and written postoperative instructions and any prescriptions that the dentist may have written. It is wise to prepare printed postoperative instructions (see box, opposite), since the patient may forget verbal instructions. After surgery has been completed, the patient's face should be washed and

---

_____ , D.D.S.                                    Telephone _____

### POSTOPERATIVE INSTRUCTIONS TO PATIENT
### AFTER PERIODONTAL SURGERY

1. Do not eat or drink for 2 hours after surgery.
2. Do not investigate dressing with tongue or fingers. This dressing serves as a bandage to protect the wound.
3. Avoid tart or spicy foods.
4. Drink fruit juices with a straw.
5. In some cases a dressing will be placed over the area. The dressing serves to protect the area of surgery and to keep you comfortable. If small pieces break off, do not be alarmed. If a large piece falls off, or if the dressing is uncomfortable, call the doctor. As an emergency measure, cover the wound with softened paraffin.
6. Some swelling may occur. This is to be expected. Place ice pack over the area that has undergone surgery and rinse frequently and gently with warm water (one glass) with one teaspoon of salt.
7. A slight amount of seepage may occur, giving your saliva a red color. Do not be alarmed. If the seepage persists, call the doctor.
8. For postoperative comfort, take pills according to instructions in prescription given to you. Take antibiotics if they are prescribed.
9. Brush parts of mouth on which surgery was not performed. Brush only the biting surfaces of the teeth where surgery was performed. Be sure to brush! When no dressing is placed, brush and use floss, but do not carry the floss under the gum line.
10. Rinse mouth carefully after eating. Clean outside of dressing with moistened cotton swab or Q-tips.

---

he/she should be conducted from the operating room by the assistant or dentist. To avoid positional syncope, the chair back should be raised gradually in several steps.

As a rule a normal diet is adequate; however, when dietary supplements such as vitamins are indicated, these should be prescribed. The patient should be instructed to avoid tart or spicy foods, since these may cause pain. Fruit juices should be taken by straw for the same reason. **Diet**

## MEDICATION

Postoperative medication for pain, sedation, hemorrhage, swelling, or infection may be needed. Analgesics and narcotics are used for relief of pain. Depending on the degree of pain, acetaminophen or codeine may be prescribed. Dosage of Tylenol is usually two 5-grain tablets every 3 hours, with smaller doses for children. Tylenol with codeine no. 3 or no. 4 or Empirin Compound no. 3 (with ¾ grain of codeine) is usually prescribed, one tablet every 4 hours as needed. Patients on anticoagulant therapy, with ulcers, or with a history of postsurgical bleeding should not be given aspirin. Ibuprofen may be prescribed.[21,40,41]

In cases of severe pain, meperidine hydrochloride (Demerol) may be administered intramuscularly (50 or 100 mg) or Demerol in 50 mg tablets or Empirin Compound no. 4 orally every 4 hours. **Pain**

Sedation after surgery may be prescribed for patients who are anxious or apprehensive or when postsurgical pain warrants. Tranquilizers or barbiturates are most frequently used. Meprobamate, 200 or 400 mg, one or two tablets four times a day; librium, 5 or 10 mg, one capsule three times a day; or Valium, 5 mg, one capsule twice a day, may be used. Phenobarbital, 0.016 gm twice a day, may be prescribed when tranquilizers are contraindicated.[21] **Sedation**

Postsurgical bleeding at home can usually be controlled by local measures unless **Bleeding** the bleeding is arterial. As a rule, lavage, pressure with a $2 \times 2$ gauze square, or a wet tea bag (tannic acid) is adequate. When the patient cannot control the bleeding, he/she should be seen promptly. Following are steps to be taken at this time:

1. Cleanse the wound.
2. Find the area of bleeding.
3. Inject local anesthetic with vasoconstrictor.[12]
4. Ligate or suture, apply pressure, or use electrocautery as appropriate.
5. Apply oxidized cellulose (Oxycel) on the wound with pressure.

**Swelling**

Swelling after surgery is best prevented by the use of ice packs. After swelling develops, hot moist packs and frequent lavage with warm saline solution are preferred. Anti-inflammatory analgesics (ibuprofen) may reduce swelling. Digestive and bacterial enzymes such as trypsin (Tryptar), papain (Papase, Ananase), and streptokinase-streptodornase (Varidase) are often helpful in reducing edema.[43] When these enzymes are used, it is advisable to protect the patient with antibiotics to reduce the possibility of spread of infection. Not all postoperative swelling is caused by inflammation; some may be caused by bleeding into tissues. This may occur after flap operations and be accompanied by discoloration under the cheek, chin, or eye.

**Antibiotics**

Antibiotics may be prescribed after surgery to treat or to prevent infections. They are used regularly when bone graft or reattachment operations are performed. Their routine use after all periodontal surgery is debatable. Broad-spectrum antibiotics are recommended, and sound pharmacologic principles should be followed in all prescriptions. Antibiotics are a necessity if there is a history of rheumatic fever, valvular heart disease or if cardiovascular or orthopedic implants are present.[44]

### CLEANING AND STERILIZING

After the patient is dismissed, the operating room must be carefully cleaned and inspected. Surgical instruments are taken to a sterilizing area where all instruments are washed, sharpened, and autoclaved. The equipment in the operating room, particularly the handles of the dental spotlight, the chair controls, handles of the handpiece, Cavitron, aspirator tubing, and water spray controls, are washed and disinfected.

### RECORDS

A full report of the operation (including number of sutures) and medications should be made in the patient's chart.

## Cooperative periodontal surgery (surgical training)

A cooperative periodontal surgical experience is gained when the surgeon and an assistant collaborate in the surgical management of a patient. The primary objective of cooperative surgery is to provide competent care for the patient. The secondary objective is to contribute to the dental student's or dentist's surgical training. Training at most schools is inadequate because of the paucity of experience provided. A summary of the obligations, objectives, and sequential steps in the surgery is given in the discussion that follows.

In the school, hospital, or training setting, two surgeons may operate together, one serving as instructor, the other as the student. The student is then referred to as the assistant surgeon. The combined procedure performed by the chief and assistant surgeons is a *cooperative surgery*.

### PREOPERATIVE EVALUATION

**Role of surgeon**

One week before surgery both the surgeon and the assistant surgeon meet with the patient so that the surgeon can examine the patient (presurgical examination), establish a surgical treatment plan, and fortify rapport with the patient. Pocket depth, radiographs, patterns of mobility, osseous defects, interdental bone morphology, occlusion, bruxism, and width of the attached gingiva should be reevaluated. After these findings are recorded on the surgical chart (see Fig. 33-1), judgment must be made as to whether surgical intervention will significantly improve the prognosis and whether phase I therapy was efficacious. The surgeon must review the following as they apply:

### Patient Considerations

1. Medical history
2. Drugs currently taken by patient
3. Need for premedication
4. Need for sedation
5. Psychologic status
6. Cosmetic considerations
7. Financial considerations (The patient should have the surgical visits, costs, and consequences fully discussed.)
8. Methods of anesthesia
9. Patient consent and patient acceptance is necessary and should be given as informed consent. The patient, knowing fully the advantages and disadvantages of the surgery, must give prior consent to having surgery done.

### Surgical Access

1. Size of mouth
2. Size and position of tongue for access to lingual arch
3. Access to mandibular retromolar area
4. Access to maxillary tuberosity area and thickness of tissue pad
5. Presence of tori
6. Access to interdental areas
7. Access to maxillary buccal vestibule when coronoid process of mandible moves forward during opening
8. Muscular hypertonicity
9. Activity of cheeks and tongue
10. Presence of a gag reflex

### Anatomic Considerations

1. Location of mental foramen
2. Location of mandibular canal
3. Location of internal and external oblique ridges
4. Location of maxillary sinus
5. Location and prominence of malar eminence
6. Location of tori
7. Depth of vestibule
8. Frenum attachments
9. Muscle pull
10. Contour of palatal vault
11. Amount of gingiva
12. Thickness of gingiva
13. Amount and quality of donor soft tissue when grafts are to be performed
14. Location and pattern of osseous defects
15. Location, amount, and quality of available bone marrow, allograft bone, etc.
16. Suspicion of dehiscences and fenestrations
17. Likelihood of long connective tissue and/or long epithelial attachments
18. Contour and position of clinical crowns
19. Root proximity
20. Crown-root ratio
21. Location and extent of furcation involvements

22. Thickness of alveolar bone
23. Width of interdental bone and morphology

### Prosthetic Considerations

1. Mobility of teeth
2. Need for stabilization
3. Restorative treatment plan
4. Assessment of abutment teeth
5. Need for crown lengthening
6. Contour of edentulous ridges
7. Desirability of placing provisional restorations or splints

### Endodontic Considerations

1. Need for endodontic treatment when root amputations and hemisections are anticipated
2. Need for endodontic treatment in endodontic-periodontal lesions

### Exodontic Considerations

1. Teeth with a hopeless or questionable prognosis

## SURGICAL DESIGN AND PLANNING

The chief and assistant surgeons must design and plan the operation. The surgery may be designed, charted, and defended during a consultation with a surgical instructor. There should be sound reasoning for the following choices:

1. The number, type, and location of incisions
2. The rationale for osseous surgery; placement of implants into bony defects
3. Root amputations
4. Hemisections
5. Methods of suturing and type of suture material
6. Methods of dressing and type of material
7. Placement of soft tissue grafts

Thus, before the day of surgery, the diagnosis, the prognosis, the treatment plan, and the surgical design should all be determined. Final therapeutic judgments may occasionally be reserved until osseous defects are exposed, but it is best if every possible problem is anticipated.

## SEQUENCE OF COOPERATIVE SURGERY

Cooperative surgery involves a set sequence of steps.

1. The assistant surgeon will do the following:
   a. Arrange instruments
   b. Take intraoperative, preoperative, and postoperative photographs
   c. Retract the tongue for *access* to lingual arch and jaw placement for access to maxillary tuberosity
2. The surgeon will do the following:
   a. Make initial buccal incision
   b. Make initial lingual or palatal incision
   c. Elevate buccal flap
   d. Elevate palatal or lingual flap
   e. Join buccal and lingual/palatal flap with distal wedge
   f. Degranulate
   g. Classify osseous defects and discuss osseous therapy
3. The surgeon will do the following as needed:
   a. Perform osseous surgery, bone grafts

b. Suture

c. Place the surgical dressing

4. The assistant participates in the following:

a. Suturing

b. Placing the dressing

5. In mucogingival surgery, the assistant may participate in these procedures:

a. Suturing

b. Placing surgical dressing

In time, as the assistant surgeon gains experience, more responsibility in the performance of the surgical sequence can be delegated to the assistant until such time as he/she can be permitted to operate independently.

## POSTOPERATIVE EXAMINATIONS

The surgical field must be observed at intervals until clinical healing has taken place. The surgeon and the assistant perform the postoperative examinations. The conscientious assistant observes the patient through the completion of periodontal treatment because only long-term observations can indicate the quality and success of the surgery. Astute clinicians observe the tissues at these intervals and evaluate teleologically their surgical skill and therapeutic judgments. The following outline may serve as a guide.

At the first and any subsequent postoperative examination, the following should be evaluated:

1. Patient considerations

a. Patient's attitude toward the procedure

b. How does the patient feel? Is there pain, root sensitivity?

c. Amount of pain medication taken by patient

d. Hygiene in other areas of the mouth

e. Evidence of swelling or infection—including elevated temperature, necrosis, halitosis, food impaction beneath flap, hematomas, trismus, flap displacement, sequestration, or retained suture fragments when discernable

f. Any parasthesia?

2. Patterns of healing

a. Do tissue color, position, and size appear normal or as anticipated?

b. Has granulation tissue altered the postsurgical gingival form?

c. Is plaque or calculus present?

d. Are sutures tense or loose?

e. Is there exudate from under the flap?

f. Has tooth mobility increased appreciably?

Following removal of dressing and/or sutures, the success of the surgery should be evaluated. If untoward patterns of healing appear, these should be addressed as noted. The aforementioned factors must be evaluated in addition to the following:

1. Evidence of or recurrence of pockets

2. Normal tissue contour

3. Absence of gingivitis

4. Accessibility to interdental areas for oral hygiene

5. Lack of muscle and frenum pulls on gingival margins

6. Adequate width of gingiva

7. Esthetics

A phase II examination is performed by the surgeon 6 to 8 weeks postoperatively, and recommendations for phase III therapy are prepared.

## REFERENCES

1. Council on Dental Therapeutics: Prevention of bacterial endocarditis: a committee report of the American Heart Association, J. Am. Dent. Assoc. **110:**98, 1985.
2. Holroyd, S.V.: Pharmacology in dentistry, Alpha Omegan **77:**53, 1984.
3. Pendrill, K., and Reddy, J.: The use of prophylactic penicillin in periodontal surgery, J. Periodontol. **51:**44, 1980.
4. Mulligan, R.: Late infections in patients with prostheses for total replacement of joints: implications for the dental practitioner, J. Am. Dent. Assoc. **101:**44, 1980.
5. Baumgartner, J.C., and Plack, W.F. III: Dental treatment and management of a patient with a prosthetic heart valve, J. Am. Dent. Assoc. **104:**181, 1982.
6. Pack, P.D., and Haber, J.: The incidence of clinical infection after periodontal surgery: a retrospective study, J. Periodontol. **54:**441, 1983.
7. Slots, J., Rosling, B.G., and Genco, R.J.: Supression of penicillin-resistant oral *Actinobacillus actinomycetemcomitans* with tetracycline: considerations in endocarditis prophylaxis, J. Periodontol. **54:**193, 1983.
8. Hillman, J.D., McFall, W.T., Jr., and Gregg, J.M.: Intravenous conscious sedation in the periodontal patient, J. Periodontol. **52:**24, 1981.
9. Saadoun, A.P.: Sedation and general anesthesia in periodontal surgery, J. West. Soc. Periodontol./Periodont. Abstr. **29:**112, 1981.
10. Cohen, C.I.: Periodontal surgery for the apprehensive patient with anesthetic management: a review of 150 patients, J. Periodontol. **50:**28, 1979.
11. Glaser, J.W., Blanton, P.L., and Thrash, W.J.: Incidence and extent of venous sequelae with intravenous diazepam utilizing a standardized conscious sedation technique, J. Periodontol. **53:**700, 1982.
12. Morgan, J., et al.: Incidence and extent of venous sequelae with intravenous diazepam utilizing a standardized conscious sedation technique. II. Effects of injection site, J. Periodontol. **54:**680, 1983.
13. Ceravalo, F.J., et al.: Full dentition periodontal surgery utilizing intravenous conscious-sedation: a report of 5200 cases, J. Periodontol. **51:**462, 1980.
14. Duncan, G.H., and Moore, P.: Nitrous oxide and the dental patient: a review of adverse reactions, J. Am. Dent. Assoc. **108:**213, 1984.
15. Small, E.W.: Preoperative sedation in dentistry, Dent. Clin. North Am. **14:**769, 1970.
16. Allen, A.L., and Organ, R.S.: Occult blood accumulation under the fingernails: a mechanism for the spread of blood-borne infections, J. Am. Dent. Assoc. **105:**455, 1982.
17. Mitchell, R., et al.: The use of operating gloves in dental practice, Br. Dent. J. **154:**372, 1983.
18. Ahtone, J., and Goodman, R.A.: Hepatitis B and dental personnel: transmission to patients and prevention issues, J. Am. Dent. Assoc. **106:**219, 1983.
19. Withers, J.A.: Hepatitis: a review of the disease and its significance to dentistry, J. Periodontol. **51:**162, 1980.
20. George, J.M., and Scott, D.S.: The effects of psychologic factors on recovery from surgery, J. Am. Dent. Assoc. **105:**251, 1982.
21. Curtis, J.W., Jr., McLain, J.B., and Hutchinson, R.A.: The incidence and severity of complications and pain following periodontal surgery, J. Periodontol. **56:**597, 1985.
22. Clinical products in dentistry, J. Am. Dent. Assoc. **109:**850, 1984.
23. Eberle, P., and Mühlemann, H.R.: Ein neuer Parodontal-Verband, Schweiz. Monatsschr. Zahnheilkd. **69:**1095, 1959.
24. Rateitschak, K.H.: Graf, H., and Guldener, P.: Periodontal pack without eugenol, J. Periodontol. **35:**290, 1964.
25. Frisch, J., and Bhaskar, S.N.: Tissue response to eugenol-containing dressings, J. Periodontol. **38:**402, 1967.
26. Baer, P.N., Sumner, C.F. III, and Scigliano, J.: Studies on a hydrogenated fat-zinc bacitracin periodontal dressing, Oral. Surg. **13:**494, 1960.
27. Ewen, S.J.: Periodontal uses of a tissue adhesive, J. Periodontol. **38:**138, 1967.
28. Bhaskar, S.N., and Frisch, J.: Use of cyanoacrylate adhesives in dentistry, J. Am. Dent. Assoc. **77:**831, 1969.
29. Binnie, W.H., and Forrest, J.O.: A study of tissue response to cyanoacrylate adhesive in periodontal surgery, J. Periodontol. **45:**619, 1974.
30. O'Neil, T.C.A.: Antibacterial properties of periodontal dressings, J. Periodontol. **46:**469, 1975.
31. Addy, M., and Douglas, W.H.: A chlorhexidine containing methacrylic gel as a periodontal dressing, J. Periodontol. **46:**465, 1975.
32. Breloff, J.P., and Caffesse, R.G.: Effect of achromycin ointment on healing following periodontal surgery, J. Periodontol. **54:**368, 1983.
33. Pihlstrom, B.L., Thorn, H.L., and Folke, L.E.A.: The effect of periodontal dressing on supragingival microorganisms, J. Periodontol. **48:**440, 1977.
34. Hildebrand, C.N., and De Renzis, F.A.: Effect of periodontal dressings on fibroblasts in vitro, J. Periodont. Res. **9:**114, 1974.
35. Hangen, E.: The effect of periodontal dressings on intact mucous membrane and on wound healing, Acta Odontol. Scand. **38:**363, 1980.
36. Nezwek, R.A., et al.: Connective tissue response to periodontal dressings, J. Periodontol. **51:**521, 1980.

37. Poulson, R.C.: An anaphylactoid reaction to periodontal surgical dressing: report of case, J. Am. Dent. Assoc. **89:**895, 1974.

38. Kalkwarf, K.L., Amerman, G.W., and Tussing, G.J.: A vinyl stent for mucogingival graft procedures and postsurgical wound protection, J. Periodontol. **45:**797, 1974.

39. Glendinning, D.E.H.: A method for retention of the periodontal pack, J. Periodontol. **47:**236, 1976.

40. Vogel, R.I.: The effects of nonsteroidal anti-inflammatory analgesics on pain after periodontal surgery, J. Am. Dent. Assoc. **109:**731, 1984.

41. Dionne, R.A., et al.: Suppression of postoperative pain by preoperative administration of ibuprofen in comparison to placebo, acetaminophen plus codeine, J. Clin. Pharmacol. **23:**37, 1983.

42. Jastak, J.T., and Yagiela, J.A.: Vasoconstrictors and local anesthesia: a review and rationale for use, J. Am. Dent. Assoc. **107:**623, 1983.

43. Accepted dental therapeutics, ed. 39, Chicago, 1982, American Dental Association.

44. Pendrill, K., and Reddy, J.: The use of prophylactic penicillin in periodontal surgery, J. Periodontol. **51:**44, 1980.

## ADDITIONAL SUGGESTED READING

Haugen, E., and Mjör, I.A.: Bone tissue reactions to periodontal dressings, J. Periodont. Res. **14:**76, 1979.

Lahiffe, B.J., Caffesse, R.G., and Nasjleti, C.E.: Healing of periodontal flaps following use of MBR 4197 (Flucrylate) in Rhesus monkeys: a clinical histologic evaluation, J. Periodontol. **49:**635, 1978.

Manson, J.D., and Millar-Danks, S.: General anesthesia for periodontal surgery, J. Clin. Periodontol. **5:**163, 1978.

Newman, P.S., and Addy, M.: A comparison of a periodontal dressing and chlorhexidine gluconate mouthwash after the internal beveled flap procedure, J. Periodontol. **49:**576, 1978.

Watts, T.L.T., and Combe, E.C.: Periodontal dressing materials, J. Clin. Periodontol. **6:**63, 1979.

# CHAPTER 34

# Gingival and subgingival curettage: curettage of the pocket wall

**Definition**     *Gingival curettage* is a planned and systematic operation to remove the ulcerated, chronically inflamed gingival lining of a pocket (Fig. 34-1).

## Objectives of gingival curettage

The objectives of gingival curettage are to eliminate inflammation, to reduce pockets, and to restore gingival health. More specifically, gingival curettage is used to reduce clinical edema, hyperemia, or cyanosis and to cause a shrinkage of the free gingiva. The elimination of inflammation and the eradication of some or all of the gingival pocket may thereby be accomplished. Frequently this leaves a physiologic gingival contour so that further surgery is unnecessary.

The procedure (called *soft tissue curettage* by some) should be differentiated from scaling and root planing, which is the instrumentation applied to the tooth surface to divest it of deposits and to smooth it. During root planing, some inadvertent gingival curettage always occurs. However, gingival curettage is a purposeful procedure that is often performed at a separate visit. The procedure should be differentiated from subgingival curettage and from surgical curettage by flap, which are procedures used in reattachment operations and intentionally extend below the bottom of the pocket to alveolar bone. The term *curettage,* as used herein, will refer only to treatment of the pocket wall. Pioneers in the field used it more frequently and more extensively than any other procedure, with the exception of root planing.[1-4]

## Indications and contraindications

When gingival inflammation and edema persist after careful and thorough root planing, the operator may attempt to curette the lining of the pocket to reduce inflammation and to encourage a shrinkage of the gingival margin. Patients with edematous and granulomatous inflammations respond better to curettage than do those with

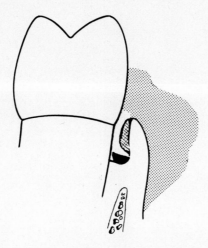

**Fig. 34-1.**   Diagram of curette removing inner wall of pocket *(cross-hatching).*

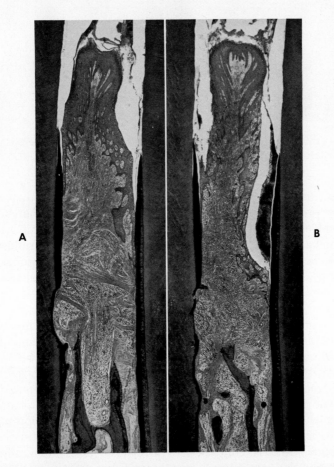

**Fig. 34-2.**   Two histologic sections of the same interproximal area in a patient with periodontitis. Note the extension of the inflammatory cellular infiltrate. **A,** Labially located section. **B,** More centrally located section.

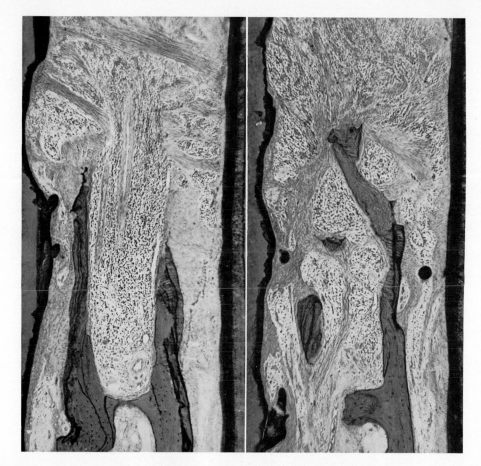

**Fig. 34-3.** *High magnification of the alveolar crestal areas shown in Fig. 34-2. Note the extension of the chronic inflammatory process into the bone marrow spaces.*

conditions characterized primarily by a fibrous hyperplasia. This treatment may also be valuable for patients in whom more extensive surgery is contraindicated because of emotional problems, resistance to surgery per se, or systemic impairment.

Fibrotic gingiva does not respond readily to curettage when shrinkage of the marginal gingiva is the aim. Wide or tortuous intra-alveolar pockets are not amenable to gingival curettage. Bony craters are treated by osseous procedures or bone grafts.

### POCKET WALL

**Chronic inflammatory tissue**

In Figs. 34-2 and 34-3, the connective tissue alongside and directly beneath the periodontal pocket is chronically inflamed. The sulcular epithelium is ulcerated and may have proliferated into the underlying connective tissue. The vessels are enlarged and increased in number. A round cell infiltrate has occurred in the lamina propria, and fibroblasts and collagen fibers are sparse. This chronically inflamed connective tissue is called *granulation tissue* although *granulomatous tissue* is more appropriate. It was once believed to be infected.[5-9] However, the term *granulation tissue* is a misnomer in this case. Granulation tissue is also found in healing wounds and is composed of fibroblasts and proliferating capillaries, which give it a granular appearance. Granulation tissue reforms into a normal fibrous connective tissue during wound healing. The chronically inflamed granulomatous tissue is not infected, however,[9] despite the occasional presence of bacteria.[10] If all the irritants are removed, it will remodel into a fibrous connective tissue.[11-13] The removal of chronic inflammatory tissue during gingival curettage may enhance the remodelling process.

## Method

Gingival curettage[14-23] excises the lining of the pocket to remove subjacent inflammatory tissue. This is a surgical procedure, and local anesthesia should be administered. The surgeon should plan to operate around a single tooth or a segment of the arch at one sitting. Whether this can be done will depend on the accessibility and topography of the pockets and the character of the tissue. One should not attempt to curette thin, friable gingiva; there is danger of perforating or tearing such tissue. The instrument should be held in a modified pen grasp, using the third or fourth finger as a rest. One should cut rather than tear or mutilate the soft tissue pocket wall. Placement of the thumb and index finger against the buccolabial or lingual surface of the gingiva during instrumentation will support the tissue and aid in performing the curettage. Using a definite pattern and short strokes, one should bring the diseased tissue to the surface and wipe the blade of the curette clean with sterile gauze. After curettage, wash the pockets with sterile normal saline solution or chlorhexidine gluconate, using a Luer-Lok syringe, with a blunt (25-gauge) needle, and inspect the surgical area to ensure that complete débridement has been achieved. Tissues should be carefully approximated to the tooth and surgical dressing applied.

Some periodontists have sets of curettes to be used only on soft tissue. These instruments are kept exquisitely sharp. They are delicate in construction, with thin blades to enter narrow, deep, and circuitous pockets. This armamentarium is made by sharpening and thinning standard curette blades to the operator's desire. The use of a curette in gingival curettage is illustrated in Fig. 34-4.

**Armamentarium**

In Fig. 34-5, *A*, an interproximal area can be seen. Calculus extends to the bottom of the pockets. The soft tissue sides of the pockets are lined with epithelium of varying thickness, ulcerated in some areas. Epithelial strands project into the lamina propria, where plasma cells, some lymphocytes, macrophages, and a few polymorphonuclear leukocytes can be seen close to the bottom of the pocket. Chronically inflamed gingival connective tissue consists mainly of plasma cells, proliferating epithelial strands, and some fibrous connective tissue elements and ground substance.

To eliminate such a pocket by gingival curettage, the surgeon should first remove all calculus by root planing (Fig. 34-5, *B*). When the root surface is thoroughly planed and smoothed and the edema has not resolved, gingival curettage is performed at a subsequent visit to remove the pocket lining and some of the inflammatory connective tissue (*C*). The result of tissue shrinkage after curettage is illustrated diagrammatically in *D*. Healing may occur in a week (Fig. 34-6).

Postoperative instrumentation in the area should be delayed for at least 2 weeks, since a longer period is necessary for connective tissue maturation.[11-14]

Reduction in edema and pocket depth is usual. However, a slight reattachment may occur.[15-18,24-26] It is possible, but not preferable, to do root planing and gingival curettage at the same visit. When this is done, the procedures are performed consecutively after lavage, not simultaneously. Root planing mobilizes fragments of calculus and cementum that may be forced into tissue during gingival curettage if the procedures are done simultaneously.

While gingival inflammation, attachment level, and pocket depth all improve when checked 4 to 9 weeks following curettage, similar results can be obtained with scaling and root planing alone.[19]

The value of gingival curettage is controversial.[20] Several authors have advocated

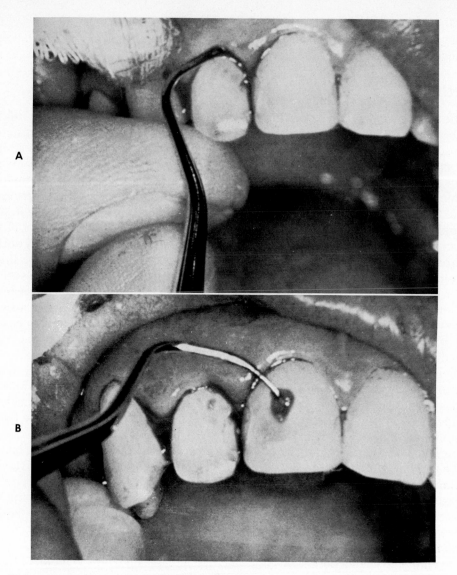

**Fig. 34-4.**  Gingival curettage. **A,** Curette in a pocket. **B,** Tissue removed by curettage. (Courtesy E. Robinson, Napa, California.)

the use of gingival curettage for pocket reduction, treatment of periodontal abscesses, presurgical débridement, and periodontal maintenance.[4,20-24]

While gingival curettage may be as successful as other forms of therapy in maintaining periodontal attachment levels,[15,17,20,25,26] the discrepancy between the reports of proponents and opponents of this technique as a method of therapy is cause for reevaluative studies of subgingival curettage.

## Other instruments and treatments

Other types of instrumentation include ultrasonic scalers, high-speed rotary diamonds, and chemicals. The ultrasonic instrument may be used for gingival curettage (Fig. 34-7). Histologic studies have shown ultrasonic scaling to be effective in the removal of ulcerated pocket epithelium. Sound energy absorbed at tissue junctions (basement membrane area) may take the form of heat, resulting in coagulation.[27] The

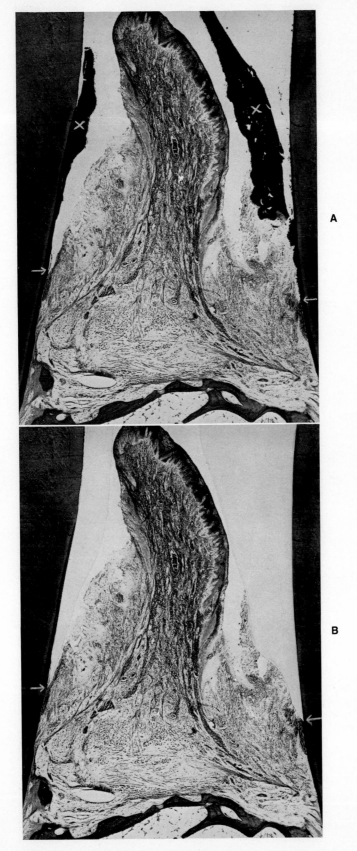

**Fig. 34-5.** Severe periodontitis in an interproximal area. *x*, Calculus. Arrows designate bottom of the pockets. **B**, Hypothetical result after calculus removed by root planing. *Continued.*

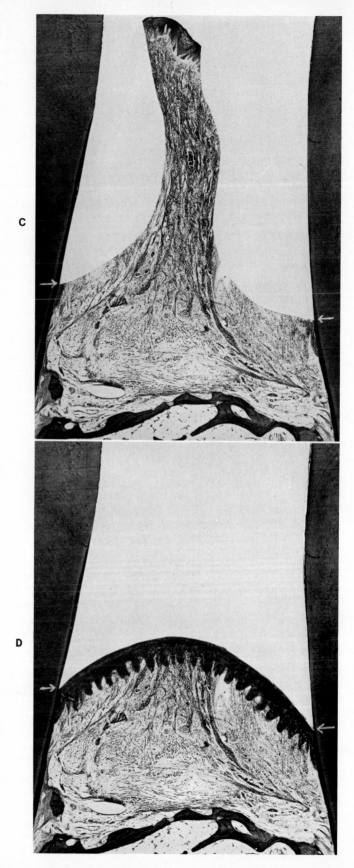

**Fig. 34-5, cont'd.** **C,** Pocket lining removed by curettage. (Simulated.) **D,** Tissue shrinkage and healing as expected after gingival curettage. (Simulated.)

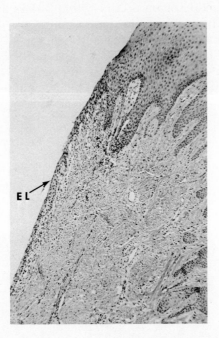

**Fig. 34-6.** Intact epithelial lining, *EL,* 8 days after gingival curettage. (Courtesy B.S. Moskow, Columbia University, New York, New York.)

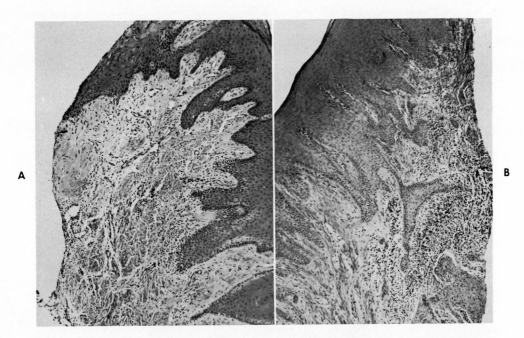

**Fig. 34-7.** **A,** Sulcular epithelium and underlying connective tissue 7 days after ultrasonic curettage. The sulcular epithelium is intact, and there is less inflammation. **B,** Seven days after hand instrumentation, epithelial continuity has not been restored, and a mild inflammation is present in the lamina propria. (Courtesy J.R. Wilson, Columbus, Ohio.)

coagulated epithelium is probably removed by the mechanical action of the vibrating tool and the lavage. Epithelization occurs within 3 days after ultrasonic curettage; fewer inflammatory cells are found in the lamina propria than are seen after hand instrumentation.[28,29] This reduction may result from the lavage.

Some operators use bipolar electrocautery (Fig. 34-8). Others use chemical treatment followed by soft tissue curettage. This old technique is the subject of renewed interest. The tissue is treated by sodium hypochlorite neutralized by citric acid. It may be equally as efficacious as soft tissue curettage described earlier but does not require anesthesia.[30]

## CASE REPORT

A localized, acute, marginal, papillary gingivitis in a 34-year-old woman (first seen at age 17) is shown in Fig. 34-9, A. Calcified deposits covered the cervical third of the

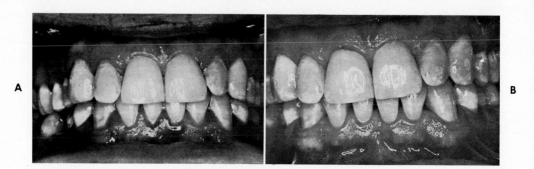

**Fig. 34-8.** **A,** Chronic, marginal, papillary gingivitis. **B,** After treatment consisting of root planing and gingival curettage with bipolar electrocautery. Tissue repair and resolution of inflammation are evident. (Courtesy W. Hiatt, Denver, Colorado.)

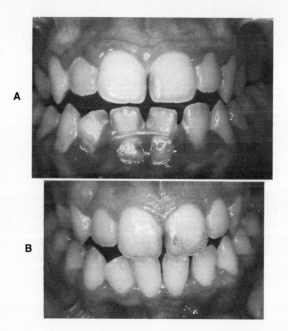

**Fig. 34-9.** **A,** Intensely inflamed gingival margins in a 17-year-old female. Inflamed gingiva has proliferated over calculus on mandibular central incisors to enclose the deposit. **B,** Following scaling, root planing, and gingival curettage, gingival enlargement has been eliminated. Gingival margins are thin, minimal probing depth is present, and effective plaque removal has enabled patient to maintain health when seen at age 34.

crowns of the mandibular central incisors. Some marginal gingiva had been destroyed, and the receded gingival margins now approximated the mucogingival junction. A periodontal probe inserted into pockets extended 1 mm beyond the mucogingival junction. The vestibular gingiva around the incisors was deep red in color and bled easily on touch. The papillae were enlarged and blunted.

Treatment consisted of root planing and plaque control. Gingival curettage was performed to remove the edematous tissue. A remarkable regeneration of tissue had taken place 3 months later ( Fig. 34-9, *B*). The gingiva throughout the mouth had the clinical characteristics of health, including shallow sulcus, physiologic form, and a functionally adequate zone of gingiva. Despite the possible mucogingival problem, cure was effected without mucogingival surgery.

## Objectives of subgingival curettage

*Closed subgingival curettage* is instrumentation by way of the lumen of the pocket   **Definition** to remove the soft tissue wall of a pocket and the connective tissue, subjacent to the level of the alveolar crest. Subgingival curettage is employed in the treatment of both suprabony and infrabony defects ( Figs. 34-10 to 34-12).

Subgingival curettage is used to cause shrinkage and to promote reattachment   **Objectives**

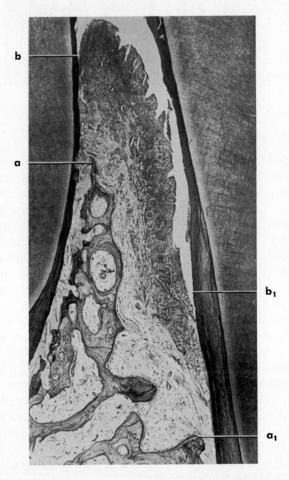

**Fig. 34-10.** Histologic section of an infrabony pocket between two molars. The alveolar bone on one molar is high, *a*, and the pocket shallow, *b*. On the other molar the pocket is deep, $b_1$, and the alveolar bone is reabsorbed, $a_1$. Opportunity for reattachment via subgingival curettage is present, but the probability of recession is minimal, since the level of the bone would prevent shrinkage.

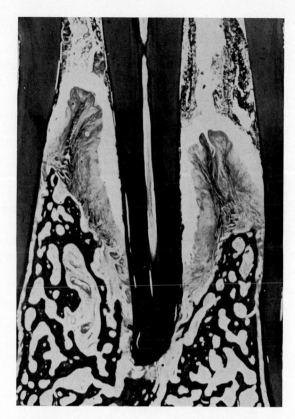

**Fig. 34-11.** Histologic section of infrabony pockets on both sides of a mandibular incisor. Such troughlike bony defects are best treated by curettage by way of flap.

(new attachment). On occasion, regrowth of bone may occur, the result of which is reduction of pocket depth and, sometimes, elimination of the pocket.[31-37] For years subgingival curettage was the classical instrumentation for reattachment.[31-32]

**Method**     Subgingival (closed) curettage requires that the area be anesthetized and surgical preparations, including sterility, be followed (Chapter 33). The instrumentation with curettes is similar to that described for gingival curettage (Fig. 34-13, *A*). For the reattachment procedure, however, all attachment epithelium must be removed, as well as some or all connective tissue adjacent and subjacent to the pocket to the level of the alveolar crest, until the curette blade contacts bone (Fig. 34-13, *B* and *C*).

The curette blade is inserted into the pocket in an exploratory closed-face position until it reaches the junctional epithelium. It is then pushed beyond the junctional epithelium until it touches the alveolar margin. The alveolar margin is usually 1 to 3 mm beyond the junctional epithelium. Next the blade is turned so its opposite edge becomes the working edge (Fig. 34-13, *C*). The soft tissues are excised with an upward curetting motion. The fingertip may be used to support the gingiva during this stroke.

The curette tip is worked circumdentally about each tooth individually. The blade is not carried across the interdental papilla to the next tooth, since this would raise a flap. Instead the instrument is removed from the lumen of the pocket of one tooth and placed in the pocket of the next tooth.

The subgingival curettage may be localized or performed about a tooth, a quadrant, or more. If more than one tooth is worked on, the interdental papilla is not reflected but is left to cover the interseptal bone to the greatest extent possible. This is characteristic of closed curettage as opposed to open curettage, in which a flap is reflected

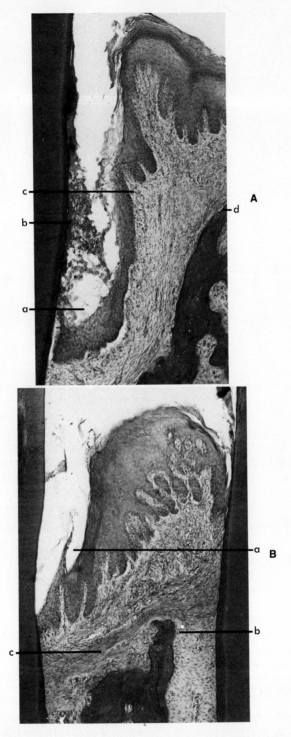

**Fig. 34-12.  A,** Histologic section demonstrating an infrabony pocket *(a)* with plaque and calculus on the root surface *(b)* and inflammation in the wall of the pocket *(c)*. *d*, Alveolar bone. Infrabony defects, such as this, may offer the opportunity for reattachment by way of closed subgingival curettage. **B,** Shallow infrabony defect offering the best opportunity for reattachment and possible new bone growth. *a*, Pocket; *b*, alveolar crest; *c*, transseptal fibers now at a more apical level.

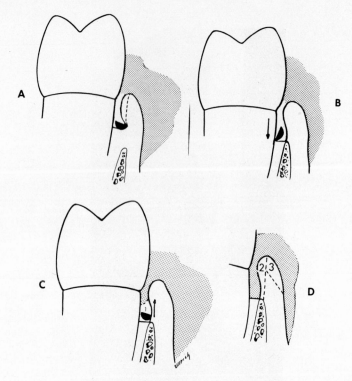

**Fig. 34-13. A,** Placement of curette at the bottom of the pocket for gingival curettage. **B,** Planing of root and curettage of connective tissue to alveolar crest in closed subgingival curettage. **C,** Removal of connective tissue and sulcular epithelium. *(Arrows indicate direction of stroke in **B** and **C.) D,** Removing the gingival wall (2). 3, Minor gingivectomy component.*

and the interdental papilla removed. Thus the gingiva is left fairly well coapted to the teeth. If it is accidentally detached, the gingiva should be pressed to the tooth. A surgical dressing should be placed. Antibiotics may be prescribed.

### STEPS

The steps of the reattachment operation by subgingival curettage are summarized as follows:

1. Remove the sulcular and junctional epithelium (Fig. 34-13, *A*).
2. Curette the underlying connective tissue to the bone (Fig. 34-13, *B* and *C*).
3. Perform a modified gingivectomy, removing some of the pocket depth as well as the marginal gingival epithelium (Figs. 34-13, *D*, and 34-14). (This step is optional and is not used by all periodontists.)
4. Approximate the gingiva to the tooth, thus reducing the size of the clot and bringing the wound into closer contact with the root.
5. Place a surgical dressing for 5 to 7 days.

### MODIFIED GINGIVECTOMY

Modified gingivectomy was added to the subgingival curettage procedure both to obtain pocket reduction and to deter migration of epithelium while the collagen fibers and a new attachment are formed. Subgingival curettage may be performed with or without the addition of the minor gingivectomy (see Fig. 34-18). In either event, the previously planed root surface should be planed and smoothed again by finishing procedures; the use of ultrasonic tips may aid in this process. Absorbed endotoxins[38] are removed, and reattachment is facilitated.[39,40] Citric acid may promote reattachment

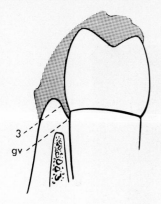

**Fig. 34-14.** *Comparison of levels of incisions in the gingivectomy. Component of subgingival curettage (3) is compared with gingivectomy (gv).*

by removing absorbed enzymes and by solubilizing superficial collagen bundles and demineralizing superficial cementum and dentin,[41-45] although the modern use of acids to assist in reattachment is by way of the open subgingival curettage procedures rather than the closed. These steps are reported to encourage the formation of a new attachment (reattachment). Tooth support previously destroyed by disease may be restored. Pocket reduction can occur even in the presence of fibrotic gingiva because of the gingivectomy component.

*A note of caution:* Use different sets of curettes for root curettage and for gingival or subgingival curettage. The latter instruments must be kept exquisitely sharp so that they function as knife blades. As they are made thinner by sharpening, they may reach inaccessible areas of circuitous pockets with greater ease.

## Summary

Although clinical observations of recession of the gingival margin after subgingival curettage were common in the past, for many years reattachment was believed to be rare or impossible to obtain.[35-36] Although clinical evidence that reattachment (new attachment) can occur is strong,[46] experimental evidence for it is sometimes subject to question.[47]

When reattachment is attempted, it may be successful, partly successful, or unsuccessful. Proper case selection and careful technique tend to increase the percentage of success ( Figs. 34-15 to 34-17).[47-50]

The clinician can evaluate the relative success of reattachment operations by careful clinical probing and roentgenograms. For investigative purposes, however, more critical criteria for evaluation are required. Reduction in pocket depth may be caused by gingival recession as well as by reattachment. Pocket closure may be effected by the formation of a new dentogingival junction after the regeneration of alveolar bone, by the formation of a long junctional epithelium or by a close adaptation of the gingiva to the tooth impeding probing (see Fig. 34-21). Growth coronal to the preexisting gingival margin may occur. This has been termed *creeping reattachment.*[51,52]

Subgingival curettage is a procedure of clinical value in obtaining pocket reduction by tissue shrinkage as well as by reattachment. It can be used locally about a single tooth or generally in both arches as by reattachment. It may provoke bone regeneration, a long epithelial attachment, or creeping reattachment. It is useful in phase I therapy coupled with procedures for débridement. Its goal in phase II therapy is bone regeneration and reattachment. When pockets recur, following properly conducted surgical interventions, and a lesser surgical procedure is needed to achieve health, subgingival curettage or gingivectomy should be considered.

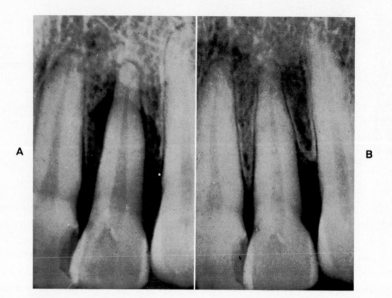

**Fig. 34-15.** **A,** Preoperative roentgenogram in a case of reattachment by subgingival curettage. Bone destruction appears in a semilunar pattern. **B,** Roentgenogram of the patient 1 year after the reattachment operation. Note the height and density of the alveolar processes.

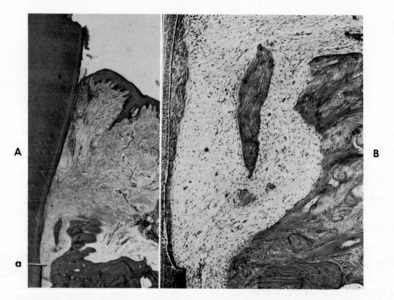

**Fig. 34-16.** **A,** Human biopsy specimen. The histologic section shows the result of an experimental reattachment operation. The notch on the surface of the cementum, *a,* and the corresponding bone defect show the extent to which curettage has been performed. **B,** Higher magnification of the apical end of the curettage showing new formation of cementum on the curetted cemental surface, with attachment of periodontal fibers and formation of new bone. This specimen may indicate only healing after surgical wounding with a curette rather than reattachment. However, it appears that there has been bone apposition lateral to the alveolar crest. (Courtesy H. Zander, Chicago, Illinois.)

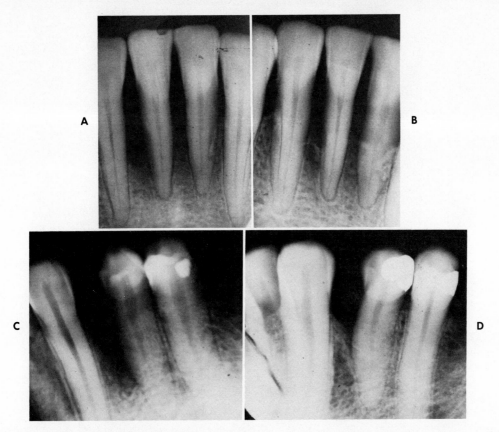

**Fig. 34-17.** **A,** Preoperative roentgenogram of bone level prior to subgingival curettage procedure. **B,** Postoperative view 2 years 8 months later. Note bone regeneration between central incisors and between central and lateral incisors accompanied by reduction in width of periodontal ligament. **C,** Preoperative view of bone level prior to subgingival curettage procedure. **D,** Postoperative view 2 years 4 months later. (**A** and **B** courtesy T. Kostaridis, Athens, Greece.)

Gingivectomy knives may be employed in gingivoplasty fashion to incise, shape, and smooth the gingival surface. This gingivectomy component of the subgingival curettage need not be performed about all teeth in a quadrant. Its use depends on the relative health of the gingiva about each tooth. In addition, it is a modified gingivectomy, and its use is limited to the marginal gingiva. Generally, it need not extend to the base of the pocket, as does the true gingivectomy (see Fig. 34-14), but it can when the pocket is shallow.

Criticism of reports of reattachment according to roentgenographs is based on the possibility of misinterpretation.

Increased density of bone may be caused by an increase in trabeculation of existing bone after treatment rather than by the formation of new bone. Roentgenograms alone cannot provide indisputable evidence of success or failure.[37,47,53] Variables in roentgenography, such as angulation, density, voltage, and amperage, make the x-ray film less than fully reliable as an evaluative tool. However, when standardized methods of taking the roentgenogram are used together with parallel projection techniques and measuring devices such as grids[53] and calibrated silver points placed in the same plane[54] (Fig. 34-18), the critically evaluated roentgenogram can be a useful clinical tool for measuring bony reattachment.[46,52,53]

Closed subgingival curettage, gingival curettage, open subgingival curettage, and the flap procedure used in more extensive periodontal surgery have certain elements in common. They produce a wounding of the marginal periodontium in which tissue

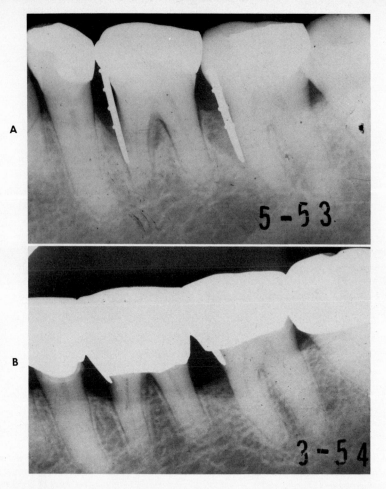

**Fig. 34-18.** Regeneration in three-walled infrabony defect after closed subgingival curettage, combining gingivectomy and curettage. Before **(A)** and after **(B)** procedure. Note the level of pockets as indicated by silver points. (Courtesy L. Hirschfeld, New York, New York.)

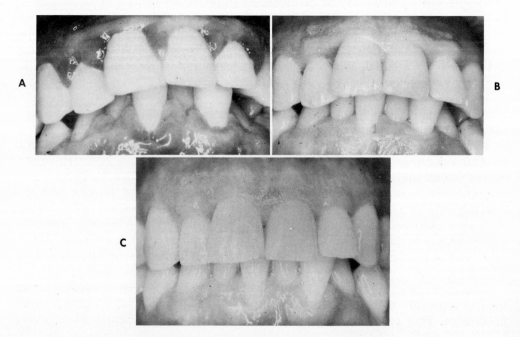

**Fig. 34-19.** **A,** Preoperative view of patient with inflammatory hyperplasia. **B,** Plaque control and curettage 3 months after scaling. **C,** Appearance 7 years after surgery.

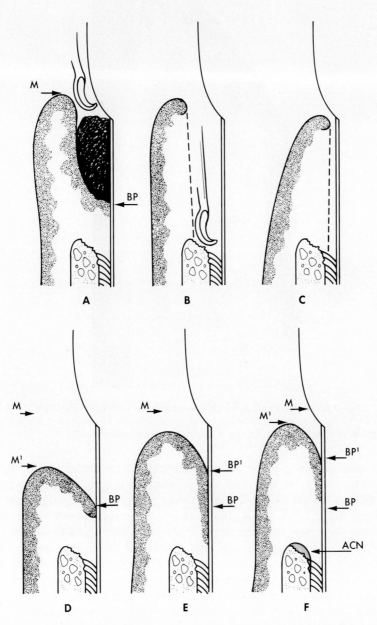

**Fig. 34-20.** **A,** Periodontal pocket with plaque and calculus prior to instrumentation. *BP*, Bottom of pocket; *M*, preoperative level of gingival margin. **B,** Subgingival curettage performed. **C,** Close apposition of wound surface to tooth. **D,** Recession of gingival margin. *M*, Preoperative level of gingival margin; *M*¹, postoperative level of gingival margin; *BP*, preoperative and postoperative attachment levels. **E,** Reattachment via long junctional epithelium. *M*, Preoperative level of gingival margin; *BP*, preoperative attachment level; *BP*¹, postoperative attachment level. **F,** Reattachment via coronal migration of junctional epithelium; connective tissue reattachment and bone apposition (regeneration). *M*, Preoperative gingival margin; *M*¹, postoperative gingival margin; *BP*, preoperative attachment level; *BP*¹, postoperative attachment level; *ACN*, new bone apposition (regeneration).

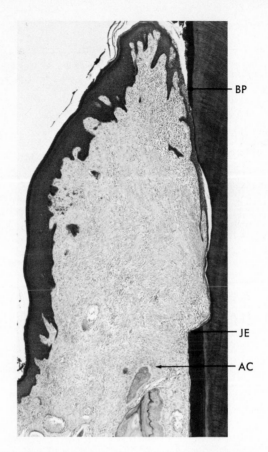

**Fig. 34-21.** Long epithelial attachment a month after subgingival curettage in a monkey. *BP,* Bottom of pocket with mild inflammation; *JE,* junctional epithelium ends in notch created by extensive root curettage; *AC,* alveolar crest with thin line of osteoid at the crest and on the periodontal ligament side.

is excised, resulting in a pocket elimination and tissue shrinkage (Figs. 34-19 and 34-20, *D*). The wounding may also lead to reattachment by way of a long junctional epithelium (Figs. 34-20 and 34-21) or to tissue regeneration through new cementum, alveolar bone, and periodontal ligament fibers[48,49,55] (Fig. 34-20, *F*). Finally, they all may encourage creeping reattachment. To a certain extent, all these phenomena will occur about the teeth in any mouth after the use of these procedures. Curettage by flap is discussed in Chapter 37. The closed subgingival curettage differs from the other procedures in various ways, perhaps the most significant of which is that it maintains the interdental papilla, whereas the others either remove it or tend to remove it.

The possible results that follow the use of closed subgingival curettage are shown diagrammatically in Fig. 34-20.

**REFERENCES**

1. Bell, D.G.: Clinical procedures in periodontal therapy, J. Periodontol. **27:**301, 1956.
2. Younger, W.J.: Pyorrhea alveolaris: remarks on the treatment, Int. Dent. J. **20:**413, 1899.
3. Sachs, H.: Die Behandlung lockerer Zähne, Berlin, 1929, Berlinische Verlagsanstalt.
4. Halik, F.J.: The role of subgingival curettage to periodontal therapy, Dent. Clin. North Am. **13:**19, 1969.
5. Zentler, A.: Suppurative gingivitis with alveolar involvement: a new surgical procedure, JAMA **71:**1530, 1918.
6. Crane, A.B., and Kaplan, H.: The Crane-Kaplan operation for the prompt elimination of pyorrhea alveolaris, Dent. Cosmos **73:**643, 1931.
7. Ward, A.: Consideration of periodontal pocket elimination, Acad. Rev. **4:**64, 1956.
8. Raust, G.T., et al.: What is the value of gingival

curettage in periodontal therapy? Periodont. Abstr. **17:**142, 1969.

9. Orban, B.: To what extent should the tissues be excised in gingivectomy? J. Periodontol. **2:**83, 1941.

10. Saglie, F.R., Newman, M.G., and Carranza, F.A., Jr.: Bacterial invasion of gingiva in advanced periodontitis in humans, J. Periodontol. **53:**217, 1982.

11. Morris, M.L.: The removal of pocket and attachment epithelium in humans: a histological study, J. Periodontol. **25:**7, 1954.

12. Moskow, B.S.: The response of the gingival sulcus to instrumentation: a histological investigation. II. Gingival curettage, J. Periodontol. **35:**112, 1964.

13. Kon, S., et al.: Visualization of microvascularization of the healing periodontal wound. II. Curettage, J. Periodontol. **40:**96, 1969.

14. Stahl, S.S., et al.: Soft tissue healing following curettage and root planing, J. Periodontol. **42:**678, 1971.

15. Ramfjord, S.P., et al.: Subgingival curettage versus surgical elimination of periodontal pockets, J. Periodontol. **39:**167, 1968.

16. Chase, R.: Subgingival curettage in periodontal therapy, J. Periodontol. **45:**107, 1974.

17. Burgett, F.G., et al.: Short term results of three modalities of periodontal treatment, J. Periodontol. **48:**131, 1977.

18. Ramfjord, S.P.: Results following three modalities of therapy, J. Periodontol. **46:**522, 1975.

19. Lopez, N. J., and Belvederesse, M.: Subgingival scaling with root planing and curettage: effects on gingival inflammation, J. Periodontol. **48:**354, 1977.

20. Chaikin, B.S.: Subgingival curettage, J. Periodontol. **25:**240, 1954.

21. Hirschfeld, L.S.: The role of subgingival curettage in periodontal therapy, Alpha Omegan **60:**115, 1962.

22. Chase, R.: Subgingival curettage in periodontal therapy, J. Periodontol. **45:**107, 1974.

23. Kenney, E.B.: Subgingival curettage, J. Mich. Dent. Assoc. **51:**295, 1969.

24. Ramfjord, S.P., et al.: Longitudinal study of periodontal therapy, J. Periodontol. **44:**66, 1973.

25. Moskow, B.S.: The response of the gingival sulcus to instrumentation. II. Gingival curettage, J. Periodontol. **35:**112, 1964.

26. Caton, J.G., and Zander, H.A.: The attachment between tooth and gingival tissues after periodontic root planing and soft tissue curettage, J. Periodontol. **50:**462, 1979.

27. Ewen, S.J.: The ultrasonic wound: some microscopic observations, J. Periodontol. **32:**315, 1961.

28. Goldman, H.M.: Histologic assay of healing following ultrasonic curettage versus hand instrument curettage, Oral Surg. **14:**925, 1961.

29. Frisch, J., Bhaskar, S.N., and Shell, D.D.: Effect of ultrasonic instrumentation on human gingival connective tissue, Periodontics **5:**123, 1967.

30. Kalkwarf, K.L., Tussing, G.J., and Davis, M.J.: Histologic evaluation of gingival curettage facilitated by sodium hypochlorite solution, J. Periodontol. **53:**63, 1982.

31. Goldman, H.M.: A rationale for the treatment of the infrabony pocket: one method of treatment, subgingival curettage, J. Periodontol. **20:**33, 1949.

32. Schaffer, E.M., and Zander, H.A.: Histological evidence of reattachment of periodontal pockets, Parodontologie **7:**101, 1953.

33. Prichard, J.: The infrabony technique as a predictable procedure, J. Periodontol. **28:**202, 1957.

34. Black, G.V.: Special dental pathology, Chicago, 1915, Medico-Dental Publishing Co.

35. Skillen, W.G., and Lundquist, G.R.: An experimental study of peridental membrane reattachment in healthy and pathologic tissues, J. Am. Dent. Assoc. **24:**175, 1937.

36. Orban, B.: Pocket elimination or reattachment, N. Y. J. Dent. **14:**227, 1948.

37. Orban, B., and Orban, T.: Three-dimensional roentgenographic interpretation in peridontal diagnosis, J. Periodontol. **31:**275, 1960.

38. Aleo, J.J., et al.: The presence and biologic activity of cementum-bound endotoxin, J. Periodontol. **45:**672, 1974.

39. Aleo, J.J., De Renzis, F.A., and Farber, P.A.: In vitro attachment of human gingival fibroblasts to root surfaces, J. Periodontol. **46:**639, 1975.

40. Register, A.A., and Burdick, F.A.: Accelerated reattachment with cementogenesis to dentin, demineralized in situ. I. Optimum range, J. Periodontol. **46:**646, 1975.

41. Register, A.A., and Burdick, F.A.: Accelerated reattachment with cementogenesis to dentin, demineralized in situ. II. Defect repair, J. Periodontol. **47:**497, 1976.

42. Stahl, S.S., and Froum, S.J.: Human clinical and histologic repair responses following the use of citric acid in periodontal therapy, J. Periodontol. **48:**261, 1977.

43. Garrett, J.S., Crigger, M., and Egelberg, J.: Effects of citric acid on diseased root surfaces, J. Periodont. Res. **13:**155, 1978.

44. Kalkwarf, K.L.: Periodontal new attachment without the placement of osseous potentiating grafts, Periodont. Abstr. **22:**53, 1974.

45. Stahl, S.S.: Repair potential of the soft tissue–root interface, J. Periodontol. **48:**545, 1977.

46. Friedman, N.: Reattachment and roentgenograms, J. Periodontol. **29:**98, 1958.

47. Moskow, B.S.: Repair potential in periodontal disease: the interproximal channel, J. Periodontol. **49:**55, 1978.

48. Register, A.A.: Bone and cementum induction by dentin, demineralized in situ, J. Periodontol. **44:**49, 1973.

49. Linghorne, W.J., and O'Connell, D.C.: Studies in the reattachment and regeneration of the supporting structures of the teeth. III. Regeneration in epithelized pockets, J. Dent. Res. **34:**164, 1955.

50. Garnick, J.J.: Long junctional epithelium: epithelial reattachment in the rat, J. Periodontol. **48:**722, 1977.

51. Goldman, H.M., et al.: Periodontal therapy, ed. 2, St. Louis, 1960, The C.V. Mosby Co.

52. Wade, A.B.: An assessment of the flap operation, Dent. Pract. **13:**11, 1962.

53. Everett, F.G., and Fixott, H.C.: Use of an incorporated grid in the diagnosis of oral roentgenograms, Oral Surg. **16:**1061, 1963.

54. Hirschfeld, L.: Calibrated silver points for periodontal diagnosis and recording, J. Periodontol. **24:**94, 1953.

55. Moskow, B.S.: Healing potential in periodontal lesions: the interdental crater, J. Periodontol. **48:**754, 1977.

### ADDITIONAL SUGGESTED READING

Beube, F.E.: The problem of reattachment, J. Periodontol. **31:**310, 1960.

Beube, F.E.: A radiographic and histologic study on reattachment, J. Periodontol. **23:**158, 1952.

Bhaskar, S.N., Grower, M.F., and Cutright, D.E.: Gingival healing after hand and ultrasonic scaling—biochemical and histologic analysis, J. Periodontol. **43:**31, 1972.

Björn, H.: Experimental studies on reattachment, Dent. Pract. **11:**351, 1960.

Carranza, F.A.: A technique for reattachment, J. Periodontol. **25:**272, 1954.

Held, A.J., and Chaput, A.: Les parodontolyses, Paris, 1959, Prelat.

Kramer, G.M., and Kohn, J.D.: Postoperative care of the infrabony pocket, J. Periodontol. **32:**95, 1961.

Lindhe, J., et al.: Clinical and structural alterations characterizing healing gingiva, J. Periodont. Res. **13:**410, 1978.

Patur, B., and Glickman, I.: Clinical and roentgenographic evaluation of the post-treatment healing of infrabony pockets, J. Periodontol. **33:**164, 1962.

Prichard, J.F.: The etiology, diagnosis and treatment of the intrabony defect, J. Periodontol. **38:**455, 1967.

Ramfjord, S.: Reattachment in periodontal therapy, J. Am. Dent. Assoc. **45:**513, 1952.

Reinhardt, R.A., Johnson, G.K., and Tussing, G.J.: Root planing with interdental papilla reflection and fiber optic illumination, J. Periodontol. **56:**721, 1985.

Rockoff, S.C., Rockoff, H.S., and Sackler, A.M.: Reattachment—a case in point, J. Periodontol. **29:**261, 1958.

Smith, T.S.: The treatment of two periodontal cases, J. Periodontol. **20:**129, 1949.

# CHAPTER 35

## Gingivectomy and gingivoplasty

**Prerequisites**

**Indications**

**Instruments**

**Method**
Gingivectomy-gingivoplasty, surgical steps
Gingivoplasty alone
Illustrative cases

**Gingivectomy-gingivoplasty procedure**
Presurgical period
Surgery
Postsurgical checklist and procedures

**Wound healing**
Aids in the healing process

**Electrosurgery**

**Evaluation of results**
Errors in surgical technique

**Contraindications**

---

*Gingivectomy* is the excision of the soft tissue wall of a pocket (Fig. 35-1, *A*). Its **Definition** objective is the elimination of pockets. *Gingivoplasty* is the recontouring of gingiva that has lost its physiologic form (Fig. 35-1, *B*). Its objective is the creation of physiologic gingival form rather than the elimination of pockets. Gingivectomy and gingivoplasty are most often performed together, although they may be considered separately for teaching purposes. The two names reflect only the two different objectives **Objectives** of the same procedure.[1-4]

In the elimination of the signs and symptoms of gingival disease, nonsurgical therapy (root planing, proper oral hygiene) or minor surgical intervention (curettage) will often suffice. In some cases inflammation and consequent periodontal disease may recur or remain unresolved. Often such failures are the result of inadequate scaling or poor performance of oral hygiene procedures. Frequently, however, recurrence relates to preexisting pocket depth that was not reduced or eliminated.[5] The pocket permits plaque accumulation and remains as a locus minoris resistentiae and predisposes to further extension of the disease. In such cases the removal of the pocket (Fig. 35-2) and proper long-term maintenance by the dentist and the patient can result in tissue health.

## Prerequisites

The gingivectomy-gingivoplasty surgical technique is used in a small number of situations. However, before gingivectomy-gingivoplasty is performed, the basic prerequisites for gingivectomy must exist:

1. The zone of gingiva must be wide enough so that the excision of part of it will still leave a functionally adequate zone.

761

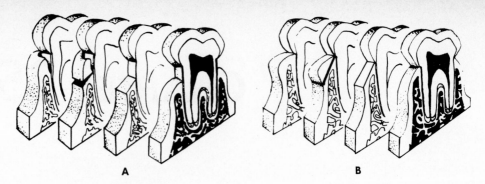

**Fig. 35-1.** **A,** Sequence in the performance of gingivectomy. **B,** Sequence in the performance of gingivoplasty. (Modified from Fröhlich, E.: Die chirurgische Behandlung der marginalen Parodontitis. In Haupl, K., Meyer, W., and Schuchardt, K.: Die Zahn-, Mund-, und Kieferheilkunde, vol. 3, pt. 1, Munich, 1957, Urban & Schwarzenberg.)

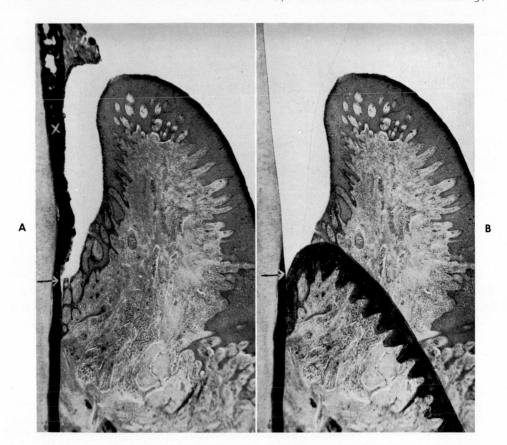

**Fig. 35-2.** Illustration to show the objective in gingivectomy. In **A,** calculus is indicated by *x;* arrow indicates the bottom of the pocket. **B,** Calculus removed by root planing and excision of gingiva, with resultant healing indicated by reduced gingival contours. (Simulated.)

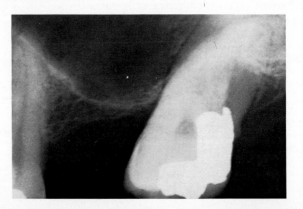

**Fig. 35-3.** The proximity of the maxillary antrum may contraindicate the performance of osseous surgery.

2. The underlying alveolar crest must be normal or nearly normal in form. If bone loss has occurred, the loss must be horizontal in nature, leaving a relatively regular crestal bone form at a lower level.[6]
3. There should be no infrabony (intra-alveolar) defects or pockets.

## Indications

If these prerequisites are met, gingivectomy-gingivoplasty may be used to do the following:

1. Eliminate supra-alveolar pockets and pseudopockets (see classification of pockets, Chapter 16, p. 357).
2. Remove fibrous or edematous enlargements of the gingiva.
3. Transform rolled or blunted margins to physiologic form.
4. Create more esthetic form in cases in which exposure of the anatomic crown has not fully occurred.
5. Create bilateral symmetry where the gingival margin of one incisor has receded somewhat more than that of the adjacent incisor.
6. Expose additional clinical crown to gain added retention for restorative purposes, to provide access to subgingival caries, or to permit a clamp to be seated in endodontic treatment.
7. Correct gingival craters.
8. Gingivectomy may be taught as a phase I method to expedite removal of tooth deposits.[7]

In addition, gingivectomy-gingivoplasty may be used as a compromise when other procedures are ordinarily indicated but are not feasible. For example, a maxillary molar (Fig. 35-3) may have an intra-alveolar defect on the mesial aspect that can ordinarily be corrected by osseous surgery. However, in this instance the proximity of the antrum can limit the extent of the osseous surgery. Still retaining the molar to serve as an abutment tooth might be advantageous. Therefore in this situation possibly gingivectomy can be used as a compromise procedure. Pocket depth will be reduced but not eliminated. The effectiveness of such a course will depend on the dentist's and the patient's ability to maintain the tooth. Sometimes long-term success will be obtained. However, it is only fair to say that compromise surgery may result in recurrence and extension of pocket depth.

## Instruments

The required instruments are discussed in Chapter 33. Gingivectomy probing is shown in Fig. 35-4; gingivectomy knives are illustrated in Fig. 35-5.

## Method

### GINGIVECTOMY-GINGIVOPLASTY, SURGICAL STEPS

Careful examination of the tissue form and measurement of probing depth will give the operator a three-dimensional picture that will permit more precise execution of the surgery.[7-10] Mark the pockets with a periodontal probe or with pocket-marking forceps. When the millimeter probe is used, measure and mark on the outer surface of the gingiva (see Fig. 35-4) by puncturing the gingiva with a probe or an explorer. When the pocket-marking forceps are used, insert the probing (straight) beak to the bottom of the pocket, and mark the depth with the puncturing beak. Mark bleeding points in all areas with probing depth, including the interdental papillae (probing depth tends to overestimate the pocket in the presence of inflammation).

Make the incision apical to the bleeding point, and extend it through the gingiva    **Incision**

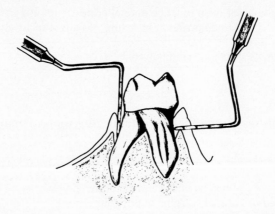

**Fig. 35-4.** Diagrammatic representation of the sounding approach to analyze alveolar bone topography by piercing the soft tissues until the bone is contacted. A systematic stepping procedure is employed until the bony architecture is ascertained. Delineate the pocket depth by marking bleeding points with a pocket probe. This will guide you in positioning the blade for the initial incision. (Courtesy G. Tussing, Lincoln, Nebraska.)

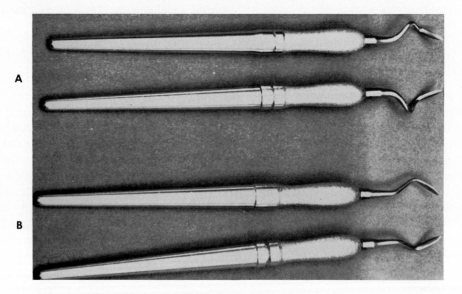

**Fig. 35-5.** **A,** Gingivectomy knives. **B,** Special knives for distal surfaces of the posterior teeth.

to end at the tooth at the level of the bottom of the pocket, that is, at the level of the bleeding point (see Fig. 35-8). Exactly how far apical to this marked point the incision should start will depend on the thickness of the gingiva and the axial inclination of the teeth. Where the gingiva is thick, the bevel may be long. Conversely, in the presence of a thin, finely textured gingiva, a short bevel will produce the desired sloping form. Undulate the incision mesiodistally in imitation of ideal scalloped form (similar to the festooning of dentures). The periodontal knife should be keenly sharp so that the incisions are made with ease and the tissues are not torn or lacerated.

You should feel the blade contacting the tooth surface at the depth of the cut. Interdentally the incision should extend deeper into the tissue. When heavy, fibrotic gingiva is present, the stroke may have to be retraced within the initial incision to sever the gingiva completely (Figs. 35-6 to 35-9).

Blend the incision with the tissues lateral to the site of operation so that good form prevails throughout the operated and adjacent areas. To do this, you may have to sacrifice a strip of adjacent normal gingiva to obtain proper blending.

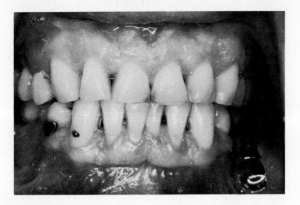

**Fig. 35-6.**   Fibrotic inflamed mandibular gingival margins are evident in a 38-year-old man. Note the tissue form in the lower anterior region.

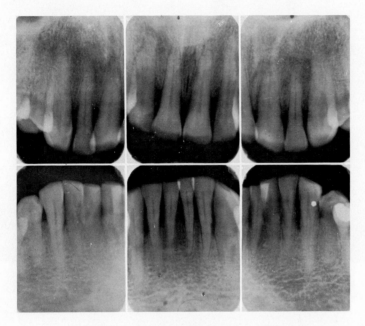

**Fig. 35-7.**   Roentgenogram showing horizontal bone loss with a regular crestal outline.

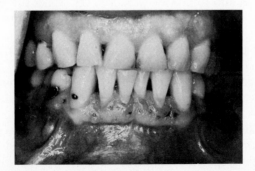

**Fig. 35-8.**   Root planing and home dental care have reduced the clinical inflammation but have failed to eliminate pocket depth or change the fibrotic gingival contours. A broad zone of gingiva is present. Pockets ranging in depth from 3 to 5 mm were present around the mandibular incisors and canines. Bleeding points illustrate the distribution of probing depths.

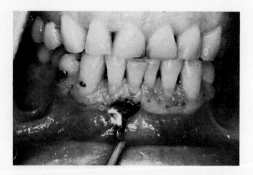

**Fig. 35-9.** A kidney-shaped knife is used to make the initial incision. Start the incision apical to the bleeding points and angulate it to eliminate pockets and to provide a coronally sloping bevel. A mesiodistal scalloped form will thus be maintained.

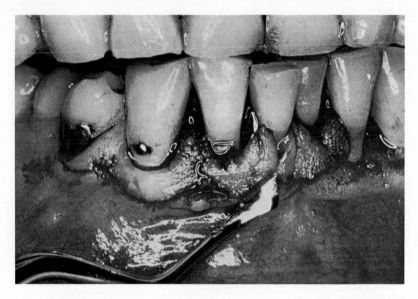

**Fig. 35-10.** The interdental papillae are severed with a thin interproximal knife and the oral (lingual) and vestibular (buccal) incisions are joined. The detached gingiva is then removed with a curette or sickle scaler.

When the surgery involves the gingiva around the last tooth in the arch, start the incision distal to this tooth. Appropriately angled knives (see Fig. 35-5) are sometimes used to incise this area and to provide proper bevel. Make the initial incision with a broad-bladed, kidney-shaped knife (using the heel of the instrument) or with similar instruments (see Figs. 33-3 and 35-9).

Use a thin-bladed gingivectomy knife such as the Orban knife to sever the interdental gingiva and to connect the incisions between the teeth (Fig. 35-10). The incised gingival tissue can then be removed by holding one end of the partially detached tissue with a tissue forceps and then severing its remaining connection with a scalpel or knife.

**Beveling and festooning**

Any additional scaling and root planing should be done at this point. If the incisions are well planned and performed, (1) pockets will be eliminated, (2) the incision will produce a surface that slopes coronally (called a bevel), (3) the bevel will end in a knife-edge margin, and (4) the remaining tissue will be scalloped about each tooth (festooned) (Figs. 35-11 to 35-14).

It is sometimes necessary to accentuate the festooning to ensure that the physiologic

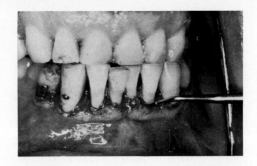

**Fig. 35-11.** A curette removes tissue tags and any remaining deposits.

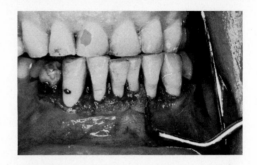

**Fig. 35-12.** A scalpel, used in a scraping motion, provides proper bevel and scalloped mesiodistal form. Interdental grooves are accentuated.

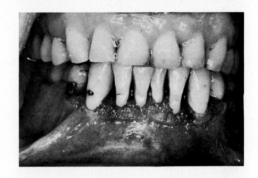

**Fig. 35-13.** Contoured wound. Note that a mucogingival problem (lack of gingiva and pull of the frenum) exists on the vestibular surface of the right canine.

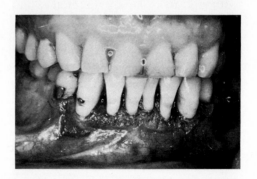

**Fig. 35-14.** An incision is made at the mucogingival junction around the right canine, and the alveolar mucosa is permitted to sag apically. The alveolar surface remains covered only by periosteum.

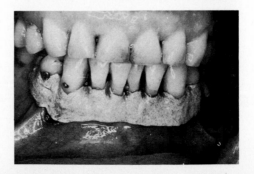

**Fig. 35-15.** After hemorrhage has been controlled, a dressing is carefully placed.

form and a shallow sulcus both are obtained.[10] Such correction can be made with the Orban knife, although some operators prefer to use surgical shears, tissue rongeurs, or electrocautery. Interdental spillways can be created with the same instruments.

The proper angulation of the initial incision in gingivectomy will create coronally sloping gingival contours and thin gingival margins. Should corrections be necessary, use kidney-shaped or interdental knives in a scraping motion to correct bevels. Scrape the edge lightly but with a firm, even pressure over the resistant fibrous tissue (see Fig. 35-12). Be careful to avoid jagged incisions. When done properly, such scraping can be used to make minor corrections, to lengthen, deepen, or blend bevels, or to help in the creation of a more prominent festooning (Figs. 35-15 to 35-20). Diamond stones are occasionally used in a similar fashion to festoon or bevel gingival surfaces when the tissue is firm[11] (Fig. 35-21).

**Electrocautery**  Electrocautery can also be used to correct gingival contours or to bevel the cut surface after the initial incision.[12-14] A number of differently shaped electrodes are available that offer access to specific areas and are designed to facilitate particular corrections of form. The electrodes can remove flat or concave tissue slices, and thin sections of tissue can be excised with ease. In addition, the cautery can be used to eliminate tissue tags and to correct ragged incisions. Be careful, however, not to touch metal restorations, bone, or periosteum because of the danger of injury to bone and pulp. Use a wooden tongue blade to retract the cheeks or to depress the tongue. To eliminate the offensive odor of burning, quickly blow air over the surgical area.

Soft tissue rongeurs (nippers) and sharp scissors are particularly useful for the creation of interdental grooves and for the removal of tissue tags.

When used correctly, within its indications, gingivectomy-gingivoplasty should not create esthetic deformity (see Fig. 35-16). Scraping knives, diamond stones, electrocautery, nippers, or scissors may improve gingival form, and their use constitutes the gingivoplasty part of the procedure.

## GINGIVOPLASTY ALONE

Gingivoplasty can be performed without gingivectomy as a procedure in its own right when the gingival margins are blunted and fibrotic and pocket depth is minimal. Although root planing, curettage, and proper oral hygiene will usually eliminate or reduce some of the deformity caused by the edema and cellular infiltrate of inflammation, fibrotic (hyperplastic) deformities may resist these measures; these deformities are best eliminated by surgery.

The relation of dentogingival form to function (i.e., the relation of tooth contour and gingival topography to the retention of plaque) is a useful concept.[10] It is assumed that these factors can make the maintenance of periodontal health easier. Where gingival margins are thick, plaque accumulation is encouraged.[15] Inflammation is encouraged, and the gingiva loses its thin margin and becomes blunted. This vicious cycle can be corrected, if necessary, by proper restorations, gingivoplasty, and oral hygiene.

## ILLUSTRATIVE CASES

Let us review some actual gingivectomy-gingivoplasty procedures.

In the first case the procedure was done in the mandible (see Figs. 35-6 to 35-16). Although the maxillary gingiva was clinically fibrotic and lacked ideal contour, particularly between the right lateral and central incisors, the clinical health of the area and the lack of pocket depth precluded the need for surgery in the upper jaw. Clinical success in maintaining health confirmed this judgment. An important therapeutic

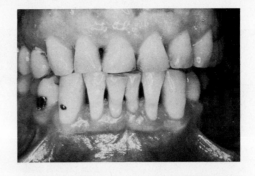

**Fig. 35-16.** Physiologic gingival form 1 year later. (See Fig. 35-15.) Maintenance procedures consisted of root planing, tooth polishing, and oral hygiene. Compare this figure with Fig. 35-6. Note that the gingival margins are apical to their original position but that tissue form is improved. An adequate width of gingiva remains.

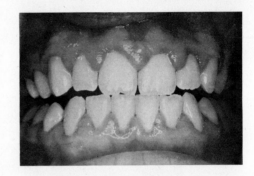

**Fig. 35-17.** Generalized, marginal, hyperplastic gingivitis in a 15-year-old girl.

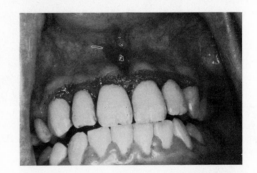

**Fig. 35-18.** Gingivectomy was performed in the upper anterior segment. The frenum was excised, since it infringed on the surgical field. Note that root planing had not corrected the gingival enlargement, still visible in the lower arch. Gingivectomy was performed later in the lower anterior region.

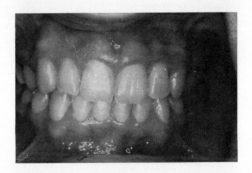

**Fig. 35-19.** Inflammation is corrected and gingival form is acceptable 6 months after therapy.

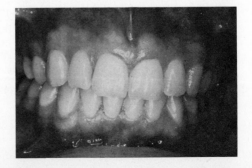

**Fig. 35-20.** Patient maintained a physiologic gingival form 5 years later.

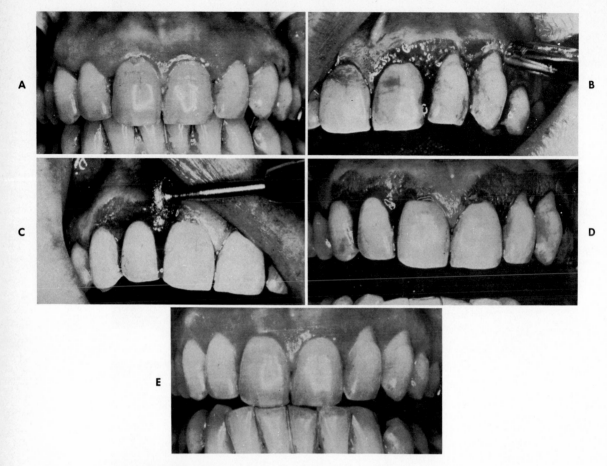

**Fig. 35-21.** Recontouring tissues by gingivoplasty. **A,** Preoperative condition. **B,** Gingivoplasty performed by scraping with a scalpel. **C,** Gingivoplasty performed by use of a coarse diamond stone. **D,** Immediately after surgery. **E,** Compare after complete healing. (Courtesy S. Schluger, Seattle, Washington.)

principle is illustrated in this case. The selection of treatment procedures is based on the individual needs of the patient, not on presumptions of ideal gingival form or on rote prescriptions of surgery.

Another illustrative case is that of a 15-year-old girl (see Figs. 35-17 to 35-20). Enlarged gingival margins and hyperplastic papillae were evident. Initial treatment consisted of root planing and oral hygiene instruction. The remaining fibrotic tissue was then removed by gingivectomy and gingivoplasty.

In still another case, gingivectomy-gingivoplasty was performed. The gingivoplasty portion was done on one side of the mouth by scraping with a knife, and on the other side by using a coarse diamond stone (see Fig. 35-21).

Gingivoplasty also is employed to correct improper gingival form that is the result of periodontitis. Such a case is seen in Fig. 35-22, showing the gingival condition of a 29-year-old man who had a chronic, hyperplastic periodontitis. There was a diastema between the mandibular left central and lateral incisors. The maxillary teeth had all been extracted. Root planing, gingival curettage, and oral hygiene instruction were carried out over a period of 2 months, leading to considerable improvement of the condition and closure of the diastema. At that time the tissues appeared fibrous, and papillary and marginal enlargement was still present. Gingivoplasty was performed.

A B

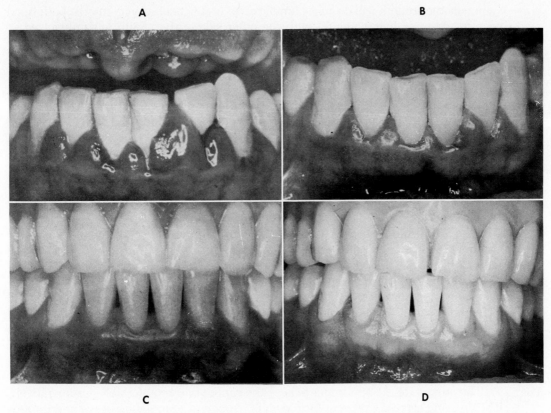

C D

**Fig. 35-22.** **A,** Hyperplastic periodontitis in a 29-year-old man. **B,** Appearance 2 months later, after root planing and gingival curettage. Note the closed contact between the mandibular left central and lateral incisors where there previously was a diastema. **C,** Six months after gingivoplasty. **D,** Six years later.

## Gingivectomy-gingivoplasty procedure

Now that the steps of the gingivectomy-gingivoplasty have been reviewed, the student is ready to proceed with surgery. Only a few additional pointers are necessary before performing a first gingivectomy-gingivoplasty.

### PRESURGICAL PERIOD

The patient's tissues must be prepared for surgery by the removal of all calcified deposits and plaque. The patient must also be taught to be effective in oral hygiene. If the patient cannot maintain proper oral hygiene before surgery, he/she will not do any better after surgery. Surely, then, surgery will not be effective.

*Scaling*

If the patient demonstrates ability in oral hygiene, most of the inflammation will have been resolved by the time of the surgery. During surgery there will be less bleeding, the tissues will have a firmer consistency, and ragged wound edges will be avoided.

*Oral hygiene*

Premedication for apprehension has been discussed in Chapter 33. In addition, antibiotic coverage[16] has been discussed. Prescriptions for premedication should be written at the visit before the surgery, when the area to be operated is examined and changes in pocket depth noted and reevaluated (see "Cooperative surgery," Chapter 31).[16]

*Premedication*

The charting and roentgenograms of the area to be operated should be studied.

*Planning surgery*

Generally the student will do only a limited area. In practice, surgery may be performed on a quadrant or half a mouth, with the other side of the mouth left uninvolved so that the patient is able to masticate comfortably.

Gingivectomy may be performed about a single tooth for access in operative procedures or to seat a clamp for endodontic procedures. Sometimes further treatment (endodontics or operative dentistry) may immediately follow the surgery. In such cases these steps should be planned in advance and the appropriate instruments be available so that the procedures may be done smoothly and without interruption.

## SURGERY

**Anesthesia**

Administer the local anesthetic by standard techniques and dosage. After anesthesia is obtained, inject a drop into each interdental papilla involved. This increases the turgor of the gingiva and makes it easier to incise. In addition, the vasoconstrictor will reduce bleeding during surgery.

After confirming that the tissues are completely anesthetized, probe the pockets, mark the pocket depths, and perform the surgery as outlined in the preceding pages.

**Control of bleeding**

Carefully inspect the wound and tooth surfaces after the surgery. Remove any remaining deposits or tissue tags. At this point it will be necessary to obtain good hemostasis before a pack is placed. This may be accomplished by rinsing the wound surfaces with sterile saline solution or water and then packing gauze sponges over the area. If this does not produce hemostasis, pack the interproximal areas with pledgets containing a dilute (no greater than 1/50,000) epinephrine. Strong epinephrine solutions could produce undesirable systemic effects.

**Placement of dressing**

The purpose of the dressing is to keep the patient more comfortable postoperatively. The dressing serves to prevent formation of exuberant granulation tissue and thereby acts as a template. It should cover the wound and protect it from mechanical trauma during chewing and from irritation by highly seasoned foods. However, the dressing itself should not become irritating; this can be ensured only if it is placed firmly. The dressing should be placed along the necks of the teeth and should not cover the occlusal surfaces. If the dressing interferes with full jaw closure, it will dislodge, become loosened, or act as an occlusal interference.

Place the dressing interdentally in cone-shaped pieces. Adapt flat strips of dressing to the buccal and lingual surfaces covering the wound. Force the pack into place by instrument and finger pressure. Inspect the dressing to be sure that it does not impinge on muscle attachments or the orovestibular mucosa. If it does, muscle trim the pack in much the same way that full denture impressions are muscle trimmed. In some cases the dressing may be covered with adhesive Burlew tinfoil. The foil helps to hold the dressing in place.

**Stents**

It is sometimes difficult to apply the pack around posterior teeth when a shallow vestibule is present. Preformed acrylic stents may be used to retain the dressing. When the surgery involves an isolated tooth, tie dental floss around the neck of the tooth, leaving dangling ends of the floss 3 to 4 mm in length. The dressing will then adhere to the floss.

## POSTSURGICAL CHECKLIST AND PROCEDURES

**Instructions to patient**

Instruct the patient to avoid eating or drinking after surgery for 1 hour or until the pack is set. Tart or spicy foods should be avoided. Brushing should be limited to occlusal and incisal tooth surfaces in the operated area. The dressing should be cleansed gently with a soft multitufted toothbrush. Frequent, gentle rinsing after meals is advisable. Any prescription for medication is made at this time (Chapter 33). Instructions for emergency situations should be presented in printed form together with the dentist's home phone number. Emergencies are infrequent, but the patient feels comforted to know that he/she can call the dentist should the need arise.

Instruct the patient to return for dressing change in 3 to 5 days or earlier if the dressing is dislodged. In minor cases the dressing may be removed at this time. Other cases may require one or two dressing changes. At each dressing change, inspect and clean the wound and root surfaces. If exuberant granulation tissue is present, it can be removed with a curette.

**Dressing changes**

On removal of the last dressing, advise the patient to resume oral hygiene in the operated area. Some patients are fearful of bleeding and let up on brushing. In these cases exuberant granulation tissue may form, or the tissue may not mature properly. Gingivectomy may fail without proper postoperative oral hygiene. Special extrasoft brushes (Butler Gum Brush, Sensodyne Gentle, Lactona Softex) may be used after dressing removal for 1 or 2 weeks.

**Dressing removal**

Internal (inverse bevel) gingivectomy is a flap procedure and is discussed in Chapter 36.

**Internal gingivectomy**

## Wound healing

Wound healing[17-24] takes place by the development of an acute inflammatory process and the formation of granulation tissue. This process occurs both in the depth of the tissue and on the surface. In the deeper tissues an acute inflammatory reaction occurs soon after surgery, consisting of dilatation of blood vessels ( Fig. 35-23, A) and migration of leukocytes into the tissue (B). This occurs during the first few days postoperatively. The connective tissue surrounding the blood vessels responds by proliferation characterized by mitotic activity in the fibroblasts (C), the endothelial cells (D), and the undifferentiated mesenchymal cells (E). This is called fibroplasia and constitutes the development of true granulation tissue.

While this process is occurring in the deeper tissues, the surface is also undergoing changes. Immediately after surgery the blood clot covers the exposed connective tissue. Two days after surgery the blood clot consists of three distinct layers ( Fig. 35-24, A). The surface of the blood clot becomes necrotic, and the innermost layer appears to be fibrinous; between these two layers is a stratum rich in leukocytes (leukocyte band), which separates the necrotic surface from the fibrinous layer. The epithelium grows under the blood clot. The necrotic surface of the blood clot is cast off (B) 4 days after the surgery, and the epithelium proceeds to cover the surface at a rate of 0.5 mm/day. At 8 days only a small part of the wound surface is unepithelized (C). The granulation tissue extends above the surface; in 14 days the entire wound is covered by the epithelium (D).

On an electron microscopic level, a new junctional epithelium with a lamina densa, lamina lucida, and hemidesmosomes has formed fully by 12 to 14 days after surgery.[20,24]

Healing proceeds by proliferation of capillaries ( Fig. 35-24, E) and fibroblasts (F) under the fibrinous inner layer of the blood clot. A large, massive blood clot has been found to delay healing, and the bacterial activity is greater. The dressing should be closely adapted, and the blood clot should be minimized.

During this process of healing (by secondary intention), infection of the granulation tissue may occur. The ever-present bacterial flora, though not virulent, grow readily on the blood clot and surface of the young granulating connective tissue. These bacteria may produce toxins that are irritating to the healing wound surface. As a reaction to this irritant and ensuing inflammatory reaction, the granulation tissue may proliferate more rapidly and grow over the surface as proud flesh or infected granulation tissue. Careful root planing, refined surgical techniques, proper placement of the dressing,

*Text continued on p. 779.*

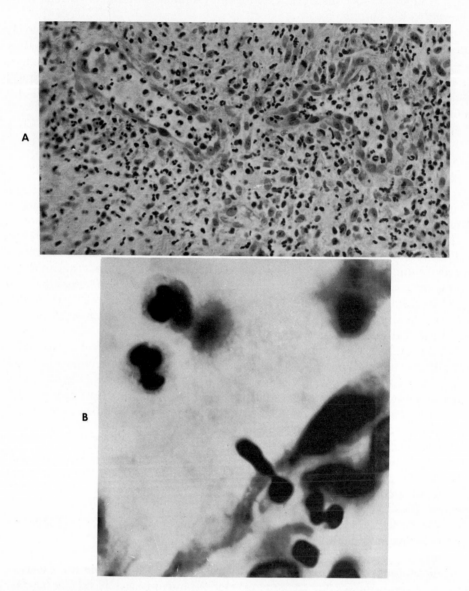

**Fig. 35-23.** **A,** Acute inflammatory reaction 2 days after gingivectomy: dilated capillaries, filled with leukocytes migrating from the capillaries into surrounding tissue. **B,** High magnification of a capillary with a leukocyte migrating through the endothelial wall.

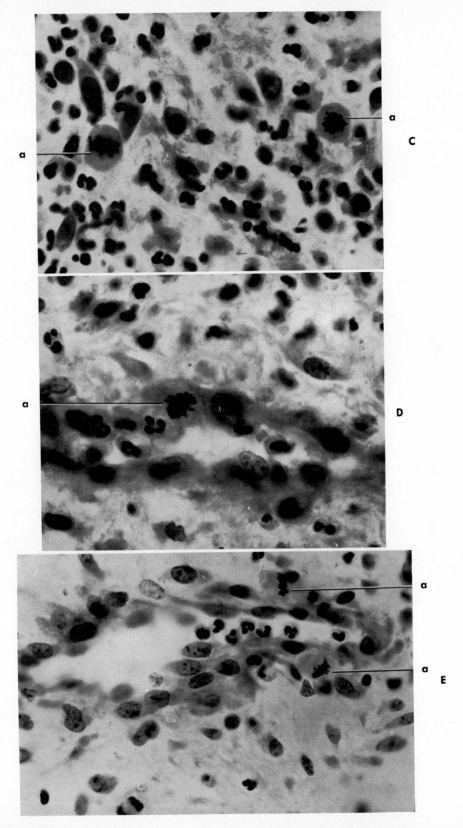

**Fig. 35-23, cont'd.** **C,** Histologic section from a healing gingivectomy wound showing mitosis, *a,* of fibroblasts. **D,** Histologic section from a healing gingivectomy wound showing mitosis, *a,* of an endothelial cell in the wall of a capillary. **E,** Histologic section from a healing gingivectomy wound showing mitosis, *a* in undifferentiated mesenchymal cells.

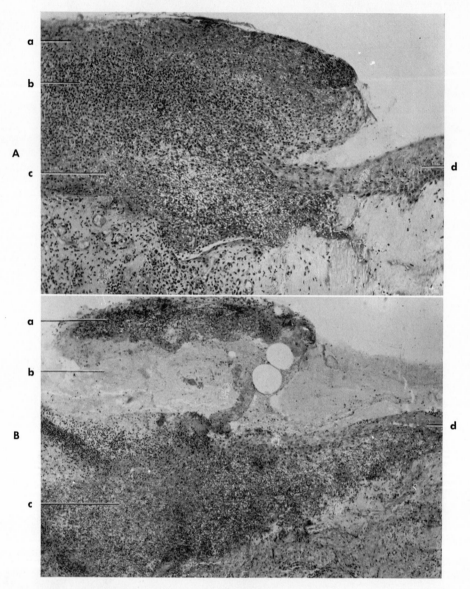

**Fig. 35-24.** **A,** Blood clot on the surface of a healing wound 2 days after gingivectomy. The blood clot is separated into three layers: the outermost, *a,* is necrotic; the innermost, *c,* is fibrinous; and the middle, *b,* consists of a wall of leukocytes limiting the outer from the inner layer. The epithelium, *d,* then proceeds to cover the wound surface. **B,** Four days after gingivectomy the outer necrotic layer, *a,* of the clot is cast off. The migration of the epithelium, *d,* progresses.

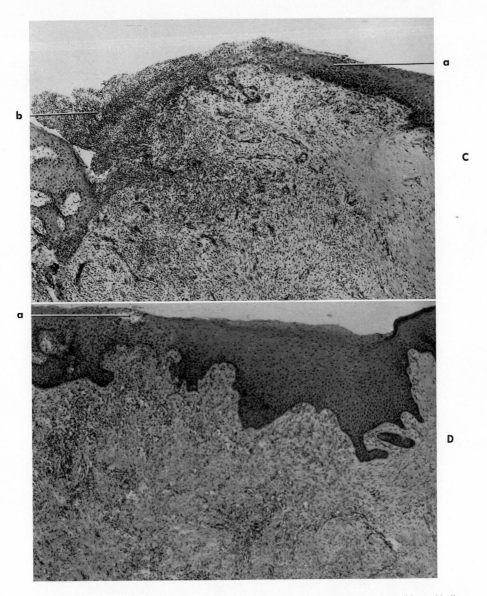

**Fig. 35-24, cont'd.   C,** Eight days after surgery, only a small area of the wound is not covered by epithelium, *a*. Granulation tissue, *b,* covers the surface. **D,** The wound surface is completely epithelized 14 days after surgery. However, there is a small area, *a,* that shows the migration of inflammatory cells to the surface.   *Continued.*

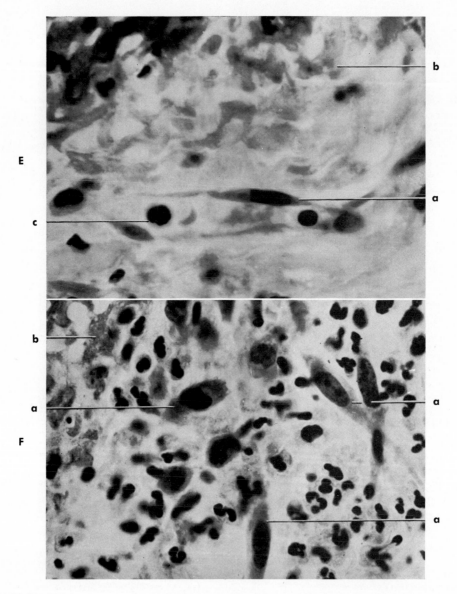

**Fig. 35-24, cont'd.** **E,** Histologic section of wound healing showing proliferation of endothelial cells, *a,* forming new capillaries. *b,* Fibrinous network; *c,* white blood cells in the new capillary. **F,** Proliferating fibroblasts, *a,* organizing remnants of the blood clot, *b.*

and proper postoperative wound care will keep surface infection to a minimum. The epithelium that must cover the exposed connective tissue can grow only if the granulation tissue is not infected and does not proliferate in an exuberant fashion.

## AIDS IN THE HEALING PROCESS

Experiments have shown that frequent change of dressing is advantageous to wound healing[25] (Fig. 35-25). The tissue underneath a dressing that had been left on without change for 10 days showed an accumulation of exudate and necrotic material and severe inflammation in the underlying connective tissue with poor epithelization

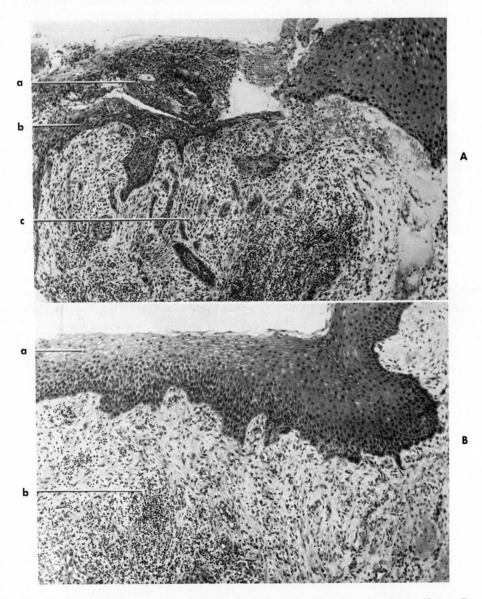

**Fig. 35-25.    A,** Wound surface in a patient in whom the surgical dressing was unchanged for 10 days. There was an accumulation of exudate and necrotic material, *a;* the epithelium was thin and proliferative, *b;* and a severe inflammatory reaction could be seen below the surface. *c.* **B,** Wound surface in a patient in whom the dressing was changed three times in 10 days. The epithelization, *a,* of the wound surface is good. There is no necrotic blood clot on the surface. The subepithelial inflammatory reaction, *b,* is moderate.

of the wound surface, whereas a postoperative wound of 10 days in which the dressing had been changed at 3-day intervals showed better healing tendency.

The following steps are helpful in aiding the healing process:

1. Use fastidious surgical technique to reduce tissue laceration and trauma.
2. Use scrupulous aseptic methods even though the oral cavity may be considered a contaminated site. Avoid the possible introduction of organisms not commonly found in the oral cavity.
3. Minimize the size of the clot.
4. Protect the wound surface with a well-placed surgical dressing.
5. Change the dressing every 3 to 5 days.
6. Remove all plaque, debris, and any remaining calculus at each dressing change. Remember, little, if anything, can be done to accelerate healing. However, infection, contamination, and debris may all retard healing.

## Electrosurgery

Some surgeons prefer to use electrosurgery for gingivectomy-gingivoplasty[12-14] This method employs either bipolar electrocoagulation or single-pole electrodes. Both can be used as adjuncts to the knife, especially in areas where access is limited and difficult. Gingivoplasty often is difficult to perform in an isolated area; electrosurgery is useful in such cases ( Fig. 35-26).

The histopathologic features of tissue healing after electrocoagulation[22] can be seen in Fig. 35-27. In A the immediate result of coagulation is seen. A blister was formed in the epithelium, and necrosis and hemorrhage could be seen in the adjacent areas. After 2 days (B) the necrotic, coagulated tissue was separated from the underlying tissue by migration of leukocytes and demarcation of the living from the dead tissue. In 14 days epithelization and shrinkage of the wound surface took place (C). In one, area, however, two small bone sequestra were found beneath the epithelium (D), which were eliminated by either sloughing or resorption. This sequestration process can delay healing considerably. It can occur whenever the current used is too strong or applied for too long a time or when the instrument is used close to bone.[14,25-28]

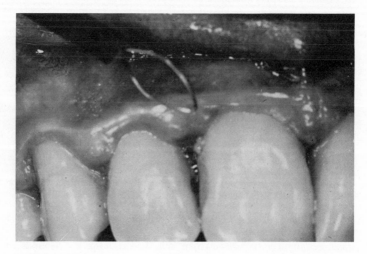

**Fig. 35-26.** Use of the unipolar electrode in the performance of gingivoplasty. (Courtesy G.P. Ivancie, Denver, Colorado.)

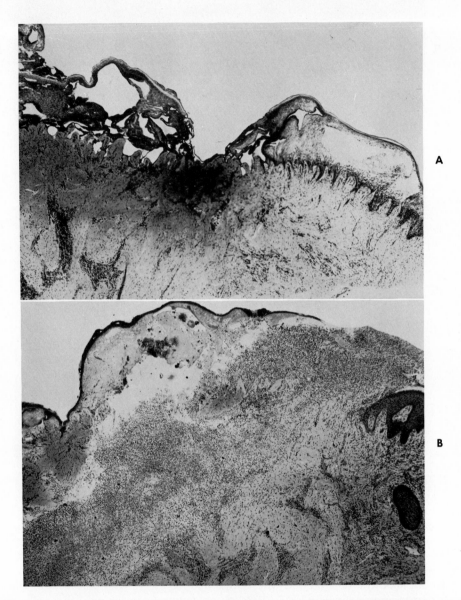

**Fig. 35-27.** Histologic features of tissue healing after electrocoagulation. **A,** Blister formation and necrosis immediately after coagulation. **B,** Demarcation of the necrotic from the viable tissue.    *Continued.*

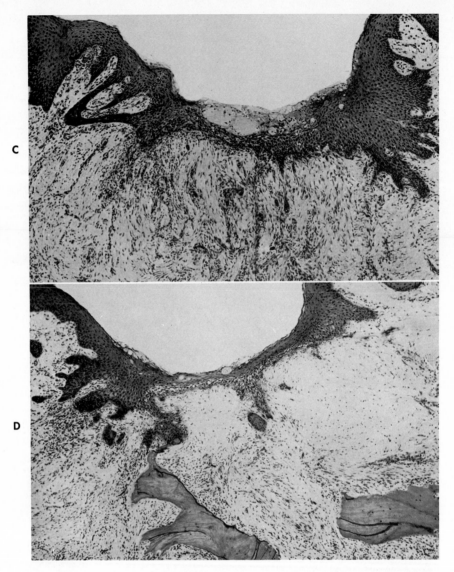

**Fig. 35-27, cont'd.** **C,** *Complete epithelization and shrinkage of the wound surface.* **D,** *Formation of sequestra, delaying the healing.*

## Evaluation of results

**Success**

If the prerequisites of gingivectomy-gingivoplasty are met and the procedure is performed as described, the results may permit long-term maintenance.

**Failure**

On occasion the desired ends are not gained, or the result cannot be maintained. Such developments are labeled failures. Such failures can occur if the basic prerequisites were not met, if the performance of the surgery was not adequate, if the procedure was used when contraindicated, if the patient's cooperation in home care was not gained, if maintenance scaling was not routinely performed, or if reinfection with organisms characteristic of progressive periodontal disease occurred at a later date.[29-31]

Approximately half the pocket depth may recur some months after gingivectomy.[15] Such regrowth may be a result of underlying bony form (infrabony defects, craters, thick ledges). In such cases the inappropriate surgical method was selected.[6]

## ERRORS IN SURGICAL TECHNIQUE

Failures or partial failures can occur immediately after healing. They may be caused by careless or inexact performance of surgery. Early failure can occur because of any of the following situations:

1. Poor and inaccurate probing and pocket marking that leads to incomplete pocket elimination
2. Timidity in making the initial and subsequent incisions so that some pocket depth remains
3. Failure to examine after surgery for residual pocket depth (If residual pockets are found, they should be eliminated.)
4. Failure to create a proper bevel leaving blunt gingival margins
5. Failure to create adequate festooning (If a mesiodistal scalloped form is not achieved, the gingival margin produced may be horizontal [without interdental papillae] or, even less desirable, one of reverse architecture. In reverse architecture the interdental tissues are lower than the oral and vestibular gingival margins. If this is pronounced, defects are produced, making oral hygiene difficult to perform.)
6. Failure to be technically proficient (If dull instruments are used, the tissue becomes lacerated and tissue tags result, which should be removed. If scaling was inadequate, calculus may remain. Any remnant of calculus must be removed at the time of operation. If the dressing is not properly mixed or placed, it may loosen and irritate the tissue. In some instances the dressing may not be placed firmly over the tissue, and clots may form. Any of these situations can lead to a coronal and lateral proliferation of granulation tissue and the reestablishment of pocket depth.)
7. Selection of inappropriate surgical method

If such a failure should result (caused by the foregoing factors), reoperation may become necessary.

Now that the dentist has learned the indications for and the methods of gingivectomy-gingivoplasty, he/she should be aware of situations in which this surgery should not be performed.

## Contraindications

Gingivectomy-gingivoplasty is not indicated in the following situations:

1. In the presence of thick oral and vestibular alveolar ledges, interdental craters, or bizarre crestal bone form. (The position of the gingival margin and the contour of the gingiva relate to the thickness of the gingiva and of the underlying bone. If the bone is too thick, it would promote coronal regrowth of gingiva. Tooth position and form also play a role in gingival morphology.)
2. If intra-alveolar (infrabony) pockets are present. (When the pocket dips below the alveolar crest, its base cannot be eliminated by gingivectomy alone. The remnant pocket will cause pocket depth to reform.)
3. If the pocket dips below the mucogingival junction, surgery will excise most or all of the gingiva and leave an inadequate zone of gingiva. (Alveolar mucosa is not an adequate substitute for gingiva.)
4. If the patient cannot or will not perform oral hygiene adequately, surgical therapy will fail.
5. If adequate patient-dentist rapport is lacking or if patient management is a problem, surgery may be eliminated. (The dentist should consider the patient's emotional status. When the patient's emotional security is threatened by proposed surgery, the dentist may elect to discontinue treatment. Such patients can be handled with empathy and with careful guidance. Consultation with the patient's physician may be necessary. If the patient is rigid and inflexible, caution is advisable and alternative treatment may be necessary. A particular concern in the management of the patient's psyche is the influence of surgically induced gingival recession (particularly around the maxillary anterior teeth,

where some patients may show a great deal of gingiva or root. When esthetic deformity is anticipated or unavoidable, the patient must be prepared for it in advance.)

6. If certain diseases and conditions exist, surgery may be contraindicated. (For example, surgery should not be performed in patients with Addison disease or uncontrolled diabetes, or in patients who are anticoagulated, weak, or debilitated or who generally respond poorly to surgery [Chapter 33]).

7. If the patient complains of tooth sensitivity before surgery. (The cause of any complaint should be investigated and treated before surgery. If the sensitivity cannot be controlled, surgery may be contraindicated.)

A good therapist knows the advantages and disadvantages of his/her treatment.[23,29] He/she recognizes limitations, knows the patient, and anticipates the patient's response.

## REFERENCES

1. Pickerill, H.P.: Stomatology in general practice, London, 1912, Henry Frowde, Hodder & Stoughton.

2. Fröhlich, E.: Die chirurgische Behandlung der marginalen Parodontitis. In Häupl, K., and Schuchardt, K., editors: Die Zahn-, Mund-, und Kieferheilkunde, vol. 3, pt. 1, Munich, 1957, Urban & Schwarzenberg.

3. Hiatt, W.H., et al.: Is the simple gingivectomy obsolete? Periodont. Abstr. **13:**62, 1965.

4. Waite, I.M.: The present status of the gingivectomy procedure, J. Clin. Periodontol. **2:**241, 1975.

5. Orban, B.: To what extent should the tissues be excised in gingivectomy? J. Periodontol. **12:**83, 1941.

6. Prichard, J.: Gingivoplasty, gingivectomy, and osseous surgery, J. Periodontol. **32:**275, 1961.

7. Glickman, I.: Fact and fad in the surgical treatment of periodontal disease, J. Am. Dent. Assoc. **59:**241, 1959.

8. Glickman, I.: The results obtained with an unembellished gingivectomy technique in humans, J. Periodontol. **27:**247, 1956.

9. Goldman, H.M.: Gingivectomy, Oral Surg. **4:**1136, 1951.

10. Goldman, H.M.: The development of physiologic gingival contour by gingivoplasty, Oral Surg. **3:**879, 1950.

11. Fox, L.: Rotating abrasives in the management of periodontal soft and hard tissues, Oral Surg. **8:**1134, 1955.

12. Sugarman, M.M.: Electrosurgical gingivoplasty—a technic, J. Periodontol. **22:**156, 1951.

13. Azzi, R.: Electrosurgery in periodontics: a literature review, J. West. Soc. Periodontol. **29:**4, 1981.

14. Azzi, R., et al.: The effect of electrosurgery on alveolar bone, J. Periodontol. **54:**96, 1983.

15. Kambiz, A.M., and Stahl, S.S.: The remodeling of human gingival tissues following gingivectomy, J. Periodontol. **48:**136, 1977.

16. Ingle, J.I.: Physical and technical considerations for periodontal surgery in the undergraduate curriculum, J. Dent. Ed. **26:**68, 1962.

17. Archer, E.A., and Orban, B.: Dynamics of wound healing following elimination of gingival pockets, Am. J. Orthod. (Oral Surg. sect.) **31:**40, 1945.

18. Ramfjord, S.P., and Costich, E.R.: Healing after simple gingivectomy, J. Periodontol. **34:**401, 1963.

19. Stahl, S.S., et al.: Gingival healing. II. Clinical and histologic repair sequences following gingivectomy, J. Periodontol. **39:**109, 1968.

20. Listgarten, M.A.: Ultrastructure of the dentogingival junction after gingivectomy, J. Periodont. Res. **7:**151, 1972.

21. Pope, J.W., et al.: Effects of electrosurgery on wound healing, Periodontics **6:**30, 1968.

22. Wennström, J.: Regeneration of gingiva following surgical excision: a clinical study, J. Clin. Periodontol. **10:**287, 1983.

23. Parham, D.: Current concepts of wound healing and healing of the excisional type of gingival wound, Periodont. Abstr. **19:**112, 1971.

24. Sabag, N., et al.: Epithelial reattachment after gingivectomy in the rat, J. Periodontol. **55:**135, 1984.

25. Aremband, D., and Wade, A.B.: A comparative wound healing study following gingivectomy by electrosurgery and knives, J. Periodont. Res. **8:**42, 1973.

26. Williams, V.D.: Electrosurgery and wound healing: a literature review, J. Am. Dent. Assoc. **108:**220, 1984.

27. Kalkwarf, K.L., Krejci, R.F., and Wentz, F.M.: Healing of electrosurgical incisions in gingiva: early histologic observations in adult men, J. Prosthet. Dent. **46:**662, 1981.

28. Orban, B.: Tissue healing following electrocoagulation of gingiva, J. Peridontol. **15:**17, 1944.

29. Orban, B.: Indications, technique and postoperative management of gingivectomy in treatment of the periodontal pocket, J. Periodontol. **12:**89, 1941.

30. Grant, D.A.: Experimental periodontal surgery: gingivectomy, excision to the alveolar crest, J. Dent. Res. **43:**790, 1964.

31. Wade, A.B.: Where gingivectomy fails, J. Periodontol. **25:**189, 1954.

## ADDITIONAL SUGGESTED READING

Bloom, J.: The justification for surgical procedures employed in periodontal therapy, Oral Surg. **15:**531, 1962.

Burch, J.G., Conroy, C.W., and Ferris, R.T.: Tooth mobility following gingivectomy—a study of gingival support of the teeth, Periodontics **6:**90, 1968.

Donnenfeld, O.W., and Glickman, I.: A biometric study of the effects of gingivectomy, J. Periodontol. **37:**447, 1966.

Hirschfeld, L., et al.: Is surgical pocket elimination necessary for successful periodontal therapy? J. West. Soc. Periodontol. **11:**88, 1963.

Hulin, C.: Les parodontoses pyorrhéiques ou pyorhées alvéolaires, Paris, 1941, Foulon.

Korn, N.A., Schaffer, E.M., and McHugh, R.B.: An experimental assessment of gingivectomy and soft tissue curettage in dogs. J. Periodontol. **36:**96, 1965.

Orban, B.: Surgical gingivectomy, J. Am. Dent. Assoc. **32:**701, 1945.

Orban, B.: Indications, technique and postoperative management of gingivectomy in treatment of the periodontal pocket, J. Periodontol. **12:**89, 1941.

Pick, R.M., Pecaro, B.C., and Silberman, C.J.: The laser gingivectomy: the use of the $CO_2$ laser for the removal of phenytoin hyperplasia, J. Periodontol. **56:**492, 1985.

Ramfjord, S.P., Engler, W.O., and Hiniker, J.J.: A radioautographic study of healing following simple gingivectomy. II. The connective tissue, J. Periodontol. **37:**179, 1966.

Stahl, S.S., and Nghiem, H.T.: Histologic response in basal cells of the crevicular epithelium to gingival surgery, J. Periodontol. **50:**36, 1979.

Supipat, N., Gjermo, P., and Johansen, J.R.: Gingival fluid flow after gingivectomy related to mechanical or chemical plaque control, J. Periodontol. **49:**542, 1978.

# Periodontal flap

Periodontal surgery is performed with a variety of techniques. The procedures are differentiated in terms of therapeutic intent and vary with the goal sought.[1-3] For instance some procedures are primarily excisional (i.e., gingivectomy) and aim to eliminate pockets. The therapeutic intentions of flap surgery go beyond pocket elimination. Flap procedures seek to gain access to bone and roots and achieve cosmetic and structural goals in addition to pocket elimination. Excisional,[4] reconstructive, and plastic surgical elements[5] are blended in an attempt to achieve the desired end result.

## Goals

Some or all of the following are included in the goals of flap surgery:

1. Gain access for root débridement and pocket reduction or elimination
2. Regeneration of alveolar bone, periodontal ligament, and cementum
3. Establishment or retention of a gingiva of adequate width
4. Establishment of an acceptable soft and hard tissue contour (physiologic architecture)[6]

These goals of flap surgery remain valid even if some bone is lost and when apical displacement of the gingival tissues is planned to eliminate pockets. The goals are not valid when they risk loss of teeth.

To gain the goals listed, the surgeon generally must employ the flap technique, which salvages rather than discards potentially useful gingiva. Today the flap has become the basic surgical procedure of periodontal therapy. A properly performed flap procedure not only provides access to the underlying tissues, but permits the surgeon the opportunity to perform a variety of interrelated osseous and grafting attachment. In addition, the flap provides a manageable unit of gingiva and alveolar mucosa that can be easily and properly manipulated during suturing to gain desired mucogingival and plastic surgical structural forms.

The flap elevates a unit of gingiva and alveolar mucosa of such dimensions as to provide the surgeon with the following: **Objectives**

1. Access to and visualization of the subgingival portion of the roots
2. Access to and visualization of the alveolar bone
3. A pliable and adaptable unit of soft tissue
4. Alveolar bone either covered with tissue or uncovered, as needed for the surgical procedure
5. The opportunity of manipulating the flexible flap during suturing to place the gingival margin at a desired position.

## Flap design

A flap is a segment of gingiva and adjoining alveolar mucosa raised from the underlying tissues by surgical means. The base of the flap is left intact to provide the flap with an adequate vascular supply. The flap must be uniformly thick, usually about 2 mm. One determinant of how the flap will be raised, that is, either as a full-thickness or as a partial- (split-) thickness flap, is the thickness of the gingiva before surgery. Generally a full-thickness flap is used where the gingiva is thin, and a split-thickness flap is used where the gingiva is thick. Among other requirements, the flap must be sufficiently thin and movable to permit proper flap positioning during suturing and of sufficient length to permit access to and visibility of the underlying tissue as needed in osseous surgery. **Definition**

### FULL-THICKNESS FLAP

A full-thickness flap includes all tissue from periosteum to the epithelial surface. It is elevated by blunt dissection after an initial inverse bevel incision from the gingival margin, within the gingiva, or through the gingival sulcus to the alveolar crest (Figs. 36-1, *A* and *B,* and 36-2, *A*). The initial incision is made with the scalpel and thins the marginal gingiva internally. With careful use of the elevator, all the tissues covering the bone, including periosteum, are then raised (Fig. 36-1, *C* to *F*). Thus tooth and bone are bared by the reflection of this type of flap. Generally the full-thickness flap is used whenever the tissue is thin, that is, 2 mm or less in width. If a full-thickness **Width** flap were to be used where the tissue is thicker, the collagen density and the thickness of the flap would diminish its pliability. This inflexibility would impede the surgeon's ability to manipulate the flap during suturing, blocking attainment of mucogingival and plastic surgical goals.

### PARTIAL-THICKNESS FLAP

A partial-thickness flap splits the gingival tissue as its name implies, leaving the alveolar bone covered by soft tissue. It is employed where the gingival tissue is thicker than 2 mm and when periosteal suturing is planned. When exposure of bone is to be avoided, as in the case of fenestrations or dehiscences, a partial-thickness flap may be employed. After an inverse bevel incision (Fig. 36-2, *B* and *C*), sharp dissection is used to produce a partial-thickness flap about 1.5 to 2 mm uniformly thick, leaving bone and periosteum covered by the remaining gingival connective tissue (Fig. 36-2, *D*). This tissue remnant may be retained for periosteal suturing (Fig. 36-2, *D* and *E*), excised (Fig. 36-2, *F*), or simply thinned out.

A thick flap cannot be manipulated during suturing to gain mucogingival structural goals. *Thus, when the gingiva is thick and fibrotic, a split-thickness flap must be*

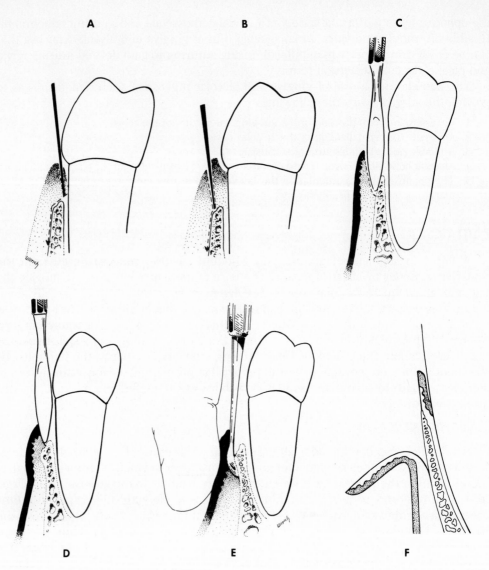

**Fig. 36-1.** A full-thickness flap is elevated to the alveolar crest after an inverse bevel incision, **A,** from the gingival margin or, **B,** within the attached gingiva. **C,** The tissues are then reflected with a periosteal elevator. **D,** When a marginal exostosis is present, the tissue can be elevated, **E,** with a Molt curette supported by finger pressure, **F,** Tooth and bone are bared by this type of flap.

*employed.* This is frequently the case in the region of the tuberosities, the retromolar pads,[7] and on the palate[4] and is almost always the case in the region of the interdental papillae. On the other hand, an excessively thin flap may become necrotic. Hence tissue that is extremely thin initially should be treated with caution, or a full-thickness flap should be used.

### FLAP LENGTH

The length of the flap should be extensive enough to permit the detached tissue to drape, that is, to be easily maneuvered so as to provide access and visualization of the underlying structures and to permit ease of placement into any desired position during suturing. Generally, the incision extends from beyond the last molar to and beyond the central incisors (Figs. 36-3 and 36-4) but may end at the canine. The

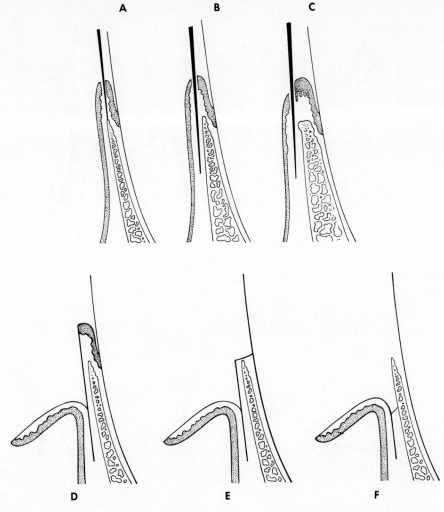

**Fig. 36-2.   A,** A full-thickness flap is used where the tissue is thin, and **B** and **C,** split-thickness flaps are used where the tissue is thicker. Note that all three flaps are made to be of equal width. The cervical wedge may be, **D,** left in place, **E,** detached to the level of the alveolar crest, or, **F,** detached to uncover the marginal alveolar bone.

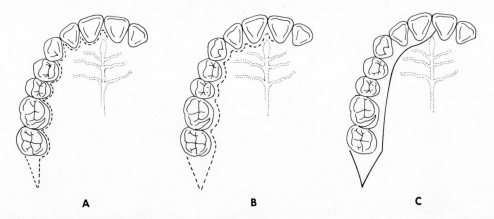

**Fig. 36-3.**   The incision may extend from the distal side of the last molar to the central incisors and may be festooned (**A** and **B**) or linear **(C).**

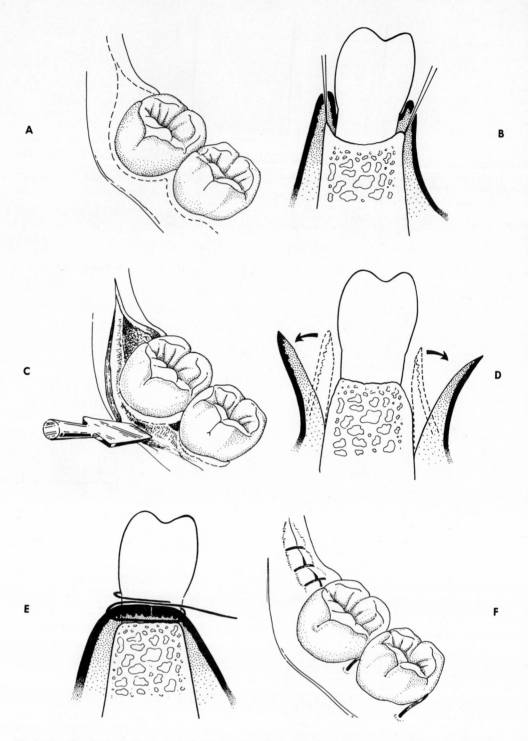

**Fig. 36-4.** Mandibular incisions generally, **A,** go to the distal of the last molar so that, **B** to **D,** the flap envelope may be retracted to expose the alveolar bone and the retromolar area. **E** and **F,** The flaps are coapted after surgery and sutured to form a butt joint.

shape that the surgeon gives to the flap will depend on specific needs, such as providing adequate surgical access for osseous surgery or repositioning the gingiva.[1-3] Flap designs are further subdivided into two categories: the full flap[8-10] and the modified flap.[11]

## FULL FLAP

Full flaps[9,10] (Fig. 36-5, *A*) are defined as having a vertical or oblique relieving incision at each lateral end. When relieving incisions are used, they should extend far enough into the gingiva and into the alveolar mucosa, where necessary, to relieve tissue tension and permit good surgical access. The relieving incisions are always made at line angles (Fig. 36-5, *B*) rather than at the midinterproximal. The incision itself is beveled and descends obliquely to the bone to provide for fine flap coaptation later. Since the relieving incision is made at the line angle, the remainder of the papilla can be reshaped by a papillary gingivoplasty if one is needed. Relieving incisions made over the root prominence often result in recessions in these areas. Lingual and palatal relieving incisions are infrequently used (see Fig. 36-3). If osseous surgery is contemplated, the relieving incision should be at least one tooth mesial or distal to the site of the osseous intervention for better access and visualization of the operative field and for ease of suturing. If a lateral transposed flap is being performed, the relieving incision may be "cut back" for greater ease of flap manipulation.[12]

Vertical incisions permit some areas to be reflected and not others. They allow two segments of a flap to be positioned independently at different levels.

## MODIFIED FLAP (ENVELOPE FLAP)

Modified flaps (Fig. 36-5, *C*) differ in that they have only one or no relieving incisions.[12] When a modified flap is employed, the incision must be sufficiently ex-

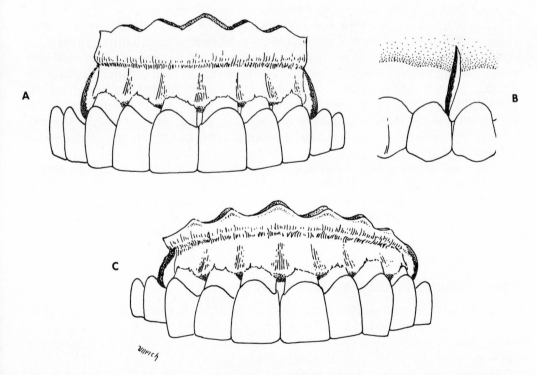

**Fig. 36-5.** **A,** The full flap has a relieving incision at each end. **B,** The relieving incision extends into the alveolar mucosa and is made at the line angle, not the midinterproximal. **C,** The modified flap has either one or no relieving incision.

tensive to permit the flap to be draped apically during surgery, thus providing the same access as would be gained by the full flap. The extension should be one or more teeth mesial and distal to the operative site. The draped flap is then termed the *flap envelope*. Thus modified flaps are also known as *envelope flaps*. They are more frequently used than the full flap.

### SURGICAL JUDGMENT

The design of the flap depends on several factors, all of which can be determined preoperatively. These include the following:

1. What is the operative site? Which teeth does it include? What are the pocket depths about these teeth? What is the roentgenographic picture of bony defects? What is the thickness of the bone over the roots? What is the topography of the bone relative to the gingiva?
2. What is the thickness of the gingival wall?
3. What are the desired mucogingival goals?
4. What are the desired osseous surgical goals?

For example, increased bone loss will require the placement of the initial incision farther apically during palatal surgery (see Fig. 36-3, *A* and *B*) so that the flap wall will cover the bone margin but not extend up over the roots. In addition, scalloping will permit better interdental coaptation. On the other hand, if thick, fibrous, or spongy tissue; palatal bony ledging; or circumferential cratering are present, the removal of tissue will be extensive and the use of a straight-line incision may be required (see Fig. 36-3, *C*).

The design and management of a flap are critical determinants in the success of periodontal surgery.[13] Knowledge of the principles of flap surgery and clinical experience will govern the selection of the type of flap and the extent of the incision. Adequate access to the underlying tissues must be obtained while simultaneously a satisfactory blood supply to the flap is maintained. The base of the flap should be at least as long as the incision. Care should be exercised to avoid cutting through or perforating the flap base. Excessive pressure on the flap base while it is retracted may embarrass circulation to the flap. Use of excessive vacuum (high vacuum) can aspirate the flap, move it, and traumatize it. Trauma produced by folding the flap should be avoided during retraction. Excessive tension, which may result if the flap incision is too narrow and too shallow, should be prevented by proper surgical design. The flap should not be allowed to desiccate during surgery. These factors all cause damage that may lead to flap necrosis.

One must always keep in mind that flap surgery is an operation in its own right.[12] One does not simply elevate the gingiva to obtain access to the underlying tissues but expertly performs a flap dissection with another procedure (e.g., mucogingival, open flap, curettage, bone grafting, or osseous surgery) intended as a sequel. The proper positioning and suturing of the flap afterward complete the surgical endeavor.

## Flap incision and elevation

### BLUNT DISSECTION (FULL-THICKNESS FLAP)

The initial incision is made by sharp dissection with a Bard-Parker blade (no. 12B, 15 or 15 C, no. 10 handle) to the alveolar crest (see Fig. 36-1, *A*). One or more blades are used for each surgery and are discarded after the surgery, since the sharpness of the blade is an important factor in surgical success.

The initial incision may be made through the sulcus or residual pocket wall as an inverse bevel incision extending to the alveolar crest (see Fig. 36-1, *A*). At this point blunt dissection is performed. Either a fine periosteal elevator (Hirschfeld, Goldman-

Fox) or a sharp Molt curette is inserted under the flap in contact with the alveolar bone. The instrument is carefully worked between the flap and the alveolus, reflecting the gingiva, alveolar mucosa, and periosteum, with care taken not to tear through the flap base. In regions where the gingiva is thin, at the mucogingival junction, or over circumferential craters or exostoses, the tissue and the instrument should be supported by finger pressure to prevent flap perforation. After the flap is elevated and depending on the goals of surgery, the remaining tissue left on the oral, vestibular, and interproximal surfaces of the roots and the alveolus may be excised by scalpel and/or curette (see Fig. 36-2, *D* and *F*). This tissue remnant is often referred to as the *cervical wedge*.

Care should be exercised to ensure that the flap is of uniform width, that is, no thicker in the region of the interdental papillae than on the buccal and lingual surfaces of the teeth. This thickness is controlled by the initial incision (Fig. 36-6, *A* to *E*). A common error occurs when the flap is completely raised by blunt dissection (Fig. 36-7, *A*); then the papillae are reflected more or less intact and are thicker than the remainder of the flap (Fig. 36-7, *B* and *C*). This may lead to rolled margins and a coarser postsurgical appearance.

## SHARP DISSECTION (PARTIAL-THICKNESS FLAP)

The Bard-Parker blade is used to incise the gingiva so as to provide an approximately 1.5 to 2-mm uniformly thick flap wall (see Fig. 36-6, *A* to *C*). The flap is extended under tension as the incision proceeds apically. It is useful to distend the flap with the back of the blade. Care must be exercised not to perforate the flap base accidentally with the scalpel. After elevation of the flap, the remaining interproximal tissue and the tissue over the alveolar crest (the cervical wedge) may be excised (see Fig. 36-2, *D* to *F*). The soft tissue over the alveolar bone may be either partially or fully excised or left intact. The tissue must be removed where osseous resection is to be employed

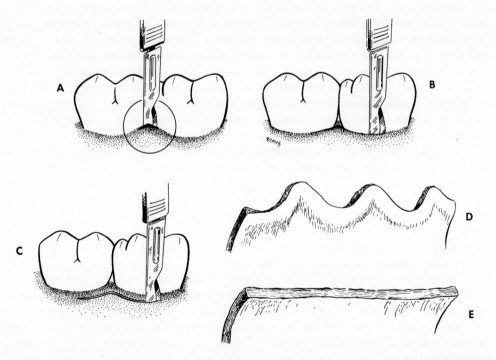

**Fig. 36-6.**   **A,** The interdental papilla must be elevated by a split-thickness incision, which is then carried, **B,** mesially and distally at the gingival margin or, **C,** further apically within the gingiva to obtain a flap, **D,** and **E,** of uniform width throughout its extent.

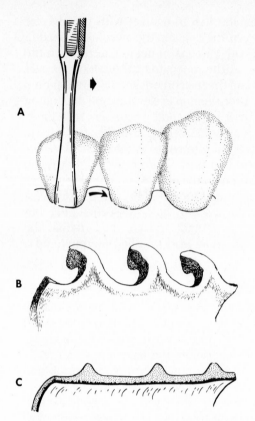

**Fig. 36-7.** If the flap is, **A,** elevated with a periosteal elevator, then most frequently the papillae are, **B,** reflected intact, and, **C,** a flap of uneven width results.

(see Fig. 36-2, *F*). The cervical wedge is most easily excised by sharp dissection along the alveolus with the blade. A second incision is made at the base of the wedge, perpendicular to the alveolus, and the wedge is further undermined with a curette and removed, holding the wedge with a mosquito forceps. Sometimes the surgeon wants to leave the bone covered with periosteum. This is desirable in the presence of thin bony plates, since exposure may result in postsurgical resorption.[14-17] The tissue is best left in place when the gingiva is repositioned or transposed. Then the gingiva can be sutured to this residual tissue with greater ease (periostial suturing)[18] (Fig. 36-8, *B* and *C*).

Combinations of split-thickness and full flaps are possible (Fig. 36-8, *D*). Portions of the remnant tissue may be excised and other portions left intact. The tissue may be left over some teeth while it is removed over others, giving rise to varying flap designs that may be termed split-full-split flaps, etc. When the remnant tissue covering the bone is fibrous and thick, the excess tissue may be removed so that the coapted flap will be thinner than the original tissue.

It may be necessary to use a split flap even where the gingival tissue is less than 2 mm thick and where a full-thickness (periosteal) flap would have been preferable (e.g., where the bone is thin). This requires considerable surgical skill but can be accomplished by an inverse bevel incision in the usual manner, continuing the incision with the flap extended by tension. One may distend the flap gently with a tissue forceps or with a periosteal elevator. In an alternative method, a releasing incision is made and the scalpel is inserted into its base. The flap is split by moving the blade upward toward the sulcus.[9,14]

The gingival margin of the flap may be either a straight line (see Fig. 36-3, *C*) or scalloped (see Figs. 36-3, *A* and *B*, and 36-4, *A*). In either case the margin should be

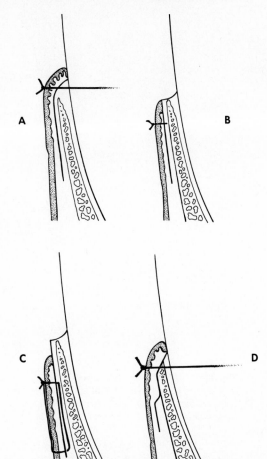

**Fig. 36-8.**  Split-thickness flaps can be sutured in a variety of ways: **A,** placed back to position and held with an interdental tie; **B** and **C,** apically positioned at different levels and sutured with periosteal sutures to the residual connective tissue; or **D,** sutured to the alveolar plate with an interdental tie. A long periosteal retention suture is shown in **C.**

thin. If it is made too thick, the coapted flap may heal with thick margins. If a flap is made thick, the situation may be retrievable, but only with difficulty. One may attempt to thin a thick flap with surgical shears, by scalpel, or with electrocautery. Holding and cutting a reflected flap for this purpose is difficult, frequently resulting in a flap cut shorter but no thinner or resulting in tissue trauma. It is simpler to perform the initial incision correctly.

## PALATAL FLAP

The flap is the procedure of choice on the palatal surfaces, since healing is generally more rapid than when the gingivectomy is used. The flap heals by first intention, the gingivectomy by second. Moreover, pockets and bony defects more often than not occur on the palatal surfaces.[19]

The position of the alveolar crest can be determined by sounding (probing horizontally and vertically with a needle or probe to the bone)[17] (Fig. 36-9, *A*) through the palatal tissue under anesthesia. The initial incision should be made at a height consistent with the alveolar margin, that is, 1 or 2 mm above the bone margin (Fig. 36-9, *B*).

In making the palatal flap incision, one should know the position of the greater palatine foramen to avoid the anterior palatine artery. One may operate in the region of the incisive foramen, since the vessels do not tend to be large.

Where the bone loss is marked and the palatal gingiva is heavy, the palatal incision may be made perpendicular to the root surface. The excess tissue is excised, since it

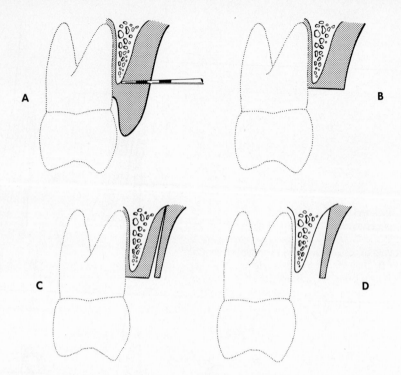

**Fig. 36-9.** *The position of the alveolar crest can be determined by,* **A,** *probing under anesthesia (sounding) and,* **B,** *making a horizontal incision at a height consistent with the bone margin, creating a flat ledge of tissue.* **C,** *The palatal tissue is elevated with an undermining incision to provide a flap of acceptable width,* **D,** *The underlying wedge of tissue is transected near the base of the flap incision and removed.*

is difficult to apically reposition the palatal tissues. Consequently, it is permissible to excise some attached gingiva by way of this perpendicular gingivectomy to remove the pocket and to approximate gingival and bone levels. The flat surface resulting from excision constitutes a ledge. The ledge provides easy access for a split-thickness incision ("ledge-and-wedge" incision). The remnant over the bone is transected near its base and removed, leaving a flap wall of proper dimensions ( Fig. 36-9, *B* to *D*).

Palatal relieving incisions are infrequently used, since they tend to cut larger vessels, which may lead to excessive bleeding.

Palatal incisions are difficult with a straight-handled blade. To make the surgery easier, one may position the patient's head turned away from one and use a long-handled Bard-Parker blade with a large photographic mirror to obtain close to a 90-degree entrance of the blade. The mesiopalatal gingiva may be overscalloped to compensate for excess tissue at the mesiopalatal line angle.

Skilled surgeons prefer different blades and knives to achieve flap reflection. The steps in the reflection of a flap 1-2 mm thick and the removal of the underlying tissue (secondary flap) to bare the bone is illustrated in Fig. 36-10, *A* to *I*.

## RETROMOLAR FLAPS

**Distal wedge**    Distal to the last standing maxillary molar, the connective tissue is dense and is generally removed en masse after the appropriate incisions are made. The mass of tissue and the procedure for removing it are called the *distal wedge*.[7,20,21] The incisions are inverse bevel incisions made by observing the previous instructions concerning width. They are joined mesially to the split- or full-thickness flaps in the buccal and palatal gingiva (see Fig. 36-3).

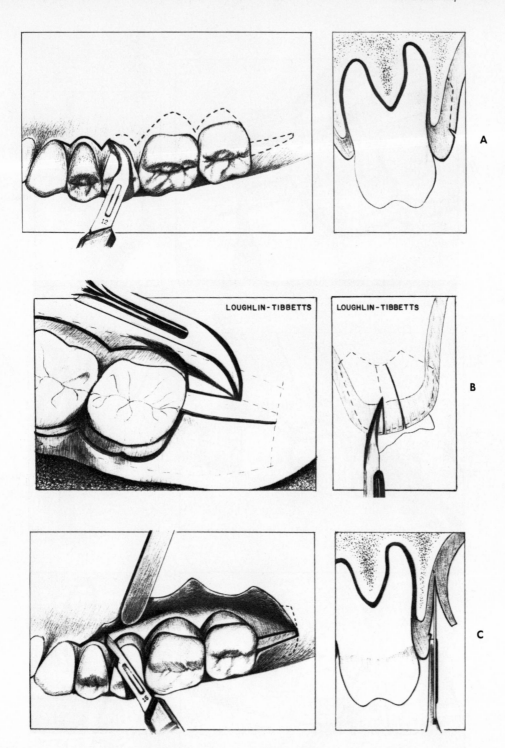

**Fig. 36-10.   A,** The outline of the flap to be reflected is shown by dotted lines. This outline should represent the anticipated form of bone following osseous surgery so that the flap margin is no more than 2 mm coronal to bone. **B,** The incision is begun anteriorly and the 12B blade is moved in a push motion posteriorly to outline the retromolar incisions. The depth of the initial outlining incision is about 1 mm. **C,** A 15C blade is used to incise the flap while it is retracted by the assistant. The incision parallels the palatal surface and the flap is 1.5 to 2.0 mm thick. When the palate is flat, the procedure is more difficult. The papillae can be thinned using a 12B blade (with mesial and distal entering incisions) or an Orban 1/2 knife or a 15C blade. The blade should not touch bone, to maintain sharpness.                                                                                    *Continued.*

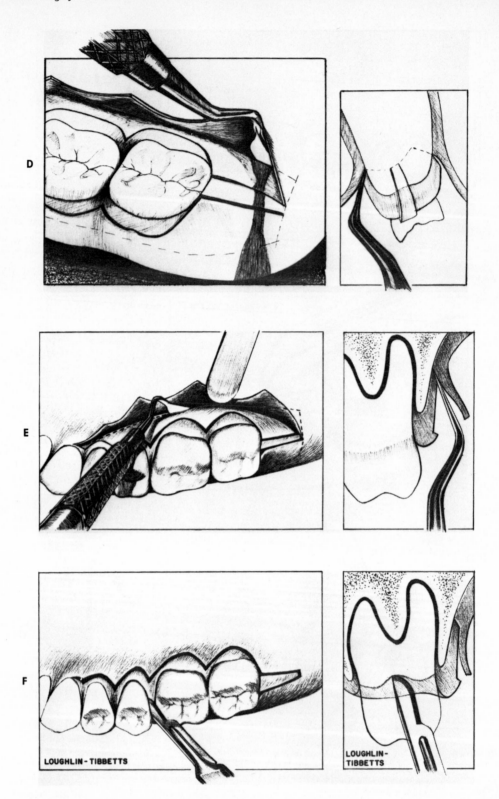

**Fig. 36-10, cont'd.** **D,** A Kirkland 15/16 knife is used to carry the incision to bone. Since the shank has no cutting edge, it can be safely drawn along the base of the flap, extending the flap as the incision is made. **E,** The flap is retracted by the assistant while the surgeon extends the incision to bone. **F,** A 15, 15C, or 12B blade is placed into the sulcus and extended to touch bone in order to separate the gingival tissue from the tooth.

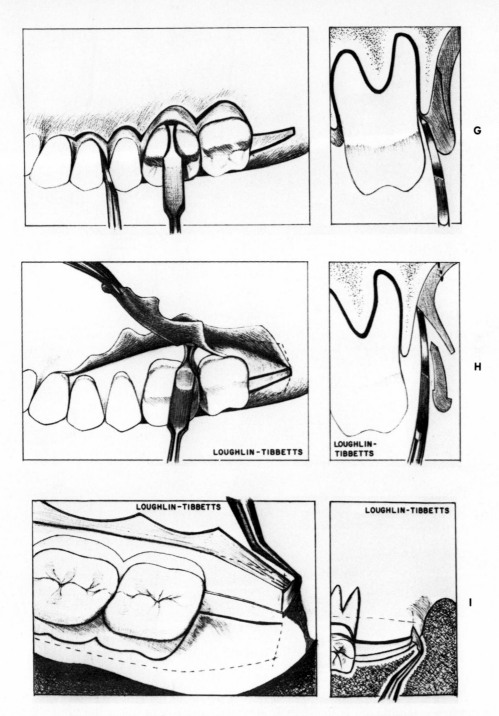

**Fig. 36-10, cont'd.   G,** The collar of tissue (secondary flap) is now removed by using an Ochsenbein #2 chisel. Starting anteriorly, the chisel is moved apically along bone to detach the secondary flap until the incision made apically with the Kirkland 15/16 knife is reached. The surgeon proceeds in an anteroposterior direction. **H,** The assistant extends the partially excised secondary flap, while the surgeon detaches this tissue with the Ochsenbein #2 chisel. **I,** The distal (retromolar) wedge is now used. While the assistant distends the primary flap with a tissue forceps or periostome, the surgeon traces and extends the incisions, joining buccal and palatal incisions near the hammular notch area. The Ochsenbein #2 chisel is then inserted to undermine and detach the distal wedge, which is grasped in a mosquito forceps by the assistant and removed. Occasionally the surgeon may place a vertical incision in the buccal flap at the distobuccal line angle of the second molar in order to obtain closure and coaptation of retromolar flap margins. (Fig. 36-10, *A to I*, courtesy D. Loughlin and L.S. Tibbetts, Arlington, Texas.)

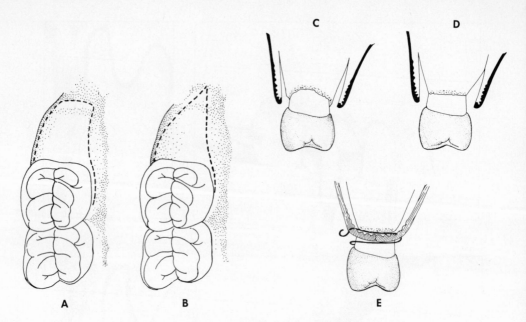

**Fig. 36-11.** **A,** Rectangular distal wedge outline, **B,** Triangular distal wedge outline. **C,** After appropriate internal bevel incisions and flap elevation, **D,** osseous correction is performed and, **E,** flap is coapted and sutured.

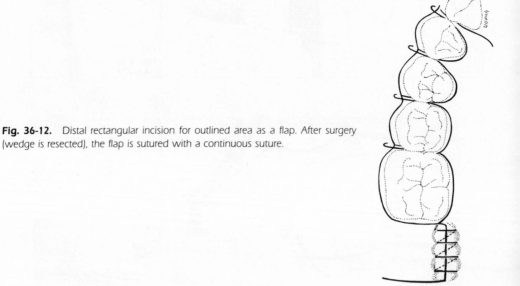

**Fig. 36-12.** Distal rectangular incision for outlined area as a flap. After surgery (wedge is resected), the flap is sutured with a continuous suture.

The design of the tuberosity incisions depends in part on the thickness of the tissues. The outline of the incisions is either rectangular, or triangular (Fig. 36-11, *A* and *B*). The triangular incisions extend to the hamular notch region posteriorly and are continuous with the buccal and palatal flap incisions anteriorly. When the rectangular outline is used, coaptation may become a problem. This can be circumvented by forming the rectangle into a pedicle flap[19] (Fig. 36-12). These pedicles are useful adjuncts to osseous grafts distal to the last molar.

It is often convenient to displace the loose wedge tissue toward the palate, holding the wedge with a mosquito forceps and undermining with a curette.

**Mandible**      The mandibular retromolar incisions are made in the same fashion, employing the triangular or rectangular outline (see Fig. 36-4). Where the tissue is of a dense fibrous consistency, this can be done with ease. When the tissue is loose mucosa, the tissue must be carefully dissected. If the external oblique ridge is prominent, the buccal incision should be made directly above it or lingual to it to provide proper access toward the buccal surface and to permit the remnant tissue to be removed with ease. A common error occurs when the surgeon attempts to use too small a triangular outline.

Retromolar flaps may be reflected by making incisions either (1) close to the buccal (over the external oblique ridge) or (2) lingual to it. The amount and position of gingiva will dictate incision design. A goal is to retain as much gingiva as possible. Avoid a postsurgical line of closure at the midline. Since it is generally easier to reflect from buccal to lingual, where gingival topography permits, make incisions on the buccal so that flap reflection may be made toward the lingual.

The incisions are joined distal to the molar and are blended with scalloped incisions at the distobuccal and distolingual. The flaps are thinned, extending incisions to bone, and a wedge is removed.

A lingually placed incision is done where a shallow vestibule is present or there is a very close proximity to the ramus.

After reflection of the flap (see Fig. 36-4, *C* and *D*), all necessary osseous procedures are performed. The flap margins are then coapted carefully to form a butt joint (Figs. 36-4, *E* and *F*, and 36-13) and are held in place by sutures.

## SURGERY UNDER PONTICS

Surgery under pontics may be done in two ways. Where the tissue is thick, incisions are made to the bone on the buccal and lingual surfaces of the pontic and inclined in toward the alveolar plate. The isolated wedge of tissue is then removed. Buccal and lingual flaps of appropriate thickness are elevated after undermining incisions are made. The remnant tissue over the bone is dissected away. In suturing, the two flap margins are coapted.

When the tissue over the bone is thin, a single incision is made to the bone on either the buccal or lingual surface of the pontic. This tissue is elevated or pushed from under the pontic as part of the flap. Later it may be passed back under the pontic and sutured.

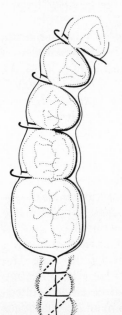

**Fig. 36-13.** Distal triangular outline after suturing.

If alveolar mucosa is present under the pontic, one may denude to bone to encourage healing with gingiva.

## Basic principles

The flap is the basic procedure for the following surgical interventions:

1. Surgical curettage (open subgingival curettage)
2. Reattachment operation
3. Osseous resection
4. Bone grafting
5. Flap grafting, that is, apical, lateral, or coronal positioning of pedicle flaps
6. Connective tissue and scleral grafting
7. Free gingival grafting

The ability to perform these procedures rests on the first steps: the design, the incision, and the elevation of the flap; the manipulation of the flap without trauma; and the later placement or positioning of the flap. In general the bone should be covered by the flap to avoid bone loss that occurs when it is left exposed after surgical procedures.[14,22-25]

Following are the basic principles of flap management:

1. Conserve the gingiva so that after healing there is an adequate width of gingiva
2. Make the flap uniformly thin so that it is pliable, easily manipulated, and sutured to place
3. Avoid flap necrosis by avoiding desiccation or otherwise maltreating the flap or injuring its blood supply
4. Design the flap sufficiently long and deep to permit it to be retracted fully and with ease. This will provide access and also proper draping while avoiding pressure injury to the flap
5. Avoid excessive use of relieving incisions coupled with narrow two-, three-, or four-tooth flaps

Surgeons are judged by the geometric neatness of their incisions, the meticulous handling of the tissue, the finesse of suturing, and the lack of tissue tags, crude margins, and inconsistent thickness of flaps.

The principles and techniques for periodontal flaps have been discussed. Illustrations of the surgery follow (Fig. 36-14, *A* to *H*).

Several problems must be faced in making palatal incisions on posterior teeth, including access and vision. Since all incisions are made from a frontomesial view, it is difficult to locate the root midpoint on the gingiva of posterior teeth (Fig. 36-14, *A*). When contra-angled knives or blades are used, incisions can be made at right angles. Incisions made with a straight handle and blade cannot be made at right angles to soft tissue or to the gingiva. As a result, the arcuate crest of the incision is likely to be placed mesial or distal to the height of the root contour (Fig. 36-14, *A*). To compensate for these access and vision problems, a large photographic mirror may be used. The patient's head should be tilted away from the surgeon, and the patient should be instructed to move the mandible away from the surgeon in a lateral excursion (Fig. 36-14, *B*). A shallow incision is then made to outline the design of the flap (Fig. 36-14, *C*). The mesial line angles of the incision should be overscalloped to compensate the thicker tissue that is usually left at mesiopalatal line angles of the flap. Once an acceptable outline is made, reflection of a split-thickness of the flap is begun with a Bard-Parker 15 or 15C blade. The thickness of the flap is established at this time. The blade is made to enter tissue and to distend the flap at the same time. The reflecting incision is started at the distal end of the flap. The blade should be angled (tilted) mesially and coronally and should not touch tooth or bone, so as to maintain sharpness (Fig. 36-14, *D*). As the interdental areas are approached, the back (noncutting) edge

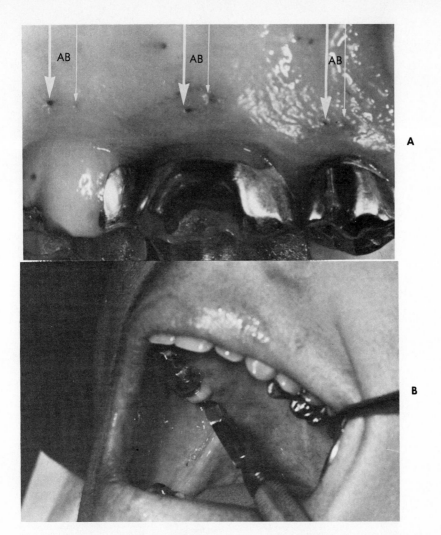

**Fig. 36-14.   A,** Flap incisions are made from a frontomesial view. At this angle, the root midcenter is difficult to locate. The crest of the scalloped incision may be inaccurately placed (A). The arcuate center is located at B. **B,** Have patient turn head away from the surgeon and move the mandible laterally to permit an incision that is closer to right angles to the gingiva.                                                          *Continued.*

of the blade is used to distend the flap and the flap is carefully dissected to maintain a 1.5- to 2-mm tissue thickness. Moving around the tooth, the blade may be flexed against the tooth, in order to distend the flap and to assist in maintaining the flap thickness. Once the incision is completed, the blade is reintroduced distally and the incision is extended to bone (Fig. 36-14, *E*). The primary flap is thus reflected. A periosteal elevator may be introduced when necessary and the flap reflected so that it can be displaced without tension. A thin-bladed, contra-angled knife (Orban) is introduced into the sulcus to separate the secondary flap from tooth and bone. The knife is then inserted apically over the interdental connection of the secondary flap. The end of the secondary flap is grasped with tissue forceps, and the periosteum is reflected via the sulcular incisions and pushed apically to detach the secondary flap. The secondary flap is discarded or used for ridge augmentation or for free gingival grafts. Remnants and tags of tissue can be removed with currettes or Rhodes chisels to bare bone. The teeth are planed with curettes and/or ultrasonic instruments.

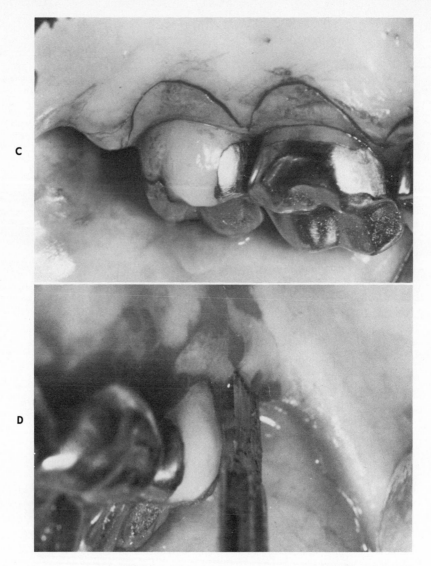

**Fig. 36-14, cont'd.** **C,** Outline the flap design with a shallow incision. **D,** Flap thickness is established at the distal terminus of the flap.

The buccal flap is incised and elevated in the same manner. Since buccal tissue is usually thinner than palatal, the secondary flap may consist of a narrow wedge of tissue (Fig. 36-14, *F*). Overscalloping of mesial line angles permits the surgeons to avoid greater tissue bulk at the mesial line angles. The crest of the arc of the incision over maxillary incisors is placed slightly distal to the midroot for esthetic reasons.[26]

Following reflection of the flap and any osseous, open curettage or grafting procedures, a trial placement of the flap is made. Coaptation of interdental margins and coverage is desirable when bone grafts are placed. For pocket elimination following open curettage or osseous surgery, the flap margins should be placed 1 mm coronal to the alveolar crest. Any corrections in flap design are made with a sharp scalpel blade or tissue scissors, and the flap is secured by suturing (Fig. 36-14, *G* and *H*). For further techniques in periodontal flap surgery see also Fig. 36-10, *A* to *I*.

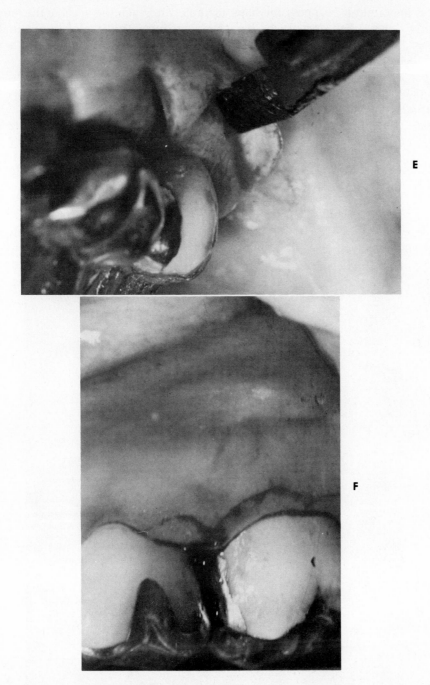

**Fig. 36-14, cont'd.    E,** The blade is directed mesially and coronally. The blade is not permitted to touch bone in order to maintain sharpness. Later, the incision is extended to bone. **F,** Accentuating the scallop over the mesial tooth surface can compensate for any greater flap thickness on the mesial surface.    *Continued.*

# Suturing

### FLAP PLACEMENT

It is important to reappose the flaps accurately to reach the goals of the surgery. A properly coapted flap encourages hemostasis, reduces the size of the wound to be repaired, selects healing by first intention over second intention, and prevents unnecessary bone exposure and consequent resorption.[2,14,15,23-25]

After the surgery has been performed, the flap should be thinned and trial fitted to its planned position to ensure that the tissues are properly adapted. There should be no residual pocket depth and tissue form, length, and thickness should be in harmony with the underlying bone form. If the initial flap was correctly designed,

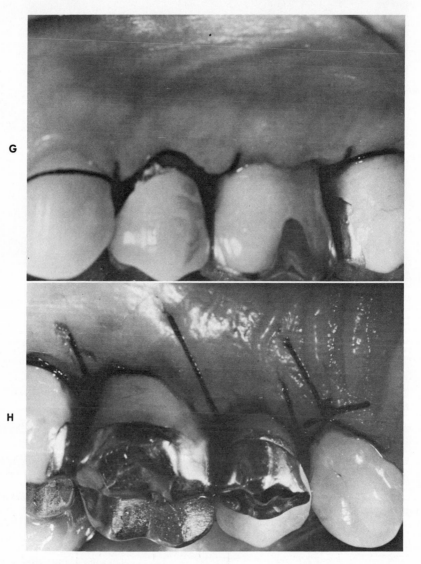

**Fig. 36-14, cont'd.** **G,** The flap is trial-fitted and sutured no more than 1 mm coronal to bone, following osseous resection. **H,** Suturing should provide proper flap adaptation and placement. (Fig. 36-14, *A* to *H,* courtesy O. Bahat, Beverly Hills, California.)

positioning is not a problem. If an excess of tissue is found coronally, the excess must be removed either by trimming the margin or by altering the position of the flap before suturing. Trimming of the flap margins may be carried out by scalpel, tissue scissors, or electrocautery. The flap margins should coapt where bony lesions have been treated by grafting and over edentulous ridges.

Suturing is used to maintain the readapted flap and the coapted wound margins in position until such time as wound healing has progressed sufficiently that the tissues remain in place.[27,28] Alternative means of holding the tissue in place, such as pinning or fixation by cyanoacrylates[29] or laser beam, exist but are not in routine use.

Apically positioned flaps may be sutured either to cover the alveolar margin or to barely expose it. Since uncovered bone tends to resorb,[14,22-25] bone is not usually left exposed.

Full flaps are sutured in place by ties that encircle the tooth (sling sutures) or by simple interdental sutures (Figs. 36-8, *A* and *D*, 36-15, and 36-16).

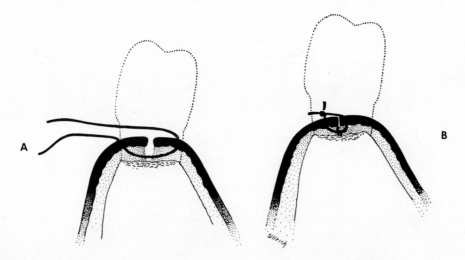

**Fig. 36-15.** **A,** Suture material passes through the buccal flap from its external surface and through the lingual flap from its internal surface. **B,** Suture is tied with a square knot, which is placed over intact tissue, not over the incision.

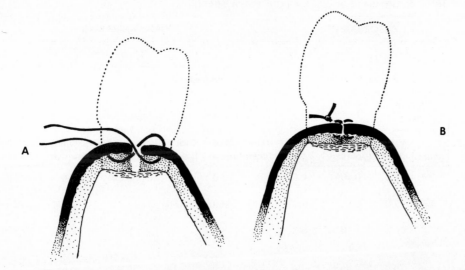

**Fig. 36-16.** **A,** In the figure-eight interdental tie, the buccal flap is pierced from the buccal side, the needle is reversed, and the lingual flap is pierced from its lingual surface. **B,** Suture is tied with a square knot.

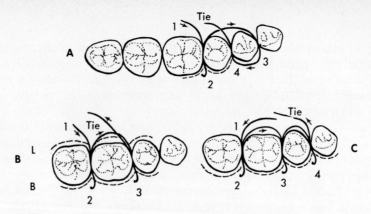

**Fig. 36-17.** Variations of sling sutures. **A,** Anchor variations. Use when only one papilla is flapped. **B,** Suspensory or sling. **C,** Modification. (Courtesy R. LaBelle, Minneapolis, Minnesota.)

**Table 36-1**  Suture materials

| Material | Company Ethicon | Davis & Geck | Deknatel |
|---|---|---|---|
| Catgut | Plain<br>Chromic | Plain<br>Chromic | Plain<br>Chromic |
| Synthetic absorbable | Vicryl* | Dexon* | — |
| Nylon | Ethilon* | Dermalon* | Nylon |
| Silk | Perma Hand*<br>Surgical silk | Silk | Silk |
| Dacron | Mersilene*<br>Ethiflex* (Teflon treated) | Ti-crom* | PolyDek* |
| Polypropylene | Prolene* | Blue linear polyethylene | — |
| Surgical steel | Surgical steel | Surgical steel | Surgical steel |
| Nylon braided | Nurolon* | Surgilon* | — |
| Cotton | Cotton | Cotton | Cotton |

*Trademark

**Table 36-2**  Suture diameter and knot-pull tensile strength*

| | ABSORBABLES | | | | NONABSORBABLES | | | | | |
|---|---|---|---|---|---|---|---|---|---|---|
| | | | | | Class I | | | | | |
| | U.S.P. requirement† | | | | U.S.P. requirement† | | | | | |
| | Diameter (mils) | | | | Diameter (mils) | | | | | |
| U.S.P. size | Min-imum | Max-imum | Knot pull (pounds) | Ethicon gut | Min-imum | Max-imum | Knot pull (pounds) | Ethicon silk (braid & twist) | Mersilene‡ (braided) | Ethiflex§ (braided) |
| 6-0 | 3.5 | 5.0 | 0.40 | 0.6 | 3.0 | 4.0 | 0.44 | 0.6 | 0.6 | 0.6 |
| 5-0 | 5.5 | 7.0 | 0.84 | 1.3 | 4.0 | 6.0 | 0.88 | 1.2 | 1.7 | 1.8 |
| 4-0 | 7.7 | 9.5 | 1.70 | 2.3 | 6.0 | 8.0 | 1.30 | 2.0 | 2.8 | 2.8 |
| 3-0 | 10.5 | 12.5 | 2.80 | 3.8 | 8.0 | 10.0 | 2.10 | 2.8 | 4.2 | 4.0 |

*Courtesy Ethicon, Inc., Somerville, N.J.
†U.S.P. XVIII diameter and/or tensile strength requirement for averages on 10-strand samples, compared with mean averages f
Ethicon sutures.
‡Trademark.
§Trademark for Ethicon‡ polyester fiber suture coated with polytetrafluoroethylene.

The outer or mucosal unit of split-thickness flaps is positioned by sutures to the residual tissue overlying the bone (periosteal retention sutures)[18] (see Fig. 36-8, *B* and *C*) or by sutures encircling the tooth (sling sutures) (Fig. 36-17).

The emphasis on flap techniques in periodontal therapy requires the dentist to be conversant with the various styles and types of suture needles, suturing materials, and needle holders, as well as the techniques employed in their use, including knotting.

## MATERIALS

The suture material may be braided silk, dermal, synthetic (polypropylene, monofilament), or catgut (Table 36-1). The silk or synthetic materials are most commonly employed and must be removed 4 to 10 days postoperatively. Synthetics are generally stronger and create less inflammation than silk, but some have an elastic memory and tend to untie unless they are triple knotted. Silk is the easiest to use. Gut sutures may be employed where the sutures cannot be removed, since they resorb within the tissue. **Suture materials**

The widths of the suture materials employed in periodontal surgery range from 000 (3-0) to 000000 (6-0) (Table 36-2). Eyeless (swaged) sutures are less traumatic than sutures knotted to the needle and are preferred. The relation of suture width to number is shown in Table 36-2.

Sometimes, particularly when the tissue is very thin, as when laterally positioned flaps or free gingival grafts are attempted, a 5-0 or 6-0 suture may be necessary. In cases in which the flap is thicker, a 4-0 suture is used.

The needles should be eyeless. Needles may be fine in diameter or large; they may be one fourth, three eighths, one half, or five eighths of a circle (see Fig. 36-18). These curved needles pierce and are passed through the tissue by rotating the wrist while holding the needle holder. **Needles**

The cutting edges of the needle may be reverse cutting, conventional cutting, Astralok, or pointed (noncutting) (Fig. 36-18).

Needle holders may be chosen from many types and sizes (Fig. 36-19, *A*). Hemostats do not make useful needle holders.[12] Incorrect choice of needle and poor handling of the needle holder can produce necrosis or can cut through the tissue. **Needle holders**

Suture pliers may be used to grasp the tissue and permit accurate insertion of the needle into the flap (Fig. 36-19, *E*). **Suture pliers**

| NONABSORBABLES | | | | | | | | | | |
|---|---|---|---|---|---|---|---|---|---|---|
| Class I | | | Class II | | | | | Class III | | |
| Prolene‡ (mono) | Ethilon‡ and Nurolon | | U.S.P.† knot pull (pounds) | Ethicon virgin and dermal silk | Ethicon cotton | Ethicon linen | U.S.P.† knot requirements (pounds) | Ethicon stainless steel | | B & S gauge |
| | Mono | Braid | | | | | | Mono | Twist | |
| 0.7 | 0.7 | — | 0.25 | — | — | — | 0.60 | 0.9 to 1.4 | — | 40 to 38 |
| 1.4 | 1.6 | 1.4 | 0.51 | 0.7 | 1.2 | — | 1.20 | 2.9 | 2.1 | 35 |
| 2.2 | 2.5 | 2.2 | 1.00 | 1.6 | 2.0 | 1.9 | 1.80 | 3.7 to 5.1 | 3.2 to 4.0 | 34 to 32 |
| 3.5 | 3.9 | 3.5 | 1.40 | 2.3 | 3.0 | 2.5 | 3.00 | 8.3 | 6.5 | 30 |

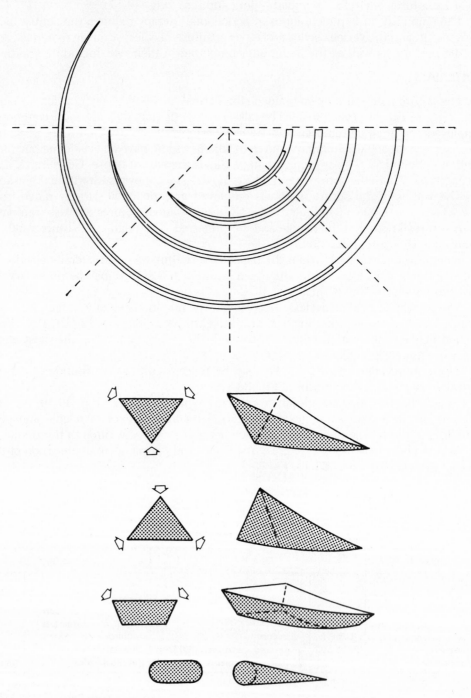

**Fig. 36-18.** Needles are described by their arc as one fourth, three eighths, one half, or five eighths of a circle. They all have a point and either three, two, or no cutting edges. The silhouettes shown are reverse, conventional, spatula, or rectangular and noncutting.

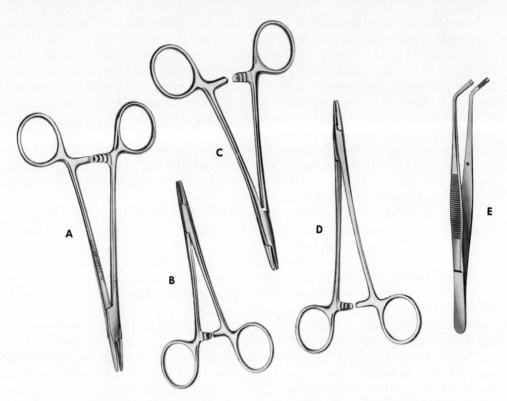

**Fig. 36-19.**   Commonly used needle holders. **A,** Mayo-Hegar (Gardner 6); **B,** Derf; **C,** Hegar-Baumgartner; **D,** Crile-Wood; **E,** Suture plier.

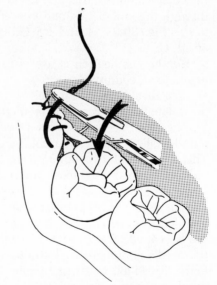

**Fig. 36-20.**   When suturing, close the needle holder firmly on the heel of the needle, engage the tissue, and rotate the wrist (and needle holder) so that the needle passes through the tissue.

## TECHNIQUES

When suturing, close the needle holder firmly on the heel of the needle. The needle and suture are passed through the tissue deeply enough and sufficiently distant from the marginal gingiva so as not to tear through the tissue (Fig. 36-20). The thread is kept apical to the contact point. Double ties (square knots) are used with silk suture material; triple ties are used with synthetic material, since this type of material has elastic memory and the knots tend to untie.

**Interdental ligation**

Interdental ligation (interrupted suturing) is a frequently used form of suturing. It has several modifications. A firm adaptation of soft tissue to underlying tooth and bone is produced and is of greatest value when both buccal and lingual flaps are to be coapted closely, under equal tension, to bone and tooth surfaces. The needle is passed through the buccal flap from the buccal or external surface and through the lingual flap from its internal surface, or vice versa. The needle is passed back again through the interdental space, and the suture is tied (see Fig. 36-15).

**Interdental tie**

Generally the needle is passed interdentally, but when the contact is open, the suture can be slipped through the contact. If the passage is slightly impeded, the suture may be forced through the contact, provided it is one of the stronger plastic materials and not silk or gut, which are too weak. Floss or tape may also be used to force the weaker materials through the contact.

Exercise care to avoid tearing the tissues with the needle or the suture. Similarly avoid breaking the suture. Do not suture too tightly, since that may cause tissue necrosis, or the suture may gradually cut through the tissue.

**Figure-eight tie**

The figure eight is a modification of the interdental ligature. The buccal flap is pierced as described before, but the needle does not enter the inner aspect of the opposite flap. Instead the needle is reversed after passing through the interdental space and pierces the lingual flap from the lingual (external) surface (see Fig. 36-16).

**Suspensory ligation**

Suspensory ligation (see Fig. 36-17) encircles the tooth and can be used when a flap is reflected only on the buccal or the lingual surface. When one flap is to be positioned apically, whereas the other is to be replaced in its original position, and when different suture tensions are required, suspensory ligation is effective. Another situation in which this suturing is sometimes used occurs when teeth are overlapped and passing the suture needle between teeth is difficult. In suspensory ligation, pass the needle through the outer surface of the flap around the neck of the tooth, through the adjacent embrasure, and insert it through the next papilla. Bring the suture back through the embrasure, and knot it on either the facial or the lingual surface of the tooth (Fig. 36-21, *A* and *B*). Other forms of anchoring the tie are shown in Fig. 36-21, *C*.

**Continuous ligation**

Continuous ligation is useful to suspend the flap at a desired level.[12,26,27] In this technique a continuous mattress type of suture is used for an entire quadrant or for an area involving several teeth. Three types of continuous sutures are used to approximate flaps to bone and teeth. The first type (Fig. 36-22) pierces the papilla from the buccal surface, crosses the interdental space and passes lingual to the tooth, returns interdentally in the next space, and exits to the buccal. Here the procedure is repeated. This occurs tooth by tooth until the last standing tooth is reached. After having passed around the most distal tooth, the suture pierces the buccal flap, may be wrapped twice around the distal tooth, and crosses back to the lingual. The lingual flap is pierced, and the suture is brought back and passed buccal to the last tooth. It is then passed interdentally, piercing the lingual papilla, and passed back interdentally and around the buccal surface of the next tooth. The procedure is repeated tooth by tooth until the needle is brought back through the first interdental space. The knot is then tied to the thread left at the first papilla. One may start the procedure at the mesial or the distal aspect of the flap. Remember to position the buccal flap (using wet gauze) to its desired position before suturing the lingual. (See discussion of apically positioned flap in Chapter 40.)

In an alternate method, the suture is knotted at the first buccal papilla and passed interdentally, piercing the lingual flap, and passed back interdentally. The suture courses around the buccal surface of the tooth and then interdentally to pierce the lingual papilla. It is brought back interdentally to pierce the buccal papilla and then back interdentally and around the lingual surface of the adjacent tooth, through the

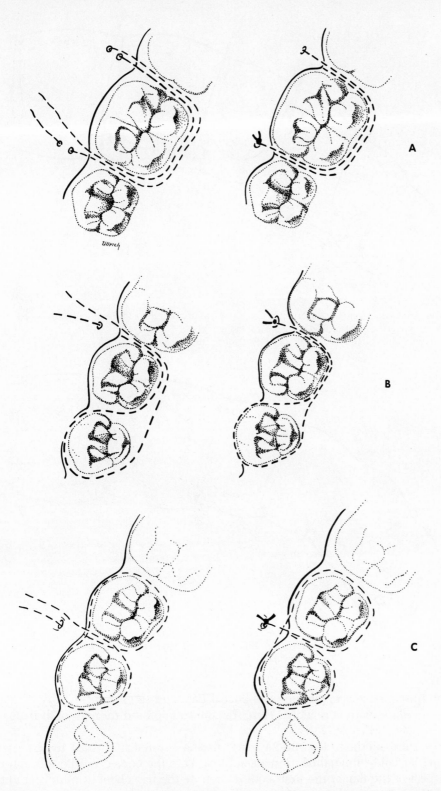

**Fig. 36-21.**  Variations in anchoring suspensory sutures involving, **A,** one adjacent tooth; **B,** the adjacent tooth and the one beyond it; and **C,** two adjacent teeth.

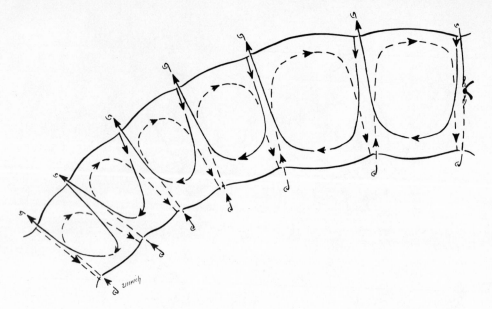

**Fig. 36-22.** Continuous suture used first to fix the buccal flap in place, then, after passing mesial to the incisor, to suture the lingual flap to place. It is knotted distal to the molar.

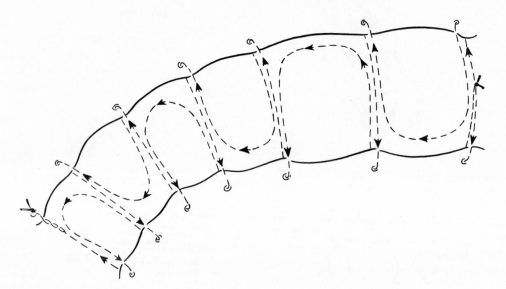

**Fig. 36-23.** A variation of a continuous suture in which buccal and lingual flaps are sutured in place at one tooth in an interrupted fashion before the needle is passed to the next distal tooth.

next interproximal space, piercing the buccal flap, and so on until the distal side of the last standing tooth is reached. Here the suture is passed through both flaps and knotted on itself (Fig. 36-23).

In the third method (Fig. 36-24) each flap is sutured and fixed to place with individual buccal or lingual continuous sutures. Pass the curved needle through the outer aspect of the flap at the first tooth. Penetrate the flap about 2 mm distal to the edge of the anterior releasing incision (if one is used), close to the mucogingival junction. The needle will enter from the outside and exit on the inside of the tissue flap. Circle the neck of the tooth with the suture, and pass the suture back at the next

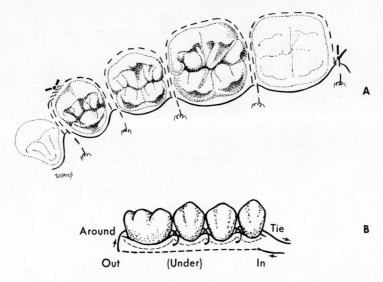

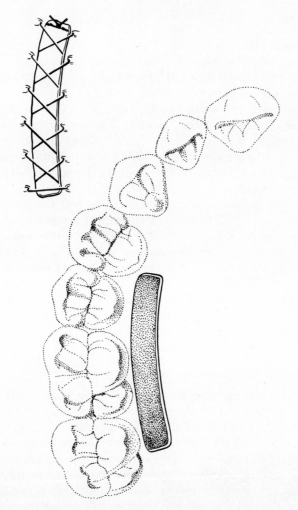

**Fig. 36-24.** **A,** Continuous suture used to fasten only one flap in place, in this case the lingual. **B,** Malamed suture: a variation in the tie of a suture affixing a single flap, in this case the buccal. (Courtesy R. LaBelle, Minneapolis, Minnesota.)

**Fig. 36-25.** "Bootlace" continuous suture, tied with two needles used for edentulous areas such as the palatal donor site for free gingival grafting.

embrasure to enter the flap on its inner aspect; then reverse the needle and repeat the procedure. Thus the entire flap is held in suspension. The tie is made at the last tooth, but alternatively the suture can be run over the necks of the teeth to tie the original strand where the tail end of the thread remains from the insertion of the needle (Fig. 36-24, *B*). Press a gauze square against the flap to position the flap accurately to the desired level. Then, while an assistant holds the flap in place with the gauze, tighten the tie and make a double (square) knot. If the opposite (lingual or buccal) area is similarly involved, use a continuous suture separately for this flap.

Two types of continuous sutures can be used for suturing edentulous areas: one is a mattress suture used like a bootlace (Fig. 36-25); the other is a continuous hem loop (Fig. 36-26). Of course, interrupted sutures may be used, as well as circumferential sutures. Relieving incisions are sutured with simple interrupted sutures.

**Periosteal suturing**

Periosteal suturing is used to fix a partial-thickness flap to the periosteum remaining on bone. It is applicable in most areas, except the buccal surface of the mandibular molars, where the periosteum is loosely adherent to bone. Flaps may be positioned apically to permit exact approximation of flap margins to bony margins by way of sutures placed apical to the mucogingival junction (Fig. 36-27) or at the gingival margin and bone crest (see Fig. 36-8). The techniques for periosteal suturing are described in Figs. 36-28 and 36-29.

## Suture removal

Sutures are usually removed between 5 and 14 days after surgery. Some practitioners place dressings over the sutured wound, although dressings are used less frequently in current periodontal surgical practice. Where the wound surface is undressed, sutures are usually removed earlier.

Before suture removal, the wound surface should be inspected and a topical anesthetic (Pontocaine) placed for patient comfort. The wound surface is débrided with moistened cotton pledgets or cotton swabs. Loose sutures are easily removed. Where sutures are in place, the suture is grasped near the tie and the suture is cut. Do not pull the knot through tissue. Gently pull and remove the suture. Reinspect the wound area for any suture material.

Sutures that might be inadvertently left in place will become readily apparent, usually within a few days to a few weeks. Postsurgical inspection will readily identify a retained suture fragment. When a suture fragment is left in tissue, acute swelling and abscess formation occur within a month or less. The area should then be anesthetized and any remnant suture material removed. Prompt removal will prevent further discomfort.

The teeth should be polished with a desensitizing prophylaxis paste, plaque control instructions repeated, and the patient should be given appointments for postsurgical examinations at 1- to 2-week intervals for from one to four visits.

## Summary

Precise flap design and suturing are necessary for accurate adaptation of the flap to tooth and bone and for accurate placement of the flap in its desired position. These factors are also necessary to coapt flaps and to position flaps coronally, apically, or laterally. Close adaptation of the flap to bone may help to reduce postoperative pain and result in an improved tissue form after surgery. Perfect coaptation of flap margins is essential in bone grafting operations to enclose the grafted material and encourage a take. Cooperation between the dentist and the assistant is necessary during the suturing procedure. Careful training and practice will permit these procedures to be performed with relative ease.

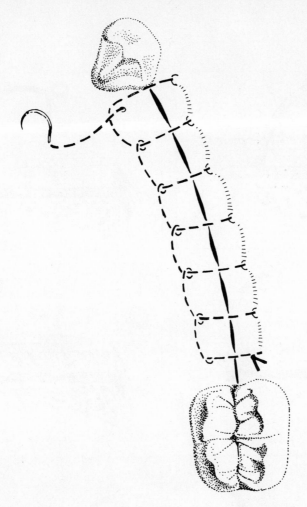

**Fig. 36-26.** Hem (eyelet) continuous suture used for edentulous areas and at times for tissue grafts.

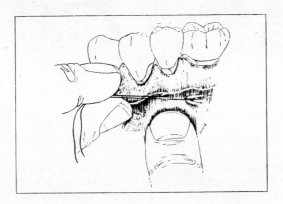

**Fig. 36-27.** Periosteal suturing at the mucogingival junction to displace flap apically and permit flap margin to parallel bone margin at crest. To test a periosteal suture to ensure that the tack has actually penetrated the periosteum and is actually holding the tissue in place, gently pull the two suture ends taut with one hand, and then move the tissue slightly in a coronal-apical direction. If the gingival margin is observed to move in the same direction, the suture must be removed and tied once more. This should be done before tying the knot to prevent wasted effort. One should leave a suture only if it will actually do the job intended; that is, it should hold the tissue in the exact place and manner that is preferred by the operator and should do so predictably. (From Chaikin, R.W.: Quintessence Int. **7:**75, 1976.)

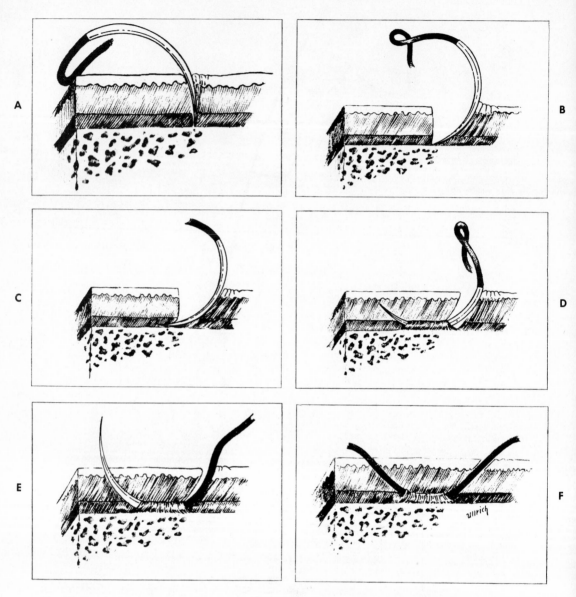

**Fig. 36-28. A,** *Penetration* is the first step when suturing to periosteum, as in this example of a mucoperiosteal tack. Note that the needle is perpendicular to the tissue, unlike the usual insertion, in which the angle may be 30 degrees. **B,** *Rotation* is a separate and distinct second movement of the needle, again quite different from the usual stroke. In this, the axis of rotation is at the point of the needle. It is the hub—the junction of the suture material and the metal needle—that moves most. Closely compare the needle position with that in **A. C,** *Glide* the needle along the surface of bone, taking care not to penetrate into a nutrient canal. **D,** As the needle glides along the bone, the hub is still rotating, so as to follow as in **C, E,** *Rotation* is again employed. However, here the axis of rotation is at the hub of the needle to exit as steeply as possible. A slow exit produces an incline of perhaps 30 degrees, which will tend to tear. **F,** The suture must be tied off very carefully with a square or surgeon's knot. (From Chaikin, R.W.: Quintessence Int. **7:**75, 1976.)

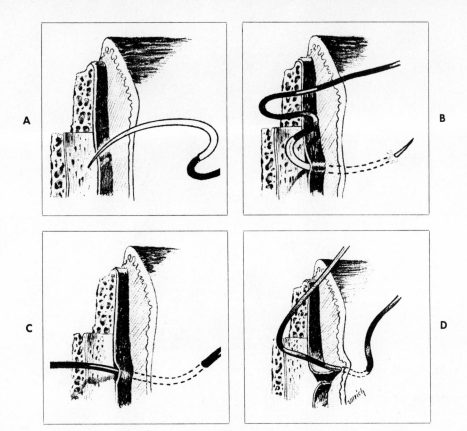

**Fig. 36-29.** *Another view of a periosteal suture. However, the penetration, rotation, glide, and exit have been applied between* **A** *and* **B.** *The suture material has been pulled slightly after* **C,** *so that now the periosteum has been torn by the suture materials, as seen in* **D.** *It is easily possible to place too much tension on the suture either by pulling on it directly with the needle or by doing so accidentally in the course of tying the knot. When pulling on the two ends of the suture material, it is important to realize that the pull is across the surface of the adjacent tissue and not at an angle to it. If, when pulling tight, the knot is raised up from the tissue surface, the underlying suture material can easily rip through the periosteum. (From Chaikin, R.W.: Quintessence Int.* **7:***75, 1976.)*

## Wound healing

There are a number of histologic reports on the healing of flaps.[14,23,24,29-33] Close reapposition of the flap is necessary. New bone, ligament, and cementum may be found in the apical part of the wound and are derived from subjacent periodontal ligament cells that migrate coronally. The new junctional epithelium is formed from oral epithelium that migrates along the inner aspect of the flap to the base of the flap and then coronally to establish a long epithelial attachment between the tooth and the flap. With good maintenance, it is possible that the long junctional epithelium may be replaced by a connective tissue junction beginning near the apical part of the junctional epithelium.

New junctional epithelium may form on either cementum or dentin[31] by the elaboration of an extracellular material composed of a protein and mucopolysaccharide complex and of hemidesmosomes.[34-37] Junctional attachment epithelium is reestablished in 1 week. By the end of the second week, a collagenous reunion with the root has formed.[38]

Resorptions may occur on both cementum and dentin. They are more prominent

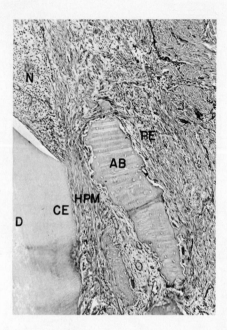

**Fig. 36-30.** Vertical section of a surgically created pocket. The healing periodontal ligament, *HPM*, consists of fibers aligned parallel to the long axis of the root between bone, *AB*, and cementum, *CE*. (Courtesy M.L. Morris, New York, New York.)

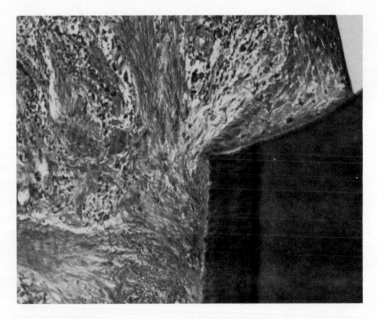

**Fig. 36-31.** Dentogingival fibers are found in functional alignment in a 120-day experimental section from a human. A full flap had been reflected. The height of the alveolar crest at the time of flap reflection is marked by a groove in the tooth. Dentogingival and dentoperiosteal fibers have been formed and are seen exiting from cementum below the crest. The parallel alignment of fibers seen in 30- and 60-day specimens has been succeeded by the functionally aligned fibers characteristic of this area. (Courtesy R.J. Rizzo, Ogden, Utah.)

in deep root concavities. However, at approximately 40 days new cementum appears in concavities and nicks.[39]

In the initial phase of collagen formation, an interlacing network of collagen fibers forms parallel to the root surface[14] ( Fig. 36-30). This arrangement may occur over dentin or old cementum before deposition of new cementum. New cementum is then deposited, Sharpey's fibers are incorporated, and the classical dentogingival fiber orientation is established ( Fig. 36-31).

In summary, the reunion of a periodontal flap and root may be successfully accomplished if firm apposition of tissues is realized. A long junctional epithelium is formed by 2-3 weeks and a collagenous attachment develops in the apical part of the wound. This area is best left unprobed for at least a month.

## REFERENCES

1. Johnson, W.N., Groat, J.E., and Romans, A.R.: The periodontal flap: literature review, Periodont. Abstr. **15:**11, 1967.
2. Nabers, C.L.: Repositioning the attached gingiva, J. Periodontol. **25:**38, 1954.
3. Dahlberg, W.H.: Incisions and suturing: some basic considerations about each in periodontal flap surgery, Dent. Clin. North Am. **13:**149, 1969.
4. Kieser, J.B.: An approach to periodontal pocket elimination, Br. J. Oral Surg. **12:**177, 1974.
5. Schluger, S.: The surgical approach to pocket elimination, N.Y. Dent. J. **22:**396, 1952.
6. Goldman, H.: Development of physiological gingival contours by gingivoplasty, Oral Surg. **3:**879, 1950.
7. Robinson, R.E.: The distal wedge operation, Periodontics **4:**256, 1966.
8. Neumann, R.: Atlas der radical-chirurgischen Behandlung der Paradentosen, Berlin, 1926, Hermann Meusser.
9. Everett, F.G., Waerhaug, J., and Widman, A.: Leonard Widman, surgical treatment of pyorrhea alveolaris, J. Periodontol. **42:**571, 1971.
10. Ariaudo, A.A., and Tyrrell, H.A.: Repositioning and increasing the zone of attached gingiva, J. Periodontol. **28:**106, 1957.
11. Kirkland, O.: Modified flap operation in surgical treatment of periodontoclasia, J. Am. Dent. Assoc. **19:**1918, 1932.
12. Kopczyk, R.A., and Young, L.L.: Principles of periodontal surgery. In Clark, J.W., editor: Clinical dentistry, ed. 3, New York, 1976, Harper & Row, Publishers.
13. Tibbetts, L.S., Jr.: The initial incision in pocket surgery. In Clark, J.W., editor: Clinical dentistry, ed. 3, New York, 1976, Harper & Row, Publishers.
14. Staffileno, H., Wentz, F.M., and Orban, B.: Histologic study of healing of split thickness flap surgery in dogs, J. Periodontol. **33:**56, 1962.
15. Hoag, P.M., et al.: Alveolar crest reduction following full and partial thickness flaps, J. Periodontol. **43:**141, 1972.
16. Prichard, J.F.: Advanced periodontal disease, ed. 2, Philadelphia, 1972, W.B. Saunders Co.
17. Easley, J.: Methods of determining alveolar osseous form, J. Periodontol. **38:**112, 1967.
18. Kramer, G.M., Nevins, M., and Kohn, J.D.: The utilization of periosteal suturing in periodontal surgical procedures, J. Periodontol. **41:**457, 1970.
19. Ochsenbein, C., and Bohannan, H.: The palatal approach to osseous surgery. I. Rationale, J. Periodontol. **34:**60, 1963.
20. Kramer, G.M., and Schwarz, M.S.: A technique to obtain primary intention healing in pocket elimination adjacent to an edentulous area, Periodontics **2:**252, 1964.
21. Saadoun, A.P.: Surgical management of the maxillary tuberosity area, Cont. Educ. **5:**34, 1984.
22. Wilderman, M.N., Wentz, F.M., and Orban, B.: Histogenesis of repair after mucogingival surgery, J. Periodontol. **31:**283, 1960.
23. Grant, D.A.: Experimental periodontal surgery: sequestration of alveolar bone, J. Periodontol. **38:**409, 1967.
24. Pfeiffer, J.S.: The reaction of alveolar bone to flap procedure in man, Periodontics **3:**135, 1965.
25. Carranza, F.A., Jr., and Carrara, J.J.: Effect of removal of periosteum on postoperative result of mucogingival surgery, J. Periodontol. **34:**223, 1963.
26. Kay, H.B.: Esthetic considerations in the definitive prosthetic management of the maxillary anterior segment, Int. J. Periodont. Rest. Dent. **3:**45, 1983.
27. Morris, M.L.: Suturing techniques in periodontal surgery, Periodontics **3:**84, 1965.
28. Malamed, E.H.: A technique of suturing flaps in periodontal surgery, Periodontics **1:**207, 1963.
29. Javelet, J., Torabinejad, M., and Danforth, R.: Isobutyl cyanoacrylate: a clinical and histologic comparison with sutures in closing mucosal incisions in monkeys, Oral Surg. **59:**91, 1985.
30. Rizzo, R.J.: Postsurgical dimensions of the

dentogingival junction, Master's thesis, Chicago, 1978, Loyola University.

31. Morris, M.L.: Healing of human periodontal tissues following surgical detachment from vital teeth: the position of the epithelial attachment, J. Periodontol. **32:**108, 1961.

32. Morris, M.L., and Thompson, R.H.: Healing of human periodontal tissues following surgical detachment: factors related to the deposition of new cementum on dentin, Periodontics **1:**189, 1963.

33. Morris, M.L.: The reattachment of human periodontal tissues following surgical detachment: a clinical and histological study, J. Periodontol. **24:**220, 1953.

34. Toto, P.D., and Sicher, H.: The epithelial attachment, Periodontics **2:**154, 1964.

35. Stallard, R.E., Diab, M.A., and Zander, H.A.: The attaching substance between enamel and epithelium—a product of the epithelial cells, J. Periodontol. **36:**130, 1965.

36. Stern, I.B.: Electron microscopic observations of oral epithelium, Periodontics **3:**224, 1965.

37. Listgarten, M.A.: Electron microscopic study of the junction between surgically denuded root surfaces and regenerated periodontal tissues, J. Periodont. Res. **7:**68, 1972.

38. Hiatt, W.H., et al.: Repair following mucoperiosteal flap surgery with full gingival retention, J. Periodontol. **39:**11, 1968.

39. Morris, M.L.: Healing of human periodontal tissues following surgical detachment: the arrangement of the fibers of the periodontal space, Periodontics **1:**118, 1963.

## ADDITIONAL SUGGESTED READING

Barkmeier, W.W., and Williams, H.J.: Surgical methods of gingival retraction for restorative dentistry, J. Am. Dent. Assoc. **96:**1002, 1978.

Cattermole, A.E., and Wade, A.B.: A comparison of the scalloped and linear incisions as viewed in the reverse bevel technique, J. Clin. Periodontol. **5:**41, 1978.

Garrett, S.: The effect of notching into dentin on new cementum formation during periodontal wound healing, J. Periodont. Res. **16:**350, 1981.

Holmes, C.H., and Strem, B.E.: Location of flap margin after suturing, J. Periodontol. **47:**674.

Hugoson, A., and Schmidt, G.: Influence of plaque control on the healing of experimentally induced bone defects in dogs, J. Periodontol. **49:**135, 1978.

Johnson, R.H.: Basic flap management, Dent. Clin. North Am. **20:**3, 1976.

Kohler, C.A., and Ramfjord, S.P.: Healing of gingival mucoperiosteal flaps, Oral Surg. **13:**89, 1960.

Kon, S., et al.: Gingival flap–split thickness flap: a combined procedure, J. Periodontol. **50:**427, 1979.

Lilly, G.E.: Reaction of oral tissues to suture materials, Oral Surg. **26:**128, 1968.

Listgarten, M.A.: Normal development, structure, physiology, and repair of gingival epithelium, Oral Sci. Rev. **1:**3, 1972.

Listgarten, M.A., et al.: Progressive replacement of epithelial attachment by a connective tissue junction after experimental periodontal surgery in rats, J. Periodontol. **53:**659, 1982.

Litch, J.M., O'Leary, T.J., and Kafrawy, A.H.: Pocket epithelium removal via crestal and subcrestal scalloped internal bevel incisions, J. Periodontol. **55:**152, 1984.

McDonald, F.L., Saari, J.T., and Davis, S.S.: A comparison of tooth accumulated materials from quadrants treated surgically and non-surgically, J. Periodontol. **48:**147, 1977.

Mormann, W., and Ciancio, S.G.: Blood supply of human gingiva following surgery, J. Periodontol. **48:**681, 1977.

Morris, M.L.: The unrepositioned muco-periosteal flap, Periodontics **3:**147, 1965.

Newman, P.S.: The effect of the inverse bevel flap procedure on gingival contour and plaque accumulation, J. Clin. Periodontol. **11:**361, 1984.

Palomo, F., and Kopczyk, R.A.: Rationale and methods of crown lengthening, J. Am. Dent. Assoc. **96:**257, 1978.

Pollack, R.P.: Modified distal wedge procedure, J. Periodontol. **51:**513, 1980.

Ramfjord, S.P.: Results following three modalities of periodontal surgery, J. Periodontol. **46:**522, 1975.

Robertson, P.D., Levy, S., and Garguilo, A.W.: Healing of reentry wounds with periosteal preservation, J. Periodontol. **42:**225, 1971.

Schallhorn, R.G.: Mucosal grafts (flaps) in pocket surgery, Clin. Dent. **3:**1, 1976.

Staffileno, H.: Significant differences and advantages between the full thickness and split thickness flaps, J. Periodontol. **45:**421, 1974.

Zamet, J.S.: A comparative clinical study of three periodontal surgical techniques, J. Clin. Periodontol. **2:**89, 1975.

# CHAPTER 37

## Open subgingival curettage: surgical curettage by flap, modified Widman flap procedure, new attachment-reattachment operations, and guided tissue regeneration

---

## Procedures

Surgical (open) subgingival curettage is a component of all flap surgery involving alveolar bone. The procedures have been employed for years.[1-7] They involve instrumentation of the root and bone, as does closed subgingival curettage. However, in open subgingival curettage a flap is used to obtain visibility and better access. Modifications by individual clinicians and teachers make it necessary to describe several techniques.

The individual variations in technique result from differences in the objectives of the surgery. The basic procedure is intended to expose difficult-to-reach root surfaces for planing and to expose bone and thereby encourage remodeling of the alveolar surface and the formation of new attachment. For purposes of convenience, other procedures that do not intentionally expose bone are included. These procedures are within the scope of open subgingival curettage and include those that retain connective tissue attachment over bone and do not expose bone, as well as those that raise a flap by split-thickness incisions and then excise some of the remaining gingiva over the bone (internal bevel gingivectomy).

The open subgingival curettage procedures include the following:

1. Those that intentionally expose the bone surface
   a. New attachment-reattachment by way of flap[8]
   b. Modified Widman flap[9,10]

**Objectives**

823

  c. Interdental denudation[11]
  d. Interdental resection[12]
  e. Surgical subgingival curettage by way of flap[2,3,6]
 2. Those that do not intentionally expose the bone surface
  a. Excisional new attachment[13-15]
  b. Internal bevel gingivectomy[16]

## New attachment-reattachment

The restoration of previously destroyed periodontal structures is the best possible treatment result for both patient and dentist. The operations to create such tissue regeneration were generally called *reattachment operations*.[1]

**New attachment**

In 1966, the World Workshop in Periodontics adopted new terminology for *reattachment* and *new attachment*.[17] *Reattachment* was defined as "the reunion of connective tissue and root separated by incision or injury." *New attachment* was defined as "the reunion of connective tissue with a root surface that had been pathologically exposed." With new attachment, a new connective tissue fiber attachment to cementoid must be achieved. New attachment to pathologically exposed roots seems to be limited to the apical portion of the defect. At the coronal aspect either a long junctional epithelium results or root resorption (ankylosis) is induced. It is possible that the long junctional epithelium may be gradually displaced by connective tissue, beginning at the apical end.

New attachment operations are performed to obtain new attachment coronal to the preoperative level. New bone and new cementum are deposited, and new periodontal ligament fibers are formed and become organized. The junctional epithelium reforms coronal to its presurgical level. The bottom of the sulcus (pocket) is shifted coronally, and pocket depth is reduced or eliminated[18-24] (Fig. 37-1).

The term *new attachment operation* is applied to two distinct surgical procedures: extension of closed subgingival curettage beyond the sulcular and junctional epithelium to bone and surgical curettage by flap of three-walled (and sometimes two-walled) infrabony craters. This section will discuss surgical curettage by flap, which has become identified as the classical procedure to induce new bone growth and attachment.

### INDICATIONS

The most favorable situation for new attachment is found in the three-walled infrabony (intra-alveolar) pocket.[8,17,18,19-24] Although new attachment may occur in any infrabony or suprabony pocket, the pocket with three bony walls yields the greatest percentage of success (Fig. 37-2).

When infrabony defects are found interdentally, one tooth has a deeper bone loss than its neighboring tooth (Fig. 37-3).

Reattachment operation by flap requires removal of all pocket epithelium, removal of chronic inflammatory tissue bordering pockets to the bone, and removal of all connective tissue over the bone defect. This may be followed by proliferation of periodontal ligament cells that can regenerate bone, ligament, and cementum. Some bone resorption and apposition can occur, and, with cementum, apposition leading to the formation of new attachment.[19-22] With the resorption of thin bony margins and spicules and some bone regeneration, irregularities tend to be corrected, and a more regular crestal alveolar form may result (Fig. 37-4). Prichard[25] recommends that the flap be cut, to leave the bone margins exposed, and then covered by foil.[26]

**Long attachment**

Depending on the extent of connective tissue regeneration and gingival shrinkage, the new junctional epithelium may be short or long.

Successful open subgingival curettage does not depend on new attachment and

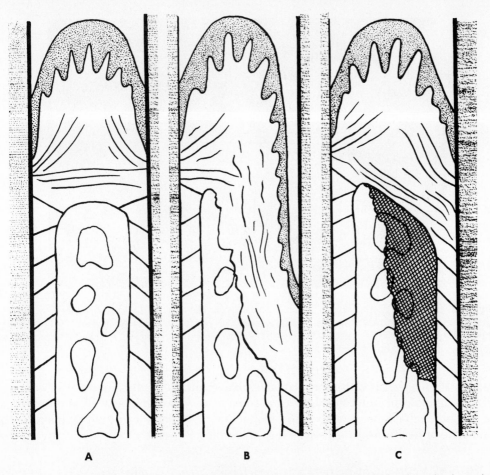

**Fig. 37-1.** Diagrammatic illustration of, **A,** healthy interdental area, **B,** development of an intra-alveolar pocket, and, **C,** postoperative result after successful new attachment operation. New periodontal ligament, new alveolar bone, and new cementum have developed where the defect once existed. The probable source of these cells are undifferentiated mesenchymal cells of the periodontal ligament.

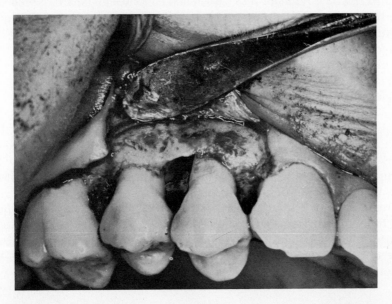

**Fig. 37-2.** Three-walled infrabony (intra-alveolar) crater between the premolars seen after the reflection of a modified full-thickness flap.

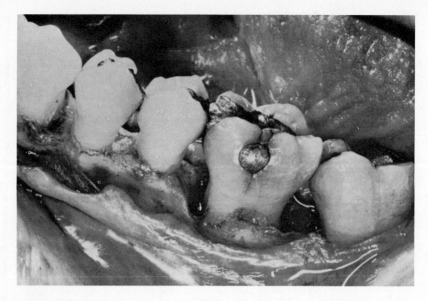

**Fig. 37-3.** Interdental osseous craters on a mandibular molar. The crater on the mesial has three walls at its greatest depth. Near the crest the buccal (vestibular) bony wall is lost, and the defect becomes two walled. On the distal a two-walled crater is found. The interdental septum has been destroyed, leaving buccal and lingual bony walls to form a deep infrabony defect.

**Creeping attachment**

regeneration alone. It can induce considerable shrinkage of the gingiva that, coupled with scrupulous plaque control, induces some bony remodeling as well as the coronal migration of attachment, or creeping reattachment. Patients can then be maintained in a state of health for long periods (i.e., exceeding 20 years).[12]

## Open subgingival curettage and modified Widman flap procedure

### FLAP DESIGN

The term *modified Widman flap*[10] was adopted to designate a flap procedure used for access for open subgingival curettage rather than surgical pocket elimination, which was the intent of the original Widman procedure.[10]

The initial incision is made parallel to the long axis of the tooth at least ½ to 1 mm from the gingival margin and extended to the alveolar crest. The incision is scalloped about the teeth. A minimal amount of the interproximal papillae is removed, sufficient to eliminate epithelium, retaining enough for coaptation in suturing. Vertical releasing incisions 2 to 3 mm long may be made at each end of the initial incision but are usually not needed. Mucoperiosteal elevators are used to elevate a full-thickness flap 1 to 3 mm or the minimal depth needed to gain access to the tooth and bone. A second incision is made from the depth of the crevice to the crest of the bone. The third and last incision is made with sharpened Orban knives following the contour of the crest and the interproximal septum to excise the loosened collar of tissue. This collar is removed with curettes. The roots are then planed, and all soft tissues are removed from the surface of infrabony lesions. The flaps are then coapted and sutured with interrupted sutures. The flaps may have to be thinned and some bone may have to be removed from the outer aspects of the alveolar processes to ensure coaption of the flaps.[9,10]

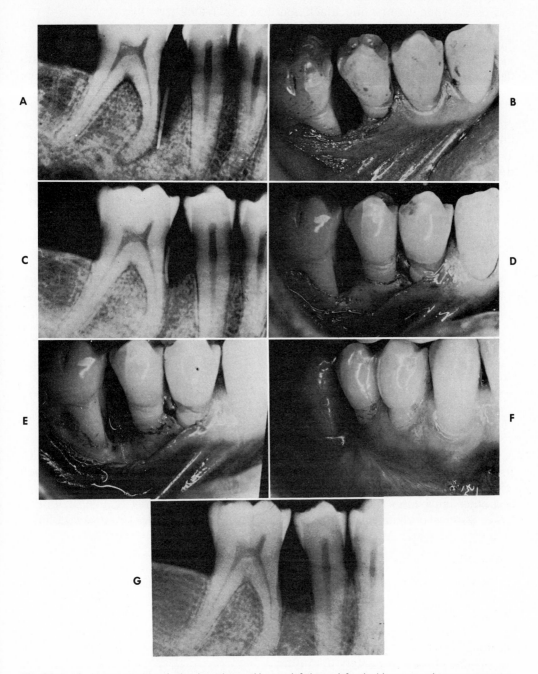

**Fig. 37-4.    A,** A gutta-percha point has been inserted into an infrabony defect in this preoperative roentgenogram. **B,** A modified flap has been reflected in a reattachment operation to reveal the three-walled osseous defect on the mesial surface of a mandibular first molar. **C,** Roentgenogram taken 6 months later shows that considerable regeneration of bone has taken place. **D,** A modified flap is reflected to reveal the residual osseous defect, a two-walled hemiseptum. **E,** Osseous surgery was performed to eliminate the defect. **F,** Clinical appearance of the area is good 2 years later. **G,** Roentgenogram confirms the elimination of the pocket. (Courtesy J. Prichard, Fort Worth, Texas.)

This procedure is recommended as an alternative to osseous surgery and sacrifices less tissue while maintaining attachment levels on a long-term basis.

Where the alveolar surface is to be exposed, full flaps are employed. Less extensive flaps are used for the modified Widman procedure, where only the crest and 1 to 2 mm apical to it are exposed. Straight-line incisions or minimally retracted flaps (mini-flaps) may be used to expose interdental bone for interdental denudation or resection.

The flap used in the excisional new attachment procedure extends only to the base of the pocket and does not involve the alveolar bone. The open surgical curettage procedures have in common an incision that extends tooth to tooth on buccal and lingual aspects, raising either a small or an extensive flap. Common to all procedures as well is the excision of some or all of the interdental tissue. The exposed root surface then is thoroughly planed along its complete submarginal extent to and including the alveolar crest. The exposed root surface is planed to a smooth, hard finish. Root conditioning has been recommended to promote new attachment.[27-30] However, clinical results are not encouraging.[31-34]

## OBJECTIVES

The primary purpose of the flap is to gain access for subgingival curettage to remove inflammatory tissue and remnants of connective tissue within the infrabony defect, as well as any remaining calcified deposits. The soft tissue contents of the bony crypt are enucleated by curettage, and the bony defect is exposed.

Following are the objectives of open subgingival curettage*:

1. Resolution of inflammation
2. Reduction of pocket depth, not only by inducing recession of the gingival wall but also by inducing regeneration and new attachment
3. A favorable remodeling of bone and gingiva, which makes possible the maintenance of health
4. Exposure of the alveolar bone for osseous resection and osseous grafting procedures
5. Exposure of the root surface for effective débridement and planing

Surgical curettage is generally used in the management of advanced periodontitis. Its intent is pocket reduction by means of shrinkage and new attachment. When extensive bone loss has occurred, scaling and gingival curettage may not be adequate, and other procedures (gingivectomy or osseous surgery) may not be indicated (Fig. 37-5). Surgical curettage may give results that are as good as or superior to other forms of surgery for pocket elimination.

## METHODS

**Reflection of full-thickness flap**

Make the initial incision with a scalpel and Bard-Parker blade along the oral and vestibular surfaces of the teeth and bisect the papillae (Fig. 37-5, *C* and *D*). Then elevate a full-thickness flap by blunt dissection using a periosteal elevator (Fig. 37-5, *D*). When the flap is elevated only as far as the mucogingival junction, it is termed a *miniflap*. Generally, however, the flap is elevated to expose bone sufficiently to permit the options of osseous surgery or grafting.

**Subgingival curettage**

The excellent access and visibility obtained will permit the removal of adherent inflammatory tissue from teeth and bone and the planing of the exposed root surfaces (Fig. 37-5, *E*). Remove inflammatory tissue from the inner surface of the reflected flaps. Then replace the flap and suture it by interdental sutures (Fig. 37-5, *F*). Fig. 37-5, *G*, shows the result 2 years later.

**Coaptation**

If flap coaptation is ideal, healing will be rapid. When the flap is poorly adapted,

---

*\*Subgingival curettage* is defined by some as root planing with either intentional or inadvertent gingival curettage. In this text, subgingival curettage denotes instrumentation with curettes to the alveolar crest.

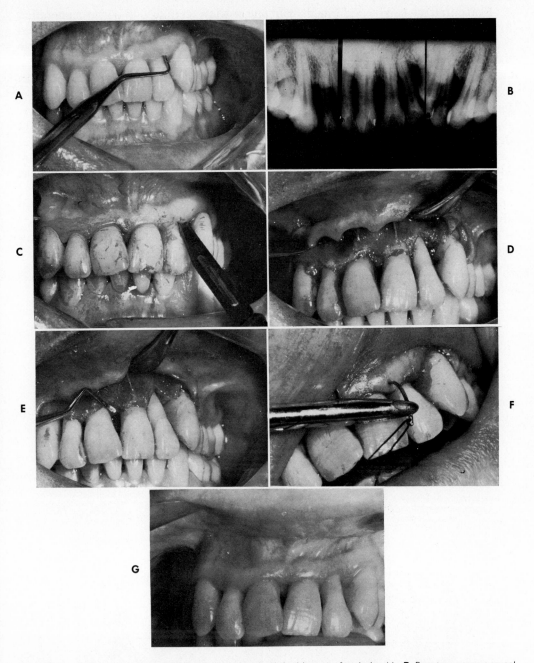

**Fig. 37-5.** **A,** A probe is inserted to illustrate pocket depth in this case of periodontitis. **B,** Roentgenograms reveal extensive alveolar resorption. **C,** A disposable surgical blade is used to incise the papillae and marginal gingiva. **D,** The flap is reflected by blunt dissection. **E,** A curette is used to remove deposits, the root surface is planed, and both tooth and bone are débrided. **F,** The flap is sutured in place. **G,** Result 2 years later. (Courtesy J. Ingle, Palm Springs, California.)

healing will be delayed and bone resorption may occur.[35] The modified Widman flap procedure requires exact coaptation of flaps by sutures that do not perforate the periosteal surface of the flap.[9] Other procedures employ standard suturing.

Flap curettage can be performed about one or a few teeth to gain bone regeneration in infrabony defects, or it can be performed in a sextant or a quadrant. Three-walled infrabony pockets have the greatest chance for fill. The procedure is most predictable in such instances (see Fig. 37-4).

Sometimes one-walled or two-walled infrabony defects are successfully treated. In a 37-year-old woman with advanced periodontal disease, vertical bone destruction was found around the mandibular right first premolar and first molar (Fig. 37-6, *A*). After repeated scaling and with good plaque control, inflammation was eliminated. Pocket depth remained (Fig. 37-6, *B*). A flap was reflected to reveal the osseous deformities (Fig. 37-6, *C*). Despite repeated presurgical scaling, some calcified deposits were found. Although the outer surface of the gingiva appeared healthy, granulomatous tissue was found in the pockets. A new attachment operation was done. A year later the gingiva appeared healthy (Fig. 37-6, *D*). Minor pocket depth remained. Reflection of a flap showed a remarkable regeneration of bone (Fig. 37-6, *E*).

In another patient with a two-walled infrabony defect, a flap operation with subgingival curettage resulted in fill and remodeling (Fig. 37-7).

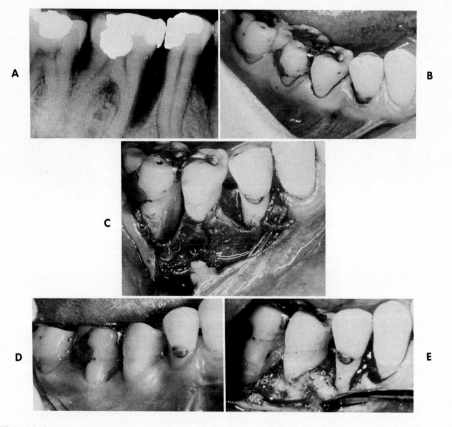

**Fig. 37-6.** **A,** Roentgenogram of the mandibular right molar and premolar area showing vertical bone destruction. **B,** After root planing and instruction in plaque control, clinical inflammation was reduced. Pocket depth remained. **C,** A modified flap was reflected for open subgingival curettage. One- and two-walled osseous defects were present. **D,** A year later a physiologic gingival form was present. **E,** A flap was reflected so that osteoplasty could be performed. A remarkable regeneration of bone had occurred.

## Comparative studies

Surgical (open) subgingival curettage has a long history; its current acceptance is an indication of its success in therapy.[1-7,9,36] Comparative studies indicate that open subgingival curettage may be as effective in pocket elimination as is the apically repositioned flap coupled with osseous contouring. However, it does not achieve equally improved tissue contours.[37,38] Subgingival curettage* produces a gain in interproximal attachment levels for up to 3 years postoperatively but is not equally effective in pocket reduction when compared with the modified Widman flap and/or pocket elimination surgery.[39] The latter eliminates pockets effectively at the expense of attachment but with improved tissue contours. The Widman flap is intermediate between the two, reducing interproximal probing depth but not gaining as much reattachment as subgingival curettage.[39,40] (For comparative studies of nonsurgical and surgical treatment, see Chapter 48.)

### EXCISIONAL NEW ATTACHMENT PROCEDURE

The excisional new attachment procedure essentially consists of a miniflap elevated with a split-thickness incision. The sulcular epithelium is excised, and the root scaled and planed. The bone is not exposed. The flap is then sutured to position. It has been reported to provide pocket reduction as well as reattachment for suprabony pockets.[13-15] An overall net gain of 1.5 mm was found 5 years after treatment.[41]

### FIBER RETENTION

Stahl and Froum[29] and Ramfjord[9,10] favor the retention of supracrestal collagen fibers for new attachment. Consequently, the question is raised as to whether thorough planing of the root below the junctional epithelium is desirable. Stahl and Froum[29] suggest that the junctional epithelium is limited by the level of the retained supracrestal

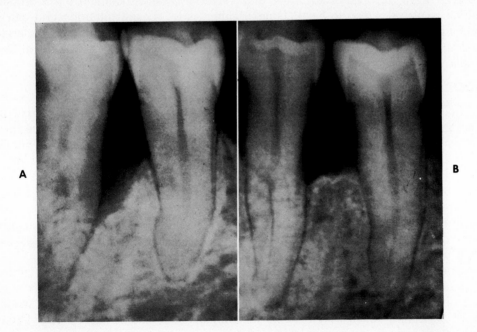

**Fig. 37-7.    A,** Roentgenogram of a mandibular premolar with a distal pocket. A flap and open subgingival curettage were performed. **B,** Roentgenogram of the patient 1 year after surgery. (Courtesy T. Messinger, Colorado Springs, Colorado.)

fiber remnants. The fiber retention procedure requires further examination and evaluation.

## INTERNAL (INVERSE BEVEL) GINGIVECTOMY

**Definitions and indications**

The internal gingivectomy is the removal of gingiva by way of flap. This procedure is useful in cases of phenytoin hyperplasia, in the presence of orthodontic bands, and where bleeding problems are exaggerated by open wounds after surgery.

**Method**

A scalloped, _inversely_ beveled incision is made coronal to the depth of the pocket, extending through the gingiva until the blade contacts tooth or bone. A thin flap (approximately 1 to 2 mm in thickness) is thus elevated. A second incision is then made adjacent to the root until the apical end of the first incision is reached. A wedge of tissue may then be excised and any tissue tags eliminated by scalpel, curette, scissors, or soft-tissue rongeurs. The exposed tooth surface may then be planed. The procedure is repeated on the opposing buccal or lingual surface, the interproximal areas carefully debrided, and the flaps coapted and fixed by interrupted sutures.

**Advantages**

The advantage of this procedure is in minimizing the exposed postsurgical wound surface. In cases of phenytoin hyperplasia, hygiene may be continued without interruption, and the irritation caused by surgery and dressings and the retention of plaque may be avoided. Postsurgical tissue hyperplasia, which is a major problem in patients receiving phenytoin, may thereby be avoided.

Similar advantages are present when tissue must be excised during orthodontic treatment. Where patients have bleeding problems, the smaller exposed wound surface is an obvious advantage.

## INTERDENTAL DENUDATION

Interdental denudation is the excision of all interproximal soft tissue in the reflection of a flap to bare the interproximal bone. The root surfaces are planed, and the flap is sutured below the crest or left apical to the alveolar crest without sutures. A dressing or foil is placed over the bared bone. Healing is by second intention and can be prolonged. Remodeling of the bared bone occurs with resorption at the coronal margins and apposition at the base of osseous craters, when the procedure is successful (Fig. 37-8).

## ROOT CONDITIONING

Root conditioning refers to chemical treatment of roots exposed by periodontal disease to encourage connective tissue healing to those surfaces.[27-30,42,43] Substances used include citric acid, phosphoric acid, formalin, citric acid–sodium hypochlorite (antiformin), phenol and various phenol preparations, sodium deoxycholate and Cohn IV human plasma fraction, citric acid and fibronectin, and fibronectin alone. Also EDTA alone and combined with citric acid followed by saline irrigation have been proposed.[43-45]

Of all the substances suggested, citric acid and citric acid–fibronectin combinations seem most promising. However, all substances have been used primarily in experimental studies,[28] and definitive conclusions cannot be made at this time regarding their use in humans.

The use of acids exposes dentinal collagen[29,30,46] (with prior removal of cementum). Presumably this promotes new connective attachment to the exposed collagen. Conditioning may induce more cementum regrowth than do control procedures without root conditioning. Citric acid is the most commonly used conditioner.[44-63] The effective range for its use is given in Table 37-1.

After reflection of a flap and instrumentation of the root surface, a saturated solution of citric acid is applied to the root surface for 5 minutes. The root surface is washed with saline solution. The flaps are then repositioned and sutured. In one study, new

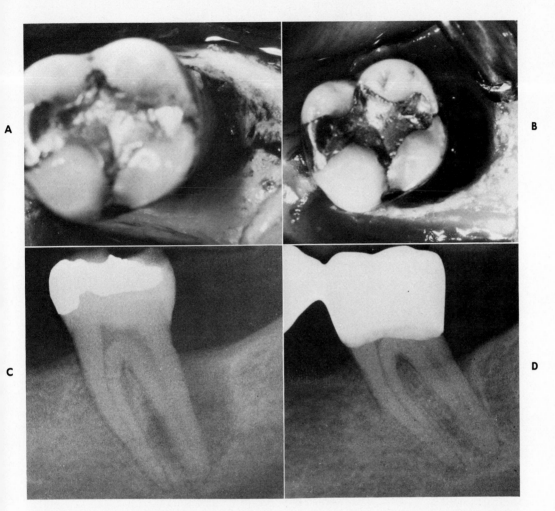

**Fig. 37-8.** **A,** Wide three-walled intrabony defect distal to the lower right second molar. The defect extended to but did not penetrate into the furcation. The defect was treated by open débridement, thorough root planing, and postsurgical bone denudation. **B,** Reentry at 11 months. The defect filled with bone. Shallow residual defect is still present. **C,** Preoperative radiograph of the lower right second molar. **D,** 5-year postoperative radiograph. Complete repair of defect. Tooth serves as a retainer for a fixed bridge. (Courtesy W. Becker, Tucson, Arizona.)

**Table 37-1**   Optimal times for various pHs that are followed by attachment with cementogenesis

| pH | Time of application (minutes) |
|---|---|
| 0.5 | 1.0 to 1.5 |
| 1.0 | 1.5 to 2.0 |
| 1.5 | 2 to 3 |
| 2.0 | 3 to 5 |
| 2.5 | 5 |

From Register, A.A., and Burdick, F.A.: Accelerated reattachment with cementogenesis, demineralized in situ. I. Optimum range, J. Periodontol. **46:**646, 1975.

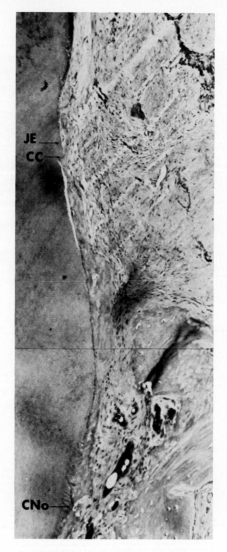

**Fig. 37-9.** New connective tissue attachment subsequent to regenerative procedure employing citric acid. New attachment extends from the apical extent of the notch to the junctional epithelium *(JE)*. The notch was placed within the previous confines of calculus. New cementum formation *(CC)* extends beyond the coronal limit of the notch *(CNo)*, approximating the junctional epithelium. (From Cole, R.T., et al.: J. Periodontol. Res. **15:**1, 1980.)

cementum and new connective tissue attachment coronal to the presurgical position appeared 4 months later (Fig. 37-9). The junctional epithelium ended 1.2 to 2.6 mm coronal to the notch placed at surgery.

## GUIDED TISSUE REGENERATION

If periodontal tissues could be regenerated[64-67] predictably and to a clinically significant level, such regeneration would be preferable to pocket elimination by excisional surgery or to attempts to maintain teeth with deep pockets. Such regeneration has been described using inert membranes (Millipore filter or Gore-Tex membrane) inserted between the primary flap and the osseous defect for 2-8 weeks.[68,69] This procedure isolates the root surface, preventing ingrowth of gingival tissues (particularly epithelium), while permitting the coronal proliferation and migration of periodontal ligament cells.[70-72] In this manner the regeneration of a new attachment is promoted.

The inert membranes act by contact inhibition,[73] to discourage apical migration of epithelium along the root surfaces while permitting ligament cells access to the root.

## Summary

The conclusion to be drawn is that scaling and root planing, gingival curettage, and subgingival curettage by either closed or open access are effective procedures. The debate concerning whether regeneration and reattachment are possible has diminished.[23,60] Current debate concerns the relative effectiveness and predictability of each of these procedures and of the bone resection and bone grafting procedures.[58] Such debate cannot be resolved until the parameters of a successful result are fully defined and generally accepted. Until that time, parochial criteria will be employed, and success will be gauged by what each group sees, perceives, and seeks. In terms of these criteria, what each practitioner can achieve will determine which measures are used.

## REFERENCES

1. Kirkland, O.: The suppurative periodontal pus pocket: its treatment by the modified flap operation, J. Am. Dent. Assoc. **18:**1462, 1931.
2. Kirkland, O.: The surgical flap and semiflap technique in periodontal surgery, Dent. Dig. **42:**125, 1936.
3. Ingle, J.L.: Periodontal curettement in the premaxilla, J. Periodontal. **23:**143, 1952.
4. Gilson, C.M.: Surgical treatment of periodontal disease, J. Am. Dent. Assoc. **44:**733, 1952.
5. Patur, B., and Glickman, I.: Clinical and roentgenographic evaluation of the post-treatment healing of infrabony pockets, J. Periodontol. **33:**164, 1962.
6. Wade, A.B.: An assessment of the flap operation, Dent. Pract. **13:**11, 1962.
7. Goldman, H.M., and Cohen, D.W.: The infrabony pocket, classification and treatment, J. Periodontol. **29:**272, 1958.
8. Prichard, J.: The infrabony technique as a predictable procedure, J. Periodontol. **28:**202, 1957.
9. Ramfjord, S.P., and Nissle, R.R.: The modified Widman flap, J. Periodontol. **45:**601, 1974.
10. Ramfjord, S.P.: Present status of the modified Widman procedure, J. Periodontol. **48:**558, 1977.
11. Prichard, J.: Present state of the interdental denudation procedure, J. Periodontol. **48:**566, 1977.
12. Beube, F.E.: Interdental tissue resection: an experimental study of a surgical technique which aids in repair of the periodontal tissues to their original contour and function, Oral Surg. **33:**497, 1947.
13. Yukna, R.A., et al.: A clinical study of healing in humans following the excisional new attachment procedure, J. Periodontol. **47:**696, 1976.
14. Yukna, R.A.: A clinical and histologic study of healing following the excisional new attachment procedure in Rhesus monkeys, J. Periodontol. **47:**701, 1976.
15. Yukna, R.A.: Longitudinal evaluation of the excisional new attachment procedure in humans, J. Periodontol. **49:**142, 1978.
16. Schluger, S., Youdelis, R.A., and Page, R.C.: Periodontal disease, Philadelphia, 1977, Lea & Febiger.
17. Ramfjord, S.P., Kerr, D.A., and Ash, M.M.: World Workshop in Periodontics, Ann Arbor, 1966, University of Michigan Press, p. 321.
18. Box, H.K.: Treatment of the periodontal pocket, Toronto, 1928, University of Toronto Press.
19. Prichard, J.: The diagnosis and management of vertical bony defects, J. Periodontol. **54:**29, 1983.
20. Polson, A.M., and Heijl, L.C.: Osseous repair in infrabony periodontal defects, J. Clin. Periodontol. **5:**13, 1985.
21. Bowers, G.M., Schallhorn, R.G., and Mellonig, J.T.: Histologic evaluation of new attachment in human infrabony defects: a literature review, J. Periodontol. **53:**509, 1982.
22. Nyman, S., et al.: New attachment following surgical treatment of human periodontal disease, J. Clin. Periodontol. **9:**290, 1982.
23. Frank, R., et al.: Gingival reattachment after surgery in man: an electron microscopic study, J. Periodontol. **43:**597, 1972.
24. Cole, R.T., et al.: Connective tissue regeneration to periodontally diseased teeth: a histological study, J. Periodont. Res. **15:**1, 1980.
25. Prichard, J.: Reattachment, presented at the Orban Seminar, Glenwood Springs, Colo., 1960.
26. Prichard, J.: Personal communication, 1979.
27. Register, A.A., and Burdick, F.A.: Accelerated reattachment with cementogenesis to dentin, demineralized in situ. I. Optimum range, J. Periodontol. **46:**646, 1975.
28. Register, A.A., and Burdick, F.A.: Accelerated

reattachment with cementogenesis to dentin, demineralized in situ. II. Defect repair, J. Periodontol. **47**:497, 1976.

29. Stahl, S.S., and Froum, S.J.: Human clinical and histologic repair responses following the use of citric acid in periodontal therapy, J. Periodontol. **48**:261, 1977.

30. Garrett, J.S., Crigger, M., and Egelberg, J.: Effects of citric acid on diseased root surfaces, J. Periodont. Res. **13**:155, 1978.

31. Cole R., et al.: Pilot clinical studies on the effect of topical citric acid application on healing after replaced periodontal flap surgery, J. Periodont. Res. **16**:117, 1981.

32. Nightingale, S.H., and Sheridan, P.J.: Root surface demineralization in periodontal therapy: subject review, J. Periodontol. **53**:611, 1982.

33. Parodi, R.J., and Esper, M.E.: Effect of topical application of citric acid in the treatment of furcation involvement in human lower molars, J. Clin. Periodontol. **11**:644, 1984.

34. Smith, B.A., et al.: The effectiveness of citric acid as an adjunct to surgical reattachment procedures in humans, J. Clin. Periodontol. **13**:701, 1986.

35. Caffesse, R.G., Ramfjord, S.P., and Nasjleti, C.E.: Reverse bevel periodontal flaps in monkeys, J. Periodontol. **39**:219, 1968.

36. Kalkwarf, K.L.: Periodontal new attachment without the placement of osseous potentiating grafts, Periodont. Abstr. **22**:53, 1974.

37. Zamet, J.S.: A comparative clinical study of three periodontal surgical techniques, J. Clin. Periodontol. **2**:87, 1975.

38. Burgett, F.C., et al.: Short term results of three modalities of periodontal treatment, J. Periodontol. **48**:131, 1977.

39. Ramfjord, S.P., et al.: Results following three modalities of periodontal therapy, J. Periodontol. **46**:522, 1975.

40. Caton, J., and Nyman, S.: Histometric evaluation of periodontal surgery. I. The modified Widman flap procedure, J. Clin. Periodontol. **7**:212, 1980.

41. Yukna, R.A., and Williams, J.E., Jr.: Five year evaluation of the excisional new attachment procedure, J. Periodontol. **51**:382, 1980.

42. Baiorunos, J.R., and Robbins, F.E.: Root demineralization as a new attachment procedure, Periodont. Abstr. **28**:84, 1980.

43. Register, A.A.: Bone and cementum induction by dentin, demineralized in situ, J. Periodontol. **44**:49, 1973.

44. Vievra, E.M., O'Leary, T.J., and Kafrawy, A.H.: The effect of sodium hypochlorite and citric acid solutions on healing of periodontal pockets, J. Periodontol. **53**:71, 1982.

45. Lasho, D.J., O'Leary, T.J., and Kafrawy, A.H.: A scanning electron microscope study of the effects of various agents on instrumented periodontally involved root surfaces, J. Periodontol. **54**:210, 1983.

46. Albair, W.B., Cobb, C.M., and Killoy, W.J.: Connective tissue attachment to periodontally diseased roots after citric acid demineralization, J. Periodontol. **53**:515, 1982.

47. Ririe, C.M., Crigger, M., and Selvig, K.A.: Healing of periodontal connective tissues following wounding and application of citric acid in dogs, J. Periodont. Res. **15**:314, 1980.

48. Daryabegi, P., Pameijer, C.H., and Ruben, M.P.: Topography of root surfaces treated in vitro with citric acid, elastase and hyaluronidase, J. Periodontol. **52**:736, 1981.

49. Wirthlin, M.R., Hancock, E.B., and Gaugler, R.W.: Regeneration and repair after biologic treatment of root surfaces in monkeys, J. Periodontol. **52**:729, 1981.

50. Wirthlin, M.R., and Hancock, E.B.: Regeneration and repair after biologic treatment of root surfaces in monkeys. II. Proximal surfaces of posterior teeth, J. Periodontol. **53**:302, 1981.

51. Renvert, S., and Egelberg, J.: Healing after treatment of periodontal intraosseous defects. II. Effect of citric acid conditioning of the root surface, J. Clin. Periodontol. **8**:459, 1981.

52. Nilvéus, R., et al.: The effect of topical citric acid application on the healing of experimental furcation defects in dogs. II. Healing after repeated surgery, J. Periodont. Res. **15**:544, 1980.

53. Nilvéus, R., and Egelberg, J.: The effect of topical citric acid application on the healing of experimental furcation defects in dogs. III. The relative importance of coagulum support, flap design and systemic antibiotics, J. Periodont. Res. **15**:551, 1980.

54. Nyman, S., Lindhe, J., and Karring, T.: Healing following surgical treatment and root demineralization in monkeys with periodontal disease, J. Clin. Periodontol. **8**:249, 1981.

55. Aukhil, I., Simpson, D.M., and Schaberg, T.V.: An experimental study of new attachment procedure in beagle dogs, J. Periodont. Res. **18**:643, 1983.

56. Selvig, K.A., et al.: Fine structure of new connective tissue attachment following acid treatment of experimental furcation pockets in dogs, J. Periodont. Res. **16**:123, 1981.

57. Proye, M., and Polson, A.M.: Effect of root surface alterations on periodontal healing. I. Surgical denudation, J. Clin. Periodontol. **9**:428, 1982.

58. Heritier, M.: Ultrastructural study of new connective tissue attachment following phosphoric acid application on human root dentin, J. Periodontol. **54**:515, 1983.

59. Cogen, R.B., Garrison, D.C., and Weatherford, T.W.: Effect of various root surface treatments on the viability and attachment of human gingival fibroblasts, J. Periodontol. **54**:277, 1983.

60. Caffesse, R.G., et al.: The effect of citric acid and fibronectin application on healing following surgical treatment of naturally occurring

periodontal disease in beagle dogs, J. Clin. Periodontol. **12:**578, 1985.

61. Woodyard, S.G., et al.: A histometric evaluation of the effect of citric acid preparation upon healing of coronally positioned flaps in non-human primates, J. Periodontol. **55:**203, 1984.

62. Cogen, R.B., et al.: Effect of various root surface treatments on the attachment and growth of human gingival fibroblasts: histologic and scanning electron microscopic evaluation, J. Clin. Periodontol. **11:**531, 1984.

63. Lopez, N.J.: Connective tissue regeneration to periodontally diseased roots, planed and conditioned with citric acid and implanted into the oral mucosa, J. Periodontol. **55:**381, 1984.

64. Ellegaard, B., and Löe, H.: New attachment of periodontal tissues after treatment of infrabony lesions, J. Periodontol. **42:**658, 1971.

65. Prichard, J.F.: The diagnosis and management of vertical bony defects, J. Periodontol. **54:**29, 1982.

66. Karring, T., Nyman, S., and Lindhe, J.: Healing following implantation of periodontitis affected roots into bone tissue, J. Clin. Periodontol. **45:**725, 1980.

67. Karring, T., et al.: New attachment formation on teeth with a reduced but healthy periodontium, J. Clin. Periodontol. **12:**51, 1985.

68. Gottlaw, J., et al.: New attachment formation as the result of controlled tissue regeneration, J. Clin. Periodontol. **11:**494, 1984.

69. Gottlaw, J., et al.: New attachment formation in the human periodontium by guided tissue regeneration, J. Clin. Periodontol. **13:**604, 1986.

70. Ellegaard, B., Karring, T., and Löe, H.: New periodontal attachment procedure based on retardation of epithelium migration, J. Clin. Periodontol. **1:**75, 1974.

71. Nyman, S., et al.: New attachment following surgical treatment of human periodontal disease, J. Clin. Periodontol. **9:**290, 1982.

72. Nyman, S., et al.: The regeneration potential of the periodontal ligament: an experimental study in the monkey, J. Clin. Periodontol. **9:**257, 1982b.

73. Winter, G.D.: Transcutaneous implants: reactions of the skin-implant interface, J. Biomed. Mater. Res. Symposium **5:**99, 1974.

**ADDITIONAL SUGGESTED READING**

Allen, D.R., and Caffesse, R.G.: Comparison of results following modified Widman flap surgery with and without dressing, J. Periodontol. **54:**470, 1983.

Crigger, M., Renvert, S., and Bogle, G.: The effect of topical citric acid application on surgically exposed periodontal attachment, J. Periodont. Res. **18:**303, 1983.

Durwin, A., et al.: Healing after treatment of periodontal intraosseous defects. IV. Effect of a non-resective versus a partially resective approach, J. Clin. Periodontol. **12:**525, 1985.

Frank, R., et al.: Ultrastructural study of epithelial and connective gingival reattachment in man, J. Periodontol. **45:**626, 1974.

Froum, S.J., Kusher, L., and Stahl, S.S.: Healing responses of human intraosseous lesions following the use of débridement, grafting and citric acid treatment. I. Clinical and histologic observations six months postsurgery, J. Periodontol. **54:**67, 1983.

Froum, S.J., et al.: Periodontal healing following open débridement flap procedures. I. Clinical assessment of soft tissue and osseous repair, J. Periodontol. **53:**8, 1982.

Hunter, R.K., O'Leary, T.J., and Kafrawy, A.H.: The effectiveness of hand versus ultrasonic instrumentation in open flap root planing, J. Periodontol. **55:**697, 1984.

Kashani, H.G., Magner, A.W., and Stahl, S.S.: The effect of root planing and citric acid applications on flap healing in humans: a histologic evaluation, J. Periodontol. **55:**679, 1984.

Listgarten, M.A., Rosenberg, S., and Lerner, S.: Progressive replacement of epithelial attachment by a connective tissue junction after experimental periodontal surgery in rats, J. Periodontol. **53:**659, 1982.

Moskow, B.S.: Healing potential in periodontal lesions: the interdental crater, J. Periodontol. **48:**754, 1977.

Nyman, S., Rosling, B., and Lindhe, J.: Effect of professional tooth cleaning on healing after periodontal surgery, J. Clin. Periodontol. **2:**80, 1975.

Polson, A.M., and Frederick, G.T.: Cell processes in dentin tubule during early phases of attachment to demineralized periodontitis-affected surfaces, J. Clin. Periodontol. **12:**162, 1985.

Polson, A.M., et al.: The production of a root surface smear layer by instrumentation and its removal by citric acid, J. Periodontol. **55:**443, 1984.

Stahl, S.S., Froum, S.J., and Kusher, L.: Periodontal healing following open débridement flap procedures. II. Histologic observations, J. Periodontol. **53:**15, 1982.

# CHAPTER 38

## Periodontal osseous resection

Objectives and rationale

Normal bony features and osseous defects

Therapeutic procedures
Presurgical preparation
Armamentarium
Surgical procedures

Contraindications

Alternative treatments

Summary
Causes of failure

Wound healing
Phases

---

**Definition**
Osseous resection includes procedures designed to eliminate morphologic defects in the alveolar bone associated with periodontitis.[1-15] Osseous surgery involves removal of bone to establish bony contours resembling those of a healthy, undamaged alveolar process. Thus gingival contours that can be maintained in health are created. Periodontal pockets are eliminated in the course of osseous resection.

**Ostectomy and osteoplasty**
Osseous resection[16] can be divided into *ostectomy* and *osteoplasty*.[17] *Ostectomy* is the reshaping of bone that provides attachment for periodontal ligament fibers.[18] *Osteoplasty* is the reshaping of bone that does not provide attachment for periodontal ligament fiber.[17,18] Osteoplasty does not result in loss of attachment.

## Objectives and rationale

The goal of osseous resection with ideal form free of bony discrepancies that predispose to recurrence of pocket depth.[19] This means that the surgery must lead to pocket elimination.

**Ideal osseous architecture**
In osseous surgery, alveolar bone is resculpted to establish an ideal osseous architecture with the following characteristics:

1. A *positive osseous architecture (scalloping)*. This occurs when the alveolar bone is more coronal interdentally and in the facial and lingual furcations than over the facial and lingual prominences of the roots (Fig. 38-1). A *flat osseous architecture* may be created in order to preserve bone and to avoid opening furcations.
2. *An alveolar crest parallel to the adjacent cementoenamel junction*. The interdental bone margins in the bicuspid and anterior regions are curved to conform to the contour of the cementoenamel junctions. In contrast, the interdental septum in the molar region is relatively flat or straight (Figs. 38-2 and 38-3).
3. *A thin alveolar margin*. The bony margin on the facial and lingual aspects of the teeth should be 0.5 to 1 mm wide. The alveolar bone becomes thicker as it progresses apically (Fig. 38-4).
4. *The bone is festooned in buccolingual contour*. Grooves are made on the facial and some

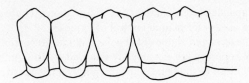

**Fig. 38-1.**   Positive osseous architecture.

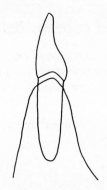

**Fig. 38-2.**   Crest of the alveolar bone parallel to the cementoenamel junction of a mandibular incisor.

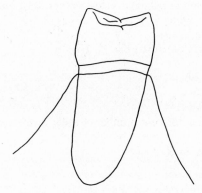

**Fig. 38-3.**   Alveolar bone parallel to a relatively flat cementoenamel junction of a mandibular molar. Compare this posterior interdental crest with the highly curved anterior interdental crest shown in Fig. 38-2.

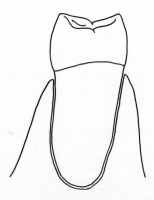

**Fig. 38-4.**   Alveolar bone that is thin at its margin and gradually becomes thicker apically.

lingual surfaces apical to interdental areas and furcations. These grooves improve gingival form and provide access for plaque control (Fig. 38-5).

5. *The contour in the level and shape of the bone is made harmonious gradually.* Precipitous changes in bony contours are not usually followed by the gingiva. Gradual changes in the height and contour of the bone allow the gingival tissues to duplicate the form of the underlying bone.

6. As a corollary, since thick, fibrotic gingiva prevents compatibility between gingiva and bone, *dense connective tissue in the tuberosity and palatal regions is thinned.*

## Normal bony features and osseous defects

In osseous surgery, the existing bony topography is changed to eliminate periodontal pockets. When a therapist performs osseous resection, there must be an awareness of normal contours and of anatomic aberrations present in the patient's osseous form.[20] The following defects may be present:

A. Vestibular, lingual, or palatal defects associated with
  1. Normal anatomic structures
     a. External oblique ridge
     b. Retromolar triangle
     c. Mylohyoid ridge
     d. Zygomatic process
  2. Exostoses and tori
     a. Mandibular lingual tori (Fig. 38-6)
     b. Buccal and posterior palatal exostoses (Figs. 38-7 and 38-8)
  3. Dehiscences (Fig. 38-9)
  4. Fenestrations (Fig. 38-9)
  5. Reverse osseous architecture (Fig. 38-10)
B. Vertical defects
  1. Three walls (Fig. 38-11)
  2. Two walls (Fig. 38-12)
  3. One wall (Fig. 38-13)
  4. Combination with a different number of walls at the various levels of the defect
C. Furcation defects
  1. Class I or incipient (Fig. 38-14)

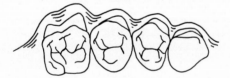

**Fig. 38-5.** Occlusal view of maxillary posterior segment showing grooving in the interdental and furcation areas and distal to the terminal tooth.

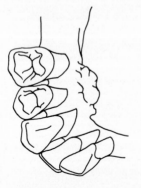

**Fig. 38-6.** Occlusal view of a mandibular segment with a lingual torus.

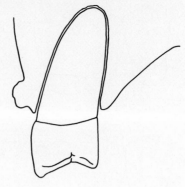

**Fig. 38-7.**   Maxillary posterior facial exostosis.

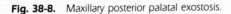

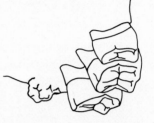

**Fig. 38-8.**   Maxillary posterior palatal exostosis.

**Fig. 38-9.**   Maxillary bicuspid with a fenestration and a maxillary molar with a fenestration on the mesial root and a dehiscence on the distal root.

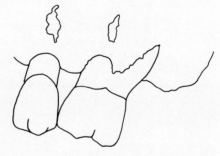

**Fig. 38-10.**   Reverse osseous architecture. Interdental bone is apical to facial bone.

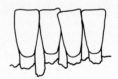

**Fig. 38-11.**   Three-wall infrabony defect on the mesial side of a mandibular molar.

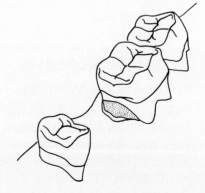

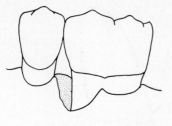

**Fig. 38-12.** Two-wall infrabony defect on the mesial side of a mandibular molar. The mesial and lingual alveolar bone comprises the remaining walls. An interproximal crater is the most common example of a two-wall defect.

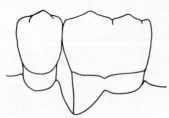

**Fig. 38-13.** One-wall infrabony defect on the mesial of a mandibular molar. This is also termed a *hemiseptum*.

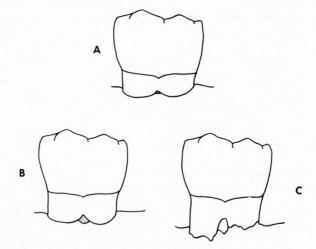

**Fig. 38-14.** **A,** Class I (incipient) furcation involvement on a mandibular molar. The indentation leading into the furcation but not the furcation itself is exposed. **B,** Class II (partial) furcation involvement. An explorer can be inserted under the roof of the furcation but not completely through. **C,** Class III (complete) furcation involvement. The tip of an explorer can be passed through the furcation.

    2. Class II or partial (Fig. 38-15)
    3. Class III or through and through (Fig. 38-16)

Facial and lingual furcation involvements are corrected more easily than are mesial and distal furcations. Mesial and distal furcations of maxillary molars and first bicuspids have a poorer prognosis.

## Therapeutic procedures

### PRESURGICAL PREPARATION

Osseous resection should not be done until initial therapy has been completed. Clinically detectable inflammation must be eliminated by scaling and root planing and by the patient's exercise of optimal plaque control. If occlusal trauma is present, it must be treated presurgically by occlusal adjustment, temporary splinting, orthodontic therapy, and/or night guards. If alteration of tooth position would create more favorable

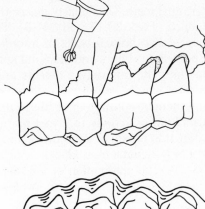

**Fig. 38-15.** Osteoplasty to remove ledges and place interdental grooves in the bicuspid region. Note the untreated molar segment.

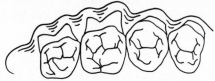

**Fig. 38-16.** Occlusal view after completion of osteoplasty.

bone contours, decrease pocket depth, or improve occlusal function, orthodontic treatment should be done beforehand.

A surgical treatment plan must be formulated before surgery because flap design is determined in part by the underlying osseous topography. A presurgical charting of pocket depths, furcation involvements, and tooth mobility must be done, since these data will have changed from the time of the original examination because of presurgical preparation. The operator may supplement this charting with roentgenograms and "sounding." The surgeon should attempt to visualize the alveolar topography in a three-dimensional view before beginning the surgery. A sketch of the anticipated defects on a surgical chart with the corrections to be made can facilitate the surgery.

## ARMAMENTARIUM

Osseous surgery requires some special instruments in addition to those presented in Chapter 33. The following list may be modified to suit the individual surgeon:

1. High-speed handpiece with fiber optics and surgical burs, which come with longer shanks (nos. 8, 6, and 4 carbide); flame-shaped and spear-shaped (carbides)
2. Bone files: Schluger, Buck, and/or Sugarman
3. Chisels: Wedelstaedt (assorted sizes), back-action, Rhodes, and Ochsenbein
4. Ultrasonic scaler

## SURGICAL PROCEDURES

After appropriate premedication and local anesthesia, incisions are made and periodontal flaps are elevated to expose the underlying alveolar bone (Chapters 33 and 36). Proper flap design and management are essential to the success of osseous surgery. After the flaps are elevated, the remaining soft tissue is removed from the teeth and from the defects. The exposed bone form should be compared with the presurgical drawing or anticipated findings. If necessary, corrections should be made in the sketch and the surgical treatment plan modified before proceeding.

Osseous resection should be done systematically so that an ideal osseous architecture can be achieved without the excessive sacrifice of bone. The surgeon should not unduly prolong the procedure, which would be traumatic. A high-speed handpiece with a no. 8 surgical bur, cooled by a water spray, is used to thin and shape the buccal and lingual alveolar housing. This initial osteoplasty is done to remove ledges, exostoses, and tori. It is also used to reduce tuberosities, to give edentulous areas a saddle shape,

**Systematic steps**

Initial osteoplasty

and to establish grooves apical to the interdental spaces and furcations and distal to terminal teeth. Osteoplasty places the bone over the roots into facial and lingual prominence (Figs. 38-17 and 38-18). This thinning of the alveolar housing narrows the buccal and lingual walls of interdental defects and thus facilitates their treatment. Spear-shaped burs and diamond stones, bone files, chisels, and curettes are employed to eliminate interdental defects and to establish an ideal bony contour. Interdental defects should be refined with hand instruments only. The use of a bur to refine the interdental septum may result in the accidental grooving of the roots. Some periodontists limit ostectomy to 2 mm marginally and use grafting for anything beyond that. After this proximal contouring and grafting, the interdental alveolar crest should be flat or horizontal mesiodistally and very slightly curved faciolingually (Figs. 38-19 and 38-20). The elimination of interdental defects often leaves small spicules of bone at the line angles of the teeth (widow's peaks). This may result in reverse osseous ar-

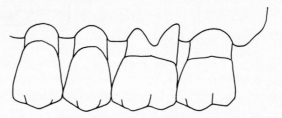

**Fig. 38-17.** Facial view of the alveolar crest after ostectomy and osteoplasty showing a positive osseous architecture.

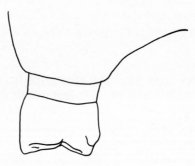

**Fig. 38-18.** Interproximal aspect after osseous resection, showing a slightly curved alveolar crest.

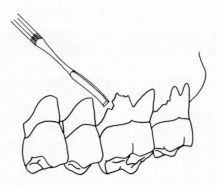

**Fig. 38-19.** Ostectomy to establish a positive osseous architecture. A chisel is shown removing a "widow's peak." Osseous resection is complete in the bicuspid region.

chitecture if the bony margin and the gingiva facial and lingual to the roots heal coronal to the interdental alveolar crest.

Osseous resection is more difficult around molars because of the presence of furcations as well as the obstacles provided by access and vision. The surgeon should not invade unopened furcations. Furcation involvements may be opened by osteoplasty for access for root planing and plaque removal (see Chapter 42 for management of furcation involvement). Thus the position of the furcations as related to osseous defects should be ascertained by x-ray, probing, and sounding. The length of the root trunk leading to the furcation should be assessed. The trunk usually varies from 2 to 5 mm in length. Trunk length will influence the amount of osseous resection that is permissible.

Mandibular molars are inclined lingually approximately 20° to 25°. The lingual furcation is more apically situated than the buccal, which influences the direction of bone removal by the surgeon. The roots of the mandibular first molar are usually more divergent than those of the second molar.

The initial osseous surgery in treating interdental osseous craters adjacent to mandibular molars is osteoplasty on buccal and lingual bone surfaces to thin thick bone, to eliminate ledges, and to slope the bone coronally, ending in a thin margin (Figs. 38-21 to 38-24). Interdental grooves are sometimes created to assist in flap replacement.

**Interdental craters next to mandibular molars**

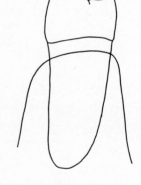

**Fig. 38-20.** Interdental view after osseous resection.

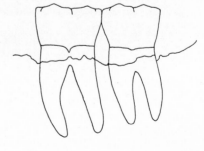

**Fig. 38-21.** The buccal surfaces of the mandibular molars show reverse architecture and intraosseous defects. There are no furcation involvements.

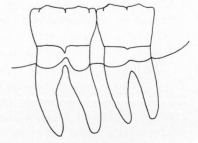

**Fig. 38-22.** Following osseous surgery, a form consistent with health has been created (positive architecture).

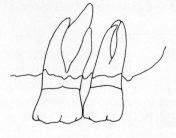

**Fig. 38-23.** The buccal region of the maxillary molars shows reverse bony architecture and intraosseous defects. There are no furcation involvements.

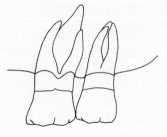

**Fig. 38-24.** Following osseous surgery, a form consistent with health has been created (positive architecture).

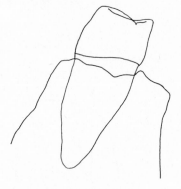

**Fig. 38-25.** An intraproximal bony crater on a mandibular molar.

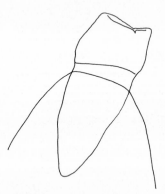

**Fig. 38-26.** The same area (as in Fig. 38-25) following osseous resection. Note the osteoplasty required to eliminate the lingual ledge of bone.

Mildly scalloped or flat buccal and lingual bony outlines may be created. A flatter outline is recommended by Ochsenbein in order to conserve bony support.[19]

The bone next to the furcation should not be reduced. The bone over the mesial and distal roots may be treated individually, like that over adjacent premolars.

The mandibular osseous crater is usually reduced or eliminated at the expense of lingual bone by sloping the interdental bone toward the lingual (Figs. 38-25 and 38-26). Minor ostectomy can be performed on the lingual crest of the crater. After the crater is eliminated, minor scalloping may be done on the lingual and buccal surfaces as appropriate. A flat buccal outline may also be created in order to preserve bone and preserve an intact furcation.

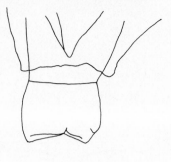

**Fig. 38-27.**  The proximal view of a maxillary molar, showing an interproximal crater.

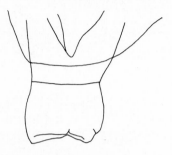

**Fig. 38-28.**  The same area (as in Fig. 38-27) following osseous resection. The bony surgery was done at the expense of palatal bone to minimize reduction of buccal bone in order to protect the buccal furcation.

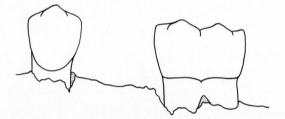

**Fig. 38-29.**  Facial view of a mandibular segment with an edentulous area, reverse osseous architecture, infrabony defects, and class II furcation involvement.

**Maxillary molar interdental craters**

Maxillary molar interdental craters should be treated via a palatal approach,[25] removing bone at the expense of the palatal bone. After thinning any ledges and after interdental grooving, the crater is corrected by sloping toward the palate. This conserves buccal bone. The buccal bone may be given a mildly scalloped or flat outline (Figs. 38-27 and 38-28).

**Facial and lingual form by ostectomy**

A scalloped (arcaded) positive architecture can now be established on the facial and lingual surfaces. This is done by ostectomy with burs, chisels, and curettes (Fig. 38-29). Care should be taken to avoid removing bone in furcations. Cavitron and root planing may be done now to smooth the roots and to remove soft tissue remnants.

The final stage of osseous resection is to again use a bur or Molt curette to thin, shape, and smooth the buccal and lingual external alveolus. The goals of this step are to establish bony margins that are 0.5 to 1 mm thick and that blend smoothly with the interdental bone (Fig. 38-30).

**Contiguous edentulous areas**

When osseous resection involves an edentulous area, the edentulous ridge should be shaped to eliminate bony defects on teeth adjacent to the edentulous area. This also provides gingival contours that facilitate the placement and cleansing of a prosthesis. This shaping is accomplished by creating a saddle area (Figs. 38-29 to 38-32).

The existence of partial and complete furcation involvements in molar or maxillary first bicuspid teeth is a unique problem, which is treated by methods such as odontoplasty, root amputation, or hemisection (Chapter 42). The goal of treatment is to provide the patient with access to the furcation for plaque control. Another alternative for furcation involvements is to attempt to maintain them by frequent root planing and

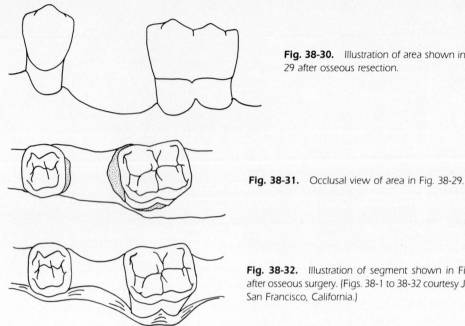

**Fig. 38-30.** Illustration of area shown in Fig. 38-29 after osseous resection.

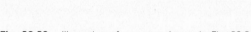

**Fig. 38-31.** Occlusal view of area in Fig. 38-29.

**Fig. 38-32.** Illustration of segment shown in Fig. 38-31 after osseous surgery. (Figs. 38-1 to 38-32 courtesy J. Bartlett, San Francisco, California.)

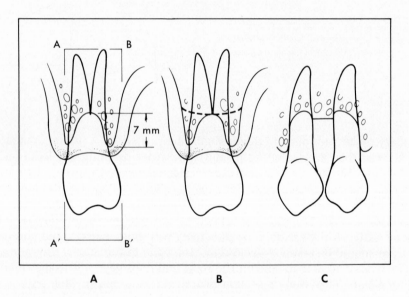

**Fig. 38-33.** Criteria for extent of ostectomy. **A,** Infrabony defect measuring 7 mm from the alveolar crest to the bottom of the defect. **B,** If bone were removed to eliminate the defect as outlined, the result would be unacceptable. **C,** Additional loss of supporting bone would create an unfavorable crown-to-root ratio and unacceptable bone contours and would threaten survival of two teeth.

meticulous plaque control. If a furcation cannot be cleansed by the patient, the prognosis for the tooth is threatened.

There are limitations on the amount of bony housing that can be removed (ostectomy). The removal of bony housing is permissible to the extent of about 2 mm. Removal of more bone is usually improper, and procedures such as bone grafting and reattachment are combined with osseous resection where deep defects are present (Figs. 38-33 and 38-34).

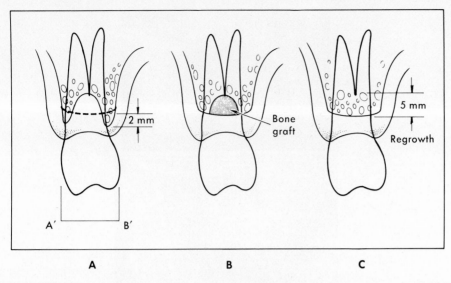

**Fig. 38-34.** *Permissible extent of osseous resection (ostectomy).* **A,** *In a bony defect as shown in Fig. 38-33, only 2 mm of bone could be resected. A bone graft* **(B)** *would then be placed to correct the remaining osseous defect* **(C).**

After the bone contouring procedures are completed, the periodontal flaps should be positioned and sutured. The margins of the flaps may be coapted, placed at the bony margins, or apically repositioned.

## Contraindications

Several factors can contraindicate the use of osseous resection to eliminate periodontal pockets[21]:

1. Anatomic features such as the close proximity of the maxillary antrum or the ramus
2. Impaired physical or emotional health of the patient
3. Advanced age
4. Inadequate oral hygiene resulting from lack of either dexterity or motivation
5. High caries index
6. Extreme root sensitivity
7. Unacceptable esthetic result
8. Advanced periodontitis
9. Any additional bone loss that would result in an unfavorable crown-root ratio and an increase in tooth mobility ( Fig. 38-35).

## Alternative treatments

Before employing osseous resection to treat an infrabony defect, the therapist should consider the following alternative treatments:

1. Maintenance with periodic root planing
2. Bone grafts
3. New attachment procedures
4. Hemisection or root amputation
5. Orthodontics
6. Extraction

Osseous resection is taught and performed differently at different schools. There is a spectrum of goals ranging from the scalloped, arcaded bone form seen in Fig.

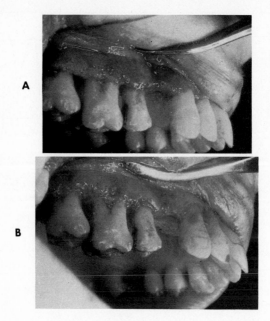

**Fig. 38-35.** Periodontitis in a 38-year-old woman. Root planing, gingival curettage, and proper oral hygiene resolved most of the clinically evident inflammation. Pockets and osseous deformities still remain. **A,** The osseous surface is exposed for access. Note the deformities present. Blunted alveolar margins, interdental craters, and a furcation involvement on the second molar can be seen. **B,** A scalloped, beveled bone form was created. Bony deformities were eliminated. Periodontal health, with minor isolated increase in pocket and probing depth has been maintained for 26 years.

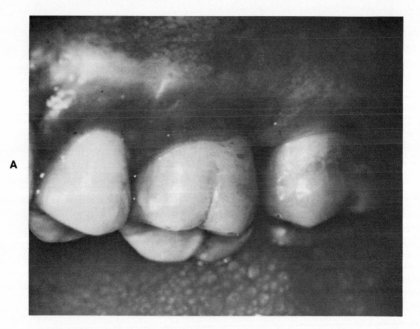

**Fig. 38-36.** **A,** The palatal approach to osseous surgery conserves buccal bone, leaving a straighter, less scalloped bone form. Such flatter bone form is seen more frequently in disease-free areas when flaps are reflected. A crater could be probed between the maxillary first and second molars.

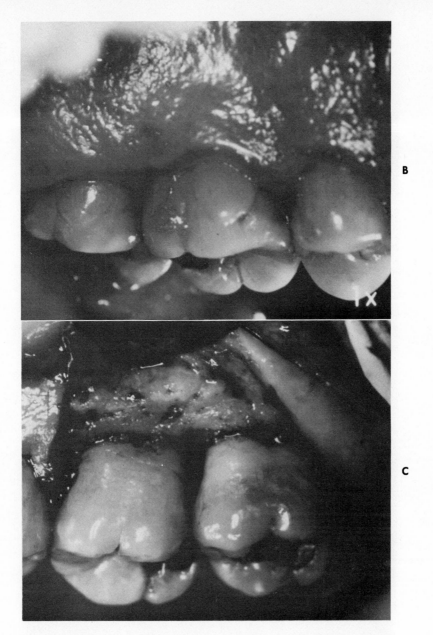

**Fig. 38-36, cont'd. B,** Palatal gingival form suggests the probing depth indicative of bone loss and pocket formation. An interdental crater is present between the first and second molars. **C,** The reflection of a modified flap reveals the interdental osseous crater. Note the relatively flat buccal bone form where no bone loss occurred.

*Continued.*

38-35 to a modest, flat architecture designed to preserve buccal bone (Fig. 38-36, *A* to *H*), to the minimal removal of bone to facilitate coaption of flap margins.[12,14,16,22] The value of osseous recontouring in restoring and maintaining periodontal health has not been established.*

---

*See references 12, 13, 15, 16, 22, and 23.

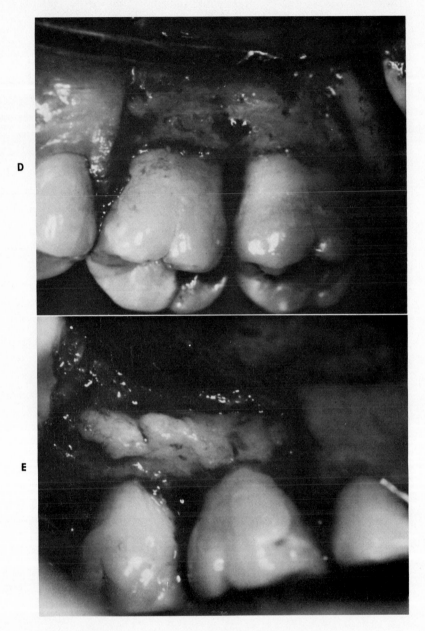

**Fig. 38-36, cont'd.   D,** Interdental grooving was performed with burs. No crestal bone was removed. **E,** The interdental crater seen from the palatal. Note the bony exostosis.

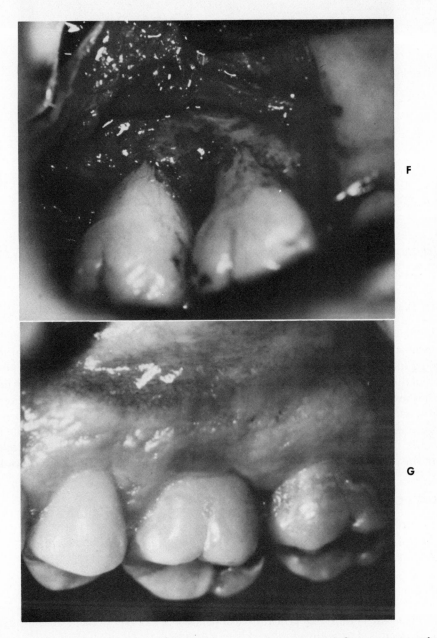

F

G

**Fig. 38-36, cont'd.    F,** The osseous crater is corrected by ramping from the palatal. Ostectomy was performed over the palatal roots. **G,** Postoperative buccal gingival form is acceptable. Interdental probing depth was less than 3 mm.                                                                                          *Continued.*

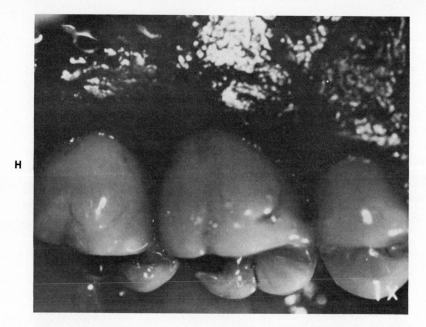

**Fig. 38-36, cont'd.** **H,** Palatal gingival form reflects the scalloped bone contour created by surgery. (Fig. 38-36, *A to H* courtesy C. Ochsenbein, Dallas, Texas.)

## Summary

Osseous resection is a relatively complicated procedure. It is a challenge to the surgeon's judgment and technical ability.[18,24-26] The operator must transform the conceptual ideal of osseous architecture into reality. Osseous surgery does not cure periodontal disease. It provides the patient with the opportunity and the access to maintain his/her own periodontium and dentition by scrupulous oral hygiene procedures. Such maintenance usually meets with long-term success. Osseous resection sometimes fails to provide long-term elimination of periodontal pockets. Recurrence is usually a result of either inadequate plaque control or undertreatment by the surgeon.[19] Undertreatment means that the conceptual ideal form is not fully understood or achieved by the surgeon.

### CAUSES OF FAILURE

Failure of osseous surgery may be the result of (1) poor postoperative plaque control, (2) incomplete pocket elimination, (3) failure to create ideal bone form. Other causes may occur:

1. Improper flap management
2. Sequestration of resorption of bone following surgery
3. Improper suturing or dressing management
4. Exposure of thin bony plates, alveolar dehiscences, or fenestrations during surgery
5. Postsurgical exposure of thinned bone margins
6. Flap necrosis
7. Postsurgical infection
8. Root caries or pulpal problems incident to the surgery

The techniques for ostectomy-osteoplasty have been discussed and the actual performance of this surgery has been illustrated in clinical photographs (Figs. 38-35 and 38-36).

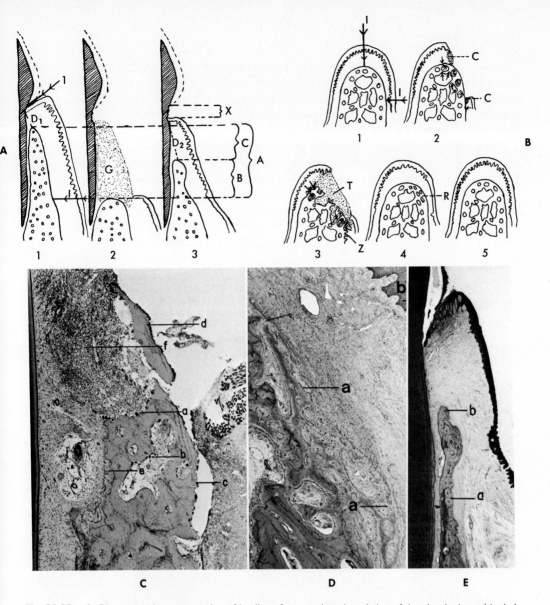

**Fig. 38-37.** **A,** Diagrammatic representation of healing after complete denudation of the alveolar bone (dog). *1,* Preoperative appearance. Between the two arrows, *1,* all epithelium and connective tissue, including the periosteum, were removed, baring the bone. *2,* Appearance 6 to 10 days postoperatively. Young connective tissue, *G,* is granulation tissue. *3,* Appearance 95 to 185 days after surgery. *A,* Extent of complete osseous exposure and resorption (5 mm); *B,* extent of bone repair (2.5 mm); *C,* extent of final loss of alveolar bone height (2.5 mm); *D₂,* original length of the connective tissue attachment; *X,* lowering of the level of the junctional epithelium below the cementoenamel junction. **B,** Diagrammatic representation of healing in the interdental area after complete denudation of alveolar bone (dog). *1,* Preoperative view. *Arrows,* Direction of the incision. *2,* Appearance 2 to 4 days postoperatively. *Small arrows,* Direction of osseous resorption; *C,* small blood clots and exposed bone. *3,* Postoperatively 6 to 10 days. *T,* Young connective tissue (granulation tissue); *Z,* formation of coarse, fibrillar bone trabeculae. *4,* Appearance 28 days after surgery. *R,* Formation of trabecular bone at the wound site. *5,* Postoperatively 95 to 185 days. Note the return to the preoperative appearance. **C,** Micrograph corresponding to **A,** *2.* Undermining resorption has occurred at the crest, *a,* and in the marrow spaces facing the periodontal ligament, *b.* Frontal resorption is evident on the surface of the vestibular bony plate below the wound edge, *c.* The crest has been resorbed. An inflammatory reaction is present in the proliferating young connective tissue that occupies the former periodontal ligament area, *f,* in the bone marrow and at the edge of the incision. **D,** Micrograph corresponding to **B,** *4.* Coarse, immature trabeculae lined with osteoid and osteoblasts indicate rapid new bone formation, *a. b,* Surface epithelium. **E,** Micrograph corresponding to **A,** *3.* The amount of regeneration of alveolar bone 93 days after bone exposure is evident between *a* and *b. a,* Alveolar crest after postoperative bone loss; *b,* highest level of regeneration of the alveolar crest 93 days after surgery. The connective tissue attachment between the alveolar crest and the apical end of the attachment epithelium is twice normal length. The junctional epithelium is on cementum. The width of the periodontal ligament has returned to normal. (Courtesy M.N. Wilderman, New Orleans, Louisiana.)

## Wound healing

Osseous surgery may be followed by further bone loss.[27,28] When bone is cut or left uncovered by soft connective tissue, varying amounts of bone extending from the surface operated on may become necrotic. Poor surgical procedures will enhance such sequelae. Necrotic bone is resorbed by osteoclasts, which differentiate from pluripotent blood-borne monocytes in adjacent marrow spaces and haversian systems.

Granulation may come from the periodontal ligament and adjacent fixed wound margins (Fig. 38-37). The osseous wound thus becomes covered with a young, proliferating connective tissue. Such granulation tissue is the product of a proliferation of undifferentiated mesenchymal cells, fibroblasts, and capillaries from vital bone, periodontal ligament, and (to a lesser extent) soft tissue wound margins. This granulation tissue resorbs, undermines, and removes necrotic bone as well as some vital bone (Fig. 38-38). Osteoblastic activity then follows and bone forms.

### PHASES

Experimental studies in dogs[29] indicate the following phases of healing (Fig. 38-39):

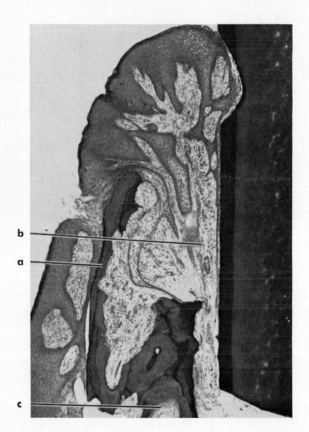

**Fig. 38-38.** Large sequestrum, *a*, in a specimen of human periodontal tissue. The notch in the tooth indicates the level of the alveolar bone at the time of surgery. At one point the necrotic bone is nearly in contact with the surface, covered by only a few degenerating epithelial cells. Extensive epithelial proliferation has taken place into the lamina propria, where the collagen fibers are being replaced by a young proliferating connective tissue, *b*. The junctional epithelium has proliferated down the root parallel to the necrotic alveolar crest. Empty lacunae are present in the bone. A few pyknotic nuclei are present in lacunae at the most apical extent of the photomicrograph, where a thin seam of osteoid, *c*, lines a marrow space. (From Grant, D.A.: J. Periodontol. **38:**409, 1967.)

1. Osteoclastic phase—2 to 10 days
2. Osteoblastic phase—10 to 28 days
3. Functional repair of dentoperiodontal unit and dentogingival junction—28 to 185 days

When flaps are coapted postsurgically, the earliest changes that follow the acute inflammation are the differentiation of osteoclasts and the resorption of bone in the wound area. This is followed by bone deposition that tends to repair the surgical area. Split-thickness flaps have been found to produce less damage to bone.[30]

In similar experiments with the periosteum retained, the phases of healing were identical but without residual deformities.[31] There is less resorption and less deformity if a thick layer of connective tissue is left over bone.

When flaps are reflected and then replaced, the sequence and time for bone healing are essentially the same. During the first few days acute inflammation occurs; a fibrin network is formed and begins to be replaced by collagen in 4 to 6 days. Junctional attachment epithelium becomes evident in about a week.[32] Bone resorption begins after several days and continues for about 2 weeks unless a sequestrum is present, in which case healing is delayed.[33] Repair (osteoblastic phase) then goes on for 3 to 4 weeks, at which time the resorption is almost completely repaired.[34] Some bone re-

**Osteoclastic phase**

**Osteoblastic phase**

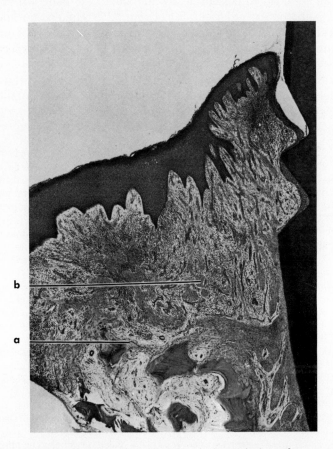

**Fig. 38-39.** Reactive and compensatory bone deposition occurs in the repair phase after osseous surgery. A large amount of osteoid, *a*, has been formed in this human specimen. The lamina propria, *b*, is filled with a highly vascular, young, proliferating connective tissue. The notches indicate the presurgical depth of the sulcus and level of the alveolar crest on the reflection of a flap.

contouring occurs with the loss of thin spines and spicules and with some bone apposition. Full maturation of the connective tissue may take as long as 6 months.[18] When flaps are loosly sutured, defects similar to those produced by bone denudation may occur.

**Functional repair phase**

Reapposition of a flap to cover bone after osseous surgery undoubtedly reduces the amount of bone resorption (or sequestration) that may take place. All osseous surgery is followed by some small bone loss[13] (see Fig. 38-38). In turn a period of reactive and compensatory bone deposition occurs, which may be called the repair phase (Fig. 38-39). The repair, however, rarely restores all the bone lost by surgical injury.[29] This means that the surgeon cannot plan to cut bone like inert clay and expect it to retain the precise form created. Osseous surgery must be planned with the full knowledge of the tissue reactions that will follow surgical manipulation.[28,34-43] Furthermore, ultimate bone contours may differ from those established during osseous surgery as a result of function.

The effects of denudation of crestal alveolar bone have been observed in dogs and humans.[28] The osteoclastic phase lasts about 10 days and is followed by a repair or osteoblastic phase that lasts up to 30 days. In the interdental area, marrow spaces provide cellular elements that contribute to restoration of lost bone. However, part of the thin bone over the roots may be lost completely. The loss may be 2.5 mm.

When flaps are coapted postsurgically, the amount of bone lost after reshaping is insignificant, being on the order of 0.5 to 1 mm.[29,34,44] The greater bone loss reported by some investigators could be caused by overheating in the use of diamond stones.[40] The least damage, with best repair, results with chisels, high-speed engines with coolant sprays, and carbide steel burs.[34,38-41,43,44]

Fibers near the tooth are found aligned parallel to the root surface 30 to 60 days after flap reflection and replacement. By 120 days classic fiber orientation has occurred and dentogingival fibers are seen exiting from cementum, coursing in classic alignment.[45]

## REFERENCES

1. Stern, I.B., Everett, F.G., and Robicsek, K.: S. Robicsek—a pioneer in the surgical treatment of periodontal disease, J. Periodontol. **36:**265, 1965.
2. Cieszynski, A.: Bemerkungen zur radikal-chirurgischen Behandlung der sogenannten Pyorrhoea alveolaris, Dtsch. Monatsschr., 1914.
3. Widman, L.: Om operativ behandling af alveolar pyorrhoe, Sven. Tandläk. Tidskr. **10:**85, 1917.
4. Zentler, A.: Suppurative gingivitis with alveolar involvement: a new surgical procedure, JAMA **71:**1530, 1918.
5. Neumann, R.: Atlas der radikal-chirurgischen Behandlung der Paradentosen, Berlin, 1926, Hermann Meusser.
6. Zemsky, J.L.: Surgical treatment of periodontal disease with the author's open view operation for advanced cases of dental periclasia, Dent. Cosmos **68:**465, 1926.
7. Ward, A.W.: The surgical eradication of pyorrhea, J. Am. Dent. Assoc. **15:**2146, 1928.
8. Crane, A.B., and Kaplan, H.: The Crane-Kaplan operation for prompt elimination of pyorrhea alveolaris, Dent. Cosmos **74:**643, 1931.
9. Carranza, F.A.: Cuando y porque sacrificiar hueso en tratamiento de al paradentosis, An. Ateneo Inst. Munic. Odontol. **3:**311, 1941.
10. Schluger, S.: Osseous resection—a basic principle in periodontal surgery, Oral Surg. **2:**316, 1949.
11. Kakehashi, S., and Parakkal, P.F.: Proceedings from the state of the art workshop on surgical therapy for periodontics, J. Periodontol. **53:**475, 1982.
12. Smith, D.H., Ammons, W.F., and Van Belle, G.: A longitudinal study of periodontal status comparing osseous recontouring with flap curettage. I. Results after 6 months, J. Periodontol. **5:**367, 1980.
13. Aeschlimann, C.R., Robinson, P.J., and Kaminski, E.J.: A short time evaluation of periodontal surgery, J. Periodont. Res. **14:**182, 1979.
14. Selipsky, H.: Osseous surgery—how much need we compromise? Dent. Clin. North Am. **20:**79, 1976.
15. Bahat, O., et al.: The influence of soft tissue on interdental bone height after flap curettage. I. Study involving six patients, Int. J. Periodont. Rest. Dent. **2:**9, 1984.
16. Ochsenbein, C.: Current status of osseous surgery, J. Peridontol. **48:**577, 1977.

17. Friedman, N.: Periodontal osseous surgery: osteoplasty and osteoectomy, J. Periodontol. **26:**257, 1955.
18. Donnenfeld, O.W., Hoag, P.M., and Wiessman, D.P.: A clinical study on the effects of osteoplasty, J. Periodontol. **41:**131, 1970.
19. Ochsenbein, C.: A primer for osseous surgery, Int. J. Periodont. Rest. Dent. **4:**8, 1986.
20. Clarke, M.A., and Bueltmann, K.W.: Anatomical considerations in periodontal surgery, J. Periodontol. **42:**610, 1971.
21. Bradin, M.: Precautions and hazards in periodontal surgery, J. Periodontol. **33:**154, 1962.
22. Hill, R.W., et al.: Four types of periodontal treatment compared over two years, J. Periodontol. **52:**655, 1981.
23. Moghaddas, H., and Stahl, S.S.: Alveolar bone remodeling following osseous surgery: a clinical study, J. Periodontol. **51:**376, 1980.
24. Tibbets, L.S., Jr., Ochsenbein, C., and Loughlin, D.M.: Rationale for the lingual approach to mandibular osseous surgery, Dent. Clin. North Am. **20:**61, 1976.
25. Ochsenbein, C., and Bohannan, H.M.: Palatal approach to osseous surgery, I. Rationale, J. Periodontol. **34:**60, 1963.
26. Seibert, J.S.: Treatment of infrabony lesions by surgical resection procedures. In Stahl, S.S., editor: Periodontal surgery: biologic basis and technique, Springfield, Ill., 1976, Charles C Thomas, Publisher.
27. Grant, D.A., Friedman, N., and Orban, B.: Response of the periodontal tissues around the alveolar crest to surgical procedures presented at a meeting of the American Academy of Periodontology, Los Angeles, 1960.
28. Pennel, B.M., et al.: Repair of the alveolar process following osseous surgery, J. Periodontol. **38:**426, 1967.
29. Wilderman, M.N., et al.: Histogenesis of repair following osseous surgery, J. Periodontol. **41:**551, 1970.
30. Staffileno, H., Wentz, F.M., and Orban, B.: Histologic study of healing of split thickness flap surgery in dogs, J. Periodontol. **33:**56, 1962.
31. Wilderman, M.N.: Repair after a periosteal retention procedure, J. Periodontol. **34:**187, 1963.
32. Hiatt, W.H., et al.: Repair following mucoperiosteal flap surgery with full gingival retention, J. Periodontol. **39:**11, 1968.
33. Grant, D.A.: Experimental periodontal surgery: sequestration of alveolar bone, J. Periodontol. **38:**409, 1967.
34. Caffesse, R.J., Ramfjord, S.P., and Nasjleti, C.E.: Reverse bevel periodontal flaps in monkeys, J. Periodontol. **39:**219, 1968.
35. Wilderman, M.N., Wentz, F.M., and Orban, B.: Histogenesis of repair after mucogingival surgery, J. Periodontol. **31:**283, 1960.
36. Lobene, R.R., and Glickman, I.: The response of alveolar bone to grinding with rotary diamond stones, J. Periodontol. **34:**105, 1963.
37. McFall, T.A., Yamane, J.M., and Burnett, G.W.: Comparison of the cutting effect on bone of an ultrasonic cutting device and rotary burs, J. Oral Surg. Anesth. Hosp. Dent. Serv. **19:**200, 1961.
38. Spatz, S.: Early reaction in bone following the use of burs rotating at conventional and ultra speeds, Oral Surg. **19:**808, 1965.
39. Moss, R.W.: Histopathologic reaction of bone to surgical cutting, Oral Surg. **17:**405, 1964.
40. Costich, E.R., Youngblood, P.J., and Walden, J.M.: A study of the effects of high-speed rotary instruments on bone repair in dogs, Oral Surg. **17:**563, 1964.
41. Boyne, P.J.: Histologic response of bone to sectioning by high-speed rotary instruments, J. Dent. Res. **45:**270, 1966.
42. Heins, P.J.: Osseous surgery: an evaluation after twenty years, Dent. Clin. North Am. **13:**75, 1969.
43. Easley, J.R.: Methods of determining alveolar osseous form, J. Periodontol. **38:**112, 1967.
44. Hoag, P.J., et al.: Alveolar crest reduction following full and partial thickness flaps, J. Periodontol. **43:**141, 1972.
45. Rizzo, R.J.: Parameters of the dentogingival junction: a postoperative healing study in humans, Master's thesis, Chicago, 1978, Loyola University.

## ADDITIONAL SUGGESTED READING

Caton, J., and Zander, H.: Osseous repair of an infrabony pocket without new attachment of connective tissue, J. Clin. Periodontol. **3:**54, 1976.
Cogswill, W.W.: Dental oral surgery, Colorado Springs, Colo., 1932, Out West Printing Co.
Goldman, H.M., and Cohen, D.W.: The infrabony pocket: classification and treatment, J. Periodontol. **29:**272, 1958.
Hugoson, A., and Schmidt, G.: Influence of plaque on the healing of experimentally induced bone defects in the dog, J. Periodontol. **49:**135, 1978.
McDonald, F.L., Saari, J.T., and Davis, S.S.: A comparison of tooth accumulated materials from quadrants treated surgically or nonsurgically, J. Periodontol. **48:**147, 1977.
Nery, E.B., Corn, H., and Eisenstein, I.L.: Palatal exostosis in the molar region, J. Periodontol. **48:**663, 1977.
Owings, J.R., Jr., and Fritz, M.E.: A technique employing metallic implants for the evaluation of periodontal surgery, J. Periodontol. **40:**661, 1969.
Vogan, W.I., and Knoell, A.C.: The biomechanical effects of simulated osseous surgery, J. Periodont. Res. **11:**360, 1976.
Walsh, T.F., and Waite, I.M.: A comparison of postsurgical healing following débridement by ultrasonic or hand instruments, J. Periodontol. **49:**201, 1978.

# CHAPTER 39

## Bone grafts and transplants

| | |
|---|---|
| **Introduction** | **Clinical experience** |
| **Classification** | **Method** |
| **Graft materials** | **Wound healing** |
| Autografts | Graft vs. nongraft regenerative procedures |
| Allografts | Advantages and disadvantages |
| **Indications** | **Summary** |

## Introduction

The ideal goal of periodontal therapy is the reconstruction of the bone and ligamentous attachment that has been destroyed by disease.[1] Several therapeutic methods may be used to reach this goal; one of these is bone grafting. The objective of bone grafting is the restoration of lost alveolar bone and the regeneration of a functional attachment apparatus.[2] Pocket depth would be reduced or eliminated.

At the present time there is evidence in humans that bone grafting is accompanied by regeneration of a new attachment composed of new bone, cementum, and a periodontal ligament coronal to the bone defect. The new attachment occurred over a previously contaminated root surface.[3] This finding has resulted in controversy.[4,5]

A recent study, comparing autogenous bone grafts with open curettage, found statistically significant increase in probing bone levels only in the deepest defects.[6] Some have suggested that the graft may act as a physical barrier to impede the apical migration of junctional epithelium.[7] Noting incomplete fill of defects, another has suggested that bone grafting may convert deep intraosseous defects into shallow ones amenable to osseous resective treatment.[8]

The success of bone grafts is not predictable. When successful, they may or may not restore all of the lost attachment or eliminate all pocket depth. Clinical evidence of reduced probing depth may be caused by a long junctional epithelium, adhesion of connective tissue fibers oriented parallel to the root surface, or a junctional epithelium interposed between bone and the root surface[9-11] rather than by the regeneration of a functional periodontal attachment complex. Nonetheless, new attachment occurs frequently enough to warrant the use of bone grafts in selected cases.[11-13] Furthermore, there is evidence that supracrestal bone formation is possible with certain bone grafting materials.[12-14]

**Definition**      A graft is a viable tissue that, after removal from a donor site, is implanted within a host tissue which is then restored, repaired, or regenerated. In the case of bone grafts the donor bone is incorporated in the healing process and remains afterward as a functioning part of the periodontium. When the transplant is bone, it does not survive indefinitely but is progressively resorbed and replaced by newly formed bone.[2] The transplant serves as a scaffold in the healing process.

## Classification

A graft is any tissue or organ used for implantation or transplantation. *Transplantation* implies surgical transfer of living tissue. The *transplant* is the tissue used. *Implantation* implies the use of nonliving tissue. An *implant* is a material inserted or grafted into intact tissue of the recipient. An *autograft* is a tissue transferred from one position to a new position in the same individual. Autogenous grafts (autografts) generally yield the best results. They do not provoke immune reactions, which can cause rejection. Periodontal autografts may be either intraoral or extraoral, depending on the site of procurement. An *allograft* is a tissue graft between individuals of the same species but with nonidentical genes. An allograft may be fresh, frozen, freeze-dried or decalcified freeze-dried. Allografts were formerly called *homografts*. A *xenograft* is a tissue graft between members of differing species. Xenografts were formerly called *heterografts*. An *alloplast* is an inert foreign body used for implantation into tissues. Calcium phosphate ceramics are examples of alloplastic implants.

**Transplant**

**Implant**

**Autograft**

**Allograft**

**Xenograft**

**Alloplast**

## Graft materials

The following materials listed and other types have been used in periodontal therapy. They can be classified as autografts, allografts, xenografts and alloplasts:

Autografts
  Cortical bone chips
  Osseous coagulum
  Bone blend (combinations of cortical and cancellous bone)
  Intraoral cancellous bone and marrow
  Extraoral cancellous bone and marrow (fresh and frozen)
Allografts
  Frozen iliac bone and marrow
  Sterilized iliac bone and marrow
  Freeze-dried bone
  Decalcified freeze-dried bone
  Merthiolated bone
  Demineralized dentin
  Lyophilized dura mater
  Sclera
  Cartilage
Xenografts
  Boplant
  Os purum
  Boiled bovine bone
  Anorganic bone
  Kiel bone
Alloplasts
  Beta tricalcium phosphate
  Hydroxylapatite
  Replamineform hydroxylapatite
  Plaster of Paris

## AUTOGRAFTS

**Cortical bone chips**

Cortical bone chips are obtained by osteoplasty and osteoectomy from sites within the surgical area. Bone fill has been reported in one- and two-wall intraosseous defects.[15] Histologic evaluation 57 months postsurgery has demonstrated replacement with new, vital bone[16] (Fig. 39-1). This type of graft has largely been replaced by osseous coagulum and bone blend techniques.

**Osseous coagulum**

For osseous coagulum, bone fragments are obtained by a round carbide bur revolving at either slow or high speed. When coated with the patient's blood these become a coagulum. Bone deformities within the surgical area such as exostoses or thick bone

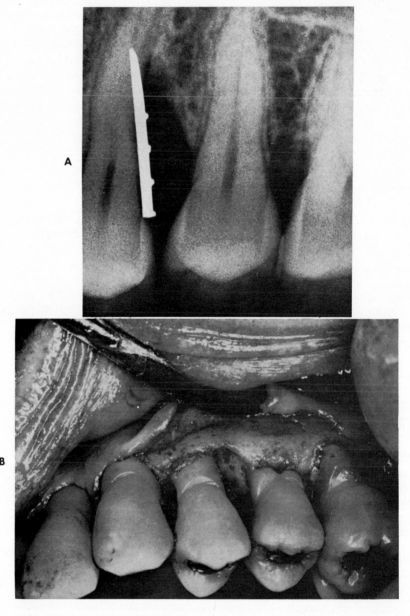

**Fig. 39-1.** **A,** Roentgenogram with a calibrated silver point illustrating the extent of the bony lesion. **B,** A modified flap has been reflected to expose a two-walled infrabony crater on the distal of the maxillary first premolar.

ledges are used as donors. The coagulum is collected and implanted directly into the bone defect. The smaller the particle size, the more certain is its resorption and replacement with new host bone.[17,18] Clinical reports suggest that many intraosseous defects can be managed with this material[17] (Fig. 39-2). The major disadvantages of osseous coagulum are the fluidity of the material, difficulty in collection and transfer, and problems in aspiration during collection. Use of a disposable filter unit is helpful.[19]

The limited amount of coagulum available has encouraged development of the bone blend technique.[20] Cortical or cancellous bone is collected from any accessible intraoral donor site, placed in a sterile amalgam capsule with a pestle, and triturated for a minimum of 10 seconds. The particle size obtained is approximately 105 to 210 μm.[21] This slushy osseous mass is then molded into the bone defect. Osseous repair has been reported[22,23] and confirmed histologically.[24,25]

**Bone blend**

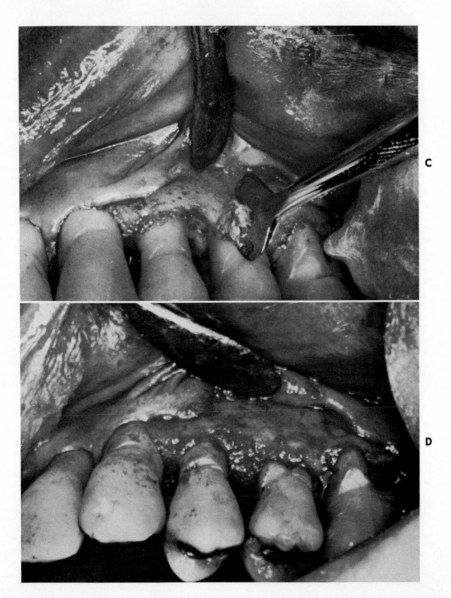

**Fig. 39-1, cont'd.   C,** Cortical bone is obtained when the alveolar surface is scraped with a Molt curette. **D,** Cortical bone scrapings (donor bone) placed in the osseous defect. The finely scraped bone particles form a mash when moistened by blood.

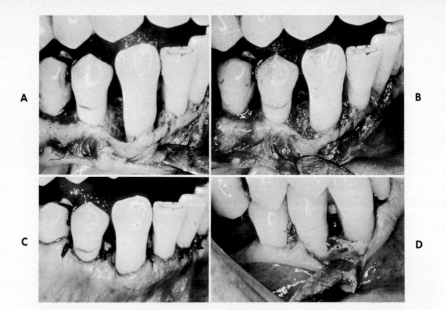

**Fig. 39-2.** **A,** Troughlike osseous crater around a tooth with grade 2 mobility. **B,** An osseous coagulum has been placed in the defect. **C,** Flap margins are coapted and sutured to place. **D,** After 6 months, bone has regenerated to eliminate the defect.

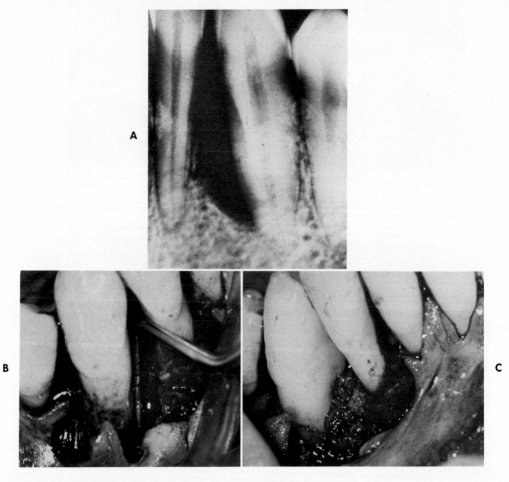

**Fig. 39-3.** **A,** Preoperative radiograph of a two-walled infrabony defect mesial of cuspid extending to within 3 mm of apex. **B,** Defect is opened and débrided of all soft tissue. Probe shows a 10-mm combination infrabony defect that becomes three-walled at its apex. **C,** Defect is filled with cancellous bone fragments taken from a molar extraction site. The molar had been extracted 7 weeks before the periodontal surgery.

Intraoral cancellous bone and marrow has been obtained from healing extraction sockets, the maxillary tuberosity, healing bone wounds, the retromolar area, and edentulous areas.[8,26-28] The healing socket can be used from 8 to 12 weeks[29] after extraction. The maxillary tuberosity, while more desirable than the remaining intraoral donor sites, may not contain much red marrow.[30] Donor material is obtained with spoon-shaped curettes or rongeurs and is fragmented before implantation. Bone repair of periodontal defects and the histologic presence of a new attachment have been reported[8,12,26-28] (Fig. 39-3).

A procedure similar to bone grafting is called *swaging* or *contiguous autogenous transplant*. It involves making a greenstick fracture of bone bordering an intraosseous defect. The bone is then displaced into the defect. Successful results have been reported but the procedure may embarrass circulation with danger of failure.[31,32]

**Intraoral cancellous bone and marrow**

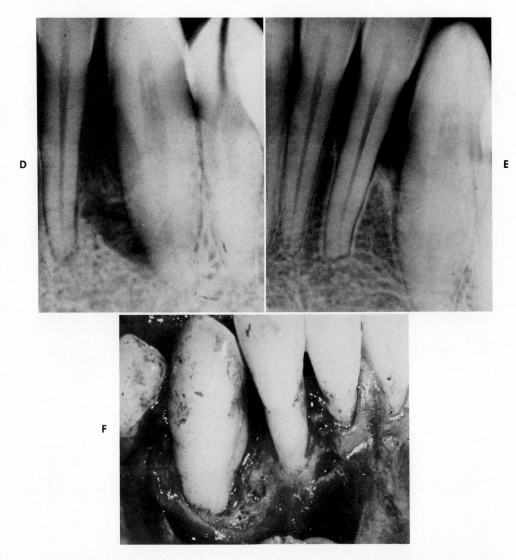

**Fig. 39-3, cont'd.** **D,** Radiograph (continuation of Fig. 39-3) 2 weeks postoperatively. Bone chips from the extraction site are in place. **E,** Radiograph 20 months postoperatively; note the formation of lamina dura and supporting bone. **F,** Reentry surgical procedure to recontour bone was performed 8 months after first procedure. Note the new bone formed on the mesial surface of the cuspid. (Courtesy E. Sugarman, Atlanta, Georgia.)

**Extraoral cancellous bone and marrow**

Iliac cancellous bone and marrow has the highest osteogenic potential.[33-35] The graft is usually obtained by a physician from either the anterior or posterior iliac crest with a biopsy needle or trephine. For short-term storage (3 hours to 1 week), the graft can be placed in Minimal Essential Medium (MEM) and refrigerated at 4° C. For longer storage (1 week to 6 months), the graft is placed in MEM with 15% to 25% glycerol and frozen.[36] Before transplantation it is rapidly thawed and fragmented. Repair of intraosseous defects of varying morphology, furcation defects, correction of a facial dehiscence, and crestal apposition of new bone and histologic new attachment have been reported[13,14,37-41] (Fig. 39-4). Iliac cancellous bone and marrow may be used either fresh or frozen. If used fresh, it should be placed in MEM, lactated Ringer's solution, or blood.[14] Iliac crest bone placed directly following acquisition may be associated with external root resorption.

## ALLOGRAFTS

The inability to obtain sufficient quantities of autogenous material at the time of surgery led to the development of several types of bone allografts.

**Frozen iliac allograft and sterilized iliac allograft**

Frozen iliac allografts are procured from donors following brain death. Extensive cross-matching between donor and recipient is necessary to reduce antigenicity. Despite such cross-matching, however, cytotoxic antibodies in the recipient have been reported.[42,43] To circumvent this potentially severe limitation, iliac allografts were ir-

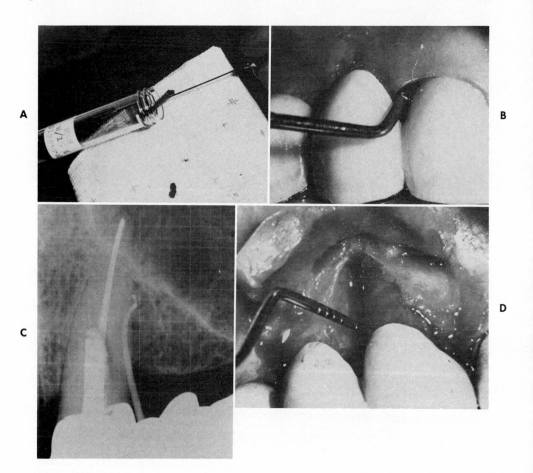

**Fig. 39-4.** **A,** Osseous core ready for implant. It was removed from the posterior iliac crest and stored in minimum essential medium with 15% glycerin. The core may be cut into small fragments. **B,** Preoperative clinical photograph of 10-mm pocket. **C,** Preoperative radiograph, with a gutta-percha point of an 8-mm infrabony defect. **D,** Defect is 7 mm from the buccal margin to the lingual margin.

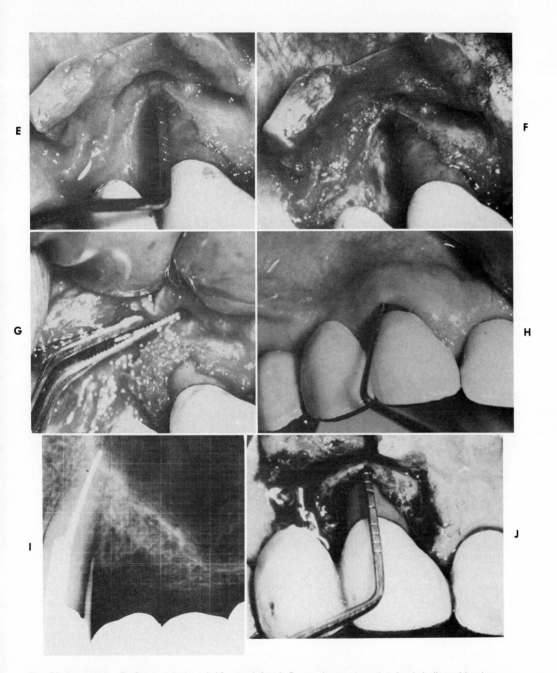

**Fig. 39-4, cont'd.** **E,** Osseous lesion. A 10-mm defect is 2 mm deeper than the depth indicated by the gutta-percha point **(C)** indicated. **F,** All soft tissue in the defect has been removed prior to grafting. **G,** Iliac crest marrow core placed into the proximal defect. **H,** One year after surgery. The clinical probing depth is 1 mm. **I,** Roentgenogram 1 year postoperatively with point in place. There is 8 mm of osseous regeneration. **J,** Reentry procedure to recontour bone 2 years after surgery shows bone regeneration and a 2-mm troughlike defect remaining. (Courtesy E. Sugarman, Atlanta, Georgia.)

radiated with 6 mega rads of gamma irradiation.[2] Although clinical and histologic results have been encouraging, the problems of antigenicity and possible disease transfer, the lag period in healing with irradiated material, and the extensive tissue bank facilities required may make these allografts impractical.

**Freeze-dried bone allograft**

Freeze-dried bone allograft is bone that has been frozen, with the water removed by sublimation in a vacuum. The allograft is usually procured and processed by a tissue bank. Recently, standards for tissue banking of allogeneic bone have been adopted.[44] The donor must be free of infectious disease, malignant disease, or diseases of unknown etiology. Tissue may be either sterile or nonsterile. A nonsterile approach requires chemical or physical sterilization, which may render the graft less desirable for human transplantation. If bone is obtained under sterile conditions, processing is begun within 24 hours of death. Cortical bone is removed and frozen in liquid nitrogen. If all bacteriologic cultures, biologic reports, serologic tests, and the results of diagnostic autopsy fail to reveal contraindications to the use of the allograft, the bone is freeze-dried. The freezing process takes approximately 14 days, during which 95% of the total water content is removed. The final product is nonviable. As a result, the freeze-dried allograft functions as a passive scaffold (osteoconduction), which is progressively replaced by new host bone. It has been demonstrated that freeze-drying markedly reduces the antigenicity of the bone allograft.[45,46] Freeze-dried bone allografts are the only periodontal grafting material that have been extensively tested.[47-49] Complete repair or greater than 50% bone repair has been reported. The addition of autogenous bone to form a composite graft significantly improves results, especially in furcation defects.[49] The addition of tetracycline to the freeze-dried bone in the treatment of patients with juvenile periodontitis is reported to enhance a "take."[50,51]

**Decalcified freeze-dried bone allograft**

Animal studies suggest that decalcified freeze-dried bone allograft is a material of high osteogenic potential.[52-54] Demineralization may be necessary because calcium is said to block the effect of the chemical-inducing agent.[55] This component of bone matrix has been called *bone morphogenetic protein (BMP)*.[56] BMP, a hydrophobic glycoprotein, apparently induces the differentiation of mesenchymal cells into osteoblasts.[57] Cortical bone contains more bone matrix and therefore more BMP than cancellous bone.[57] Successful clinical results with decalcified freeze-dried bone allograft have been reported[58-61] (Fig. 39-5). However, there is no routinely accepted method for processing this material other than demineralization in 0.6 N hydrochloric acid. Histologically, new attachment and new supracrestal bone formation have been reported[62] (Fig. 39-6).

**Other bone allografts**

Cancellous bone removed during hip surgery or from amputated limbs or ribs and stored in merthiolate solution has been used infrequently in periodontal surgery. A case report suggests that some degree of bone repair is possible.[63] It should be noted that merthiolate is toxic to host tissue. Although demineralized dentin has been advocated as a possible graft,[64] it has not gained widespread acceptance because clinical results have been somewhat disappointing.[65,66] The use of lyophilized allogeneic dura mater in periodontal osseous defects has resulted in gain of clinical (probing) attachment and reduction in probing depth. Histologically, bone has been seen alongside but never in the implant.[67] Success has been reported with preserved sclera,[68] but there were no signs of osteogenesis within the sclera and it remained encapsulated at the site.[65,69] Cartilage allografts provide no statistically significant advantage in bone or soft tissue repair over flap débridement alone.[70]

**Xenografts**

Xenografts (heterografts) used to treat human periodontal bone defects include: (1) boplant (calf bone that is detergent-extracted with chloroform-methanol, sterilized in propiolactone, and freeze-dried); (2) os purum (cow bone soaked in potassium hydroxide, acetone, and salt solution); (3) anorganic bone (cow bone extracted by

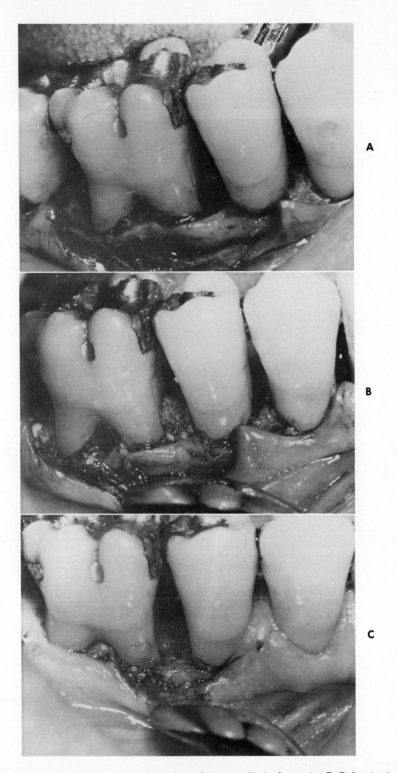

**Fig. 39-5.** **A,** A two-wall defect on the mesial surface of the mandibular first molar. **B,** Defect implanted with decalcified freeze-dried bone allograft. **C,** A six-month postoperative reentry procedure demonstrating the extent of osseous repair—minimal crestal resorption and complete resolution of the defect. (From Quintero, G., et al.: J. Periodontol. **53:**276, 1982.)

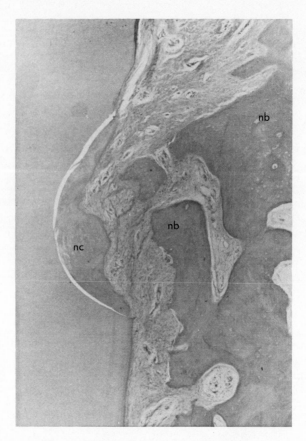

**Fig. 39-6.** One-year postoperative block section illustrating new attachment following placements of decalcified freeze-dried bone allograft. *nc,* New cementum in notch, which was placed in calculus; *(nb)* new bone, and *(pdl)* new periodontal ligament. (Courtesy of Dr. G.M. Bowers.)

means of ethylenediamine and sterilized by autoclaving); (4) boiled bone (cow bone that is boiled and autoclaved); (5) kiel bone (cow bone denatured with hydrogen peroxide, dried with acetone, and sterilized with ethylene oxide). These graft materials have had limited clinical trials.[68-75] Most are no longer used because of rejection and failure. Kiel bone may have some promise.[76] However, xenografts are generally not acceptable for human use because of possible immunologic complications.

**Alloplasts— bone substitutes**

Sterile plaster of Paris is rapidly resorbed and does not induce bone formation but is tolerated as a graft.[77] However, because plaster of Paris is so rapidly resorbed, it is questionable whether it is of any benefit.

Two types of calcium phosphate ceramics are available for clinical use: tricalcium phosphate (resorbable) and hydroxylapatite (nonresorbable).[78] The tricalcium phosphate ceramics are biocompatible and bioresorbable. Control sites heal in 4 weeks, and the ceramic implant site heals in 22 weeks.[79,80] An increase in bone height may occur.[81-83] Human biopsies most often show graft particles encapsulated in fibrous connective tissue with no new bone formation.[84] Hydroxylapatite acts as a biocompatible foreign body.[85,86] Nonetheless, significant repair of bone defects may occur with this material.[87-89] Chemically processed hydroxylapatite replamineform has been used for periodontal grafting.[90] It may have an advantage over other forms of hydroxylapatite in that it possesses a coral-like structure with a uniform pore diameter and interconnections into which new bone may grow.

The future role of the alloplastic materials has not been determined. They may serve as expanders (fillers) for either autogenous or allogeneic bone or they may be combined with bone-inductive proteins to stimulate osteogenesis.

## Indications

The indications for bone grafting include but are not limited to the following:

1. Deep intraosseous defects of varying morphology; narrow three-wall defects may be excluded because they may respond to débridement procedures alone (Fig. 39-6)
2. Shallow intraosseous defects, especially in the anterior area of the mouth where resective surgery may create an esthetic problem
3. Need for added support about critical teeth
4. Anatomic limitations that exclude other procedures
5. Furcation and shallow-wide crater defects
6. Ridge augmentation

## Clinical experience

The use of a bone graft does not ensure clinical success. A number of factors influence clinical results.[91] These factors have been divided into major and minor prerequisites. The major prerequisites include:

1. Patient selection; only medically noncompromised patients should be selected
2. Morphology of the defect; generally, the greater the number of osseous walls, the greater the amount of bone repair
3. Root preparation; meticulous root planing is indispensable
4. Type of graft; autografts are preferable to allografts and allografts are preferable to alloplasts
5. Effective plaque control
6. Patient's healing potential
7. Periodontal maintenance program, type, and frequency

The minor prerequisites are:

1. Type of flap
2. Placement of graft
3. Epithelial retardation
4. Occlusal problems and tooth mobility
5. Suture technique and flap coaptation
6. Use of antibiotics
7. Postoperative care

## Method

Bone grafting involves several steps. A sulcular or internal bevel incision is placed ½ mm from the free gingival margin. Maximum tissue preservation to facilitate primary closure and complete graft coverage is necessary. Full-thickness flaps are reflected to permit adequate visualization and instrumentation of root surfaces and bony defects. The bony defect is denuded of all soft tissue. Ultrasonic and hand instrumentation may be used to plane the root surface. The root surface should be hard, smooth, and free of detectable deposits. Some clinicians decorticate and penetrate the bone defect wall with burs to (theoretically) enhance the ingress of mesenchymal cells.

**Autograft**

A site for graft material is selected, such as an edentulous ridge, healing extraction socket, or a torus or exostosis, to obtain autogenous bone. After gaining access, bone is removed with a rongeur, curette, trephine, or bur. It is fragmented when necessary and placed into the defect to the height of the existing bony walls (Fig. 39-7). The material should be firmly packed into the defect, allowing for ingrowth of blood vessels.

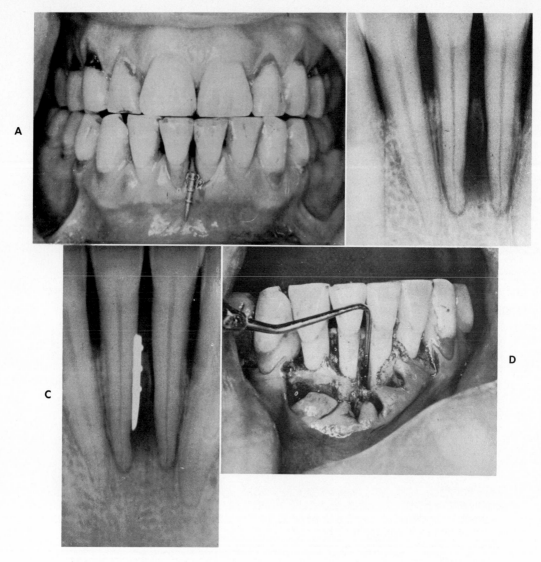

**Fig. 39-7.** **A,** Clinical appearance before bone grafting. A calibrated silver point indicates pocket depth. **B,** Roentgenogram indicates bone loss. **C,** The calibrated silver point in the pocket shows a depth of 9 mm. **D,** A modified flap is reflected to reveal a two-walled osseous defect.

**Allograft**     The advantage of an allograft is that a secondary surgical site is unnecessary and a sufficient quantity of bone is available to fill deeper or multiple sites. Cortical freeze-dried bone allograft is supplied in sterile ½ oz glass bottles. Usually each bottle contains enough bone to fill several defects. The freeze-dried bone may be reconstituted with sterile saline and inserted directly into the defect to completely fill it. Some clinicians overfill to enhance crestal apposition. However, overfilling the defect may impede adequate flap coaptation or encourage exfoliation of graft material. The interproximal papillae may gap, failing to enclose the graft. If primary closure cannot be obtained, osteoplasty of the interproximal bone may be necessary to enhance flap closure. The flaps are sutured with 4-0 or smaller suture material. An interrupted or vertical mattress suture may be used. Gentle but firm finger pressure on moistened gauze is applied to the flap for 2 or 3 minutes to maximize the blood clot. When coaptation of flap margins cannot be obtained, a free gingival graft or foil may be used to enclose the bone graft. A periodontal dressing may be placed to help protect the wound. Postoperative instruc-

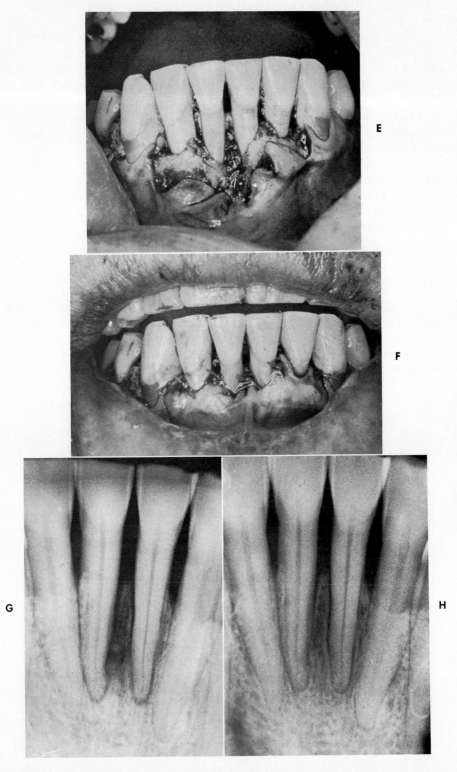

**Fig. 39-7, cont'd.   E,** Donor bone is placed in the recipient bed. **F,** The flap margins are coapted and then sutured to place. **G,** Roentgenogram showing the graft in place 1 week after surgery. **H,** Seventh-month postoperative roentgenogram. The graft has taken and the pocket is eliminated. (Courtesy J. Nabers, Wichita Falls, Texas.)

tions are given and medications prescribed. Tetracycline, 1 gm per day for 10 days beginning the day of surgery, is popular.

The patient is initially seen 1 week following surgery for dressing change, suture removal, plaque removal, and irrigation of the surgical site with saline and hydrogen peroxide. A new periodontal dressing is placed where necessary and removed the following week. Additional dressing changes are usually not necessary. The patient should resume the daily regimen for plaque control when the dressing has been removed. Chlorhexidine rinses are useful postsurgically. Biweekly postoperative visits are suggested until the regular maintenance interval is reestablished. The maintenance interval is tailored to the individual needs of the patient and is based on the level of effectiveness in plaque removal. The recall interval may vary from several weeks to months but rarely beyond 3 months. Monitoring plaque control is important. A plaque index and diagrammatic charts are beneficial motivating tools. Occlusion is reevaluated to eliminate postsurgical mobility. Radiographs of periodic probing of attachment levels are made and compared to baseline records. Short- and long-term results ultimately hinge on maintenance.

## Wound healing

In the healing sequence of an autogenous bone graft, new bone formation is seen at 7 days, cementogenesis at 21 days, and new periodontal ligament at 3 months.[13,92] By 8 months the graft should have been incorporated in the healing process with functionally oriented fibers coursing between new bone and new cementum[13,93] (Figs. 39-8, 39-9, and 39-10). However, maturation may take up to 2 years.[93]

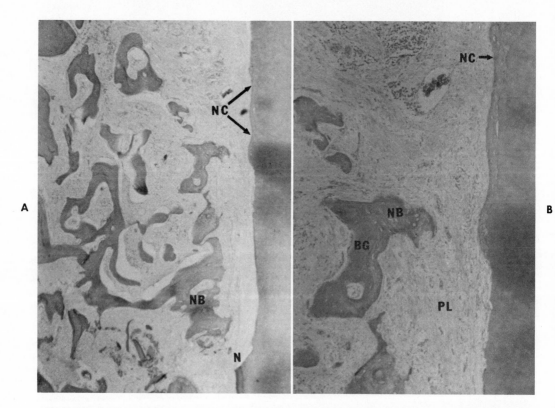

**Fig. 39-8. A,** Two-month block section illustrating new bone *(NB)* and new cementum *(NC)* above the notch *(N)*, which was placed at the base of the intrabony defect. **B,** High-power photograph of 2-month block section illustrating periodontal ligament *(PL)*, new cementum *(NC)*, and new bone *(NB)* deposited on a bone graft *(BG)*. (From Dragoo, M.R., and Sullivan, H.C.: J. Periodontol. **44:**599, 1973.)

Root resorption may follow implantation of fresh iliac cancellous bone and marrow. The resorption may extend into dentin and the pulp chamber.[14,94-96] The resorptive area may fill with new bone, producing an ankylosis. Other possible postoperative wound-healing sequelae include infection, exfoliation, tooth devitalization, prolonged healing, recurrence of the defect, exophytic granulation, and pulp necrosis.[95-97]

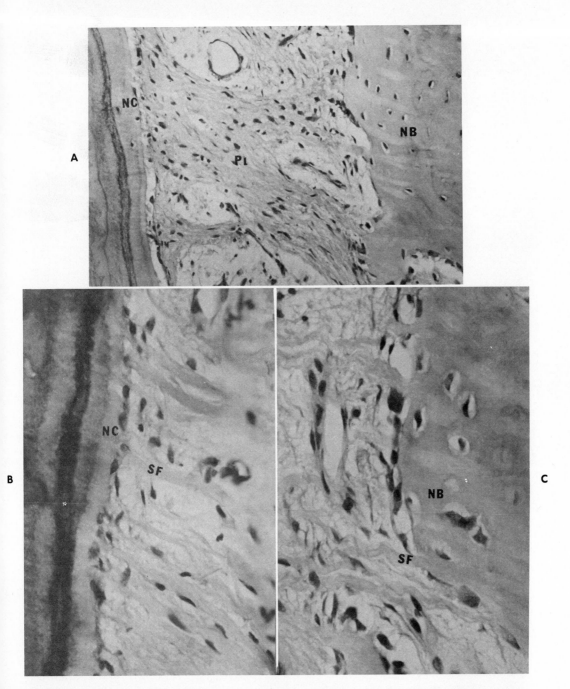

**Fig. 39-9.** **A,** Three-month block illustrating functional orientation of the periodontal ligament *(PL)*, new bone *(NB)*, and new cementum *(NC)*. **B,** Higher power photograph of 3-month block section. Note Sharpey's fibers *(SF)* embedded in new cementum *(NC)* and the presence of prominent cementoblasts. **C,** Higher power micrograph of 3-month block section. Note Sharpey's fibers *(SF)* embedded in new bone *(NB)* surrounded by osteoblasts. (From Dragoo, M.R., and Sullivan, H.C.: Periodontol. **44:**599, 1973.)

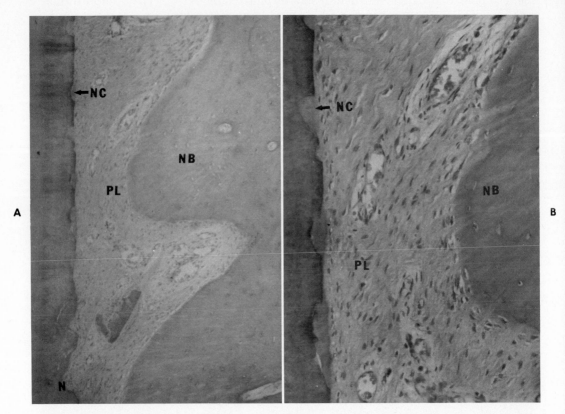

**Fig. 39-10. A,** Eight-month block section illustrating new bone *(NB)*, periodontal ligament *(PL)*, notch *(N)*, and new cementum *(NC)*. **B,** Higher power photograph of 8-month block section. Note functional orientation of new bone *(NB)*, periodontal ligament *(PL)*, and new cementum *(NC)*. (From Dragoo, M.R., and Sullivan, H.C.: J. Periodontol. **44:**599, 1973.)

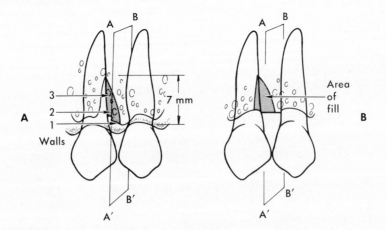

**Fig. 39-11. A,** Bony defects may show three walls at the most apical extent, then become two walled, and finally have one bony wall at the most coronal extent. Any attempt to eliminate a bony defect by ostectomy would seriously weaken the supportive tooth or teeth in the area. **B,** Ostectomy not to exceed 2 mm may be performed, and bone grafts then employed to correct the remaining osseous defect.

**Table 39-1** Grafting compared with open flap débridement in human studies

| Graft material | Results | |
| --- | --- | --- |
| | Graft | Control |
| **AUTOGRAFT** | | |
| Osseous coagulum-bone blend[23] | 2.98 mm (71%) fill | 0.66 mm (22%) fill |
| Intraoral cancellous bone and marrow[102] | 3.07 mm gain clinical attachment in two-wall, 2.35 mm in one-wall | 2.15 mm gain clinical attachment in 2-wall, 2.25 mm in 1-wall |
| Intraoral cancellous bone and marrow[27,36] | No significant difference | |
| Intraoral cancellous bone and marrow[66] | 3.2 mm gain clinical attachment | 2.0 gain clinical attachment |
| Intraoral cancellous bone and marrow, iliac cancellous bone and marrow, frozen iliac allograft[12] | Histologic new attachment consistently found | Commonly associated with lack of cementogenesis and bone formation |
| Intraoral cancellous bone and marrow, frozen iliac allograft[10] | Histologic new bone and cementum | Little if any new cementum or bone fill |
| Iliac cancellous bone and marrow[38] | Graft improved results of treatment | |
| Iliac cancellous bone and marrow[42] | 4.36 mm (61%) fill | 0.66 mm (22%) fill |
| Iliac cancellous bone and marrow[6] | 1.2 mm gain probing bone level; statistically significant only for deepest defects | 0.8 mm gain probing bone level |
| **ALLOGRAFT** | | |
| Freeze-dried bone allograft[96] | 60% of defects >50% bone fill | 60% of defects >50% bone fill |
| Freeze-dried bone allograft[51] | 1.9 mm (39%) fill | 1.0 mm (31%) fill |
| Freeze-dried bone allograft and tetracycline[51] | 2.8 mm (61%) fill | 1.4 mm (36%) fill |
| Decalcified freeze-dried bone allograft[61] | 2.57 mm (65%) fill | 1.26 mm (38%) fill |
| Decalcified freeze-dried bone allograft[60] | 1.38 mm bone fill (radiographic) | 0.33 mm bone fill (radiographic) |
| Cartilage allograft[70] | 1.0 mm gain of clinical attachment | 0.6 mm gain of clinical attachment |
| Freeze-dried dura mater allograft[65] | 1.4 mm increase in probing bone level | 0.9 mm increase in probing bone level |
| Demineralized dentin allograft[66] | 2.8 mm gain of clinical attachment | 2.0 mm gain of clinical attachment |
| **ALLOPLAST** | | |
| Hydroxylapatite (Periograf)[88] | 1.1 mm gain of clinical attachment | 0.6 mm gain of clinical attachment |
| Hydroxylapatite (Periograf)[87] | 1.7 mm bone fill | 0.5 mm bone fill |
| Hydroxylapatite (Calcitite)[89] | 3.36 mm (54%) fill of defect | 0.45 mm (20%) fill of defect |
| Hydroxylapatite (Interpore 200)[90] | 3.53 mm bone fill | 0.73 mm bone fill |

**Table 39-2** Grafting materials for repair of periodontal bone defects

| Materials | Advantages | Disadvantages | No. of defects | Mean bone repair |
|---|---|---|---|---|
| AUTOGRAFT COMPARED WITH OPEN FLAP DÉBRIDEMENT IN HUMANS | | | | |
| Cortical bone chips | Easy procurement from surgical field, complements osseous resection | Sequestration of large fragments, low osteogenic potential | 8 | No quantification, marked coronal increase in bone height reported[15] |
| Osseous coagulum-bone blend | Easy procurement, rapid technique | Extensive defects may require more graft material than technique can provide; difficult to manage material | 25 | 2.93 mm (73%) bone fill[22] |
| Intraoral cancellous bone and marrow | Relative ease of procurement, good osteogenic potential | Additional surgical procedure may be necessary; extensive defects may require more material than can be obtained | 90 / 166 / 400 | 80% of three-wall, 70% of two-wall[99] / 3.65 mm (up to 12 mm bone fill in some lesions)[27] / >50% on predictable basis[8] |
| Iliac cancellous bone and marrow | Excellent osteogenic potential, sufficient quantities for extensive defects, may be stored | Additional surgical procedure necessary, possible extensive morbidity from marrow procurement, logistic problems, additional expense, potential root resorption with fresh material | 7 / 182 | 4.36 mm (60.7%) bone fill[22] / 3.33 mm (2.54 mm bone apposition in crestal defects)[14] |
| ALLOGRAFT COMPARED WITH OPEN FLAP DÉBRIDEMENT IN HUMANS | | | | |
| Freeze-dried bone allograft (FDBA) | Tissue bank procurement, adequate material, obviates second surgical procedure to procure bone | Expense, availability, poor osteogenic potential | 97 / 189 / 272 | 64% of defects treated showed >50% bone repair[47] / 60% of defects treated showed >50% bone repair[48] / 63% of defects treated showed >50% bone repair[49] |
| Freeze-dried bone allograft and autogenous bone | Autograft expander, enhanced osteogenic potential as composite graft | Second surgical site usually necessary to procure donor bone | 109 | 80% of defects treated showed >50% bone repair[49] |
| Freeze-dried bone allograft and tetracycline | Same as for FDBA alone, enhanced osteogenic potential (?) | Evaluated in juvenile periodontitis patients only | 12 | 3.51 mm (80%) bone fill[51] |
| Decalcified freeze-dried bone allograft (DFDBA) | Tissue bank procurement, adequate material for extensive defects, good osteogenic potential | Availability, processing protocol not standardized among tissue banks, expense | 27 / 3 | 2.40 mm (65%) bone fill[59] / 4-10 mm bone fill[58] |

**Table 39-2**  Grafting materials for repair of periodontal bone defects—cont'd

| Materials | Advantages | Disadvantages | No. of defects | Mean bone repair |
|---|---|---|---|---|
| ALLOGRAFT COMPARED WITH OPEN FLAP DÉBRIDEMENT IN HUMANS—cont'd | | | | |
| Frozen iliac allo-graft | Adequate material for extensive grafting, good osteogenic potential, tissue bank procurement | Possible transmission of disease, antigen-icity, laboratory tests necessary | 194 | 3.07 mm bone fill (2.06 mm in crestal lesions)[42] |
| Sterilized iliac allo-graft | Adequate material, no disease transfer, tissue bank procurement, laboratory testing probably unnecessary | Questionable osteogenic potential, availability | 27 | 3.5 mm bone fill[2] |
| ALLOPLAST | | | | |
| Tricalcium phosphate | Availability, bone graft expander potential | Expense, negligible osteogenic potential | 10 13 | 2.8 mm bone fill[81] 1.8 mm (radiographic) bone fill[84] |

## Graft vs. nongraft regenerative procedures

Some grafts produce remarkably successful results ( Fig. 39-11), while others give results no different from open curettage. A graft may simply act as an agent to prevent the downgrowth of junctional epithelium.[7,67] Grafting may convert a deep bony defect into a shallow one that is later amenable to ostectomy and osteoplasty.[8] Open curettage may repair a bony defect.[98-100] However, the results are unpredictable and fill may not occur. Open curettage alone may result in about 1.0 mm of alveolar crestal resorption and 1.0 mm of bone fill.[101] A comparison of bone grafting and open flap curettage (control) indicates that both interventions may produce bone fill. In most studies, however, the graft is superior[102,103] to the control and the control never achieves greater fill than the graft (Table 39-1).

### ADVANTAGES AND DISADVANTAGES

The advantages and limitations of the various grafting materials as well as reported levels of bone repair are presented in Tables 39-1 and 39-2. Note that bone fill or clinical attachment gain is not necessarily equivalent with the histologic demonstration of gain of attachment (i.e., new bone, ligament, and cementum).

## Summary

The future realization of periodontal reconstruction may depend on the implantation of a substance with a high potential for osteoblastic formation. Only controlled experiments will be able to determine the proper biologic additive that will not only grow bone but also stimulate the formation of the highly specialized periodontal apparatus and eliminate the possibility of root resorption. Root conditioning may be another element to encourage colonization of the root surface by fibroblasts and impede proliferation of epithelium. Inert membranes ( guided tissue regeneration) may impede epithelial proliferation and encourage periodontal ligament cell ingrowth into the defect (see Chapter 37). The grafting of bone for restoring lost bone is a feasible operation. Autogenous cancellous bone offers the best opportunity for success. However, the procedure requires careful case selection, precise instrumentation, and proper postoperative care for best results.

## REFERENCES

1. Zander, H.A, Polson, A.M., and Heijle, C.D.: Goals of periodontal therapy, J. Periodontol. **47:**261, 1976.
2. Schallhorn, R.G.: Present status of osseous grafting procedures, J. Periodontol. **48:**570, 1977.
3. Bowers, G.M., Schallhorn, R.G., and Mellonig, J.T.: Histologic evaluation of new attachment in human intrabony defects: a literature review, J. Periodontol. **53:**509, 1982.
4. Gara, G.G., and Adams, D.F.: Implant therapy in human intrabony pockets: a review of the literature, J. West. Soc. Periodont. Abstr. **29:**32, 1981.
5. Ramfjord, S.P.: Changing concepts in periodontics, J. Prosthet Dent. **52:**781, 1984.
6. Renvert, S., et al.: Healing after treatment of periodontal osseous defects. III. Effect of osseous grafting and citric acid conditioning, J. Clin. Periodontol. **12:**441, 1985.
7. Melcher, A.H.: On the repair potential of periodontal tissues, J. Periodontol. **47:**256, 1976.
8. Rosenberg, M.M.: Free osseous tissue autografts as a predictable procedure, J. Periodontol. **42:**195, 1971.
9. Stahl, S.S.: Repair potential of the soft tissue-root interface, J. Periodontol. **48:**545, 1977.
10. Listgarten, M.A., and Rosenberg, M.M.: Histological study of repair following new attachment procedures in human periodontal lesions, J. Periodontol. **50:**333, 1979.
11. Moskow, B.S., Karsh, F., and Stein, S.D.: Histological assessment of autogenous bone graft: a case report and critical evaluation, J. Periodontol. **50:**291, 1979.
12. Hiatt, W.H., Schallhorn, R.G., and Aaronian, A.J.: The induction of new bone and cementum formation. IV. Microscopic examination of the periodontium following human bone and marrow autograft, allograft, and nongraft periodontal regenerative procedures, J. Periodontol. **46:**495, 1978.
13. Dragoo, M.R., and Sullivan, H.C.: A clinical and histologic evaluation of autogenous iliac bone grafts in humans. I. Wound healing 2 to 8 months, J. Periodontol. **44:**599, 1973.
14. Schallhorn, R.G., Hiatt, W.H., and Boyce, W.: Iliac transplants in periodontal therapy, J. Peridontol. **41:**566, 1970.
15. Nabers, C.L., and O'Leary, T.J.: Autogenous bone transplants in the treatment of osseous defects, J. Periodontol. **36:**5, 1965.
16. Nabers, C.L., Reed, O.M., and Hammer, J.E.: Gross and histologic evaluation of an autogenous bone graft 57 months postoperatively, J. Periodontol. **43:**702, 1972.
17. Robinson, R.E.: Osseous coagulum for bone induction, J. Periodontol. **40:**503, 1969.
18. Rivault, A.F., et al.: Autogenous bone grafts: osseous coagulum and osseous retrograde procedures in primates, J. Periodontol. **42:**787, 1971.
19. Hutchinson, R.A.: Osseous coagulum collection filter, J. Periodontol. **44:**688, 1973.
20. Diem, C.R., Bowers, G.M., and Moffitt, W.C.: Bone blending: a technique for osseous implants, J. Periodontol. **43:**295, 1972.
21. Zanner, D.J., and Yukna, R.A.: Particle size of periodontal bone grafting materials, J. Periodontol. **55:**406, 1984.
22. Froum, S.J., et al.: Osseous autografts. I. Clinical responses of bone blend or hip marrow grafts, J. Periodontol. **46:**516, 1975.
23. Froum, S.J., et al.: Osseous autografts. III. Comparison of osseous coagulum-bone blend implants with open curettage, J. Periodontol. **47:**287, 1976.
24. Froum, S.J., et al.: Osseous autografts. II. Histologic responses to osseous coagulum-bone blend grafts, J. Periodontol. **46:**656, 1975.
25. Froum, S.J., Kushner, L., and Stahl, S.S.: Healing responses of human intraosseous lesions following the use of débridement, grafting and citric acid root treatment. I. Clinical and histologic observations six months postsurgery, J. Periodontol. **54:**67, 1983.
26. Halliday, D.G.: The grafting of newly formed autogenous bone in the treatment of osseous defects. J. Periodontol. **40:**511, 1969.
27. Hiatt, W.H., and Schallhorn, R.G.: Intraoral transplants of cancellous bone and marrow in periodontal lesions, J. Periodontol. **44:**194, 1973.
28. Ross, S.E., and Cohen, D.W.: The fate of a free osseous tissue autograft: a clinical and histologic case report, Periodontics **6:**145, 1968.
29. Evian, C.I., et al.: The osteogenic activity of bone removed from healing extraction sockets in humans, J. Periodontol. **53:**81, 1982.
30. Kucaba, W.J., and Simpson, D.M.: Incidence and distribution of hematopoietic marrow in human maxillary tuberosity, J. Dent. Res. (Special Issue A) **57:**141, 1978.
31. Ewen, S.J.: Bone swaging, J. Periodontol. **36:**57, 1965.
32. Ross, S.E., Malamed, E.H., and Amsterdam, M.: The contiguous autogenous transplant: its rationale, indications and technique, Periodontics **4:**246, 1966.
33. Amler, M.H.: The effectiveness of regenerating versus mature marrow in physiologic autogenous transplants, J. Periodontol. **55:**268, 1984.
34. Bierly, J.A., et al.: An evaluation of the osteogenic potential of marrow, J. Periodontol. **46:**277, 1975.
35. Cushing, M.: Autogenous red marrow grafts: potential for induction of osteogenesis, J. Periodontol. **40:**492, 1969.
36. Schallhorn, R.G.: Osseous grafts in the treatment of periodontal osseous defects. In Stahl, S.S., editor: Periodontal surgery: biologic ba-

sis and technique. Springfield, Ill. 1976, Charles C Thomas.

37. Haggerty, P.C., and Maeda, I.: Autogenous bone grafts: a revolution in the treatment of vertical bone defects, J. Periodontol. **42:**626, 1971.

38. Patur, B.: Osseous defects: evaluation of diagnostic and treatment methods, J. Periodontol. **45:**523, 1974.

39. Schallhorn, R.G.: Eradication of bifurcation defects utilizing frozen autogenous hip marrow implants, J. West. Soc. Periodontol. **15:**101, 1967.

40. Schallhorn, R.G.: The use of autogenous hip marrow biopsy implants for bony crater defects, J. Periodontol. **39:**145, 1968.

41. Seibert, J.S.: Reconstructive periodontal surgery: case report, J. Periodontol. **41:**113, 1970.

42. Schallhorn, R.G., and Hiatt, W.H.: Human allografts of iliac cancellous bone and marrow in periodontal osseous defects. II. Clinical observations, J. Periodontol. **43:**67, 1972.

43. Hiatt, W.H., and Schallhorn, R.G.: Human allografts of iliac cancellous bone and marrow in periodontal osseous defects. I. Rationale and methodology, J. Periodontol. **42:**642, 1971.

44. American Association of Tissue Banks: Standards for tissue banking, 1984, Arlington, Va.

45. Friedlaender, G.E., et al.: Studies on the antigenicity of bone. I. Freeze-dried and deep frozen bone allografts in rabbits, J. Bone Joint Surg. **58A:**854, 1976.

46. Turner, D.W., and Mellonig, J.T.: Antigenicity of freeze-dried bone allograft in periodontal osseous defects, J. Periodontol. Res. **16:**89, 1981.

47. Mellonig, J.T., et al.: Clinical evaluation of freeze-dried bone allograft in periodontal osseous defects, J. Periodontol. **47:**125, 1976.

48. Sepe, W.W., et al.: Clinical evaluation of freeze-dried bone allografts in periodontal osseous defects. Part II. J. Periodontol. **49:**9, 1978.

49. Sanders, J.J., et al.: Clinical evaluation of freeze-dried bone allograft in periodontal osseous defects. III. Composite freeze-dried bone allografts with and without autogenous bone grafts, J. Periodontol. **54:**1, 1983.

50. Yukna, R.A., and Sepe, W.W.: Clinical evaluation of localized periodontosis defects treated with freeze-dried bone allografts combined with local and systemic tetracycline, Int. J. Periodont. Rest. Dent. **2**(5):9, 1982.

51. Mabry, T.W., Yukna, R.A., and Sepe, W.W.: Freeze-dried bone allografts combined with tetracycline in the treatment of juvenile periodontitis, J. Periodontol. **56:**74, 1985.

52. Urist, M.R.: Bone formation by autoinduction, Science **150:**893, 1965.

53. Urist, M.R., et al.: Inductive substrates for bone formation. Clin. Orthop. **59:**59, 1968.

54. Mellonig, J.T., Bowers, G.M., and Baily, R.C.: Comparison of bone graft materials. I. New bone formation with autogenous autografts and allografts determined by strontium-85, J. Periodontol. **52:**291, 1981.

55. Urist, M.R., and Strates, B.S.: Bone formation in implants of partially and wholly demineralized bone matrix, Clin. Orthop. **71:**271, 1970.

56. Urist, M.R., and Strates, B.S.: Bone morphogenetic protein, J. Dent. Res. **50:**1392, 1972.

57. Urist, M.R., and Twata, H.: Preservation and biodegradation of the morphogenetic property of bone matrix, J. Theor. Biol. **38:**155, 1973.

58. Libin, B.M., Ward, H.L., and Fishman, L.: Decalcified, lyophilized bone allograft for use in human periodontal defects, J. Periodontol. **46:**51, 1975.

59. Quintero, G., et al.: A six-month clinical evaluation of decalcified freeze-dried bone allograft in human periodontal defects, J. Periodontol. **53:**726, 1982.

60. Pearson, G.E., Rosen, S., and Deporter, D.H.: Preliminary observations on the usefulness of a decalcified freeze-dried cancellous abone allograft material in periodontal surgery, J. Periodontol. **52:**55, 1981.

61. Mellonig, J.T.: Decalcified freeze-dried bone allograft as an implant material in human periodontal defects, Int. J. Periodont. Rest. Dent. **4**(6):41, 1984.

62. Bowers, G.M., et al.: Histologic evaluation of new attachment in humans, J. Periodontol. **56:**381, 1985.

63. Haggerty, P.C.: Human allografts—the efficient therapeutic approach to the infrabony defect, J. Periodontol. **48:**743, 1977.

64. Register, A.A., et al.: Human bone induction by allogeneic dentin matrix, J. Periodontol. **43:**459, 1972.

65. Dragoo, M.R.: Clinical and histologic evaluation of alloplasts and allografts in regenerative periodontal surgery in humans, Int. J. Periodont. Rest. Dent. **3**(2):8, 1983.

66. Movin, S., and Borring-Moller, G.: Regeneration of infrabony periodontal defects in humans after implantation of allogeneic demineralized dentin, J. Clin. Periodontol. **9:**141, 1982.

67. Busschop, J., and De Boever, J.: Clinical and histologic characteristics of lyophilized allogeneic dura mater in periodontal bony defects in humans, J. Clin. Periodontol. **10:**399, 1983.

68. Klingsberg, J.: Periodontal scleral grafts and combined grafts of sclera and bone: two-year appraisal, J. Periodontol. **45:**262, 1974.

69. Feingold, J.P., et al.: Preserved scleral allografts in periodontal defects in man—histologic evaluation, J. Periodontol. **48:**4, 1977.

70. Chodroff, R.E., and Ammons, W.F.: Periodontal repair after surgical débridement

with and without cartilage allografts, J. Clin. Periodontol. **11:**295, 1984.

71. Beube, F.E., and Silvers, H.F.: Further studies on bony ageneration with the use of boiled heterogenous bone, J. Periodontol. **7:** 17, 1936.

72. Beube, F.E.: A radiographic and histologic study on reattachment, J. Periodontol. **23:** 158, 1952.

73. Cross, W.G.: Bone implants in periodontal disease—a further study, J. Periodontol. **28:**184, 1957.

74. Forsberg, H.: Transplantation of os purum and bone chips in the surgical treatment of periodontal disease (preliminary report), Acta Odontol. Scand. **13:**235, 1956.

75. Scopp, I.W., et al.: Bovine (boplant) implants for infrabony oral lesions, Periodontics **4:**169, 1966.

76. Nielson, I.M., Ellegaard, B., and Karring, T.: Kiel bone in new attachment attempts in humans, J. Periodontol. **52:**723, 1981.

77. Shaffer, C.D., and App, G.R.: The use of plaster of Paris in treating infrabony periodontal defects in humans, J. Periodontol. **42:**685, 1971.

78. Han, T., Carranza, F.A., and Kenney, E.B.: Calcium phosphate ceramics in dentistry, J. West. Soc. Periodontol. **32:**88, 1984.

79. Levin, M.P., et al.: Biodegradable ceramic in periodontal defects, Oral Surg. **38:**344, 1974.

80. Levin, M.P., et al.: Healing of periodontal defects with ceramic implants, J. Clin. Periodontol. **1:**197, 1974.

81. Snyder, A.J., Levin, M.P., and Cutright, D.E.: Alloplastic implants of tricalcium phosphate ceramic in human periodontal osseous defects, J. Periodontol. **55:**273, 1984.

82. Nery, E.B., and Lynch, K.L.: Preliminary clinical studies of bioceramic in periodontal osseous defects, J. Periodontol. **49:**523, 1978.

83. Strub, J.R., Gaberthuel, T.W., and Firestone, A.R.: Comparison of tricalcium phosphate and frozen allogeneic bone implants in man, J. Periodontol. **50:**624, 1979.

84. Baldock, W.T., et al.: An evaluation of tricalcium phosphate implants in human periodontal osseous defects of two patients, J. Periodontol. **56:**1, 1985.

85. Froum, S.J., et al.: Human clinical and histologic responses to Durapatite implants in intraosseous lesions, J. Periodontol. **53:**719, 1982.

86. Moskow, B.S., and Lubarr, A.: Histologic assessment of human periodontal defect after durapatite ceramic implant: report of a case, J. Periodontol. **54:**455, 1983.

87. Rabalais, M.L., Yukna, R.A., and Mayer, E.T.: Evaluation of Durapatite ceramic as an alloplastic implant in periodontal osseous defects. I. Initial six-month results, J. Periodontol. **52:**680, 1981.

88. Yukna, R.A., Mayer, E.T., and Brite, D.V.: Longitudinal evaluation of Durapatite ceramic as an alloplastic implant in periodontal osseous defects after three years, J. Periodontol. **55:**633, 1984.

89. Meffert, R.M., et al.: Hydroxylapatite as an alloplastic graft in the treatment of human periodontal osseous defects, J. Periodontol. **56:**63, 1985.

90. Kenney, E.B., et al.: The use of a porous hydroxylapatite implant in periodontal defects. I. Clinical results after six months, J. Periodontol. **56:**82, 1985.

91. Schallhorn, R.G.: Long-term evaluation of osseous grafts in periodontal therapy, Int. Dent. J. **30:**109, 1980.

92. Dragoo, M.R.: Clinical and histologic evaluation of autogenous bone grafts, J. Periodontol. (Abst). **44:**123, 1972.

93. Sullivan, H.C., and Dragoo, M.R.: Regenerative techniques in periodontal therapy, Dent. Clin. North Am. **20:**131, 1976.

94. Dragoo, M.R., and Sullivan, H.C.: A clinical and histologic evaluation of autogenous iliac bone grafts in humans. II. External root resorption, J. Periodontol. **44:**614, 1973.

95. Hoffman, I.D., and Flanagan, P.: Exophytic granulation reactions associated with autogenous iliac marrow transplantation into periodontal defects, J. Periodontol. **45:**586, 1974.

96. Burnette, E.W.: Fate of the iliac graft, J. Periodontol. **43:**88, 1972.

97. Schallhorn, R.G.: Postoperative problems associated with iliac transplants, J. Periodontol. **43:**3, 1972.

98. Ellegaard, B., and Löe, H.: New attachment of periodontal tissues after treatment of intrabony lesions, J. Periodontol. 42:648, 1971.

99. Polson, A.M., and Heijle, L.D.: Osseous repair in infrabony periodontal defects, J. Clin. Periodontol. **5:**13, 1978.

100. Rosling, B., et al.: The healing potential of the periodontal tissues following different techniques of periodontal surgery in plaque-free dentitions, J. Clin. Periodontol. **3:**233, 1976.

101. Froum, S.J., et al.: Periodontal healing following open débridement flap procedures. I. Clinical assessment of soft tissue and osseous repair, J. Periodontol. **53:**8, 1982.

102. Carraro, J., Sznajder, N., and Alonso, C.A.: Intraoral cancellous bone autografts in the treatment of infrabony pockets, J. Clin. Periodontol. **3:**104, 1976.

103. Altiere, E.T., Reeve, C.M., and Sheridan, P.J.: Lyophilized bone allografts in periodontal osseous defects, J. Periodontol. **50:**510, 1979.

# CHAPTER **40**

# Mucogingival surgery

**Definitions**
Functional zone of gingiva

**Etiology of problems**

**Indications and objectives**

**Surgical techniques**
Free gingival graft
Free connective tissue autograft
Freeze-dried skin allografts
Pedicle grafts
Frenum procedures

## Definitions

Mucogingival surgery consists of procedures that are designed for the following purposes:

1. To create a widened zone of gingiva
2. To retain such a zone after a pocket has been eliminated
3. To prevent or to remedy gingival defects produced by recession
4. To alter the position of or to eliminate a frenum pull where the band of gingiva is narrow
5. To deepen the vestibule where it is associated with too narrow a zone of gingiva

### FUNCTIONAL ZONE OF GINGIVA

A "functionally adequate" zone of gingiva is defined as one that is keratinized, firmly bound to tooth and underlying bone, and resistant to probing and gaping when the lip is distended.

The gingiva bound to tooth and bone contains cornified (keratinized) epithelium and a lamina propria of dense, well-organized fiber bundles with few elastic fibers. It is firmly joined to the root of the tooth and to bone. It is structured to withstand the frictional stresses of mastication and brushing. *Gingiva*

The alveolar mucosa, on the other hand, functions as a lining tissue; it has a thin, nonkeratinized epithelium, is loosely textured, has elastic fibers in the mucosa and submucosa, and is loosely bound to the periosteum of the alveolar bone. The alveolar mucosa appears to be well adapted to permit movement but not frictional stresses.[1] *Alveolar mucosa*

The narrowest band of gingiva is found on the facial surfaces of the canines and first bicuspids and the lingual surfaces of the mandibular incisors.[2] Narrow gingival zones may occur also at the mesiobuccal root of maxillary first molars, associated with prominent roots and sometimes with bony dehiscences, and at the mandibular third molars.

Since recession and narrow zones of gingiva are interrelated and one may lead to the other, the presumption that a narrow gingiva is more vulnerable to recession has not stood up to scientific scrutiny. Nonetheless surgery to restore the width of the gingiva may be advisable in some cases. Recession is cosmetically and otherwise disturbing to some patients.

883

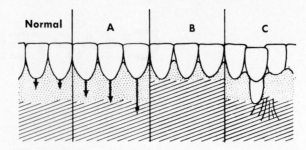

**Fig. 40-1.** Diagram of mucogingival problems. **A,** Pockets that do not encroach on the mucogingival junction can be treated by an apically positioned flap or by open subgingival curettage and a replaced flap; **B,** pockets encroaching on the mucogingival junction with little or no gingiva can be treated with a free gingival graft; **C,** recession to the mucogingival junction can be treated with either a laterally positioned flap or a free gingival graft along with a frenectomy.

Mucogingival problems requiring treatment may develop as a consequence of bone loss and pocket formation in periodontitis or may develop where some teeth had little or no gingiva from the time of eruption (Fig. 40-1, *B*). Such problems may or may not require treatment. Treatment will be necessary when bone loss and recession occur in a mouth that has little or no gingiva or where the gingiva present has receded owing to cleft formation. It is believed that clefts occur when proliferating oral and sulcular epithelia fuse and a cleft or recession then results from minor wounding (e.g., toothbrush abrasion).

Although mucogingival procedures are not primarily excisional, they may be combined with procedures designed to reduce probing depth (i.e., osseous resection, bone grafts, and new attachment operations). Much of mucogingival surgery is concerned with problems that center around the position of the gingiva and the alveolar mucosa and, in turn, their relationship to the root and crown of the tooth.[2-12]

The width of gingiva that is attached to root is determined by measuring with a periodontal probe from the margin of the gingiva to the mucogingival junction and subtracting the sulcus or pocket depth (Fig. 40-1). The precise minimal number of millimeters that is functionally adequate has not been established, and in some cases patients do well without a keratinized gingiva. An "inadequate" zone of gingiva is said to exist when its width is not great enough to withstand recession in the opinion of the dentist. Lang and Löe[2] concluded that "2 mm of keratinized gingiva is adequate to maintain gingival health." The use of the 2-mm figure as a guideline for determining "adequacy" is questionable.

Recession may occur in susceptible areas even in elderly patients. When a narrow band of attached gingiva is present, the position of the margin and the mucogingival junction, the probing depth of the sulcus, and the number of millimeters of recession should be recorded. If recession progresses, grafting should be considered. If the condition can be documented as stable, grafting may be unnecessary.

The width of gingiva may be constant in health. However, in disease, as pockets deepen or gingiva recedes, the pocket eventually encroaches on the mucogingival junction.

Inflammation seems more evident when the gingiva is very narrow (see Fig. 40-1) than when the gingiva is of normal dimension. There may be increased plaque accumulation leading to increased inflammation.[2] Inflammation may secondarily lead to further plaque accumulation, food impingement, and retention, all of which can result in pocket formation and further recession. As a result the marginal tissue may become poorly suited to withstand trauma (e.g., toothbrushing).

Margins of alveolar mucosa may occasionally remain stable, particularly in molar regions. However, width is not the only measure of adequacy. A functionally adequate

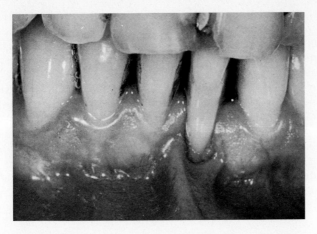

**Fig. 40-2.** Frenum pull in a lower central incisor. Note the prominence of the root.

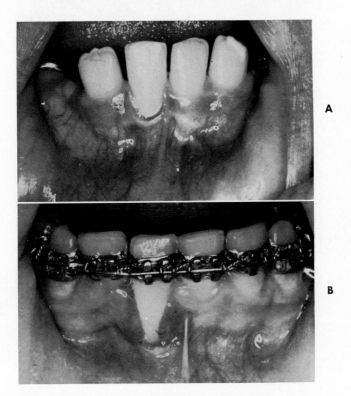

**Fig. 40-3.** Individual gingival recession in two brothers, **A,** 9 years old and, **B,** 13 years old. (Courtesy W.B. Hall, San Francisco, California.)

zone of gingiva is one that does not gape under pull and will remain in health without further recession.[5-7] Pull is gauged by extending the lips and cheeks by pulling on them and thus stretching the mucosa[5-7] (Figs. 40-2 and 40-3) and frenula. If the gingival margin moves or blanches, the frenum may contribute to the recession.

## Etiology of problems

Mucogingival problems may be the result of the following:

1. *Tooth malposition.* Some problems of inadequate gingival width relate to malposition and crowding of teeth.[11] Teeth that are lingually or labially malpositioned will have a narrower

band of gingiva on their prominent surface (Figs. 40-2 and 40-3). Prominent roots may contribute to the etiology.

2. *Developmental anomalies.* These include (a) lack of gingiva, (b) high frenum, and (c) shallow vestibule. A tooth may erupt without gingiva. The frenum may develop close to the gingival margin, or a shallow vestibule may be present.

3. *Pocket formation.* Pockets may extend to and beyond the mucogingival junction.

4. *Recession related to inflammation, trauma, toothbrush abrasion, or food impaction* (Figs. 40-4 and 40-5). Dental procedures can be irritating and produce recession.[13] When crowns, bridges, splints, or partial dentures are made, there should be adequate gingiva. A crown's margin should be nonirritating and should end at or above the gingival margin. The same is true for class V restorations (Fig. 40-6). Preparatory procedures (rubber dam clamps, burs, chisels) may produce trauma. During full-crown preparations, trauma may be caused by high-speed burs and diamonds, impression procedures, cord packing, and electrocautery. Clasps of partial dentures may traumatize the gingiva of abutment teeth

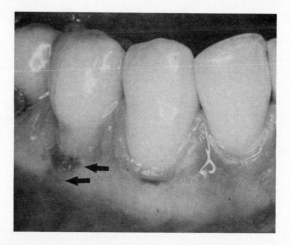

**Fig. 40-4.** Repeated toothbrush injury has produced gingival recession. The traumatized tissue is evident. A shallow pocket extends beyond the mucogingival junction.

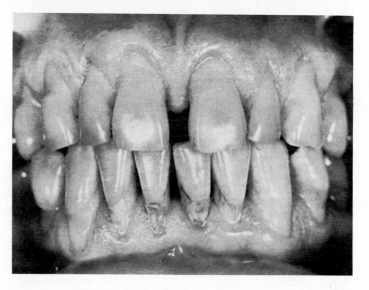

**Fig. 40-5.** Recession of the gingiva and abrasion of the teeth brought about by overly vigorous and incorrect brushing or the use of a brush with sharp, hard bristles. Note the narrow zone of gingiva at the mandibular right canine. Extensive cervical abrasion is present in the incisors, the canine, and the first premolar.

(Fig. 40-7). Lingual bars of partial dentures may compress the gingiva (Figs. 40-7 and 40-8). Improperly constructed night guards can impinge on gingival margins and cause recession. Overdentures can traumatize the gingival tissue of the abutment teeth. Trauma sometimes is produced by orthodontic bands. If the gingiva is too thin and too narrow before treatment, these traumatic events may produce recession.

5. *Periodontal surgery.* Excisional surgery (gingivectomy) may result in a diminished and sometimes inadequate gingival width.

6. *Orthodontic tooth movement.* At times bone dehiscences and gingival recession follow orthodontics (Fig. 40-9). If the problem is present before orthodontic movement, corrective surgery should be performed beforehand. Bands may be irritating to a thin gingiva and may produce recession. A tooth may be moved too far lingually or labially and thus be followed by recession.

## Indications and objectives

The indications for and the objectives of mucogingival surgery follow:

1. To eliminate pockets extending to or beyond the mucogingival junction
2. To cover roots exposed by recession
3. To add to gingiva of diminished width

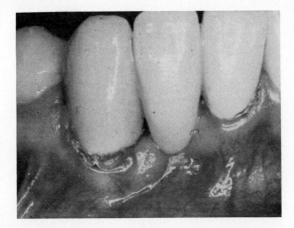

**Fig. 40-6.** Inflamed, receded gingival margin apical to an inadequate margin on a ceramic crown.

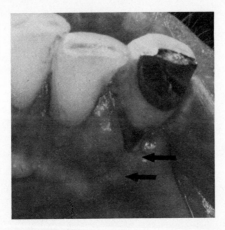

**Fig. 40-7.** Pressure from a lingual bar of a partial denture has produced soft tissue and bone fenestration. The gingival margin has receded.

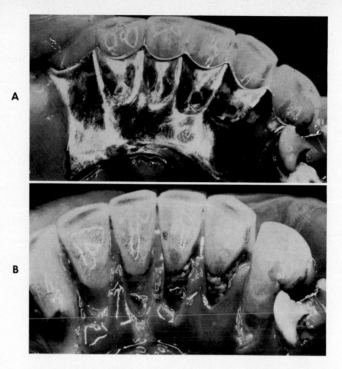

**Fig. 40-8.** **A,** Lower partial denture with lingual apron. The apron presses against the gingival margins. **B,** Denture removed. The gingiva has receded owing to the settling metal apron.

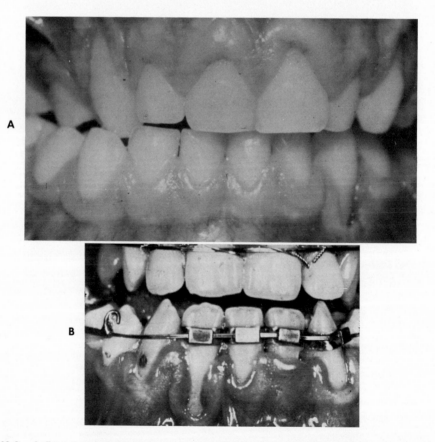

**Fig. 40-9.** **A,** Extensive gingival recession over the maxillary canines and the mandibular left canine is seen after the orthodontic bands are removed. Blunted, fibrotic gingival margins are seen throughout. **B,** Recession of the gingiva brought about during orthodontic therapy when a tooth was removed too rapidly or too far in a labial direction.

4. To create a gingival form resistant to damage from the patient's home care procedures
5. To replace alveolar mucosa adjacent to the gingival margin by gingiva
6. To stop gaping of gingival pockets caused by frenum pull

If mucogingival conditions are to be treated, one must take the following factors into consideration:

**Clinical judgment**

1. Cause of the recession
2. Treatment plan and prognosis
3. Quality of previous dental treatment and home care
4. Age of patient
5. Cosmetics
6. Root sensitivity

For instance, in cases in which dental restorations are poor and patient motivation toward improved care is lacking, one would not correct gingival width. Surgery should be performed only if the patient has a history of good home care or demonstrates improvement. Do not consider surgery for the patient who cannot or will not cooperate.

The need for surgery may be questioned where a narrow zone of gingiva has persisted for years without receding. Unless restorative needs demand more gingiva, the tissue may require only special oral hygiene (soft toothbrush, low abrasive quality, and nontraumatic stroke).

## Surgical techniques

The following outline includes present and previous techniques:

1. Free grafts
   A. Gingival including epithelium[13-54]
   B. Connective tissue[55-64]
   C. Freeze-dried skin homografts[65-72]
2. Pedicle grafts
   A. Laterally positioned[73-95]
   B. Rotated papilla
      1. Single papilla[75]
      2. Double papilla[79,96]
3. Coronally positioned flaps[62,90,97-104]
4. Apically positioned flaps[105-118]
5. Frenectomy, frenotomy[83,119-124]
6. Vestibular extension[125-142]
   A. Periosteal retention
   B. Periosteal fenestration
   C. Denudation

### FREE GINGIVAL GRAFT

The free gingival graft is used to create or to increase the width of gingiva on either buccal or lingual surfaces[13-47] (Fig. 40-10). It can also be used to cover root surfaces (preferably those with a narrow denudation) and in some instances to correct frenum problems[124] and to extend the vestibule.[16,17]

Absence of an adequate band of gingiva is not necessarily by itself an indication for a free gingival graft. Other factors must be considered before making a decision including the fact that further recession may not occur.[143-146]

The procedure is almost always successful when used to augment the zone of gingiva (Fig. 40-11). A free gingival graft may be used *therapeutically* to widen the gingiva after recession has occurred. It has been used prophylactically to prevent

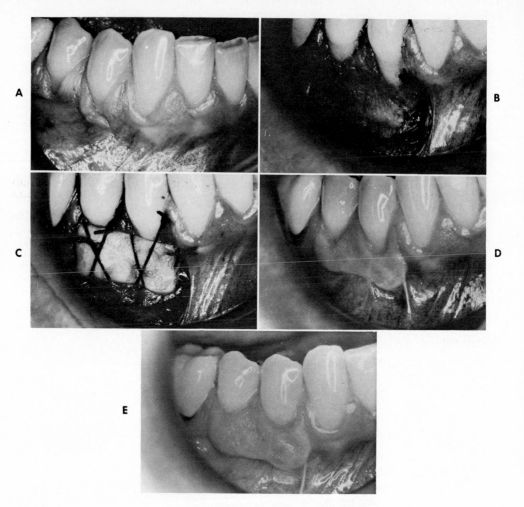

**Fig. 40-10.** **A,** Almost complete absence of gingiva on buccal side of mandibular premolars. Band of gingiva bordering canine is very narrow. **B,** Epithelium and connective tissue are dissected away, leaving a thin covering of connective tissue and periosteum. **C,** Palatal donor tissue is sutured to place at recipient site. In this instance two retention sutures secure the graft. **D,** Postoperative result, showing increased width of gingiva. **E,** Two years later creeping attachment has further increased the width of gingiva. (Courtesy I. Speckman, Mexico City, Mexico.)

further recession where the band of gingiva is narrow and of a thin, delicate consistency. In some instances it may also be used when fillings, crown fillings, crowns, or orthodontic bands will contact a narrow, thin gingiva.[2,147,148] The evidence in support of prophylactic grafting is not convincing.

Free gingival grafts to cover denuded roots may or may not yield a completely successful result. Partial root coverage can occur. The graft may be used to correct localized, one-surface, narrow recessions or clefts, but success is less predictable in deep, wide recessions. Predictability may be defined as the success-failure ratio or as the number of successes in the total number of operations. In deep, wide recessions, the laterally positioned flap or combined techniques may be more predictable.[9,48-51] "Creeping attachment" may occur on a previously denuded root surface several months after grafting[45,51,149,150] (Fig. 40-10). The term *creeping attachment* is used to describe a gradual coronal migration of the gingival margin.

The first step in grafting is the preparation of the recipient bed. There are two types of bed preparations.

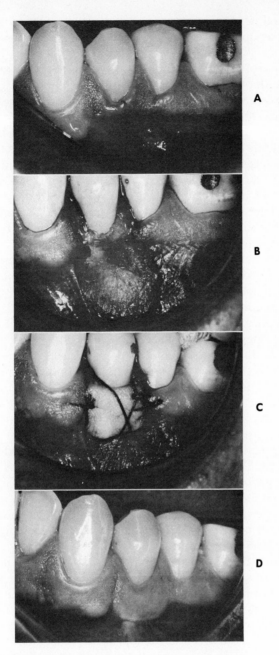

**Fig. 40-11.**  *Gingival augmentation.* **A,** *The gingival margin and the mucogingival junction are at the same level on the first premolar. The gingival margin is inflamed despite relatively good oral hygiene.* **B,** *The recipient bed is prepared to the gingival margin.* **C,** *Donor tissue is sutured to cover the cementoenamel junction.* **D,** *A widened gingiva is present after surgery. (Courtesy I. Speckman, Mexico City, Mexico.)*

In the first type the incision is made along the mucogingival junction and extended several millimeters to either side of the teeth involved in order to compensate for graft contraction. The incision is carried apically, leaving the periosteum and a thin layer of connective tissue over bone. Where connective tissue is to be left, it should be thin, smooth, and firm and without tissue tags, muscle, or loose connective tissue. Some prefer to totally denude the recipient bed with the intent of binding the graft.[40,51,149-152] Others prefer to perform periosteal fenestrations at the base of the recipient site to improve graft stability.[125,153,154] Generally speaking, if the receptor bed is properly prepared no additional steps are required. A slight beveling of the gingiva above the incision will permit an overlapping of the graft tissue, which will improve the appearance of the end result.

The second type of incision is made at the free margin of the gingiva and is extended apically as a split-thickness flap. Some surgeons excise and discard the flap, whereas others apically position it and suture it to the most apical portion of the bed with resorbable sutures. The second type generally yields a more acceptable gingival form; it permits root coverage and avoids a line of alveolar mucosa between the marginal gingiva and the graft after vertical contraction of the graft has taken place.

If root coverage is a goal of surgery the prepared bed must be free of all epithelium. The root surfaces should be planed smooth. Prominent roots should be reduced by curettes, chisels, or diamond burs and then planed smooth. Some clinicians have suggested conditioning of the root surface with citric acid to promote connective tissue attachment,[52-54] but further research is needed to verify the effectiveness of citric acid conditioning. The graft should be placed so that its margins are at the level of or slightly coronal to the cervical lines of the teeth. If interproximal recession has occurred the graft should be placed at the level of the most coronal portion of the papillae.

The next step involves obtaining the donor tissue. The tissue to be grafted is usually taken from the gingival or peripheral zone of the palatal tissue, but it may be taken from edentulous sites or from the mandibular gingiva.[47] One may use the probe as a ruler to measure the dimensions of the recipient site. Alternatively, a template of adhesive foil is cut to fit the size and shape of the recipient site. In either case the dimensions are transferred to the donor site, the first by direct measurement, the second by outlining the template with shallow incisions. The donor tissue is undermined at a depth of 1 mm in the same manner as forming a split-thickness flap. Apicocoronal height should be approximately one-third greater than the ultimately desired height to compensate for shrinkage.[37,68]

The appropriate thickness of the graft can be gauged by introducing only the beveled edge of the scalpel. The tissue should be of uniform thickness, and it does not necessarily need a covering epithelium.[56]

Some operators prefer to use the Paquette or Detsch knife or similar instruments for donor tissue excision. The graft must be shaped after its excision. If thickness is not uniform, it will taper from the center to the borders. Such tissue is useful for gingival augmentation, but not for root coverage.

Before the donor tissue is detached the aspirator tip must be changed to the narrowest one available so that the graft is not aspirated. Some operators continue to use the same suction tip, but, by passing a suture through the free end of the graft, they hold it and prevent its inadvertent loss. The graft is picked up with a fine tissue forceps and fitted to place over the receptor bed where bleeding has been controlled. It is sutured to place with a 5-0 or 6-0 suture and an atraumatic swaged ophthalmic needle. Sutures may be placed at both ends of the graft coronally and at each interdental space. No sutures need be placed apically, although they are sometimes necessary for stabilization. Alternatively, stabilizing sutures in the form of a continuous sling or mattress suture have been used. In addition to the sling sutures, Holbrook and Ochsenbein use suturing to stretch the graft mesiodistally.[155] A cyanoacrylate spray or simple pressure may eliminate the need for sutures.[156,157] Retaining sling sutures that do not pass through the graft may also be used[56] (Fig. 40-12). Other inert materials have also been suggested as dressings.[158]

Pressure is applied to the graft for a few minutes with a wet gauze sponge. This serves to obtain a fibrinous adherence, preventing blood from pooling under the graft; to achieve a good adaptation to the receptor bed; and to obtain hemostasis.

The wound may be covered with a surgical dressing, Stomahesive or Orahesive bandage, reconstituted collagen sponge, or freeze-dried skin. The donor site may be

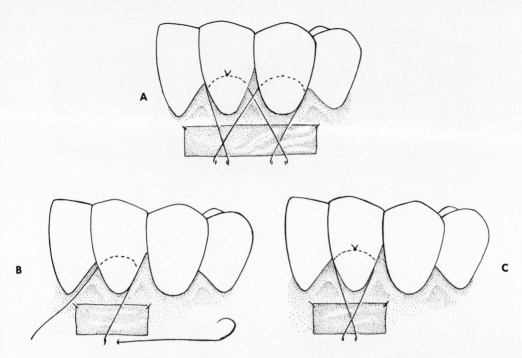

**Fig. 40-12.** **A,** Retaining sutures suspended from two teeth secure a free gingival graft. **B,** Suture is passed around a tooth, crossing the flap diagonally; is passed through the mucosa or periosteum; and, **C,** crosses diagonally over the free gingival graft and is tied. The graft is thus secured. Such suturing can be used for more than one tooth.

sutured if it is bleeding; if not, it may be covered with a surgical dressing. If Orahesive bandage is used the patient must be given additional pieces to replace the first one after it has dissolved. In rare cases an acrylic palatal stay-plate (stent) may be used to cover the site. If the patient is edentulous the denture can serve to cover the palatal site. Some surgeons place dry foil under the pack to keep the suture ends from becoming embedded. Others put the foil above the pack to hold the dressing in place while it sets. The surgical pack should be kept in place for about 5 to 8 days and need not be replaced unless necessary.[159]

The first 2 days after a free graft is placed are probably the most critical. The graft is in contact with a fibrin net through which plasma diffuses (Fig. 40-13, *A*). Vascularization is evident in about 48 hours. Adequate vascularization is present in about a week.[159] Collagen attachment begins approximately 4 days after grafting, and the graft becomes firm by the tenth day.[20] The surface of the epithelium desquamates during the first 3 to 5 days.[24] A new epithelial surface is derived from the adjacent epithelium and possibly from surviving basal cells (Fig. 40-13, *B* and *C*). The time necessary for complete reepithelization depends on the size of the gingival graft. In 2 weeks the tissue appears to have reformed, but maturation is not complete for 10 to 16 weeks (Fig. 40-13, *D*). Keratinization will be evident about 28 days after surgery.[24] Contraction of the tissue is also related to the thickness of the graft. The thicker the graft, the greater the primary contraction.[20] The free graft retains its histologic characteristics even when surrounded by alveolar mucosa. The surgeon may occasionally transplant palatal rugae. Gingivoplasty may be performed to improve the final gingival contour.

## FREE CONNECTIVE TISSUE AUTOGRAFT

Dense connective tissue from the palate, gingiva, or tuberosities, may be transplanted to replace alveolar mucosa. The surgical procedure is quite similar to free gingival grafting and is shown in Fig. 40-14. It differs in that the transplant is connective

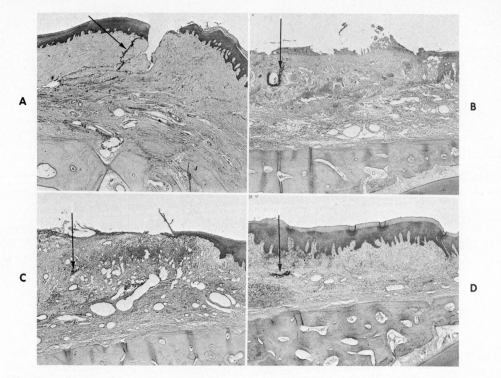

**Fig. 40-13. A,** Free gingival graft in a monkey at 0 hours. Note the approximation between graft tissue and receptor bed. The absence of a clot or a minimal clot is essential to retention and maturation of the graft. The donor tissue is palatal gingiva. Before the transport operation was performed the donor area was tattooed *(arrows).* **B,** At 4 days. Note the necrosis of surface epithelium, the dilatation of vascular channels, and the cellular disorganization in the grafted tissue. The epithelium from the adjacent host margins is beginning to migrate over the graft. **C,** At 7 days. The graft tissue is continuing to mature, and epithelium from the adjacent receptor site continues to migrate over the graft. **D,** At 3 weeks. There is almost complete maturation. The surface epithelium is continuous with the adjacent receptor site and appears normal. The connective tissue also appears normal. (From the collection of W.H. Wright.)

tissue without epithelial covering. Epithelium derived from the adjacent tissue migrates over the connective tissue graft, which induces it to keratinize.[59-62] Thus grafting with dense connective tissue taken from keratinized areas results in the formation of keratinized tissue even when the graft is transplanted to nonkeratinized zones.

This procedure is more desirable than free gingival grafting because it permits primary closure at the donor site, diminishes postoperative pain and risk of bleeding, and avoids the need for surgical packs that are difficult to maintain. Connective tissue grafts may be used in combination with free gingival grafts when large areas are involved.

### FREEZE-DRIED SKIN ALLOGRAFTS

One major advantage of freeze-dried skin allografts is the avoidance of an additional wound to obtain donor tissue. There is an adequate amount of material instantly available, and the material can be stored indefinitely at room temperature, while retaining its inductive capacity[79,80] (Fig. 40-15).

The recipient bed preparation is similar to that for free gingival grafts. The lyophilized tissue is placed in saline solution for about 30 minutes for rehydration and is sutured to place.

Freeze-dried skin grafts are biologically compatible and nonimmunogenic.[77-79] They have been used successfully to increase vestibular depth and to create or widen gingiva.[78,79,81] The grafted site retains some dermal characteristics.

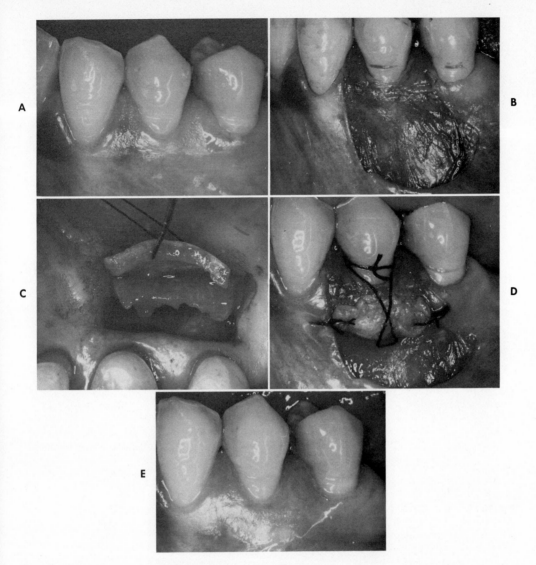

**Fig. 40-14.**   *Connective tissue graft.* **A,** *Narrow collar of gingiva is present around the mandibular first premolar.* **B,** *Recipient bed is prepared.* **C,** *Graft of connective tissue is obtained from the palate, after which the palatal flap is sutured back to place.* **D,** *Graft is sutured to place over the recipient site.* **E,** *Postoperative result.* (Courtesy I. Speckman, Mexico City, Mexico.)

## PEDICLE GRAFTS
### Laterally positioned flap

The laterally positioned flap (pedicle graft) is gingival mucosa that is laterally transposed to an adjacent area lacking this tissue. The graft remains attached at its base. It is used to correct recession, providing root coverage and creating a broader band of gingiva.[73-94] It is also used to treat localized recession or clefts on buccal or lingual surfaces (Fig. 40-16). The procedure may be used in the absence of recession to widen the zone of gingiva.

The laterally positioned flap, originally described as the sliding flap procedure, is illustrated in Fig. 40-17. A localized defect was present on the mandibular incisor. There was adequate gingiva on the adjacent incisor. Beveled incisions were made, and the tissue bordering the defect was trimmed free of pocket epithelium. The root was thoroughly planed. A full-thickness flap one and one half to two times as wide as the

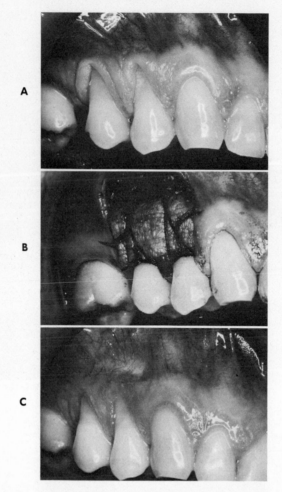

**Fig. 40-15.** **A,** Preoperative view of receded gingiva. **B,** Freeze-dried skin allograft in place. **C,** Healed freeze-dried skin allograft showing a widened but thin gingiva in place but with no clinical improvement in recession. (Courtesy I. Speckman, Mexico City, Mexico.)

defect was reflected to the mucogingival junction and extended as a split-thickness flap for several millimeters. It was moved laterally to cover the exposed root, leaving the donor site partially denuded. The flap was sutured with 5-0 or 6-0 suture and an atraumatic needle. The flap was pressed into place with a wet gauze sponge for several minutes to minimize clot thickness and to encourage fibrinous adherence of the flap to the exposed root. The technique may be modified in several minor aspects:

1. The receptor site may be beveled so that the flap with its beveled incision will overlap the adjacent bevel (Fig. 40-17, *D*). This permits a more rapid vascular union of flap and receptor tissue.
2. A collar of gingiva may be left around the donor tooth margin (Fig. 40-17, *C*), thus decreasing the likelihood of root exposure on the donor tooth.
3. Vertical incisions may be cut back (angled toward the receptor site), facilitating closure of the wound without tension (Fig. 40-17, *C* and *D*).
4. Where the donor tissue is sufficiently thick, the flap may be of partial thickness (Fig. 40-17, *D*), leaving periosteum and some connective tissue covering the donor area and thus avoiding exposed bone.

Localized recessions often occur on buccally positioned teeth. Where the exposed root is prominent it may be flattened with a curette, chisel, or bur. When successful,

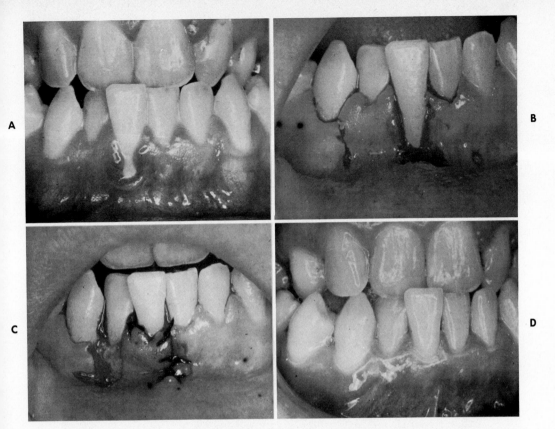

**Fig. 40-16.** Result of a laterally positioned flap after 8 years. **A,** Preoperative view. **B,** Operative view. **C,** Immediate postoperative view. **D,** Appearance 8 years after surgery. Note that the malposition of the involved tooth was not corrected. (From the collection of H.E. Grupe.)

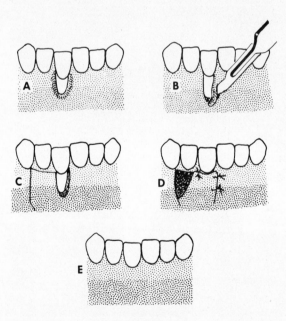

**Fig. 40-17.** Laterally positioned flap. **A,** Severe gingival recession on the lower right central incisor. **B,** Excision of the margin of the lesion, including the junctional epithelium. On the left side of the defect the incision is beveled externally and on the right side internally. The most prominent part of the exposed root surface is planed with a stone and very sharp curettes. **C,** The width of the flap is one and a half teeth. The horizontal incision leaves a collar of gingiva on the lateral incisor. **D,** The flap is reflected by sharp dissection, leaving periosteum intact. It is sutured to the recipient site without tension. The internal bevel of the one side and the external bevel of the other then form a lap joint. **E,** Appearance of the operative site after a year. (Modified from Grupe, H.E.: J. Periodontol. **37:**491, 1966.)

**Root conditioning with citric acid**

the laterally positioned flap heals with new attachment to the exposed root. The attachment may be a connective tissue attachment, a "long" epithelium attachment, or a combination of these.[74,95] Although conditioning of the root with citric acid has been suggested as a promoter of connective tissue attachment for laterally transposed flaps,[124,160-162] its value remains to be demonstrated. Probing should be avoided for about 6 months. Later, probing usually reveals a shallow sulcus.

When an adjoining edentulous area with adequately wide and thick attached gingiva is present, it may be used as the donor site[73-88] (Fig. 40-18).

Placing a laterally positioned flap should not be attempted in the presence of pocketing and osseous defects without simultaneously correcting these as well. The laterally positioned flap cannot be used when donor sites are inadequate (e.g., narrow gingiva, thin gingiva). The laterally positioned pedicle graft is reported to achieve 69% root coverage, at the expense of minor recession at the donor site.[92]

Since the pedicle graft has an intact blood supply, healing is rapid.[163] Where connective tissue has been left exposed at the donor site, the wound heals more slowly. Some shrinkage[92] may occur in the first months but may be compensated for by "creeping attachment."

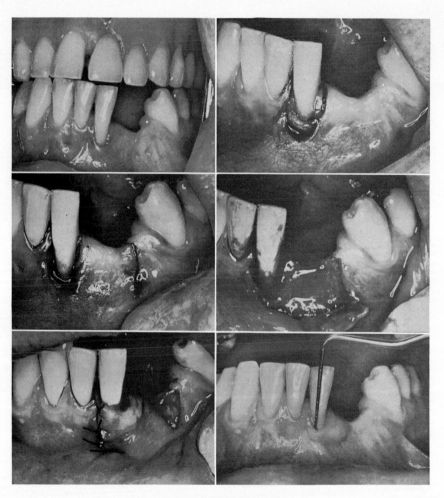

**Fig. 40-18.** The laterally positioned flap may use an adjoining edentulous donor site. The result after 1 year is shown in the bottom right illustration. (From the collection of H.E. Grupe.)

## Rotated papilla flap

The rotated single papilla flap is a variation of the laterally positioned flap.[75] It may be used for localized gingival recession where the adjacent papilla provides sufficient tissue. A single full- or split-thickness pedicle is formed and rotated to cover the root (Figs. 40-19 and 40-20).

**Single rotated papilla**

The major advantage of a rotated papilla flap (and other laterally positioned flaps) is that the color matches that of adjacent gingiva (unlike transplants of palatal mucosa).

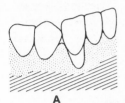 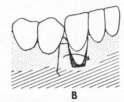 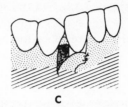 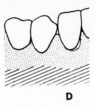

A       B       C       D

**Fig. 40-19.** Single rotated flap procedure. **A,** Preoperative view. Gingival recession in the lower right canine. **B,** Margin of the receded gingiva excised. The view also shows the incision line. **C,** Flap mobilized and sutured to its new position. **D,** Postoperative result.

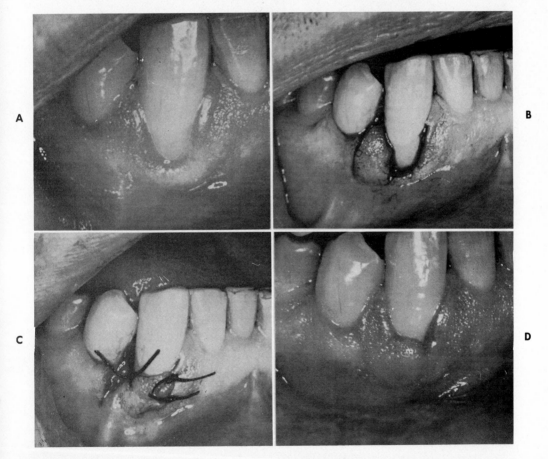

**Fig. 40-20.** Rotated single papilla flap. The 1-year result is shown in the lower right illustration. (Courtesy W.B. Hall, San Francisco, California.)

### Double papilla flap

The double papilla flap uses two adjacent papillae to cover a denuded root[79,96] (Fig. 40-21). The papillae mesial and distal to a tooth with recession are undermined by split-thickness incisions and rotated to cover the receptor bed. The two pedicles must be mitered to fit precisely. The papillae are sutured to each other and to the receptor bed. A successful result depends on the flaps joining, with healing across the mitered union.

### Coronally positioned flap

A coronally positioned flap is a split-thickness pedicle flap moved coronally to gain root coverage[90,97-104] (Fig. 40-22). This requires attached gingiva of adequate thickness, which may not exist where recession is present. A free gingival graft may be placed

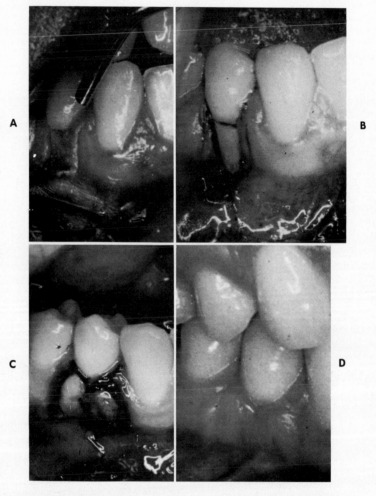

**Fig. 40-21.** Rotated double papilla flap. **A,** A broad gingival cleft may be seen denuding the root of a mandibular premolar. The base of the cleft is bordered by alveolar mucosa, and a blast of air has caused the mucosa to retract, revealing a pocket. The root is planed, and the friable tissue bordering the cleft is excised. **B,** A single papilla flap is not wide enough to cover the cleft. **C,** Papillae mesial and distal to the cleft are rotated laterally and sutured together. Finger pressure is applied to obtain a fibrin adherence. The pedicles are ligated to the neck of the tooth by a suspensory ligature. **D,** Result 2 years after surgery reveals a firmly attached gingiva with sulcular depth of less than 1 mm.

apical to the recession to create gingiva of sufficient thickness. Then a coronally positioned flap may be created as a second-step procedure. Alternatively, a split-thickness flap may be moved coronally, and a free gingival graft may be sutured to its base. Another procedure encloses the base of a free connective tissue graft that has been placed over a root in an envelope flap.[62]

### Apically positioned flap

The apically positioned flap is most often used in conjunction with other surgical procedures such as osseous surgery (Figs. 40-23 and 40-24). This flap employs a full- or split-flap incision. It is rarely used as a procedure in its own right.

The significance of the apically positioned flap is that the flap is sutured to place at a more apical level. It may cover or expose the alveolar margin. In the latter instance additional attached gingiva granulates from the periodontal ligament to form a broader zone of gingiva.

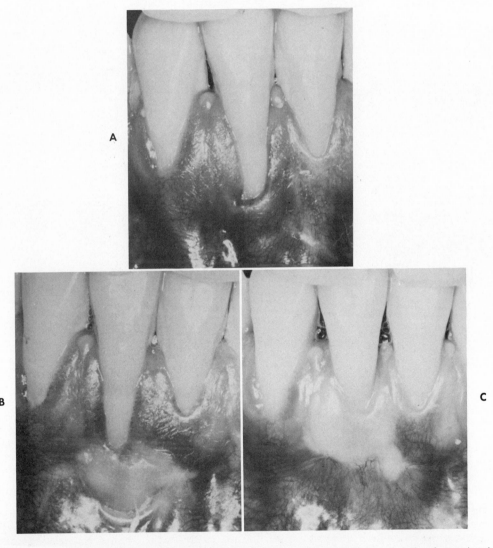

**Fig. 40-22. A,** Localized gingival recession on mandibular right central incisor. **B,** A free gingival graft was placed to create a zone of gingiva. **C,** The widened gingiva was positioned coronally to correct the recession. (From Caffesse, R.G., and Guinard, E.A.: J. Periodontol. **49:**357, 1978.)

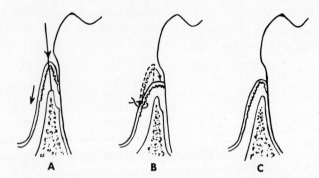

**Fig. 40-23.** Apically positioned flap. **A,** Initial reverse bevel incision. **B,** Tissue adhering to the tooth is curetted away, the bony defect is exposed and treated, and the flap is positioned and sutured apically. **C,** Postoperative result.

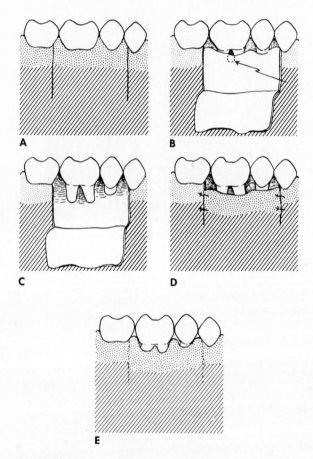

**Fig. 40-24.** Diagram of an apically positioned flap after osseous resection. **A,** Mandibular first molar with a pocket in the bifurcation. The pocket extends below the mucogingival junction. Relieving incisions are placed. **B,** Alveolar bone and interradicular crater *(arrow)* are exposed. **C,** Osseous surgery treating the crater. Bone ramping accomplished. **D,** Flap sutured apically. **E,** Postoperative view.

The surgeon may use the outer unit of a split flap as its own pedicle graft. A split-thickness flap is dissected, leaving the underlying connective tissue bed intact. The split-thickness flap is sutured to the recipient bed but positioned apically.

## FRENUM PROCEDURES

Localized gingival recessions may be found on labially positioned teeth or on teeth with prominent roots. Bony dehiscences may accompany such recessions. Localized recessions are sometimes associated with frena, sometimes as a cause and at other times as a result. Thus mucogingival problems may be present when frenum attachments and the marginal gingiva (high frenum attachment) approach each other[83,119-124] (see Fig. 40-1, *D*).

Persistence of the mandibular labial frenum is the most common problem. The problem may first be noticed when the permanent incisors erupt or may develop later in life. It should be treated when first observed (Fig. 40-25). A prominent maxillary labial frenum may recede when the permanent canines erupt. If it persists beyond that time or if the maxillary frenum is attached to the incisive papilla, removal is indicated (Fig. 40-26).

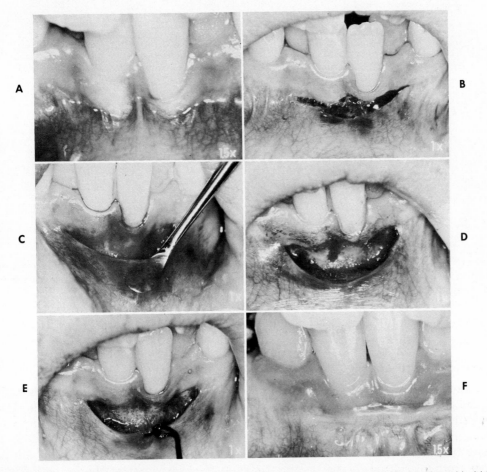

**Fig. 40-25.   A,** The frenum is attached close to the gingival margin, which has receded. **B,** A horizontal incision is made at the mucogingival line. The incision must extend to at least one tooth on either side of the area to undergo operation. **C,** The mucosa is undermined. **D,** A narrow horizontal band of periosteum is scraped to expose bone (periosteal fenestration). **E,** The undermined mucosa is sutured to the periosteum below the periosteal fenestration. **F,** Postoperative view.

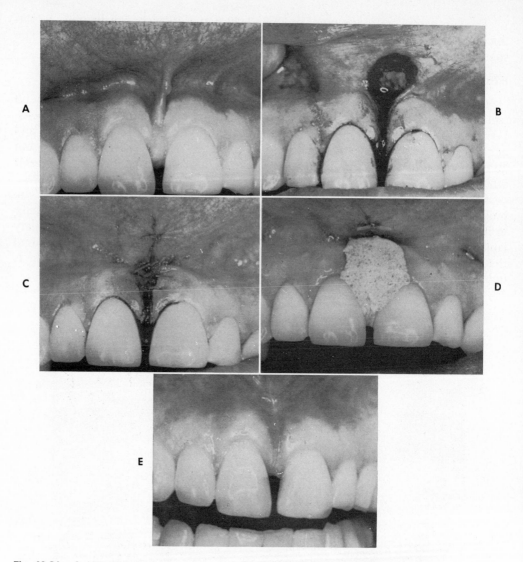

**Fig. 40-26. A,** Heavy maxillary frenum extending interproximally. **B,** Incisions are made parallel to the frenum, and the frenum is excised. **C,** Edges of the wound are sutured. **D,** The wound is protected by surgical dressing. **E,** Postsurgical view.

Other frena include the mandibular lingual frenum and buccal frena in the premolar regions.

### Frenotomy, frenectomy

Frenotomy is the incision of a frenum to detach it from bone and simultaneously induce scar formation. Frenectomy is the excision of a frenum. A frenotomy is illustrated in Fig. 40-27. A mandibular labial frenum extends nearly to the free margin of the gingiva, and gingival recession is evident. After anesthesia is induced, the lip is pulled out firmly and an incision is made at the mucogingival line, extending at least one tooth to each side of the frenum parallel to the alveolar plate. The mucosal flap is freed from the periosteum by blunt or sharp dissection, exposing 6 to 8 mm of periosteum at a more apical level. A scar forms that binds the tissue down and eliminates the frenum pull. It is common practice today to cover the denuded area with a free gingival graft[123] (Fig. 40-28).

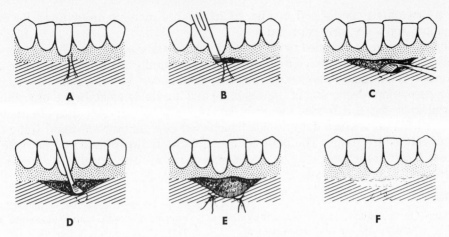

**Fig. 40-27.** Frenotomy. **A,** Preoperative appearance. The frenum inserts into the marginal gingiva. The gingiva gapes when pull is exerted on the frenum. **B,** An incision is made along the mucogingival line in an attempt to preserve a collar of tissue around the involved tooth. **C,** The mucosal flap is dissected from the underlying periosteum. **D,** The mucosal flap is undermined. **E,** The mucosal flap is sutured to the underlying periosteum. **F,** Postoperatively a scar forms, separating the frenum from the gingiva.

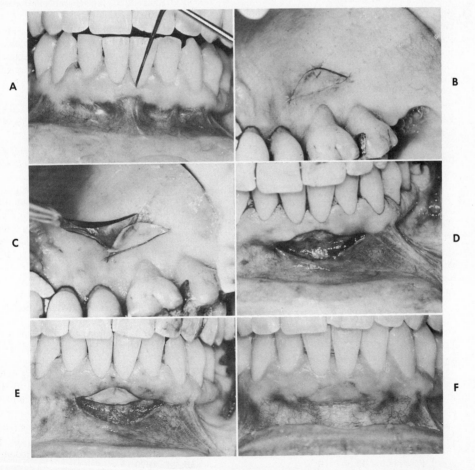

**Fig. 40-28.** Frenotomy with free gingival graft. **A,** Preoperative view. **B,** Donor tissue from the palatal gingiva. **C,** Donor tissue being dissected. **D,** Receptor site being prepared. **E,** Donor tissue inserted. **F,** Result 1 year after surgery. (Courtesy W.B. Hall, San Francisco, California.)

A frenectomy is performed in Fig. 40-26. Wound margins are sutured for close adaptation, and a dressing is placed.

**Periosteal retention and fenestration**

This procedure is intended to eliminate problems associated with a narrow zone of gingiva that cannot be corrected because of the proximity of the vestibule. The vestibuloplasty techniques of periosteal retention, denudation, or fenestration do not produce a permanent deepening of the vestibule and are rarely used. In the procedure a split-thickness flap is extended into a shallow vestibule. Any muscle fibers in the path of the incision are dissected away. The bone is left covered by periosteum and a thin layer of connective tissue. The periosteum is fenestrated (perforated to the bone) at its base. A soft tissue graft may be placed over the bone. The apically positioned flap coupled with a free graft yields a more predictable result.

## REFERENCES

1. Stern, I.B.: Oral mucous membrane. In Bhaskar, S.N., editor: Orban's oral histology and embryology, ed. 8, St. Louis, 1976, The C.V. Mosby Co.
2. Lang, N.P., and Löe, H.: The relationship between the width of the attached gingiva and gingival health, J. Periodontol. **43:**623, 1972.
3. Goldman, H.M.: Periodontia, ed. 3, St. Louis, 1953, The C.V. Mosby Co.
4. Bowers, G.M.: A study of the width of attached gingiva, J. Periodontol. **34:**201, 1963.
5. Parfitt, G.J., and Mjör, I.A.: Clinical evaluation of local gingival recession in children, J. Dent. Child. **31:**257, 1964.
6. Vincent, J.W., Machen, J.B., and Levin, M.P.: Assessment of attached gingiva using the tension test and clinical measurements, J. Periodontol. **47:**412, 1976.
7. Guastamacchia, C., Hoter, F., and Peccatori, G.: Studio statistico sulla frequenza di anomalie del frenulo neila populazione scolastica (6-11 Anni) di Milano, Rass. Int. Stomatol. Prat. **14:**23, 1963.
8. Nery, E.B., and Davies, E.E.: The historical development of mucogingival surgery, J. West. Soc. Periodontol./Periodont. Abstr. **24:**149, 1976.
9. Guinard, E.A., and Caffesse, R.G.: Localized gingival recessions. I. Etiology and prevalence, J. West. Soc. Periodontol./Periodont. Abstr. **25:**3, 1977.
10. Gartrell, J.R.: Influence of the classifications of oral mucosa on the development of mucogingival surgery, J. West. Soc. Periodontol./Periodont. Abstr. **24:**143, 1976.
11. Beagrie, G.S., Thompson, G.N., and Basu, M.K.: Tooth position and anterior bone loss in skulls, Br. Dent. J. **129:**471, 1970.
12. Baker, D.L., and Seymour, G.J.: The possible pathogenesis of gingival recession. A histological study of induced recession in the rat, J. Clin. Periodontol. **3:**2089, 1976.
13. Hall, W.B.: Present status of soft tissue grafting, J. Periodontol. **48:**587, 1977.
14. Björn, H.: Free transplantation of gingiva propria, Sven. Tandlak. Tidskr. **55:**684, 1968.
15. Cowan, A.: Sulcus deepening incorporating mucosal graft, J. Periodontol. **36:**188, 1965.
16. Nabers, J.M.: Extension of vestibular fornix utilizing a gingival graft, Periodontics **4:**77, 1966.
17. Nabers, J.M.: Free gingival grafts, Periodontics **4:**243, 1966.
18. Wennström, J.L.: Status of art in mucogingival surgery, Schweiz. Monatsschr. Zahnmed. **95:**290, 1985.
19. Gargiulo, A.W., and Arrocha, R.: Histoclinical evaluation of free gingival grafts, Periodontics **5:**285, 1967.
20. Sullivan, H.C., and Atkins, J.H.: Free autogenous gingival grafts. I. Principles of successful grafting. II. Histology of the graft site. III. Utilization of grafts in the treatment of gingival recession, Periodontics **6:**121, 130, 152, 1968.
21. Bressman, E., and Chasens, A.I.: Free gingival graft with periosteal fenestration, J. Periodontol. **39:**298, 1968.
22. Frisch, J., and Bhaskar, S.N.: Free mucosal graft with tissue adhesives; report of 17 cases, J. Periodontol. **39:**190, 1968.
23. Calandriello, M.: Free mucosal grafts in mucogingival surgery, Parodontol. Acad. Rev. **2:**74, 1968.
24. Oliver, R.C., Löe, H., and Karring, T.: Microscopic evaluation of the healing and revascularization of free gingival grafts, J. Periodont. Res. **3:**84, 1968.
25. Hangorsky, U., and Bissada, N.: Clinical assessment of free gingival graft effectiveness on the maintenance of periodontal health, J. Periodontol. **51:**274, 1980.
26. Levin, M.P., Frisch, J., and Bhaskar, S.N.: Tissue conditioner dressing for free tissue grafts, J. Periodontol. **40:**271, 1969.
27. Caffesse, R.G., et al.: Healing of free gingival grafts with and without periosteum. I. Histologic evaluation, J. Periodontol. **50:**586, 1979.
28. Caffesse, R.G., et al.: Healing of free gingival grafts with and without periosteum. II. Radioautographic evaluation, J. Periodontol. **50:**595, 1979.
29. Sullivan, H.C., and Atkins, J.H.: The role of free gingival grafts in periodontal therapy, Dent. Clin. North Am. **13:**133, 1969.
30. Staffileno, H., and Levy, S.: Histologic and

clinical study of mucosal (gingival) transplants in dogs, J. Periodontol. **40:**311, 1969.

31. Hawley, C.E., and Staffileno, H.: Clinical evaluation of free gingival grafts in periodontal surgery, J. Periodontol. **41:**105, 1970.

32. Brackett, R.C., and Gargiulo, A.W.: Free gingival grafts in humans, J. Periodontol. **41:**581, 1970.

33. Matter, J.: Free gingival grafts for the treatment of gingival recession, J. Clin. Periodontol. **9:**103, 1982.

34. Mlinek, A., Smukler, J., and Buchner, A.: The use of free gingival grafts for the coverage of denuded roots, J. Periodontol. **44:**246, 1973.

35. Wiggins, Jr., H.E., and Engel, L.D.: Free palatal mucosa grafts. An evaluation of twenty-six cases, Oral Surg. **35:**35, 1973.

36. Vandersall, D.C.: Management of gingival recession and a surgical dehiscence with a soft tissue autograft: 4 year observation, J. Periodontol. **45:**274, 1974.

37. Egli, V., Vollmer, W.H., and Rateitschak, K.H.: Follow-up studies of free gingival grafts, J. Clin. Periodontol. **2:**98, 1975.

38. Snyder, M.B.: Gingival recession: a review of causative factors and treatment. II. Use of free gingival grafts, Compend. Contin. Educ. Dent. **3:**263, 1982.

39. Brasher, W.J., Rees, T.D., and Boyce, W.A.: Complications of free grafts of masticatory mucosa, J. Periodontol. **46:**133, 1975.

40. Dordick, B., Coslet, J.G., and Seibert, J.S.: Clinical evaluation of free autogenous gingival grafts placed on alveolar bone, I. Clinical predictability, J. Periodontol. **47:**559, 1976.

41. Dordick, B., Coslet, J.G., and Seibert, J.S.: Clinical evaluation of free autogenous gingival grafts placed on alveolar bone. II. Coverage of nonpathologic dehiscences and fenestrations, J. Periodontol. **47:**568, 1976.

42. Mörmann, W., Schaer, F., and Firestone, A.R.: The relationship between success of free gingival grafts and transplant thickness: revascularization and shrinkage—a one year clinical study, J. Periodontol. **52:**74, 1981.

43. Schokking, C.C.: Free grafts of palatal mucosa on the lingual aspects of the mandible: a report of two cases, J. Clin. Periodontol. **3:**251, 1976.

44. Ellegaard, B., Karring, T., and Löe, H.: Retardation of epithelial migration in new attachment attempts in infrabony defects in monkeys, J. Clin. Periodontol. **3:**23, 1976.

45. Matter, J., and Cimasoni, G.: Creeping reattachment after free gingival grafts, J. Periodontol. **47:**574, 1976.

46. Irwin, R.K.: Combined use of the gingival graft and rotated pedical procedures: case reports, J. Periodontol. **48:**38, 1977.

47. Saadoun, A.P., and Farnoush, A.S.: Alternatives to palatal mucosa as donor sites for free gingival grafts, Quintessence Int. **15:**533, 1984.

48. Casullo, O.P., and Hangorsky, U.: The use of free gingival grafts in periodontics and restorative dentistry, Compend. Contin. Educ. Dent. **2:**138, 1981.

49. Farnoush, A., and Schonfeld, S.E.: Rationale for mugogingival surgery: a critique and update, Periodont. Abstr. **31:**125, 1983.

50. Fritz, M.E., and Shuster, A.: Current status of mucogingival surgery, Alpha Omegan **76:**61, 1983.

51. Shiloah, J.: Complications of free autogenous gingival grafts placed on denuded alveolar bone, Periodont. Case Rep. **2:**15, 1980.

52. Miller, P.: Root coverage using the free soft tissue autograft following citric acid application. I. Technique, Int. J. Periodont. Rest. Dent. **2:**65, 1982.

53. Miller, P.: Root coverage using the free soft tissue autograft following citric acid application. II. Treatment of the carious root, Int. J. Periodont. Rest. Dent. **3:**39, 1983.

54. Miller, P.: Root coverage using the free soft tissue autograft following citric acid application. III. A successful and predictable procedure in areas of deep-wide recession, Int. J. Periodont. Rest. Dent. **5:**15, 1985.

55. Karring, T., Lang, N.P., and Löe, H.: The role of gingival connective tissue in determining epithelial differentiation, J. Periodont. Res. **10:**1, 1974.

56. Speckman, I.: El transplante de tejido conectivo libre, Rev. Assoc. Dent. Mex. **35:**521, 1978.

57. Stambaugh, R., and Gordon, H.P.: Connective tissue influence on mucosal keratinization, I.A.D.R. Abstr. No. 355, p. 147, 1973.

58. Edel, A.: Clinical evaluation of free connective tissue grafts used to increase the width of keratinized gingiva, J. Clin. Periodontol. **1:**185, 1974.

59. Broome, C.W., and Taggart, J.E.: Free autogenous connective tissue grafting—report of two cases, J. Periodontol. **47:**480, 1976.

60. Botero, A., Ruben, M.P., and Kramer, G.: Connective tissue grafts induction of formation of gingiva in mucosal receptor sites, J. Periodontol. **46:**630, 1975.

61. Donn, B.: The free connective tissue autograft: a clinical and histologic wound healing study in humans, J. Periodontol. **49:**253, 1978.

62. Raetzke, P.: Covering localized areas of root exposure employing the "envelope" technique, J. Periodontol. **56:**397, 1985.

63. Karring, T., Ostergaard, E., and Löe, H.: Conservation of tissue specificity after heterotopic transplantation of gingiva and alveolar mucosa, J. Periodont. Res. **6:**282, 1971.

64. Karring, T., Lang, N.P., and Löe, H.: Role of connective tissue in determining epithelial specificity, J. Dent. Res. **51:**1303, 1972.

65. Yukna, R., et al.: Evaluation of the use of freeze-dried skin allografts in the treatment

of human mucogingival problems, J. Periodontol. **48:**187, 1977.

66. Yukna, R., and Sullivan, W.: Evaluation of resultant type following the intraoral transplantation of various lyophilized soft tissues, J. Periodont. Res. **13:**177, 1978.

67. Yukna, R., et al.: Comparative clinical evaluation of freeze-dried skin allografts and autogenous gingival grafts in humans, J. Clin. Periodontol. **4:**191, 1976.

68. Rateitschak, K.H., Egli, W., and Fringeli, G.: Recession: a 4 year longitudinal study after free gingival grafts, J. Clin. Periodontol. **6:**158, 1979.

69. Ouhayoun, J.P., et al.: Freeze-dried skin allografts. A human clinical and histological study, J. Periodontol. **54:**463, 1983.

70. Gher, M.E., et al.: Evaluation of the immunogenicity of freeze-dried skin allografts in humans: cell-mediated response, J. Periodontol. **53:**325, 1982.

71. Yukna, R., Turner, D., and Robinson, L.: Variable antigenicity of lyophilized allogeneic and lyophilized xenogeneic skin in guinea pigs, J. Periodont. Res. **12:**197, 1977.

72. Gher, M., et al.: Evaluation of the immunogenicity of freeze-dried skin allografts in humans, J. Periodontol. **51:**571, 1980.

73. Corn, H.: Edentulous area pedicle grafts in mucogingival surgery, Periodontics, **2:**229, 1964.

74. Wilderman, M.N., and Wentz, F.M.: Repair of a dentogingival defect with a pedicle flap, J. Periodontol. **35:**218, 1965.

75. Pennel, B.M., et al.: Oblique rotated flap, J. Periodontol. **36:**305, 1965.

76. Grupe, H.E.: Modified technique for the sliding flap operation, J. Periodontol. **37:**491, 1966.

77. McFall, W.T.: Laterally repositioned flap—criteria for success in periodontics, Periodontics **5:**89, 1967.

78. Caffesse, R.G., et al.: Revascularization following the lateral sliding flap procedure, J. Periodontol. **55:**352, 1984.

79. Cohen, D.W., and Ross, S.E.: The double papillae repositioned flap in periodontal therapy, J. Periodontol. **39:**65, 1968.

80. Moskow, B.S.: Repair of gingival clefts, J. Am. Dent. Assoc. **98:**940, 1979.

81. Pfeifer, J.S., and Heller, R.: Histologic evaluation of full and partial thickness lateral repositioned flaps: a pilot study, J. Periodontol. **42:**331, 1971.

82. Björn, H.: Coverage of denuded root surfaces with a lateral sliding flap; use of free gingival grafts, Odontol. Rev. **22:**37, 1971.

83. Miller, Jr., P.D.: The frenectomy with a laterally positioned pedicle graft, J. Periodontol. **56:**102, 1985.

84. Albano, E., et al.: Estudio biometrico de colgajos des plazzapas lateralmente, Rev. Odontol. Argent. **61:**12, 1973.

85. Smukler, J.: Laterally positioned mucoperiosteal pedicle grafts in the treatment of denuded roots. A clinical and statistical study, J. Periodontol. **47:**590, 1976.

86. Patur, B.: The rotation flap for covering denuded root surfaces—a closed wound technique, J. Periodontol. **48:**41, 1972.

87. Grupe, H.E., and Warren, Jr., R.F.: Repair of gingival defects by a sliding flap operation, J. Periodontol. **27:**92, 1956.

88. Robinson, R.E.: Utilizing an edentulous area as donor site in the lateral repositioned flap, Periodontics **2:**79, 1964.

89. Caffesse, R., and Espinel, M.: Lateral sliding flap with a free gingival graft technique in the treatment of localized gingival recessions, Int. J. Periodont. Rest. Dent. **1:**23, 1981.

90. Espinel, M., and Caffesse, R.: Comparison of the results obtained with the laterally positioned pedicle sliding flap revised technique and the lateral sliding flap with a free gingival graft technique in the treatment of localized gingival recessions, Int. J. Periodont. Rest. Dent. **1:**31, 1981.

91. Carvalho, J.C., Pustiglioni, F., and Kon, S.: Combination of a connective tissue pedicle flap with a free gingival graft to cover localized gingival recession, Int. J. Periodont. Rest. Dent. **2:**27, 1982.

92. Guinard, E.A., and Caffesse, R.G.: Treatment of localized gingival recessions. I. Lateral sliding flap, J. Periodontol. **49:**351, 1978.

93. Janson, W.A., et al.: Development of the blood supply to split-thickness free gingival autografts, J. Periodontol. **40:**707, 1969.

94. Wilderman, M.N., and Wentz, F.M.: Repair of a dentogingival defect with a pedicle flap, J. Periodontol. **35:**218, 1965.

95. Common, J., and McFall, Jr., W.T.: The effects of citric acid on all attachments of laterally positioned flaps, J. Periodontol. **54:**93, 1983.

96. Marggraf, E.: A direct technique with a double lateral bridging flap for coverage of denuded root surface and gingiva extension, J. Clin. Periodontol. **12:**69, 1985.

97. Kalmi, J., et al.: The solution of the aesthetic problem in the treatment of periodontal disease of the teeth; gingivoplastic operation, Paradontologie **3:**53, 1959.

98. Patur, B., and Glickman, I.: Gingival pedicle flaps for covering roots denuded by chronic destructive periodontal disease—a clinical experiment, J. Periodontol. **29:**50, 1958.

99. Bernimoulin, J.P., Lüscher, B., and Mühlemann, H.R.: Coronally repositioned periodontal flap. Clinical evaluation after one year, J. Clin. Periodontol. **2:**1, 1975.

100. Caffesse, R.G., and Guinard, E.A.: Treatment of localized gingival recessions. II. Coronally repositioned flap with a free gingival graft, J. Periodontol. **49:**357, 1978.

101. Guinard, E.A., and Caffesse, R.G.: Treatment of localized gingival recessions. III. Comparison of results obtained with lateral sliding and coronally repositioned flaps, J. Periodontol. **49:**457, 1978.

102. Tenenbaum, H., Klewansky, P., and Roth, J.J.: Clinical evaluation of gingival recession treated by a coronally positioned flap technique, J. Periodontol. **51:**686, 1980.

103. Matter, J.: Free gingival graft and coronally repositioned flap: a 2-year follow-up report, J. Clin. Periodontol. **6:**437, 1979.

104. Matter, J.: Free gingival grafts for the treatment of gingival recession—a review of some techniques, J. Clin. Periodontol. **9:**103, 1982.

105. Nabers, C.L.: Repositioning the attached gingiva, J. Periodontol. **25:**38, 1954.

106. Friedman, N.: Mucogingival surgery: the apically repositioned flap, J. Periodontol. **33:** 328, 1962.

107. Staffileno, H., Wentz, F.M., and Orban, B.: Histologic study of healing of split thickness flap surgery in dogs, J. Periodontol. **33:**56, 1962.

108. Donnenfeld, O.W., Marks, R.M., and Glickman, I.: Apically repositioned flap, J. Periodontol. **35:**381, 1964.

109. Wright, W.H.: The scalloped reverse bevel incision in mucogingival surgery, Odontol. Tidskr. **73:**515, 1965.

110. Hiatt, W.H. et al.: Repair following mucoperiosteal flap surgery with full gingival retention, J. Periodontol. **39:**11, 1968.

111. Levine, H.L.: Periodontal flap surgery with gingival fiber retention, J. Periodontol. **43:**91, 1972.

112. Fagan, F., and Freeman, E.: Clinical comparison of the free gingival graft and partial thickness apically positioned flap, J. Periodontol. **45:**3, 1974.

113. Pustiglioni, F.E., et al.: Split thickness flap, apically replaced, with protected linear periosteal fenestration, J. Periodontol. **46:**742, 1975.

114. Maynard, G.J., and Ochsenbein, C.: Mucogingival problems, prevalence and therapy in children, J. Periodontol. **46:**543, 1975.

115. Holmes, C.H., and Strem, B.E.: Location of flap margin after suturing, J. Periodontol. **47:**674, 1976.

116. Kohler, C.A., and Ramfjord, S.P.: Healing of gingival mucoperiosteal flaps, Oral Surg. **13:**89, 1960.

117. Staffileno, H.: Significant differences and advantages between the full thickness and split thickness flaps, J. Periodontol. **45:**421, 1974.

118. Zamet, J.S.: A comparative clinical study of three periodontal surgical techniques, J. Clin. Periodontol. **2:**89, 1975.

119. Gottsegen, R.: Frenum position and vestibule depth in relation to gingival health, Oral Surg. **7:**1069, 1954.

120. Bork, K.C., and Weiler, J.F.: Frenum reduction, as a treatment for periodontal atrophy, Oral Surg. **11:**370, 1958.

121. Hileman, A.: Repositioning the vestibule and frenum as adjunctive periodontal treatment procedures, Dent. Clin. North Am., p. 55, March 1960.

122. Dewel, B.F.: The labial frenum, midline diastema, and palatine papilla: a clinical analysis, Dent. Clin. North Am., p. 175, March 1966.

123. Ward, V.J.: A clinical assessment of the use of the free gingival graft for correcting localized recession associated with frenal pull, J. Periodontol. **45:**78, 1974.

124. Ibbott, C.G., Oles, R.D., and Laverty, W.H.: Effects of citric acid treatment on autogenous free graft coverage of localized recession, J. Periodontol. **58:**662, 1985.

125. Corn, H.: Periosteal separation—its clinical significance, J. Periodontol. **33:**140, 1962.

126. Ivancie, G.P.: Experimental and histologic investigation of gingival regeneration in vestibular surgery, J. Periodontol. **28:**259, 1957.

127. Rosenberg, M.M.: Vestibular alterations in periodontics, J. Periodontol. **31:**231, 1960.

128. Wilderman, M.N., Wentz, E.M., and Orban, B.: Histogenesis of repair after mucogingival surgery, J. Periodontol. **31:**283, 1960.

129. Staffileno, H., Wentz, F., and Orban, B.: Histologic study of healing of split thickness flap surgery in dogs, J. Periodontol. **33:**56, 1962.

130. Ramfjord, S.P., and Costich, E.R.: Healing after exposure of the periosteum on the alveolar process, J. Periodontol. **39:**199, 1968.

131. Bohannan, H.M.: Studies in the alteration of vestibular depth. I. Complete denudation. II. Periosteum retention. III. Vestibular incision, J. Periodontol. **33:**120, 354, 1962; **34:**209, 1963.

132. Edlan, A., and Mejchar, B.: Plastic surgery of the vestibulum in periodontal therapy, Int. Dent. J. **13:**593, 1963.

133. Pfeifer, J.S.: The growth of gingival tissue over denuded bone, J. Periodontol. **34:**10, 1963.

134. Wilderman, M.N.: Repair after a periosteal retention procedure, J. Periodontol. **34:**487, 1963.

135. Pennel, B.M., et al.: Retention of periosteum in mucogingival surgery, J. Periodontol. **36:**39, 1965.

136. Carranza, Jr., F.A., et al.: Effect of periosteal fenestration in gingival extension operations, J. Periodontol. **37:**335, 1966.

137. Staffileno, H., Levy, S., and Gargiulo, A.W.: Histologic study of cellular mobilization and repair following a periosteal retention via split thickness mucogingival flap surgery, J. Periodontol. **37:**117, 1966.

138. Grant, D.A.: Experimental periodontal surgery: sequestration of alveolar bone, J. Periodontol. **38:**409, 1967.

139. Allen, D.L., and Shell, J.H.: Clinical and radiographic evaluation of a periosteal separation procedure, J. Periodontol. **39:**290, 1968.

140. Wade, B.A.: Vestibular deepening by the technique of Edlan and Mejchar, J. Periodont. Res. **4:**300, 1969.

141. Hilming, F., and Jervoe, P.: Surgical extension of vestibular depth, Tandlaegebladet **74:**329, 1970.

142. Bergenholtz, A., and Hugoson, A.: Vestibular sulcus extension. Surgery in the mandibular front region. The Edlan-Mejchar method—a five year follow-up study, J. Periodontol. **44:**309, 1973.

143. Miyasato, M., Crigger, M., and Egelberg, J.: Gingival condition in areas of minimal and appreciable width of keratinized gingiva, J. Clin. Periodontol. **4:**200, 1977.

144. De Trey, E., and Bernimoulin, J.: Influence of free gingival grafts on the health of the marginal gingiva, J. Clin. Periodontol. **7:**381, 1980.

145. Dorfman, H., Kennedy, J., and Bird, W.: Longitudinal evaluation of free autogenous gingival grafts, J. Periodontol. **53:**349, 1982.

146. Schoo, W.H., and Van der Velden, J.: Marginal soft tissue recessions with and without attached gingiva: a five year longitudinal study, J. Periodont. Res. **20:**209, 1985.

147. Ochsenbein, C., and Maynard, G.: The problem of attached gingiva in children, J. Dent. Child. **41:**263, 1974.

148. Maynard, G., and Wilson, D.K.: Physiologic dimensions of the periodontium significant to the restorative dentist, J. Periodontol. **50:**170, 1979.

149. Matter, J.: Creeping attachment of free gingival grafts. A five-year follow-up study, J. Periodontol. **51:**681, 1980.

150. Pollack, R.: Bilateral creeping attachment using free mucosal grafts, J. Periodontol. **55:**670, 1984.

151. William, J., and McFall, W.: Placement of free gingival grafts on denuded alveolar bone. I.

Clinical evaluations, J. Periodontol. **49:**283, 1978.

152. William, J., McFall, W., and Burkes, J.: Placement of free gingival grafts on denuded alveolar bone. II. Microscopic observations, J. Periodontol. **49:**291, 1978.

153. Robinson, R.E.: Periosteal fenestration in mucogingival surgery, J. West. Soc. Periodontol. **9:**107, 1961.

154. Zingale, J.: Observations on free gingival autografts, J. Periodontol. **45:**748, 1974.

155. Holbrook, T., and Ochsenbien, C: Complete coverage of the denuded root surface with a one stage gingival graft, Int. J. Periodont. Restorative Dent. **3:**9, 1983.

156. Hoexter, D.L.: The sutureless free gingival graft, J. Periodontol. **50:**75, 1979.

157. Miller, N.: Sutureless gingival grafting, J. Clin. Periodontol. **9:**171, 1982.

158. Levin, M.P., Tsaknis, P.J., and Cutright, D.E.: Healing of the oral mucosa with the use of collagen artificial skin, J. Periodontol. **50:**250, 1979.

159. Speckman, I., Noyola, E., and Cuauhtecontzi, G.: Respuesta del tejido conectivo a diferentes apositos quirurgicos, Pract. Odontol. **5:**10, 1984.

160. Liu, J.-L., and Solt, C.W.: A surgical procedure for the treatment of localized gingival recession in conjunction with root surface citric acid conditioning, J. Periodontol. **51:**505, 1980.

161. Shiloah, J.: The clinical effects of citric acid and laterally positioned pedicle grafts in the treatment of denuded root surfaces, J. Periodontol. **51:**652, 1980.

162. Oles, R.D., et al.: Effects of citric acid treatment on pedicle flap coverage of localized recession, J. Periodontol. **56:**259, 1985.

163. Busschop, J., de Boever, J., and Schautteet, H.: Revascularization of gingival autografts placed on different receptor beds: a fluorangiographic study, J. Clin. Periodontol. **10:**327, 1983.

# CHAPTER 41

# Interrelated endodontics-periodontics

**Classification**
Periodontal pulpal disease (periodontal origin with secondary endodontic involvement)
Pulpal periodontal disease (primary endodontic origin with secondary periodontal involvement)

**Diagnosis**

**Treatment sequence**

**Summary**

## Classification

A close relationship exists between disease of the dental pulp and periodontal disease, and it expresses itself in several ways[1-4] ( Fig. 41-1):

1. Pulpal disease causing periodontal disease (endodontic origin)
2. Periodontal disease causing pulpal disease (periodontal origin)
3. Combined periodontal and pulpal disease (concurrent)
4. Endodontic failures in periodontally diseased teeth
5. Vertical cracks and fracture

Depending on the origin of the disease, one may speak of pulpal periodontal disease or of periodontal pulpal disease. The following diagram illustrates various possible periodontal pulpal disease interrelationships*:

| Pulpal disease | → | Combined disease of pulp and periodontium | ← | Periodontal disease | **Primary disease** |
| ↓ | | | | ↓ | |
| Pulpal periodontal disease | | | | Periodontal pulpal disease | **Secondary disease** |

### PERIODONTAL PULPAL DISEASE (PERIODONTAL ORIGIN WITH SECONDARY ENDODONTIC INVOLVEMENT)

Atrophic changes in the pulp of teeth with severe periodontal disease are common. One third of such teeth have inflammatory pulp disease; 10% have pulp necrosis. Exposed lateral canals and accessory foramina form the basis for this finding.[1-5] The frequency of such aberrant canals is considerable and is underestimated by the profession.[1] Progressive periodontal disease with bone and attachment loss can expose accessory canals.[6-12] When such a lateral or accessory canal becomes exposed to oral flora, pulpal damage may occur. In some instances the lateral or the accessory canal is obliterated by calcification, but in many cases some entry to the pulp exists.[12] If

---

*Modified from Simon, J.H.S., Glick, D.H., and Frank, A.L.: The relationship of endodontic-periodontic lesions, J. Periodontol. **43:**202, 1972.

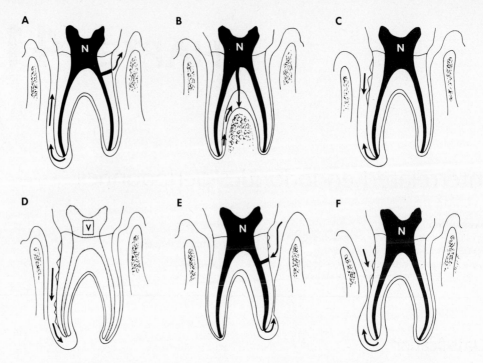

**Fig. 41-1. A** and **B,** Pulpal periodontal disease. Pulps are nonvital, and disease ultimately extends into periodontal tissues. **C,** Combined lesion with initiation in pulpal tissues and periodontal disease occurring secondarily. **D** and **E,** Periodontal pulpal disease. Pulp is vital at first, but bacteria gain access through apical or lateral foramina, and pulp death follows. **F,** "True" combined disease in which both pulpal and periodontal pathologic conditions form a coalescence. (From Simon, J.H.S., Glick, D.H., and Frank, A.L.: J. Periodontol. **43:**202, 1972.)

pulpitis and pulp necrosis results, toxic products then exit into the periodontium, aggravating and extending the periodontal lesion. This mode of aggravation of periodontal disease can also occur in primary pulpal disease.

Experimental periodontitis in monkeys has evoked pathologic pulp changes ranging from irregular secondary dentin and inflammation to necrosis of the pulp.[11] Scaling can expose patent and calcified dentinal tubules and can permit direct communication between the pulp and the pocket even in the absence of lateral canals.[13] Deep scaling may also sever previously uninvolved blood vessels in the vicinity of the periodontal pocket, further compromising the pulpal blood supply. Pulp necrosis can occur when the principal blood supply to the pulp is compromised.[8,9]

### PULPAL PERIODONTAL DISEASE (PRIMARY ENDODONTIC ORIGIN WITH SECONDARY PERIODONTAL INVOLVEMENT)

The floor of the pulp chamber in molars may have numerous small vascular channels to the periodontium[10,12,14-16] (Fig. 41-2). Toxic products of a necrotic pulp may lead to loss of the crest of the interradicular septum[17] (Figs. 41-3 and 41-4).

Occasionally an apical abscess may drain through the gingival sulcus and cause the precipitous appearance of a deep pocket. In such cases root canal treatment can eliminate the pocket and lead to complete bone regeneration. If, on the other hand, severe pocket formation precedes the apical abscess, combined endodontic-periodontal therapy (see Figs. 21-7 and 21-8) will be necessary. The reason for this difference lies in the fact that the root surface of a deep pocket is encrusted with calculus and coated with plaque. The chronicity of the periodontal lesion has a bearing on the difference in the behavior of these two similar lesions.[18] The endodontic situation may appear

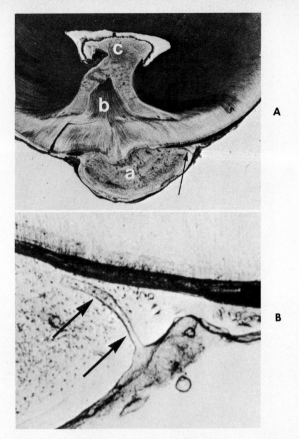

**Fig. 41-2.** **A,** Buccolingual section through the bifurcation of a lower first molar. Note the bifurcational ridge, *a.* A basilar cone of disturbed dentin formation, *b,* can be seen forming a dentin plug, *c,* in the pulp chamber. An accessory canal *(arrow)* can be seen in the intermediate ridge. **B,** Higher magnification of the accessory canal (ground sections).

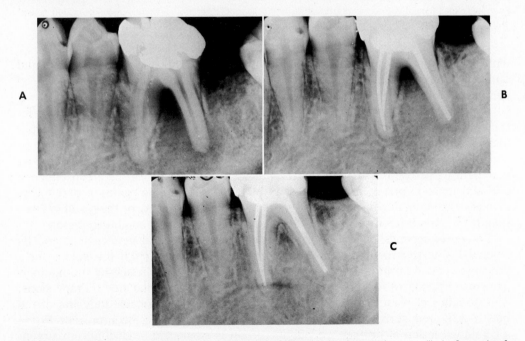

**Fig. 41-3.** Roentgenographic report of the treatment of a bifurcation involvement in a mandibular first molar. **A,** Large area of rarefaction in the bifurcation involving the apex of the distal root. There was a dull, intermittent pain as well as swelling and a discharging fistula. No response to electric pulp testing could be elicited. Root canal treatment was completed on May 31, 1966. **B,** The area of rarefaction in the bifurcation and around the distal apex has decreased in size. An incipient furcation involvement on the buccal side (2 mm deep) was noted. Routine periodontal therapy was performed in 1967. **C,** Follow-up roentgenogram taken in 1968 shows complete disappearance of the bifurcation rarefaction. (Courtesy University of Washington School of Dentistry, Department of Endodontics, Seattle, Washington.)

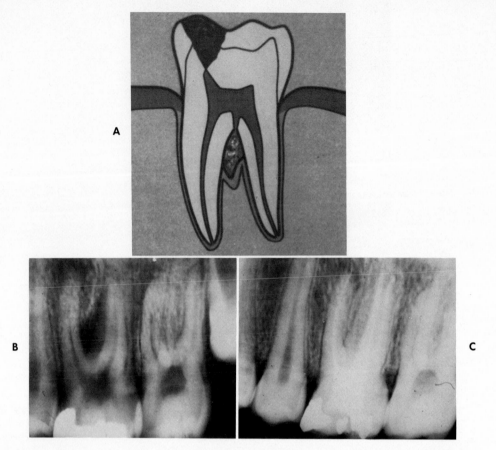

**Fig. 41-4.** **A,** Diagram of bone destruction in the furcation of a molar by inflammation by an accessory canal. **B,** Endodontic involvement with bone destruction in the furcation. **C,** After root canal therapy the lesion has healed, and bone has regenerated. (Courtesy P. Ziegler, San Diego, California.)

with acute symptoms, and then the pocket appears suddenly, whereas the periodontal problem exhibits chronicity, and pulp death occurs as a consequence of advanced periodontal disease.

Other causes of combined pulpal-periodontal disease exist. Accidental root perforation during endodontic therapy may also aggravate the periodontal picture, particularly if the perforation is not sealed quickly and the perforation is close to the periodontal pocket. Persistent hypersensitivity to hot and cold after extensive root planing may indicate mild inflammatory pulpal changes.[19] Pulp death can be a consequence of desensitization procedures (e.g., use of 30% sodium fluoride paste) or may follow extensive grinding during occlusal adjustment. Pulp disease may be the result of tooth fracture.[20-23] Such fractures may lead to pulpal, periodontal, or combined disease.

Prognosis depends on the degree of secondary periodontal involvement and its amenability to treatment. Draining of endodontic lesions through the sulcus for a prolonged period permits secondary involvement of the root surface by the microorganisms of periodontitis,[3] and the lesions may not yield to endodontic therapy alone. The presence of plaque and calculus on the root is a more reliable indicator of the health of the root surface than the length of time the fistula has been present. When a combined lesion of primary endodontic origin is suspected, endodontic treatment should precede any periodontal therapy by about 2 weeks. If the pocket is no longer probeable no further treatment may be necessary.

# Diagnosis

Diseases of pulpal or periodontal origin involving the other tissue secondarily or in combination are found when the patient has pain or an abscess. On occasion, however, the situation may be uncovered during a routine examination. When the patient has an emergency, proper diagnosis and treatment are required for the relief of the complaint. One must pulp test, examine for caries, do diagnostic roentgenography (with probes or gutta-percha points in the pockets or fistulous tracts), explore the sites of suppuration, check for mobility, examine the tooth and roentgenograms for fracture lines, and take a history of the symptoms present. If an abscess is present drainage must be established, and appropriate antibiotic and analgesic medication prescribed.

It is important to determine whether the primary lesion may be pulpal or periodontal[3,10,24-28]; otherwise the wrong treatment may be chosen or there may be unnecessary overtreatment.

**Vitality**

The first step would be to examine for vitality by pulp testing and with heat and cold. A nonvital tooth may indicate primary pulpal involvement, although it can at times indicate secondary pulpal disease. Root canal therapy is necessary. A vital tooth indicates primary periodontal involvement and does not require endodontic therapy. Pulp testing can give false positive results when part of the pulp is vital, and the therapist should be alert to this possibility. When irreversible pulpal changes have occurred, endodontic therapy must be started.

**Pulp testing**

Teeth should be well isolated and dried to prevent false positive reactions to electrical stimulation. Adjacent and contralateral teeth should be tested to determine the normal range of response. A rapid response at lower levels than seen in control teeth may indicate a hyperactive pulp, whereas delayed response at a higher level than in controls may indicate a degenerating pulp.[1] A positive response in single-rooted teeth generally means they are vital. The same response in multirooted teeth is suspect because one or more of the root canals may contain vital tissue. No response to an electric pulp test is normally a good indicator of pulpal necrosis.[29] Teeth with full-coverage restorations require alternate forms of testing because the restoration prevents proper electric pulp tests.

A hot-and-cold test will give some indication of the condition of the pulp. No response to temperature may indicate a nonvital pulp, whereas exaggerated and prolonged responses usually indicate pulpitis. Finally, drilling into the tooth without first inducing anesthesia may indicate pulpal necrosis if no response is elicited.

**Roentgenogram**

The roentgenogram may show loss of bone at the alveolar crest, an apical radiolucency, or a continuous bone loss involving both sites. Apical radiolucency indicates primary pulpal disease. Bone loss confined to the coronal one third of the tooth is associated with primary periodontal disease. When the loss involves both sites there is more difficulty in ascribing causation. If the tooth has a large carious lesion, large restoration, or pins that approach the pulp, the presence of primary pulpal disease is likely. If the tooth is free of caries then primary periodontal disease is probable. If the tooth has a roentgenographic furcation involvement that cannot be detected clinically, look for pulpal involvement. Gutta-percha points used as probes in sinus tracts can be a valuable aid in tracing the origin of a draining lesion.[30] Inability to probe a roentgenographically apparent lesion suggests a nonperiodontal origin.

**Pain and/or abscess formation**

Clinical signs and symptoms will help to differentiate endodontic and periodontal lesions. It is important to establish whether the lesion is of short or of long duration. Pulpal necrosis may involve a complaint of pain with heat, relieved by cold. An acute pulpitis or hyperemia in a vital tooth produces a complaint of pain with cold. As the pulpal situation worsens there may be complaints of pain with heat and cold or even of pain at room temperature. A periodontal abscess may produce a dull, more even pain accompanied by a feeling of fullness in the area or of a "high" tooth. It is not made more intense by heat or cold.

The pulpal lesion may be difficult to localize when the symptoms start, but localization of the pain to a specific tooth occurs as the infection becomes more acute. The periodontal lesion is usually easy to localize.

During acute abscess formation both pulpal and periodontal abscesses may drain into the mucobuccal fold, but if the lesion is localized, suppuration from the pulpal lesion is by way of a fistula through the alveolar mucosa or gingiva. It only rarely fistulates through the sulcus. The periodontal abscess usually drains through the lumen of the pocket. Endodontic lesions are generally associated with more severe symptoms. Acute pain of rapid onset and severe discomfort to percussion and mastication indicate an endodontic lesion that has not established drainage. Extrusion of the affected tooth may result. The extruded tooth is then traumatized during mastication, intensifying discomfort. Once drainage is established discomfort is reduced.

**Probing**

Probing of the affected teeth is usually necessary for differential diagnosis. Probing should be done with a searching motion and with light force. Excessive force in probing may penetrate the connective tissue and enter an endodontic lesion even if no communication existed beforehand.[13]

When the presenting condition has occurred suddenly and the patient's previous periodontal charting indicates that there was no pocket present, then the situation is pulpal. On the other hand, if charting notations indicate that a pocket was present, then the causation is probably periodontal.

**Pocket depth**

A long, narrow pocket in a single tooth in a mouth generally free of periodontal disease is usually associated with primary pulpal disease. A pocket that does not extend to the apical one third of the root in a periodontally diseased mouth indicates primary periodontal origin. Sometimes treatment is diagnostic. Periodontal treatment of an abscess about such a tooth followed by resolution would confirm the diagnosis. An endodontically involved tooth would still require endodontic therapy. Failure of both periodontal and endodontic treatment would signify a split root. Mandibular molars have the highest frequency of split roots. The presence of a split root would cause both approaches to fail. Such teeth have a hopeless prognosis (Fig. 41-5).

A blending of all findings and considerations leads to the proper conclusion and diagnosis of periodontic and endodontic problems. Treatment is determined by proper diagnosis.

## Treatment sequence

In general, when primary disease of one tissue (pulp or periodontium) is present and secondary disease is just starting in the other, treatment of the primary disease will cure the secondary. When the secondary disease is established and chronic, both primary and secondary diseases must be treated. If primary pulpal disease forms a narrow fistula through the sulcus of a tooth that is otherwise in good health, the pocket will be eliminated after endodontic treatment. This is also true of furcal bone loss resulting from primary pulp disease. On the other hand signs of a mild pulpitis (e.g., sensitivity to cold or sweet) will be eliminated by successful periodontal treatment, if the pulpitis was caused by the periodontal disease process.

Lesions of endodontic origin with secondary periodontal involvement should first be treated endodontically to take advantage of the normally excellent healing potential of an endodontic lesion (Fig. 41-6). Residual periodontal lesions can then be treated after the response to endodontic therapy is evaluated. Combined periodontal-endodontic lesions should also undergo endodontic therapy first. When in doubt as to whether the lesion is endodontic or periodontal in origin, endodontic therapy should generally

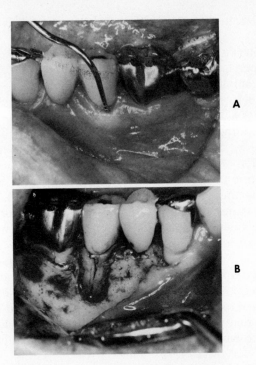

**Fig. 41-5.   A,** A periodontal probe penetrates to 8 mm in an apparently deep periodontal pocket. The tooth tested nonvital. **B,** The reflection of a flap revealed a cracked root. Extraction was necessary. (Courtesy M.E. Gher, U.S. Navy.)

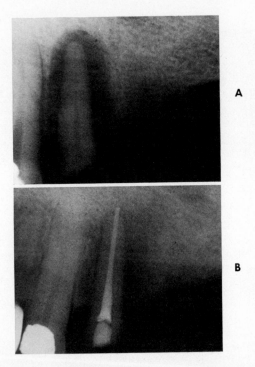

**Fig. 41-6.   A,** A continuous nonprobeable radiolucency encompasses a tooth with primary endodontic etiology. **B,** After endodontic therapy bone regeneration has restored alveolar height. The radiolucency has considerably diminished in size. (Courtesy M.E. Gher, U.S. Navy.)

be performed first because of its significantly better prognosis and minimal posttreatment sequelae.

In an upper anterior tooth a chronic deep pocket may exist that communicates with an involved periapical area. In such a case endodontic-periodontal combined therapy may be accomplished in a single session by the use of a flap approach to gain access to the root surface and the apex (see Figs. 21-7 and 21-8). A labial involvement has the best prognosis, a lingual involvement the worst. The pulp of a tooth testing vital may be degenerating, thus contributing to a periodontal pulpal defect. When such teeth receive combined therapy dramatic results sometimes ensue (Fig. 41-7).

**Root resection**

A special situation exists when one or two roots of a firm, multirooted tooth are untreatable by routine endodontic or periodontal measures. For instance, in a firm mandibular molar a single canal may be untreatable, a single root may have lost all bone, or extensive caries may almost have severed a root or involved the exposed bifurcation. The treatment of choice in such cases is root amputation (removal of one or two roots in an upper molar) or hemisection (buccolingual sectioning of a mandibular molar).[31-36] Hemisection also involves the crown and is discussed in Chapter 42.

**Root transplants**

Autogenous root transplants into edentulous areas can provide abutments at needed sites.[37,38] The technique involves the preparation of a socket by surgical means. The endodontically treated root is transplanted into the socket, and the flap sutured closed over the root for approximately 6 months. Then the root is surgically exposed and fitted with a postcoping crown. Endosseous implants are rapidly replacing root transplants (Chapter 48).

**Forced root eruption**

Orthodontic root eruption is another valuable technique in which roots with trans-

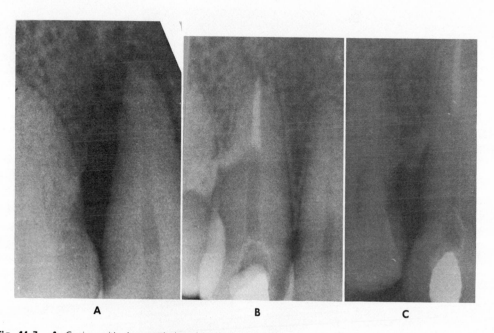

A          B          C

**Fig. 41-7. A,** Canine with deep periodontal pockets and radiolucency on distal and palatal surfaces. Pockets could be probed close to the apex. No caries restorations were present. The tooth tested vital. Root planing and curettage had been performed regularly during the previous 30-month period. **B,** Six months after root canal therapy and open curettage, the radiolucency is not visible. **C,** Two years after treatment regeneration of bone is evident. (Courtesy H. Staffelino, Jr., Chicago, Illinois.)

verse fractures, perforations, or external resorptions in the coronal one third of the root are treated endodontically. Then orthodontic treatment is used to bring the root into a position in which it is accessible for restorative dentistry. The technique is quite useful when a cusp has fractured below the gingiva or where caries extends below the gingiva at a level where periodontal surgical procedures would produce a result that would not be cosmetic (see chapter on Preprosthetic Surgery).[39]

## Summary

Combined endodontic-periodontal therapy is widely used because of the close proximity of pulp and periodontal structures and their mutual involvement in disease. In most cases of this nature endodontic procedures are performed first and when necessary are followed by periodontal measures. However, in some cases both procedures may be done at a single session.

Some rather rare pseudoperiodontal situations may, in fact, be due to *primary* pulp disease and may clear up after endodontic treatment alone: (1) the suddenly appearing deep pocket that is in reality a fistulous tract from the periapical area to the gingival sulcus and (2) the roentgenographically diagnosed furcation involvement that cannot be probed and may be a result of discharge from a necrotic pulp through a bifurcational accessory canal. Endodontic treatment alone may cure both these conditions. When advanced, chronic periodontal disease or periodontal treatment has exposed lateral canals or the apical foramen leading to *secondary* pulpitis or pulp death, the chances of curing the condition by endodontic treatment alone are slim. This is a more common situation than the two preceding. Root canal therapy and periodontal intervention (combined endodontic-periodontal therapy) are indicated.

The value of precise pocket probing and correct appraisal of the vitality of the pulp is therefore evident. In some doubtful cases the better part of wisdom is to wait until after the root canal therapy is completed to see whether spontaneous resolution (pocket closure and osseous fill-in) will occur before surgical periodontal procedures are begun. The clinical experience and acumen of the dentist must be of the highest degree to enable choosing the procedure that will bring healing with the appropriate intervention.

Properly treated teeth remain firm and can be maintained in health without increase in pocket probing depth for considerable periods of time.[40-42]

**REFERENCES**

1. Weine, F.S.: Endodontic therapy, St. Louis, 1982, The C.V. Mosby Co.
2. Simring, M., and Goldberg, M.: The pulpal pocket approach: retrograde periodontitis, J. Periodontol. **35:**22, 1964.
3. Hiatt, W.H.: Pulpal periodontal disease, J. Periodontol. **48:**598, 1977.
4. Simon, J.H.S., Glick, D.H., and Frank, A.L.: The relationship of endodontic-periodontic lesions, J. Periodontol. **43:**202, 1972.
5. Hess, W.: The anatomy of the root-canals of the teeth of the permanent dentition, London, 1925, John Bale, Sons & Danielsson Ltd.
6. Vertucci, F.J., and Williams, R.G.: Furcation canals in the human mandibular first molar, Oral Surg. **38:**308, 1974.
7. Burch, J.G.: A study of the presence of accessory foramina and the topography of molar furcations, Oral Surg. **38:**451, 1974.
8. Bender, I.B., and Seltzer, S.: The effect of periodontal disease on the pulp, Oral Surg. **33:**458, 1972.
9. Langeland, K., Rodrigues, H., and Dowden, W.: Periodontal disease, bacteria, and pulpal histopathology, Oral Surg. **37:**257, 1974.
10. Seltzer, S., Bender, I.B., and Ziontz, M.: The interrelationship of pulp and periodontal disease, Oral Surg. **16:**1474, 1963.
11. Bergenholtz, G., and Lindhe, J.: Effect of experimentally induced marginal periodontitis and periodontal scaling on the dental pulp, J. Clin. Periodontol. **5:**59, 1978.
12. Lowman, J.V., Burke, R.S., and Pelleu, G.B.: Patent accessory canals: incidence in molar furcation region, Oral Surg. **36:**580, 1973.
13. Harrington, G.W.: The perio-endo question: differential diagnosis, Dent. Clin. North Am. **23:**673, 1979.
14. Everett, F.G., et al.: The intermediate bifurcational ridge, J. Dent. Res. **37:**162, 1964.
15. Kovacs, I.: Contribution à l'étude des rapports entre le development et la morphologie des racines des dents humains, Bull. Group. Int. Rech. Sci. Stomatol. Odontol. **7:**85, 1964.

16. Orban, B., and Mueller, E.: The development of the bifurcation of multirooted teeth, J. Am. Dent. Assoc. **16:**297, 1929.

17. Johnston, H.B., and Orban, B.: Interradicular pathology as related to accessory root canals, J. Endodont. **3:**21, 1948.

18. Hiatt, W.H.: Regeneration of the periodontium after endodontic therapy and flap operation, Oral Surg. **12:**1471, 1959.

19. Everett, F.G., Hall, W.B., and Phatak, N.M.: Treatment of hypersensitive dentin, J. Oral Ther. Pharm. **2:**300, 1966.

20. Ritchey, B., Mendenhall, R., and Orban, B.: Pulpitis resulting from incomplete root fracture, Oral Surg. **10:**665, 1957.

21. Hiatt, W.H.: Incomplete crown-root fracture in pulpal-periodontal disease, J. Periodontol. **44:**369, 1973.

22. Polson, A.M.: Periodontal destruction associated with vertical root fracture: report of four cases, J. Periodontol. **48:**27, 1977.

23. Silvestri, A.R.: The undiagnosed split-root syndrome, J. Am. Dent. Assoc. **92:**930, 1976.

24. Simon, P., and Jacobs, D.: The so-called combined periodontal-pulpal problem, Dent. Clin. North Am. **13:**45, 1969.

25. Blair, H.A.: Relationships between endodontics and periodontics, J. Periodontol. **43:**209, 1972.

26. Sharp, R.E.: The relationship of the pulp and periodontium, J. West. Soc. Periodontol./Periodont. Abstr. **25:**130, 1977.

27. Ross, I.F.: The relation between periodontal and pulpal disorders, J. Am. Dent. Assoc. **84:**134, 1972.

28. Chacker, F.M.: The endodontic-periodontic continuum, Dent. Clin. North Am. **18:**393, 1974.

29. Mullaney, T.P., Howell, R.M., and Petrick, J.D.: Resistance of nerve fibers to pulpal necrosis, Oral Surg. **30:**690, 1970.

30. Sugarman, M.M., and Sugarman, E.F.: The differential diagnosis of periodontic-endodontic problems, J. Ala. Dent. Assoc. **53:**16, 1969.

31. Messinger, T.F., and Orban, B.: Elimination of periodontal pockets by root amputation, J. Periodontol. **25:**213, 1954.

32. Amen, C.R.: Hemisection and root amputation, Periodontics **4:**197, 1966.

33. Hiatt, W.H.: The repositioned alveolar ridge mucosal flap, Periodontics **5:**132, 1967.

34. Black, G.V.: In Litch, W., editor: The American system of dentistry, Philadelphia, 1886, Lea.

35. Everett, F.G.: Bifurcation involvement, J. Ore. Dent. Assoc. **28:**2, 1959.

36. Staffileno, H.I.: Furcation treatment in periodontics, Dent. Radiogr. Photogr. **38:**83, 1965.

37. Natiella, J.R., Armitage, J.E., and Greene, G.W.: The replantation and transplantation of teeth, Oral Surg. **29:**397, 1970.

38. Yuodelis, R.A., and Filipchuk, C.E.: A technique for autogenous root transplantation, J. Prosthet. Dent. **35:**307, 1976.

39. Simon, J.H.S., et al.: Extrusion of endodontically treated teeth, J. Am. Dent. Assoc. **97:**17, 1978.

40. Hamp, S.E., Nyman, S., and Lindhe, J.: Periodontal treatment of multi-rooted teeth. Results after 5 years, J. Clin. Periodontol. **2:**126, 1975.

41. Klaven, B.: Clinical observations following root amputation in maxillary molar teeth, J. Periodontol. **46:**1, 1975.

42. Ross, I.F., and Thompson, R.H., Jr.: A long term study of root retention in the treatment of maxillary molars with furcation involvement, J. Periodontol. **49:**238, 1978.

## ADDITIONAL SUGGESTED READING

Abou-Rass, M.: Endodontics, Alpha Omegan **75:**18, 1982.

Basaraba, N.: Root amputation and tooth hemisection, Dent. Clin. North Am. **13:**121, 1969.

Bender, I.B., and Freedland, J.B.: Adult root fracture, J. Am. Dent. Assoc. **107:**413, 1983.

Bergenholtz, A.: Radectomy of multirooted teeth, J. Am. Dent. Assoc. **85:**870, 1972.

Feldman, G., et al.: Endodontic treatment of periodontal problems, Dent. Radiogr. Photogr. **54:**1, 1981.

Guldener, P.H.A.: Die Beziehung zwischen Pulpa- und Parodontalerkrankungen, Dtsch. Zahnarztl. Z. **30:**377, 1975.

Gutmann, J.L.: Prevalence, location and patency of accessory canals in the furcation region of permanent molars, J. Periodontol. **49:**21, 1978.

Hiatt, W.H., and Amen, C.R.: Periodontal pocket elimination by combined therapy. Dent. Clin. North Am., p. 133, March 1964.

Kirkham, D.B.: The location and incidence of accessory pulpal levels in periodontal pockets, J. Am. Dent. Assoc. **91:**353, 1973.

Lommel, T.J., et al.: Alveolar bone loss associated with vertical root fractures, Oral Surg. **45:**863, 1978.

Rosenberg, E.S., et al.: A combined endodontic-periodontal lesion: its management and resolution, J. Clin. Periodontol. **8:**369, 1981.

Rubach, W.C., and Mitchell, D.F.: Periodontal disease, accessory canals, and pulp pathosis, J. Periodontol. **36:**34, 1965.

Seltzer, S., Sinai, I., and August, D.: Periodontal effects of root perforations before and during endodontic procedures, J. Dent. Res. **49:**332, 1970.

Sicher, H.: Ueber Pulpaerkrankungen als Folge von Paradontose, Z. Stomatol. **34:**819, 1936.

Stahl, S.S.: Pathogenesis of inflammatory lesions in pulp and periodontal tissues, Periodontics **4:**190, 1966.

# CHAPTER 42

# The periodontally diseased furcation

One of the more serious complications of periodontal disease is the involvement of the bifurcations and trifurcations of multirooted teeth. Such situations at one time were considered untreatable and an indication for extraction. Pockets in such areas were not amenable to treatment. They deepened and led to abscesses. Root caries was a frequent occurrence. As understanding of the pathogenesis of periodontal disease has improved, and as the anatomy of furcations has been clarified, effective treatment methods have been developed.

## Furcation anatomy

Furcal areas of the tooth can be divided into three parts (Fig. 42-1). One is the area of the root separation, the portion of the tooth where adjacent roots forming the furcation are not in contact with each other and are separated by alveolar bone. Another is the surface of the tooth just coronal to the root separation. This area is usually concave, grooved, or fluted. The final portion is the roof of the furcation (Fig. 42-1).

The flute of the tooth and the area of root separation are both areas of plaque retention (Fig. 42-2). In addition the flute area may contain an enamel projection. The roof contains furcation ridges[1,2] (Figs. 41-2 and 42-3, *B*). These ridges run mesiodistally in lower and buccolingually in upper molars. There may be one or more ridges, which tend to make plaque control difficult. The inner surfaces of the roots of the lower molars and the mesiobuccal root of the upper molars usually contain developmental grooves (see Fig. 41-2), further complicating the situation.

Maxillary molars generally have three roots. The roots separate from the root trunk approximately 5 to 5.5 mm apical to the cementoenamel junction (CEJ).[3] These root separations are preceded by root trunk concavities (furcation entrances) that deepen as they merge to reach the furcation (see Fig. 42-1 and 42-2). The furcation entrances are the earliest areas of furcation involvement. They are located 3.6, 4.2, and 4.8 mm apical to the CEJ on the mesial, facial, and distal surfaces (Table 42-1). The roof of the furcation is concave in about 50% of maxillary first molars and is located 4.5 mm

**Maxillary molars**

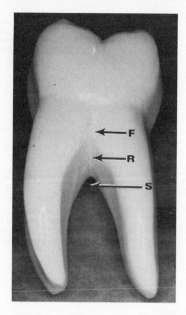

**Fig. 42-1.** *F,* Flute; *R,* root of furcation; *S,* root separation. (Courtesy B. Klavan, Phoenix, Arizona.)

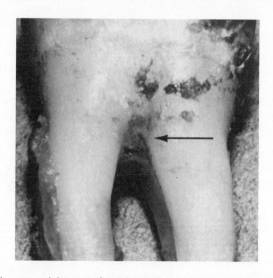

**Fig. 42-2.** The flute of the root and the area of root separation are both areas of plaque retention. Note plaque and calculus in flute and root furcation. (Courtesy B. Klavan, Phoenix, Arizona.)

apical to the CEJ.[3] The roof is 0.5 to 1.0 mm coronal to the root separations. Access to this area is extremely difficult for instrumentation of deep pockets (Fig. 42-3, *A*). Furcation ridges further complicate instrumentation (Fig. 42-3, *B*). These cementum ridges also impede plaque removal.

The palatal root is the longest and most massive of the three roots. The mesiobuccal root is the widest, extending for two thirds of the width of the crown buccolingually.[4,5] The surface area of the mesiobuccal root is equal to that of the palatal root because of its shape (Table 42-2). The distal root provides a smaller (19%) yet significant surface for attachment. *The root trunk provides 32% of the total root surface area of the maxillary first molar. Horizontal attachment loss involving the root trunk that extends to the level of the furcation (5.0 mm apical to the CEJ) results in a loss of one third of the total support of the tooth.*

**Attachment surface**

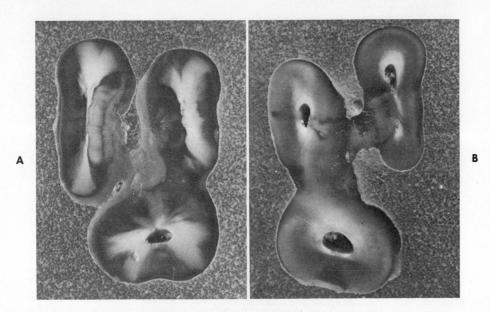

**Fig. 42-3.** **A,** Cross section of maxillary first molar at the level of the roof of the furcation. Note the roof is domed and is coronal to the furcation entrance. **B,** Cross section of maxillary first molar. Note the ridge of cementum extending between the mesiobuccal and distobuccal roots. (Courtesy M.E. Gher, U.S. Navy.)

**Table 42-1**  Maxillary first molar: mean distances of root structures apical to CEJ junction (mm)*

| Furcation entrances | Root separations | Furcation roof |
|---|---|---|
| Mesial 3.6 ± 0.8 | Mesiobuccal 5.0 ± 0.7 | 4.6 ± 0.6 |
| Facial 4.2 ± 1.0 | Distobuccal 5.5 ± 0.8 | |
| Distal 4.8 ± 0.8 | | |

From Gher, M.E., et al.: Linear variation of the root surface area of the maxillary first molar, J. Periodontol. **56**:39, 1985.
*Mean and standard deviation figures for 20 maxillary first molars.

**Table 42-2**  Surface area measurements of the maxillary first molar

| Root area | Appropriate root surface area (mm²)* | Comparative relationships (% of root surface area) | | Length (mm)* |
|---|---|---|---|---|
| | | Three roots | Three roots + root trunk | |
| Distobuccal | 91.22 | 28% | 19% | 8.65 |
| Mesiobuccal | 117.74 | 36% | 25% | 8.78 |
| Palantal | 114.52 | 35% | 24% | 9.15 |
| Root trunk | 152.95 | 35% | 32% | 4.32 |

From Gher, M.E., et al.: Linear variation of the root surface area of the maxillary first molar, J. Periodontol. **56**:39, 1985.
*Mean values for 20 samples.

Where the roots diverge access is limited.[5] Most curettes are too wide to properly instrument this area. The separation of the roots is approximately 0.75 mm at the level of the furcation,[5] and curette blades are usually wider. Narrowed curettes may be used for proper instrumentation (Fig. 42-4).

Concave root surfaces further complicate instrumentation. Ninety-four percent of mesiobuccal roots of maxillary first molars have a furcation concavity (Fig. 42-5). Thirty-one percent of distobuccal roots and 17% of palatal roots have similar concavities.[6] Access is also limited by the angulation, shape, and relationship of the three roots[7] (Fig. 42-5).

**Root concavities**

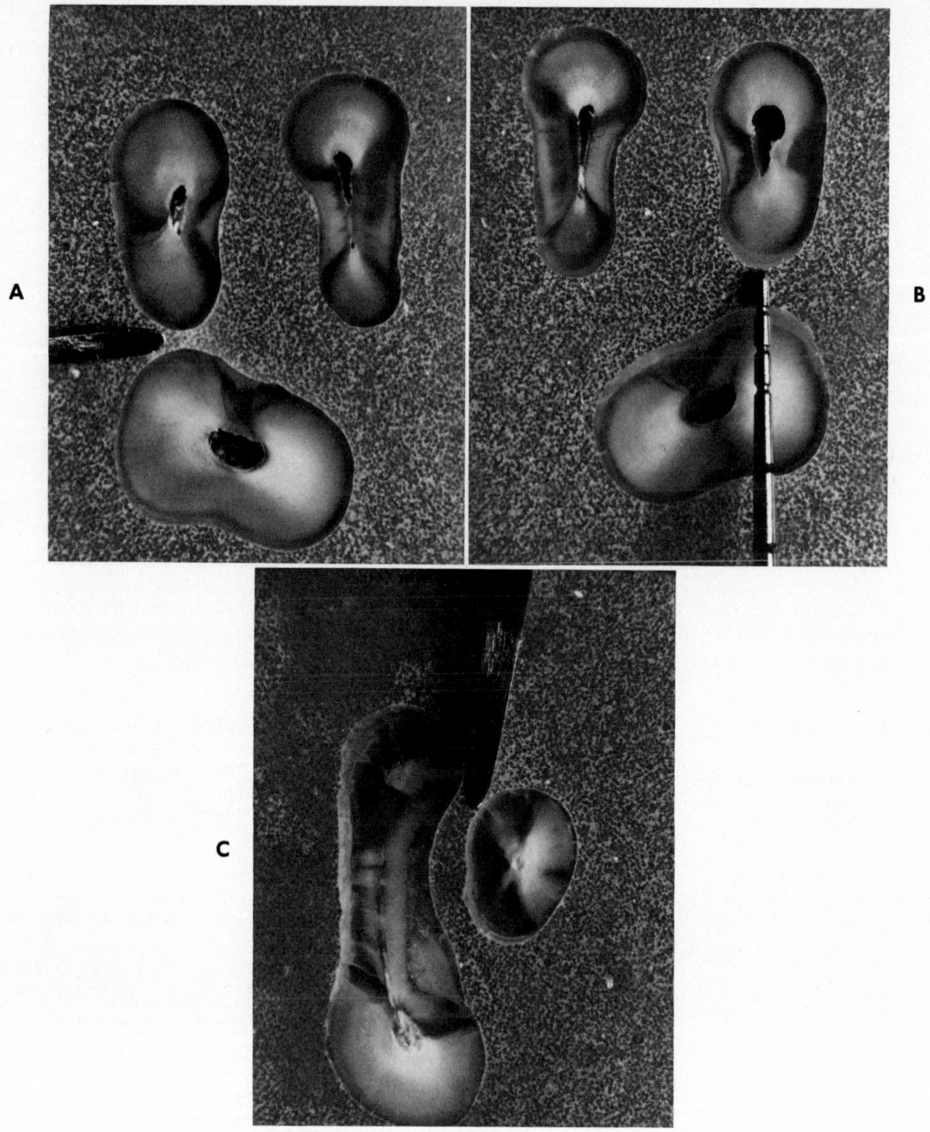

**Fig. 42-4.** **A,** Cross section of maxillary first molar just apical to furcation entrance. Note that the curette blade is wider than the furcation entrance. **B,** Periodontal probe illustrates the narrow furcation width between the distobuccal and palatal roots, 2 mm below the furcation entrance. **C,** The curette is too wide and improperly shaped to enter the facial furcation. (Courtesy M.E. Gher, U.S. Navy.)

Thirty-two percent of the total support of the maxillary first molar is located 2 mm above and 2 mm below the furcation area (Fig. 42-6).

**Maxillary second molar**

The maxillary second molar has similar anatomic characteristics except that the roots are in closer proximity and are more often fused.

**Mandibular molars**

Mandibular molars generally have two roots of similar size and length (Table 42-3).[8,9] The root trunk of the mandibular first molar supplies 31% of the total attachment area, whereas the mesial and distal roots supply 37% and 32%, respectively.[8] The mesial root has a barbell-shaped cross section owing to mesial and distal concavities[6] (Fig. 42-7). The distal root has mesial and less frequently, distal concavities.[6] It also has a smaller buccolingual dimension.[6] Thus the mesial root has a slightly greater surface area.

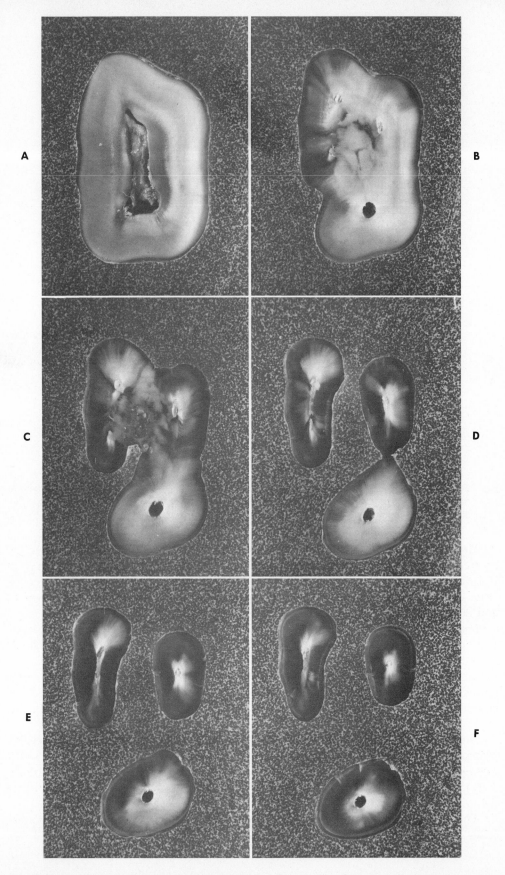

**Fig. 42-5.** **A** to **F,** Starting at the cementoenamel junction of the maxillary first molar, the variation in root form, the concavities, and the furcation entrances can be seen in cross-sections. These are illustrated proceeding apically in 2-mm increments. (Courtesy M.E. Gher, U.S. Navy.)

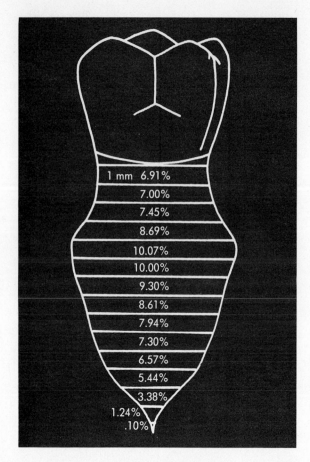

1 mm  6.91%
7.00%
7.45%
8.69%
10.07%
10.00%
9.30%
8.61%
7.94%
7.30%
6.57%
5.44%
3.38%
1.24%
.10%

**Fig. 42-6.**  *The root surface area of the maxillary first molar is shown in 1-mm increments. If this tooth had a single root, its form would be as depicted. The greatest root surface area is at a level from 2 mm above to 2 mm below the furcation.* (Courtesy M.E. Gher, U.S. Navy.)

Molar furcations are complicated by the presence of fused roots, *cervical enamel projections, enamel pearls,* and *furcation ridges.*[10-18] The intermediate bifurcation ridge is a ridge of cementum extending across the furcation in a mesial to distal direction (Fig. 42-8). *Cervical enamel projections* are reported in 17% of maxillary first molars and 29% of mandibular first molars (Fig. 42-9).

**Maxillary first premolar**

Most maxillary first premolars are bifurcated at the middle third of the root trunk.[19] A deep, broad mesial root trunk concavity becomes deeper as it progresses apically to merge with the furcation. The distal furcation entrance is more precipitous. This entrance merges with the *buccal furcation groove,* a groove present on the furcation surface of the buccal root in most bifurcated maxillary first premolars.[20] Buccal furcation grooves apparently represent an attempt at multiple root formation (Fig. 42-10). A small number of maxillary first premolars have three roots (Fig. 42-11).

Deep mesial concavities and limited interproximal space between the maxillary first premolar and the maxillary cuspid often limit access. Once the pocket extends to the middle third of the root, furcation involvement is likely, contributing to poor prognosis. The inaccessibility of this area seriously inhibits plaque removal and root surface débridement.[21]

**Mandibular first premolar**

The formation of cul-de-sacs or bifurcations in mandibular premolars is infrequent (Fig. 42-12); however grooves may be present on the mesiolingual surface.

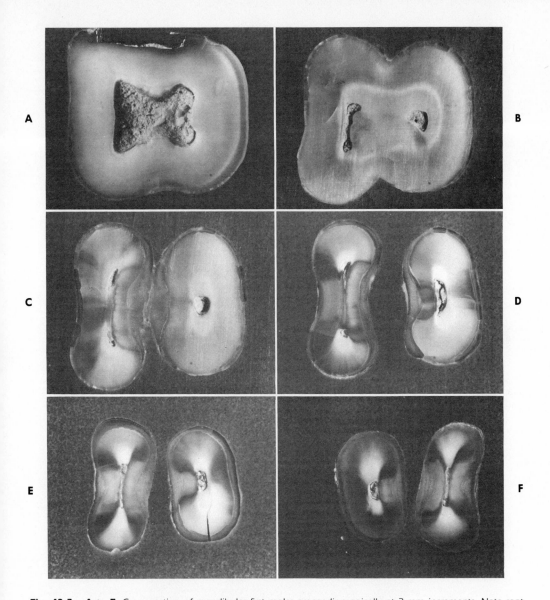

**Fig. 42-7.** **A** to **F,** Cross section of mandibular first molar proceeding apically at 2-mm increments. Note root concavities and narrow furcation entrance at **C.** (Courtesy M.E. Gher, U.S. Navy.)

**Table 42-3**   Mandibular first molar root surface area (RSA) values for 20 teeth

|  | RSA (mm²)* | % total RSA† | % RSA† for 2 roots |
|---|---|---|---|
| Mesial root | 161.5 | 37.0 | 53.2 |
| Distal root | 141.8 | 32.4 | 46.7 |
| Root trunk | 133.5 | 30.5 | |
| Total RSA | 436.8 | | |

From: Gher, M.E., et al.: Linear variation of the root surface area of the maxillary first molar, J. Periodontol. **56:**39, 1985.
*Mean for 20 mandibular molars.
†% RSA values rounded to the nearest 0.1%
$t = 5.50$ for mesial vs. distal RSA, $P = 0.01$.

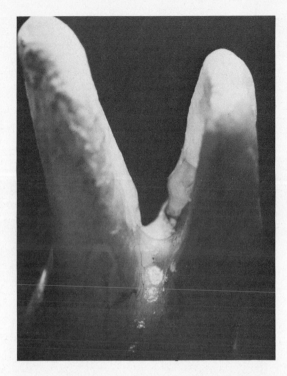

**Fig. 42-8.** The mandibular first molar has an intermediate bifurcation ridge extending between the roots in approximately 75% of teeth. (Courtesy M.E. Gher, U.S. Navy.)

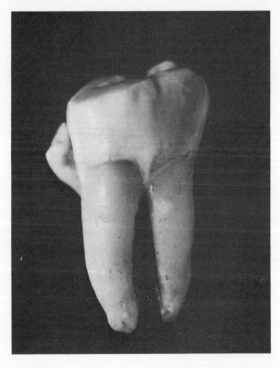

**Fig. 42-9.** A cervical enamel projection in the furcation of a mandibular first molar. This tooth also has an accessory cusp. (Courtesy M.E. Gher, U.S. Navy.)

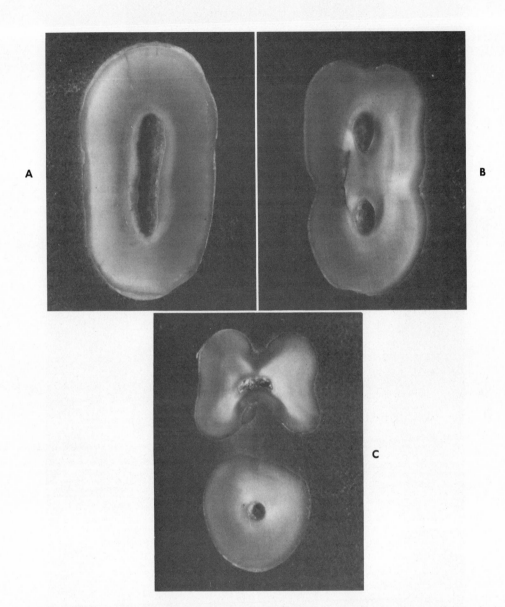

**Fig. 42-10.   A** to **C,** The maxillary first premolar is bifurcated 56% of the time. The furcation usually starts in the middle third of the root. **C,** The buccal root may show a buccal concavity and a concavity on the furcation surface called the *buccal furcation groove*. (Courtesy M.E. Gher, U.S. Navy.)

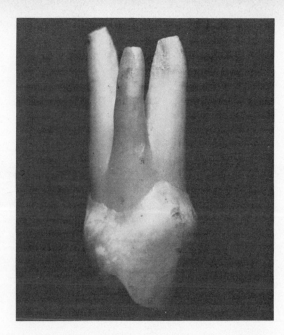

**Fig. 42-11.** A three-rooted maxillary first premolar. Three roots occur in 4% of these teeth. (Courtesy M.E. Gher, U.S. Navy.)

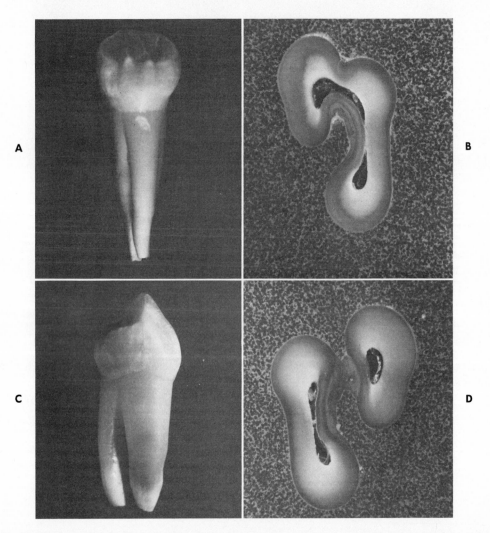

**Fig. 42-12.** **A** and **B,** Mandibular first premolar showing a deep cul-de-sac on the mesial root surface and a concavity on the buccal aspect of the root. **C** and **D,** A bifurcated mandibular first premolar. This occurs rarely. (Courtesy M.E. Gher, U.S. Navy.)

## Classification

Furcation involvement is classified according to the severity of the attachment loss. Degree I involves the *furcation entrance* (Fig. 42-13, *A*). Degree II involvement extends under the *roof of the furcation* but not through and through (Fig. 42-13, *B*). Degree III is a through-and-through involvement (Fig. 42-13, *C*).

Subclassification[22-24] is necessary to permit a more accurate description. The subclassification measures probeable vertical depth from the roof of the furcation. Class A is a probing depth of 1 to 3 mm, Class B is 4 to 6 mm, and Class C is 7 or more mm (Table 42-4). The subclassification is an important indicator of prognosis.

## Diagnosis

Treatment methods are chosen to match the degree of involvement, so accurate perception is of great importance. Roentgenograms are necessary to gauge the degree of bone loss,[26,27] but they may be imprecise and ambiguous (Fig. 42-14). Periodontal probes are useful for determining the probing depth in a vertical direction (pocket depth) but are less useful for determining the degree of horizontal involvement. For this purpose either curved explorers or curettes (Fig. 42-15, *A*) are very useful. The curvature of these instruments allows them to be passed under the roof of the furca and to measure the degree of involvement. Roentgenograms may be taken with probes, explorers, or curettes in place (Fig. 42-15, *B*).

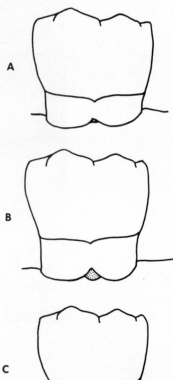
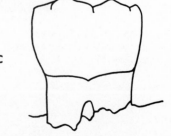

**Fig. 42-13.** Classification of furcation involvement, horizontal component. **A,** Class I. **B,** Class II. **C,** Class III. (Courtesy B. Klavan, Phoenix, Arizona.)

**Table 42-4** Classification of furcation invasions

| Horizontal component[22] | Vertical component[23,24] |
|---|---|
| Degree I: horizontal loss of periodontal tissue support is less than 3 mm | Class A: vertical destruction up to one third of the total interradicular height (1-3 mm) |
| Degree II: horizontal loss of support exceeds 3 mm but does not encompass the total width of the furcation area | Class B: vertical destruction reaching two thirds of the interradicular height (4-6 mm) |
| Degree III: horizontal through-and-through destruction of the periodontal tissue in the furcation | Class C: interradicular osseous destruction into or beyond the apical third (>7 mm) |

Standlee, J.P., et al.: Analysis of stress distribution by endodontic posts, Oral Surg. **33:**952, 1972.

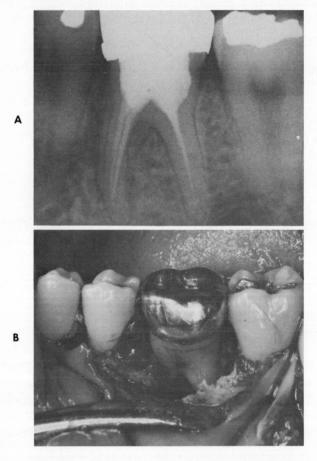

**Fig. 42-14. A,** Roentgenogram of mandibular first molar does not demonstrate the severity of the furcation involvement actually present (see **B**). **B,** Clinically, a class II B furcation involvement was apparent during surgery. (Courtesy M.E. Gher, U.S. Navy.)

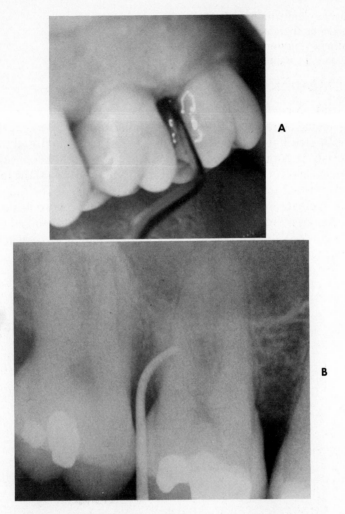

**Fig. 42-15.    A,** Periodontal probe in distal furcation of maxillary right first molar. **B,** X-ray study of curette in same furcation. (Courtesy B. Klavan, Phoenix, Arizona.)

## Treatment

The major principle of treatment of involved furcas is to eliminate the involvement whenever possible.

A variety of methods are available for treatment. Not all of them provide for elimination of the furcation: Some provide only for increased accessibility for plaque removal[28]; some reduce the susceptibility of the tooth to caries. These methods include odontoplasty, osteoplasty, root amputation, hemisection, root separation, the tunneling procedure, and extraction.[29-37]

Many factors must be taken into consideration when deciding on a mode of therapy:

1. Degree of involvement
2. Crown-root ratio
3. Length of roots
4. Degree of root separation
5. Strategic value of the tooth or teeth in question
6. Root anatomy of the involved tooth
7. Residual tooth mobility

8. Ability to eliminate the defect
9. Endodontic therapy and complications
10. Prosthetic requirements
11. Periodontal condition of adjacent teeth

## INITIAL PREPARATION

Scaling and proper oral hygiene are the first treatment procedures.[38] Defective restorations should be replaced, since they complicate therapy and may impede plaque removal.[39-43] Degree I and mild degree II involvements respond well to initial therapy.

**Odontoplasty**     Odontoplasty is defined as the reshaping of a tooth. Odontoplasty can eliminate class I and mild class II furcation involvements. The fluted area of the tooth is reshaped. In a sense the flute is extended toward the occlusal surface. The rationale behind the technique is to create improved access for plaque control.[5] At times odontoplasty can be performed as an individual procedure.[44] At other times it is coupled with the surgical procedure (Fig. 42-16). Odontoplasty can contribute to increased sensitivity and should be used judiciously.

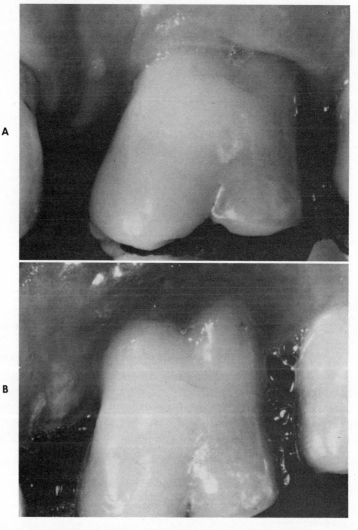

**Fig. 42-16.** **A,** Class I furcation involvement in maxillary molar. **B,** After odontoplasty the area is accessible for cleansing. (Courtesy B. Klavan, Phoenix, Arizona.)

Osteoplasty may be used with class I and mild class II involvements to tuck the gingiva into the furcation in order to provide better gingival form, as well as to eliminate sulcular depth. The procedure may be combined with odontoplasty (Fig. 42-17). Incomplete bifurcation involvements of mandibular molars are treated by grooving the bone between the roots and then festooning and beveling the bone over the roots.[45]

## CLASSES II AND III FURCATION INVOLVEMENTS

Moderate and severe furcation involvements require additional methods of treatment when the disease process is not controlled by initial preparation. Such treatment may include tunneling.

### Root amputation

Root amputation is the removal of one or more roots from a multirooted tooth. The primary benefit gained from root amputation is improved access. This benefit must outweigh the loss of support of the amputated root. In addition, the need for endodontic and restorative care should also be considered. Indications for root amputation include:

1. Severe and disproportionate attachment loss around the affected root
2. Furcation defects that can be eliminated by root amputation
3. Improved prognosis for adjacent teeth
4. Retention of a tooth with strategic value

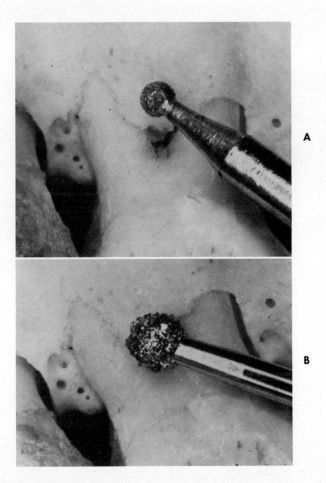

**Fig. 42-17.** Osteoplasty **(A)** and odontoplasty **(B)** being performed in mild class II furcation. (Courtesy B. Klavan, Phoenix, Arizona.)

5. Elimination of an endodontically untreatable root
6. Elimination of cracked or deeply fissured roots
7. Pockets in areas of root proximity of adjacent multirooted teeth
8. Recession exposing most or all of a root in a multirooted tooth
9. Inoperable root caries

An abutment molar may become periodontally diseased. Its loss would mean loss of the bridge. Root amputation may permit retention of the tooth and the bridge (Fig. 42-18).

Root amputation will permit retention of a tooth that would otherwise be lost owing to a cracked root, caries, deep developmental fissures, and periodontal involvement, provided the remaining roots are functional (Fig. 42-19). In addition, involved teeth with endodontic perforations or nonnegotiable canals can be retained.

Root amputation can be performed in teeth with severe gingival recession without raising a flap (Fig. 42-20). However, most root resections require a flap. This permits access, visualization, osteoplasty, and contouring of the root trunk.

Ideally, endodontic therapy should precede amputation. Sometimes the initial periodontal-endodontic lesion will heal, precluding the need for root amputation. Where an amputation is planned, amalgam may be placed in the canal of the root to be amputated to permit contouring.[44] When the therapist is uncertain as to which root will be amputated, or when a combined periodontal-endodontic lesion is suspected, all canals should be filled. Factors determining selection for root amputation include:

1. Bone levels in the furcation
2. Accessibility for plaque removal

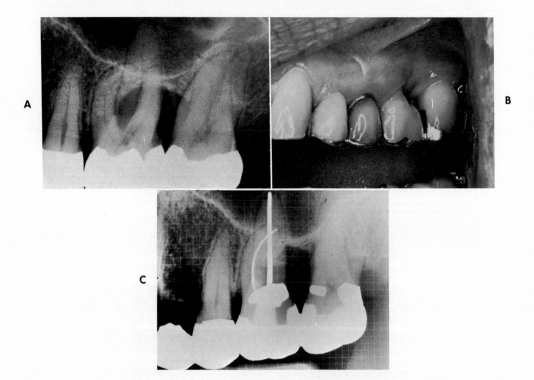

**Fig. 42-18.** **A,** Preoperative roentgenogram. Maxillary first molar with large trifurcation involvement. The distobuccal root suffers from severe alveolar bone loss. The tooth is included in an extensive splint. Root canal therapy was performed, and the distobuccal root was resected. **B,** Clinical appearance 1 year later. Note the reshaping of the crown in the area where the amputation was performed. **C,** Roentgenogram 15 years after surgery. The tooth is firm and in good periapical and periodontal health.

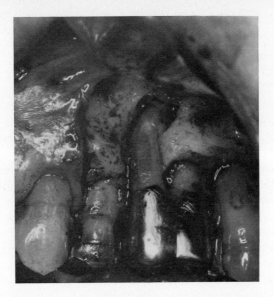

**Fig. 42-19.** This maxillary first molar with a vertical fracture of the mesiobuccal root and accompanying bone loss may be retained after the root is amputated. (Courtesy M.E. Gher, U.S. Navy.)

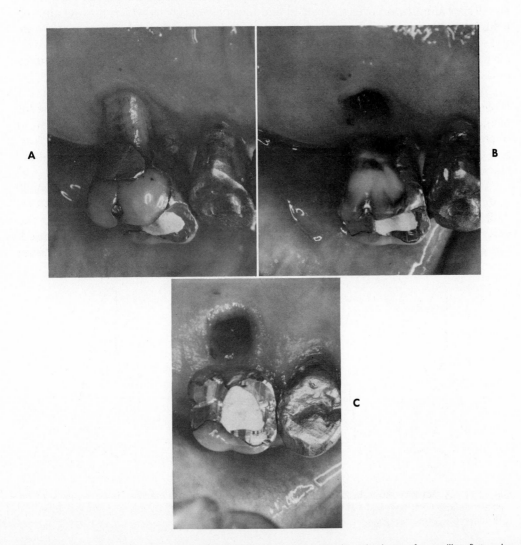

**Fig. 42-20.** **A,** Severe gingival recession and localized bone loss around a palatal root of a maxillary first molar. **B,** Root amputation performed without flap surgery. **C,** Occlusal table narrowed after root amputation. (Courtesy M.E. Gher, U.S. Navy.)

3. Root proximity
4. Position of the root in the arch
5. Root morphology
6. Endodontic complications

**Root selection**

Normally, the root with the greatest bone loss should be considered for amputation. Removal of any root on a maxillary molar will improve access to the furcation. Removal of a mesiobuccal root, for example, provides access for removal of plaque on remaining roots. Hemisection of a mandibular molar eliminates the furcation. In either case the prognosis of the remaining roots is improved. Root amputation is facilitated by divergent roots. When roots do not diverge or are partially fused, amputation is complicated or impossible. When the distobuccal root of the maxillary first molar contacts or is close to the mesiobuccal root of the second molar, removal of the distobuccal root is preferred. Access to both teeth and their prognosis are improved. The buccal roots of maxillary molars are more centrally located in the arch, in line with the premolars, and therefore they are more readily crowned or used as abutments than the palatal root. Amputation of the palatal root facilitates access to the buccal furcation. Removal of a buccal root makes maintenance of a furcation more difficult.

Root surface area should be considered before a root is amputated. In maxillary molars distobuccal roots provide the least support and should be considered preferentially for amputation over the palatal and mesiobuccal roots, which provide approximately equal support. When removal of a palatal or mesiobuccal root is considered, the arch position favors the retention of the mesiobuccal root; however, access for plaque control is complicated by a distal concavity. Access to this area (proximal surface of molars) is improved by palatal root amputation.

Mandibular molar roots are approximately the same size, although the mesial root is slightly larger.[8,9] However, the concavities on the mesial root are less accessible for plaque removal. The two narrow pulp canals of the mesial root are more difficult to treat endodontically than the single, larger canal on the distal root (Fig. 42-7). Post-and-core restorations are more easily constructed on the distal root.[46] Root perforation, cracked roots, and nonnegotiable canals are indications for amputation.

**Root amputation technique**

After the flap is elevated and soft tissue is debrided, amputation of the root is accomplished with a tapered carbide or diamond bur in a high-speed handpiece (Fig. 42-21). The cut is designed to contour the root trunk and crown while separating the root from the tooth. The initial cut is made at the expense of the root being amputated. The root is carefully elevated and removed without placing pressure on the remaining

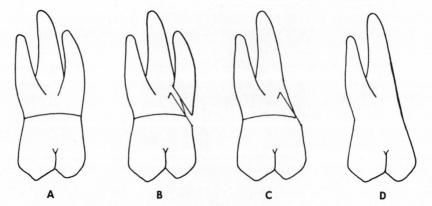

**Fig. 42-21.** **A,** Maxillary molar. **B,** Proper technique for root resection on a maxillary molar involves a cut to separate the root from the root trunk, **C,** Extraction of the separated root, and, **D,** final recontouring of the root trunk to remove all overhanging root structure, creating a smooth contour.

tooth. Removal of the root may require additional removal of root structure and overlying bone. The root trunk is then shaped to ideal contour. This includes removal of spurs and contouring of the root trunk to eliminate inaccessible portion of the furcation. If a palatal root is amputated the buccolingual width of the crown should be narrowed from the lingual surface to the approximate width of a premolar (see Fig. 42-20, *C*).

Remaining roots should be planed and osteoplasty completed to enhance pocket elimination and flap closure. Sutures are used to maintain flap adaptation, and a dressing is placed as desired. Where needed, a restoration is placed to seal the exposed root canal.

Vital root amputation may be performed with the intention of maintaining pulp vitality or with the intention of completing endodontic therapy subsequently. Vital amputation may be done when removal of a root has not been planned but is considered necessary during periodontal surgery. Unexpected patterns of bone loss, root fracture, root caries, external resorption, and root anomalies may require vital root amputation during periodontal surgery.[47] There is little or no pain for about a month after surgery.[48] Capping of the exposed pulp stump is not necessary if a root canal filling will be placed postoperatively. The patient may experience discomfort to hot or cold stimuli, and pulp polyps may develop in the area of the exposure. The primary disadvantage is the increased difficulty in gaining profound anesthesia for subsequent pulp extirpation.[47]

**Vital root amputation**

Long-term maintenance of pulp vitality requires pulp capping at the time of root amputation.[36] A small preparation is made in the exposed root canal with an inverted cone bur. The pulp is capped with calcium hydroxide followed by an amalgam restoration. A success rate of 70% over 5 years has been reported.[36]

Retention of the pulpal vitality may decrease the susceptibility of root-resected teeth to fracture.[48] However, endodontic therapy before or immediately after root amputation remains the treatment of choice.[49]

### Tooth sectioning

Sectioning is the surgical sectioning of a tooth into segments consisting of the root and overlying crown. An individual section may be extracted or retained. Hemisectioning generally applies to mandibular molars but may be performed on any multirooted tooth. Endodontic treatment is completed before sectioning is attempted. Hemisection may be performed for the same reasons as root amputation. Hemisection is contraindicated in teeth where:

**Hemisection**

1. The remaining periodontal support is inadequate
2. The tooth cannot be treated endodontically
3. Adequate restoration of the remaining tooth including splinting cannot be performed

### Hemisection technique

After endodontic therapy is completed the pulp chamber can be filled with amalgam. When possible, hemisection can be completed without flap elevation. A flap is required when visibility is limited, bone loss is irregular, and osseous defects require access for treatment (Fig. 42-22). Exploratory surgery may be necessary to confirm suspected problems such as cracked roots, caries, or resorption. A flap is elevated and granulation tissue removed to provide access for sectioning. The sectioning is done with a carbide bur or tapered diamond. The involved root is carefully extracted. The retained root is contoured to remove remnants of the furcation roof and to obtain a smooth, even contour. Minimal osteoplasty may be performed to enhance flap closure. Sutures and dressing are placed. Mobility may be increased after the operation.[50] The occlusion should be relieved to reduce trauma. The tooth should become firm within 6 months. If the tooth doesn't become firm, splinting is necessary.[50,51]

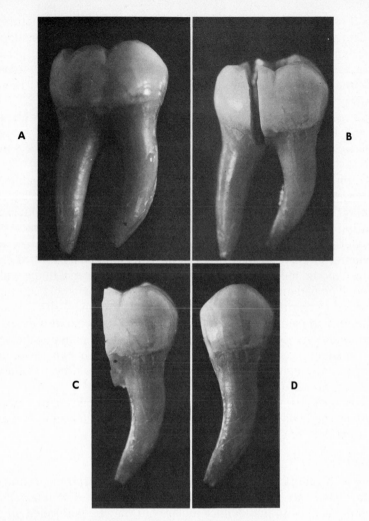

**Fig. 42-22. A,** Mandibular first molar. **B,** The tooth is sectioned with a fissure bur, at the expense of the tooth segment to be removed, before contouring. **C,** Retained tooth segment before contouring. **D,** Sectioned tooth after contouring. (Courtesy M.E. Gher, U.S. Navy.)

### Root separation

Root separation is the process of dividing a mandibular molar into two separate teeth (bicuspidization).[22] The rationale is that by separation of the roots, plaque control is enhanced, and the part of the tooth most susceptible to caries is changed from a dentin or cementum surface to a metallic one. The tooth fragments may be joined by one metallic restoration or converted into two separate teeth by the construction of two crowns (Figs. 42-23 and 42-24). The procedure is indicated when there is a class III involvement, the tooth is a strategic tooth, and the roots are well supported and sufficiently separated from each other to allow construction of restorations. The procedure may be combined with osteoplasty to correct defective bone contour.

When there is space mesial or distal to a strategically important mandibular molar with moderate interradicular destruction, the tooth can be hemisected after endodontic therapy, and the two halves moved apart orthodontically.[45] The sections can be moved apart 3 to 4 mm, and the furcation problem is solved. The two halves of the tooth are treated restoratively—splinted like two bicuspids—and a new papilla forms (see Fig. 42-23). The restoration must meet the requirements of sufficient embrasure space,

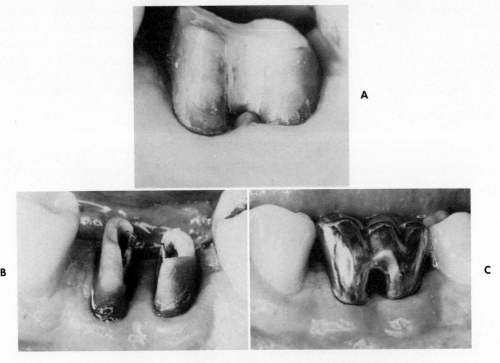

**Fig. 42-23.** **A,** Hemisected crown with temporary restoration before root separation. **B,** Orthodontic screws employed in root separation. **C,** Splinted crowns in place. (Courtesy B. Klavan, Phoenix, Arizona.)

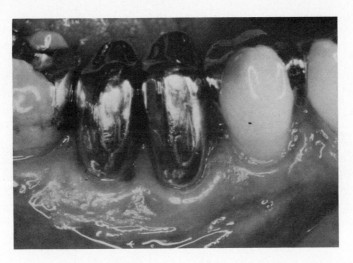

**Fig. 42-24.** Individual crowns placed on separated mesial and distal roots of a mandibular first molar (bicuspidization). (Courtesy R.W. Dunlap, U.S. Navy.)

margins without overhangs, and creation of a new contact point or solder joints that permit adequate interradicular cleaning. Teeth with deep furcation defects and unaffected mesial and distal surfaces are poor candidates for sectioning.

## Tunneling

Tunneling is a more rarely used procedure available for treatment of teeth with class II or III furcation involvement. The furcation is opened more widely to improve access for plaque control by proximal brushes, yarn, or pipe cleaners. However, the furca remains vulnerable to root caries, and plaque accumulation is encouraged by the reverse architecture that results from the procedure (Figs. 42-25 and 42-26). Topical application of fluoride solutions may assist in caries control. Tunneling is generally limited to mandibular molars but may be combined with root amputation in maxillary molars. Odontoplasty can be used to raise the roof of the furcation for increased access for plaque removal.[11,20] Tunneling should not be used in caries-prone individuals.[22]

## Bone grafting

Bone grafts have relatively little effectiveness in furcations. Although there have been occasional reports of success,[52-54] bone grafting in a furcation has a poor prognosis.[55] When two- or three-walled defects are present, one may attempt bone grafting.

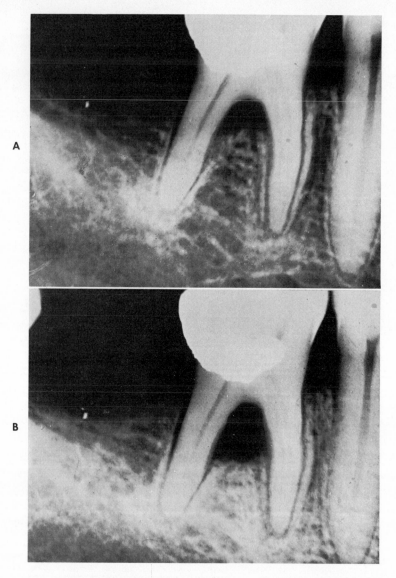

**Fig. 42-25.** **A,** Roentgenogram showing bifurcation involvement of a mandibular molar. The mesial and distal alveolar crests are not involved. **B,** Roentgenogram showing enlargement of the space in the bifurcation after surgery (tunneling) which has produced a reverse architecture. Maintaining the health of a tooth with an exposed bifurcation can be a problem because of the difficulty of plaque control and the danger of root caries incident to inadequate oral hygiene procedures.

## New attachment procedures

Root conditioning with citric acid may have potential for a new connective tissue attachment.[56-57] Successful closure of periodontally involved furcations has been demonstrated with citric acid demineralization in animal studies[58] but not in humans.[59,60]

## Guided tissue regeneration

Promising results have been reported with guided tissue regeneration (see Chapter 37).

## Maintenance

The treatment of classes II and III furca involvements usually requires a combination of procedures that may include endodontics, surgical procedures, crown restoration, and splinting. These procedures are of benefit to the patient when the tooth is required as an abutment or plays a strategic role or if other treatment is more involved or less predictable. However, the treatment of a furcation may be complex and expensive, and extraction should be considered. On the other hand, teeth with furcation involvements can be maintained for years by meticulous plaque control, regular maintenance, and other appropriate therapeutic measures.

## Extraction

Extraction is the treatment of choice when:

1. The patient's oral hygiene will not maintain the tooth
2. The patient does not choose to comply with restorative recommendations without which the tooth cannot survive
3. Adjacent teeth would serve as adequate abutments
4. Financial considerations preclude acceptance of treatment
5. Extraction will improve the prognosis of the adjacent teeth by improving bone levels resulting from socket fill
6. If an otherwise heroic effort for a tooth with a questionable prognosis would be better handled by an implant

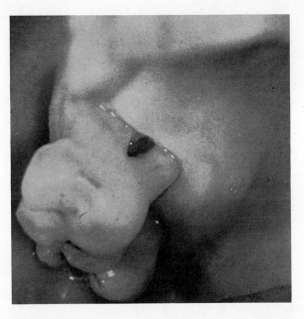

**Fig. 42-26.**   Trifurcation involvement in a maxillary first molar exposed by surgery. The furcation is made accessible because of extraction of the second premolar.

## Failures in furcation therapy

Inadequate plaque control and maintenance, poor root resection technique, improper restoration after initial periodontal therapy, endodontic failures, cracked roots, root caries, and patients who respond poorly despite the best treatment efforts all contribute to failures subsequent to furcation therapy.[21,37,61]

Endodontic failure and root fracture are the most frequent causes of failure.[37,61] Endontically treated teeth become brittle, making them more susceptible to fracture.[61,62,63] Gutta-percha condensation and the forcing of dowels, pins and posts, and inlays may cause root fracture.[25,64-66] Proper endodontic management and restorative treatment associated with root-resected teeth are extremely important for overall success of treatment (Fig. 42-27).[67]

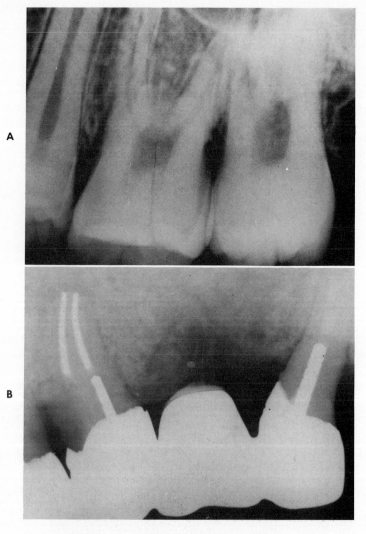

**Fig. 42-27. A,** Root proximity of distobuccal root of maxillary first and mesiobuccal root of maxillary second molar makes pocket elimination impossible. **B,** Mesial root of first molar and distal root of second molar have been removed and the teeth splinted after hemisectioning of both teeth. (Courtesy B. Klavan, Phoenix, Arizona.)

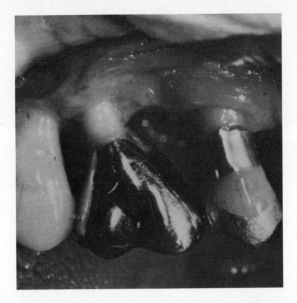

**Fig. 42-28.** Restoration after amputation of the mesiobuccal root of the maxillary first molar. Crown is tapered to follow form created in amputation, eliminating undercuts that hamper removal of plaque. (Courtesy R.M. Dunlap, U.S. Navy.)

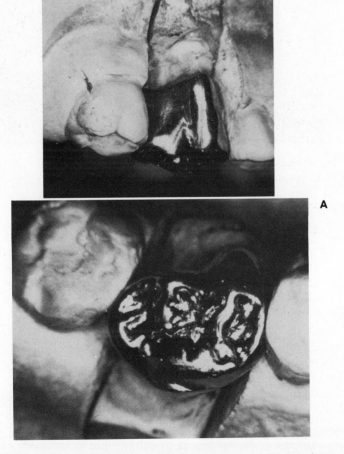

**A**

**Fig. 42-29.  A,** Form of crown restoration after amputation of distobuccal root.

*Continued.*

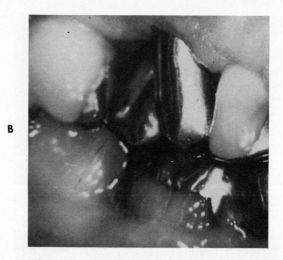

**Fig. 42-29, cont'd.** **B,** Crown with altered form. (Courtesy M. Pann, Los Angeles, California.)

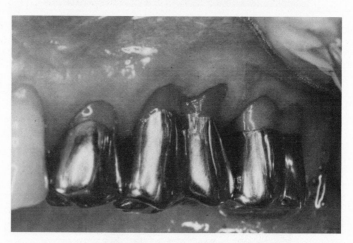

**Fig. 42-30.** Access to furcation is provided by proper contour of restorations. (Courtesy R.L. Duell, U.S. Navy.)

## Restorative management

Crowns used to restore root-resected teeth should follow the form created during the amputation procedure described previously. Proximal walls should taper evenly into the remaining root surface (Figs. 42-28 and 42-29). No spurs or overhangs should remain to complicate maintenance. Interproximal areas should be open to facilitate cleaning. Root concavities in the furcation area should be reproduced in the restoration.[68] Contours should be flat for access for effective plaque removal (Fig. 42-30). Hemisected teeth should not be cantilevered unless supported by splinting.

Endodontic therapy should be conservative, with minimal enlargement of the root canal for root strength.[37] Condensation should not be excessive. Gutta-percha permits the placement of posts without disturbing the apical seal.

Badly broken-down teeth may be built up with a post and core before final restoration is attempted. Post design should include:

1. Minimum enlargement of the root canal
2. Extension for most of the root length, to within 3 mm of the apex[69]
3. Parallel walls for maximal retention and to decrease lateral forces

4. A shoulder with a positive seat directing occlusal forces in the long axis
5. Serrated or coarse posts for increased retention
6. Close, even adaption of the post walls to the root canal
7. A mechanical lock in the coronal area to prevent torquing/twisting forces; a flat plane parallel to the long axis of the tooth is most effective in resisting rotational forces[70]
8. Passive seating during cementation[37]
9. Use of a noncorrosive alloy to prevent post corrosion[71]

When placing posts use the palatal roots of maxillary molars and distal roots of mandibular molars.[46] If pins are placed use new, sharp drills and passive cementation.[66]

## Summary

The treatment of osseous problems involving furcated teeth will depend on the type of tooth, the extent and pattern of bone loss, the anatomy of the affected areas, and accessibility to treatment and oral hygiene. Prognosis will depend on the extent and pattern of bone destruction in the furcation, the width of the space, root length, and tooth mobility.[21,37,62,72]

The following factors should be considered in the prognosis of teeth with furcation involvements:

1. *Extent of involvement.* Is the involvement partial or total? What is the apical extent of bone loss? Examine clinically and correlate with roentgenograms.
2. *Status of adjoining interproximal, buccal, and lingual areas.* If these areas are relatively sound or treatable, the effort to save the tooth is justified.
3. *Mobility.* Class II or III mobility makes for an unfavorable prognosis unless this mobility can be eliminated. The root length and crown-to-root ratio should be considered.
4. *Angulation of root spread.*
5. *Health of neighboring teeth.* When good abutment teeth are present mesial and distal to the involved tooth, extraction may be considered.
6. *Position of tooth in the arch.* Isolated teeth or those most distal in the arch may be retained and treated if retention of the tooth is desirable for prosthetic reasons.
7. *Age and health of the patient.* The life expectancy of the patient and of the tooth should be considered.
8. *Oral hygiene and caries index.* Treatment is indicated only when oral hygiene performance is acceptable and caries incidence is low.
9. *Failure of endodontic therapy or complications.* Root resection may be necessary to remove roots that have failed endodontically because of perforations, cracks, or inability to negotiate or obturate the canal.[22,61,71]

Bifurcated teeth, in general, are more amenable to treatment than are trifurcated teeth, with the exception of maxillary first premolars. Their root anatomy and poor accessibility for plaque control make for a guarded or poor prognosis. The mandibular first molar has a better prognosis, in general, than the second molar because of better access and more divergent roots.

**REFERENCES**

1. Everett, F.G., et al.: The intermediate bifurcational ridge, J. Dent. Res. **37:**162, 1964.
2. Everett, F.G.: Bifurcation involvement, J. Ore. Dent. Assoc. **28:**2, 1959.
3. Gher, M.E., et al.: Linear variation of the root surface area of the maxillary first molar, J. Periodontol. **56:**39, 1985.
4. Hermann, D.W., et al.: The potential attachment area of the maxillary first molar, J. Periodontol. **54:**431, 1983.
5. Bower, R.C.: Furcation morphology relative to periodontal treatment: furcation entrance architecture, J. Periodontol. **50:**23, 1979.
6. Bower, R.C.: Furcation morphology relative to periodontal treatment: furcation root surface anatomy, J. Periodontol. **50:**366, 1979.
7. Jepsen, A.: Root surface measurement and a method for x-ray determination of the root surface area, Acta Odontol. Scand. **21:**35, 1963.
8. Dunlap, R.W., and Gher, M.E.: Root surface measurements of the mandibular first molar, J. Periodontol. **56:**234, 1985.

9. Anderson, R.W., et al.: Root surface measurements of mandibular molars using stereophotogrammetry, J. Am. Dent. Assoc. **107:**613, 1983.

10. Masters, D.H., and Hoskins, S.W.: Projections of cervical enamel into molar furcations, J. Periodontol. **35:**49, 1964.

11. Everett, F.G., et al.: The intermediate bifurcation ridge: a study of the morphology of the bifurcation of the lower first molar, J. Dent. Res. **37:**162, 1958.

12. Burch, J.G., and Hulen, S.: A study of the presence of accessory foramina and the topography of molar furcations, Oral Surg. **38:**451, 1974.

13. Waerhaug, J.: Current concepts concerning gingival anatomy: the dynamic epithelial cuff, Dent. Clin. North Am. p. 715, 1960.

14. Schroeder, H.E., and Listgarten, M.A.: Fine structure of the developing epithelial attachment of human teeth. In Monographs in developmental biology, ed. 2, New York, 1977, S. Karger, vol. 2, pp. 104-106.

15. Lieb, A.M., Berdon, J.K., and Sabes, W.R.: Furcation involvements correlated with enamel projections from the cementoenamel junction, J. Periodontol. **38:**330, 1967.

16. Grewe, J.M., Meskin, L.H., and Miller, T.: Cervical enamel projections: prevalence, location and extent; with associated periodontal implications, J. Periodontol. **36:**460, 1965.

17. Bissada, N.F., and Abdelmalek, R.G.: Incidence of cervical enamel projections and its relationship to furcation involvement in Egyptian skulls, J. Periodontol. **44:**583, 1973.

18. Swan, R.H., and Hurt, W.C.: Cervical enamel projections as an etiologic factor in furcation involvement, J. Am. Dent. Assoc. **93:**342, 1976.

19. Wheeler, R.C.: Dental anatomy and physiology, ed. 4, Philadelphia, 1968, W. B. Saunders Co.

20. Gher, M.E., and Vernino, A.R.: Root morphology—clinical significance in pathogenesis and treatment of periodontal disease, J. Am. Dent. Assoc. **101:**627, 1980.

21. Hirschfeld, L., and Wasserman, B.: A long term survey of tooth loss in 600 treated periodontal patients, J. Periodontol. **49:**225, 1978.

22. Hamp, S.-E., Nyman, S., and Lindhe, J.: Periodontal treatment of multirooted teeth: results after 5 years, J. Clin. Periodontol. **2:**126, 1975.

23. Tarnow, D., and Fletcher, P.: Classification of the vertical component of furcation involvement, J. Periodontol. **55:**283, 1984.

24. Eskow, R.N. and Kapin, S.H.: Furcation invasions: correlating a classification system with therapeutic considerations. I. Examination, diagnosis, and classification, Compend. Contin. Educ. Dent. **5:**487, 1984.

25. Newell, D.H.: Current states of the management of teeth with furcation invasions, J. Periodontol. **52:**559, 1981.

26. Ross, I.F., and Thompson, R.H.: Furcation involvement in maxillary and mandibular molars, J. Periodontol. **51:**450, 1980.

27. Bender, I., and Seltzer, S.: Roentgenographic and direct observation of experimental lesions in bone, J. Am. Dent. Assoc. **62:**152, 1961.

28. Waerhaug, J.: The furcation problem. Etiology, pathogenesis, diagnosis, therapy and prognosis, J. Clin. Periodontol. **7:**73, 1980.

29. Saxe, S.R., and Carmen, D.K.: Removal or retention of molar teeth: the problem of the furcation, Dent. Clin. North Am. **13:**783, 1969.

30. Farrar, J.N.: Radical and heroic treatment of the alveolar abscess by amputation of roots of teeth, Dent. Cosmos **26:**79, 1884.

31. Messinger, T.F., and Orban, B.: Elimination of periodontal pockets by root amputation, J. Periodontol. **26:**213, 1954.

32. Lloyd, R.S., and Baer, P.W.: Periodontal therapy by root resection, J. Prosthet. Dent. **10:**362, 1960.

33. Amen, C.R.: Hemisection and root amputation, Periodontics **4:**197, 1966.

34. Abrams, L., and Trachtenberg, D.I.: Hemisection—technique and restoration, Dent. Clin. North Am. **18:**415, 1974.

35. Van Swol, R.L., and Whitsett, B.D.: Root amputation as a predictable procedure: report of a case, Oral Surg. **43:**452, 1977.

36. Haskell, E.W., Stanley, H., and Goldman, S.: A new approach to vital root resection, J. Periodontol. **51:**217, 1980.

37. Langer, B., Stein, S.D., and Wagenberg, B.: An evaluation of root resections: a ten-year study, J. Periodontol. **52:**719, 1981.

38. Ross, I.F., and Thompson, R.H.: A long-term study of root retention in the treatment of maxillary molars with furcation involvement, J. Periodontol. **49:**238, 1978.

39. Sackett, B.P., and Gildenhuys, R.P.: The effect of axial crown overcontour on adolescents, J. Periodontol. **47:**320, 1974.

40. Gilmore, N., and Sheiham, A.: Overhanging dental restorations and periodontal disease, J. Periodontol. **42:**8, 1971.

41. Silness, J.: Periodontal conditions in patients treated with dental bridges. III. The relationship between the location of the crown margin and the periodontal condition, J. Periodont. Res. **5:**225, 1970.

42. Lang, N.P., Kiel, R.A., and Vanderhalden, K.: Clinical and microbiological effects of subgingival restorations with overhanging or clinically perfect margins, J. Clin. Periodontol. **10:**563, 1983.

43. Gorzo, I., Newman, H.N., and Strahan, J.D.: Amalgam restorations, plaque removal and periodontal health, J. Clin. Periodontol. **6:**98, 1979.

44. Kirchoff, D.A., and Gerstein, H.: Presurgical crown contouring for root amputation procedures, Oral Surg. **27:**379, 1969.

45. Goldman, H.M., Shuman, A.M., and Isenberg, G.A.: Management of the partial furcation involvement, Periodontics **6:**197, 1968.

46. Abou-Rass, M., et al.: Preparation of space for posting: effect of thickness of canal walls and incidence of perforation in molars, J. Am. Dent. Assoc. **104:**834, 1982.

47. Smukler, H., and Tagger, M.: Vital root amputation: a clinical and histologic study, J. Periodontol. **47:**324, 1976.

48. Newell, D.H.: Current status of the management of teeth with furcation invasion, J. Periodontol. **52:**559, 1981.

49. Gerstein, K.A.: The role of vital root resection in periodontics, J. Periodontol. **48:**478, 1977.

50. Galler, C., et al.: The effect of splinting on tooth mobility. II. After osseous surgery, J. Clin. Periodontol. **6:**317, 1979.

51. Selipsky, H.: Osseous surgery—how much need we compromise? Dent. Clin. North Am. **20:**79, 1976.

52. Dragoo, M.R., and Sullivan, H.C.: A clinical and histological evaluation of autogenous iliac bone grafts in humans. I. Wound healing 2 to 8 months, J. Periodontol. **44:**599, 1973.

53. Hiatt, W.H., Schallhorn, R.G., and Aaronian, A.J.: The induction of new bone and cementum formation. IV. Microscopic examination of the periodontium following human bone and marrow allograft, autograft and nongraft periodontal regenerative procedures, J. Periodontol. **49:**495, 1978.

54. Robinson, R.E.: Osseous coagulum for bone induction, J. Periodontol. **40:**503, 1969.

55. Hiatt, W.H., and Schallhorn, R.G.: Intraoral transplants of cancellous bone and marrow in periodontal lesions, J. Periodontol. **44:**194, 1973.

56. Register, A.A., and Burdick, F.A.: Accelerated reattachment with cementogenesis to dentin, demineralized in situ. II. Defect repair, J. Periodontol. **47:**497, 1976.

57. Garrett, S., Crigger, M., and Egelberg, J.: Effects of citric acid on diseased root surfaces, J. Periodont. Res. **13:**538, 1978.

58. Crigger, M., et al.: The effect of topical citric acid application on the healing of experimental furcation defects in dogs, J. Periodont. Res. **13:**538, 1978.

59. Stahl, S.S., and Froum, S.J.: Human clinical and histologic repair responses following the use of citric acid in periodontal therapy, J. Periodontol. **48:**261, 1977.

60. Polson, A.M., and Proye, M.P.: Effect of root surface alterations on periodontal healing. II. Citric acid treatment of the denuded root, J. Clin. Periodontol. **9:**441, 1982.

61. Gher, M.E., et al.: Clinical survey of fractured teeth, J. Am. Dent. Assoc. **114:**174, 1987.

62. Blair, H.A.: The role of endodontics on restorative dentistry, Dent. Clin. North Am. **15:**619, 1971.

63. Helfer, A.R., Melnick, S., and Schilder, H.: Determination of the moisture content of vital and pulpless teeth, Oral Surg. **34:**661, 1972.

64. Meister, F., Lommel, T.J., and Gerstein, H.: Diagnosis and possible causes of vertical root fracture, Oral Surg. **49:**243, 1980.

65. Wechsler, S.M., et al.: Iatrogenic root fracture; a case report, J. Endodont. **4:**251, 1978.

66. Standlee, J.P., Collard, E.W., and Caputo, A.A.: Dentinal defects caused by some twist drills and retentive pins, J. Prosthet. Dent. **24:**185, 1970.

67. Morris, M.L.: Artificial crown contours and gingival health, J. Prosthet. Dent. **12:**1146, 1962.

68. Yuodelis, R.A., Weaver, J.E., and Sapkos, S.: Facial and lingual contours of artificial complete crown restorations and their effects on the peridontium, J. Prosthet. Dent. **29:**61, 1973.

69. Johnson, J.K., Schwartz, N.L., and Blackwell, R.T.: Evaluation and restoration of endodontically treated posterior teeth, J. Am. Dent. Assoc. **93:**597, 1976.

70. Kantor, M.E., and Pines, M.S.: A comparative study of restorative techniques for pulpless teeth, J. Prosthet. Dent. **38:**405, 1977.

71. Peterson, K.B.: Longitudinal root fracture due to corrosion of an endodontic post, J. Can. Dent. Assoc. **37:**66, 1971.

72. Becker, W., Berg, L.: and Becker, B.E.: Untreated periodontal diseases: a longitudinal study, J. Periodontol. **50:**234, 1979.

# CHAPTER 43

## Preprosthetic surgery

## Introduction

During the performance of surgery, alteration of tissues for later prosthetic treatment must be considered. The preparation of the maxilla and the mandible for complete and partial dentures is often the responsibility of the oral surgeon. Preparatory surgery for fixed prosthodontics relates more to periodontics than to oral surgery.[1] In the course of periodontal surgery the periodontist may, because of the proximity or involvement of teeth and adjacent tissues, need to become involved in such preprosthetic treatments as:

1. Crown lengthening and cosmetic and apical positioning of gingival margins[2,3]
2. Ridge preservation or augmentation[4-25]
3. Ridge reduction, alveoloplasty, removal of undercuts, retromolar tissue reduction[26,27]
4. Removal of tori and exostoses[26]
5. Gingival grafting[28-47]
6. Access flaps for tooth preparation and for endodontics[46,47,64,65]
7. Vestibuloplasty and vestibular extension to accommodate denture flanges[61,63]
8. Frenectomy[40,41]
9. Extractions
10. Cosmetic correction of gingival margins for "smile-line" enhancement

When necessary, preprosthetic surgery is done with periodontal surgery, otherwise it is performed in the absence of periodontal disease to satisfy prosthetic needs.

## Crown lengthening

Crown-lengthening procedures remove gingiva, bone, or both to create a longer clinical crown or to move gingival margins apically. Crown lengthening may be done in the following situations:

1. When esthetic considerations call for correction of excessive display of gingiva caused by familial, inflammatory, or drug-induced hyperplasia; "altered or delayed" passive eruption; or gingival deformity (Fig. 43-1, *A-C*)
2. Tooth over-eruption (in order to make gingival margins harmonious with those of adjacent teeth)
3. Crown fracture in proximity to the gingival margin or at or below the alveolar crest (Fig. 43-2, *A-D*)
4. Interproximal and cervical caries, or external root resorptions above or below bone
5. Post or pin perforations
6. Short clinical crowns offering inadequate retention for restorations or clasps
7. Loss of tooth structure (occlusal [Fig. 43-3] or lateral or cervical wear) resulting from chemical, abrasive, or traumatic factors
8. Need to revise tooth preparation to carry margins farther apically

The prosthetic dentist requires sufficient sound tooth structure to restore a crown reduced by caries, trauma, or earlier dentistry. It is suggested that 4.0 to 5.0 mm of sound tooth structure coronal to the gingival margin is needed to provide retention. Approximately 2 mm is required for connective attachment of tissue and epithelium at the dentogingival junction for attachment[48-50,57,58] and a shallow sulcus.

Where an adequate band of gingiva is present, a gingivectomy may be done for crown lengthening or for esthetics if the problem is caused by the position of the gingival margin. Before gingivectomy, one must "sound" through the gingiva to ensure that bone is not involved. If the alveolar bone is involved, gingivectomy is precluded and flap procedures and osseous surgery are needed (see Chapters 36 and 38).

## Preservation of ridges and reconstruction of deformed edentulous ridges

Extraction of teeth is followed by resorption of the alveolus and may result in an altered, deformed ridge. This alteration in ridge form is more extensive when teeth with advanced periodontal disease are extracted. Extractions involving periapical pathology, root fracture, or fracture of the labial plate of bone may be followed by ridge deformation. Postextraction healing may be accompanied by further resorption of the ridge. Yearly losses of 0.1 mm of bone for the edentulous maxillary ridge and 0.4 mm for the mandibular ridge have been reported.[51]

The deformed ridge may show a mesiodistal concavity (or saddle), a buccolingual concavity (collapsed ridge), or both. When a collapsed, deformed ridge is present, esthetic problems complicate the construction of a removable or fixed bridge. These problems must be addressed by the restorative dentist. Possible solutions include the placement of a long pontic, the addition of pink-colored plastic at the apical end of the pontic to simulate normal gingiva, the fabrication of a removable pontic in a fixed prosthesis,[4] or a gingival mask. Food retention, difficulties with speech, and dissatisfaction with esthetics are common patient complaints.

Ridge deformity may be prevented in some cases. Teeth or roots may be orthodontically erupted to create increased ridge height before extraction.[52] In addition, root retention (submerged roots) or the placement of ceramic implants in the extraction sockets may be used to prevent or limit postextraction ridge shrinkage.[10-19]

For vital root retention, a full flap is reflected and the clinical crown and the root above the alveolar ridge are removed with a fissure bur. The remaining root is left flush with or slightly below the alveolar crest. Where periodontal bone defects are present, these are débrided of soft tissue and the contiguous root surfaces are planed. Bone grafts may be placed where appropriate. The flap margins are then coapted over

**Root retention techniques**

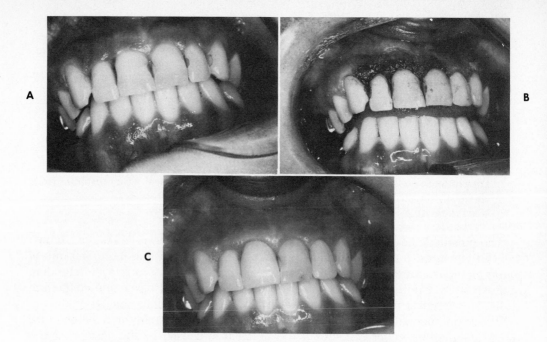

**Fig. 43-1.** **A,** Interdental crater between right central incisors and lateral incisors. A porcelain crown was planned for the central incisor. **B,** Gingivoplasty was performed to correct the gingival contour. **C,** Following healing and crown placement, the gingival contour is normal.

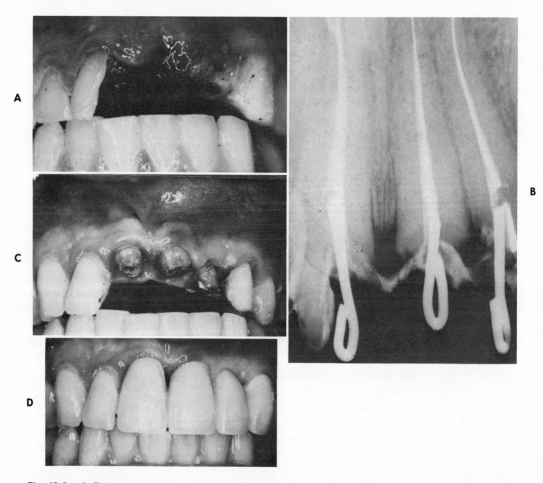

**Fig. 43-2.** **A,** This patient slipped on the ice and fractured several teeth. **B,** Vital endodontics was performed after obtaining surgical access. **C,** Root elongation procedures exposed the roots. **D,** Porcelain crowns were fabricated.

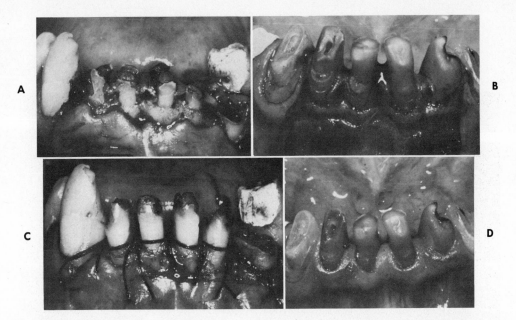

**Fig. 43-3.** **A,** Modified flap is reflected around the clinical crown of mandibular incisors shortened by caries and retrograde wear. **B,** Ostectomy and osteoplasty were performed to lengthen the clinical crowns. **C,** Flap was positioned apically and secured by continuous ligation. **D,** Postoperatively adequate crown length was created to receive porcelain jacket crowns. (Courtesy A. Saadoun, Los Angeles, California.)

the retained roots. Healing must be monitored to assure that gingiva has covered the submerged roots (Fig. 43-4, A-D). Vital submerged roots remain submerged, maintaining ridge height and form.[16,18,19] The pulpal tissue in these roots becomes fibrous and continuous with that of the overlying gingival connective tissue. Alveolodental fibers continue to course between cementum and bone and the periodontal ligament is maintained in a functional form[11,12] (Fig. 43-4, E).

When the root is permitted to extrude or is exposed at the ridge margin, denture attachments may be placed directly on the exposed portion of the root, or the root may be covered first with a gold cap. In such cases, plaque removal and regular scaling and root planing are important. Orthodontic tooth eruption may be used to salvage fractured or extensively decayed teeth.[52] As the tooth is forced to erupt, bone is formed at the crest and the gingival margin moves with the bone. Later, root exposure and gingival margin correction is achieved surgically (Fig. 43-5).

*Orthodontic eruption*

## Ridge augmentation

Deformed ridges may be restored to esthetic and functional form by surgical reconstruction of the ridge.[53-56] Techniques for such reconstruction include:

1. Full masticatory mucosal grafts placed over or on the deformed ridge (onlay graft)[7]
2. Submucosal connective tissue grafts under a flap or in a pouch[5,6]
3. Submucosal implants of hydroxylapatite or bone chips[20-25,55,56,59,60]
4. A doubled-under (roll under) flap[4,9]

Before performing the graft, inspect and measure the recipient site and make sure that adequate donor tissue or implant material is available. The graft measurement in both buccolingual and apicocoronal dimensions should be planned taking into consideration the following:

*Technique*

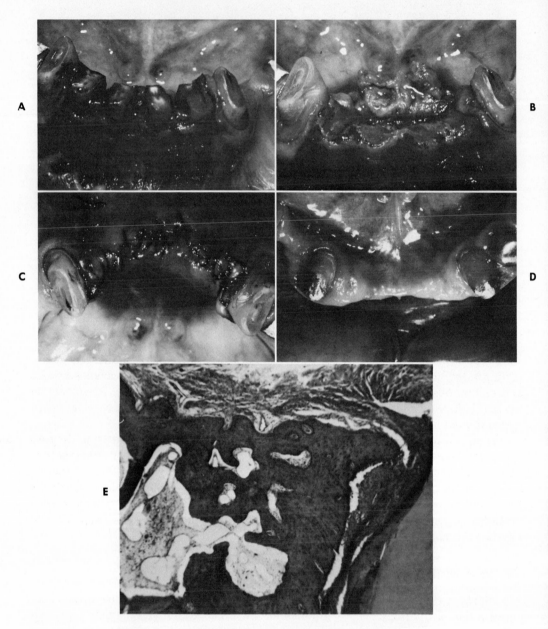

**Fig. 43-4.   A,** A flap was reflected and the mutilated mandibular incisors exposed. **B,** The roots were ground flush with bone or slightly apical to the alveolar crest. **C,** Flap margins were coapted and sutured over the roots. **D,** Following healing, ridge form has been retained. Fixed or removable prosthesis may be constructed. **E,** A root that was submerged has bone to its margin. Corrected tissue covers the submerged root. Bone was opposed to the root margin. (**A** to **D** courtesy A. Saadoun, Los Angeles, California; **E** courtesy G. Bowers, Baltimore, Maryland.)

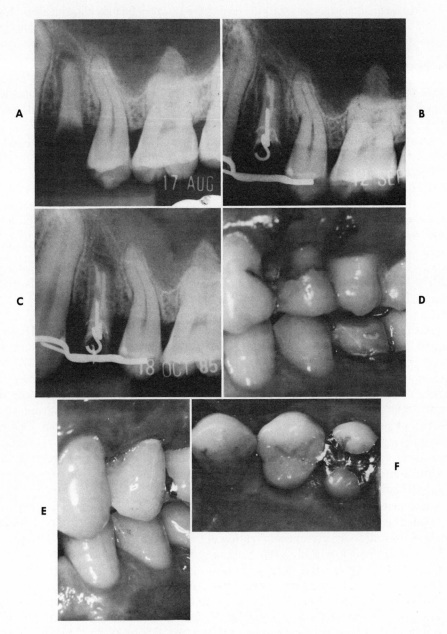

**Fig. 43-5.   A,** A 40-year-old patient desired restoration of the left maxillary bicuspid but did not want to lose the tooth. **B,** A hook was placed in the canal after root canal therapy. **C,** A bar was placed between the cuspid and second bicuspid and using rubber elastics the root was extruded. In 3 weeks 4 mm of extrusion was obtained. **D,** Periodontal surgery was performed to correct osseous and gingival contour. **E,** One week postoperatively. **F,** A porcelain crown on a metal base fabricated with a distal male attachment joining an inlay with a precision mesial attachment in the second bicuspid was cemented. This was done to compensate for the less favorable crown-root ratio on the first bicuspid (Courtesy K. Mori, Tokyo, Japan.)

1. The length of pontic teeth to be used
2. The embrasure dimensions between pontic teeth and abutment teeth
3. Arch contour and vestibular form of the arch
4. Axial inclination of abutment teeth and proposed axial inclination of pontic teeth. It should be a goal to make the axial inclination of the pontic teeth compatible with that of a normal ridge form and with adjacent abutment teeth.

## FREE MASTICATORY MUCOSAL GRAFT

It is sometimes possible to restore a deformed ridge by placing a free masticatory mucosal graft, a full-thickness onlay graft, on the reduced ridge.[54,58,61] A sufficient bulk of tissue must be available from the donor site (palate or tuberosities).

**Technique**      To restore normal ridge and gingival contour it is necessary to create a thicker ridge over the extraction sites to compensate for postsurgical shrinkage so that subsequent gingivoplasty may create convex labial surfaces and simulate root eminences, interdental grooves, and papillae.

**Site preparation**      Anesthetic without epinephrine should be administered to the recipient (deformed ridge) site. A de-epithelized wound surface is created in the recipient site either with a large oval diamond stone or by scraping with a kidney-shaped knife. At this time a second anesthetization is performed, using anesthetic with epinephrine (1:100,000) to control any excessive bleeding of the recipient site and to anesthetize the donor site. The recipient bed is measured with a periodontal probe and the measurements are transferred to the donor site by bleeding points, indelible pencil, or via a foil template.

**Donor site**      Graft dimensions, including mesiodistal, apicocoronal length and thickness must planned. Some loss of tissue contour should be anticipated, because contraction and shrinkage of the graft in the first 4 weeks may result in as much as a 30% loss in dimension for a thick graft and in greater loss for a thin graft.[56] It is therefore important to place a larger, thicker graft in anticipation of shrinkage. The ridge should be overbuilt. Later, it is simple to reduce size or contour the ridge by gingivoplasty. The presence of submucosa and fatty tissue in the donor tissue is acceptable. The vascularity of these tissues is good.[66] A thin palatal tissue may limit availability of an adequate donor tissue for a graft, in which case extraoral donor sites may be used (i.e., dermal collagen from the buttocks). Following selection of an appropriate donor site the graft is excised and hemostatic or gauze sponges are placed to stem bleeding.

**Recipient site**      A trial placement of the graft to the recipient site is made to check dimensions for any adjustments that may be required. The graft is sutured in place. Up to 10 sutures may be required[9] to assure immobilization of the graft over the deformed ridge. Dressings are unnecessary over the graft when a provisional prosthesis is available to serve as a surgical covering. The pontic of the provisional bridge should be trimmed by grinding to prevent impingement and pressure on the grafted tissue.

A dressing may be placed on the oral donor site or freeze-dried human skin may be sutured over the site, which considerably lessens patient discomfort. The sutures are removed 7 to 10 days later. The surgical sites are cleaned and oral hygiene measures reviewed (Fig. 43-6).

Four to 6 weeks later gingivoplasty may be performed with a diamond stone to create pseudopapillae, root eminences, and concavities mimicking gingival crown contours. Sloughing and loss of free masticatory mucosal grafts may occur, particularly where a thick onlay graft has been placed.

## SUBMUCOSAL CONNECTIVE TISSUE GRAFT

**Technique**      Deficient ridge contour (mutilated pontic area) may be restored by a connective tissue graft placed beneath a full- or partial-thickness flap reflected over the deformed

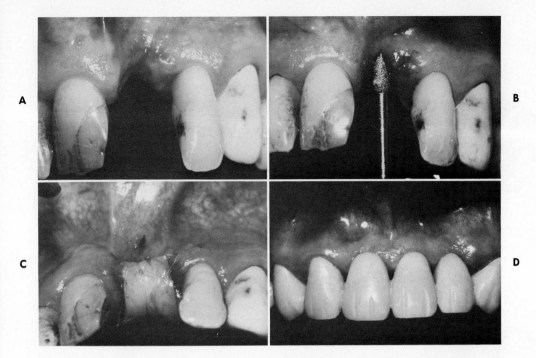

**Fig. 43-6.   A,** A ridge with a buccolingual concavity and a mesiodistal saddle. **B,** The ridge was de-epithelialized with a diamond stone. **C,** The onlay graft was sutured into place. **D,** The healed, restored ridge. (Courtesy A. Saadoun, Los Angeles, California.)

ridge.[5,6] Vertical incisions should be angled distoapically and placed so that the final tissue contours will blend with those of the adjacent abutment teeth. Papillae of adjacent abutment teeth should not be incised. The horizontal incision connecting the vertical incisions may be made at the crest of the ridge, or more often palatally, to enhance increased height of the ridge after the placement of the transplanted connective tissue. The donor tissue is obtained from the palate by reflecting primary and secondary flaps, and excising the secondary flap to bone. Similarly, during periodontal surgery for pocket elimination, the secondary flap, which would normally be discarded, may be used as donor tissue. The donor tissue is then stored on gauze moistened with normal saline or placed immediately.

Overbuilding the ridge should be planned to compensate for postsurgical shrinkage. Beveled margins of the palatal primary flap are coapted to the beveled coronal edge of the donor site and sutured to place. Pressure is placed over the flap to control bleeding.

The donor tissue is then placed on the recipient bed and trimmed to size. The flap is positioned over the tissue transplant and sutured to place. A gap will remain on the palatal surface of the recipient bed, which may be covered with a freeze-dried skin graft or left to heal by second intention (Fig. 43-7).

*Recipient site*

*Suturing donor site*

## PENTOGRAPHIC LIP EXTENSION PROCEDURE

Several limitations accompany the use of the submucosal fibrous connective tissue graft. These include (1) the availability of sufficient donor tissue and (2) the flap design itself. This design limits the amount of implant that can be placed submucosally and still coapt and close the lateral flap margins postsurgically. In many cases buccolingual enlargement of the ridge is possible, although apicocoronal augmentation cannot be achieved because the flap or pouch cannot be extended coronally.

The use of an advancement flap, bringing mucosa from the vestibule and lip forward

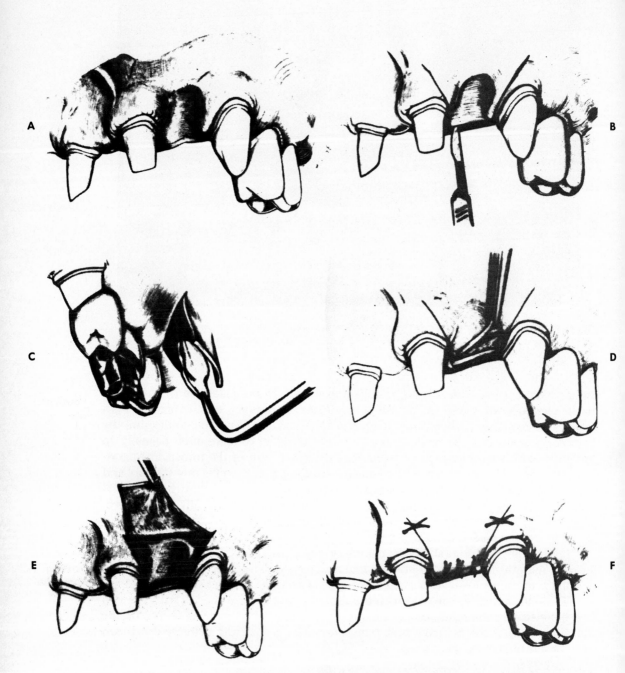

**Fig. 43-7.** **A,** A deformed, collapsed ridge. **B,** A split-thickness flap was prepared with a No. 15 surgical blade. **C,** A connective tissue graft was removed from a prepared palatal donor site. **D,** Reflection of the split-thickness flap seen in the recipient site. **E,** The recipient site was prepared to receive the graft. **F,** The split-thickness flap was sutured over the inserted graft to augment the ridge and correct the deformity. (From Langer, B.: J. Prosthet. Dent. **44:**363, 1980.)

and coronally, may permit placement of sufficient material such as allograft bone in order to correct ridge defects.

The *pentographic lip extension procedure*[6a] uses the extensibility of the alveolar mucosa of the lip or cheek mucosa to permit the implantation of sufficient material to permit apicocoronal and buccolingual augmentation that restores ridge form. Bone or ceramic implant materials are most often used, although fibrous connective tissue can also be implanted.

By extending the incisions into lip or cheek mucosa apicocoronal extension of the ridge is made possible. In some cases a secondary free gingival graft is placed over the mucosa after healing, in order to provide a surface of masticatory mucosa. The technique is described in Fig. 43-8.

## POUCH PROCEDURE

When a buccolingual ridge deformity is found, a connective tissue transplant, bone, or bioceramic material may be placed by means of a pouch procedure. The pouch may have either a single entrance at the mesial or distal end of the deformed ridge or openings at both ends.[9,25,27,56] The incisions are similar for the single or double pouch.

In the double pouch, vertical incisions are placed starting near the vestibular fornix and extending into the gingiva. Papillae bordering the ridge are not included. A periostome is inserted into the incision and moved subperiostally in a mesiodistal direction along bone to create a pouch. The procedure is repeated at the incision made at the opposite end of the ridge deformity. When a high frenum is present, it is usually not included. The connective tissue transplant is then drawn through the pouch and sutured to the overlying flap with resorbable suture to prevent displacement.[54,55] Bio- **Ceramic** compatible hydroxylapatite may be placed instead of connective tissue transplants. **implants** These ceramic particles may be introduced into the pouch with a syringe adapted for this purpose or with a periostome. The pouch orifices must be carefully sutured for coaptation without gaps. Complications observed include loss of particles, dehiscences at incision sites, transient paresthesia, migration of material from implanted site into contiguous loose connective tissues and the necessity to remove small amounts of material. Tricalcium phosphate and hydroxylapatite implants are biocompatible. These implants are better used to restore buccolingual width of a ridge, which is called, "plumping out." They are much less effective for restoring ridge height (Fig. 43-9).

## ROLL TECHNIQUE

A procedure called the *roll technique*[4] involves the doubling under of a flap to **Technique** restore coronoapical ridge height and buccolingual thickness to a collapsed ridge. Palatal tissue of adequate thickness is a prerequisite. The thickness of palatal tissue is assessed by sounding with a periodontal probe or with the injection needle, and the amount of roll under is planned. At least 3-mm thickness of palatal tissue is necessary where rugae are present; the measurement is made from the valley between rugae. Anesthetic without epinephrine is injected. The dimension of the flap to be rolled under is de-epithelized with a coarse, football-shaped diamond stone. Vertical incisions are made to bone on the palate and then extended over the ridge, to diverge in a coronoapical direction on the vestibular surface, ending in alveolar mucosa. The tissue is detached and the de-epithelized margins of the flap are rolled under (Fig. 43-10). Resorbable sutures are placed to hold the doubled-under tissue together. Nonresorbable sutures are then placed to secure the doubled-under flap in place. Freeze-dried skin or periodontal dressing may be placed over the exposed portion of the palatal wound. Sutures may be removed at 10 days.

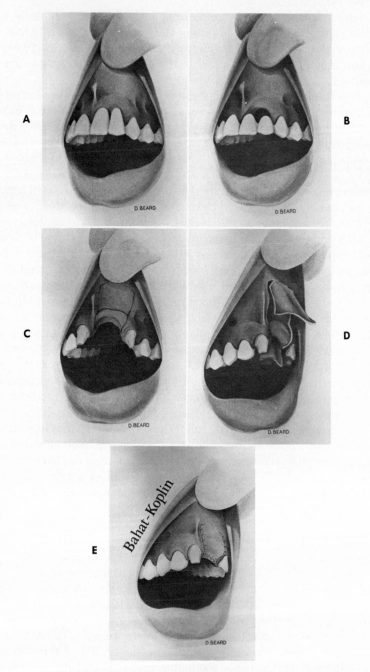

**Fig. 43-8. A,** Elongated pontics have been used to compensate for ridge collapse, producing an unesthetic and poorly functional prostheses. **B,** The pontics were reduced in preparation for ridge augmentation. **C,** An incision was made in alveolar mucosa near the mucogingival junction and vertical incisions were made into the lip mucosa, apically, and over the ridge to the palate, coronally. **D,** The flaps were reflected and hemostasis obtained. Bone was placed for ridge augmentation. **E,** The apical flap was sutured first, tacking the corners initially. The coronal flap was sutured to oppose flap margins. Ridge augmentation was obtained. (Courtesy O. Bahat, Beverly Hills, California.)

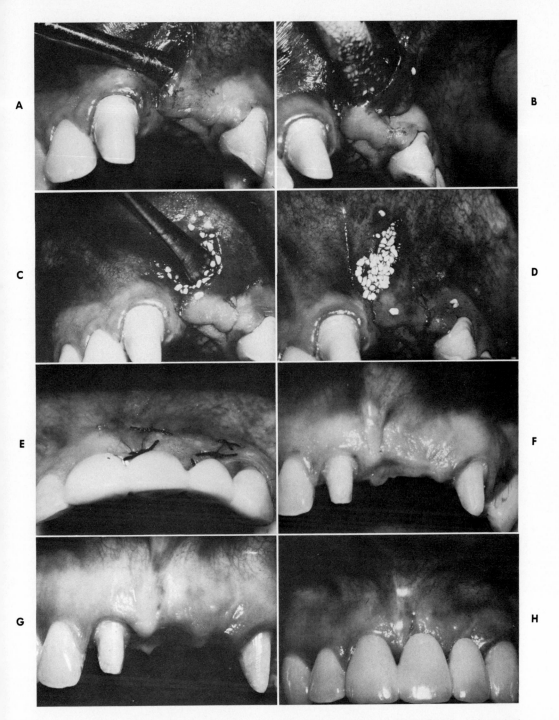

**Fig. 43-9.** **A,** The buccolingual and mesiodistal dimensions of the partially edentulous ridge make esthetic restorations difficult. A single incision was made from the crest of the ridge, extending into the alveolar mucosa and a periostome was inserted to create a pouch. **B,** Hydroxylapatite particles were inserted into the pouch with a syringe. **C,** The hydroxylapatite fragments were pushed into the pouch with an elevator. **D,** The augmented ridge before suturing. **E,** The pouch was sutured to enclose the ceramic implant. **F,** The expanded ridge before gingivoplasty. **G,** Eminences and papillae. **H,** The restored ridge with fixed bridge in place. (Courtesy A. Saadoun, Los Angeles, California.)

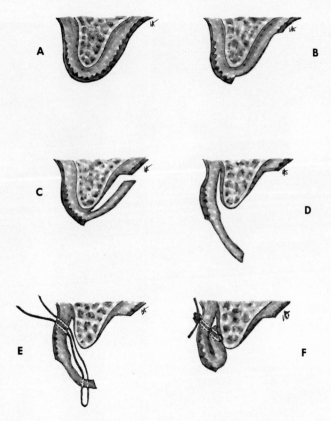

**Fig. 43-10.** **A,** Cross-section of a deformed ridge. **B,** De-epithelialization of the palatal segment of the proposed flap. **C,** Elevation of the flap. **D,** The flap was elevated over the buccal segment of the ridge. **E,** Sutures were placed through the mucogingival junction and the tip of the flap. **F,** The flap was secured to restore the ridge concavity. (Courtesy L. Abrams, Philadelphia, Pennsylvania.)

## Ridge reduction

Ridge reduction may be needed when a large ridge would prevent or interfere with the placement of a pontic because of insufficient coronoapical space. Less frequently, bulbous ridges may need buccolingual reduction to harmonize with alveolar form over abutment teeth.[26,27]

The techniques of flap reflection and osteoplasty are applied to the edentulous ridge, either reducing coronoapical height or narrowing buccolingual contours.

## Removal of tori and exostoses

Tori and exostosis may be removed by techniques similar to those employed in ridge reduction in such situations where these bony prominences would interfere with the seating of a partial denture[26,47] (Fig. 43-11).

### GINGIVAL GRAFTING

**Increasing gingival width or thickness**

The periodontist is often called on to augment the zone of gingiva for prosthetic reasons. The need for a specific width of gingiva is not mandatory, yet there are situations where firmly attached gingiva appears to be necessary for plaque control performance without tissue injury.[57,58] In other situations, a masticatory mucosal graft may be needed to eliminate ridge undercuts that would interfere with denture inser-

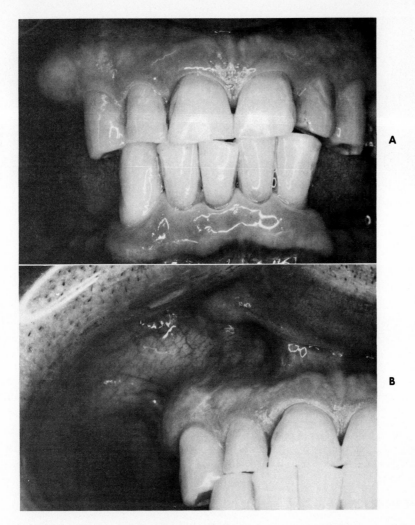

**Fig. 43-11.** **A,** Exostosis over the cuspid would prevent partial denture from seating. **B,** After removal of exostosis, tissue over cuspid conforms with contour of the edentulous ridge.

tion.[28-46,62,63] The techniques for augmentation of gingiva by free grafting and pedicle flaps are identical with those discussed in Chapter 40.[28-46,62,63]

## GINGIVAL RETRACTION AND ACCESS FLAPS

Surgical gingival retraction is sometimes necessary for rubber dam clamp placement for class V restorations and for endodontics. This is usually done by gingivectomy, miniflap, or envelope flap, as appropriate.[64,65]

## VESTIBULAR EXTENSION

Vestibular extension is more often required for a full-denture prosthesis. The techniques for localized vestibular extension to accommodate partial denture bars and flanges are those of free gingival grafting (see Chapter 40).

## FRENECTOMY

Frenectomy may be performed to accommodate partial dental flanges to expedite oral hygiene procedures or for esthetics (see Chapter 40).

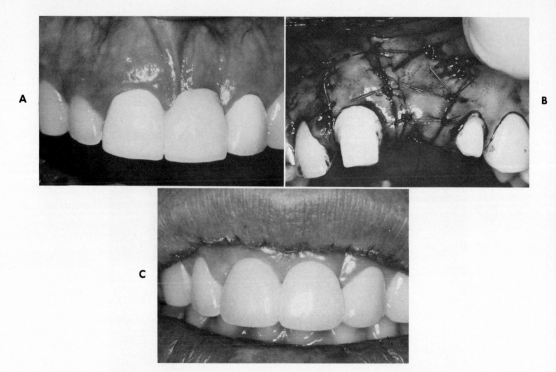

**Fig. 43-12.** **A,** There is a temporary bridge extending from the right central to the left lateral incisor. The crowns of the right lateral and central incisors are short and too much gingiva is displayed. They require root-lengthening procedures. The ridge below the left central incisor is partially collapsed and the pontic is butted against the ridge. This area needs ridge augmentation. **B,** The procedures are performed using osseous surgery over the right central and lateral incisors to gain root length. Ceramicized hydroxylapatite was placed over the edentulous left central incisor area "to plump it out." The pontic was shortened to permit healing without pressure. **C,** Smile line showing cosmetic improvement with the final bridge in place. Note the more uniform tissue contour. (Courtesy H. Israelson, Richardson, Texas.)

## EXTRACTIONS

Extraction of hopeless teeth or of teeth whose uncertain prognosis might endanger the lifespan of fixed or partial dentures is the joint diagnostic responsibility of the periodontist and the prosthodontist. The treatment of defects incident to third molar extraction requires periodontal treatment, including bone grafting, bone denudation, free gingival grafts and apically positioned flaps as appropriate[8-72] (see Chapters 30 and 36 to 40).

## COSMETICS

An important facet of preprosthetic surgery is creation of an esthetic conformation of the gingival tissues to the teeth. This includes a scalloped margin that extends symmetrically and barely shows the gingiva when the patient smiles (smile line). Such results can be obtained by a combination of grafting and excisional techniques[72] (Fig. 43-12).

## Summary

Although periodontal surgery is performed with the aim of treating periodontal disease, some surgical procedures may be done in the absence of disease. The surgery is performed, for cosmetic or functional purposes to optimize the adaptation of prosthetic restorations to the mucosal topography. This type of surgery is referred to as *preprosthetic surgery.* The term has been expanded to include prosthetic surgical and cosmetic prosthetic goals.

## REFERENCES

1. Starshak, T.J.: Preprosthetic oral surgery, St. Louis, 1971, The C.V. Mosby Co.
2. Saadoun, A.P., et al.: Surgical treatment of the short clinical crown in an area of inadequate keratinized gingiva, Compend. Cont. Educ. Dent. **4(1):**71, 1983.
3. Rosenberg, E.S., et al.: Tooth lengthening procedures, Compend. Cont. Educ. Dent. **1:**161, 1980.
4. Abrams, L.: Augmentation of the deformed residual edentulous ridge for fixed prosthesis, Compend. Cont. Educ. Dent. **1:**205, 1980.
5. Langer, B., and Calagna, L.: The subepithelial connective tissue graft, J. Prosthet. Dent. **44:**363, 1980.
6. Langer, B., and Calagna, L.: The subepithelial connective tissue graft: a new approach to the enhancement of anterior cosmetic, Int. J. Periodont. Rest. **2:**23, 1982.
6a. Bahat, O., and Koplin, L.: Pentographic lip extension in ridge augmentation. (In press.)
7. Seibert, J.: Reconstruction of deformed partially edentulous ridges, using full thickness grafts. I. Technique and wound healing, Comp. Cont. Educ. Gen. Dent. **4:**437, 1983.
8. Seibert, J.: Reconstruction of deformed partially edentulous ridges, using full thickness grafts. II. Prosthodontic/periodontal interrelationships, Comp. Cont. Educ. Gen. Dent. **4:**549, 1983.
9. Saadoun, A.P., and Farnoush, A.: Esthetic reconstruction of residual deformed ridges for restorative purposes, Calif. Dent. Assoc. J. :39, 1984.
10. Dungan, D.J., Getz, J.B., and Epker, B.N.: Root banking to preserve alveolar bone: a review and clinical recommendation, J. Am. Dent. Assoc. **103(5):**737, 1981.
11. Whitaker, D.D., and Shangle, R.J.: A study of the histologic reaction of submerged root segments, Oral Surg. **37:**919, 1974.
12. Plata, R.L. and Kelly, E.E.: Intentional retention of vital submerged roots in dogs, Oral Surg. **42:**100, 1976.
13. Guyer, S.E.: Selectively retained vital roots for partial support of overdentures: a patient report, J. Prosthet. Dent. **33:**258, 1975.
14. Cook, R.T., Hutchens, L.H., and Burkes, J.J. Jr.: Periodontal osseous defects associated with vitally submerged roots, J. Periodontol. **48:**249, 1977.
15. Evian, C.I.: The effect of submerging roots with periodontal defects, Compend. Cont. Educ. Gen. Dent. **4:**37, 1983.
16. Garver, D.G., et al.: Vital root retention in humans: a final report, J. Prosthet. Dent. **43:**368, 1980.
17. Murray, C.G. and Adkins, K.F.: The elective retention of vital roots for alveolar bone preservation: a pilot study, J. Oral Surg. **37(8):**650, 1979.
18. Masterson, M.P.: Retention of vital submerged roots under complete dentures: report of 10 patients, J. Prosthet. Dent. **41(1):**12, 1979.
19. Bowles, W.H. and Daniel, R.E.: Reevaluation of submerged vital roots, J. Am. Dent. Assoc. **107(9):**429, 1983.
20. Nery, E.B.: Alveolar ridge augmentation with tricalcium phosphate ceramic, J. Prosth. Dent. **40(6):**668, 1978.
21. Rabalais, M.L., et al.: Evaluation of durapatite ceramic as an alloplastic implant in periodontal osseous defects, J. Periodontol. **52:**68, 1981.
22. Cohen, D.W.: Report of a clinical conference on a new implant material for ridge augmentation, Compend. Cont. Educ. Gen. Dent. Sup. **2:**545, 1982.
23. Kent, J.N., et al.: Correction of alveolar ridge deficiencies with non-resorbable hydroxyapatite, J. Am. Dent. Assoc. **105:**993, 1982.
24. Jarcho, M.: Calcium phosphate ceramic as hard tissue prosthetics, Clin. Orthop. **157:**259, 1981.
25. Rosenberg, S., et al.: Use of ceramic materials for augmentation of the partially edentulous ridge: a case report, Comp. Cont. Educ. Gen. Dent. **5:**279, 1984.
26. Kaldahl, W.B., Becker, C.M., and Wentz, F.M.: Periodontal surgical preparation for specific problems in restorative dentistry, J. Prosth. Dent. **51:**36, 1984.
27. Garber, D.A., and Rosenberg, E.S.: The edentulous ridge in fixed prosthodontics, Compend. Contin. Educ. Gen. Dent. **11:**212, 1981.
28. Dorfman, H., et al.: Longitudinal evaluation of free autogenous gingival grafts, J. Clin. Periodontol. **7:**316, 1980.
29. Dorfman, H., et al.: Longitudinal evaluation of free autogenous gingival grafts: four year report, J. Periodontol. **53:**349, 1982.
30. De Trey, E., and Bernimoulin, J.: Influence of free gingival grafts on the health of the marginal gingiva, J. Clin. Periodontol. **7:**381, 1980.
31. Grupe, H.E., et al.: Repair of gingival defects by sliding flap operation, J. Periodontol. **27:**290, 1956.
32. Grupe, H.E.: Modified technique for the sliding flap operation, J. Periodontol. **37:**491, 1966.
33. Corn, H.: Edentulous area pedicle grafts in mucogingival surgery, Periodontics **2:**229, 1964.
34. Pennel, B.M., et al.: Oblique rotated flap, J. Periodontol. **36:**305, 1965.
35. Cohen, D.W., et al.: The double papillae repositioned flap in periodontal therapy, J. Periodontol. **39:**65, 1968.

36. Rubelman, P.A.: Interdental papilla grafts, Alpha Omegan **70:**66, 1977.
37. Bjorn, H.: Free transplantation of gingiva propris, Sven. Tandläk. Tidskr. **22:**684, 1963.
38. Sullivan, H.C., et al.: Free autogenous gingival graft. I. Principles of successful grafting, Periodontics **6:**121, 1968.
39. Coslet, J.G., et al.: The free autogenous gingival graft, Dent. Clin. North. Am. **24:**651, 1980.
40. Dordick, B., Coslet, J.G., and Seibert, J.S.: Clinical evaluation of free autogenous gingival grafts placed on bone. I. Clinical predictability. J. Periodontol. **47:**559, 1976.
41. Mormann, W., et al.: The relationship between success of free gingival grafts and transplant thickness—revascularization and shrinkage—one year clinical study, J. Periodontol. **52:**74, 1981.
42. James, W.C., McFall, W.T., and Burkes, E.J.: Placement of free gingival grafts on denuded alveolar bone. II. Microscopic observations, J. Periodontol. **49:**291, 1978.
43. James, W.C., and McFall, W.T.: Placement of free gingival grafts on denuded alveolar bone. I. Clinical evaluations, J. Periodontol. **49:**283, 1978.
44. Dordick, B., Coslet, J.G., and Seibert, J.S.: Clinical evaluation of free autogenous gingival grafts placed on alveolar bone. II. Coverage of nonpathologic dehiscences and fenestrations, J. Periodontol. **47:**568, 1976.
45. Mlinek, A., Smukler, H., Buchner, A.: The use of free gingival grafts for coverage of denuded roots, J. Periodontol. **44:**248, 1973.
46. Hall, W.: The current status of mucogingival problems and their therapy, J. Periodontol. **52:**569, 1981.
47. Hall, W.: Periodontal preparation of the mouth for restoration, Dent. Clin. North. Am. **24:**195, 1980.
48. Gargiulo, A.E., et al.: Dimension and relation of the dentogingival junctions in humans, J. Periodontol. **32:**261, 1961.
49. Ingber, J.S., et al.: The "biological width": a concept in periodontics and restorative dentistry, Alpha Omegan **70:**62, 1977.
50. Maynard, G., and Wilson, R.: Physiologic dimension of the periodontium significant to restorative dentistry, J. Periodontol. **50:**170, 1979.
51. Atwood, D.A., and Coy, W.A.: Clinical cephalometric and densitometric study of reduction of residual ridges, J. Prosthet. Dent. **26:**280, 1971.
52. Ingber, J.: Forced eruption: a method of treating isolated one and two wall infrabony defects: rationale and case report, J. Periodontol. **45:**199, 1974.
53. McHenry, K.R., Smutko, G.E., and McMullen, J.A.: Restructuring the topography of the mandibular ridge with gingival autografts, J. Am. Dent. Assoc. **104:**478, 1982.
54. Kaldahl, W.B., et al.: Achieving an esthetic appearance with a fixed prostheses by submucosal grafts, J. Am. Dent. Assoc. **104:**449, 1982.
55. Greenstein, G., et al.: Repair of anterior gingival deformity with durapatite: a case report, J. Periodontol. **56:**200, 1985.
56. Allen, E.T., et al.: Improved techniques for localized ridge augmentation: a report of 21 cases, J. Periodontol. **56:**195, 1985.
57. Lang, N.P., et al.: The relationship between the width of the keratinized gingiva and gingival health, J. Periodontol. **43:**623, 1972.
58. Miyosoto, M., et al.: Gingival conditions in areas of minimal and appreciable width of keratinized gingiva, J. Clin. Periodontol. **4:**200, 1977.
59. Rothstein, S.F., Paris, D., and Sage, B.: Use of durapatite for the rehabilitation of resorbed alveolar ridges, J. Am. Dent. Assoc. **109:**511, 1984.
60. Cohen, H.V.: Localized ridge augmentation with hydroxylapatite: report of a case, J. Am. Dent. Assoc. **108:**54, 1984.
61. Amphlett, J., and Colwell, W.C.: Edentulous vestibuloplasty using the palatal graft technique, J. Prosth. Dent. **48:**8, 1982.
62. Corn, H.: Periosteal separation: its clinical significance, J. Periodontol. **33:**140, 1962.
63. Dello Russo, N.M.: Gingival autografts as an adjunct to removable partial dentures, J. Am. Dent. Assoc. **104:**179, 1982.
64. Barkmeier, W.W., and Williams, H.J.: Surgical methods of gingival retraction for restorative dentistry, J. Am. Dent. Assoc. **96:**1002, 1978.
65. Simring, M., and Collins, J.F.: The periodontal access flap for restorative dentistry, N.Y. Dent. J. **47:**138, 1981.
66. Grant, D.A.: Presentation at American Academy of Periodontics Meeting, New Orleans, 1983.
67. Ash, M.M., Jr., Costitch, E.R., and Hayward, J.R.: A study of periodontal hazards of third molars, J. Periodontol. **33:**209, 1962.
68. Zeigler, R.S.: Preventive dentistry—new concepts preventing periodontal pockets, Va. Dent. J. **52:**11, 1975.
69. Szmyd, L., and Hester, W.: Crevicular depth of the second molar in impacted third molar surgery, J. Oral Surg. **21:**185, 1963.
70. Groves, B.J., and Moore, J.R.: The periodontal implications of flap design in lower third molar extractions, Dent. Pract. Res. **20:**297, 1970.
71. Grondahl, H.G., and Lekholm, U.: Influence of mandibular third molars on related supporting tissues, Int. J. Oral Surg. **2:**137, 1973.
72. Kay, H.B.: Esthetic considerations in the definitive periodontal prosthetic management of the maxillary anterior segment, Int. J. Perio. Rest. Dent. **3:**45, 1983.

# PART SEVEN

## Occlusal and Reconstructive Aspects of Therapy

# Treatment of periodontal trauma

The proper management of occlusion is not merely a problem of periodontics—it is a problem of dentistry. The functional relationship of the dentition should be of paramount concern to all dentists.

To discuss occlusion from the periodontal point of view, we must have a clear understanding of the concepts and terminology that are basic to occlusion. Then we may proceed to the consideration of periodontal trauma and its treatment.

Probably no other phase of dentistry is so confused by divergence of terminology and definitions as is the field of occlusion. The reader must have some insight into this problem and also a vocabulary to facilitate learning the techniques of treatment for occlusal traumatism. Without a vocabulary, explanation of occlusion and its correction is difficult. With a common vocabulary and defined terms, communication and understanding are possible. Since no universally accepted terminology is used by those who discuss occlusion,[1] it is necessary to define the terms as used in this text.

## Terminology in occlusion

Occlusion is the relationship of the teeth when they are in contact, regardless of jaw position. Therefore the full range of jaw positions within which the teeth can make contact is included in this term.

**Occlusion**

The mandible is in *rest position* when the jaw is held in a relaxed state and is not being used in speech, swallowing, mastication, or parafunctional movements. Although the jaw is at rest, the muscles are active, since rest position is controlled by muscle tonus. The teeth are not involved in rest position. There is an average space of 2 to 3 mm between the upper and lower teeth, which is known as the *freeway space* or the

**Rest position of mandible**

*interocclusal clearance.*[2-5] After a person swallows or speaks, the mandible automatically assumes this position. However, since it is a postural position, it can vary with the way in which the person holds the head or body. Although rest position is considered to be relatively stable, it can be influenced by fatigue, nervous tension, or any of the physiologic or pathologic factors that influence muscle length and tonus.

**Centric**

There are a variety of definitions and usages of the term *centric*. Some authors think that when all the teeth are in occlusal contact the position is centric. Others believe that centric occurs with the mandible in its most retruded position. Still others believe that centric occurs slightly anterior to this point. Each group considers its defined position to be *true* centric. Terms such as *false centric, acquired centric, habitual centric,* or *functional centric* illustrate the divergence of opinions. Finally,

**Centric relation**

some practitioners believe centric to be a relationship (rather than a position) of the jaws throughout the range of a certain border movement, with centric occlusion occurring at closure. These various usages are almost indelibly imprinted in our literature and language. In reading, you must try to assess which definition applies when the author uses the term *centric*.

**Centric occlusion**

Ramfjord states: "Centric occlusion is a tooth to tooth and jaw to jaw relationship, in which the teeth are in ideal intercuspation and all components of the masticatory system—the temporomandibular joint, the neuromuscular elements and the occlusal surfaces are in a harmonious relationship."[6]

To understand occlusion, the reader must accept centric as an *ideal* position without defining its precise location and then focus on the terminal hinge relationship of the mandible.

**Terminal hinge position**

The terminal hinge position is the most retruded physiologic position of the condyle in the glenoid fossa that the patient can achieve by the activity of his/her own musculature (Fig. 44-1). The term relates to movement of the mandible with the head of the condyle in the most retruded position in the fossa. In this movement the mandible

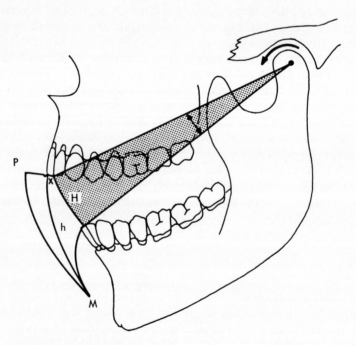

**Fig. 44-1.** The terminal hinge relation of the mandible, *H,* is the rotational path that the mandible makes about an axis in the condyles. This path is the most retruded rotational movement the patient can make under the control of his/her own musculature. *P,* Maximal protrusion; *M,* maximal open position; *h,* habitual closing movement.

turns without any translatory component in an arc whose axis lies in the condyle.

The importance of this movement is that the edentulous patient or the patient deprived of cuspal guidance can be trained to repeatedly go through the movement while points along the path of the movement are registered and reregistered. At a given degree of opening, a fixed, repeatable reference point can be established and used in mounting casts on an articulator. The opening of the mandible in the terminal hinge relation is a trained movement. Humans can move their mandibles in the hinge relationship when trained to do so. Properly instructed, they can duplicate the movement. Terminal hinge relation is called *centric relation* by some authors.[5] Terminal hinge position is sometimes referred to as *hinge position, centric occlusion,* or *retruded position.*

If one closes the jaws with the lower incisors protruded beyond the upper incisors (*P* in Figs. 44-1 and 44-2) and then draws the lower jaw slowly backward, the maxillary incisors will soon be contacted; then opening slightly so that the incisal edges clear each other, one will come to a point known as the terminus of the hinge relation. In this position terminal hinge occlusion (or retrusive contact) (Fig. 44-2) is achieved.

**Terminal hinge occlusion**

*Occlusal position* may describe any position in which there is full contact of the teeth. This term refers to any of the terms used earlier for centric, whether false or true, to describe acquired or habitual position.

The intercuspal position is the firm intermeshing of a maximal number of cusps and fossae of the mandibular teeth touching tightly against the maxillary teeth. The position of the condyle in the glenoid fossa in the intercuspal position is thus determined by the maximal intercuspation of the teeth. Since the intercuspation can be altered by many factors (extractions, restorations), the position of the condyle in the glenoid fossa may not be the same as when it is determined by an ideal relationship of other components of the masticatory system (i.e., the temporomandibular joint, neuromuscular elements, and surrounding tissues).

**Intercuspal position**

When occlusal contact is made in the median plane, it is called the median occlusal position.[7] This distinction is particularly important because there are other occlusal positions. Sicher[1] stated, "If one opens the jaws wide and then snaps them shut, the closing muscles pull the jaw unerringly and unhesitatingly into the median occlusal position." This is a directed movement and is not unique to the jaws. Neurologists, testing proprioceptive nerves and neural pathways, have long used a similar movement in their battery of tests. The patient is asked to touch the tip of the nose with the tip of the forefinger with the eyes closed. If there is no disease of the nervous system, the patient is able to do so without difficulty, although there may be some variation in

**Median occlusal position (median jaw relation)**

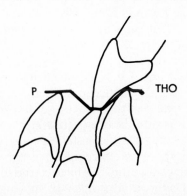

**Fig. 44-2.** Path described by the mandible as it is moved backward from its most protruded position, *P,* in full closure to the most retruded position that the patient can voluntarily assume. *THO,* Terminal hinge occlusion, which is the closure in terminal hinge relation.

many normal individuals. Proprioceptive signals play a role in guiding the shoulder, elbow, wrist, and finger into an efficient, almost precise pattern of movement. The impulses that guide this recognizable and repeatable movement arise in all the participating muscles and joints. The pattern of control (engram) is retained in the "memory banks" of the brain.

A similar memory of proprioceptive impulses also guides the mandibular muscles by reflex feedback when the jaw snaps shut. However, this movement is extraordinarily precise because neural stimuli arising in the periodontium are added to those arising in muscles and joints. The periodontal memory (engram) is subject to change with time. Eruptive and migratory tooth movements and attrition bring about changes in proprioception that, even in a completely healthy dentition, require revision of the engram to changes. Therefore the proprioceptive memory is a fleeting memory that may be recaptured or reestablished repeatedly. This occurs whenever the teeth meet in the median occlusal position.[1,8]

Edentulous persons who have lost their periodontal ligaments and, consequently, the related proprioceptive nerve impulses, must depend mainly on proprioceptive receptors in the capsule of the joint and the masticatory muscles.

**Protrusive and lateral occlusal positions**

An anterior occlusal position (protrusive position) and a right or left lateral occlusal position also exist. If the median occlusal position is slightly anterior to the most retruded or terminal hinge position, then we can also speak of a posterior or retrusive occlusal position. The movement into each position from median occlusal position can be termed protrusive movement, right or left lateral movement, and retrusive movement. Sometimes these movements are referred to as glides or excursive movements. The teeth also occlude in other positions intermediate between the lateral and protrusive positions and the median occlusal position.

## Range of mandibular movements

Similar mechanisms operate when one places the incisors edge to edge (in protrusive position) or is told to touch a lower canine to an upper canine. A patient may voluntarily assume an occlusal position within the limits set by his/her dentition, the form of the maxilla and mandible, the mobility of the temporomandibular joints, and the ability of the musculature. In fact, one may also move the mandible with the mouth open within limits set by these same structures. You may explore these borders by opening your mouth as wide as possible, protruding the jaw as far as possible, and moving to the limits of right and left lateral excursive movements with and without the teeth in contact. If a solid construction of these limits as described by the tips of the lower incisors were made, it would form a three-dimensional structure with some degree of bilateral symmetry. If it were then bisected, you could examine the range of movement in a median plane. Reexamine Figs. 44-1 and 44-2. Fig. 44-1 shows the range of movement of the mandible in the median sagittal plane.

The lateral borders of movement may be noted in Fig. 44-3. A tracing plate is bisected to show the interrelationship between the horizontal and vertical borders that gives the three-dimensional extent of the envelope of motion.

**Gothic arch tracing**

The technique of using a central bearing screw and a tracing plate (Gothic arch tracing) temporarily simulates the edentulous state because tooth contact is prevented. When such a device is used, there are no coordinated nerve impulses from the periodontal ligament to guide the patient into the most retruded position. If, during hinge axis registration, a tracing (Gothic arch) is made by moving into right and left lateral position from the median occlusal position (Fig. 44-4), the apex of the angle is formed when the condyles are in the most retruded position.[9]

These Gothic arch tracings made at different degrees of opening can be super-

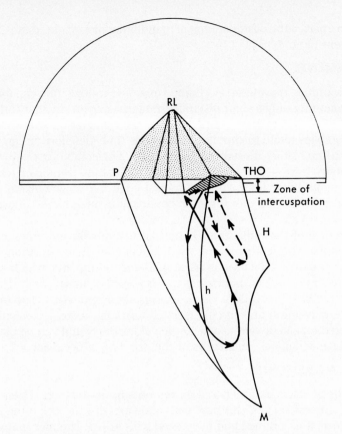

**Fig. 44-3.** A tracing plate has been used to describe the horizontal limits of mandibular movement *(stippled)* and the relationship to the limits of motion in a median plane. Half the plate has been removed, and only those movements to the right of the median plane are shown. Arrows indicate chewing, which will be explained later in the text. *h,* Habitual closing movement; *THO,* terminal hinge occlusion; *P,* maximal protrusion; *H,* hinge movement; *M,* maximal open position.

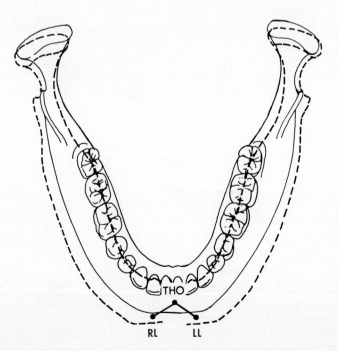

**Fig. 44-4.** Movement of the mandible from the most retruded position, *THO,* to the right lateral, *RL,* and left lateral, *LL,* positions (dotted outlines show the movement made), forming a Gothic arch tracing *(solid line).*

imposed to form part of the posterior limit of mandibular movement, that is, the terminal hinge movement (Fig. 44-5).

## HINGE MOVEMENTS

**Rotatory and translatory movements**

The terminal hinge movement is a limited one. The condyles are capable of a purely rotatory movement for only a short distance through a narrow arc that can be recorded at the edge of the lower incisors (see *H* in Figs. 44-1 and 44-3). If the jaws continue to open, the condyles rotate further but at the same time glide forward on the articular eminences in a translatory movement (Fig. 44-6). The combined rotatory and translatory movements have a projected and more generalized center of rotation in the region of the mandibular foramen. The incisal edge moves downward and forward from the widest portion of the posterior boundary of mandibular movement (Fig. 44-6).

**Border movements**

The importance of these diagrams is that all mandibular movements must occur within their limits. The teeth may be used functionally in mastication, swallowing, and speech. They may also be used in parafunctional movements, which are discussed later. The border movements themselves are not used in mastication. Habitual mastication occurs within the borders (see *h* in Figs. 44-1 and 44-3). The importance of terminal hinge movement and the interrelated terminal hinge occlusion is that they can be registered repeatedly with some degree of accuracy and can be used as a point of reference for mechanical articulators or the grinding of occlusion.

## FUNCTIONAL MOVEMENTS

**Mastication**

Consider the physiologic functional movements in mastication. These movements start with biting into food and continue with chewing, during which the food bolus is reduced in size as it is softened and moistened with saliva. The movements terminate with swallowing.

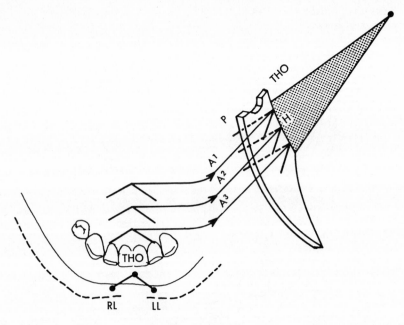

**Fig. 44-5.** Schematic drawing that relates Gothic arch tracings made in a horizontal plane with the hinge movement made in the median plane. Tracings *A¹*, *A²*, and *A³* can be made at different degrees of opening. Their apices contact the hinge movement or hinge relation, which is made up of an infinite number of superimposed Gothic arches. *P*, Most protruded position; *H*, hinge movement; *THO*, terminal hinge occlusion.

When one bites into food, arm and shoulder muscles are pitted against neck and masticatory muscles, by which means a piece of food is torn away. Considerable forces may be exerted on the teeth, yet the teeth do not make contact.

After the bite, the initial chewing strokes are large and more protrusive in position (see Fig. 44-3). The later strokes are smaller because the bolus is reduced, and the mandible moves toward the terminal hinge position (Fig. 44-7). The size of the bolus prevents the teeth from occluding in the early strokes, but with successive strokes the teeth come closer to each other; contact generally occurs before swallowing[10] (Fig. 44-7).

The opening movement is performed more quickly than the closing movement, which is slower, more deliberate, and dependent on proprioceptive feedback signals.[11]

**Opening and closing movements**

The path of movement is described as being teardrop in shape[11] (Figs. 44-7 and 44-8) and is directed from the cusp incline toward the central fossa. Although much variation exists in the teardrop pattern, the range of movement away from the median occlusal position is limited. The border occlusal movements that one performs with articulators do not generally occur in mastication.

The opening and closing motions per se are isotonic and are not associated with

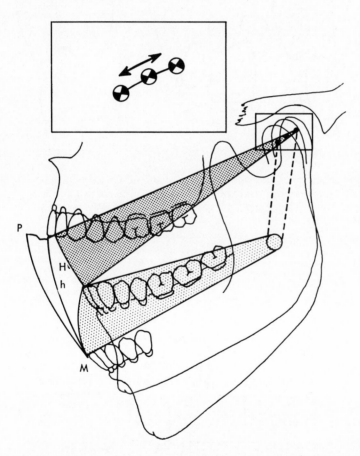

**Fig. 44-6.** In opening, the heavily stippled area represents hinge movement about a center of rotation in the condyle. In opening wider, the condyles continue to rotate beyond the limit of purely rotatory movement (see marking of magnified centers of rotation in inset) but also glide forward on the eminentia. These two movements, that is, further rotation and translation, have a projected center of rotation in the vicinity of the mandibular foramen. The opening beyond the limit of hinge rotation is indicated by the lightly stippled sector formed about the secondary center of rotation. The incisal point moves downward and forward, and the chin point moves downward and backward as the center of rotation is carried forward by the translatory movement *(inset).*

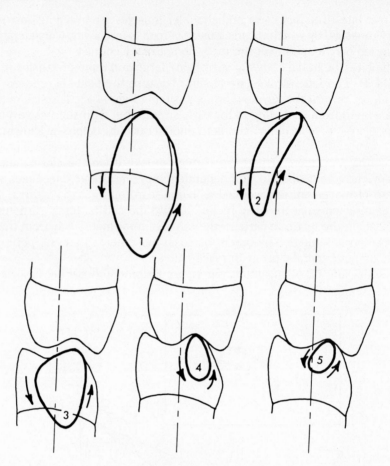

**Fig. 44-7.** Diagrams depicting five successive masticatory strokes, each made in the teardrop pattern. The first stroke is the largest, and the later strokes successively smaller. The teeth do not contact in strokes *1* through *3*, but light tooth contact is made in strokes *4* and *5* just before swallowing. (Modified from Beyron, H.: Acta Odontol. Scand. **22:**597, 1964.)

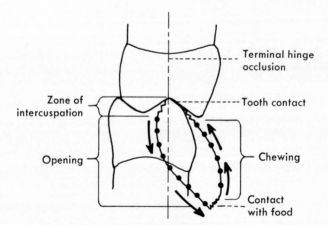

**Fig. 44-8.** Diagram depicting opening and closing movements between two opposing molars. The opening movement is performed quickly as the depressors of the mandible contract isotonically. When contact with food is made, isometric and isotonic elements combine under proprioceptive guidance, and the mandible closes more slowly. Zigzag lines indicate influence of proprioceptive impulses. Chewing strokes are short of full closure. Tooth contact is made just before swallowing close to terminal hinge occlusion. Note the teardrop pattern and the stroke directed toward the median plane rather than toward the lateral position. *Dots,* Actual recordings. (Modified from Murphy, T.R.: Arch. Oral Biol. **10:**981, 1965.)

strong forces. When resistance is met, isometric components develop. These are associated with greater forces but are controlled by proprioceptive impulses. Consequently heavy pressures are not generated unless the initial biting into food is especially forceful, the food is unusually coarse and resistant, the teeth are used to split hard objects (e.g., nuts), or a piece of bone or other hard material is unexpectedly encountered in the softer bolus.

## PARAFUNCTIONAL MOVEMENTS

If mastication does not generate heavy pressures, if the teeth do not contact during mastication in general, and if masticatory movements do not resemble articulator excursive glides, how then are the wear facets produced? They are distant from the median occlusal position and very common ( Fig. 44-9). They are the result of bruxism.

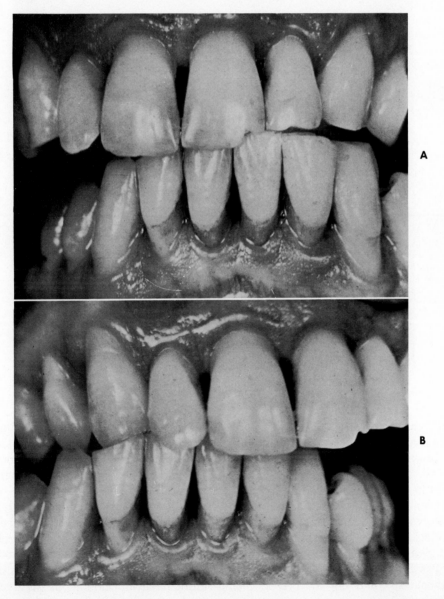

**Fig. 44-9.**   Dentition of a 30-year-old man. The wear facets of the incisors fit the opposing teeth in extreme lateral positions, **A** and **B**.                                                                                 *Continued.*

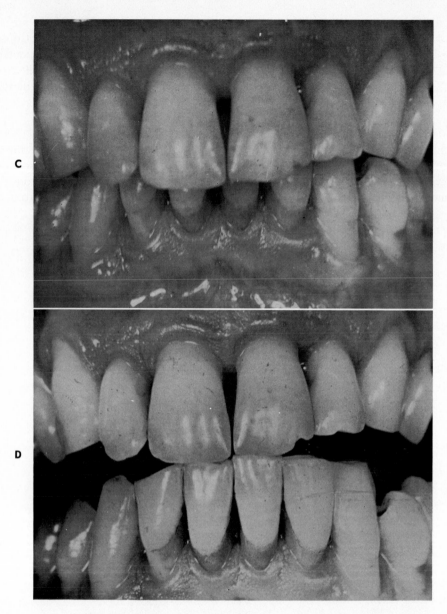

**Fig. 44-9, cont'd.** **C,** Median occlusal position. **D,** Protrusive position.

Bruxism,[12] clenching, and rocking of teeth are parafunctional movements.[13] The term *parafunction* (outside or beyond function) was first suggested by Drum.[13]

**Bruxism**    Bruxism[14] is the habit of grinding the teeth. It may occur during sleep or while awake. The patient is usually unaware of the habit, which consists of rubbing the teeth in protrusive and lateral occlusal movements.

**Clenching and clamping**    Clenching and clamping are produced through isometric contraction of the masticatory muscles while the teeth are in contact, usually in the median jaw relation.

**Rocking**    Rocking of the teeth, which is most deleterious, results when a slight lateral force is added to clenching.

Parafunctional movements are practically universal. They need not be abnormal or pathogenic.[15] It is not the presence of parafunctional movement but the excessive degree, frequency, and duration of these strong isometric contractions that contribute to pathologic conditions. Certainly if trauma does not result, the presence of parafunction is not pathologic. One could say that pathologic conditions result in only a percentage of those who brux and clench. Indeed, parafunction may be useful in the dissipation of tension or of pent-up energy.

Causes for these habits are not fully known, but the habits may be psychologic, neurologic, occupational, or occlusal.[6,15,16] The psychologic causes may be tension or the unconscious expression of hate or displeasure[17,18] (see the discussion on psychologic factors in Chapter 26). When these emotions are portrayed by actors, the play of their masticatory musculature may be easily observed. Tetany (active or latent), meningitis, epilepsy, and parkinsonism constitute some of the neurologic causes for these phenomena, which may lead to hypertonicity of the masticatory musculature and to bruxism or clenching. Occupational bruxism or clenching can be seen in truck drivers[19,20] and in individuals performing feats of great strength. Sometimes bruxism may be related to stimuli from irregularities in the occlusion such as premature contacts or dental restorations that are too high; the patient tries to remove the annoying high point by compensatory parafunction.[17] Bruxism is also common in children and may permit the secondary teeth to erupt in proper position. Possibly, from a phylogenetic viewpoint, bruxism is a primate tooth-honing mechanism.[21]

Persons who brux are often completely unaware of their habit and will often deny bruxing when asked by the dentist. However, spouses may comment about the noises produced during bruxing in sleep; once the question is raised, the patient may become aware of the habit. The diagnosis should not be made in the form of an accusation implying disease or abnormality. When some persons who brux awaken, they may feel the fatigue of the jaw muscle, pain in the temporomandibular joint, or limitation of ability to open wide (see discussion of subjective indications of periodontal traumatism).

Bruxism may lead to the formation of wear facets. The occlusal situation is aggravated as one tooth meets its opponent on flat planes and grips it more intimately during contact, thus contributing to the leverage and intensity of force application.

The importance of ongoing regeneration of the periodontium has been discussed. There is sufficient time for reparative turnover to compensate for tissue damage incident to mastication during the periods between meals when the masticatory organ is at rest. What might be significant in bruxism is that the regeneration period is reduced. When these habits occur in the presence of periodontal disease, additional stress and strain are put on the inflamed or dystrophic tissues, and the chances for tissue breakdown may be increased. Koivumaa, Landt, and Nyquist[22] have found a definite correlation between bruxism and temporomandibular joint and muscle disorders. The relationship between bruxism and periodontal disease, although likely, has not been fully established.[23]

Before the treatment of traumatism by occlusal adjustment, the dentist must examine and classify the type of occlusion and tooth to tooth relationships (intercuspation) (Figs. 44-10 to 44-13).

## Occlusions

### IDEAL OCCLUSION

A picture of ideal occlusion has been provided by orthodontic concepts. This is useful in describing various occlusal relationships. The intercuspation of the teeth as defined by Angle is such that the mesiobuccal cusp of the upper first molar occludes with the mesiobuccal groove of the lower first molar.[24] The upper canine intercuspates with the distal incline of the lower canine and the mesiobuccal cusp incline of the premolar; the other premolars and molars intercuspate perfectly between the inclines

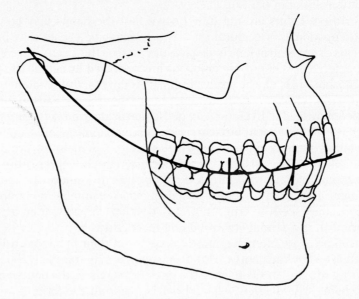

**Fig. 44-10.** Ideal occlusion. Line drawn through the occlusal plane indicates the curve of Spee. Alignment markers drawn perpendicular to this curve indicate the correct first molar and canine relationships according to Angle.

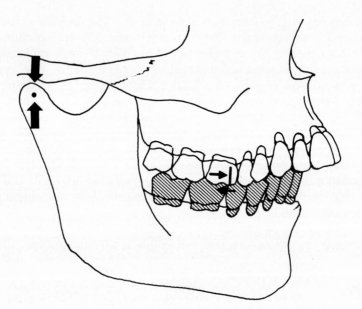

**Fig. 44-11.** Angle class II, division 1, malocclusion. The mesiobuccal cusp of the maxillary first molar intercuspates anterior to the mesiobuccal groove of the mandibular first molar. The maxillary canine is similarly anterior to the position that it occupies in the ideal occlusion. The overjet is pronounced. Large arrows indicate that the mandible is in terminal hinge position.

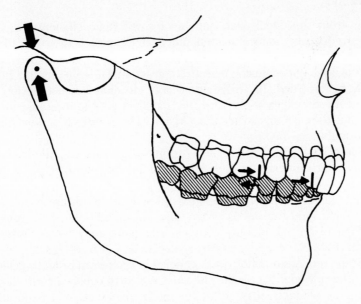

**Fig. 44-12.**   Angle class II, division 2, malocclusion. The mesiobuccal cusp of the maxillary first molar intercuspates anterior to the mesiobuccal cusp of the mandibular first molar. The maxillary canine is anterior to the ideal position. Note the deep overbite. Large arrows indicate that the mandible is in terminal hinge position.

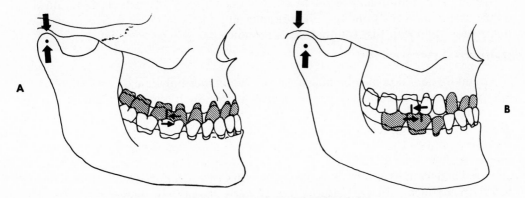

**Fig. 44-13.**   Class III malocclusion. **A,** All the mandibular teeth are in mesioversion to the maxillary teeth. The jaw is prognathic. The mandibular teeth are buccal and labial to the maxillary teeth. **B,** Pseudoclass III occlusion. The anterior mandibular teeth are in mesioversion. The jaw (condyle) is brought forward to allow full intercuspation in closure. This produces a situation of habitual occlusion in class III relationship. The crossing of the posterior teeth that change from buccoversion to linguoversion is termed a *crossbite*. Large arrows indicate the terminal hinge position, **A,** and lack thereof, **B.**

distal to these landmarks (Fig. 44-10). In addition, the occlusal plane is relatively flat, and the curve of Spee and the curve of Monson are not steep.

## MALOCCLUSIONS

Deviations from this ideal occlusion are termed malocclusions. Ideal occlusion occurs only infrequently; malocclusion of one or more teeth is the rule rather than the exception. Angle[24] classified malocclusions into three types: classes I, II, and III.

**Angle class I and Angle class II-1**

An Angle class I malocclusion has the correct molar relationship; however, the anterior teeth are crowded. In an Angle class II, division 1 malocclusion the mesio-buccal cusp of the maxillary molar and the maxillary canine intercuspate anterior to the position that they occupy in ideal occlusion. The overjet is pronounced, but the overbite is normal (Fig. 44-11).

**Angle class II-2**

In an Angle class II, division 2 malocclusion the maxillary teeth also occlude with the mandibular teeth anterior to their ideal position, but the overbite is pronounced (Fig. 44-12).

**Angle class III**

In the Angle class III malocclusions the mandibular teeth are in mesioversion to the maxillary teeth, and the jaw is prognathic. All mandibular teeth may be in mesioversion (Fig. 44-13, *A*), or only the posterior teeth may be in mesioversion, as happens when there is a pseudoclass III malocclusion (Fig. 44-13, *B*).

Malocclusions related to major discrepancies in arch form or tooth position should be treated by the orthodontist. Malocclusions related to occlusal form discrepancies, such as premature contacts, may be treated by the periodontist or restorative dentist. In fact, many of the malocclusions that are treated by the periodontist in conjunction with the restorative dentist are actually major malocclusions. Occlusal therapy then is an important part of periodontal therapy and is as difficult as the treatment of major malocclusions by conventional orthodontic methods.

This chapter discusses occlusal adjustment by grinding. The methods for occlusal adjustment can be and sometimes are applied even if traumatism is not present. For example, if many inlays are being prepared or bridgework is planned, you may want to adjust the occlusion before doing the reconstruction. On the other hand, if there is no evidence of trauma and reconstruction is not required, then there is no need to adjust an occlusion by grinding. The presence of a major or minor malocclusion does *not* necessarily mean that traumatism is present.

## MUTILATED OCCLUSIONS

An entire dentition may be maloccluded. Sometimes only one or a few teeth of an otherwise normal dentition may be in malocclusion. Such teeth may be described by the terms supraclusion, infraclusion, mesioclusion, distoclusion, tilted, or rotated. These situations frequently develop in dentitions in which teeth have been extracted and not replaced. The occlusions are then termed mutilated. There may be mutilated normal occlusions or mutilated class I, II, or III malocclusions. When mutilations have occurred and teeth have moved, you may have to surmise how the teeth were arranged before the extractions were performed to properly classify the occlusion.

## Clinical diagnosis

Ideal occlusion does not have the same connotation to a prosthodontist as it does to an orthodontist. An orthodontist is usually most concerned with the positional relationship of the teeth and jaws to the cranium and the esthetic arrangement of the teeth. The prosthodontist also considers jaw relations; however, the prosthodontist is more concerned with the occlusal anatomy and its relation to tooth contacts.

The orthodontic concept of an ideal occlusion is useful in describing various jaw relationships.

Just as it is necessary in the course of the examination to inspect the color, texture, and consistency of the gingival tissues, to measure the pocket depths, and to examine the teeth and occlusion, so it is necessary to examine for signs of trauma.

Since a biopsy examination of the periodontal ligament, cementum, and bone cannot be done on patients, and since intraoral telemetry and electromyography are primarily research tools, how can you determine whether periodontal trauma is present? You must depend on clinical examination. Periodontal trauma is more easily diagnosed when a systematic and disciplined order of history and examination is used.

## SUBJECTIVE INDICATIONS

During the interview the patient may make one or more of the following complaints:

1. My bite seems wrong.
2. My teeth are sore when I close.
3. This tooth seems to hit before the others; it's longer.
4. My teeth and gums feel "itchy."
5. My jaws hurt (muscles or mastication).
6. My teeth are sensitive (pulpal irritation).
7. My jaw joints hurt; they make cracking noises.
8. I grind my teeth.
9. My teeth have loosened.
10. My teeth have moved.
11. I find it hard to open my mouth in the morning.
12. My face hurts.

Such remarks should lead you to suspect that trauma may have occurred. Periodontal trauma can occur when an excessive or misdirected masticatory force is transmitted through the tooth to the periodontium, causing tissue injury. Frequently such a force arises when two opposing teeth occlude before all other teeth meet. Such prematurities can be the direct result of malocclusion. The malocclusions may be minor (when one or two teeth are malposed) or major. However, what appears as pathologic from an orthodontic point of view (Angle class II relation, crossbite) may function physiologically without destroying periodontal tissues. On the other hand, an occlusion that appears nearly perfect from the orthodontic view may be less than perfect from the aspects of occlusion and articulation, or parafunctional habits may contribute to the breakdown of supporting structures of the tooth.

## OBJECTIVE SIGNS AND TESTS

In the course of the examination, you should record the following data:

1. *Mobility—passive.* How loose are the teeth on palpation? Rock each tooth with instrument handles while the patient's head is in a relatively steady position.
2. *Mobility—dynamic.* How loose are the teeth during functional and parafunctional movements? Ask the patient to open and close the jaws and also to move the closed jaws into the lateral and protrusive positions. Test the teeth for mobility and heavy contacts. You may do this by holding your fingertips lightly half on the teeth and half on the gingiva. The patient should clench and rock the teeth while you carefully observe for visual or tactile (fremitus) signs of mobility.
3. *Migration.** Have the teeth migrated? Have some teeth elongated beyond the occlusal plane? Have others drifted forward, opening diastemata? Have teeth rotated?

---

*Pathologic migration may also be a symptom of juvenile periodontitis. However, juvenile periodontitis is a relatively rare disease, whereas traumatism is encountered frequently.

4. *Palpation of the masticatory muscles.* How large and powerful are these muscles? In some cases hypertrophy of the muscles may be indicative of bruxism.
5. *Roentgenographic signs.* Have the periodontal ligament spaces widened? Is there any change in the lamina dura? Is any radiolucency present in the furcation areas? Are there periapical zones of radiolucency about vital teeth? Do signs of root resorption exist? Has the pulp chamber become smaller? Remember that buccal and lingual widening of the periodontal ligament space may not be evident in the roentgenogram that represents a mesiodistal profile.
6. *Wear facets.* Are wear facets present on the teeth beyond what you would expect for the patient's age?

Perhaps the most important signs to look for are *mobility* of teeth, *widening* of the periodontal ligament space in roentgenograms, and pathologic tooth *migration*. These are symptoms of actual damage. Wear facets indicate what the patient is doing in parafunctional movements; they may also signify potential damage, but in the absence of other objective signs, they do not necessarily show that traumatism is occuring.

If actual damage from occlusal traumatism has been diagnosed, the source of the trauma must be determined. Examine the occlusion for disharmonies as well as to see how the force application may be contributing to the trauma. In addition, try to gain some idea of the types of mandibular movements the patient is capable of making. Following are areas to check in examination of occlusion:

1. Type of occlusion
   A. Normal
   B. Angle class I
   C. Angle class II
   D. Angle class III
2. Teeth present—number and position
   A. Alignment
   B. Tilting
   C. Crowding
   D. Drifting
   E. Crossbite relationships
   F. Diastemata
   G. Relationship to occlusal plane
3. Missing teeth
4. Crown-to-root ratio of teeth
5. Buccolingual width of teeth
6. Form of the occlusal plane
   A. Type of curve of Spee (normal, exaggerated, horizontal, reverse)
   B. Mutilations caused by extrusion
   C. Double plane of occlusion (i.e., posterior teeth and anterior teeth on different planes)
7. Degree of anterior overbite and overjet
   A. Deep overbite
   B. Incisal edges contacting gingival or palatal tissue
   C. Anterior teeth in nonocclusion
8. Extent of zone of intercuspation
   A. Cusp inclination
   B. Cusp-fossa relationship
   C. Locked bite
9. Functional relations*
   A. Premature contacts in terminal hinge position
   B. Form and range of hinge movement
   C. Premature functional (working) side contacts in lateral occlusal positions and movements
   D. Nonfunctional (nonworking) side contact in lateral occlusal position and movements
   E. Premature contacts in protrusive occlusal position and movements

10. Parafunctional relations*
    A. Premature contacts in lateral occlusal positions and movements
    B. Nonfunctional side contact in lateral occlusal position and movements
    C. Premature contacts in protrusive occlusal position and movements
    D. Form and range of lateral and protrusive movements
11. Rest position of the mandible and extent of the freeway space*
12. Deviations in the path of opening and closing*
13. Palpation of the temporomandibular joints during functional movements

When the treatment plan includes reconstruction, other data may be needed. Some of these must be provided by an examination of well-articulated diagnostic (study) casts, especially when missing teeth or many carious teeth are present. At times the mobility will involve so many teeth that occlusal grinding alone is not sufficient. When the treatment plan includes reconstruction as well as occlusal adjustment, additional factors must be known:

**Examination for reconstruction**

1. Position and number of missing teeth
2. Position, number, and periodontal status of abutment teeth
3. Degree of involvement of carious teeth
4. Alignment of teeth in terms of parallelism
5. Presence of food impaction and retention areas
6. Diastemata (old or newly formed)
7. Operative quality and periodontal adequacy of existing restorations
8. Esthetics or absence thereof
9. Plaque retention score

Once these factors are understood, the amount and degree of restorative dentistry necessary and the occlusal morphology of the reconstruction can be planned, and the degree of the risk gauged (Chapters 46 and 47).

In evaluating occlusal traumatism determine the direction, frequency, distribution, and intensity of functionally occurring forces (as in mastication, deglutition, and speech) and parafunctional forces (as in bruxism, clenching, tongue thrusting, and other oral habits).[5,25] Perhaps the strongest of these forces are the parafunctional, where isometric muscle contraction is the rule.

Understanding occlusion is a necessary adjunct to full denture and partial denture construction, in fixed bridgework and restorative dentistry, and in orthodontic therapy. Rules for adjusting occlusions have developed in some of these clinical disciplines, which are predicated on the presence of occlusal discrepancies. Such rules provide a foundation for the type of adjustment required to treat periodontal trauma.

Remember that a malocclusion or occlusal abnormalities do not necessarily mean that traumatism is present. Trauma is a tissue lesion. There are many instances in which tooth malpositions are present without trauma, and trauma is present without tooth malpositions.

## Occlusal disharmonies and their treatment

Therapy of occlusal trauma can be accomplished in the following ways[26]:

1. Occlusal adjustment by grinding
2. Orthodontic treatment
3. Splinting
4. Prosthetic reconstruction
5. Construction of bite guards
6. Extraction of extruded teeth

---

*Some clinicians maintain that such observations can be made only with instruments.

Often more than one of these steps must be performed. The ensuing discussion deals mainly with correction by grinding and alleviation of parafunctional habits with night guards.

## PRINCIPLES

Earlier in this chapter the term *premature contact* was used. What are premature contacts? They are initial contacts of opposing tooth surfaces that are made before the remaining teeth come into contact. When do they occur? They can occur during functional and parafunctional movements. What do they do? If the premature contact occurs in centric (terminal hinge occlusion), the mandible is deflected into some other occlusal position (habitual occlusion). If the prematurity occurs during a glide movement, the adjacent teeth may be prevented from making contact during the glide. Consequently prematurities are known as interceptive or deflective contacts; the terms *cuspal interferences* or *occlusal interferences* that prevent occlusal harmony and *occlusal disharmonies* are also used.

Prematurities often occur in conjunction with malocclusions, but malocclusion per se does not necessarily mean that premature contacts are present. Deflective contacts can and do occur in some grossly normal occlusions. Therefore do not judge whether a prematurity is present on the basis of tooth arrangement, alignment, or irregularity. Rather, examine the functional and parafunctional movements of the mandible. Although trauma is not a necessary sequel of disharmony, premature contacts and trauma often exist in a cause-effect relationship. If such a cause-effect relationship exists, correct the occlusion by grinding in periodontal treatment. In the fabrication of partial dentures and fixed bridges or in the restoration of a dentition with inlays, eliminate all prematurities before the restorations are made so as not to perpetuate the disharmony. There are good and sufficient reasons for the establishment of a harmonious occlusion in such cases. Nevertheless in the absence of trauma, prophylactic adjustment of occlusions is not a justifiable procedure.[27]

**Occlusal adjustment**

Occlusal adjustment is the establishment of an occlusion according to some ideal plan by grinding the occluding and other surfaces of the teeth. In the establishment of an ideal occlusion, occlusal disharmonies are eliminated. The ideal occlusion is believed to permit function that is physiologically compatible with the periodontium, the temporomandibular joints, and the muscles of mastication. Then the stomatognathic system is said to be in harmony.

Several concepts of occlusion have been described: bilateral balance, group function, and canine protection or disclusion-occlusion. In addition, many dentists believe that only centric harmony is essential; yet most agree on the need for a simultaneous bilateral intercuspation of the posterior teeth in the terminal hinge position.

Regardless of the ideal articulation, occlusal adjustment must obtain centric free of premature contacts. Most of the variation between the concepts occurs in the handling of eccentric movements.

The question may be asked, why should the teeth be made to intercuspate well in hinge position? Although this position is not assumed often during rest or in ordinary chewing, it is apparently used during parafunctional movements such as bruxism and clenching as well as during some functional movements. The dentist's aim is not to reposition the mandible but rather to avoid premature contacts in any position in which the patient may intercuspate the teeth in functional or parafunctional activities.

**Bilateral balance**

*Bilateral balance* is essentially a full denture concept maintaining that occlusal forces should be equally distributed to all teeth.[28-32] In this way each tooth carries a proportionate share of the load. In centric the cusp tip should enter the fossa to the full depth of the fossa. In lateral excursions functional and nonfunctional (working and balancing) sides are ground to make bilateral contact (equilibration). Although this method has been superseded in periodontal therapy by other methods, it is still used occasionally (e.g., when all maxillary teeth distal to the canine are missing on one side).

In a group function type of occlusion the buccal slopes of mandibular buccal cusps and the lingual slopes of maxillary buccal cusps are shaped so that the load is equally distributed among these cusps at all times during lateral movement.[32-37] Clinical observations indicate the premature contacts on the nonfunctional side may be the most destructive of all premature contacts. Consequently, nonfunctional side contacts are deliberately avoided or removed. The load in lateral excursion is borne only by the functional side.

*Group function*

However, nonfunctional interferences are also possible on the functional side. The chewing stroke may pass beyond the median occlusal position and the lingual cusps of the functional side may come to carry the load and thus act as premature balancing contacts.[34] These contacts must then be removed. After such corrections, function is borne by groups of teeth (canines to molars of one side) in lateral excursions and by the anterior teeth in protrusive excursion.

The aim of *canine-protected occlusion* is that the maxillary and the mandibular canines carry the occlusal load in lateral excursions, causing the other teeth to become disoccluded.[38,39] The root length and bone support of the canines are believed to be well suited for carrying such a heavy load. Since the posterior teeth are disoccluded in excursions, they cannot be stressed by premature forces. A variant of this type of approach requires, in addition, that the posterior teeth become slightly disoccluded in protrusive glides while the anterior teeth bear the load. In centric the posterior teeth carry the load while the anterior teeth are slightly disoccluded. Such a mechanical plan is termed disocclusion.[40-43] In a disclusion-occlusion, contact on posterior teeth occurs only when the mandible is in terminal hinge occlusion (centric relation occlusion); in this position the anterior teeth are slightly out of occlusion. The canines and incisors disocclude the posterior teeth in all lateral excursive movements. Proper ridge, cusp, and groove direction must be established so that when the cusps leave centric relation, they will be immediately disoccluded and pass without contact along shearing or escape grooves, depending on which is the functional and which the nonfunctional side.

*Canine protection (disclusion-occlusion)*

Most dental schools teach occlusal adjustment by way of either group function or canine protection.

## GENERAL OBJECTIVES

Objectives in occlusal adjustment are outlined as follows[23,26,43-46]:

1. To distribute forces in median occlusal position to the largest possible number of teeth.
2. To coordinate the median occlusal position with the terminal hinge position of the mandible, either by making them coincide or by establishing freedom of movement between the two positions (long centric).
3. To eliminate prematurities in excursive movements to either gain a group function occlusion or disclusion-occlusion. (Chewing should be possible on the right and left side with equal ease. This is facilitated by the simultaneous gliding contact between the teeth on the functional side.[23])
4. To direct occlusal forces, as far as possible, centrally along the long axis of the tooth.[47] (As a corollary, tilting or torquing forces should be minimized.)
   A. In median occlusal position the lingual cusps of the maxillary teeth and the buccal cusps of the mandibular teeth should project into the central fossae of their antagonists.
   B. Related harmonious cusp inclines should be established in all teeth of a group, and their cuspal inclinations should be reduced so that lateral vectors are minimized and long axis vectors are maximized (Fig. 44-14).

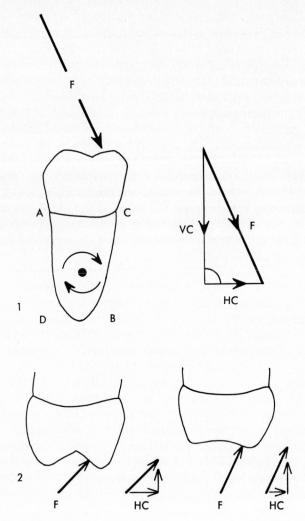

**Fig. 44-14.** **1,** A known force, *F,* directed perpendicular to a cusp surface may be divided by means of vector analysis into a vertical component, *VC,* and a horizontal component, *HC.* In the vector analysis each line represents the true magnitude of the force. The vertical component is conducted in an axial direction. The horizontal component produces a torque about the center of rotation of the tooth *(dot).* This causes compression at *C* and *D* and tension at *A* and *B.* **2,** Comparison of vector diagrams for forces of equal magnitude, *F,* applied to a steep-cusped tooth and a less steep-cusped (after grinding) tooth. The vertical component is increased in the shallow-cusped tooth. The horizontal component, *HC,* is decreased. Consequently this tooth receives less torque.

5. To improve or maintain masticatory performance, since better-related occlusal surfaces are presumed to require less force.
   A. Establish static relationships between cusps and fossae of opposing teeth to minimize tooth mobility during function. Then reshape plunger cusps that wedge antagonist teeth apart (see Fig. 44-20).
   B. Retain cusp sharpness, establish occlusal grooves and sluiceways, and smooth tooth surfaces because these are conducive to improved masticatory performance.
   C. When open contacts exist, reestablish proximal tooth contact, since the mutual support that contact provides enhances tooth stability and prevents food impaction.
   D. When the width of the occlusal table of a tooth has been increased by wear or by grinding, narrow it.
6. To accomplish the occlusal adjustment without reducing vertical dimension and by retaining an acceptable interocclusal clearance.
7. To reduce or eliminate fremitus.

## FIVE STEPS IN OCCLUSAL ADJUSTMENT

Occlusal adjustment consists of the following five steps: (1) initial grinding, (2) harmonization in terminal hinge occlusion, (3) harmonization in protrusive position and movement, (4) harmonization in lateral occlusal position and lateral excursion, and, finally, (5) reestablishment of physiologic occlusal anatomy and careful polishing of all ground surfaces. These steps presume that the patient has a relatively normal occlusion or an Angle class I or class II, division 1, occlusion. Details vary for an Angle class II and a class II, division 2, and a class III occlusion and also in various crossbite and open-bite relationships.

If occlusal adjustment is undertaken, it is not a simple task that can be performed hurriedly and without planning.[26,43,44] There are simple cases, to be sure, but even these should be carefully considered. Some practitioners study the occlusion in the mouth; others take diagnostic study casts and mount them on an anatomic articulator. In either case a fairly complete study should be made. Some operators adjust the occlusion on articulator-mounted casts and prepare a grinding list of the corrections performed.

Initial grinding may include the following:

**Initial grinding**

1. Narrowing of buccolingual diameters
2. Shortening of extruded teeth
3. Improvement of esthetics
4. Correction of marginal ridge relationships
5. Reduction of plunger cusps
6. Correction of rotated, malposed, or tilted teeth
7. Correction of facets and abraded teeth
8. Rounding of sharp edges when indicated

Such grinding should precede adjustment in hinge position, since many interferences are eliminated during this step, and often further adjustment may become unnecessary. In fact, this grinding may be all that is required to remove the disharmonies.

In initial grinding, try to recarve the teeth to obtain as ideal an arch and occlusal plane as possible. Once this is obtained, the steps in a definitive grinding tend to become easier.

1. *Buccolingual narrowing.* By narrowing the buccolingual diameter of the teeth, you will make the occlusal table smaller, and consequently the rounded extreme edges of the occlusal surface will be unable to participate in transmitting torquing forces. Occlusal forces will become centered over the tooth and will tend to be transmitted along the long axis of the tooth (Figs. 44-15 and 44-16). This step is indicated only when such narrowing would neither disturb vertical dimension by removing cusp tips that contact in centric nor induce cheek biting.
2. *Shortening of extruded teeth.* Teeth frequently extrude after they have lost their antagonists or have migrated. The elongated tooth becomes unesthetic and may be the premature tooth in many movements. Moreover, the plane of occlusion is disturbed, and, unless the tooth is shortened, good occlusion in restorative or reconstructive dental procedures cannot be obtained. In such cases exposure of the dentin in grinding is permissible (Fig. 44-17).
3. *Improvement of esthetics.* Although shortening of extruded teeth will improve esthetics, there are some cases in which other factors require attention. For instance, the anterior teeth may not be symmetric in length or may have ragged, abraded incisal surfaces and may be rotated or slightly overlapped. Such teeth can be ground to a more symmetric and regular form (Figs. 44-18 and 44-21).
4. *Correction of marginal ridge relationships.* Marginal ridges may exhibit three types of variation: they may be unequal in height; they may not meet at the contact area (because of rotation or malposition); or they may have faulty marginal ridge and sluiceway form (because of poor restoration or grinding). In some cases, grind these defects. When grinding cannot be done, correct them by restorative dentistry (Fig. 44-19).

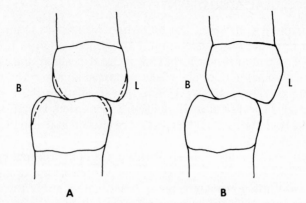

**Fig. 44-15.** **A,** Buccolingual narrowing. Area to be ground is outlined. **B,** Buccolingual narrowing as completed.

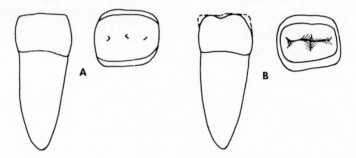

**Fig. 44-16.** **A,** The tooth is worn, obliterating the occlusal anatomy and making the occlusal surface broad. **B,** Reshaping narrows the occlusal table and restores the anatomy. (See also Fig. 44-19, C). (Modified from Miller, S.C.: Textbook of periodontia, ed. 2, Philadelphia, 1943, The Blakiston Co.)

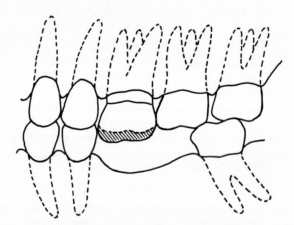

**Fig. 44-17.** An extruded tooth has been shortened *(shaded area)* to create a normal occlusal plane. A fixed bridge can be fabricated to restore the lower missing teeth. Had the maxillary molar been left as it was, the resultant bridge would have had a distorted occlusal plane.

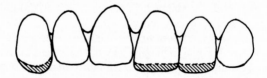

**Fig. 44-18.** When individual anterior teeth are disproportionately longer than the same teeth on the other side of the mouth, they may be ground *(shaded area)* to a more regular length.

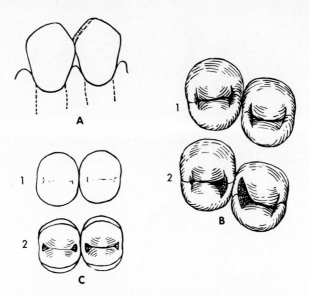

**Fig. 44-19.** Correction of marginal ridge relationships. **A,** Dotted line shows correction in teeth that are of unequal height. **B,** Rotated teeth that have, *1,* the marginal ridge of one tooth adjacent to the buccal or lingual cusp incline of the other and, *2,* the marginal ridges corrected by grinding shown by cross-hatching. **C,** Worn, ground, or poorly carved tooth with faulty marginal ridge and sluiceway form, *1;* corrected, *2.*

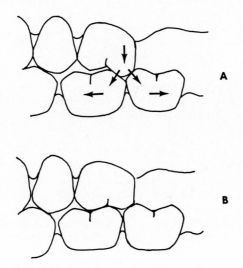

**Fig. 44-20.** **A,** The elongated distobuccal cusp of the maxillary molar wedges the lower molars and forces them apart. Food impaction occurs during mastication. **B,** The distobuccal cusp of the maxillary molar is rounded, and both wedging and food impaction are eliminated.

5. *Plunger cusps and food impaction.* If a tooth has a prominent cusp that meets the marginal ridges of the pair of opposing teeth, it may wedge the opposing teeth apart. This is especially true when the opposing teeth are mobile and the antagonist is firm. Such wedging is conducive to food impaction. The wedging cusp is termed a plunger cusp. Shorten and round it without taking the tooth out of centric occlusion, since such cuspal relationships are often the sites of centric prematurity (Fig. 44-20).

6. *Rotated, malposed, or tilted teeth.* Rotated teeth have been mentioned in relation to esthetics. Careful grinding will improve the crown form of individual rotated, tilted, or malposed teeth (Fig. 44-21).

7. *Wear facets and abraded teeth.* Teeth subject to masticatory and parafunctional activity tend to wear. Such areas are known as *wear facets.* Abraded teeth require more force in

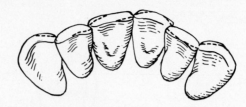

**Fig. 44-21.** Rotated lower incisors and the indicated correction *(dotted lines)* that may improve esthetics and occlusion. (Modified from Beube, F.E.: Periodontology: diagnosis and treatment, New York, 1953, The Macmillan Co.)

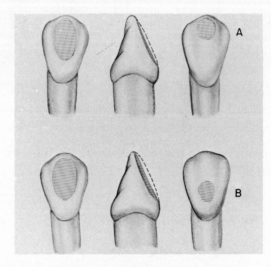

**Fig. 44-22.** A long-wear facet is present, which should be reduced by recontouring the tooth. The recontouring may preserve the incisal, **A,** or cervical, **B,** region of the wear facet to preserve contact in the median occlusal position. The lower end of the wear facet is preserved in exceptional instances such as in cases of deep overbite.

mastication; their wear facets should be reduced (Fig. 44-22). You may also recarve occlusal anatomy (see Fig. 44-16) at this time, unless further steps in occlusal adjustment are planned.

8. *Sharp edges.* If the buccal surfaces of the upper teeth or the lingual surfaces of the lower teeth have worn to sharp edges, round them. Sharp edges can be irritating to the tongue and cheek. If restorations have sharp margins protruding beyond the enamel surface, or if the enamel has been undermined and chipped exposing sharp edges, round such edges and polish them smooth.

The next step is to establish multiple-contact closure and to coordinate it with terminal hinge position.

**Harmonization in terminal hinge occlusion**

1. *Disharmony between cusp inclines.* If a disharmony exists between the hinge position and the median occlusal position, the interference most frequently is between the mesial cusp inclines of the maxillary teeth (usually the lingual cusp of the first premolar) and the distal cusp inclines of the mandibular teeth. Depending on the steepness of the cuspal inclination, grind either the mesial inclines of the maxillary teeth or the distal inclines of the mandibular teeth (never both) (Figs. 44-23 and 44-24). (This is sometimes referred to as the MU-DL rule.) Reduce the steeper incline by grinding until the less steep cusp tip has a definite cusp seat located at the occlusal plane. This should be a centric stop. If this cannot be achieved by grinding, then restorative dentistry is an alternative approach.

2. *Disharmony between cusp and fossa.* If in closure of the mandible on the hinge a disharmony exists between a cusp and the opposing fossa and there is no cuspal interference

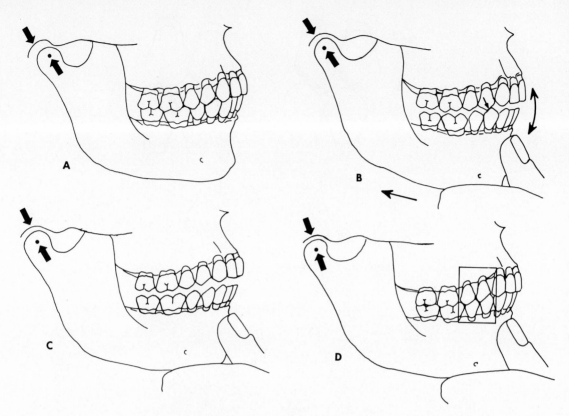

**Fig. 44-23.** **A,** In ordinary closure into maximal intercuspation, a premature contact causes displacement of the condyle from the fossa. **B,** The interference is located by movement in the hinge relation *(small arrows).* **C,** Premature contact is ground away. **D,** Now maximal intercuspation occurs with the condyle in its most retruded position, as well as in habitual closure. Generally, more than one or two such interferences must be eliminated before **D** is obtained. Large arrows show terminal hinge position, **B** to **D,** and lack thereof, **A.**

    in excursive movements, deepen the fossa. If a cusp interference exists, reshape the cusps as noted in Fig. 44-25. Do not grind away the centric holding contact.
3. *Disharmony between the anterior teeth.* When occlusal interference exists between the anterior teeth in the hinge position (Fig. 44-26), correct the incisal edges of the mandibular incisors. Maxillary teeth should be ground when the protrusive relationship is premature.

    In Angle class II, division 2 (deep overbite), no grinding of posterior teeth can be performed. Such grinding will reduce vertical dimension, and the anterior teeth will be increasingly forced into premature contact. In such cases the anterior relationship may be improved by grinding both upper and lower incisors if possible or, better, by orthodontics before other grinding steps are undertaken.

    In Angle class III habitual relationship (pseudoclass III), both upper and lower incisors may have to be ground to establish a stop in terminal hinge occlusion. The posterior teeth still may not make contact in terminal hinge position. However, you can either wait 6 to 12 months for them to erupt into position or build up the teeth with crowns or onlays to establish contact.

    These steps properly performed should bring about a harmony between median occlusal and terminal hinge positions. You are now ready to consider eccentric positions and excursive movements.

    Only after cuspal interferences in the hinge position have been eliminated should you proceed to correct eccentric disharmonies. Once terminal hinge position is estab-

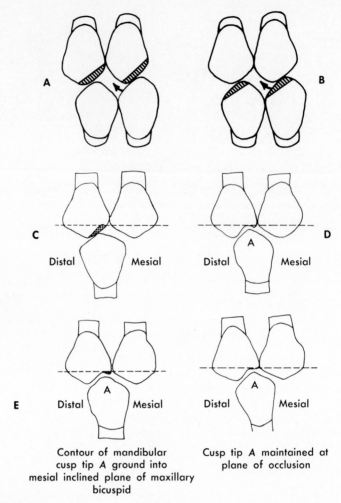

Distal  Mesial          Distal  Mesial

Distal  Mesial          Distal  Mesial

Contour of mandibular
cusp tip **A** ground into
mesial inclined plane of maxillary
bicuspid

Cusp tip **A** maintained at
plane of occlusion

**Fig. 44-24.**  Enlargement of the box in Fig. 44-23, **D,** corresponds to Fig. 44-23, **B,** before correction. Depending on cusp steepness, grind either, **A,** the mesial inclines of the maxillary teeth or, **B,** the distal inclines of the mandibular teeth, permitting the mandible to move back into terminal hinge occlusion. Area to be reshaped is shaded. **C,** Shaded area indicates additional tooth structure to be removed to eliminate the small area of restraint left on the marginal ridge area (*A* in **D**). **D,** Occlusion after removal of tooth structure on incline of the maxillary tooth. **E,** If additional tooth structure *(shaded area)* is removed, the mandibular cusp will enter the terminal hinge position and can glide protrusively into the habitual centric position without interference. The ability to glide from terminal hinge position into habitual centric is termed *long centric*. If the mandible is deflected laterally, it may be necessary to create a *wide* centric in combination with the long centric.

lished, be extremely careful not to disturb it in the grinding steps that follow.

**Harmonization in protrusive position and movement**

Usually protrusive position and excursion are ground before lateral excursions, but the order may be reversed. Grind the protrusive position first to deal with the special problems that relate to deep overbite cases. If the order is reversed and you inadvertently reduce vertical dimension in such a case, you may not be able to correct the resultant anterior relationship by grinding; reconstruction will then become a necessity.

1. *Establishment of incisor group contact in edge-to-edge relationship.* Bring as many incisors as possible into occlusion in edge-to-edge position. Grind the upper incisal edges to achieve this, except in classes II and III malocclusions. For these situations the lower incisors do not make contact, and they (the lower incisal edges) should be ground. Another instance in which lower incisal edges may be ground is when individual incisors have

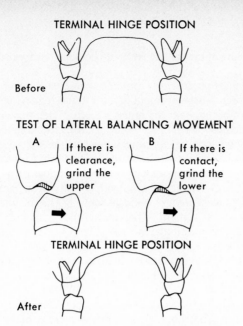

**TERMINAL HINGE POSITION**

Before

**TEST OF LATERAL BALANCING MOVEMENT**

A — If there is clearance, grind the upper

B — If there is contact, grind the lower

**TERMINAL HINGE POSITION**

After

**Fig. 44-25.** If there is premature contact between a fossa and an opposing cusp in the terminal hinge position, test the excursive movement. If no cuspal interference exists in lateral excursions on the balancing side, deepen the fossa, A. If cuspal interference exists on the balancing side, reshape the mandibular buccal cusp, B, to obtain freedom from the premature contact on closure in the terminal hinge position.

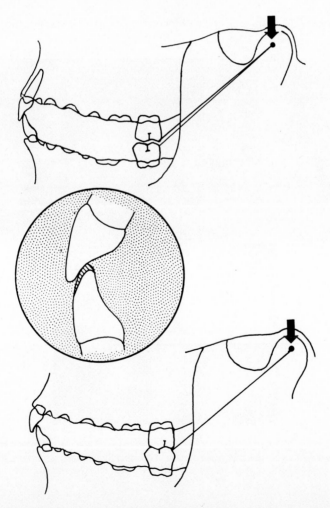

**Fig. 44-26.** Reshape the incisal edges of the mandibular incisors when there is an interference with the maxillary teeth, depending on which are steeper. Where possible, try to maintain cusp height relationship.

extruded. No grinding of incisal edges should be done in cases of anterior open bite (Fig. 44-27).

2. *Incisor disharmony in protrusive excursion (establishment of incisal guidance).* Premature contact in protrusive movement in the anterior region may be caused by steepness of the lingual slopes of the maxillary anterior teeth. When this occurs, reduce the incisal guidance of the maxillary teeth (Fig. 44-28, *A*). If the mandibular tooth were shortened, it would lose static contact in the terminal hinge position and eventually erupt into contact again. The mandibular incisor can be ground in protrusive interference if there is a long contact (frequently a facet is present) between the lingual surface of the maxillary tooth and the labial surface of the mandibular tooth (*B*). Tooth structure can then be reduced incisally to the most apical point of occlusal contact. The maxillary tooth may be ground for a smooth protrusive movement. When there is no contact, as in class II malocclusion, grind either maxillary or mandibular incisors or both (*C*). As you repeat this step, gradually more and more of the anterior teeth will be brought into function during protrusive glide. The objective is to bring as many anterior teeth as possible into contact. The ideal situation is attained when the distal slope of the canine carries some of the load in protrusive excursion (Fig. 44-29).

3. *Posterior disharmony in protrusive excursion.* Premature contacts of posterior teeth in protrusive movements usually occur on the mesial inclines of the mandibular cusps (Fig. 44-30, *A*) (usually on the lingual) and on the distal inclines of the maxillary cusps (Fig. 44-30, *B*) (usually on the buccal), depending on which is the steeper incline. Eliminate these by reducing the steepest interfering inclines. The elongated third molar is often the offender in such situations.[25] When grinding these areas would result in excessive loss of tooth structure, groove the opposing inclined plane to allow cuspal freedom in protrusive excursion.

4. *Anterior open bite.* Many cases of anterior open bite caused by tongue thrust (a swallowing

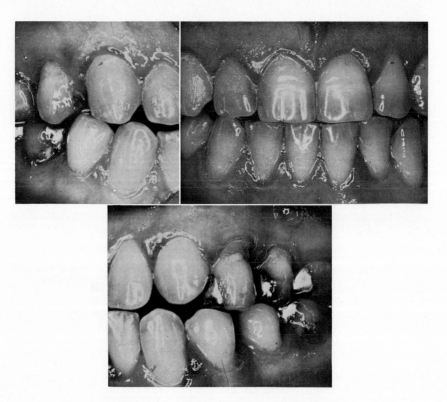

**Fig. 44-27.** No grinding of incisal edges should be done in cases of anterior open bite. Some cases are very deceptive, and the anterior teeth appear to make contact. If grinding for esthetics were done, the open bite would be increased.

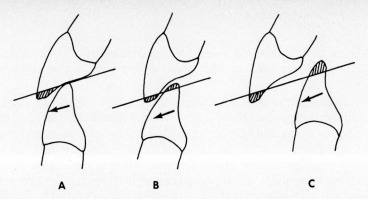

**Fig. 44-28.** Premature contacts in protrusive movement *(arrows)*. **A,** Grind the maxillary tooth *(shaded area)* unless as in **B.** If there is a long region of contact, then grind both the maxillary tooth and the mandibular tooth. If, as in **C,** the teeth do not contact in median occlusal position, grind either tooth or both teeth. The plane established by grinding should harmonize with the incisal guidance.

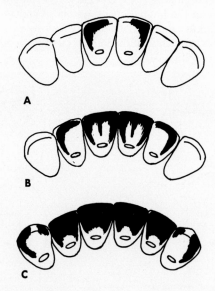

**Fig. 44-29.** The shaded area represents teeth marked during protrusive glide. In **A** only the central incisors bear the load. Grinding next brings the lateral incisor into contact too, **B.** Finally, the canines are engaged. The distal slopes of the canines should come into functional contact during protrusive excursion, **C.**

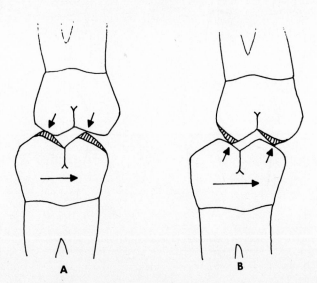

**Fig. 44-30.** If in protrusive movement premature contacts exist between opposing posterior teeth, grind either, **A,** the mesial cusp inclines of the mandibular teeth or, **B,** the distal cusp inclines of the maxillary teeth, depending on which are steeper. Where possible, try to maintain cusp height and centric relations established in a previous step. *Large arrows,* Direction of protrusive glide; *small arrows,* prematurities; *shading,* area to be ground.

habit) are seen.[48] Treatment directed solely at grinding the posterior teeth to bring the anterior teeth into contact is contraindicated in such cases as long as the basic problem remains.

Harmoniza-
tion in lateral
occlusal posi-
tion and lat-
eral excursion

Group functional grinding is advocated for lateral excursions in accordance with many of Schuyler's principles. However, in healthy dentitions you may prefer to use canine guidance or a mutually protected occlusion. In such instances, except when the canines carry the load in lateral excursions, coordinate the inclines of the other teeth as if they were ground for group function. Then if the canine wears until the posterior teeth occlude, there will be no posterior disharmonies in lateral excursions. The amount of canine guidance and posterior disocclusion should be small; otherwise the torquing force on the canine (Fig. 44-31, *A*) may be excessive.

1. *Disharmony of cuspal inclinations of opposing teeth on the working side.* It is desirable to have harmonious inclinations of the cusps of the maxillary and mandibular teeth in group function type of occlusion. If in right lateral movement of the mandible the buccal cusps are in contact but the lingual cusps are out of contact (Fig. 44-31, *B*), grind the lingual incline of the buccal cusps of the maxillary tooth so that its plane will be the same as that of the buccal incline of the lingual cusp of the mandibular tooth (*C*). In this

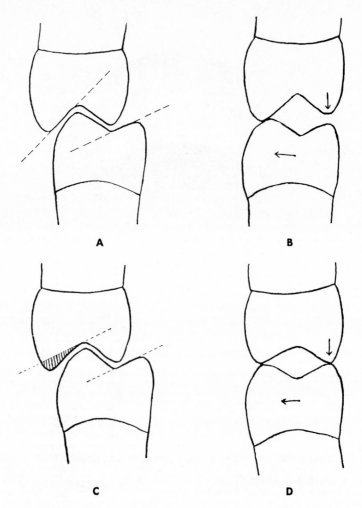

**A**

**B**

**C**

**D**

**Fig. 44-31.** If there are differences in inclination of cusps of opposing or adjacent teeth, **A,** steep inclines take cusps out of function. **B,** Reduce the steeper inclination to conform with the flatter one, **C.** This will permit good functional contact of both cusps, **D.**

manner the cusps and fossae will remain in static relation, and the buccal and lingual cusps will be in functional contact in right lateral excursive movement (*D*). If the buccal cusp of the mandibular tooth had been ground, the cutting efficiency of the tooth would have been reduced. These same rules apply when cusps of adjoining teeth have different inclinations. If you do not follow these rules, the tooth with the steeper cusps will take over the occlusal position in excursive movement, and the adjoining tooth with the flatter incline will be out of contact.

2. *Disharmony of cuspal inclinations of adjacent teeth on the working side.* If the inclination of cusps of oposing teeth is the same but there is an interference in lateral excursion, you may have to reshape the buccal upper and lingual lower cusps (BU-LL, Fig. 44-32, *A*). If the buccal lower and lingual upper cusps are ground (*B*), the tooth would be taken out of terminal hinge occlusion and thus would be able to migrate again into a disharmonious relationship. The buccal cusps of the mandibular teeth and the lingual cusps of the maxillary teeth are responsible for keeping the teeth in their proper position and for determining the vertical dimension of the dentition. If these cusps have heavy, bulging buccal or lingual surfaces, reshape them (*C*), but be careful not to grind the respective cusp tips.

3. *Disharmonies of cuspal inclinations between the functional and nonfunctional sides (balancing side prematurities).* Proper occlusal contact may be present in the terminal hinge position, but in right lateral excursive movement, for example, a premature contact may exist on the nonworking side. In this situation the teeth do not contact on the working side (Fig. 44-33), and the condyle may be malpositioned in the fossa. To evaluate this situation before grinding is done, you must bring the teeth into working excursive contact at the opposite (left) side (Fig. 44-33). The decision as to which cusp will be ground is determined by the excursive position of the mandibular buccal and the maxillary lingual cusps. If the mandibular buccal cusp is in proper functional contact with the maxillary buccal cusp and the lingual cusp is out of contact, reshape the maxillary lingual cusp. If the lingual cusp is in good functional relation and the buccal cusp is out of contact, reshape the mandibular buccal cusp. If, under similar circumstances, in left lateral excursion both lingual and buccal cusps are in good functional contact, reshape either the maxillary lingual or the mandibular buccal cusp, but never both. The cusp to be preserved is one that directs forces more closely within the long axis of the tooth. Contact on the nonfunctional side is neither necessary nor desirable in the natural dentition.[37] Prematurities on the nonfunctional side transmit torsional forces to the periodontium that may be damaging to the temporomandibular articulation.

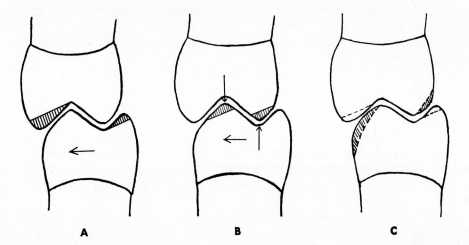

**A**          **B**          **C**

**Fig. 44-32.**  If in lateral excursions there is cuspal interference, reduce the buccal upper and lingual lower cusps (BU-LL), **A.** If the buccal lower and lingual upper cusps were reduced, the tooth would be taken out of static contact, **B.** If the buccal surface of the buccal cusps of the mandibular teeth and the lingual surface of the lingual cusps of the maxillary teeth are very heavy, reduce the bulge, **C,** but do not touch the tips of the cusps.

Right                          Left

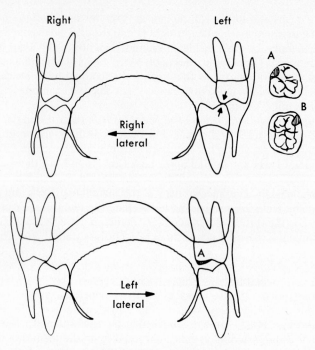

**Fig. 44-33.**  In right lateral excursion a premature contact exists on the opposite, nonfunctional side *(arrows),* preventing tooth contact on the functional side. Note the space between the teeth of the right side. Should the upper prematurity, *A,* or the lower prematurity, *B,* be ground? To determine which, move the mandible to left lateral excursion and study the cusp relationship. Grind the cusp that is out of functional contact (in this case *A)* to correct the prematurity and permit functional contact in right lateral excursion.

**Reestablishment and polishing**

When occlusal grinding is completed, reestablish occlusal tooth anatomy. Form sluiceways and embrasures and round sharp edges slightly. Polish all tooth surfaces that were ground, and make them comfortable to tongue and cheek.

## UNUSUAL SITUATIONS

**Tipped, tilted, or rotated teeth**

When a tooth is tipped lingually or buccally, great care should be exercised in deciding on a corrective procedure. Such teeth can be very easily taken out of static contact, and migration of the tooth that has been reshaped may occur. The tooth with static cuspal contact in the hinge position should not be reshaped under any circumstances (Fig. 44-34).

**Class III malocclusions and crossbite**

Cases with class III malocclusions and crossbite require grinding in lateral excursions that is the reverse of BU-LL. In other words the lingual cusp of the upper and the buccal cusp of the lower should be ground. However, the principles of grinding are unchanged.

**Micrognathia**

In cases in which the mandible is disproportionately smaller than the maxilla, occlusion may depend on the extreme outer tip of the occlusal surface of the mandibular teeth catching the inner tip of the maxillary teeth. Any grinding of these points would disocclude the teeth and cause the mandibular teeth to miss the maxillary teeth either partially or completely, collapsing the bite.

**Problems**

Problems arise whenever the buccolingual relation of the teeth is abnormal, the teeth are in crossbite, teeth are missing and have not been replaced, or prosthetic appliances are present that do not comply adequately with periodontal specifications. On occasion, particularly in the presence of extreme overjet, patients have trained themselves to habitually close in a second convenient protrusive position. Such patients have a dual bite. Occlusal correction may be necessary for either or both positions.

**Dual bite**

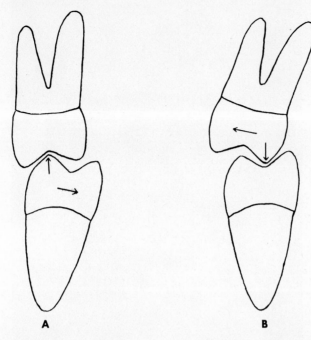

**Fig. 44-34.   A,** If a mandibular tooth is inclined lingually and its buccal cusp is in static contact with the fossa of the maxillary tooth, grind all eccentric premature contacts by reshaping the maxillary tooth. **B,** If a maxillary tooth is inclined buccally and its lingual cusp is in static contact with the fossa of the mandibular tooth, eliminate all prematurities by reshaping the mandibular tooth.

In some situations it may be desirable to establish a group function type of occlusion on one side and a disclusion type on the other.

**Dual occlusion**

## PRACTICAL PROCEDURES

Armed with an understanding of the rules for occlusal adjustment, you are now ready to proceed with a practical case. There are two approaches. In one you will work directly in the mouth. In the other you will first do the grinding on articulator-mounted study casts; this procedure is better for students.

If you use the articulator procedure, obtain good casts of the patient's dentition. Establish the centers of rotation (hinge) for both temporomandibular articulations, then mount the stone casts in hinge position, according to the Frankfort horizontal plane, with a face-bow paralleling the occlusal plane to the Frankfort plane. The articulator should reasonably duplicate opening-closing, protrusive, and lateral excursions.

**Articulator procedure**

You should now have mounted casts of the patient that can be studied and that to a certain degree can reproduce tooth-to-tooth relationships. Realize, however, that no machine, no matter how ingeniously constructed, is capable of completely reproducing the mandibular movements of an individual. Realize also that the direction, magnitude of force, and frequency of tooth contact cannot be gauged from the articulator. Many clinicians therefore prefer to correct the occlusion without any articulator mounting.

Nevertheless, those who use the articulator correct the occlusion on the casts first, according to the rules for occlusal adjustment (Figs. 44-35 and 44-36). They then note the procedure step by step on a grinding list, which serves as a guide when the grinding is done in the mouth.

The studying, marking, and cutting of the stone casts does not ensure that the

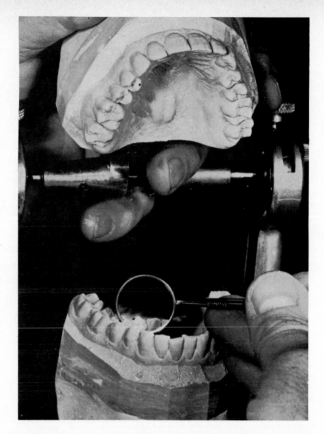

**Fig. 44-35.** Place thin, silk typewritter ribbon on the occlusal surfaces of casts in the articulator, and tap the teeth gently together. (Elevate the incisal guidance pin so that it does not touch.)

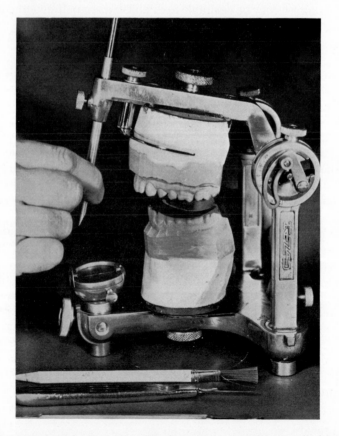

**Fig. 44-36.** Mark contacts between the right maxillary first premolar, lingual cusp, and mesiobuccal incline and the mandibular first premolar, buccal cusp, and distolingual incline.

spots will be corrected to the same degree in the mouth. In fact, on the stone casts much larger portions of the teeth can be cut away than can be done later in the mouth. The grinding list is only a blueprint of what can be expected in occlusal adjustment. This procedure familiarizes the operator with the occlusion of the patient and frequently helps to avoid problems that would otherwise arise.

The procedures to be followed will be determined by the objectives for each patient. Occlusal adjustment is not an all-or-nothing measure. One patient might require only the narrowing of the buccolingual diameters of the teeth, whereas another might require more extensive adjustment. The distribution and extent of lesions present and their relation to the occlusal problem will determine the amount and type of occlusal adjustment to be done. This, however, cannot excuse crude or haphazard attempts to occlusal adjustment. The method used and the desired objectives must be precisely planned (box, below). It is useful for students to fill out occlusal and examination

---

### OCCLUSAL ANALYSIS AND DIAGNOSIS

Student _____         Patient's name and record number _____

**A. Pertinent items abstracted from medical and dental history**

1. Chief complaint (related to occlusion) _____
2. History of orthodontic treatment or previous occlusal adjustment:

   ☐ No   ☐ Yes   Date _____

3. Mobile teeth (circle)

| 1 | 2 | 3 | 4 | 5 | 6 | 7 | 8 | 9 | 10 | 11 | 12 | 13 | 14 | 15 | 16 |
|---|---|---|---|---|---|---|---|---|----|----|----|----|----|----|----|
| 32 | 31 | 30 | 29 | 28 | 27 | 26 | 25 | 24 | 23 | 22 | 21 | 20 | 19 | 18 | 17 |

4. Furcas (circle)

| 1 | 2 | 3 | 4 | 5 | 6 | 7 | 8 | 9 | 10 | 11 | 12 | 13 | 14 | 15 | 16 |
|---|---|---|---|---|---|---|---|---|----|----|----|----|----|----|----|
| 32 | 31 | 30 | 29 | 28 | 27 | 26 | 25 | 24 | 23 | 22 | 21 | 20 | 19 | 18 | 17 |

**B. Radiographic findings**

1. Angular bone loss (circle)

| 1 | 2 | 3 | 4 | 5 | 6 | 7 | 8 | 9 | 10 | 11 | 12 | 13 | 14 | 15 | 16 |
|---|---|---|---|---|---|---|---|---|----|----|----|----|----|----|----|
| 32 | 31 | 30 | 29 | 28 | 27 | 26 | 25 | 24 | 23 | 22 | 21 | 20 | 19 | 18 | 17 |

2. Significant horizontal bone loss (circle)

| 1 | 2 | 3 | 4 | 5 | 6 | 7 | 8 | 9 | 10 | 11 | 12 | 13 | 14 | 15 | 16 |
|---|---|---|---|---|---|---|---|---|----|----|----|----|----|----|----|
| 32 | 31 | 30 | 29 | 28 | 27 | 26 | 25 | 24 | 23 | 22 | 21 | 20 | 19 | 18 | 17 |

3. Widened PDL or funneling (circle)

| 1 | 2 | 3 | 4 | 5 | 6 | 7 | 8 | 9 | 10 | 11 | 12 | 13 | 14 | 15 | 16 |
|---|---|---|---|---|---|---|---|---|----|----|----|----|----|----|----|
| 32 | 31 | 30 | 29 | 28 | 27 | 26 | 25 | 24 | 23 | 22 | 21 | 20 | 19 | 18 | 17 |

4. Changes in alveolar bone density
   a. Overall trabeculation: Increased ☐   Decreased ☐

   b. Lamina dura thickening ___|___   Crestal lamina dura indistinct ___|___
5. Evaluation of teeth

   a. Root form: Conical, clubbed, divergent (specify) _____|_____

   b. Crown-root ratio: Adequate ☐   Disproportional (specify) _____|_____

*Continued.*

**C. Static analysis from study casts**

   1. Angle's classification (circle): Normal   I   II   II, Div. 1   II, Div. 2   III

   2. Midline position (mandibular to maxillary central incisors):
      Normal □   Mandibular teeth displaced to right □   or left □   _____ mm

   3. Arch form
      a. Symmetric □   Asymmetric □   Describe _____
      b. Occlusal plane configuration (curve of Spee):
         Normal □   Exaggerated □   Flat (horizontal) □   Reverse □

   4. Missing teeth: Distribution _____|_____

   5. Positions of groups of teeth
      a. Open bite (indicate opposing teeth not in contact) _____|_____

      b. Anterior overbite (vertical overlap):
         Normal to slight □    Moderate □    Severe □    Very severe □
         (incisal one third)    (middle one    (cervical one    (mandibular incisors
                         third)         third)       occlude with maxillary
                                                palatal gingiva)

         Edge-to-edge _____

      c. Anterior overjet (horizontal overlap): _____ mm (Measure with probe.)   □ (1 to 2 mm)

      d. Teeth in cross bite _____|_____ Crowding _____|_____
   6. Position of individual teeth (note on patient's clinical charting)
      a. Rotation
      b. Inclinations
      c. Extrusion
      d. Drifting
      e. Pathologic migration
   7. Morphology of teeth
      a. General morphology
         Cusps: Steep □   Shallow □
      b. Marginal ridge relations (note uneven ridges with arrow)

         Relation to restorations _____
      c. Occlusal and/or incisal wear
         (1) General: Slight □   Moderate □   Severe □

         (2) Facets _____ (Correlate
            with parafunctional; see section E.)
   8. Observe lingual aspect of teeth with casts in occlusion
      a. Severe anterior overbite with contact of mandibular incisor with

         lingual of maxillary gingiva? _____

      b. Plunger cusps _____

**D. General appraisal**

   1. Facial form: Normal □   Asymmetry □   Hypertrophy right □   Hypertrophy left □

   2. Habits (describe) _____
   3. Tension

**E. Parafunctional tooth contacts**

   1. Habits: Bruxism □   Clenching □   Tapping □   Tongue thrust □   Mouth breathing □
      Lip, tongue, or cheek biting □

      Other (explain) _____
   2. Patient awareness of habits
      a. Bruxism:   None □   In sleep □   On awakening □   Daytime □   Under tension □
      b. Clenching: None □   In sleep □   On awakening □   Daytime □   Under tension □

   3. Wear facets (circle)

| 1 | 2 | 3 | 4 | 5 | 6 | 7 | 8 | 9 | 10 | 11 | 12 | 13 | 14 | 15 | 16 |
|---|---|---|---|---|---|---|---|---|----|----|----|----|----|----|----|
| 32 | 31 | 30 | 29 | 28 | 27 | 26 | 25 | 24 | 23 | 22 | 21 | 20 | 19 | 18 | 17 |

**F. Musculature**
   1. Function
      a. Maximal opening: _____ mm (incisal edge to incisal edge at midline)

      b. Restrictions on opening? Yes ☐   No ☐   · Describe _____
      c. Jaw manipulation: Easy ☐   Difficult ☐
         (1) Inhibited voluntary movement: To right lateral ☐   Left lateral ☐   Protrusive ☐
         (2) Deflections on opening or closing (specify—right, left, S, etc.)
   2. Spasm and/or pain (circle): None   On palpation: R L   Temporal area: R L   Masseter area:
      R L   Pterygoid: R L

   3. Freeway space _____ mm

   4. Occlusion/disocclusion ratio (in laterals) _____

**G. Summary of evidence for occlusal adjustment**
   1. Based on the interpretation of the accumulated data:
   2. Is an occlusal adjustment indicated? Yes ☐   No ☐
   3. Defend your answer _____
   _____

   If your answer is yes, proceed with face-bow transfer and mounting of study casts.

**H. Functional analysis with study casts mounted on an adjustable articulator after face-bow transfer**
   (Make following notations after using green wax or articulating paper or tape; correlate with Fig. 40-37):
   1. Centric pathway prematurity
      a. Guide articular into centric relation.
         (1) Mark and observe slide. Repeat to confirm.
         (2) Record location of centric pathway prematurity _____

         (3) Record slide: ☐ None   Anterior: _____ mm   Lateral: _____ mm   Left: _____
         mm
      b. Confirm in mouth. Have patient close in centric relation to initial contact; ask patient to point to side where contact is located. This contact is the centric pathway prematurity. Place green wax (shiny side toward tooth) over maxillary molar and premolar areas; guide patient to touch spot to record in wax.
   2. Protrusive
      a. Guide articulator into protrusive movement and record markings.
      b. Confirm in mouth.
   3. Lateral movements
      a. Move articulator into lateral movements. Check for working and balancing contacts and record them.
      b. Confirm in mouth.

Prematurities in centric (circle)

| 1 | 2 | 3 | 4 | 5 | 6 | 7 | 8 | 9 | 10 | 11 | 12 | 13 | 14 | 15 | 16 |
|---|---|---|---|---|---|---|---|---|----|----|----|----|----|----|----|
| 32 | 31 | 30 | 29 | 28 | 27 | 26 | 25 | 24 | 23 | 22 | 21 | 20 | 19 | 18 | 17 |

Prematurities in protrusive (circle)

| 1 | 2 | 3 | 4 | 5 | 6 | 7 | 8 | 9 | 10 | 11 | 12 | 13 | 14 | 15 | 16 |
|---|---|---|---|---|---|---|---|---|----|----|----|----|----|----|----|
| 32 | 31 | 30 | 29 | 28 | 27 | 26 | 25 | 24 | 23 | 22 | 21 | 20 | 19 | 18 | 17 |

Right lateral—working and balancing (circle)

| 1 | 2 | 3 | 4 | 5 | 6 | 7 | 8 | 9 | 10 | 11 | 12 | 13 | 14 | 15 | 16 |
|---|---|---|---|---|---|---|---|---|----|----|----|----|----|----|----|
| 32 | 31 | 30 | 29 | 28 | 27 | 26 | 25 | 24 | 23 | 22 | 21 | 20 | 19 | 18 | 17 |

Left lateral—working and balancing (circle)

| 1 | 2 | 3 | 4 | 5 | 6 | 7 | 8 | 9 | 10 | 11 | 12 | 13 | 14 | 15 | 16 |
|---|---|---|---|---|---|---|---|---|----|----|----|----|----|----|----|
| 32 | 31 | 30 | 29 | 28 | 27 | 26 | 25 | 24 | 23 | 22 | 21 | 20 | 19 | 18 | 17 |

**I. Occlusal adjustment**
   1. List the steps of occlusal adjustment in sequence.

   2. Make a grinding list and do an occlusal adjustment on articulator-mounted study models.

   3. Repeat grinding in mouth (consult grinding list).

**Occlusal analysis and diagnosis**

analysis forms before performing occlusal adjustment. Items A and B of the occlusal analysis and examination form are obtained from the patient's dental history chart and roentgenograms; item C is obtained from the patient's diagnostic study casts; items D to F are obtained by direct examination of the patient; item G is the clinical conclusion; and items H and I are the steps to be performed in the occlusal adjustment (grinding list) and should be indicated on the chart in Fig. 44-37.

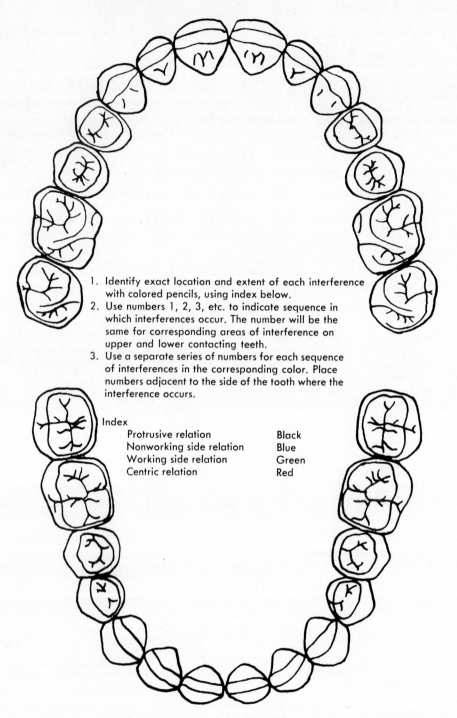

1. Identify exact location and extent of each interference with colored pencils, using index below.
2. Use numbers 1, 2, 3, etc. to indicate sequence in which interferences occur. The number will be the same for corresponding areas of interference on upper and lower contacting teeth.
3. Use a separate series of numbers for each sequence of interferences in the corresponding color. Place numbers adjacent to the side of the tooth where the interference occurs.

Index

| | |
|---|---|
| Protrusive relation | Black |
| Nonworking side relation | Blue |
| Working side relation | Green |
| Centric relation | Red |

**Fig. 44-37.** Occlusal adjustment chart for sequence of grinding steps. (Courtesy A. Solnit, University of Southern California School of Dentistry, Los Angeles, California.)

Selective grinding is contraindicated in the following situations: when pulp chambers are large, in the presence of tooth sensitivity, when major occlusal discrepancies may require orthodontics or reconstruction, and in patients who are poor candidates for mouth reconstruction because of psychologic factors. These patients become tooth conscious after such procedures and are unhappy with the results.

**Contraindications to selective grinding**

After teaching the patient to close in terminal hinge position, establish the premature contacts by marking with thin articulating paper or typewriter ribbon after the teeth have been dried with cotton rolls. Encourage the patient to relax and tap the teeth lightly together with the carbon paper, typewriter ribbon (special inking), or special wax in place. One or more points may be marked by the articulating paper. After consulting the grinding list, you will be able to establish easily whether the first point of contact found in the articulator is identical with the finding in the patient's mouth. If the mounting of the casts was correct and the patient closed on the hinge, there will be little question that the first points of premature contact are identical. The first premature contact can be eliminated by grinding the spot that was determined on the articulator. This will save considerable chair time and fatigue to the patient by eliminating indecision and establishing a definite goal.

**Occlusal adjustment in oral cavity**

After the first premature contact has thus been eliminated, dry the surfaces of the teeth once more, and place the articulating paper or wax on the occlusal surfaces. The teeth are tapped together as before. Then find the next point of contact and, after consulting the grinding list, eliminate it. Previously ground spots may again come into premature contact, which indicates that insufficient tooth structure was removed.*

In this way the entire occlusion can be corrected, and all premature contacts and irregularities eliminated. The rules for reshaping should be observed carefully, but exceptions can be made when necessary.

After the reshaping is finished, tapping should produce an unmuffled, solid, single sound. The patient often will comment on the improvement in the occlusion—not just after it is finished but even shortly after the first prematurities have been eliminated. After the worst premature contacts have been eliminated, the patient will often be able to help in finding any remaining premature contacts by tapping the teeth lightly together on the hinge and putting a finger on the offending tooth. Most patients adapt readily to the changes in occlusion.

In correcting functional occlusal disharmonies, adjust the occlusion only to the range of functional movement. In correcting for parafunctional movement, adjust the occlusion to the range of such movement as evidenced by wear facets.

**Adjusting to lateral excursions**

Occlusal adjustment is not intended to relocate the mandible but rather to enable the patient to use the different jaw positions and movements with good intercuspation and to chew efficiently with comfort and without damage to the periodontium. Occlusal adjustment is complete when these aims have been accomplished.[49]

**Completion of occlusal adjustment**

Before the completion of the discussion of occlusal adjustment, consider the method of grinding advocated by Jankelson[50,51] and employed by some dentists. It is interesting because it is at variance with the previous methods.

**Jankelson's method**

In the Jankelson method major emphasis is placed on the cusp-fossa relationship of the teeth in terminal hinge occlusion. Deflective contacts are believed to create a physiologic instability during swallowing.

In the removal of interferences, the buccal surface of the mandibular teeth and the lingual surfaces of the maxillary teeth are ground. Excursive movements are not considered to be physiologic; therefore no grinding of excursive movements is performed. Instead the relationship of the teeth is examined, and the types of prematurities

---

*Needless to say, when the grinding is done directly in the mouth, the procedure is in no way different from what it would be if the articulator-mounted procedure were used, except that there is no grinding list to consult.

are classified. Premature contacts in centric are classfied as types I, II, and III (Fig. 44-38) as defined below.

1. *Type I.* The buccal surfaces of the lower teeth are in premature contact with the buccal cusps of the upper teeth. A corresponding relationship holds for the anterior teeth.
2. *Type II.* The lingual surfaces of the upper posterior teeth are in premature contact with the lingual cusps of the lower teeth.
3. *Type III.* The lingual cusps of the upper teeth are in premature contact with the buccal cusps of the lower teeth.

These prematurities are detected by the use of 30-gauge wax strips while the mandible is moved in hinge relation by the therapist. The prematurities are evidenced by a tearing or thinning of the wax. Thin or torn wax areas are marked with a pencil; such areas are then reduced by grinding. Reduction of premature contacts produces a better cusp-fossa relationship in centric. The correction of type I and type II prematurities is in reality buccolingual narrowing (see Fig. 44-15). Sometimes, as a result of these corrections, teeth that are in a poor cusp-fossa relationship are freed of restrictions and tend to shift into a better relationship. After the type I and II prematurities are corrected, the patient is dismissed to permit time for this uprighting to occur.

At the next visit the patient is again tested for new type I and type II premature contacts that may have developed as a result of tooth shifting. Then type III prematurities are corrected. On completion of the correction, only the mandibular buccal cusp tips and the maxillary lingual cusp tips make registrations in the wax.

The occlusion is tested again in a week and periodically thereafter to determine whether further eruption and uprighting has produced additional prematurities.

It is possible to combine elements of Jankelson grinding with the Schuyler type of grinding (see Fig. 44-32, C).

## Periodontal occlusal adjustment

The adjustment discussed thus far is for the correction of occlusal disharmonies and malocclusion. In the discussion of function and tissue structure, a good masticatory organ was said to be one that functions comfortably and, in functioning, preserves the integrity of its component tissues. A pathologic condition cannot be inferred simply because teeth do not come together as we would like them to do. A disorder exists only when there is a lesion in the periodontium and possibly also when there is a

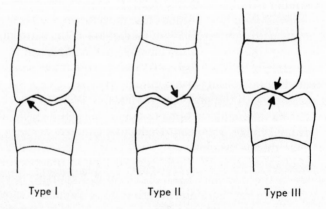

Type I          Type II          Type III

**Fig. 44-38.** Jankelson classification of prematurities. In type I the buccal surfaces of the lower teeth are in premature contact with the buccal cusps of the upper teeth. In type II the lingual surfaces of the upper teeth are in premature contact with the lingual cusps of the lower teeth. In type III the lingual cusps of the upper teeth are in premature contact with the buccal cusps of the lower teeth. Arrows indicate the areas to be corrected by grinding.

malfunctioning of the temporomandibular joints or the muscles of mastication accompanied by spasm and pain.[52]

Grinding to correct occlusal disharmonies is often quite useful in general and reconstructive dentistry. No positive case has been made, however, to prove that disharmonies, per se, produce periodontal disease. You cannot inspect an occlusion and decide on the basis of its arrangement that traumatism has occurred.

Correction of occlusal disharmonies is not done to prevent or cure inflammatory or dystrophic periodontal disease. No one has cured a periodontal pocket or even a gingivitis simply by grinding the occlusion or by reconstructing a bad bite. To give undue emphasis to the grinding of occlusion as a primary or exclusive treatment of periodontal disease would constitute complete neglect of the known facts of biology.

On the other hand, periodontal trauma may be a significantly aggravating factor when periodontal diseases are present.[53-57] When periodontal trauma exists with occlusal traumatism, occlusal adjustment is indicated in the treatment program because the improvement in function may permit a beneficial tissue response to occur. You must depend on clinical findings and on roentgenograms to correctly diagnose periodontal trauma. If trauma exists, it may not be adequately treated by a simple following of the rules for the grinding of the disharmonies. Such an approach, which focuses on the disharmony rather than on the periodontium, may be missing the point.

Thus do not be surprised to find that trauma and traumatism may occur in mouths that have previously had occlusal disharmonies removed by grinding. Even when the grinding has achieved previously described norms or malocclusions have been well corrected by the orthodontist, or even in some cases in which the mouths have been well reconstructed or splinted, traumatism may still occur. How can this be? The answer is merely that trauma does not necessarily stem from disharmonies alone but rather from the influences of parafunction. The treatment of disharmonies alone does not automatically correct parafunction and parafunctionally induced periodontal trauma.

Periodontal trauma should be treated in the absence of marginal (inflammatory) periodontal disease. Such symptoms as tooth mobility, tooth soreness, and the opening of proximal tooth contacts should be corrected.

## ADDED OBJECTIVES

In cases of overt, severe trauma, you may reshape the occluding surfaces of the teeth to reduce disharmonies, as in grinding; however, in addition, the following objectives become much greater in importance:

1. To immediately neutralize, minimize, or eliminate mobility.
2. To reduce the zone of intercuspation, thus reducing cusp inclines so that horizontal vectors of force are minimized (see Figs. 44-14 to 44-16). (In the correction of disharmonies, even when group function is gained, the resultant cusp inclination still may not be sufficiently shallow and the whole group of teeth may remain in trauma in lateral excursions. In these situations, continue to grind to reduce cusp inclination even though group function was obtained earlier.)
3. To establish cusp-fossa contact that holds a tooth in position but does not lock the mandible. (In this way tooth shifting and migration are prevented; yet, since the teeth glide past each other, they cannot be pitted against each other as in rocking. Isometric parafunctional forces cannot be built up. The forces generated during movements are mostly isotonic. The isometric component of force does not build up until the mandible stops moving. Isometric forces are much stronger than isotonic forces and consequently are more damaging. If the patient cannot gain purchase (grasp) on a tooth, both shearing forces and isometric contraction will be minimized.)
4. To encourage tooth eruption to obtain reduction or elimination of angular bone defects by repeated grinding of morsal surfaces.

## TIMING IN RELATION TO SURGERY

Occlusal adjustment for trauma must be integrated with the course of periodontal treatment. At three times in the course of periodontal treatment, occlusal interventions may be undertaken: (1) preliminary grinding, (2) definitive grinding, and (3) check grinding.

**Preliminary grinding**

Preliminary grinding is a necessity as the first step early in treatment when the patient complains of pain or discomfort or when normal function is prevented by excessive mobility. Such complaints merit immediate attention.

If an individual tooth is involved, the grinding is referred to as spot grinding. Examples are the relieving of a tooth during endodontic treatment, the adjustment of a high spot shortly after a new restoration is placed, and the shortening of a tooth with a periodontal abscess or inflammation of the periodontal ligament pericementitis.

In some instances, when an individual tooth is quite loose, the tooth may be relieved by spot grinding over many successive visits before it begins to stabilize. In other instances, as in juvenile periodontitis, successive grinding visits may result in a further eruption of the tooth, which, as it erupts, brings the bone along with it, resulting in the elimination of subcrestal defects.[58]

In general, however, preliminary grinding is a treatment of immediate need and stops short of complete occlusal adjustment.

**Definitive grinding**

Definitive grinding, or complete occlusal adjustment, is usually performed later in treatment. If the initial examination reveals tooth mobility and roentgenographic signs of trauma, the treatment plan must contain occlusal adjustment. This step will follow root scaling, since inflammation often displaces a tooth from its position. Thus the position seen at the time of examination may not be the normal position. After scaling and the resolution of inflammation, the tooth may move back to its normal position. The decision that must be made is whether to do the adjustment before or after surgery when both steps are necessary. The timing depends on how loose the teeth are. If some teeth have mobilities of 1½ degrees or more, do the adjustment first. Fabrication of night guards may also be necessary because surgery often produces an increased looseness of teeth.[59] Postsurgical mobility is generally transient; however, if it is superimposed on teeth that are already quite loose, it may become permanent. In instances when mobility is of less significance, the occlusal adjustment can be done after surgery. In this case definitive and check grinding can be done at the same time. On occasion the elimination of high spots on restorations is useful. Often bruxism is minimized after such steps.

**Check grinding**

Check grinding is generally performed as a final measure (during phase III therapy) after all other therapy has been completed and before the dismissal of the patient. Usually a month is allowed to elapse after surgery, and the mouth is checked for trauma that may have resulted from a slight shifting of the teeth. Such shifting frequently follows a total course of periodontal treatment. It can, in fact, occur because of changes in the periodontal tissues months and years after treatment.

## REEVALUATION AND REPEATED OCCLUSAL ADJUSTMENT

Shifting of the teeth may occur subsequent to treatment. For this reason the teeth are checked for trauma and, if necessary, are adjusted at each recall visit. Teeth move, particularly periodontally involved teeth. Unless the teeth are held by fixed splints, further minor adjustments are often necessary at a later time. (See discussion on the maintenance phase in Chapter 49.) In instances of extreme malocclusion, particularly if the patient's plane of occlusion is very steep (exaggerated curve of Spee or deep overbite), orthodontics may be necessary before occlusal adjustment can be undertaken.

**Benefits**

Clinical experience has shown that after successful repeated occlusal adjustments many or all of the following benefits may be expected:

1. Loose teeth may tighten.[60]
2. Life of the dentition may be extended.
3. Food impaction, impingement, and retention may be minimized.
4. Esthetics may be improved.
5. Bruxism and clenching may become less forceful and less frequent.
6. Reconstruction of the dentition may be facilitated.
7. Temporomandibular joint conditions may disappear.
8. Hypertonicity or spasm of facial, masticatory, or neck muscles may diminish.
9. Diastemata may close spontaneously.
10. Teeth may move into better alignment.

*To repeat:* Complete occlusal adjustment is neither necessary nor indicated in every patient. Under certain conditions the elimination of disharmonies may not be as necessary as recontouring some of the teeth. The occlusal table can be narrowed and sluiceways improved. Sometimes the objective may be limited to the improvements of esthetics.

Occlusal adjustment is complete when the signs of trauma have been eliminated. If the trauma cannot be eliminated by occlusal adjustment, then resort to splinting as a sequel to treatment. In cases in which occlusal adjustment is or would be obviously unsuccessful, you may splint directly. When there is doubt, a waiting period of 6 to 12 months after occlusal adjustment should suffice to disclose whether the teeth have tightened.

**Completion of occlusal adjustment for periodontal trauma**

Since parafunctional forces are the most common of the factors that produce trauma, a reconsideration of the treatment of trauma from the standpoint of the treatment of parafunction may be called for.

**Therapy for parafunction**

The Mandibular Kinesiograph uses electronic instrumentation to trace the movement of the mandible. Conventional assessment of occlusion may either employ articulated study casts gnathologically mounted or establish closed position with guided retrusion of the mandible. Pressure produces tension in the musculature, which induces muscular hyperactivity. Such hyperactivity may later relate to traumatism.

**Mandibular Kinesiograph**

The neuromuscular concept of Jankelson and colleagues[61,62] requires that the musculature be "relaxed" during the recording of occlusal position. The Myo-Monitor, an electrical stimulator, applies stimulation to the fifth and seventh nerves and the masticatory and facial musculature. The occlusal relationship obtained during the ensuing contractions is the reference point for a "neuromuscular occlusion."[61,62] The Mandibular Kinesiograph monitors the contractions to determine vertical dimension and interocclusal space. These parameters help determine whether occlusal adjustment is indicated or whether reconstruction of the occlusion would be preferable. If occlusal adjustment is indicated, the Myo-Monitor permits identification of initial contact. The Myo-Monitor bypasses proprioceptive influences on muscle contraction. The contractions are very rapid, and the forces produced are light. These small forces are not sufficient to drive the mandible beyond initial contact.

**Myo-Monitor**

**Neuromuscular occlusion**

## Muscle therapy

Gottlieb[63-64] believed that a patient should be taught to relax the masticatory muscles consciously and to keep the mandible in rest position at all times except when masticating. Another approach to the treatment of bruxism is positive suggestion.[65-66] A patient may be instructed to awaken at night if he/she starts to grind or grit the teeth during sleep. During the day he/she may remind himself to keep the teeth apart. Another method is to teach the patient the habit of forcefully contracting the depressors of the mandible.[67]

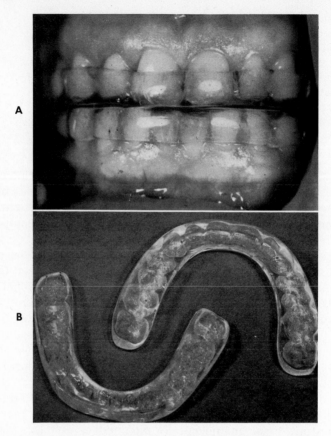

**Fig. 44-39.** Therapy for parafunction: night guard splints to prevent damage to the periodontium. **A,** In the mouth. **B,** Tooth surface view of splints.

## Night guards

Smooth-surfaced splints may also be indicated in the treatment of periodontal trauma.[68] Such horseshoe-shaped splints, which are called night guards or bite stabilizers, may be constructed for one or both jaws, freeway space permitting.[69-71] They are usually constructed for the maxilla. (Fig. 44-39). They cover all occlusal surfaces and permit the patient to move the mandible freely in all excursions. They are usually worn at night but may be worn during the day.

Many patients become so accustomed to wearing splints that they can hardly sleep without them. They may wear deep indentations in the acrylic material, thus giving evidence of the force and persistence of the bruxing movements. Wearing the splints may modify the nature of the habit or redirect the forces into a nontraumatic pattern. Other patients may have great difficulty in adjusting to the night guards and may give up wearing them.

The splints should be thin enough so that they are comfortable to wear, but the palate should not be covered. There must be no sharp edges to irritate the tongue or cheek, although the night guards should make complete contact in all excursions (bilateral balance). Care should be so exercised in the fitting that the splint does not encroach on the freeway space, although in many instances night guards that do this are successfully tolerated by the patient. The splints may be kept moist when not worn so that they do not warp.

Some patients do not tolerate the night guards well because they cannot fall asleep

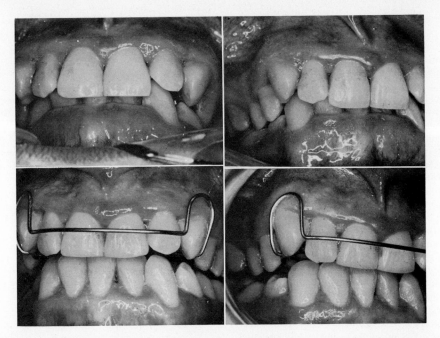

**Fig. 44-40.** When a deep overbite and an exaggerated curve of Spee exist, the patient cannot be fitted with upper and lower night guards unless the dentist opens the bite excessively. In such cases a Hawley appliance with a bite platform against which the lower incisors occlude may be used.

with the night guards or they object to the interference with their normal bruxing and clenching patterns. Considerable patience must be exercised in treating these patients. The importance of night guards must be carefully explained; if necessary, the night guards may have to be worn during the day rather than at night. In other cases only one guard at a time can be worn.

In patients with a deep overbite or an exaggerated curve of Spee, you may not be able to prescribe night guards. In these cases a bite plane (Hawley retainer) may be used (Fig. 44-40) if the health of the lower anterior teeth permits. These uses should be carefully monitored, to prevent extrusion of the mandibular incisors. An occlusal platform may be incorporated in the appliance to occlude with the mandibular incisor.

**REFERENCES**

1. Sicher, H.: Positions and movements of the mandible, J. Am. Dent. Assoc. **48:**620, 1954.
2. Thompson, J.R.: Rest position of the mandible and its significance to dental science, J. Am. Dent. Assoc. **33:**151, 1946.
3. Thompson, J.R.: Rest position of the mandible and its application to analysis and correction of malocclusion, Angle Orthod. **19:**162, 1949.
4. Thompson, J.R., and Craddock, F.W.: Functional analysis of occlusion, J. Am. Dent. Assoc. **39:**404, 1949.
5. Ramfjord, S.P., and Ash, M.M., Jr.: Occlusion, ed. 2, Philadelphia, 1971, W.B. Saunders Co.
6. Ramfjord, S.P.: Bruxism, a clinical and electromyographic study, J. Am. Dent. Assoc. **62:**21, 1961.
7. Denton, G.B.: The vocabulary of dentistry and oral science, Chicago, 1958, American Dental Association.
8. Sicher, H.: Oral anatomy, ed. 4, St. Louis, 1965, The C.V. Mosby Co.
9. Orban, B.: Biologic basis for correcting occlusal disharmonies, J. Periodontol. **25:**257, 1954.
10. Beyron, H.: Occlusal relations and mastication in Australian aborigines, Acta Odontol. Scand. **22:**597, 1964.
11. Murphy, T.R.: The timing and mechanism of the human masticatory stroke, Arch. Oral Biol. **10:**981, 1965.
12. Nadler, S.C.: The effects of bruxism, J. Periodontol. **37:**311, 1966.
13. Drum, W.: Ueber Parafunktionen, Zahnaerztl. Rundsch. **59:**257, 1950.
14. Nadler, S.C.: Detection and recognition of bruxism, J. Am. Dent. Assoc. **61:**742, 1960.

15. Belting, C.M., and Gupta, O.P.: The influence of psychiatric disturbances on the severity of periodontal disease, J. Periodontol. **32:**219, 1961.

16. Engelberger, A., Rateitschak, K.H., and Mühlemann, H.R.: Diagnostik und Therapie der funktionellen Störungen in Kausystem, Schweiz. Monatsschr. Zahnheilikd. **70:**586, 1960.

17. Drum, W.: Parafunktionen und Autodestruktionsprozesse, Berlin, 1969, Quintessenz.

18. Nadler, S.C.: Bruxism, a classification; critical review, J. Am. Dent. Assoc. **54:**615, 1957.

19. Ingle, J.I.: Occupational bruxism and its relation to periodontal disease, J. Periodontol. **23:**7, 1952.

20. Natkin, E., and Ingle, J.I.: Further report on alveolar osteoporosis and pulpal death associated with compulsive bruxism, Periodontics **1:**260, 1963.

21. Zingeser, M.R.: Cercopithecoid canine tooth honing mechanisms, Am. J. Phys. Anthropol. **31:**205, 1969.

22. Koivumaa, K.K., Landt, H., and Nyquist, G.: Investigations on the incidence of periodontal disease and disorders of the temporomandibular point in cases of bruxism, Tandläk. Sällsk. Förhandl. **56:**328, 1960.

23. Posselt, U.: Occlusion related to periodontics. In Ramfjord, S.P., Kerr, D.A., and Ash, M.M., editors: World workshop in periodontics, Ann Arbor, Michigan, 1966, University of Michigan Press.

24. Angle, E.H.: Malocclusion of the teeth, ed. 7, Philadelphia, 1907, S.S. White Co.

25. Thielemann, K.: Die Biomechanik der Paradentose, ed. 2, Munich, 1956, Johann Ambrosius Barth.

26. Posselt, U.: Physiology of occlusion and rehabilitation, ed. 2, Philadelphia, 1968, F.A. Davis Co.

27. Reeves, R.L.: Is prophylactic occlusal adjustment a justifiable procedure? J. Periodontol. **28:**272, 1957.

28. McCollum, B.B.: Fundamentals involved in prescribing restorative dental remedies, Dent. Items Interest **61:**522, 641, 724, 852, 942, 1939.

29. Schuyler, C.H.: Fundamental principles in the correction of occlusal disharmony, natural and artificial, J. Am. Dent. Assoc. **22:**1193, 1935.

30. Schuyler, C.H.: Correction of occlusal disharmony of the natural dentition, N.Y. Dent. J. **13:**445, 1947.

31. Miller, S.C.: Textbook of periodontia, ed. 2, Philadelphia, 1943, Blakiston Division, McGraw-Hill Book Co.

32. Schuyler, C.H.: Factors of occlusion applicable to restorative dentistry, J. Prosthet. Dent. **3:**772, 1953.

33. Beyron, H.: Physio-pathologic correlations between function of the masticatory system and periodontics, Parodontologie **20:**61, 1966.

34. Schuyler, C.H.: Factors contributing to traumatic occlusion, J. Prosthet. Dent. **11:**708, 1961.

35. Weinberg, L.A.: Rationale and technique for occlusal equilibration, J. Prosthet. Dent. **14:**74, 1964.

36. Zachrisson, B.U., and Mjör, I.A.: Remodeling of teeth by grinding, Am. J. Orthod. **68:**545, 1975.

37. Youdelis, R.A., and Mann, W.V.: The prevalence and possible role of nonworking contacts in periodontal disease, Periodontics **3:**219, 1965.

38. D'Amico, A.: The canine teeth-normal functional relation of the natural teeth of man, J.S. Calif. Dent. Assoc. **26:**6, 49, 127, 175, 194, 239, 1958.

39. D'Amico, A.: Functional occlusion of the natural teeth of man, J. Prosthet. Dent. **11:**899, 1961.

40. Stuart, C.E., and Stallard, H.: Principles involved in restoring occlusion to natural teeth, J. Prosthet. Dent. **10:**304, 1960.

41. Stallard, H., and Stuart, C.E.: Eliminating tooth guidance in natural dentitions, J. Prosthet. Dent. **11:**474, 1961.

42. Stallard, H., and Stuart, C.E.: Concepts of occlusion. What kind of occlusion should recusped teeth be given? Dent. Clin. North Am., p. 591, Nov. 1963.

43. Beyeler, K.: Beschleifen der Zähne bei Paradentose, Bern, 1944, Paul Haupt.

44. Kiefer, E.: Paradentosebehandlung mit besonderer Berücksichtigung der Entlastung, Munich, 1951, Carl Hanser Verlag.

45. Schuyler, C.H.: Intra-oral methods of establishing maxillomandibular relations, J. Am. Dent. Assoc. **19:**1012, 1932.

46. Ramfjord, S.P.: Die Voraussetzungen für eine ideale Okklusion, Dtsch. Zahnaerztl. Z. **26:**106, 1971.

47. Ross, F.I.: Occlusion: a concept for the clinician, St. Louis, 1970, The C.V. Mosby Co.

48. Ray, H., and Santos, H.A.: Consideration of tongue thrusting as a factor in periodontal disease, J. Periodontol. **25:**250, 1954.

49. Glickman, I., et al.: When and to what extent do you adjust the occlusion during periodontal therapy? J. Periodontol. **41:**536, 1970.

50. Jankelson, B.: Physiology of human dental occlusion, J. Am. Dent. Assoc. **50:**664, 1955.

51. Jankelson, B.: Considerations in occlusion in fixed partial dentures, Dent. Clin. North Am., March 1959.

52. Fröhlich, F.: Die okklusionbedingten Schmerzen im Kiefer-/Gesichts-Bereich, Schweiz. Monatsschr. Zahnheilkd. **76:**764, 1966.

53. Macapanpan, L.C., and Weinmann, P.: The influence of injury to the periodontal membrane on the spread of gingival inflammation, J. Dent. Res. **32:**665, 1953.

54. Glickman, I.: Effect of excessive occlusal bones upon the pathway of gingival inflam-

mation in humans, J. Periodontol. **36**:141, 1965.

55. Orban, B.: Traumatic occlusion and gum inflammation, J. Periodontol. **10**:39, 1939.
56. Glickman, I.: Inflammation and trauma from occlusion, co-destructive factors in periodontal disease, J. Periodontol. **34**:5, 1963.
57. Stahl, S.S.: The responses of the periodontium to combined gingival inflammation and occluso-functional stresses in four human surgical specimens, Periodontics **6**:14, 1968.
58. Everett, F.G.: A preliminary report on the treatment of the osseous defect in periodontosis, J. Periodontol. **35**:429, 1964.
59. Glickman, I., et al.: The effect of occlusal forces on healing following mucogingival surgery, J. Periodontol. **37**:319, 1966.
60. Mühlemann, H.R., Herzog, H., and Rateitschak, K.H.: Quantitative evaluation of the therapeutic effect of selective grinding, J. Periodontol. **28**:11, 1957.
61. Jankelson, B., et al.: Kinesiometric instrumentation: a new technology, J. Am. Dent. Assoc. **90**:834, 1975.
62. Jankelson, B., et al.: Neural conduction of the Myo-Monitor stimulus: a quantitative analysis, J. Prosthet. Dent. **34**:245, 1975.
63. Gottlieb, B.: Histologic considerations of the supporting tissues of the teeth, J. Am. Dent. Assoc. **30**:1872, 1943.
64. Gottlieb, B.: Traumatic occlusion and the rest position of the mandible, J. Periodontol. **18**:7, 1947.
65. Boyens, P.J.: Value of autosuggestion in the therapy of "bruxism" and other biting habits, J. Am. Dent. Assoc. **27**:1773, 1940.
66. Leof, M.: Clamping and grinding habits: their relation to periodontal disease, J. Am. Dent. Assoc. **31**:184, 1944.
67. Ackerman, J.B.: A new approach to the treatment of bruxism and bruxomania, N.Y. Dent. J. **32**:259, 1966.
68. Karolyi, M.: Beobachtungen über Alveolarpyorrhoe, Oest. Ung. Vjschr. Zahnheilkd. **17**:259, 1901.
69. Gottlieb, B.: Schmutzpyorrhoe, Paradentalpyorrhoe und Alveolaratrophie, Berlin, 1925, Urban & Schwarzenberg.
70. Allen, D.L.: Accurate occlusal bite guards, Periodontics **5**:93, 1967.
71. Berliner, A.: Ligatures, splints, bite planes and pyramids, Philadelphia, 1964, J.B. Lippincott Co.

**ADDITIONAL SUGGESTED READING**

Anderson, D.J., and Picton, D.C.A.: Tooth contact during chewing, J. Dent. Res. **36**:21, 1957.
Buckley, L.A.: The relationships between malocclusion, gingival inflammation, plaque and calculus, J. Periodontol. **52**:35, 1981.
Butler, J.H., and Zander, H.A.: Evaluation of two occlusal concepts, Parodontol. Acad. Rev. **2**:5, 1968.
Chasens, A.: Occlusion: current concepts and its role in periodontal therapy, Alpha Omegan **76**:68, 1983.
Clark, G.T., and Love, R.: The effect of gingival inflammation on nocturnal masseter muscle activity, J. Am. Dent. Assoc. **102**:319, 1981.
Courant, P.: Use of removable acrylic splints in general practice, J. Can. Dent. Assoc. **33**:494, 1967.
Ericsson, I., and Lindhe, J.: Lack of significance of increased tooth mobility in experimental periodontitis, J. Periodontol. **55**:447, 1984.
Eschler, J.: Bruxism and function of the masticatory muscles, Parodontologie **15**:109, 1961.
Frisch, J., Katz, L., and Ferreira, A.J.: A study on the relationship between bruxism and aggression, J. Periodontol. **31**:409, 1960.
Fröhlich, E.: Die Parafunktionen, Symptomatologie, Aetiologie und Therapie, Dtsch. Zahnaerztl. Z. **21**:536, 1966.
Geiger, A.: Occlusion in periodontal disease, J. Periodontol. **36**:387, 1965.
Gibbs, C.H., et al.: Comparison of typical chewing patterns in normal children and adults, J. Am. Dent. Assoc. **105**:33, 1982.
Glickman, I.: Clinical significance of trauma from occlusion, J. Am. Dent. Assoc. **70**:607, 1965.
Glickman, I., and Smulow, J.B.: Further observations on the effects of trauma from occlusion, J. Periodontol. **38**:280, 1967.
Graber, G.: Psychisch motivierte Parafunktionen auf Grund von Aggressionen und Myoarthropathien des Kauorgans, Schweiz. Monatsschr. Zahnheilkd. **81**:713, 1971.
Guggenheim, P., and Cohen, L.: The nature of masseteric hypertrophy, Arch. Otolaryngol. **73**:15, 1961.
Hofman, M., and Diemer, R.: Die physiologische Zahnbewegung, Dtsch. Zahnaerztl. Z. **12**:707, 1966.
Jernberg, G.R., Bakdash, M.B., and Keenan, K.M.: Relationship between proximal tooth open contacts and periodontal disease, J. Periodontol. **54**:529, 1983.
Kepic, T.J., and O'Leary, T.J.: Role of marginal ridge relationships as an etiologic factor in periodontal disease, J. Periodont. Res. **49**:570, 1978.
Koral, S.M., Howell, T.H., and Jeffcoat, M.K.: Alveolar bone loss due to open interproximal contacts in periodontal disease, J. Periodontol. **52**:447, 1981.
Lemmer, J., Lewin, A., and van Rensburg, L.B.: The measurement of jaw movement. I. J. Prosthet. Dent. **36**:211, 1976.
Lewin, A., Lemmer, J., and van Rensburg, L.B.: The measurement of jaw movement. II. J. Prosthet. Dent. **36**:312, 1976.
Mejias, J.E., and Mehta, N.R.: Subjective and objective evaluation of bruxing patients undergoing short-term splint therapy, J. Oral Rehab. **9**:279, 1982.
Moozeh, M.B., Suit, S.R., and Bissada, N.F.: Tooth mobility measurements following two methods

of eliminating nonworking side occlusal interferences, J. Clin. Periodontol. **8:**424, 1981.

Mühlemann, H.R.: Ten years of tooth mobility measurements, J. Periodontol. **31:**110, 1960.

Murphy, T.R.: The progressive reduction of tooth cusps as it occurs in natural attrition, Dent. Pract. **19:**8, 1968.

O'Leary, T.J., Rudd, K.D., and Nabers, C.L.: Factors affecting horizontal tooth mobility, Periodontics **4:**308, 1966.

O'Leary, T.J., et al.: The effect of mastication and deglutition on tooth mobility, Periodontics **5:**26, 1967.

Perry, H.T., et al.: Occlusion in a stress situation, J. Am. Dent. Assoc. **60:**626, 1960.

Picton, D.C.A.: A study of normal tooth mobility and the changes with periodontal disease, Dent. Pract. **12:**167, 1962.

Posselt, U.: Studies in the mobility of the human mandible, Acta Odontol. Scand. **10**(suppl.):19, 1952.

Posselt, U., and Emslie, R.D.: Occlusal disharmonies and their effect on periodontal diseases, Int. Dent. J. **9:**367, 1959.

Posselt, U., and Wolff, I.B.: Treatment of bruxism by bite guards and bite plates, J. Can. Dent. Assoc. **29:**773, 1963.

Rateitschak, K.H., Fistarol, A.F., and Wolf, H.F.: Parafunctionen, Schweiz. Monatsschr. Zahnheilkd. **76:**289, 1966.

Reding, G.R., Rubright, W.C., and Rechtschaffen, A.: Sleep pattern of tooth grinding: its relationship to dreaming, Science **145:**725, 1964.

Ross, I.F.: Coronal reshaping, Alpha Omegan **73:**35, 1980.

Rugh, J.D., and Johnson, R.W.: Temporal analysis of nocturnal bruxism during EMG feedback, J. Periodontol. **52:**263, 1981.

Schireson, S.: Grinding teeth for masticatory efficiency and gingival health, J. Prosthet. Dent. **13:**337, 1963.

Shapiro, S., and Shanon, J.: Bruxism as an emotional reactive disturbance, Psychosomatics **6:**427, 1965.

Sheppard, I.M., and Markus, N.: Total time of tooth contacts during mastication, J. Prosthet. Dent. **12:**460, 1962.

# CHAPTER 45

# Orthodontic measures in periodontal therapy

## Indications

Orthodontic measures taken to correct tooth malpositions are often necessary in periodontal treatment. When the disease increases in severity, there is a tendency for teeth to loosen and migrate. These migrations may range from slight to extensive. Teeth also migrate, tilt, and extrude after extraction and nonreplacement. Bony defects and pockets may result. Periodontics has traditionally included measures for the treatment of tooth migrations.[1] Periodontal and orthodontic techniques and concepts can be employed[2] in such areas as (1) the elimination of bony defects and pockets incident to tilting of teeth, (2) the correction of malpositions that might predispose to periodontal disease,[3] (3) the preparation of the mouth for reconstruction if correction of rotated and tilted teeth and collapsed or mutilated arches is necessary, and (4) the improvement of esthetics as well as the repositioning of periodontally diseased teeth.

Orthodontic treatment for individuals with periodontal disease may be indicated in the following situations[4-7]:

1. If a basic malocclusion exists and further promotes periodontal disease or affects its course
   A. Mouths with crowded teeth
   B. Deep overbites
   C. Close proximity of roots
2. If tooth migrations occur such as flaring caused by disease, parafunction, or because of tooth extraction, which can increase the severity of disease
   A. Tooth migrations caused by habits such as tongue thrusting

B. Tooth migrations seen in inflammation or encountered in juvenile periodontitis
C. Tooth migrations resulting from trauma, loss of teeth, or other mutilation of the dentition (tilted teeth, flared teeth, extruded teeth)
D. Tooth migrations in gingival hyperplasias
3. If better alignment of teeth for such purposes as axial force distribution, parallelism of abutments, tooth contact, spacing, and pontic design is necessary before reconstruction
4. If esthetic improvement would result

## BASIC MALOCCLUSIONS

Class I malocclusions involve malpositions of teeth when the molars and cuspids are in ideal relationship. Class II malocclusions involve the distal positioning of the mandibular first molars (and cuspids) relative to the maxillary first molar (and cuspid), but tooth position can be normal in the mandible, and the maxillary teeth can be in mesial position. In class II, division 1, there is an overjet and protrusion. In class II, division 2, there is a deep bite—the overjet is not present. In class III malocclusions, the mandibular first molars (and cuspids) are mesial to their normal positions, and the mandible is prognathic (see Figs. 44-10 to 44-13).

**Crowded teeth**

Crowded, malposed teeth may result in poor gingival form.[8] Hygiene is difficult for even the conscientious patient. When periodontitis is present, osseous defects may be difficult to treat because of proximity of roots. Such problems can occur throughout the mouth but are conspicuous in the mandibular anterior teeth. When fixed splinting is necessary, tooth preparation is difficult and, in the mandibular anterior teeth, may be virtually impossible. Replacement with an adequate bulk of restorative material may cause impingement on gingiva, closed contacts, plaque harbors, and unesthetic appearance.

**Crowded mandibular anterior teeth**

**Deep overbite**

Deep overbites are often accompanied by (1) trauma to maxillary palatal gingiva; (2) trauma to mandibular labial gingiva; (3) locked bite anteriorly, directing excessive force on the maxillary incisors, often with migration and/or mobility as a result; and (4) excessive wear on the labial surfaces of the mandibular incisors and the lingual surfaces of the maxillary incisors.

## MIGRATION
### Causes

When migration is caused by periodontal disease, it is accelerated with the loss of alveolar bone. Teeth drift away from the pocket side and move toward areas of greatest attachment. Chronic inflammatory connective tissue is found in the area from which the tooth has migrated. The presence of inflammation, edema, exudate, and capillary proliferation tends to increase tooth mobility and migration.

Physical forces can act on the tooth in a manner similar to that of an orthodontic appliance. These forces may be physiologic or nonphysiologic. Forces may be exerted by such factors as the actions of the tongue, lips, and cheeks[9,10]; various habits; newly placed fillings; and rocking partial dentures. Tooth position depends on the balance of forces acting on the tooth coupled with the resistance of the tooth and the periodontium to these forces. Drifting occurs only when the forces are unbalanced (e.g., mesial migration or continuous eruption).

Physiologic tooth movements occur in most dentitions into old age. Although they may influence the migration of periodontally involved teeth, they are responsible for the drifting of uninvolved teeth as well. Nonphysiologic tooth movements are those caused by thumb sucking, drifting into the space of an extracted molar (Fig. 45-1), and tongue thrusting.

Finally, changes in the patient's metabolism may influence the periodontium.[11,12] Pregnancy, scurvy, and altered carbohydrate metabolism have been associated with increased tooth mobility; their effects have not been adequately studied.[13] In disorders

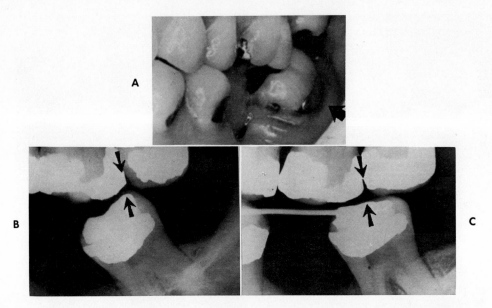

**Fig. 45-1.** Early loss of the mandibular first molar resulted in the mesial tipping of the second molar. Tooth movement to upright and parallel the abutment teeth was needed. **A,** Preoperative clinical view. **B,** Original bitewing film demonstrating the mesial tipping of the mandibular left second molar in relation to the maxillary molars. **C,** After tooth movement. The second molar is in a more favorable position. (Courtesy M.H. Marks and G, Wisor, Levittown, Pennsylvania.)

such as acromegaly, phenytoin-induced hyperplasia, and Paget disease, the growth of tissues can move teeth. Such aberrations may contribute to migrations caused by periodontal disease.

### Migration as a cause of disease

Tooth migration can contribute to further periodontal breakdown by producing alterations in occlusion. Posterior bite collapse may occur with loss and nonreplacement of posterior teeth. Anterior teeth may flare and loosen as a result. Tongue thrust habits may be encouraged. Contacts between teeth may open and permit food impaction. Buccal and lingual alveolar walls may become perforated or completely resorbed. Craters or infrabony defects may occur where thick bony ledges exist. Buckling may result in gingivae with bulbous or unphysiologic form, which encourages plaque retention and food impaction. Tipping of molar teeth after extraction of first or second molars can result in angular bony defects on the mesial surface of the remaining molar. Loss of vertical dimension may follow ( Figs. 45-2 and 45-3). Moreover, the migrating tooth may alter patterns of mastication and parafunction, thus bringing about periodontal traumatism. The reverse is also true since traumatism may be responsible for migration.

Not all malpositions are caused by migration. Some occur as the result of the development and eruption of the teeth. Others occur as a result of skeletal growth abnormalities. Repositioning such malposed teeth is indicated if a relationship to periodontal disease can be demonstrated. Repositioning may also be warranted in the absence of periodontal disease if esthetic needs or reconstructive requirements dictate or if conditions potentially hazardous to the periodontal health of the patient become apparent.

### TREATMENT OF BONY DEFECTS

Bony defects, as in the following examples, sometimes are treated better by combined periodontal-orthodontic measures than by periodontal treatment alone:

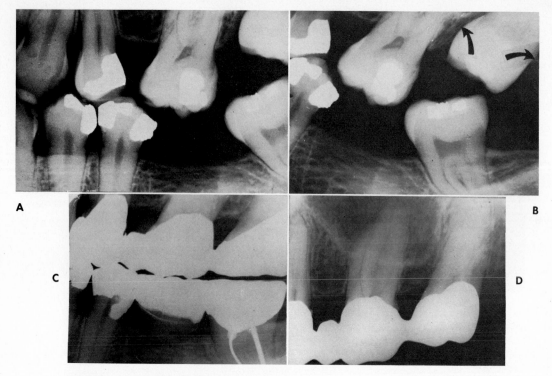

**Fig. 45-2. A** and **B,** Preoperative bite-wing films of an occlusion mutilated by extractions. The molars have drifted mesially. There are deep pockets about the maxillary molar *(arrows)*. Posterior bite collapse and flaring of the anterior teeth has occurred. **C** and **D,** After orthodontics, the teeth have been uprighted, parallelism for bridgework has been achieved, and the occlusal plane is more normal. The maxillary alveolar bone has become level, and the pocket has thus been eliminated.

1. Mesial infrabony defects and pockets on tilted teeth
2. One- and two-walled infrabony defects on a single tooth
3. Furcation defects (Fig. 45-4)
4. Bony defects existing because of stage of eruption, axial inclination of teeth, or tooth rotations

The uprighting of a tilted tooth may eliminate most of the bony defect by remodeling of the bone. Ostectomy and osteoplasty can then be used to eliminate the residual defect. Without orthodontic treatment, osteoplasty and ostectomy are ineffective in eliminating pockets mesial to severely tilted teeth.

Changing the axial inclination of roots can alter crestal bone form. As the bone is remodeled, bony defects are reduced or eliminated.

The incisal or occlusal surface of a tooth may be ground to permit eruption.[14-15] As the tooth erupts, bone is deposited at the crest, and angular defects are reduced[4,5,7] (Fig. 45-5). Orthodontically forced eruption[7] can also be used to reduce or eliminate angular bone defects (Fig. 45-6).

Furcation involvements have been successfully eliminated and regrowth of supporting tissues is induced by use of eruption preceded by open subgingival curettage. Regeneration of supporting tissues is made possible by proliferation of periodontal ligament cells into the previously open furcation. Apposition of bone during eruption may be an osteogenic inductive force.

## PREPARATION FOR RECONSTRUCTION

Dentitions that have been mutilated by missing and migrated teeth frequently

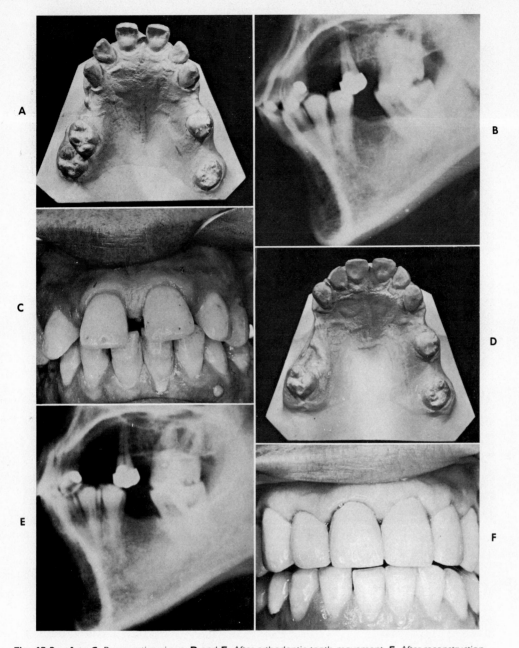

**Fig. 45-3.** **A** to **C,** Preoperative views. **D** and **E,** After orthodontic tooth movement. **F,** After reconstruction.

require extensive reconstruction.[3] The more complex the reconstruction needed, the greater the likelihood that some preliminary orthodontic treatment will be needed (see Figs. 45-1 to 45-3). The reason for this is that fixed splinting requires parallel abutments, pontic spaces of sufficient width, open embrasures, and an esthetic and harmonious occlusion. To bring about these conditions, the dentist must upright tilted and protruded teeth. When teeth are properly positioned, torque is minimized, and forces are transmitted in the long axis of the tooth. In addition, parallel preparations are obtained with more ease, and there is less chance of pulp exposure. The repositioning of grossly malposed teeth may permit the retention of these teeth in the restorative plan, whereas

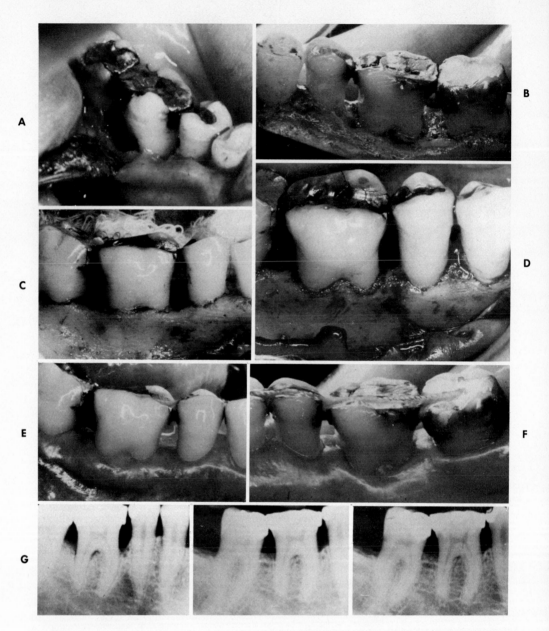

**Fig. 45-4.** **A,** A full-thickness flap was reflected for open subgingival curettage. A class II furcation involvement can be seen on the lingual surface of the mandibular first molar. The bony defect communicates with angular bony defects on both proximal surfaces of this tooth. The flap was sutured to place. The occlusal surface of the first molar was extensively ground to take the tooth more than 1 mm out of occlusion. **B,** Surgical reentry 18 months later, with eruption of the first molar, reveals that new bone apposition has repaired the bony defects (mirror view). The furcation is filled with bone. **C,** The buccal surface shows minor residual deformities remaining. The two- and three-walled bony defects originally present on the mesial and distal proximal surfaces have been almost eliminated by new bone apposition. **D,** Osteoplasty-ostectomy is performed to create a physiologic crestal bone form. Postsurgical views of the **E,** buccal, and **F,** lingual, surfaces show physiologic gingival contour. **G,** Left roentgenogram shows bony defects (4/16/73). By 2/13/74 *(middle),* some bony repair is evident. At 10/10/74 *(right),* new bone apposition has repaired most of the defects seen at start of treatment. (Courtesy H. Corn and M.H. Marks, Levittown, Pennsylvania.)

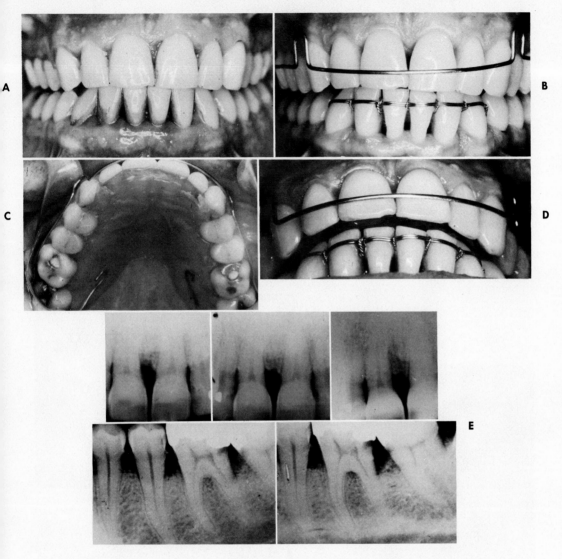

**Fig. 45-5.** Posterior eruption of the dentition in the treatment of angular bone defects and furcation involvement. **A,** Inflammation and tissue deformities are present. A 7-mm pocket can be probed on the mesial surface of the maxillary left central incisor. There is very little overjet. The mandibular teeth show mobility ranging from 1½ to 2½ degrees. Fremitus occurs in lateral and protrusive excursive movements. **B,** A maxillary Hawley bite plane was constructed that creates a 1-mm clearance between the posterior teeth. The plane is inclined to eliminate trauma from occlusion on the anterior teeth and to create a greater overjet. The mobile mandibular teeth have been ligated with stainless steel wire. Note that prior root planing and subgingival curettage coupled with good oral hygiene has eliminated the inflammation and gingival deformities. The gingival margins have receded. **C,** Occlusal view of the Hawley appliance. The palatal acrylic does not extend on the lingual aspects of the posterior teeth. The acrylic does not contact the lingual tooth surfaces, allowing them freedom for eruption. **D,** After 9 months of active Hawley appliance use, a 2.5-mm overjet was created. **E,** Radiographs show, *left,* bony defect associated with a pocket on the mesial surface of the maxillary left central incisor; *middle,* after 9 months, significant repair with new bone apposition, *right,* bony defect almost entirely eliminated 18 months later. No pocket remains.          *Continued.*

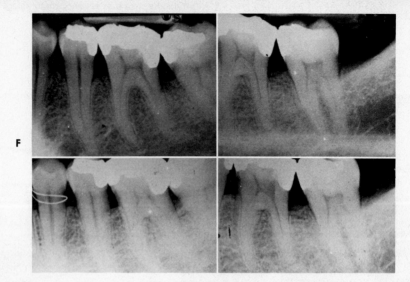

**Fig. 45-5, cont'd.   F,** Periapical radiographs. *Top,* Crestal radiolucency, lingual furcation involvement, and a 7-mm pocket on the distal surface of the mandibular molar with an associated infrabony defect; *middle,* significant repair in the furcation and the distal surface of the first molar has occurred after 9 months of posterior eruption; *bottom,* less than 1-mm infrabony defect remains after 18 months. The furcation is closed, and the density at the alveolar crest is apparent. (Courtesy H. Corn and M.H. Marks, Levittown, Pennsylvania.)

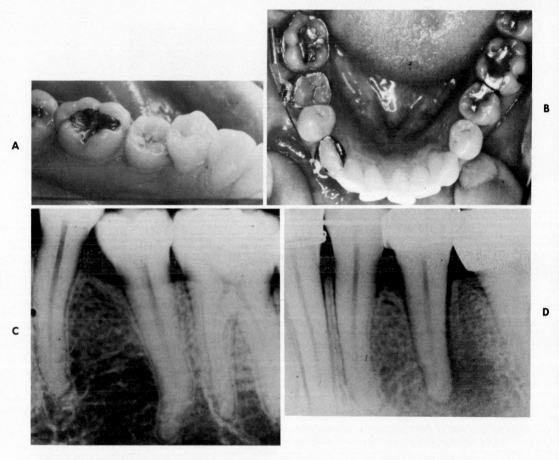

**Fig. 45-6.**   Forced eruption of a tooth, changing axial inclination of roots. **A,** A mandibular premolar is locked in infraocclusion. A pocket is present on the mesial surface of this second premolar. **B,** A fixed orthodontic appliance is placed to create space for the locked tooth and to *force* its eruption. A maxillary Hawley bite plate was constructed to free the posterior occlusion and permit eruption of the second premolar. **C,** Pretreatment x-ray film shows the tooth in infraocclusion with an angular bone outline resulting from infraocclusion of the second premolar. **D,** Posttreatment x-ray study shows the elimination of the bony defect by forced eruption of the second premolar. The widened periodontal ligament space around this tooth is a common occurrence in active orthodontic treatment. (Courtesy H. Corn and M.H. Marks, Levittown, Pennsylvania.)

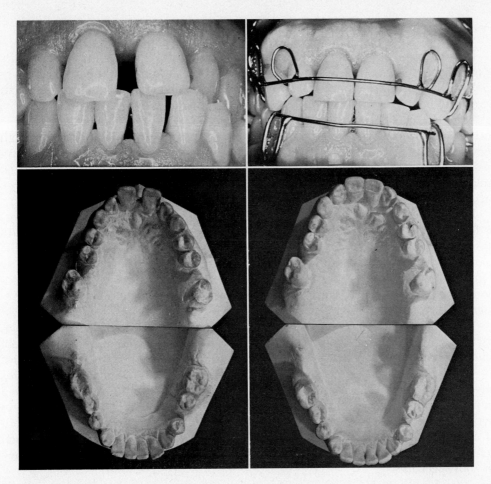

**Fig. 45-7.**  Periodontal orthodontics involving retraction of the incisors with a labial arch wire. Note that the left lateral incisors and cuspids are in crossbite. The upper incisors have been moved mesially with finger springs. Retention is necessary to prevent relapse. The arch wires have been used to correct the crossbite.

the teeth might otherwise have to be extracted.[15,16] In addition, the uprighting of tilted teeth may eliminate pockets brought about by the relationship of the tilted tooth to the adjacent alveolar ridge (see Figs. 45-2 and 45-3). Forced eruption may produce a more coronal level of alveolar bone, thereby reducing or eliminating infrabony defects.

## ESTHETIC IMPROVEMENT

Migration, which is often the first sign of periodontal disease evident to the patient, tends to be unsightly. Embarrassment and a sense of impending tooth loss may compel the patient to seek treatment. We are all familiar with the patient who screens the teeth with a hand or who draws the upper lip over protruding teeth. The correction of such conditions ( Figs. 45-3 and 45-7) is of considerable emotional value. A positive mental attitude may lead to a better maintenance of oral health by more diligent oral hygiene.

## Periodontal orthodontics

**Adult orthodontics**

In the past the public and the profession at large did not fully recognize the benefits of orthodontic treatment in adults, but we are now beginning to be much more aware of them. The majority of malposed periodontally diseased teeth in adult patients can be treated by a combination of orthodontic and periodontal measures.

Reitan[17] showed that the adult periodontium is capable of responding to orthodontic forces after an initial lag of 8 days. Therefore age is not a contraindication for tooth movement. Moreover, a tooth with some bone loss is as suitable a candidate for movement as is a tooth without bone loss. On the other hand, most authorities agree that inflammation is a hindrance to orthodontic progress and should be resolved before orthodontic therapy.[5]

**Minor tooth movement**

Periodontal orthodontics may use simplified techniques (minor tooth movement) or full orthodontic therapy. When full orthodontic therapy is employed, it adheres to the teachings of modern-day orthodontics. When the distances through which the teeth are to be moved are small and the objective of treatment is limited to securing a functional and esthetic occlusion, but not necessarily an ideal one, minimal orthodontic measures are employed. Such interventions have been termed minor tooth movement.[18]

When full orthodontic treatment is indicated, either the orthodontist or the periodontist may accept responsibility for treatment. Although most orthodontists will accept adult patients for full treatment and are fully aware of periodontal and reconstructive interrelationships, some are unwilling to treat patients whose periodontal structures have been damaged by disease. Some orthodontists are reluctant to become involved in minor tooth movement if the goals of total treatment are less than ideal. Therefore periodontists have assumed increasing responsibility for adult orthodontic treatment of a minor nature, and this has been reflected in a changing curriculum in dental schools. In addition, a small but increasing number of dentists have now been trained in both specialties.

## Diagnosis and treatment planning

Diagnosis and treatment planning require study models, roentgenograms, and a periodontal charting. To perform orthodontic movement, anchorage must be adequate, space in the arch must be adequate for the movement, and the orthodontic forces must be continuous and of proper magnitude. Desired space can be created by occlusal grinding, interproximal stripping, extraction, orthodontic movement of adjacent teeth, or expansions.

Decisions to treat or not to treat can be made only after a careful study of the case; they imply that the practitioner has an adequate knowledge of the proposed appliances as well as of the biologic response of the tissues to orthodontic forces. The charting, roentgenograms, and study models must be carefully studied.[19]

Clinical judgment must be employed in the development of a treatment plan. The chief question that must be answered is "to move or not to move the teeth." This requires careful examination, study, and evaluation of projected treatment with regard to the results that might be obtained.

1. Which teeth must be moved and which teeth retained in position? Will these latter teeth provide adequate anchorage?
2. Can the repositioning be accomplished? Is adequate space available? Can this space be obtained by stripping, extraction, or arch expansion?
3. Will the tooth movement create occlusal interferences? If so, can these be eliminated or avoided? Was the malposition originally caused by an occlusal interference?

4. Will the repositioning cause a loss of tissue?
5. What is the prognosis now, and what will it be after treatment?
6. Are the teeth in question sound enough to warrant movement? Are their furcations involved?
7. Will adjacent teeth have to be extracted, or will they be damaged? How close are their roots?
8. Will the repositioning prevent periodontal disease?
9. What force or appliance design will best serve the needs of the patient and the treatment plan?
10. If the teeth must be splinted after movement, can the patient afford the prosthesis? Can the practitioner provide adequate prosthetic treatment?

When periodontal fibers are moderately stressed, a physiologic adaptation of the alveolar housing results, with bone formation occurring in areas of tension and bone resorption in areas of compression. The remodeling of bone brings about a new positioning of the tooth as long as the periodontium is maintained in health. Since all tooth movements, migratory or orthodontic, are mediated by the cells of the periodontium, an understanding of the biology of the periodontium is essential.[20-27] (See the section on experimental occlusal traumatism in Chapter 25.)

Clinical observations have indicated that bone levels may be improved by moving teeth into defects, by producing forced eruptions, or by uprighting teeth. The remodeling of bone and periodontal ligament during orthodontic movements may eliminate defects and contribute to elimination of pockets.

## Appliances

Teeth can be repositioned by the creation of controlled forces acting on the tooth, which is the essence of orthodontics. Although spontaneous repositioning of migrated teeth sometimes follows periodontal therapy[28-30] (see Fig. 35-22), tooth movement generally requires the use of appliances. These specialized implements must be carefully controlled to do the work for which they are intended.

An orthodontic appliance is an implement designed to place pressure against a tooth to produce movement. The two types of appliances, removable and fixed, have numerous variations. An intermittent, tipping force is produced by removable appliances, whereas a continuous, multidirectional (torque, intrusion, rotation, bodily movement) application of force is provided by the fixed type. Although a majority of orthodontists in the United States prefer the fixed appliances, some orthodontists and many periodontists and general practitioners use the removable kind, which can be effective with a cooperative patient and in cases in which the scope of treatment is limited (Figs. 45-8 and 45-9). Either type may be used with success. Occasionally the patient's fixed bridgework or partial denture can be adapted to serve as an appliance by such means as the addition of springs, hooks, and so on.

### FIXED APPLIANCES

The primary advantage of the fixed appliance[31-33] is that it provides greater control of tooth movement. Because of its constant force, treatment time may be shortened. Fixed appliances are essential where bodily movement or root torque is required. However, compared with tooth movement in a child, the degree of discomfort is greater, the rate of movement is slower, and root resorption is believed to be more frequent in adults. Moreover, the adult no longer has the growth potential that orthodontists employ in the treatment of children. The nonorthodontist using fixed appliances may feel more at ease with simpler types of treatment, such as those involved in closing diastemata

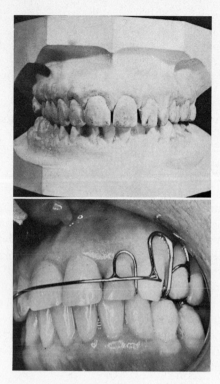 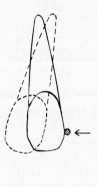

**Fig. 45-8.** Mesial movement of the left central and lateral incisors with finger springs. The clasp and arch wire are separated in this appliance to provide ease in the adjustment of each. The arch wire was made of .028-inch wire; the finger spring, of .020-inch wire.

and aligning abutment teeth, reducing anterior protrusions, relieving crowding, rotating teeth, uprighting tipped teeth, correcting crossbites, or bringing in impacted teeth. The correction of skeletal malocclusions (classes II and III) are best handled by the orthodontist. In some instances orthodontics and surgery may be combined in the treatment of skeletal malocclusions.

In fixed appliance therapy, the teeth are banded, and force-producing devices (e.g., wires and elastics) are caused to act on the banded teeth through such connections as tubes, brackets, hooks, eyelets, or buttons. Direct cementation of the apparatus to enamel is possible.[34-37]

**Anchorage**

Appliances are designed to provide both anchorage and orthodontic force. A force pitted against a tooth will be transmitted equally in the opposite direction. The appliance distributes the force to the tooth to be moved and to the anchorage teeth. The resultant movement is proportionate to the relative strength of attachment of each. Therefore the anchorage should be strong and stable to ensure movement of the proper tooth. Theoretically some reciprocal movement of the anchorage, however slight, must occur even when a minimal force is applied.

**Bodily movement**

Bodily movement implies the movement of crown and apex in the same direction and generally requires the use of a fixed appliance. The tooth is fastened to the arch wire by means of a bracketed band. The activated appliance then delivers a "force couple" and moves the tooth bodily rather than by tipping it.

## REMOVABLE APPLIANCES

Since special training is necessary to use fixed appliances, the removable appliances have become more commonly used where the scope of tooth movement is limited. These devices have their advantages: they afford ease in case management, are not

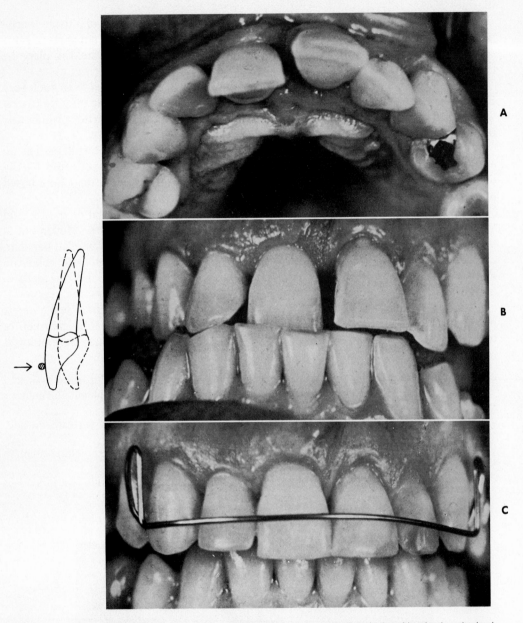

**Fig. 45-9.** **A,** Dentition of a 40-year-old woman with a protruding left maxillary incisor. Her dentist mistakenly thought that this malposition was caused by periodontosis. No pocket could be demonstrated on this tooth. **B,** The position of the right lateral incisor *(arrow)* may be caused by tooth contact during right lateral bruxing. **C,** After orthodontic repositioning of the teeth and occlusal correction. The appliance was worn at night as a passive retainer to prevent the teeth from moving back into their former protruded positions.

very irritating, and do not interfere with oral hygiene. Adults who feel conspicuous and uncomfortable with fixed appliances find removable appliances, which can be taken out at work and for social engagements, more to their liking. Furthermore, they have sufficient motivation and maturity to cooperate by replacing the appliance regularly.[38-43]

**Schwarz appliance**

One such appliance, the Schwarz appliance, is simple, consisting of a tissue-borne palatal or lingual acrylic base that is festooned about the teeth and supports various springs, hooks, arch wires, and spurs[10,38] (Fig. 45-10). The device is held in place by two to four clasps.

**Hawley appliance**

These appliances resemble a Hawley retainer and are often referred to as such (see Figs. 45-7 to 45-10). Nevertheless, they are active appliances, as is the all-wire Crozat appliance[44,45] and the Jackson appliance, whereas the retainer used after orthodontic treatment is a passive appliance designed for retention.

Occasionally the patient's fixed bridgework or partial denture can be adapted as an appliance by such additions as springs. Other appliances that are activated by the orofacial musculature are called *functional appliances*. The orthodontic school based on this concept is called functional jaw orthopedics.[46,47]

Removable appliances may be used to move teeth in buccolingual or mesiodistal directions and also to rotate, intrude, or extrude teeth (see Fig. 45-9). Movement is produced by the activation of springs, rubber bands, and the arch wire. Rubber dam elastics may be used in conjunction with the appliances. The rubber resembles the tooth in color and is esthetic. Elastics are stretched between hooks and the teeth to be moved and may even be used in place of an arch wire.

**Bite plate and bite plane**

A platform added to the palatal anterior portion of a Hawley appliance will convert it to a bite plate or bite plane useful in freeing the occlusion of contact or in directing tooth movement along an inclined plane.[45] The bite plate or plane may be employed in a number of situations:

1. To free the occlusion and permit repair of traumatized periodontal supporting tissues
2. To facilitate eruption of a posterior tooth or teeth and the depression of mandibular anterior teeth
3. To facilitate tooth movement in buccolingual or mesiodistal directions; to rotate, intrude, or facilitate eruption of a tooth or teeth
4. As an appliance for attachments to correct landmark relationships and tooth position
   A. By facilitating mandibular tooth movements
   B. By permitting retraction of anterior teeth and changing the crown-to-root ratio
5. To permit testing of changes in vertical dimension

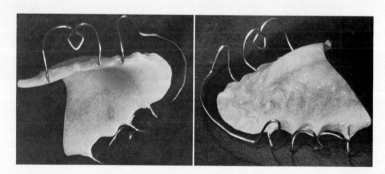

**Fig. 45-10.** Schwarz appliance (labial wire, .028 inch; lugs, .036 inch; arrowhead clasps, .020 inch) held in place by the arrowhead clasps, which engage the tooth interproximally below its greatest convexity to allow for continuous eruption.

6. To permit repair of bony defects
   A. Changes in crestal form
      1) By eruption of a tooth
      2) By changing the axial inclination of roots
   B. Infrabony (angular) defects
      1) By uprighting tilted teeth
      2) By permitting or encouraging eruption of a tooth

The bite plate should create a 1-mm space between occluding surfaces of posterior teeth. When alteration of cusp relationships or the plane of occlusion of a posterior tooth is planned, the teeth must be freed of occlusal contact. This may be done with a bite plate, to which a platform is added to the anterior palatal portion of the Hawley device (Fig. 45-10). If the platform is inclined, the occluding teeth will migrate along its slope, and the device may be termed an inclined bite plane. Some appliances may be split and have expansion screws incorporated for the expansion of the arch. An adequate freeway space should be present, and mandibular anterior teeth should be firm when bite plates and bite planes are used.

The bite plane aids in the restoration of lost occlusal vertical dimension by permitting or encouraging posterior teeth to erupt. Posterior eruption is most successful in adults when the bite plates are worn continuously except for eating (approximately 21 hours a day). Bite plane therapy has been used to treat occlusal trauma and temporomandibular joint (myofacial pain) syndrome, as well as in preparation for periodontal prosthesis.

The Hawley bite plane is not a satisfactory approach when a class III malocclusion with an edge-to-edge bite is present. Depressing the lower incisors and allowing the tongue to thrust into the space between the maxillary and mandibular anterior teeth can create an anterior open bite.

**Contra-indications**

Insertion of the maxillary Hawley bite plane provides the necessary mechanical advantage for the treatment of primary and secondary occlusal trauma. Following are advantages of this choice of therapy:

**Advantages**

1. Biologic correction of osseous defects caused by periodontal disease
2. Eruption of posterior teeth, resulting in reduction of the anterior overbite and an increase in overjet
3. Occlusal adjustment with repair of the attachment tissues; changes in cuspal inclination to eliminate fremitus patterns
4. Reduction or elimination of mobility patterns
5. Avoidance of unnecessary splinting

Frequently a patient may have an occlusal arrangement with a deep overbite and no overjet. The teeth may have significant mobility (2 to 2½ degrees) and fremitus in excursive movements. Unless eruption of the posterior teeth can be induced, occlusal adjustment by selective grinding is impossible to achieve. An alternative treatment is the immediate placement of provisional splinting.

When the appliance is used to move teeth, treatment wires need careful adjustment. Loops that connect the treatment wires to the base of the appliance are used to activate the wires. Activation is produced when the loops are opened and closed. The proper position of a wire can be maintained only if compensating bends are made in the loop during adjustments, as indicated in Fig. 45-11.

**Adjusting the appliance**

The acrylic base must be trimmed so that it does not prevent movement by its contact with the tooth. Generally only 1 mm at a time is trimmed; the base thus serves to limit the movement to 1 mm. The festooned margin of the base acts as a stop and should be relieved when necessary to free a tooth so that the tooth may be moved. In addition, the acrylic should be undermined adjacent to the area of movement to permit

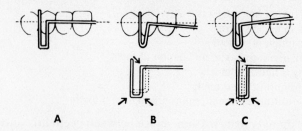

**Fig. 45-11.** **A,** Loop before adjustment. **B,** As the loop is opened, the arch wire is displaced. Proper position can be maintained only by making compensating bends at arrows altering the loop form *(dotted version)*. **C,** Loop closed and arch wire displaced. Position of the arch wire can be maintained by making compensating bends at the arrows, altering the loop form *(dotted lines)*.

space for the gingiva and for apposition of bone on the palatal surface of the maxillary alveolar plate (Fig. 45-12).

**Tipping movement**

Removable appliances generally produce tipping movements in which the crown is moved a greater distance than the apex (see Figs. 45-8 and 45-9). Although the apex may remain in place when very gentle forces are used, usually the crown and apex move in opposite directions about the center of rotation of the tooth. In teeth with undamaged alveolar support, this center is located near the cervical third of the root. As alveolar bone is lost in periodontal disease, the center moves closer to the apex, thus facilitating tipping or tilting of the tooth.

## Other treatment modalities

### LIGATION

Tooth movement of a limited scope, such as the closing of a diastema or the rotation of an individual tooth, sometimes can be achieved without fabricated appliances. In these instances rubber dam elastics, elastic ligatures, grassline ligatures, wire ligation, tongue depressors, and even finger pressure may be used. Such methods do not afford precision in control, and close observation is necessary. However, they appeal to the operator because they require no preparation and they take seemingly little chair time. Their use occurs less and less frequently as time passes.

**Rubber dam elastics**

Rubber dam elastics, which come in various widths, are stretched around teeth for repositioning (Fig. 45-13). The piece of elastic is removed by the patient at mealtime and replaced with a new one afterward. These maneuvers require cooperation and dexterity. If the bands slip apically, they may cause severe damage (Fig. 45-14); therefore the dentist and patient must be alert and perceptive. Slipping may be prevented if ligature wire loops are placed on the teeth, and the twisted ends used as guards (Fig. 45-15). Notches cut into the tooth or buttons of bonded plastic restorative or cementing material will serve the same purpose. Orthodontic bands with soldered spurs can also be used.

Since the force of the elastic acts equally, two teeth with similar support can be drawn together (see Fig. 45-13). If movement is intended for only one tooth, the anchorage tooth and the malposed tooth must have disproportionate support. This can be arranged by pitting the tooth to be moved against several other teeth by means of elastic wrapped about the anchoring teeth (see Fig. 45-13) or by the splinting of several anchor teeth with ligature wire (Fig. 45-15), welded bands,[18] or self-curing plastic.

**Elastic nylon thread**

Elastic nylon thread is available in light, medium, and heavy.[48] Medium thread is used as the arch wire, and light thread is used interproximally in the manner of wire ligation (Fig. 45-16). The thread is placed by the dentist, not the patient. Its management in all other respects is similar to that of a rubber dam elastic, since it forms

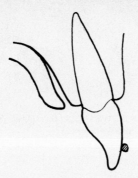

**Fig. 45-12.** Undermining of the appliance's palatal aspect to provide room for movement of tooth and apposition of bone.

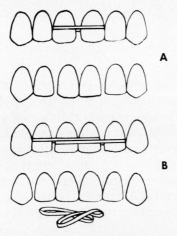

**Fig. 45-13.** **A,** Placement of a rubber dam elastic or orthodontic rubber band around two central incisors to draw them together. **B,** Use of two rubber bands to draw the lateral incisors toward the central incisors, which are used for anchorage.

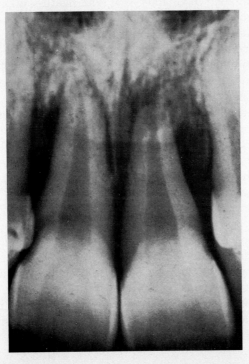

**Fig. 45-14.** Extensive resorption of bone around two maxillary central incisors of a 10-year-old girl. The tissue had been traumatized by an orthodontic rubber band that had slipped below the gingiva.

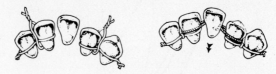

**Fig. 45-15.** Central incisor moved into alignment with rubber dam elastic *(shading)* while the two adjacent teeth on each side are ligated with wire ligature to provide anchorage.

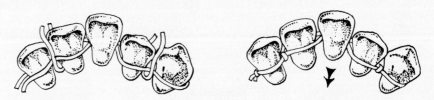

**Fig. 45-16.** Application of elastic nylon thread for minor tooth movement.

a large elastic band once the ends are tied together. It has the advantage of being esthetic but many of the disadvantages of the fixed appliance.

**Grassline ligatures**

Grassline ligatures are twisted threads of unwaxed silk that shrink approximately 25% when wet. Their mode of action differs from elastic deformation. The grassline is knotted about several contiguous anchor teeth, which serve to counteract the forces of shrinkage on them, and a long unknotted strand is placed about the tooth to be moved, which therefore receives the full effect of the shrinkage (Fig. 45-17). Although grassline may be effective, precise control is not possible, and care must be exercised. Grassline may become foul smelling; the ligatures must be replaced frequently because they loosen after shrinking.[18]

**Wire ligatures**

Wire ligatures can be used to produce an almost immediate movement if the teeth are sufficiently loose. The wire is dead soft and therefore is practically inelastic. Movement is obtained by digital pressure while the interproximal loops are being tightened (see section on wire ligation in Chapter 47). Wire ligature improperly applied during temporary splinting to immobilize teeth may result in an unexpected movement of teeth. Rubber dam elastics, elastic nylon thread, and grassline and wire ligatures all give a rather limited control and require great care in their use.

**Grassline and wire ligation**

Ligatures usually produce tipping movements. However, when wire ligation is used to stabilize the teeth—that is, the clinical crowns—grassline ligatures tied to the roots will produce a bodily movement of the roots.[49]

Orthodontic treatment should follow initial periodontal therapy, and the patient should be able to minimize plaque formation and inflammation.[50] To the extent that orthodontics produces a more normal occlusion and reduces bony defects, it is an integral step in therapy. Definitive occlusal adjustment is generally performed after the tooth movement has been completed, whereas selective grinding is performed in the course of orthodontics to provide space.

## RETENTION

Movement may loosen teeth, and there is a tendency for teeth to return to their old positions. They should therefore be held in position long enough to preclude relapse.[51,52] In cases in which splinting is part of the treatment plan, there is no further problem. In other instances, such aids as wire ligation, a splint, welded bands, direct bonding, Hawley retainers, or night guards may be needed for retention (Figs. 45-7, 45-10, and 45-18). Occlusal adjustment and procedures to break habits are often necessary to maintain the newly gained positions.

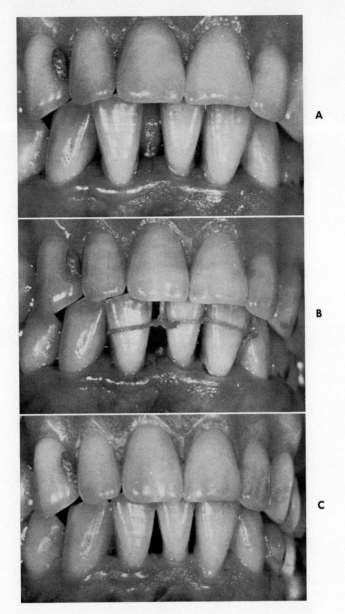

**Fig. 45-17.   A,** Lingual displacement of the mandibular central incisor. **B,** The malaligned tooth was extracted, and the remaining teeth were moved by grassline ligature. **C,** The three incisors have been moved into good alignment.

## SULCULAR INCISION

The period of retention permits remodeling of alveolar bone and connective tissue to meet the new functional status of the teeth. The relapse that often follows orthodontic movement may be a result of forces exerted by the musculature and to occlusal discrepancies. It is also believed that the fibers of the gingival group become stretched during the orthodontic movement and tend to return the teeth to their old positions. When these fibers are severed by inserting a Bard-Parker blade into the sulcus on the palatal/lingual and proximal surfaces to 3 mm below the alveolar crest (sulcus slice), there is apparently less relapse. Moreover, no noticeable recession of the gingiva

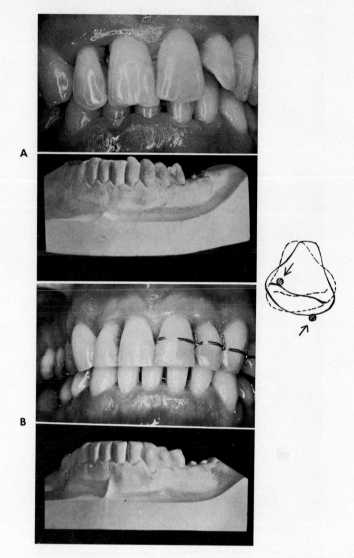

**Fig. 45-18.   A,** Drifting and rotation of an upper left lateral incisor that occluded with the projecting lower left canine. **B,** The lower canine was shortened, the lateral and central incisors were stripped to provide space, and the lateral incisor was rotated back into position. After treatment, wire ligation served as a temporary retainer during the retention period. Such corrections of rotations in adult patients may require permanent retention.

occurs, and the sulcus depth does not appear to be altered by this technique[48,53-59] (Fig. 45-19).

The comparative roentgenograms are the only means by which the response of the bone to orthodontic tooth movement and retention may be monitored.[60,61] Consequently, roentgenograms must be taken in the course of treatment, on completion of treatment, and 2 years subsequent to treatment. Moreover, photographs, posttreatment study models, and periodontal charting must be obtained.

## Results of treatment

**Beneficial results**

Kronfeld[62] repositioned the drifted teeth of a patient with juvenile periodontitis. With scaling and root planing, the teeth became firm, and the condition improved. Similar results have been noted by others.

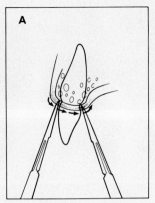 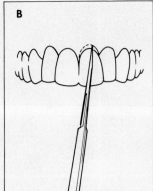 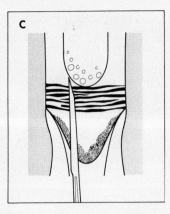

**Fig. 45-19.** **A,** Insertion of blade into gingival crevice through sulcular epithelium and gingival fibers to crest of alveolar bone. The incision is made circumferentially. **B,** Labial view of incision. **C,** Blade resects dentogingival and transseptal fibers.

When migrated teeth are repositioned, beneficial changes may result from the improved relationship of teeth to each other and to the alveolar bone.[63-73] When tilted teeth are uprighted, pocket depth may be reduced[74-77] (see Figs. 45-7 and 45-8). The apparent increased level of bone that is observed at times when teeth are moved into or away from defects or toward each other suggests a possible osteogenic response incident to the tissue remodeling that occurs during orthodontic movement. Occlusal traumatism may be reduced. Reestablished mesiodistal contact relationships minimize food impaction and provide intrinsic support. Improved tooth and gingival contour combine to eliminate plaque-harboring areas and food impingement and to provide functional stimulation of the attached gingiva. Reconstruction may be aided, and esthetics can be improved.[71-73]

## Orthodontics and advanced periodontal disease

In patients with advanced periodontal disease, either of the rapidly progressing periodontitis type or the very slowly progressing type, orthodontics can be helpful treatment (Figs. 45-20 to 45-22). The strategy in such cases is to avoid multiple extractions and restore arch integrity, reducing anterior flaring, spacing of the teeth, and correcting bite collapse, since these patients may have a variety of malocclusions that interfere with the stabilization and function of the teeth.

Classical orthodontic appliances were originally designed to treat young healthy patients and can be used with equal effectiveness on periodontally healthy adults. Periodontal disease patients are different. They may be seen with as much as 70% alveolar bone loss. This bone loss modifies the crown/root ratio and changes the location of the center of rotation. On the other hand, bone turnover is almost unmodified, but bone density is reduced.

Normal orthodontic forces move teeth *through* bone. In the patient with periodontal disease these forces may move teeth *out of* the remaining bone. Instead, orthodontics in these patients should move teeth *with* their remaining bone. This kind of predictable tissue remodeling might be achieved with very light forces, with minimal force activation, and with constant force-to-moment ratio. Plaque and disease control must be of a superlative degree.

Disease activity should be controlled with careful scaling and root planing every 4 to 6 weeks. Antibiotic therapy is necessary during acute episodes. Subgingival irrigation with a chlorhexidine solution may be prescribed to control bacterial proliferation within

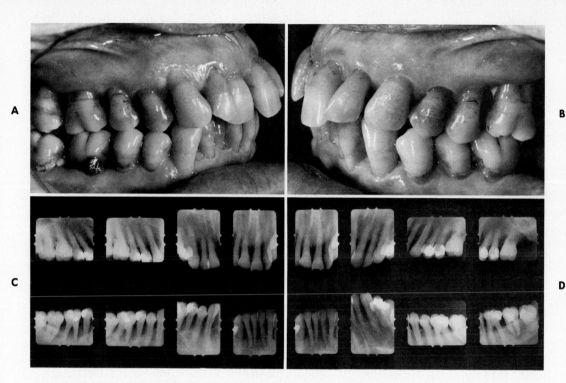

**Fig. 45-20.  A** to **D,** In 1978, a 54-year-old woman was seen with a primary malocclusion and secondary migration of the teeth. There was alveolar bone loss of approximately 60% to 70%. Class III furcation involvements were present on the first molars. (Courtesy D. Etienne, M. Laviec, and A. Fontanelle, Paris, France.)

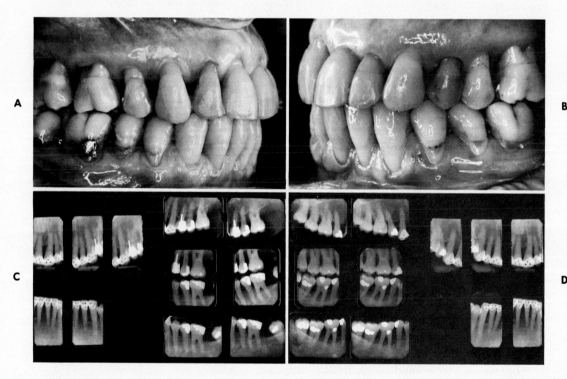

**Fig. 45-21.  A** to **D,** In 1985, after periodontal and orthodontic treatment and the extraction of the upper right first bicuspid, lower left second molar, and the lower right central incisor, gingival form has improved and the occlusion has stabilized. Acid etch splints were placed from cuspid to cuspid in the maxilla and mandible. (Courtesy D. Etienne, M. Laviec, and A. Fontanelle, Paris, France.)

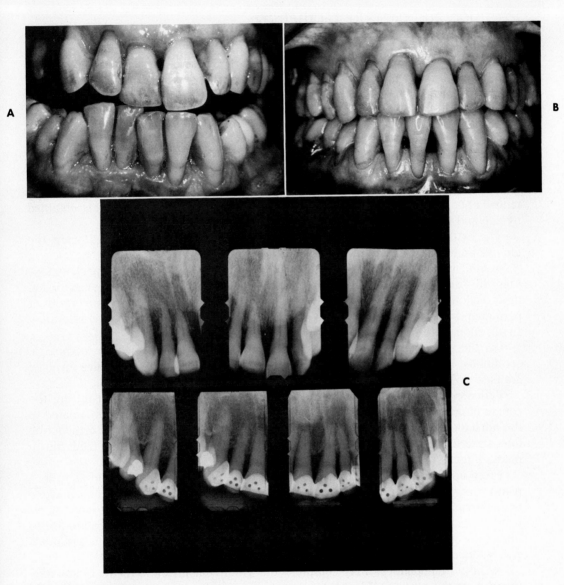

**Fig. 45-22.**   **A** to **C,** Anterior teeth in 1978 (**A** and **C** *[top]*) and in 1985 (**B** and **C** *[bottom]*). (Courtesy D. Etienne, M. Laviec, and A. Fontanelle, Paris, France.)

deep pockets or furcations. Sometimes visits at a 2-week interval will be necessary during tooth movement of questionable teeth or intrusion. Plaque control is reinforced at every session.

When arch spaces are closed and teeth are aligned, multiple extractions are avoided and acid-etched splints constitute a reasonable and conservative alternative to full mouth reconstruction of compromised teeth.

## Extrusion and periodontal therapy

Extrusion of fractured teeth and of endodontically involved roots has become an acceptable mode of saving teeth that would otherwise be extracted. The therapy involves endodontic treatment followed by forced extrusion by means of rubber elastics extending from a hook placed in the canal to a bar bonded to the adjacent teeth (see Fig. 43-4). Such extrusion normally takes only a few weeks to perform. Periapical lesions appear to be left behind by the extrusion. They repair more rapidly than usual when extrusion is performed. Repair appears to be accompanied by proliferation of periodontal ligament cells stimulated by the extrusion.

Extrusions of 3.5 mm or more can be obtained in about 3 weeks with the use of heavy force. Since bone and gingiva move occlusally with the extruded roots, simultaneous fiberotomy, minor osseous reshaping, and further root exposure are obtained by flap and minor osseous surgery.

The extrusion can be performed to salvage teeth fractured or decayed below the gingiva and at times below the alveolar crest (Fig. 45-23).[74-76]

A similar form of extrusion[63,77,78] can be used to eliminate infrabony pockets (see Figs. 45-4 and 45-5), but in those cases a lighter force is applied for a longer extrusion time. Following extrusion it is often necessary to splint teeth either temporarily or permanently because of diminished crown-root ratio or for postorthodontic retention. In all, such tooth movements can be of decided therapeutic value.

**Pathologic results**

On the other hand, injudicious treatment may inadvertently lead to pathologic conditions. Perception, dexterity, and knowledge of the biology of the tissues involved are basic to the use of orthodontics for the periodontal patient.

Periodontal lesions may be produced as a consequence of treatment during the course of orthodontic tooth movement.[20,27,79-82] Such lesions are commonly related to the appliance per se. However, periodontal trauma may be the result of orthodontic forces exerted on the teeth, or occlusal traumatism may occur during the tooth movement (jiggling) or uncorrected infantile swallowing patterns.[83]

Fixed appliances tend to promote inflammation because food retention as well as plaque and deposit formation are increased, and proper performance of oral hygiene procedures is hindered. An appliance may directly traumatize the tissues when wires bend or settle into the gingiva. Ill-fitting bands are irritating; when bands are forced under the gingiva, pockets may be formed. Adult patients tolerate such irritations poorly; children apparently are able to better tolerate them.

Removable appliances may compress the gingiva against the teeth; clasps may impinge on the gingiva. Wires that are occlusal to the contact point may settle and separate the teeth. Rubber bands may slip and be lost under the gingiva, causing exfoliation of teeth (see Fig. 45-14). Thus appliances can initiate and perpetuate periodontal disease.

Orthodontic forces produce movement by causing bone and connective tissue to resorb and reform. A small amount of tooth resorption and bone loss may occur in the most properly managed case. When excessive (unphysiologic) pressures are used for long periods, bone loss tends to increase. Dramatic bone loss and root resorption can occur in such cases. If orthodontic therapy is performed on a patient who has or develops juvenile periodontitis, considerable complications may develop.[4,14]

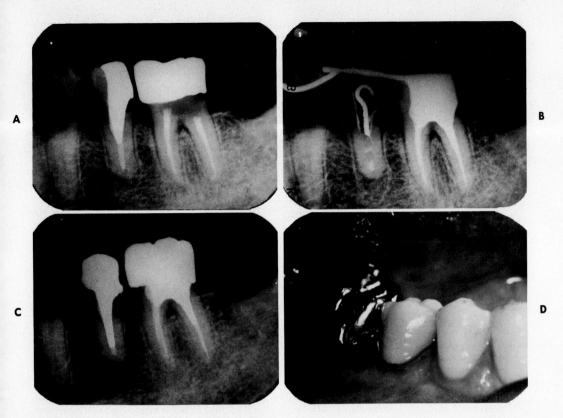

**Fig. 45-23.    A,** An open contact and food impaction were present between the lower left second bicuspid and first molar. Distal decay was present on the bicuspid. The tooth had previously had endodontic treatment; however periapical rarification was present. **B,** Orthodontic eruption was performed. **C,** A post and crown were placed. Notice the repair of the periapical lesion. **D,** Mirror view of the final restorations. (Courtesy K. Mori, Tokyo, Japan.)

Occlusal traumatism may result from orthodontic tooth movement. To reposition teeth, they may have to be moved counter to the forces of occlusion. Traumatism tends to occur, particularly when teeth are moving through cusp-to-cusp relationships. Jiggling, a situation in which orthodontic forces move the tooth in one direction and occlusal forces move the tooth in the opposite direction, is especially damaging. Jiggling occurs more frequently with removable appliances, since the patient may have occlusal relationships that differ when he/she wears the appliance and when he/she takes it off to eat. It is advisable to have the patient wear the appliance while eating.

At the completion of therapy, even when ideal intercuspation is achieved, minute occlusal discrepancies may exist. Moreover, maximal intercuspation may occur in an eccentric position (i.e., away from terminal hinge occlusion). These premature contacts should be corrected by occlusal adjustment. Standard periodontal procedures may be used in the treatment of other lesions that develop during orthodontic treatment.

## Summary

In general, the practitioner should be able to do an adult periodontal-orthodontic diagnosis, to recognize each type of malocclusion, and to determine how it came to be. The practitioner should be prepared to determine whether the malocclusion is skeletal or migrational in origin. He/she should be able to treat some migrational malocclusions with fixed and removable appliances and be aware of the difficulties involved in the treatment of the skeletal malocclusions.[82,84] The dentist should be able to assess the periodontal status of the patient and to gauge whether orthodontic treatment will be an asset or a liability to the patient.[85]

To gain these ends it is necessary that periodontal orthodontics be taught at the undergraduate level to present-day students and that practitioners avail themselves of postgraduate courses.

## REFERENCES

1. Stern, I.B.: Tooth malpositions and periodontal pathosis: an evaluation of etiology and considerations in treatment, J. Periodontol. **29:**253, 1958.
2. Morris, M.L.: Orthodontic-periodontic relationship. In Horowitz, S.L., and Hixon, E.H., editors: The nature of orthodontic diagnosis, St. Louis, 1966, The C.V. Mosby Co.
3. Marks, M.H., and Corn, H.: The role of tooth movement in periodontal therapy, Dent. Clin. North Am. **13:**229, 1969.
4. Goldstein, M.C., and Fritz, M.E.: Treatment of periodontosis by combined orthodontic and periodontal approach: report of a case, J. Am. Dent. Assoc. **93:**985, 1976.
5. Marks, M.H., and Corn, H.: Periodontics and orthodontics: coordinating the disciplines for optimal treatment planning, Alpha Omegan **76:**76, 1983.
6. Gianelly, A.A.: Orthodontic considerations in periodontal therapy, J. Periodontol. **41:**119, 1970.
7. Ingber, J.S.: Forced eruption. I. A method of treating one and two wall infrabony osseous defects: a rationale and case report, J. Periodontol. **45:**199, 1974.
8. Van der Linden, I.P.G.M.: Theoretical and practical aspects of crowding in the human dentition, J. Am. Dent. Assoc. **89:**139, 1974.
9. Breitner, C.: Tooth-supporting apparatus under occlusal changes, J. Periodontol. **13:**72, 1942.
10. Schwarz, A.M., and Gratzinger, M.: Removable orthodontic appliances, Philadelphia, 1966, W.B. Saunders Co.
11. Cheraskin, E., et al.: Resistance and susceptibility to oral disease. III. A study in clinical tooth mobility and carbohydrate metabolism, J. Calif. Dent. Assoc. **41:**416, 1965.
12. Priester, E.A.: Die endogenen Ursachen der Zahnlockerung, Dtsch. Zahnaerztl. Z. **15:**132, 1961.
13. Mühlemann, H.R.: Tooth mobility, J. Periodontol. **38:**686, 1967.
14. Baer, P.N., and Everett, F.G.: Periodontosis: a problem in orthodontics, J. Periodontol. **46:**559, 1975.
15. Langer, B., and Wagenberg, B.D.: Methods of altering crestal bone levels: clinical case reports, J. Periodontol. **50:**520, 1979.
16. Bernstein, M.: Orthodontics in periodontal and prosthetic therapy, J. Periodontol. **40:**577, 1969.
17. Reitan, K.: The inital tissue reaction incident to orthodontic tooth movement as related to the influence of function, Acta Odontol. Scand. **9**(suppl.), 1951.
18. Geiger, A., and Hirschfeld, L.: Minor tooth movement in general practice, ed. 3, St. Louis, 1974, The C.V. Mosby Co.
19. Gianelly, A.A.: Diagnosis, case selection and treatment planning, Dent. Clin. North Am. **16:**413, 1972.
20. Schwarz, A.M.: Tissue changes incidental to orthodontic tooth movement, Int. J. Orthod. **18:**331, 1932.
21. Oppenheim, A.: Die Veränderungen der Gewebe inbesondere des Knochens bei der Verschiebung der Zähne, Oest. Ung. Vjschr. Zahnheilkd. **27:**302, 1911.
22. Reitan, K.: Tissue behavior during orthodontic tooth movement, Am. J. Orthod. **46:**881, 1960.
23. Orban, B.: Biologic problems in orthodontia, J. Am. Dent. Assoc. **23:**1849, 1936.
24. Furstman, L., Bernick, S., and Aldrich, D.: Differential response incident to tooth movement, Am. J. Orthod. **59:**600, 1971.
25. Goldman, H.M., and Gianelly, A.A.: Histology of tooth movement, Dent. Clin. North Am. **16:**439, 1972.
26. Storey, E.: The nature of tooth movement, Am. J. Orthod. **63:**292, 1973.
27. Edwards, J.G.: A study of the periodontium during orthodontic rotation of teeth, Am. J. Orthod. **54:**441, 1968.
28. Ross, I.F.: Endogenous tooth movement, J. Am. Dent. Assoc. **60:**738, 1960.
29. Ross, I.F.: Tooth movement and repositioning of the mandible without appliances, J. Prosthet. Dent. **31:**290, 1973.
30. Manor, A., Kaffe, I., and Littner, M.M.: "Spontaneous" repositioning of migrated teeth following periodontal surgery, J. Clin. Periodontol. **11:**540, 1980.
31. Grewe, J.M., Little, R.M., and Chavoor, A.G.: Fixed appliances, Dent. Clin. North Am. **16:**525, 1972.
32. Gordon, L.: Band construction and application, Dent. Clin. North Am. **16:**515, 1972.
33. Hyman, S.C., and Schlossberg, A.: Technique selection for adult tooth movement, Dent. Clin. North Am. **16:**467, 1972.
34. Silverman, E., et al.: A universal direct bonding system for both metal and plastic brackets, Am. J. Orthod. **62:**236, 1972.
35. Silverman, E., and Cohen, M.: Current adhesives for indirect bracket bonding, Am. J. Orthod. **65:**76, 1974.
36. Rensch, J.A.: Direct cementation of orthodon-

tic attachments, Am. J. Orthod. **63:**156, 1973.

37. Dietz, V.S.: A technique for direct bonding of orthodontic attachments, J. Clin. Orthod. **6:**681, 1972.

38. Adams, C.P.: The design and construction of removable orthodontic appliances, Baltimore, 1964, The Williams & Wilkins Co.

39. Coote, J.D.: Removable appliance therapy: patient co-operation and its assessment, Br. Dent. J. **134:**91, 1973.

40. Lewis, H.G., and Brown, W.A.B.: The attitude of patients to the wearing of a removable orthodontic appliance, Br. Dent. J. **134:**87, 1973.

41. Norton, L.A., and Wickwire, N.A.: The use of removable partial dentures in tooth movement, Dent. Clin. North Am. **16:**505, 1972.

42. Sage, D.L.: Modified removable appliances from prefabricated components, Dent. Surv., p. 32, May, 1974.

43. Schlossberg, A.: The removable orthodontica appliance, Dent. Clin. North Am. **16:**487, 1972.

44. Wiebrecht, A.T.: Crozat appliances in interceptive maxillofacial orthopedics, Milwaukee, 1969, E.F. Schmidt Co.

45. Fedi, P.F., Jr.: The high labial appliance in periodontal therapy, Dent. Clin. North Am. **16:**497, 1972.

46. Andresen, V., Häupl, K., and Petrik, L.: Functions-Kieferorthopädie, ed. 6, Munich, 1957, Johann Ambrosius Barth Verlagsbuchhandlung.

47. Cunat, J.J.: Activators: an orthopedic puzzle, Am. J. Orthod. **65:**16, 1974.

48. Goldstein, M.C.: Adult orthodontics and the general practitioner, J. Can. Dent. Assoc. **24:**261, 1958.

49. Wank, G.S.: The use of grassline ligature in periodontal therapy, Dent. Clin. North Am. **6:**473, 1972.

50. Krampf, J.I.: Multidisciplinary treatment: orthodontics-periodontics-restorative dentistry, Dent. Clin. North Am. **16:**583, 1972.

51. Riedel, R.A.: A review of the retention problem, Angle Orthod. **30:**179, 1960.

52. Levin, M.A.: Postorthodontic maintenance in the adult patient, Dent. Clin. North Am. **16:**559, 1972.

53. Crum, R.E., and Andreasen, G.F.: The effect of gingival fiber surgery on the retention of rotated teeth, Am. J. Orthod. **65:**626, 1974.

54. Boese, L.R.: Increased stability of orthodontically rotated teeth following gingivectomy in *Macaca nemestrina,* Am. J. Orthod. **56:**273, 1969.

55. Strahan, J.D., and Mills, J.R.E.: A preliminary report on the severing of gingival fibers following rotation of teeth, Dent. Pract. **21:**101, 1970.

56. Walsh, E.A.: Precision: an aid to the reduction of rotational relapse in clinical dental practice? An assessment, Br. J. Orthod. **2:**135, 1975.

57. Kaplan, R.G.: Clinical experience with circumferential supracrestal fiberotomy, Am. J. Orthod. **70:**146, 1976.

58. Kaplan, R.G.: Supracrestal fiberotomy, J. Am. Dent. Assoc. **95:**1127, 1977.

59. Rinaldi, S.A.: Changes in the free gingival level and sulcus depth of the human periodontium following circumferential supracrestal fiberotomy, Am. J. Orthod. **75:**46, 1979.

60. Catena, D.L.: Radiologic changes associated with tooth movement, Dent. Clin. North Am. **16:**549, 1972.

61. Sjolien, T., and Zachrisson, B.U.: A method for radiographic assessment of periodontal bone support following orthodontic treatment, Scand. J. Dent. Res. **81:**210, 1973.

62. Kronfeld, R.: Zur Therapie der pathologischen Wanderung, Z. Stomatol. **27:**765, 1929.

63. Ingber, J.S.: Forced eruption. I. A method of treating isolated one and two wall infrabony osseous defects: rationale and case report, J. Periodontol. **45:**199, 1974.

64. Kramer, G.M., and Reiser, G.M.: The tipped lower molar: therapeutic considerations, Alpha Omegan **66:**33, Dec. 1973.

65. Burns, M.H.: Orthodontic management of tipped abutment molars, J. Am. Dent. Assoc. **87:**843, 1973.

66. Brown, I.S.: The effect of orthodontic therapy of certain types of periodontal defects. I. Clinical findings, J. Periodontol. **44:**742, 1973.

67. Ross, S., Dorfman, H.S., and Palcanis, K.G.: Orthodontic extrusion: a multidisciplinary approach, J. Am. Dent. Assoc. **102:**189, 1981.

68. Garrett, G.B.: Forced eruption in the treatment of transverse root fracture, J. Am. Dent. Assoc. **111:**270, 1985.

69. Tuncay, O.C., et al.: Molar uprighting with T-loop springs, J. Am. Dent. Assoc. **100:**863, 1980.

70. Simon, R.L.: Rationale and practical technique for uprighting mesially inclined molars, J. Prosthet. Dent. **52:**256, 1984.

71. Andreasen, G.F.: Treatment approaches for adult orthodontics, Am. J. Orthod. **62:**166, 1972.

72. Miller, C.J.: Minor tooth movement in general practice, Alpha Omegan **75:**23, 1982.

73. Marks, M.H., and Corn, H.: The importance of adult orthodontics in the management of occlusal problems, Alpha Omegan **73:**58, 1980.

74. Mori, K.: Interdisciplinary approach in general practice, Nippon Dental Review **499:**147, 1984.

75. Ross, S., et al.: Orthodontic extrusion: a multidisciplinary treatment approach, J. Am. Dent. Assoc. **102:**189, 1981.

76. Tuncay, O.C., and Cunningham, C.J.: 7-loop appliance in endodontic-orthodontic interactions, J. Endodontol. **8:**367, 1982.

77. Oppenheim, A.: Artificial elongation of teeth, Am. J. Orthodont. Oral Surg. **26:**931, 1940.

78. Ingber, J.S.: Forced eruption. Part II. A method

of treating nonrestorable teeth: periodontal restorative considerations, J. Periodontol. **47:** 203, 1976.

79. Atherton, J.D., and Kerr, N.W.: Effect of orthodontic tooth movement on the gingivae, Br. Dent. J. **124:**555, 1968.

80. Tirk, T.M., Guzman, C.A., and Nalchajian, R.: Periodontal tissue response to orthodontic treatment studied by panoramix, Angle Orthod. **37:**94, 1967.

81. Zachrisson, S., and Zachrisson, B.U.: Gingival condition associated with orthodontic treatment, Angle Orthod. **42:**26, 1972.

82. Formicola, A.J., and Binder, R.E.: Commonly encountered problems, Dent. Clin. North Am. **16:**573, 1972.

83. Prichard, J.F.: The effect of bicuspid extraction orthodontics on the periodontium (findings in 100 consecutive cases), J. Periodontol. **46:**534, 1975.

84. Bond, J.A.: The child versus the adult, Dent. Clin. North Am. **16:**401, 1972.

85. Chasens, A.I.: Indications and contraindications for adult tooth movement, Dent. Clin. North Am. **16:**423, 1972.

**ADDITIONAL SUGGESTED READING**

Albino, J.E., et al.: Variables discriminating individuals who seek orthodontic treatment, J. Dent. Res. **60:**1661, 1981.

Årtun, J., Osterberg, S.K., and Kokich, V.G.: Long-term effect of thin interdental bone on periodontal health after orthodontic treatment, J. Periodontol. **57:**341, 1986.

Bekeny, A.R., and DeMarco, T.J.: The effects of the rubber tooth positioner on the gingiva of orthodontic patients during retention, J. Periodontol. **42:**300, 1971.

Bryant, R.A., McNeill, R.W., and West, R.A.: Orthodontics and orthognathic surgery: adjuncts to restorative and periodontal therapy, J. Am. Dent. Assoc. **108:**33, 1984.

Iyer, V.S.: Biting platforms in orthodontic appliances, Dent. Pract. **15:**194, 1965.

Karring, T., et al.: Bone regeneration in orthodontically produced alveolar bone dehiscences, J. Periodontol. Res. **17:**309, 1982.

Kessler, M.: The bite plate: an adjunct in periodontic and orthodontic treatment, J. Periodontol. **51:**123, 1980.

Kessler, S.J., and Zweig, J.M.: Adult orthodontics and mouth reconstruction, J. Am. Dent. Assoc. **69:**572, 1964.

Kraal, J.H., et al.: Periodontal conditions in patients after molar uprighting, J. Prosthet. Dent. **43:**156, 1980.

Lamons, F.F.: The Crozat removable appliance, Am. J. Orthod. **50:**265, 1964.

Polson, A.M., and Reed, B.E.: Long-term effect of orthodontic movement on crestal alveolar bone levels, J. Periodontol. **55:**28, 1984.

Polson, A., et al.: Periodontal response after tooth movement into intrabony defects, J. Periodontol. **55:**197, 1984.

Rateitschak, K.H.: Reaction of periodontal tissue to artificial (orthodontic) forces. In Eastoe, J.E., Picton, D.C.A., and Alexander, A.G., editors: The prevention of periodontal disease, London, 1971, Henry Kimpton.

Reed, B.E., Polson, A.M., and Subtelny, J.P.: Long-term periodontal status of teeth moved into extraction sites, Am. J. Orthod. **88:**203, 1985.

Ross, I.F.: Reactive positioning of the teeth; a reappraisal, Periodontics **2:**172, 1964.

Sadowski, C., and BeGole, E.A.: Long term effects of orthodontic treatment in periodontal health, Am. J. Orthod. **80:**156, 1981.

Speckman, I.: La relación periodoncia, ortodoncia, Rev. Assoc. Dent. Mex. **36:**393, 1979.

Stallard, H.: Survival of the periodontium before and after orthodontic treatment, Am. J. Orthod. **50:**583, 1964.

Steiner, G.G., Pearson, J.K., and Ainamo, J.: Changes of the marginal periodontium as a result of labial tooth movement in monkeys, J. Periodontol. **52:**314, 1981.

Trosello, V.K., and Gianelly, A.A.: Orthodontic treatment and periodontal status, J. Periodontol. **50:**665, 1979.

Vanarsdall, R., and Corn, H.: Soft tissue management of labially positioned unerupted teeth, Am. J. Orthod. **72:**53, 1977.

Wagenberg, B.D., Eskow, R.N., and Langer, B.: Orthodontic procedures that improve the periodontal prognosis, J. Am. Dent. Assoc. **100:**370, 1980.

Wisth, P.J.: Periodontal status of neighboring teeth after orthodontic closure of mandibular extraction sites, Scand. J. Dent. Res. **83:**307, 1975.

Wisth, P.J., Norderval, K., and Boe, O.E.: Periodontal status of orthodontically treated impacted maxillary canines, Angle Orthod. **46:**69, 1976.

Zachrisson, B.U., and Alnaes, L.: Periodontal condition in orthodontically treated individuals. I. Loss of attachment, gingival pocket depth and clinical crown height, Angle Orthod. **43:**402, 1973.

Zachrisson, S., and Zachrisson, B.U.: Gingival condition associated with orthodontic treatment, Angle Orthod. **42:**26, 1972.

# CHAPTER 46

## Restorative and prosthetic dentistry

**Individual restorations**
Fixed appliances
Precision attachments

**Partial denture design**

**Fixed vs. removable prosthesis**

---

Operative and prosthetic dentistry have an important interrelationship with periodontal health and therapy. Properly constructed restorations are of therapeutic value. Restorations, when improperly constructed, can become etiologic factors in periodontal disease, since they constitute plaque harbors. Carious lesions and their sequelae become additional etiologic factors.

The outer surface of a restoration is of significance from the periodontal viewpoint.[1] Proper contact, contour, occlusion, marginal adaptation, and surface finish are as important to periodontics as they are to restorative dentistry.[2-8] These factors influence the course and direction of masticatory forces, the deflection of the food bolus, and the collection and retention of deposits and debris.

When carious lesions are present during periodontal therapy, particularly if they are advanced, it is important that they be excavated and temporary fillings be placed. Before final fixed restorations are placed, however, it is mandatory that frank periodontal disease be eliminated. The reason is that the position of the gingival margin cannot be properly anticipated if the gingiva is diseased. In fixed bridgework the same reason prevails; in addition, it is difficult to estimate what the degree of mobility will be after therapy and thus to appraise whether a slightly mobile tooth will be capable of serving as an abutment.

## Individual restorations

When planning individual restorations, one should have a clear understanding of the anatomic features of the area. Damage to the periodontium may occur during cavity and crown preparation and impression taking,[9,10] through careless use of separating disks, and from overfilled or overextended temporary fillings and crowns. Injudicious use of epinephrine (Adrenalin) string retraction and of electrocautery to expose margins of preparations must be avoided.[11,12]

The interdental embrasures are the diverging tooth surfaces that open toward the **Contact areas** vestibule, the oral cavity, the occlusal surface, and the gingiva. The proximal surfaces of the teeth form the sides, and the contact area forms the peak of the gingival embrasure. In health the papilla fills the gingival embrasure and the interdental papilla has the shape of a "sagging pup tent." With recession a space opens between the tip of the papilla and the contact point and the papilla may become convex or cratered. If the contact area is improperly restored, pathologic changes may follow (Fig. 46-1). Open contacts lead to food impaction; inadequate embrasures may lead to inflammation of the papilla by retaining plaque (plaque harbor).[13,14] Embrasure form should facilitate cleaning by the patient.

**Contour**

Buccal and lingual contours of restorations are equally important. They should protect the gingival margin from injury caused by food particles. The cervical contour should neither direct food into the gingival sulcus (Fig. 46-2) nor prevent stimulation by preventing the passage of the bolus over the gingiva[15]; overcontour, on the other hand, leads to plaque retention.[16]

**Occlusion**

The restorations should be in good occlusal relationship.[17] They should not predispose to occlusal traumatism. The rules for occlusal adjustment of natural dentitions also apply to restorations. Strive for occlusal relationships that are within the range of physiologic tolerance of the periodontium. Narrow the buccolingual diameters. Design sluiceways and marginal ridges to carry the bolus from the occlusal table, preventing food impaction. Each individual restoration must conform with the topographic relations of the dentition. Natural dentitions that require occlusal adjustment, however, should be corrected before the tooth is restored. Complete reconstructions require occlusal preplanning. Use any appropriate anatomic articulator as an aid to the planning and development of the occlusion. An occlusion devoid of interferences should be developed. Grasping contacts, plunger cusps, and balancing side interferences should be avoided. A harmony should exist among hinge position, median occlusal position

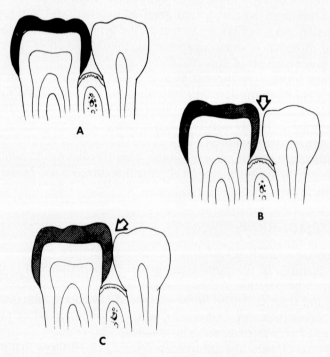

**Fig. 46-1.** **A,** Correctly placed contact. **B,** Open contact, conducive to food impaction. **C,** Unequal height of the marginal ridges, which guides food into the occlusal embrasure and may cause the contact to open.

(habitual centric), and excursive positions of the mandible. In young persons the cusp height may be steeper than in older persons who exhibit occlusal wear.

The restoration must blend at its margin into the tooth structure without catches.[18,19] **Margins** If you guide a sharp explorer over the margin, you should not be aware of passing from tooth to restoration. Composite or plastic fillings seldom permit satisfactory gingival margins and contact points may be deficient. Composite restorations with excellent margins are well tolerated by gingival tissues.[20] Overhanging margins are associated with interproximal bone loss. Poor margins lead to plaque retention and tend to harbor a microbiota like that in periodontitis.[15,21-25]

Gottlieb[6-8] taught that margins of restorations in caries-resistant persons should not be placed below the gingiva. This opinion has been supported in numerous studies showing that margins below the gingival sulcus can lead to gingival irritation.[26-36] Plastic fillings make poor subgingival margins.[37-39] Well-condensed and well-polished amalgam, gold foil, and composites are well tolerated. Well-made full gold crowns were

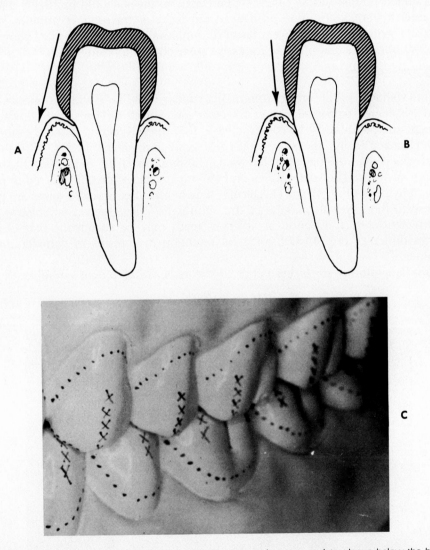

**Fig. 46-2.** Diagrammatic illustrations of, **A,** overcontour that tends to accumulate plaque below the height of contour (plaque harbor) and, **B,** undercontoured crown without deflecting contours may lead to food impaction. **C,** Model of the ideal tooth-to-tissue (gingiva) relationship. *Dotted lines,* Proper height and degree of contour; *x's,* self-cleansing areas.

constructed, with one half of their circumference below and the other half coronal to the gingival margin. The side on which the crown margin was supragingival showed better health.[35] Margins placed subgingivally often fit poorly. Gingivitis often occurs around a porcelain crown with poor margins (Fig. 46-3). Some patients can tolerate a considerable amount of irritation without breakdown. Gingival margins in caries-resistant persons are better placed above rather than below the gingival margin. Under no circumstances should any subgingival overhangs or deficiencies be permitted.

**Overhangs**

Overhangs should be removed at the time of root planing. Files, gold and amalgam knives, and enamel shavers are helpful (Rhein trimmer No. 31 to 32, chisel No. 24 and 25, No. 12 surgical blade, and EVA prophylaxis system[40] are all equally effective). When an overhang cannot be removed, the restoration should be replaced.

**Surface finish and texture**

Another important factor is surface texture—the polish of the restoration. The higher the polish and the less porous the material, the healthier the surrounding tissues. Smooth surfaces are better tolerated than rough ones, since bacterial deposits do not attach themselves as easily.[41-43] Porcelain surfaces should be highly glazed.[38] Composite materials are often used to repair decay or fractures of anterior teeth.[44] Composite structures tend to wear faster than natural teeth. Quartz-filled composites can act as abrasives and produce excessive wear on the opposing teeth.[45]

## FIXED APPLIANCES

**Pontic form and solder joints**

Pontics should fulfill form requirements similar to those of the abutments. They should be shaped to permit proper hygienic measures.[46,47] The space between the abutment and pontic must be constructed so that the interdental gingival embrasure can be cleansed easily. These principles also apply to fixed splints. Fig. 46-4 shows a case in which this rule has been followed. The margins of the fillings are flush with the tooth surfaces. The solder joints and embrasure forms are constructed to permit good oral hygiene (Fig. 46-5). These rules may be modified if solder joints are placed too close to the gingival margins of the abutments. The gingival embrasure space between abutment and pontic or adjacent tooth may be so narrow that cleaning becomes difficult (Fig. 46-4, *B*). Plaque retention may result in periodontitis and also caries.

Many laboratories stress cosmetics at the expense of proper contour. All fixed

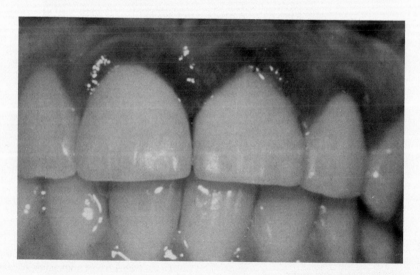

**Fig. 46-3.** *Acute gingival inflammation at the margins of ceramic crowns.*

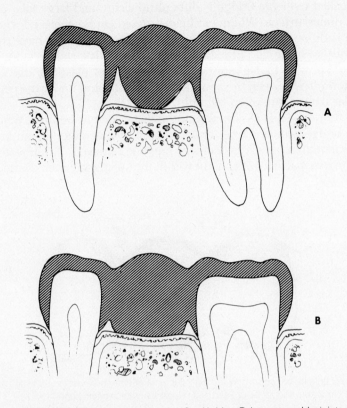

**Fig. 46-4.** **A,** Proper solder joints and embrasure spaces in a fixed bridge. **B,** Improper solder joints and embrasures.

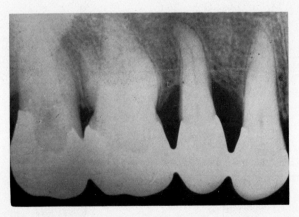

**Fig. 46-5.** Roentgenogram of proper contour, good solder joint, and good embrasure form in a fixed periodontal splint. (From the collection of M. Cattoni.)

bridges should be checked for contour of the pontic and abutment teeth. If faults in these areas exist, the pontics should be reshaped and reglazed before cementation. Temporary crowns, bridges, and splints are subject to similar considerations.

**Plaque**

The so-called hygienic bridge is difficult to clean, and large food particles adhere easily to its undersurface. When an ill-constructed pontic is placed, keeping the abutment clean is difficult (Fig. 46-6). The best arrangement is to have the pontic touch the ridge with an ovate tip (Fig. 46-7, *A*) and not with a saddle[48] (Fig. 46-7, *B*). The patient should be able to use interdental stimulators or plastic bridge cleaners, dental tape, or cotton yarn between the abutment and pontic and under the pontic. The Water Pik or similar devices are often helpful.

**Mobility**

In a fixed bridge, it is essential that the distal anchor be firm. When this tooth is mobile, the bridge acts as a lever or spring and may damage the anterior anchor.

**Excess cement**

After cementation, all excess cement must be removed. When restorations extend below the gingiva, particles of cement within the sulcus are often overlooked and cause damage.[49,50]

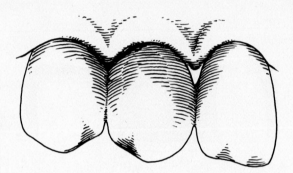

**Fig. 46-6.** Upper anterior bridge constructed with the gingival embrasure between the first premolar and canine obliterated. The embrasure should be opened and reglazed before cementation.

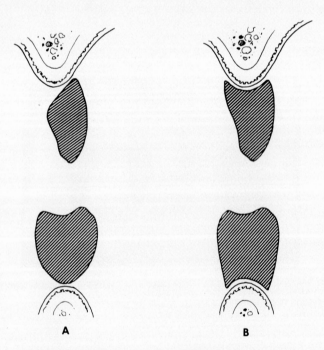

A                                    B

**Fig. 46-7.** **A,** Proper construction of pontic. Note the convex form against the ridge. **B,** Improper construction of pontic, a saddle that makes cleaning difficult.

Even the most expertly performed dentistry cannot repair the lesions of periodontitis if periodontitis is uncontrolled. Occlusal dysfunction does not cause periodontal disease; it only contributes to it. Periodontal health depends on the elimination of inflammation. Then the restoration of proper function becomes important.

**PRECISION ATTACHMENTS**

When design factors demand it, one may be forced to make a sectional fixed bridge. This can be done by a dovetail occlusal rest, a ball-socket arrangement, a fixed solderless joint, or a precision attachment. The female part can be placed in one of the abutments and the male part on the pontic or on an abutment, according to specific conditions.

## Partial denture design

Partial dentures are used to replace missing teeth and to restore function.[51-57] One **Stress** of the principal considerations in partial denture construction is the method of securing **breakers** the denture to the teeth. Teeth that are weakened may be of questionable value as single abutments. Splinting to create multiple abutments might be of great benefit. Broken stress arrangements between the abutment and the partial denture may also be useful. Whatever construction is used, stress should be distributed, and abutments should not be overloaded.

In securing a partial denture to the anchor tooth, precision attachments[58] may be used to minimize torque. Most clasps produce some torque during insertion and removal of the appliance. When weak, anchor teeth *must* be clasped; bent, wrought wire clasps are preferred to cast clasps, unless swing-lock fabrication is employed.

Lingual bars can do extensive damage to the gingiva. A lingual bar impinging on the gingiva can cut into the tissue and shear it, causing rapid gingival recession (see Fig. 23-9). Partial prostheses, their aprons, clasps, and lingual bars may also damage the periodontium after settling.[1] The partial denture should not touch the marginal gingiva of the abutment tooth.[59] Compression and subsequent damage can also occur in other situations where the denture contacts gingival margins. Palatal bars (Fig. 46-8) are probably one of the safest designs, whereas the horseshoe-shaped partial denture can be the most damaging. It is essential when inserting a partial, removable, tissue-borne prosthesis to impress on the patient that this appliance has to be examined annually to intercept damage from settling.[4]

## Fixed vs. removable prosthesis

For years controversy has existed regarding the superiority of fixed or removable prosthesis.[51-54] Most operators prefer fixed bridgework because a superior splinting effect is possible, torquing forces are minimized, and some mouths may be kept cleaner.

Some operators prefer partial dentures because they believe that oral hygiene measures can be more easily performed. Partial dentures are also used when fixed bridgework is not possible or practical.

Some clasped, single-abutment teeth are difficult to keep clean. This may be a result of wearing the denture at night. All appliances should be thoroughly cleaned daily, preferably after each meal.

The choice of prosthesis requires the evaluation of (1) the number and position of the remaining teeth, (2) the periodontal status of these teeth, (3) the clinical crown and root length, and (4) the patient. The personal preferences and abilities of the operator are also involved in this choice. A favorable influence of the prosthesis on the periodontal status of the remaining teeth is of paramount importance.[57]

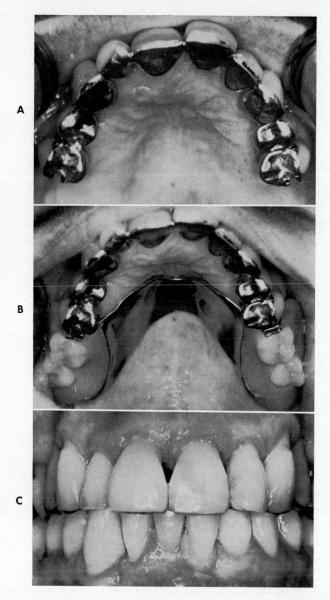

**Fig. 46-8.  A,** Fixed permanent splint employing three-quarter crowns and pin ledges. **B,** Construction of a partial denture with stress breakers and wide palatal bar. **C,** Satisfactory cosmetic appearance. Embrasures are sufficiently broad to permit proper cleansing.

The major threats to the longevity of a prosthesis are the recurrence of periodontal disease, loss of pulp vitality, and root caries. When a prosthesis has been placed in a patient previously treated for advanced periodontal disease, recall prophylaxis at 3-month intervals, examination annually, and daily plaque control (home care and germicidal therapy) are recommended.

Realignment of tilted and malposed teeth by orthodontic means will permit parallelism, pontic spaces of adequate width, open embrasures, and a normal curve of Spee.[60] Other benefits such as extrusion of fractured teeth and avoidance of pulp exposure may result from adjunctive orthodontic therapy. Moreover, teeth with a normal axial inclination and normal arch and occlusal relationships are more likely to have forces applied along their long axes.

A reduction of plaque accumulation may result from prostheses placed in a "normally" arranged dentition as opposed to a mutilated dentition. Choice of margin placement and pontic design is made easier.[61] Restorative procedures are also simplified by the use of preprosthetic surgery for ridge design, crown lengthening, provision of an appropriate gingival width,[62] endodontic therapy, and root amputation (see Chapters 41 and 43).

## REFERENCES

1. Romine, E.R.: Relation of operative and prosthetic dentistry to periodontal disease, J. Am. Dent. Assoc. **44**:742, 1952.
2. Terkla, L.G.: Crown morphology in relation to operative and crown and bridge dentistry, Oregon Dent. J. **25**:2, Dec. 1955.
3. Cripps, S.: Periodontal disease and restorative dentistry, Dent. Pract. **18**:199, 1968.
4. Motsch, A.: Parodontale Gesichtspunkte bei der konservierenden und prothetischen Planung und Behandlung, Parodontologie **24**:109, 1970.
5. Ross, I.F.: The relation between periodontal therapy and fixed restorative care, J. Periodontol. **42**:13, 1971.
6. Gottlieb, B.: Schmutzpyorrhoe, Paradentalpyorrhoe und Alveolaratrophie, Berlin, 1925, Urban & Schwarzenberg.
7. Gottlieb, B., and Orban, B.: Zahnfleischentzündung und Zahnlockerung, ed. 2, Berlin, 1936, Berlinische Verlagsanstalt.
8. Gottlieb, B., and Orban, B.: Biology and pathology of the teeth and its supporting mechanism, transl. by M. Diamond, New York, 1938, The Macmillan Co.
9. O'Leary, T.J., Standish, S.M., and Bloomer, R.S.: Severe periodontal destruction following impression procedures, J. Periodontol. **44**:43, 1973.
10. Clark, S.M.: Rubber-base foreign body, J. Prosthet. Dent. **31**:439, 1974.
11. Löe, H., and Silness, J.: Tissue reaction to string packs used in fixed restorations, J. Prosthet. Dent. **13**:318, 1963.
12. Knolle, G.: Gefahren bei der Anwendung des Adrenalinfadens, Dtsch. Zahnaerztl. Z. **21**:348, 1967.
13. Einfeldt, H.: Zur Hygiene des Interdentalraumes, Dtsch. Zahnaerztl. Z. **25**:490, 1970.
14. Motsch, A.: Der Interdentalkontakt, Dtsch. Zahnaerztl. Z. **28**:170, 1973.
15. Wilcox, C.E., and Everett, F.G.: Friction on the teeth and the gingiva during mastication, J. Am. Dent. Assoc. **66**:513, 1963.
16. Jameson, L.M., and Malone, W.F.P.: Crown margins and gingival response, J. Prosthet. Dent. **47**:620, 1982.
17. Patur, B.: The role of occlusion and the periodontium in restorative procedures, J. Prosthet. Dent. **21**:371, 1969.
18. Ogilvie, A.L.: Vital factors interrelating periodontology and restorative dentistry, J. Am. Acad. Gold Foil Oper. **4**:15, 1961.
19. Gilmore, N., and Sheiham, A.: Overhanging dental restorations and periodontal disease, J. Periodontol. **42**:8, 1971.
20. Dunkin, R.T., and Chambers, D.W.: Gingival response to Class V composite resin restorations, J. Am. Dent. Assoc. **106**:482, 1983.
21. Jeffcoat, M.K., and Howell, T.H.: Alveolar bone destruction due to overhanging amalgam in periodontal disease, J. Periodontol. **51**:599, 1980.
22. Hakkarainen, K., and Ainamo, J.: Influence of overhanging posterior tooth restorations on alveolar bone height in adults, J. Clin. Periodontol. **7**:114, 1980.
23. Gorzo, I., Newman, H.N., and Strahan, J.D.: Amalgam restorations, plaque removal and periodontal health, J. Clin. Periodontol. **6**:98, 1979.
24. Lang, N.P., Kiel, R.A., and Anderhalden, K.: Clinical and microbiologic effects of subgingival restorations with overhanging or perfect margins, J. Clin. Periodontol. **10**:563, 1983.
25. Keszthelyi, G., and Szabo, I.: Influence of Class II amalgam fillings on attachment loss, J. Clin. Periodontol. **11**:81, 1984.
26. Waerhaug, J.: Histologic considerations which govern where the margins of restorations should be located in relation to the gingiva, Dent. Clin. North Am. p. 161, March 1960.
27. Renggli, H.H.: Einfluss subgingival liegender Füllungsränder auf die Gingiva, Dtsch. Zahnaerztl. Z. **28**:169, 1973.
28. Renggli, H.H.: Auswirkungen subgingivaler approximaler Füllungsränder auf den Entzündungsgrad der benachbarten Gingiva (eine klinische studie), Schweiz. Monatsschr. Zahnheilkd. **84**:1, 181, 1974.
29. Mörmann, W., Regolati, B., and Renggli, H.H.: Gingival reaction to well-filled subgingival proximal gold inlay, J. Clin. Perodontol. **1**:120, 1974.
30. Noble, W.H., Tueller, V.M., and Douglass, G.D.: Margin placement in restorative dentistry, J. Am. Soc. Prev. Dent. **3**:49, 1973.
31. Silness, J.: Periodontal conditions in patients treated with dental bridges. II. The influence of full and partial crowns on dental plaque accumulation, development of gingivitis and pocket formation, J. Periodont. Res. **5**:219, 1970.
32. Silness, J.: Periodontal conditions in patients treated with dental bridges. III. The relationship between the location of the crown margin and the periodontal condition, J. Periodont. Res. **5**:225, 1970.

33. Kröncke, A.: Der Füllungs- und Kronenrand aus parodontologischer Sicht, Dtsch. Zahnaerztl. Z. **28:**161, 1973.

34. Eichner, K.: Untersuchungen über den Füllungs- und Kronenrand, Dtsch. Zahnaerztl. Z. **28:**166, 1973.

35. Richter, W.A., and Ueno, H.: Relationship of crown margin placement to gingival inflammation, J. Prosthet. Dent. **30:**156, 1973.

36. Newcomb, G.M.: The relationship between the location of subgingival crown margins and gingival inflammation, J. Periodontol. **45:**151, 1974.

37. Larato, D.C.: Influence of a composite resin restoration on the gingiva, J. Prosthet. Dent. **28:**402, 1972.

38. Björn, A.L., Björn, H., and Gkrovic, B.: Marginal fit of restorations and its relation to periodontal bone levels, Odontol. Rev. **20:**311, 1969.

39. Löe, H.: Reactions of marginal periodontal tissue to restorative procedures, Int. Dent. J.: **18:**759, 1968.

40. Vale, J.D., and Caffesse, R.G.: Removal of amalgam overhangs: a profilometric and scanning electron microscopic evaluation, J. Periodontol. **50:**245, 1979.

41. Clayton, J.A., and Green, E.: Roughness of pontic materials and dental plaque, J. Prosthet. Dent. **23:**407, 1970.

42. Knowles, J.W., and Snyder, D.T.: The effect of roughness on supragingival and subgingival plaque formation, I.A.D.R. Abstr. no. 345, p. 135, 1970.

43. Waerhaug, J.: Effect of rough surfaces upon gingival tissues, J. Dent. Res. **35:**323, 1956.

44. Jordan, R.E., et al.: Esthetic and conservative restoration of the fractured incisor by means of microfilled composite materials, Alpha Omegan **74:**50, 1981.

45. Chapman, R.J., and Nathanson, D.: Excessive wear of natural tooth structure by opposing composite restorations, J. Am. Dent. Assoc. **106:**51, 1983.

46. Stein, R.S.: Pontic-residual ridge relationship: a research report, J. Prosthet. Dent. **16:**251, 1966.

47. Podshadley, A.G.: Gingival response to pontics, J. Prosthet. Dent. **19:**51, 1968.

48. Silness, J., Gustavsen, F., and Mangersnes, K.: The relationship between pontic hygiene and mucosal inflammation in fixed bridge recipients, J. Periodont. Res. **17:**434, 1982.

49. Donaldson, D.: Gingival recession associated with temporary crowns, J. Periodontol. **44:**691, 1973.

50. Donaldson, D.: The etiology of gingival recession associated with temporary crowns, J. Periodontol. **45:**468, 1974.

51. Posselt, U.: Physiology of occlusion and rehabilitation, ed. 2, Philadelphia, 1968, F.A. Davis Co.

52. Fenner, W., Gerber, A., and Mühlemann, H.R.: Tooth mobility changes during treatment with partial denture prosthesis, J. Prosthet. Dent. **6:**520, 1956.

53. Grieder, A., and Cinotti, W.R.: Periodontal prosthesis, St. Louis, 1968, The C.V. Mosby Co.

54. Krogh-Poulson, W.: Partial denture design in relation to occlusal trauma and periodontal breakdown, Int. Dent. J. **4:**847, 1954.

55. Koivumaa, K.K.: Changes in periodontal tissues and supporting structures connected with partial dentures, Suom. Hammaslääk. Toim. **52**(suppl.), 1956.

56. Koivumaa, K.K., Hedegard, B., and Carlson, G.B.: Studies in partial denture prosthesis. I. An investigation into dentogingivally supported partial dentures, Suom. Hammaslääk. Toim. **56:**248, 1960.

57. Waerhaug, J.: Periodontology and partial prosthesis, Int. Dent. J. **18:**101, 1968.

58. Cohn, L.A.: Physiologic basis for tooth fixation in precision-attached partial dentures, J. Prosthet. Dent. **6:**220, 1956.

59. Bissada, N.F., Ibrahim, S.I., and Barsoum, W.M.: Gingival response to various types of removable dentures, J. Periodontol. **45:**651, 1974.

60. Evans, C.A., and Nathanson, D.: Indications for orthodontic-prosthodontic collaboration in dental treatment, J. Am. Dent. Assoc. **99:**825, 1979.

61. Giangrego, E., et al.: Restorative dentistry and total oral health: advances in tissue management, J. Am. Dent. Assoc. **111:**551, 1985.

62. Maynard, J.G., and Wilson, R.D.K.: Physiologic dimensions of the periodontium significant to the restorative dentist, J. Periodontol. **50:**170, 1979.

**ADDITIONAL SUGGESTED READING**

Coelho, D.H., and Brisman, A.S.: Gingival recession with modeling-plastic copper band impressions, J. Prosthet. Dent. **31:**647, 1974.

Frölich, E.: Pathologic-anatomical aspects of the relationship between gingival margin and artificial crowns, Dtsch. Monatsschr. Zahnheilkd. **22:**1258, 1967.

Gottlieb, B.: Die Prinzipien der Stumpfpreparation, Z. Stomatol. **22:**473, 1924.

Highfield, J.E., and Powell, R.N.: Effects of removing posterior overhanging metallic margins upon the periodontal tissues, J. Clin. Periodontol. **5:**169, 1978.

Kramer, G.M.: Reconstruction first, or periodontal treatment first, J. Am. Dent. Assoc. **64:**199, 1962.

Long, A.C.: Acrylic resin veneered crowns: the effect of tooth preparation and crown fabrication on periodontal health, J. Prosthet. Dent. **19:**370, 1968.

Marcum, J.S.: The effect of crown marginal depth

on gingival tissue, J. Prosthet. Dent. **17:**479, 1967.

Noble, W.H., Tueller, V.M., and Douglas, G.P.: Gingival margin placement in periodontal disease, J. Am. Soc. Prev. Dent. **3:**49, 1973.

Ross, J.F.: Problems connected with combined periodontal therapy and fixed restorative care, Dent. Clin. North Am. **16:**47, 1972.

Stibbs, G.D.: The role of operative dentistry in the prevention of periodontal disease, J. Am. Dent. Assoc. **45:**645, 1952.

Veldkamp, D.F.A.: The relationship between tooth form and gingival health, Dent. Pract. **14:**158, 1963.

Wei, S.H.Y.: Report on symposium: root surface caries, Council on Dental Research and Council on Dental Therapeutics, J. Am. Dent. Assoc. **106:**496, 1983.

# CHAPTER 47

## Splinting and stabilization

Periodontal disease impairs tooth support and permits secondary traumatism to occur. As a consequence, teeth may loosen, and the alveolar bone may be subjected to additional damage. Thus the reduction of mobility is an important objective of periodontal therapy. Root planing, curettage, oral hygiene, and surgery may cause teeth to tighten as inflammation is resolved.[1,2,3] However, a transient increase in mobility may occur immediately after surgery.[4] Occlusal adjustment, periodontal orthodontics, and restorative dentistry may alter occlusal relationships and redirect forces, thereby reducing traumatism. This may result in the teeth becoming firmer. Increasing the support of loose teeth may also increase their firmness; the device used for such treatment is the splint.[5-12]

**Definition**
A splint is any appliance that joins two or more teeth to provide support. Splints, like bridges, may be fixed, removable, or a combination of both. They may be temporary, provisional, or permanent, according to the type of material and duration of use. They may be internal or external, depending on whether tooth preparation is required. Permanent splinting of teeth that have been treated periodontally is also referred to as periodontal prosthesis.

## Theoretical aims

The theoretical aims of splinting are as follows:

1. Rest is created for the supporting tissues, permitting repair of trauma.
2. Mobility is reduced immediately and, it is hoped, permanently.[14] In particular, jiggling movements are reduced or eliminated.
3. Forces received by any one tooth are distributed to a number of teeth.
4. Proximal contacts are stabilized, and food impaction (but not retention) is prevented.
5. Migration and overeruption are prevented.
6. Masticatory function may be improved.
7. Discomfort and pain are eliminated.
8. Appearance may be improved.

Certain qualifications identify the ideal splint.[10] It should (1) be simple, (2) economic, (3) stable and efficient, (4) hygienic, (5) nonirritating, (6) not interfere with treatment, (7) esthetically acceptable, and (8) not provoke iatrogenic disease.

## Mode of action

Loose teeth splinted to adjacent firm teeth may become stabilized.[13-16] When many teeth are loose, adjacent sextants should be included in the splint. Teeth tend to loosen buccolingually yet may remain firm mesiodistally. Adjacent sextants therefore have complimentary strengths. Cross-arch splinting (Fig. 47-1) reduces mobility to the least common denominator. Teeth are thus immobilized and occlusal forces are better distributed.[11] Traumatism is minimized, repair is enhanced, and teeth may become firm again. Even when teeth do not tighten, the splint serves as an orthopedic brace that permits useful function of loose teeth. Teeth with reduced support often are hypermobile. This mobility may gradually increase if the teeth are not splinted.[17] Hypermobility decreases bone density in the coronal interproximal periodontium but does not change the level of the crest.[18]

## Indications

Splinting is indicated when moderate to advanced mobilities (2 degrees or more) are present and cannot be treated by any other means.[12] There is no reason for splinting nonmobile teeth or teeth with a slight, nonprogressive mobility as a preventive measure. Splinting should only be used with other necessary measures such as root planing, oral hygiene instruction, pocket elimination, and occlusal adjustment. When preprosthetic surgery or orthodontic measures are called for they should be completed before splinting whenever possible.

## Temporary splinting

Temporary splinting is a useful adjunct in many areas of treatment.[13] External splints are preferable because they are disposable. They may be used to facilitate

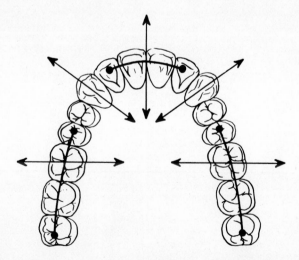

**Fig. 47-1.** Arrows indicate direction of mobility of loosened teeth. Lines with dots at each end indicate direction of stability of the same teeth. Splinting should include at least two groups of teeth so that the groups of teeth will be reciprocally stabilized by the addition of the directions of stability. (Modified from Roy, M.: Dent. Cosmos **72:**390, 1930.)

instrumentation (root planing, curettage, occlusal corrections) that might be difficult on loose teeth. They are of benefit in periodontal surgery, particularly when bone grafts or new attachment is attempted. They may serve as anchorage during, or provide retention after, orthodontic movement.

**Choice of splint**

Because several types of splints are available, a type must be selected as soon as the decision has been made to proceed with temporary splinting. The choice depends on the severity of mobility, the stage of treatment involved, and the anticipated outcome. Other considerations, such as location and distribution of missing and carious teeth, functional and esthetic needs, and cost, are also important. Any splint may be chosen if it is equal to the task. The specific advantages and disadvantages of the method and material must be weighed against the needs of the patient.

## EXTERNAL SPLINTS

External temporary splints include the following: ligatures, tooth-bonding plastic splints,[8] welded band splints, continuous clasps, and night guards.

**Ligature splints**

Ligatures are a satisfactory means of stabilizing anterior teeth.[14,15] Fig. 47-2 demonstrates the fabrication and use of a wire ligature splint. Dead-soft stainless steel wire

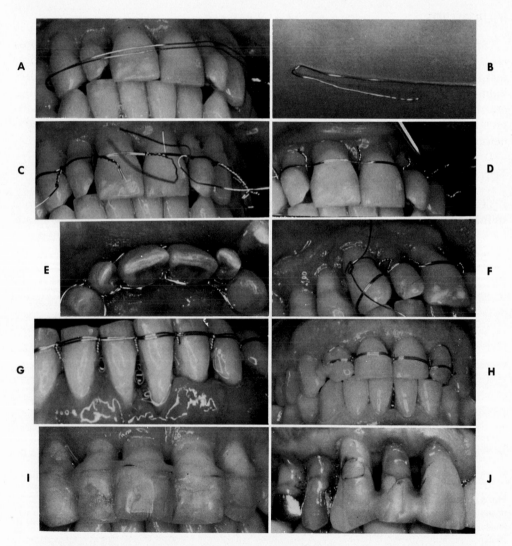

**Fig. 47-2. A** to **J,** Steps in wire ligation for temporary splinting. (See text for explanation.)

0.007 to 0.010 inch (0.175 to 0.25 mm) thick is used. Brass or silk ligatures are not as desirable. Double a 12-inch (30.5-cm) length for use as an arch wire, and bend it about the six anterior teeth. Position it apical to the contact points and incisal to the cingula, then loosely twist one end (Fig. 47-2, *A*). Provide for edentulous spaces by twisting the buccal and lingual strands of the arch wire together. Place single, hairpin-bent wires (Fig. 47-2, *B*) interdentally around the arch wires and below the contact points. Tighten them by twisting clockwise with a needle holder or Howe pliers. The interdental strands (Fig. 47-2, *C*) should not be so tight that they bring the arch wires into contact or produce tooth movement. To properly distribute force, tighten the last interdental ligature after all the other interdental ligatures and the arch wire have been tightened. Clip the ends of the wires (Fig. 47-2, *D, E,* and *G*) short (2 to 3 mm), and bend them into the interdental space to minimize catching food and to prevent injuring soft tissues (Fig. 47-2, *E*). When the wires are properly positioned, both splint and teeth are held fast. However, be careful that the splint does not slip incisally or gingivally. Slippage can be controlled by additional cervical loops (below the cingulum) (Fig. 47-2, *F* and *H*) or incisal loops (above the contact points). These oppose the direction of slippage and keep the splint in place.

Check the occlusion for interferences before dismissing the patient. Instruct the patient in oral hygiene procedures around the splinted teeth.[16] Self-cure acrylic or composite-acid etch resin may be placed over the wires.[19,20] This will improve esthetics, reduce irritation, and tend to prevent displacement (Fig. 47-2, *I*). Although ligation is a form of temporary splinting, ligatures may be retained for several months if they are tightened and replaced periodically. Ligation is useful only for anterior teeth.

A simple method of external temporary splinting employs tooth-bonding material: self-polymerized, ultraviolet light polymerized,[21] and white light polymerized composite resins. Such splints are cosmetic, fairly durable, and well tolerated by the patient. They are not able to resist heavy interocclusal forces and fractures often occur. If the bond between two teeth fractures, it can be repaired easily. The composite material is bonded to the lingual and interproximal surfaces of anterior teeth. Composite may also be placed on the facial surfaces of the teeth to increase the strength of the splint. Care must be taken to provide for adequate interproximal spaces. **Splints of enamel-bonding material**

The composite can be reinforced with a variety of materials such as wire, monofilament line, or orthodontic grid material,[21-24] or fiberglass placed along the lingual surfaces of the teeth (Fig. 47-2, *J*).

The incisal edge splint is used for mandibular incisors. A wire is placed in a prepared groove along the incisal edge of the teeth and bonded in place with a composite resin.

Welded band splints are useful for the temporary stabilization of posterior teeth (Fig. 47-3). Adapt a strip of stainless steel 0.003 to 0.005 inch (0.075 to 0.125 mm) thick to a tooth, and weld it to form a band. Weld the next strip to the mesial surface of the first band. Seat the two pieces while adapting the second strip to the tooth, then weld the second strip to form a band. Several strips can be added and formed into bands for successive teeth. The contact points must permit the band material to slip between the teeth. If necessary, you can separate the teeth by placing brass wire ligatures interdentally for 24 hours before splinting. **Welded band splints**

A modification of the welded band splint permits a single-band thickness in the contact area by the welding of a second band to the distobuccal and distolingual line angles of the first band, and so on. Another modification uses a combination of the welded band with a wire splint.[25] Enamel-bonded orthodontic brackets, connected by a ligated arch wire, have occasional use, particularly where edentulous spaces intervene between teeth to be splinted.

Be careful that the bands do not impinge on the gingiva. Also, check the occlusion for interferences. Sometimes adaptation can be improved by the use of contouring pliers and burnishers. It is possible to coat the splint with acrylic for esthetic appear-

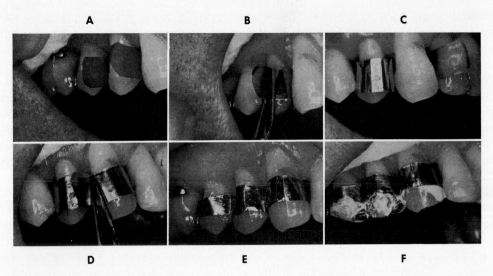

**Fig. 47-3.** Fabrication of a welded splint. **A** to **C,** Adapt a strip of stainless steel 0.003-0.005 inch (0.075-0.125 mm) to the tooth, weld to form a band. **D,** Form band on the next tooth and weld to mesial surface of first band. **E,** Several strips can be added for successive teeth and cemented (**F**) to place with temporary cement.

ance. Be additionally careful not to perform accidental minor tooth movements with the splint. Special attention should be given to plaque control, because temporary splints frequently interfere with oral hygiene. Preformed bands may also be used with the technique. Welded band splints are most useful for posterior teeth.

**Continuous clasps**

Continuous clasps may be made of acrylic, gold, or cast stainless steel[26-28] (Fig. 47-4). These simple splints may be seated and removed in the fashion of a partial denture, or they can be ligated to place. Using them as freely removable appliances is advantageous, since adequate oral hygiene is possible. They afford protracted temporary stabilization, yet they can be removed for social engagements. They may also be used at night only. They are not esthetic and may impede speech. Care should be taken to avoid irritating sharp edges and occlusal interferences. More elaborate continuous clasps can be used as permanent splinting devices, although removable splints generally do not contribute to a permanent decrease in mobility.[29-31]

**Night guards**

Night guards are special splints used for the alleviation of bruxism and clenching, as well as their deleterious influences[32-37] (Fig. 47-5). Night guards are made of heat-cured acrylic and completely cover the occlusal surfaces of the teeth. They can be constructed for one or both jaws. If freeway space permits, both arches can be covered. However, they are most often made for the maxilla. These splints can be made thin enough to be quite comfortable while worn. When a single splint is to be worn, fabricate it and adjust the occlusal contact so that a smooth maximal contact in gliding movement is achieved. The same contact should be sought for upper and lower splints when both are to be worn. The acrylic should extend just over the height of tooth contour and be finished with a thin edge for ease of insertion and removal and for retention when worn. Many patients become so accustomed to wearing night guards that they cannot sleep *without* them. Others find difficulty in adjusting to these devices. Consequently alternative methods must be sought. At times Hawley appliances may be substituted with favorable results (see p. 1013, Chapter 44).

In general, the night guard tends to stabilize mobile teeth. Care must be taken that the night guard does not rock and is not flexible. When single guards are used, the patient may pit the occlusal surface of the guard against one or more opposing teeth and cause them to loosen. If this is the case, two (opposing) night guards should be employed, or the use of the night guard should be discontinued.

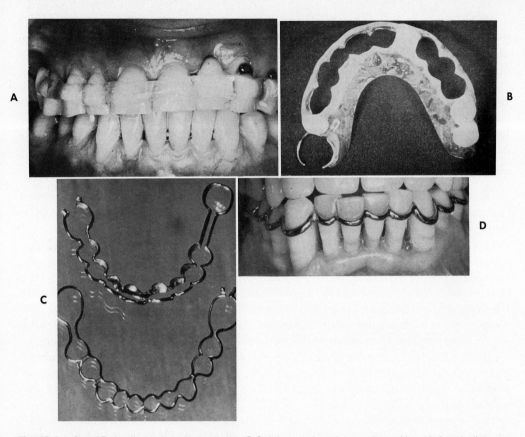

**Fig. 47-4.** **A** and **B,** Acrylic continuous clasp splint. **C,** Stainless steel continuous clasp with studs for wire ligatures. **D,** Gold continuous clasp. (**A** and **B** courtesy A. Krause, Leipzig, East Germany; **D** courtesy A. Gargiulo, Chicago, Illinois.)

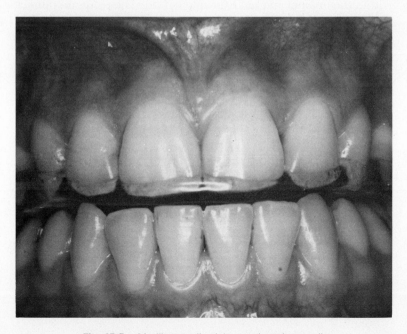

**Fig. 47-5.** Maxillary acrylic night guard used as a splint.

**Evaluation of external temporary splints**

Some external temporary devices tend to be unesthetic or unhygienic. They lack durability, rigidity, dimensional stability, or fit. The materials of other devices may stretch, warp, or loosen, and retention is poor. These conditions may permit decay or, on occasion, cause the teeth to shift. Some splints tend to break and may not last long. On the other hand, external splints are prepared easily and economically. They can be removed and replaced readily. Some may cause gingival irritation but not pulpal damage. Tooth structure is not removed, and, if the teeth become firm, the device may be discarded. Temporary splints have a definite place in the periodontal therapeutic armamentarium.

## INTERNAL SPLINTS

Internal temporary splints include acrylic, composite resin with or without embedded wire or amalgam with an embedded wire, nylon fishing line,[38] and acrylic or acrylic-and-gold provisional splints.[5,12,27,39-46]

Internal temporary splints should be used only when permanent splinting is to follow. Such splints are useful in the transition to permanent splinting. They may also be used on a provisional basis when tooth prognosis is guarded. Thus treatment is possible while final judgment is being deferred. Even when splinting cannot save teeth, it can provide a gradual and less distressing transition to full dentures. Once an internal temporary device has been used, the patient may be committed to periodontal prosthesis. You must advise the patient of this commitment before undertaking treatment.

**Acrylic splints (A splints)**

Acrylic internal temporary splints (A splints) (Fig. 47-6) require the preparation of a channel approximately 3 mm wide and 2 mm deep in several teeth. The preparations should be slightly undercut for retention. The pulpal surfaces should be coated with a protectant.

Lay a piece of platinized knurled wire (22 to 16 gauge [0.64 to 1.3 mm in diameter]) in the channel. Place self-cure acrylic to fix the wire in the channel (Fig. 47-6). Adjust the occlusion and polish the splint. Sometimes proper interproximal contour and marginal adaptation can be ensured by the use of matrices.[39-41]

**Composite splints**

The teeth to be splinted with composite resin are isolated with a rubber dam. A narrow, beveled groove is placed circumferentially around each tooth. This groove should be within the enamel and not exposing dentin. The teeth are pumice-polished.

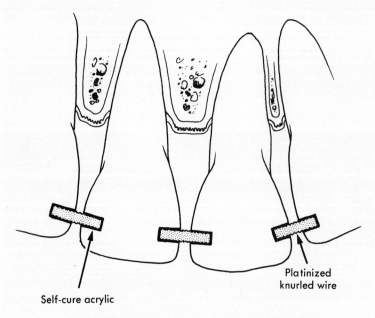

Platinized knurled wire

Self-cure acrylic

**Fig. 47-6.** Diagram of an acrylic (A) splint. Lingual view.

A 0.010 dead-soft single or double wire,[39] polyester filament yarn,[40] or nylon monofilament line is placed in the grooves, ligating the teeth with continuous figure-eight loops. The enamel is then etched with a 37% phosphoric acid solution for 60 seconds, rinsed thoroughly, and dried. Self-polymerizing or light polymerizing composite resin is then placed, cured, and polished.

The amalgam splint (Fig. 47-7) is similar to the A splint.[42-44] It has less strength **Amalgam** than that of cast gold. Its use is limited to the posterior teeth. Prepare the teeth in **splints** accordance with sound operative principles. Because commercial steel matrix bands cannot be used, make a matrix of self-cure acrylic. Condense the amalgam in one unit. Two to five teeth may be splinted in this fashion. A wire may be used for reinforcement. Amalgam splints tend to fracture easily.

Fixed temporary bridges may be made of acrylic crowns and pontics and may also **Acrylic full** serve as temporary splints[41,45,46] (Fig. 47-8). They are used when permanent fixed **crowns**

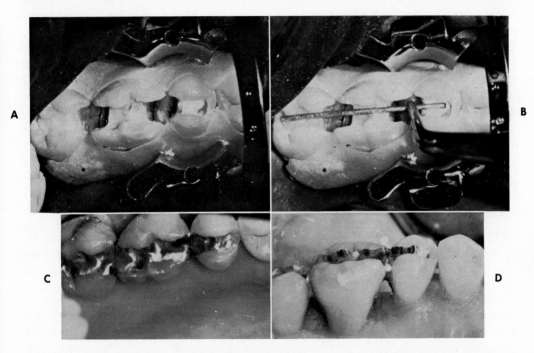

**Fig. 47-7.** Steps in the fabrication of an amalgam splint. **A,** Cavity preparation. **B,** Placement of supporting bar or wire. **C,** Finished splint, occlusal view. **D,** Lateral view to show the marginal finish and open embrasures. (Courtesy J. Atkins, Phoenix, Arizona.)

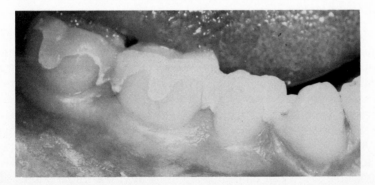

**Fig. 47-8.** Fixed temporary splint made of acrylic. Proper margins and embrasure forms help maintain gingival health. (Courtesy T. Tanaka, San Diego, California.)

splints will ultimately replace them. Many ways exist to make acrylic splints. One simple method employs duplicates of the patient's study models. The temporary acrylic splint is then made on the models of the prepared teeth. Another method uses a pressure-molded splint. Either is rebased in the mouth after the teeth are prepared.

With time, acrylic wears, and breakage becomes a problem. Consequently some clinicians prefer cast occlusals; others are concerned with the cervical relationship of the acrylic and prefer metal copings, which are less irritating to the gingiva and less likely to permit caries because of cement washout.

**Evaluation of internal temporary splints**

Internal temporary splints tend to be more serviceable than the external temporary splints, yet they have many of the same shortcomings. Their value varies with their rigidity and accuracy of fit and the patient's susceptibility to caries. The materials tend to wear and break and are dependent on the strength of the bonding medium. The position of the splint, marginal adaptation, and interproximal joints tend to create plaque harbors, which lead to caries, calculus deposition, and inflammation. Thus maintenance needs are increased, and oral hygiene procedures are made more difficult. When only part of the occlusal surface is covered by the splint, occlusal contacts may displace individual teeth from the splint. Extensive gingival recession, root indentations, and furcations make tooth preparation more difficult, and pulp involvement may result. Nevertheless, internal temporary splints have a definite place in periodontal treatment, provided they are used in situations for which they are suited. When the need for temporizing ceases, there should be no hesitation about conversion to definitive splinting. A delay may serve only to magnify the hazards involved in temporary splinting. A major cause of failure in periodontal treatment is the lack of, or delay in executing, adjunctive prosthesis or permanent splinting in the patient who requires it.

## Permanent splinting: periodontal prosthesis

### OBJECTIVES

Complete dental treatment includes periodontal and restorative aspects, which are extensively interrelated. Successful treatment most often requires both types of therapy. In many instances one cannot succeed without the other. The interdependence applies as much to a single tooth as it does to the whole dentition. The importance of stabilizing loose teeth has been discussed. Permanent splinting is indicated whenever periodontal treatment does not reduce mobility to the point at which the teeth can function without added support. Such devices serve *to stabilize loose teeth, to redistribute occlusal forces, to reduce traumatism,* and *to aid in the repair of the periodontal tissues.* Permanent splints are fabricated after periodontal treatment has been completed, when their use will extend the functional lifetime of the teeth. Such appliances must be constructed according to specifications listed in the following discussion.

### PROVISIONAL SPLINTING

Provisional restorations serve to stabilize a permanently mobile dentition from the time of initial tooth preparation until the time the dentition is periodontally stable enough for permanent restorations. It provides stability, occlusal function, and a good esthetic result. In addition, it allows the dentist to determine the optimum esthetic and functional design to be incorporated into the future permanent splint.

The provisional acrylic splint allows flexibility in case of future tooth loss. If a tooth included in the splint requires extraction, it can be separated from the splint, extracted, and the acrylic crown filled in with self-curing acrylic. Additional teeth can be crowned and added to the existing splint if additional support becomes necessary.

The provisional splint can be placed any time after the initial periodontal therapy is complete. If the splint is seated using temporary cement, it can be removed during periodontal treatment, thus facilitating access to the root surfaces ( Fig. 47-9).

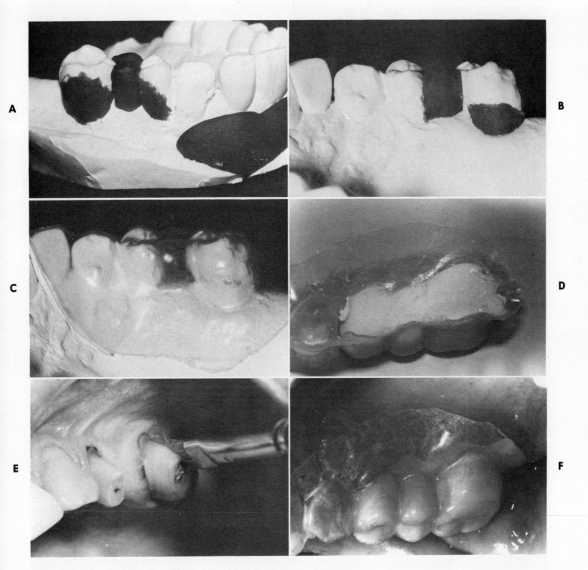

**Fig. 47-9.** **A** and **B,** The diagnostic cast should be prepared and, **C,** a vacuum-formed template fabricated. **D,** The vacuum-formed template is filled with autopolymerizing acrylic resin, and, **D,** then seated on the prepared teeth **(E),** which have been lubricated with silicone jelly **(F).** *Continued.*

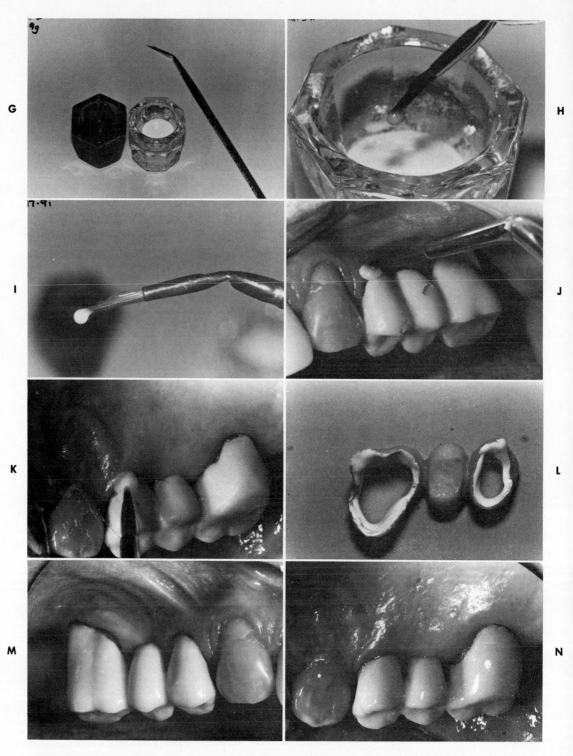

**Fig. 47-9, cont'd. G,** Dappen dishes are filled with acrylic resin monomer and polymer. **H** and **I,** A sable brush that has been dipped in monomer is used to pick up a bead of polymer. **J** and **K,** After initial trimming of the provisional restoration, liquid resin is applied with the stable brush to fill any voids. **L,** After the provisional restoration is trimmed and polished a small amount of temporary cement is applied to the margins and the cervical third of the internal aspect. **M** and **N,** All excess cement should be removed from the seated provisional restoration. The splint may be removed periodically to inspect tissue responses and esthetics, either reducing or adding to crown contours. Embrasure forms may be changed and occlusal adjustments made. (Courtesy R. Simon, Anaheim, California.)

## CLASSIFICATION

Permanent splints may be classified as follows:

1. Removable—external
   A. Continuous clasp devices
   B. Swing-lock devices
   C. Overdenture (full or partial)
2. Fixed—internal
   A. Full coverage, three-fourths coverage crowns and inlays
   B. Posts in root canals
   C. Horizontal pin splints
3. Cast-metal resin-bonded fixed partial dentures (Maryland splints)
4. Combined
   A. Partial dentures and splinted abutments
   B. Removable—fixed splints
   C. Full or partial dentures on splinted roots
   D. Fixed bridges incorporated in partial dentures, seated on posts or copings
5. Endodontic

Removable permanent devices incorporate continuous clasps and fingers that brace loose teeth[47-52] (Fig. 47-10). They strongly resemble partial dentures, and their features may be included in partial dentures. They support the teeth from the lingual surface and may incorporate additional support from the labial surface or use intracoronal rests. Palatal bars may also be added to provide a cross-arch splinting effect. Some partial dentures use pins that fit into grooves or holes in inlays[53] (Fig. 47-11).

The cosmetic disadvantages of labial continuous clasping can be overcome by use of the swing-lock appliance,[52] which tends to conceal the metal of the splint and avoid

**Removable permanent splints—external**

Swing-lock devices

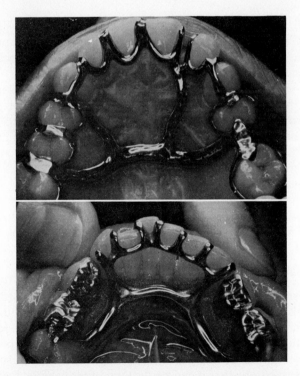

**Fig. 47-10.** Permanent removable splints for maxillary and mandibular arches. Finger clasps extend over incisal or occlusal contacts to fix the teeth in place. (Maxillary splint courtesy D.E. Erickson, El Cajon, California; mandibular splint courtesy H.E. Greenlee, Walnut Creek, California.)

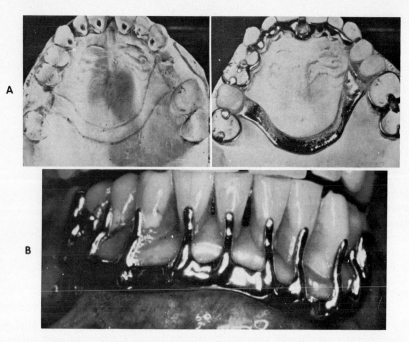

**Fig. 47-11.** **A,** Permanent removable splint for maxillary arch employing gold tubes (hollow inlays) cemented in the anterior teeth and pins that are part of the partial denture for support of the mobile teeth. **B,** Swing-lock partial denture. Mobile anterior teeth are fixed by the labial and lingual bars. A distal extension partial denture is attached to the splint by a stress breaker. (**A** courtesy E. Munch-Hansen, Virum, Denmark; **B** courtesy M. Rosa, San Diego, California.)

torque (Fig. 47-11, *B*). Swing-lock appliances may also be useful in situations in which fixed splinting is not possible or desirable: for example, in advanced age, in poor physical or mental status, or when the prognosis is questionable, the dentist chooses to avoid full coverage.

**Overdenture**

When a few teeth with questionable prognoses remain, an overdenture may be used.[54-57] The teeth are treated endodontically. They are then shortened close to the gum and fitted with a round nonanatomic gold dome, which may incorporate retention devices. A full or partial denture is then constructed over these remaining abutments. Among the advantages are a more favorable crownroot ratio and retention of alveolar bone around the roots.

The major problem in the long-term use of overdentures is the high incidence of recurrent periodontal disease,[56] although failure may be caused by endodontic and prosthetic failures.[57] The patient must carry on adequate plaque control measures and the dentist must regularly monitor the patient's periodontal status and adequacy in plaque control.[58]

## CAST-METAL RESIN-BONDED FIXED PARTIAL DENTURES

Cast-metal resin-bonded fixed partial dentures[58-61] are used with intact or very slightly altered enamel surfaces. This type of fixed prosthesis is functional, esthetic, reversible, and economic. It consists of a metal frame bonded with resin to tooth enamel. It may carry pontics. Retention is enhanced by perforations or by slots. The success rate is good[61] (see Figs. 45-21 and 45-22). Although the original use was for anterior teeth, this type of fixed prosthesis can be designed for posterior teeth.[61] The enamel bond is fairly strong; however excessively mobile teeth under a strong occlusal load can break loose from the metal framework.

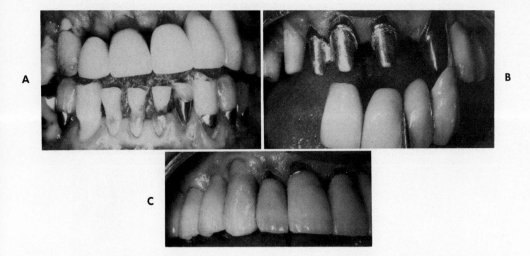

**Fig. 47-12.** **A,** Extensive periodontal disease, tooth mobility, and receded gingival margins. **B,** After treatment, splinting was necessary to control tooth mobility. Because of problems in tooth alignment, telescope crowns were prepared, and the maxillary right central and lateral incisors were splinted via the telescope arms. **C,** Fixed splint inserted, providing fixation and control of mobility. (Courtesy A. Solnit, University of Southern California School of Dentistry, Los Angeles, California.)

Fixed permanent devices may incorporate a series of soldered castings, such as crowns, three-quarter crowns, telescope crowns (Fig. 47-12), inlays, horizontal pin splints and pin ledges.[5,7,8,62-64] The splint is cemented to place. Full coverage is simple to perform if recession is not extensive and teeth are parallel. Otherwise, inlays or pin ledges may be more conserving of tooth structure and simpler to use. It is important that these splints be rigid. They should be of narrow buccolingual diameter. The interproximal solder joint should not impinge on the interdental papilla. The occlusal relationships should be harmonious. Ideally, the teeth and splint should be reciprocally stabilized in all directions (i.e., mesial, distal, vestibular, and apical). Otherwise the splint may still move about some fulcrum point, and traumatism may result.[57] Traumatism can also occur in the presence of improper occlusion.

A palatal bar connecting two fixed bridges in the upper molar and premolar areas is useful. This palatal bar is secured to the bridges on both sides by means of precision attachments and provides cross-arch splinting. Where the span of one or both of these bridges is large or when one of the bridges is weak, such palatal bars provide added stabilization.

When all segments cannot be paralleled, jeweler's screws or internal attachments may be used to combine segments of the splint (Fig. 47-13). Sectional splinting or splinted telescope crown copings also can overcome divergent parallelism (see Fig. 47-12).

The teeth must be capable of supporting a splint. The fixed splint, properly made, is one of the most effective dental restorations for the stabilization of teeth. It is comfortable and esthetic (Fig. 47-14).

Despite the advantages inherent in fixed splinting, instances occur of periodontally weakened dentitions, in which a combination of fixed splinting and partial dentures will best answer the needs of the patient.[65] These instances are governed by the distribution of remaining teeth. When partial dentures are used, the abutment teeth are best splinted[66] where feasible, with clasps and rests so placed that stabilization is afforded in all directions (Fig. 47-15). Recessed retainers and precision attachments are extremely useful in this regard. When the teeth are mobile, they may be jeopardized

**Fixed permanent splints— internal**

**Palatal bar**

**Combined permanent splints**

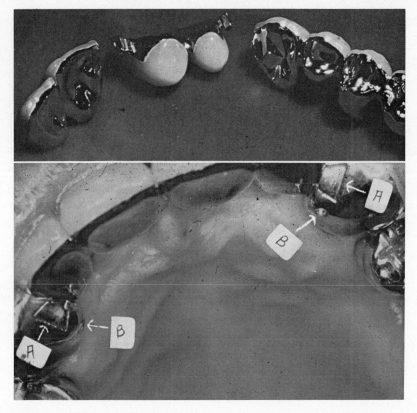

**Fig. 47-13.** Fixed removable splint. Where problems of tooth alignment or guarded prognosis for a tooth is present, a splint with precision attachments, *A*, fixed by means of a screw, *B*, may be used. The unit is preformed so that it may be incorporated in the wax-up. Screws may loosen because of torque forces and may require periodic tightening. (Courtesy D.E. Erickson, El Cajon, California.)

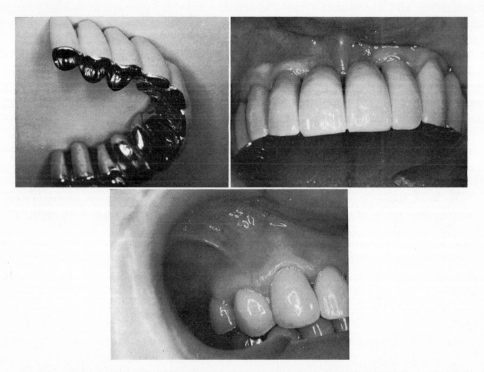

**Fig. 47-14.** Fixed bridge splinting employing full coverage. (Courtesy H. Schwartz, Seattle, Washington.)

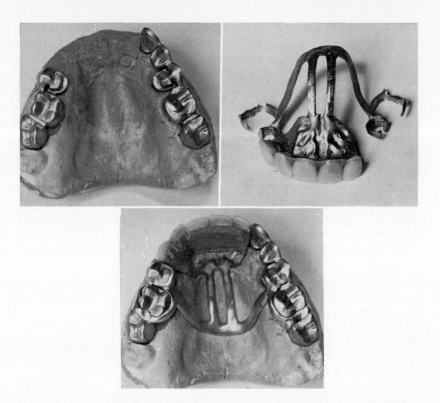

**Fig. 47-15.** *Partial denture with splinted abutments. (Courtesy J. Rotzler, Basel, Switzerland.)*

if the partial denture is completely dependent on the abutments. In these cases stress breakers may be used. On occasion, tissue-borne appliances may be necessary.

Sometimes a partial denture can be supported by crowns or endodontically treated roots splinted by a bar. The cross-section of the bar is elliptical, with the longer diameter oriented vertically. The bar must be 1 to 2 mm above the gingival margin for good hygiene. The denture is constructed over the bar.[67-69] When a few teeth remain, a partial denture partly supported by means of telescope crowns[66-68] can be used. The partial denture then serves as the splint.

## Summary

Considerable confusion exists concerning the need for periodontal prosthesis. Many popular indications for rehabilitation do not depend on existing lesions but are based on theoretical premises of conceptualized occlusal relationships. This sometimes encourages a degree of reconstruction when reconstruction is not really indicated. Splinting should not be performed unless indicated by clinical or roentgenographic manifestations (e.g., mobility, migration, or loss of bone). On the other hand, there may be a tendency to undersplint when an actual pathologic condition is present. We have all seen one mobile tooth splinted to one firm tooth and find that, before long, mobility has developed in the sound tooth as well.

*Periodontal prosthesis*

Splinting is generally effective therapeutically and achieves its objectives. In addition, there are positive emotional values that relate to the tightening and retention of loose teeth.

The question often is asked whether splinting interferes with the physiologic functional movements of the teeth. Remember that considerable loss of supporting structure has occurred, and even normal stresses might be too much for the supporting tissues.

*Splinting and functional stresses*

The movement of mobile teeth is not physiologic.[70] Under such conditions stress should be reduced. Splinting does not completely eliminate occlusal stress. Lateral stresses might be reduced by splinting, but vertical stresses are not eliminated. Functional stimuli exerted in the long axes of the teeth in a splint supply functional stimulation.[70] The purpose of a splint is to distribute and redirect functional and parafunctional forces to bring them within the tolerance of the supporting tissues and to eliminate mobility.

The ability of compromised teeth to support fixed bridgework is good providing the total area of attachment is equal to or greater than the occlusal area of the pontics they support.[71] Because bruxism may continue as a problem even after splinting, occlusal splints (night guards) might be necessary in some cases. Arch integrity, biomechanics, and the prosthesis itself may all be improved if tooth alignment is improved by orthodontics prior to reconstruction.[72]

Following reconstruction, abutment teeth have a greater tendency to become non-vital than do nonabutment teeth. More frequently than not, this loss of vitality is asymptomatic. Therefore measures for the prevention of caries and periodontal disease must be accompanied by check-ups on pulp vitality.[73]

Almost all splints demand an extra measure of motivation and diligence from the patient in plaque control. Splinting should be undertaken only in patients who have proved their willingness and ability to perform these measures.[74]

## REFERENCES

1. Rateitschak, K.H.: The therapeutic effect of local treatment on periodontal disease assessed upon evaluation of different diagnostic criteria, J. Periodontol. **34:**540, 1963.
2. Kegel, W., Selipsky, H., and Phillips, C.: The effect of splinting on tooth mobility. I. During initial therapy, J. Clin. Periodontal. **6:**45, 1979.
3. Kerry, C.J.: Effect of periodontal treatment on tooth mobility, J. Periodontol. **53:**635, 1982.
4. Galler, G., et al.: The effect of splinting on tooth mobility. II. After osseous surgery, J. Clin. Periodontol. **6:**317, 1979.
5. Lindhe, J., and Nyman, S.: The role of occlusion in periodontal disease and the biologic rationale for splinting in the treatment of periodontitis, Oral Sci. Rev. **10:**11, 1977.
6. Posselt, U.: Physiology of occlusion and rehabilitation, ed. 2, Philadelphia, 1969, F.A. Davis Co.
7. Gottlieb, B., and Orban, B.: Zahnfleischentzündung und Zahnlockerung, ed. 2, Berlin, 1936, Berlinische Verlagsanstalt.
8. Grieder, A., and Cinotti, W.B.: Periodontal prosthesis, St. Louis, 1968, The C.V. Mosby Co.
9. Cross, W.G.: The importance of immobilization in periodontology, Parodontologie **8:**119, 1954.
10. Simring, M., and Thaller, J.L.: Temporary splinting for mobile teeth, J. Am. Dent. Assoc. **53:**429, 1956.
11. Weinberg, L.A.: Force distribution in splinted anterior teeth, Oral Surg. **10:**484, 1268, 1957.
12. Stern, I.B.: The status of temporary fixed-splinting procedures in the treatment of periodontally involved teeth, J. Periodontol. **31:**217, 1960.
13. Amsterdam, M., and Fox, L.: Provisional splinting—principles and technics, Dent. Clin. North Am. p. 73, March 1959.
14. Hirschfeld, L.: The use of wire and silk ligatures, J. Am. Dent. Assoc. **41:**647, 1950.
15. Rothner, J.T.: Non-buckling metal ligation, J. Periodontol. **34:**437, 1963.
16. Ehrlich, P., Frisch, J., and Nedelman, C.: Hygienic esthetic anterior splinting, J. S. Calif. Dent. Assoc. **36:**225, 1968.
17. Nyman, S., and Lindhe, J.: A longitudinal study of combined periodontal and prosthetic treatment of patients with advanced periodontal disease, J. Periodontol. **50:**163, 1979.
18. Perrier, M., and Polson, A.: The effect of progressive and increasing tooth hypermobility on reduced but healthy periodontal supporting tissues, J. Periodontol. **53:**152, 1982.
19. Stoller, N.H., and Green, P.A.: A comparison of a composite restorative material and wire ligation as methods of stabilizing excessively mobile mandibular anterior teeth, J. Periodontol. **52:**451, 1981.
20. Greenfield, D.S., and Nathanson, D.: Periodontal splinting with wire and composite resin: a revised approach, J. Periodontol. **51:**465, 1980.
21. Polson, A.M., and Billen, J.R.: Temporary splinting of teeth using ultraviolet light-polymerized bonding materials, J. Am. Dent. Assoc. **89:**1137, 1974.
22. Friskopp, J., Blomlöf, L., and Söder, P.-O.: Fiberglass splints, J. Periodontol. **50:**193, 1979.
23. Schmid, M.O., Lutz, F., and Imfeld, T.: A new reinforced intracoronal composite resin splint: clinical results after one year, J. Periodontol. **50:**441, 1979.
24. Rosenberg, S.: A new method for stabilization

of periodontally involved teeth, J. Periodontol. **51:**469, 1980.

25. Block, P.L.: Wire-band splint for immobilizing loose posterior teeth, J. Periodontol. **39:**17, 1968.

26. Friedman, N.: Temporary splinting, an adjunct to periodontal therapy, J. Periodontol. **24:**229, 1953.

27. Baer, P.N., Malone, F.J., and Boyd, C.R.: A removable-fixed periodontal splint, Oral Surg. **9:**1057, 1956.

28. Krause, A.: Beitrag zur Behandlung des parodontal geschädigten Gebisses mit Kunststoff-schienen, Dtsch. Stomatol. **11:**904, 1961.

29. Waerhaug, J.: Periodontology and partial prosthesis, Int. Dent. J. **18:**101, 1968.

30. Fenner, W., Gerber, A., and Mühlemann, H.R.: Tooth mobility changes during treatment with partial denture prosthesis, J. Prosthet. Dent. **6:**520, 1956.

31. Renggli, H.H., and Schweizer, H.: Splinting of teeth with removable bridges—biological effects, J. Clin. Periodontol. **1:**43, 1974.

32. Karolyi, M.: Beobachtungen über Pyorrhea alveolaris, Oest. Ung. Vjschr. Zahnheilkd. **17:**259, 1901.

33. Gottlieb, B, and Orban, B.: Die Veränderungen der Gewebe bei übermässiger Beanspruchung der Zähne, Leipzig, 1931, George Thieme Verlag.

34. Gottlieb, B.: Schmutzpyorrhoe, Paradental-pyorrhoe und Alveolaratrophie, Berlin, 1925, Urban & Schwarzenberg.

35. Grupe, H.E., and Gromek, J.J.: Bruxism splint, J. Periodontol. **30:**156, 1959.

36. Posselt, U., and Wolff, I.-B.: Bite guards and bite plates: follow-up examination of their effect on bruxism and temporomandibular symptoms, Parodontopathies, p. 326, 1963.

37. Berliner, A.: Ligatures, splints, bite planes and pyramids, Philadelphia, 1964, J.B. Lippincott Co.

38. Friedman, H.: Perioprosthetic splinting for the geriatric patient, Quintessence Inter. **12:**805, 1981.

39. Obin, J.N., and Arvins, A.N.: The use of self-curing resin for temporary stabilization of mobile teeth due to periodontal involvement, J. Am. Dent. Assoc. **42:**320, 1951.

40. Kothe, J., and Taatz, H.: Die intrakoronale Kunststoffdraht-Schiene, Zahnaerztl. Welt **65:**426, 1964.

41. Ribbons, J.W., Pearson, G.J., and Davies, W.I.R.: Use of a composite filling material in periodontal splinting and the construction of post-crowns, Dent. Pract. **22:**316, 1972.

42. Alloy, J., and Motohiko, K.: Amalgam splints, J. Am. Dent. Assoc. **65:**381, 1962.

43. Lloyd, R.S., and Baer, P.N.: The amalgam splint, Dent. Clin. North Am., p. 213, March 1964.

44. Liatukas, E.L.: The amalgam splint, J. Periodontol. **38:**392, 1967; **41:**272, 1970.

45. Talkov, L.: Temporary acrylic fixed bridgework and splint, J. Prosthet. Dent. **2:**693, 1952.

46. Rudick, G.S.: Fabrication and duplication of a temporary acrylic resin splint, J. Prosthet. Dent. **28:**318, 1972.

47. Heintz, U.: A new type of periodontal splint to be attached to partial dentures, Dent. Abstr. **3:**425, 1958.

48. Loos, S.: Die Bedeutung der Teilprothetik für die Behandlung der Parodontose, Z. Stomatol. **45:**513, 1948.

49. Elbrecht, H.J.: Die prothetische Behandlung mit abnehmbaren Schienen. In Münch, J., editor: Die prothetische Behandlung des parodontal-geschädigten Gebisses, Munich, 1968, Banaschewski.

50. Wupper, H.: Die parodontal abgestützte Prothese, Heidelberg, 1967, Dr. Alfred Hüthig Verlag.

51. Dail, R.A., and Kopczyk, R.S.: Removable partial dentures and oral health: a literature review, Periodont. Abstr. **25:**122, 1977.

52. Gomes, B.C., et al.: A clinical study of the periodontal status of abutment teeth supporting swinglock removable partial dentures: a pilot study, J. Prosth. Dent. **46:**7, 1981.

53. Munch-Hansen, E.: The pinsplint, a removable splint fixation; a modification of von Weissenfluh's "Hülsen-Stiftschiene," J. Periodontol. **32:**322, 1961.

54. Brewer, A.A., and Morrow, R.M.: Overdentures, St. Louis, 1975, The C.V. Mosby Co.

55. Renner, R.P., et al.: Periodontal health of patients with overdentures, J. Prosthet. Dent. **51:**593, 1984.

56. Reitz, P.V., Weiner, M.G., and Levin, B.: An overdenture survey: preliminary report, J. Prosth. Dent. **37:**246, 1977.

57. Robbins, J.W.: Success of overdentures and prevention of failure, J. Am. Dent. Assoc. **100:**858, 1980.

58. Rochette, A.L.: Attachment of a splint to enamel of lower anterior teeth, J. Prosth. Dent. **30:**418, 1973.

59. Yanover, L., Croft, W., and Pulver, F.: The acid-etched fixed prosthesis, J. Am. Dent. Assoc. **104:**325, 1982.

60. Williams, V.D., et al.: Acid-etch retained cost metal prosthesis: a seven year retrospective study, J. Am. Dent. Assoc. **108:**629, 1984.

61. Levaditis, G.J.: Cast metal resin-bonded retainers for posterior teeth, J. Am. Dent. Assoc. **101:**926, 1980.

62. Burgess, J.K.: Modern attachments for bridgework and stabilizers for loose teeth, Dent. Cosmos **57:**1335, 1915.

63. Singer, H.: Der festsitzende Zahnersatz im parodontal geschädigten Lückengebiss, Dtsch. Stomatol. **11:**767, 1961.

64. Baumhammers, A.: Fixed permanent splints, J. Prosthet. Dent. **15:**351, 1965.

65. Stewart, K.L., and Rudd, K.D.: Stabilizing

periodontally weakened teeth with removable partial dentures, J. Prosthet. Dent. **19:**475, 1968.

66. Schär, E.: Die Eingliederung von Kronenschienen in Verbindung mit partiellen Prothesen bei parodontalen Erkrankungen, Parodontopathies, p. 335, 1966.

67. Gilmore, S.F.: A method of retention, J. Allied Dent. Soc. **8:**118, 1913.

68. Dolder, E.: Bar dentures, Int. Dent. J. **14:**249, 1964.

69. Preiskel, H.W.: Precision attachments in dentistry, ed. 2, St. Louis, 1973, The C.V. Mosby Co.

70. Glickman, I., Stein, R.S., and Smulow, J.B.: The effect of increased functional forces upon the periodontium of splinted and nonsplinted teeth, J. Periodontol. **32:**290, 1961.

71. Nyman, S., and Ericsson, I.: The capacity of reduced periodontal tissues to report fixed bridgework, J. Clin. Periodont. **9:**409, 1982.

72. Evans, C.A., and Nathanson, D.: Indications for orthodontic-prosthodontic collaboration in dental treatment, J. Am. Dent. Assoc. **99:**825, 1979.

73. Bergenholtz, G., and Nyman, S.: Endodontic complications following periodontal and prosthetic treatment of patients with advanced periodontal disease, J. Periodontol. **55:**63, 1984.

74. Schärer, P.: Patient motivation in periodontal prosthesis, Parodontologie **25:**60, 1971.

**ADDITIONAL SUGGESTED READING**

Lawell, L., and Lundgren, D.: Periodontal ligament areas and occlusal forces in dentitions restored with cross-arch bilateral end abutment bridges, J. Clin. Periodontol. **12:**850, 1985.

Simonsen, R.J.: Application of etched cost restorations to gerodontics, Gerodontol. **4:**2, 1985.

# CHAPTER 48

# Implants

**Osseointegration**
Indications
Surgical procedures
Prosthetic procedures
Impression procedures
Follow-up and complications
Preventive maintenance
Results

**Other implant systems**

**Case presentations**
Maxillary implant-supported full prosthesis
Mandibular partial endentulism: periodontal-osseointegration case

---

## Osseointegration

There are patients who cannot tolerate a removable prosthesis for psychologic or physiologic reasons. For others partial dentures or fixed bridges may not be possible because of the location, inadequate number, or distribution of abutment teeth.[1] Transmucosal implants have been tried for many years to circumvent these problems. No statistically supportable success rate with more than 5 years' follow-up data has been reported except for Biotes, Brånemark's "osseointegration,"[2] which now has 20 years of data.[3]

Brånemark demonstrated that bone has the ability to predictably integrate with a titanium (oxide) surface without an intervening layer of fibrous connective tissue. This makes it possible for a prosthesis to be anchored directly to living bone. Previous types of implants often resulted in the growth of fibrous tissue between the implant and the bone.[4] The presence of this "pseudoperiodontal ligament" was associated with epithelial downgrowth and pocket formation in the presence of bacterial colonization. Abscesses, loosening, and extrusion of the implant resulted.[5] This produced loss of bone at the alveolar crest and interfered with prosthetic treatment.

The Harvard conference on implants held in 1978 defined a successful implant as providing functional survival for 5 years in 75% of the cases, bone loss no greater than one third the height of the implant, mobility of less than 1 mm, gingival inflammation accessible to treatment, no infection, and no paresthesia.[6] No implant system was approved for unrestricted use since no one submitted data necessary for panel review despite this rather limited definition of success.

In September, 1985, the ADA Council on Dental Materials, Instruments, and Equipment granted provisional acceptance to the Biotes implant system for use in selected cases. The ADA stated that responsibility for proper patient selection, adequate training and experience in placement of the implant, and providing appropriate information for informed consent rests with the dentist.

## INDICATIONS

Osseointegrated oral implants should be recommended based on the findings of a preoperative analysis of the patient's physical, psychologic, and oral status. The patient should be partially or completely edentulous and, in addition, suffer from insufficient retention or other physical or social problems arising from the use of conventional removable prostheses. This may include such functional disturbances such as nausea or gagging elicited by the wearing of dentures.

For a patient to be accepted for treatment, certain criteria must be met: (1) the patient's physical status must be such as to permit an operation lasting about 2 hours under general or local anesthesia, (2) the mucosa at the site of the operation must be healthy and any extractions in the area must be thoroughly healed, because residual epithelium or granulomatous tissue could preclude osseointegration, (3) any pathology, such as periodontitis in either jaw, must have been treated with no overt infection present at the time of implant surgery, and (4) the patient must be able to maintain a good standard of oral hygiene.

Preoperative evaluation consists of the standard clinical examination and is carried out by those involved in the therapy. In certain cases a psychologic evaluation is advised. A patient who is psychotic should not be accepted for this treatment. In addition, a thorough radiographic analysis should include stent-indexed CT scans, orthopantographs, head films, and periapical radiographs. If the patient exhibits extreme resorption of the jaw, certain bone-grafting operations can be performed before implantation to augment the osseous crest at the site of fixture installation. This is, however, only necessary in rare instances.

## SURGICAL PROCEDURES

The method of anchoring a bridge in the jawbone is carried out in two phases. The first is called fixture installation, the fixture being the part of the titanium implant that is submerged endosseously. The second stage involves the exposure of the fixture and its connection to the abutment, the part of the titanium implant that protrudes through the mucosa (Figs. 48-1 and 48-2). Both procedures are performed under local anesthesia with intravenous sedation when necessary. Aseptic discipline and meticulous contamination control are necessary so that the titanium fixture is placed into bone atraumatically and immaculately clean. If the fixture touches anything, except another titanium instrument or tissues, it is discarded. The same basic operation is used in both jaws. A fully equipped hospital-type operating room with the patient as an outpatient is recommended (Fig. 48-3).

**Fixture installation**

At specifically selected sites, a combined split- and full-thickness mucosal flap is dissected and elevated with an incision in the lip mucosa about 1 cm from the vestibular

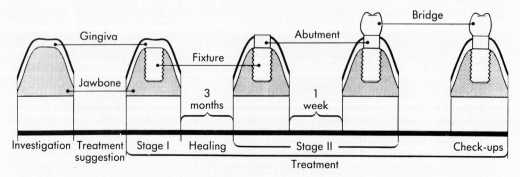

**Fig. 48-1.** Schematic representation of the different stages of the osseointegration system in intraoral applications. For the maxilla, a mean integration time of 5 months is normal. (Courtesy P.-I. Brånemark, Göteborg,)

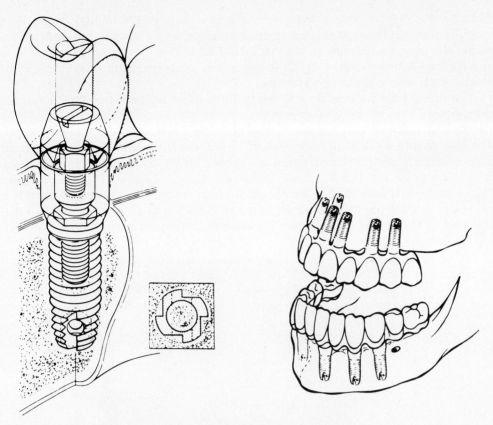

**Fig. 48-2.** Diagram of a single post, indicating the relationship with the periodontal tissues. The jaw bone corticalization increases progressively with time. The abutment passes through the soft tissues. On the right side of the drawing the bridges can be seen in a totally edentulous case, supported by five or six fixtures in between the mental foramina or maxillary sinuses. Note the cantilever bridges. (Courtesy P.-I. Brånemark, Göteborg,)

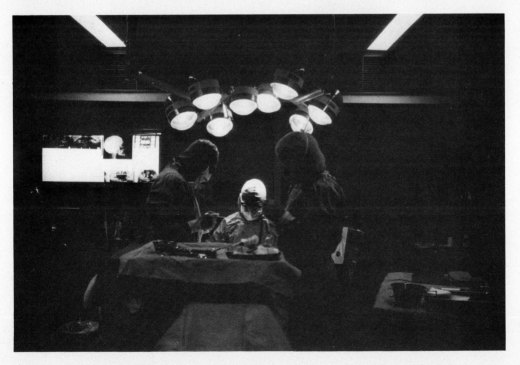

**Fig. 48-3.** The operation theater where the necessary sterility measures can be taken.

fold and the alveolar bone is exposed avoiding trauma to the mental nerve. With specially designed stainless steel spiral drills, holes are prepared with copious irrigation within the bone to the dimensions (width and length) of the fixtures (Fig. 48-4, *A* and *B*). Finally, the entrance of the fixture site is countersunk to accommodate the head of each fixture and its cover screw.

The sites for the fixtures are selected with regard to anatomic and prosthetic considerations. These sites are marked with a round bur. They are then extended with the steel spiral drills rotating at a maximum of 2000 RPM under profuse saline coolant. The sites should be at least 3.5 mm apart (7 mm center to center) to permit proper access for manipulation during surgery and later on for plaque control. Parallelism, which is not essential but is useful, is achieved with the help of direction indicators placed in the first hole(s). The fixture should extend to cortical bone and often it is necessary to go to the inferior border of the mandible or to angle the fixture so that the apex of the fixture rests on the buccal lingual internal surface of the alveolar

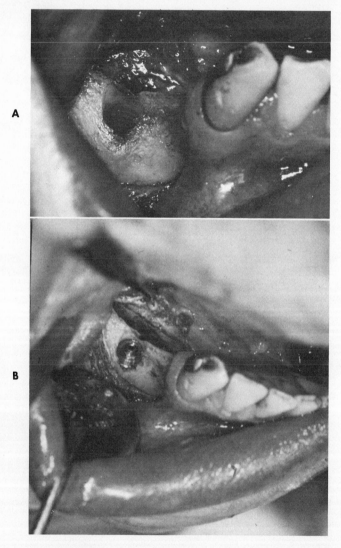

**Fig. 48-4.** **A,** The threads can clearly be seen during the fixture site preparation. **B,** A fixture is installed in this partially edentulous patient for whom no classical bridge could be provided because of the lack of a posterior abutment.

process. Normally, six fixtures are placed in between the mental foramina or in between the maxillary sinuses. A minimum of four fixtures should be used for complete edentulousness. In partial cases, the number and localizations have to be adapted to each patient individually (Figs. 48-4, *B,* and 48-5).

Once the fixture locations have been prepared, the steel instruments are set aside and a set of pure titanium instruments is used. This avoids contamination of the titanium fixtures by accidental metal ion transfer.[7] At this time a very low speed (maximum 15 RPM under profuse cooling) handpiece is used to thread the fixture

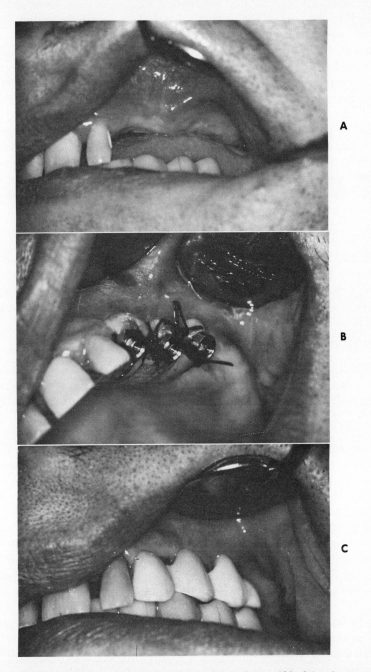

A

B

C

**Fig. 48-5.**  Another partially edentulous case after installation of three fixtures **(A)** of the abutments **(B)** of the provisional bridge **(C).**

canal with titanium tap and to install the fixture. Profuse irrigation is used because any heating above 47° C results in bone necrosis and scar tissue rather than bone repair around the fixture.[8] Once the fixtures are installed, cover screws are placed in the inner threading of the fixtures and the mucoperiosteum is carefully closed.

After a few hours of soft tissue compression by means of a gauze roll, the patient can be dismissed. An antibiotic is prescribed and the patient is restricted from using the denture during the first 2 weeks to keep from overloading the fixtures or developing fenestrations. Sutures are removed after 1 week. A special diet is prescribed.

**Fixture exposure**

Following an average healing period of 3 months for the lower and 6 months for the upper jaw, the second stage of the surgical procedure is undertaken. The cover screws are located through the gingiva rather than through the loose alveolar mucosa to obtain a better soft tissue adaptation around the abutments. An incision is made, often lingual to the abutment sites, by sounding with an explorer.

The cover screws may be partly or even completely covered by overgrowing bone. This bone must be removed so that the cover screws can be removed. The cylindric abutment can be screwed to the fixture via abutment screws if integration has been achieved. The presence of mobility indicates that fibrous tissue is interposed and that the fixture has failed to integrate. Such fixtures must be removed. The flaps are coapted and sutured. A surgical dressing is placed and retained by small healing caps or a transitional prosthesis placed on the abutments. After 1 week the sutures are removed and after a few days of further healing, the patient can be referred for prosthodontic treatment.

## PROSTHETIC PROCEDURES

Before the final prosthetic phase is undertaken, a careful reassessment must be made. During this final stage, a metallic framework is fabricated on which prosthetic teeth and a plastic base can be affixed. This prosthesis is then connected to the abutments by means of small gold screws that fit through the prosthesis. The screw holes are then sealed with an appropriate cement or plastic.

## IMPRESSION PROCEDURES

A custom tray is made with an open top so that access to the impression guide pins is possible. After the impression materials have set, each impression coping is disconnected from the abutment and the impression is removed. A working cast is poured with brass fixture analogues attached to the impression copings by reinserting the original guide pins.

Wax occlusal rims are fabricated, which are stabilized in the jaw by screwing them to the abutments. Jaw relation registrations are then obtained. A framework is cast, which connects the precision attachment precious metal cylinders. These will connect the bridge to the abutments by means of small gold screws. The teeth are set into the wax-up for a preliminary try-on. After the casting has been inspected, it is tried in the mouth of the patient to ensure that it fits precisely. The prosthetic teeth are then attached to the framework with heat-cured acrylic resin and the completed prosthesis is checked on the articulator. The prosthesis is then inserted in the mouth and attached to the abutments by the small gold screws. The occlusion is then rechecked and the patient is reinstructed in oral hygiene procedures and placed on a maintenance program.

In totally edentulous patients, a bridge of ten elements is routinely constructed and screwed on the four to six anterior abutments[3] (Figs. 48-6 and 48-7). The bridge connection system allows a divergence from parallellism for the abutments. A conversion or other transitional prosthesis can be installed while the definitive bridge is being made.[9] If only two fixtures have been installed in the lower jaw, a Hader bar or

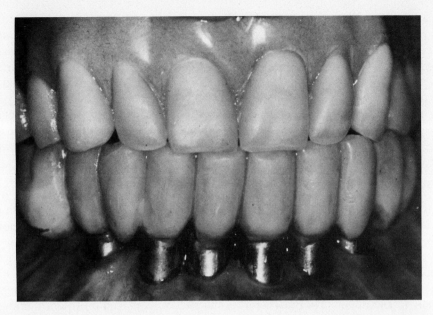

**Fig. 48-6.** A completely edentulous lower jaw, which has been rehabilitated. The esthetics are good since the lower lip always covers the abutments during normal function. Note the interproximal spaces left for an easy access for plaque control. Gingival health is present.

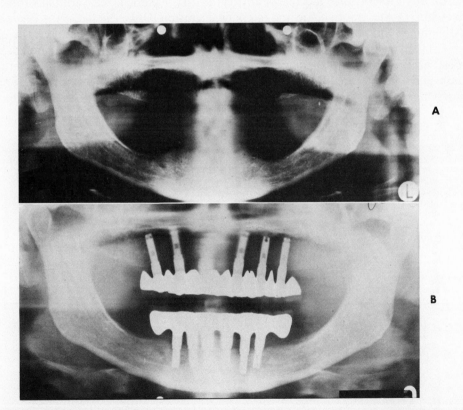

**Fig. 48-7.** Radiologic picture before **(A)** and after **(B)** installation of osseointegrated fixture-supported bridges in both upper and lower jaw.

a rare earth magnet system can be installed with an overdenture. For partially edentulous patients, the bridges can be connected with natural teeth by means of sleeve connectors so as to avoid fractures resulting from the lack of resiliency of the osseointegrated fixtures (Fig. 48-8). For this reason also, resin is used for the occlusal surfaces. Rigid connections seem to function well but long-term follow-up data is needed.

While interproximal spaces should be sufficient to permit proper plaque control, lisping or salivary spraying may occur in maxillary reconstructions if the spaces are too broad. The fixtures must be covered by the lips since they would otherwise show and are unesthetic. A removable heat-cured silicone false gingiva has been used for this problem.

### FOLLOW-UP AND COMPLICATIONS

In the immediate postoperative period there may be complications such as a transitory loss of sensation in the mental area because of injury to the nerve bundle, swelling, and hematoma. Sometimes the denture can cause a traumatic ulcer after the first surgery. This should be dealt with quickly since any communication with the oral environment can hamper the osseointegration of a fixture. At the time of the abutment installation nonintegration may be found in a small percentage of fixtures, especially in the upper jaw. Prosthetic reconstruction is placed on the remaining fixtures. Furthermore, after about one year a failed site can be used again for a new fixture installation when the bone has regenerated in the fixture socket.

### PREVENTIVE MAINTENANCE

All patients are recalled regularly for clinical and radiographic follow-up. These check-ups are scheduled repeatedly during the first year and at least annually thereafter to ensure proper oral hygiene and to check occlusion. Once the patient is treated, the osseointegration team (periodontist/oral surgeon and prosthodontist) has, in effect, undertaken a lifelong responsibility for the maintenance of the jawbone-anchored prosthesis. At each recall appointment the clinical condition of the marginal periodontium and the abutment tissues and prosthesis is determined and the presence of gingivitis, prosthetic instability, and the state of the occlusion are noted. The fixtures

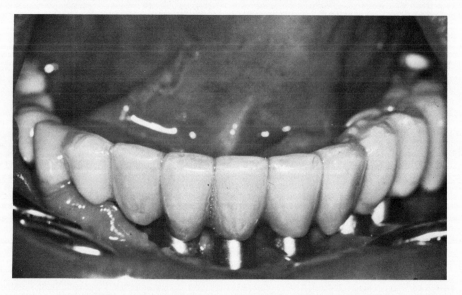

**Fig. 48-8.** A bridge made on both implanted abutments and natural teeth.

are checked annually radiographically as well, using a strictly parallel technique. This approach makes it possible to measure the marginal bone levels and to check for radiolucency around the fixture (Fig. 48-9). If necessary, oral hygiene reinstruction and minor prosthetic readjustments are done at the recall. Scraping of the titanium abutments with classic steel periodontal curettes should be avoided, because that would damage the smooth surface. Such scratches favor plaque growth. Plastic instruments are preferred. The patient should not scratch the abutments with interdental brushes.

If inflammation, significant pocket formation, or infection occurs because of plaque retention at the interface between abutments and bridge, periodontal treatment is essential. The placement of a longer abutment can be considered but the prosthesis would have to be recast. The bridge can be unscrewed for replacement of an abutment or for evaluation of fixture mobility. A fractured fixture can also be removed. The bridge can be replaced on the remaining fixtures. Four remaining fixtures can support a full prosthesis. In a partially edentulous patient with a bridge on two or three fixtures, the loss of one fixture is a more complicated problem. This often requires that a new fixture be installed.

After some 3 years there is no further need to take x-rays annually unless clinical examination indicates a need. Indeed, once integration has occurred and an equilibrium has been reached, almost no marginal bone loss will occur.[3]

## RESULTS

The Biotes osseointegration technique has been extensively investigated. More than 35,000 fixtures have been implanted in more than 9000 patients by more than 70 teams around the world. The ages of the patients range from 13 to 82 with a mean of 53 years. Some bridges have been in place for more than 20 years. A 5-year survival rate of 95% and 85% for the individual fixtures is reported for the lower and upper jaw respectively. However, as indicated above, bridges can survive even when one or two fixtures fail. Thus the survival rate is 100% and 95% *for the bridges* in the lower and upper jaw respectively over a 5- to 12-year period.[3] Results are comparable in

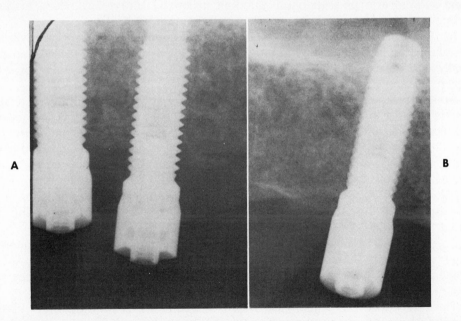

**Fig. 48-9.**   To evaluate the adaptation of bone and fixtures, proper angulation of the x-ray beam is essential. The threads should be visible as in **(A)** and not blurred as in **(B)**. (Figs. 48-3 to 48-9 courtesy D. van Steenberghe, Leuven.)

different countries.[10] However, the importance of careful technique should be stressed to avoid higher failure rates.

**Role of peri-odontics**

Because of their role in maintenance and treatment of partially edentulous patients, periodontists have played a prominent role in the placement and maintenance of implants. The Executive Council of the American Academy of Periodontology has proposed that the definition of *periodontics* be changed to read: "Periodontics is that branch of dentistry which deals with the diagnosis and treatment of the supporting and surrounding tissues of the teeth *or their substitutes and the implantation or transplantation of teeth or their substitutes.* The maintenance of the health of these structures and tissues, achieved through periodontal procedures, is also considered to be the responsibility of the periodontist. Scope shall be limited to preclude permanent restorative care."[11] Before this alteration can be finally adopted, it must be approved by the Commission on Dental Accreditation of the American Dental Association Council on Dental Education. However, periodontists are increasingly involved in implantology, particularly when the system permits the restoration of function and the retention of teeth that otherwise might have been removed. The osseointegration technique has a very high predictability and meets and surpasses the NIH requirement.[6]

## Other implant systems

Osseointegration is a prerequisite for long-term survival of permucosal oral implants. It can be predictably achieved by using the principles defined by Brånemark. Whether the high success rate obtained is bound to the use of a particular material (pure titanium) remains to be demonstrated. Some other hardware systems can achieve osseointegration when the previously mentioned biologic principles are respected. So far, however, high success rates with a satisfying statistical analysis have not been reported for these other systems.

These other systems can be grouped according to material and design: aluminum oxides, hydroxylapatite sprayed on titanium, titanium alloys, pure titanium, titanium flame sprayed over pure titanium, titanium hollow basket-type cylinders, titanium plasma sprayed over screw-type titanium, and titanium blades.

**Aluminum oxide**

In 1972, a Japanese patent was obtained for an aluminum oxide sapphire cylindric crystal root implant called *Bioceram*. It is a one-piece system that is placed transmucosally at the initial surgical visit.[12-15] It is reported to be more biocompatible than other implant materials.

In 1976, a German $Al_2O_3$ implant called *Tuebingen*[16-17] was reported. Its claims include that it can be placed in post-extraction sockets and that it may be prepared with conventional instruments to act like a tooth and thus be esthetic anteriorly. In a case described by Schulte[16] it would seem that a very long junctional epithelium resulted following anterior implant placement in extraction sockets where previously very deep pockets were present.

**Hydroxylapa-tite tricalcium phosphate**

Integral and Neodontics are two-part systems of hydroxylapatite or tricalcium phosphate sprayed over titanium.[18-21] The basic biology of both systems is promising, but neither has provided adequate sequential data.

**Titanium alloys**

Core-Vent and Titanodont are titanium alloys.[22] They have not published sequential results and refer to Brånemark's and associates' data in their advertisements. Anecedotal case reports are made but their success will ultimately be judged by acceptable data.

**Flame plasma sprayed over titanium**

The IMZ system[23] is flame plasma sprayed titanium over pure titanium. Plasma spraying titanium increases the surface area of the oxide layer. It is also claimed that it roughens the surface. Provisional data seem positive but further documentation studies on consecutive implants are needed.

The ITI is a hollow basket-type cylinder implant with design features[24] somewhat similar to Core-Vent. The TPS system is a screw-type implant with plasma-sprayed titanium over titanium.[25-27] The 5-year data for the ITT seem to be better than the criteria set by the Harvard consensus.

Blades have been part of the implant scene for 30 years or more. Fibrous encapsulation, infectious perioimplantitis, and the loss of large amounts of bone often occur (Fig. 48-10, *A* and *B*). While some blades have been noted to have long-term longevity, there are no sequential studies to document their predictable success.   **Blades**

Blades fail for a number of complex reasons:

1. Inadequate congruity of bone and implant at the time of surgical insertion
2. Improper biomaterials
3. Contamination of the implant surfaces and infection
4. Surgical overheating of bone with high speed instrumentation
5. Structural design that does not transmit forces evenly to the bone

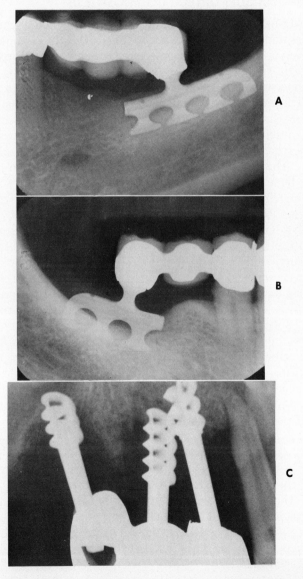

**Fig. 48-10.   A** and **B,** Examples of nonintegrated blade implants are shown with the radiolucency clearly indicating periodontal breakdown. **C,** Breakdown of an older type of implant with threads and central vent.

6. Premature loading with occlusal forces during the healing phase
7. Transmucosal penetration at the time of implant insertion

There were other early systems that resulted in bone loss (Fig. 48-10, C) and were abandoned. As implantology developed, redesigned implants and new materials were frequently introduced.

Some implants such as the Biotes successfully support bridgework, a denture, or an overdenture. Others appear to require the support of a fixed bridge to be retained.

## Case presentations

We shall now present two cases, one concerning maxillary full prosthesis and one concerning a mandibular partial prosthesis.

### MAXILLARY IMPLANT-SUPPORTED FULL PROSTHESIS

A 32-year-old single female with maxillary edentulism had 9 years of anxiety related to this body loss and was constantly preoccupied with the thought that her "defect" would be discovered. The anxiety had interfered with her social functioning. She sought to have an implant-supported prosthesis.

The evaluation was performed by a team: a prosthodontist, periodontist, and psychotherapist. The evaluation was assisted by orthopantographs, stent-indexed CT scans,[28] and the usual other radiographs and records. A new complete denture was fabricated that closely approximated the anticipated final tooth position. It was duplicated in clear acrylic. Gutta-percha cones were affixed to the cingula and central fossa (Fig. 48-11, A). This served as a radiopaque reference guide on the CT scans (Fig. 48-11, B). The bone location and height was measured on the scan and the fixture location corresponding to the above was marked on the stent. The maxillary left bicuspid scan demonstrated that the osseous anatomy allowed only for the placement of a fixture with a severe labial angulation. The anterior palatal aspect of the stent was removed up to the second bicuspid to provide room for flap displacement and the positioning of surgical drills (Fig. 48-11, C). Using the Brånemark Biotes system[3] six fixtures were inserted (Fig. 48-11, E), five in alignment with the cingula and occlusal fossa, and the left terminal fixture with a severe labial tilt. An effort was made to place the longest fixtures consistent with anatomy, the goal being to rest the fixture apex on the cortical bone of the floor of the nose. It is not uncommon to slightly penetrate the sinus or nasal floor; neither appears to be a problem if the fixture is immobile. Titanium cover screws were inserted into the fixtures and the surgical site closed with 000 nylon sutures (Fig. 48-11, F). The sutures were removed in 1 week and the denture relieved and relined at the second week.

Following a 6-month period while the fixtures were left covered and unloaded, the fixtures were exposed, the cover screws removed, and titanium transepithelial abutments screwed to place. The fixtures were tested physically and radiographically and for immobility. A 12-unit fixed prosthesis was fabricated (Figs. 48-11, G and H). As predetermined in the stent, five of the six fixture points coincided with the tooth alignment and the left terminal fixture exited within the labial "gingival" acrylic of the prosthesis. The gingiva about the abutments is now healthy and free of inflammation and pocket depth (Fig. 48-11, I). The patient says it feels like her natural dentition and claims to have benefitted dentally and psychologically, with a new sense of self-confidence. She no longer is anxious about discovery of her "defect" but talks about it in a relaxed manner.

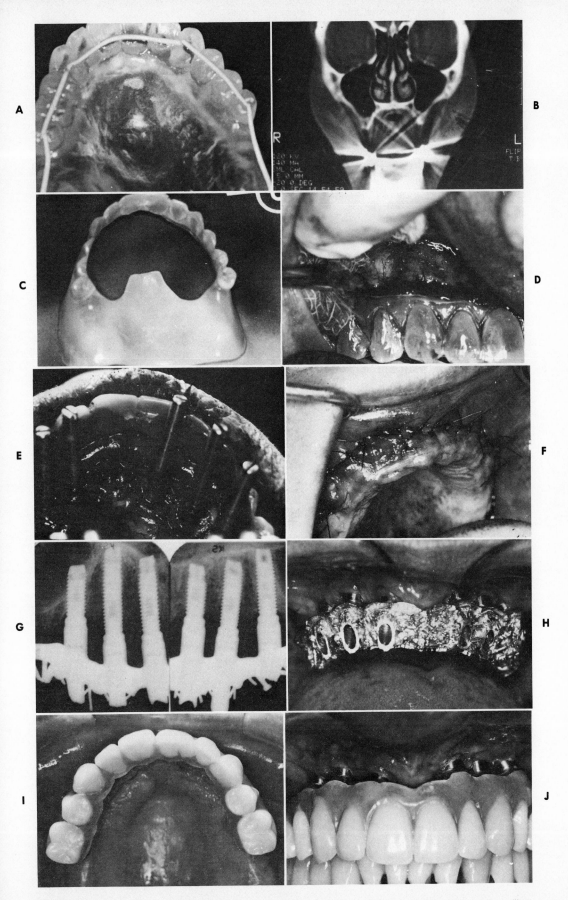

**Fig. 48-11.** **A** to **J,** A Brånemark Biotes system of implants successfully osseointegrated, supporting a full maxillary prosthesis. (Courtesy C. Berman, R. Jaffin, C. Kopp, L. Berman, and L. Marotta.)

## MANDIBULAR PARTIAL EDENTULISM: PERIODONTAL-OSSEOINTEGRATION CASE

A 65-year-old single male was referred for periodontal treatment of a deep pocket on the distal side of tooth number 27 (Fig. 48-12, A). He was edentulous except for teeth numbers 27, 28, and 29 (Fig. 48-12, B). An interview revealed that the impending and previous loss of teeth represented a significant psychologic threat; he actually looked forward to a second chance with respect to periodontal treatment and the associated natural tooth and implant-supported fixed partial prosthesis.

The pocket on the distal surface of tooth number 27 was treated periodontally and a hydroxylapatite graft placed. At the time of fixture implant surgery, soft tissue attachment was present (Fig 48-12, C).

Before implant fixture placement, a team evaluated the patient. Three 13-mm by 3.7-mm fixtures were placed in the position of teeth numbers 22, 23, 25 (Fig. 48-12, D), and a 10-mm by 3.75-mm fixture was placed in the position of tooth 21. The apex of that fixture was tipped anteriorly to avoid impingement on the mental canal.

A second-stage transepithelial abutment surgery was performed 4 months later. Coping crowns were then fabricated and cemented on 27, 28, and 29 (Fig. 48-12, E). A removable precision attachment fixed prothesis was then inserted that had three gold coping and four precision cylinders (Fig. 48-12, F). The bridge was attached to the Brånemark abutments by the means of gold screws. No cement was used under the bridge copings (Figs. 48-12, G and H).

The titanium transepithelial abutments were placed lingual to the mandibular incisors so that the screws exited on the lingual of the lower incisors (Fig. 48-12, F). The esthetic result was very good (Fig. 48-12, G). Hygiene was maintained with a proximal brush under the copings and abutments and a 3-month prophylaxis. Prophylaxis is done with a jet prophylaxis unit and plastic scalers so that the titanium abutments are not scratched with steel instruments (Fig. 48-12, H).

The pre- and postoperative radiographs represent the therapeutic result (Fig. 48-12, A, I, and J). The radiographic appearance of the bone about the fixtures is normal and there is no radiolucent zone that would indicate the presence of a fibrous capsule. There is no mobility, and the patient has the feeling of his original teeth.

Psychologically and physiologically, the treatment represented a new beginning for the patient, who had suffered from discomfort and disappointment produced by dental and periodontal disease all his life.

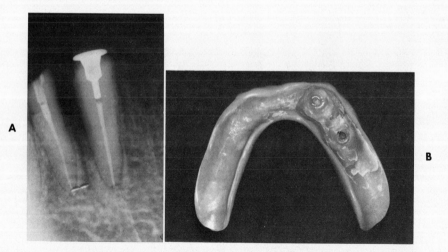

**Fig. 48-12. A** to **J,** A Brånemark Biotes system of implants successfully osseointegrated, supporting a partial mandibular prosthesis. (Courtesy G. Barrack, C. Berman, R. Jaffin, L. Berman and L. Marotta.)

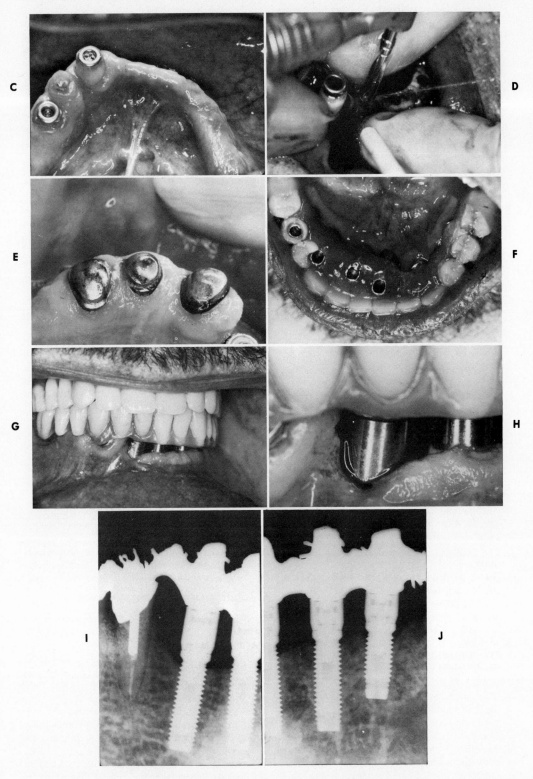

**Fig. 48-12, cont'd.** For legend, see opposite page.

## REFERENCES

1. Glantz, P.O., and Nyman, S.: Technical and biophysical aspects of crown and bridge therapy in patients with reduced amounts of periodontal tissue support. In Lindhe, J., editor: Textbook of Clinical Periodontology. Copenhagen, 1983, Munksgaard Co.
2. Brånemark, P.-I. Osseointegration and its experimental background, J. Prosthet. Dent. **50:**399, 1983.
3. Brånemark, P.-I., Zarb, G.A., and Albrektsson, T.: Tissue-integrated prostheses. Chicago, 1985, Quintessence Publishing Co.
4. Babbush, C.A.: Endosseous blade-vent implants: a research review, Oral Implantol. **3:**261, 1973.
5. Smithloff, M., and Fritz, M.E.: The use of blade implants in a selected population of partially edentulous adults, J. Periodontol. **47:**19, 1976.
6. Schnittman, P.A., and Shulman, L.B.: Recommendations of the consensus development conference on dental implants, J. Am. Dent. Assoc. **98:**373, 1979.
7. Kasemo, B., and Lausmaa, J.: Preparation and characterisation of titanium implant surfaces. In Steenberghe, D. van, editor: Tissue integration in oral and maxillo-facial reconstruction, Amsterdam, 1986, Elsevier Science Publication.
8. Eriksson, R.A., and Albrektsson, T.: The effect of heat on bone regeneration, J. Oral Maxillofac. Surg. **42:**705, 1984.
9. Balshi, T.J.: The conversion prosthesis: a provisional fixed prosthesis supported by osseointegrated titanium fixtures. In Steenberghe, D. van, editor: Tissue integration in oral and maxillo-facial reconstruction, Amsterdam, 1986, Elsevier Science Publication.
10. Steenberghe, D. van, Verbist, D., and Calberson, L.: A two and a half year follow-up report on osseointegrated fixture supported bridges and dentures, J. Head Neck Pathol. **4:**108, 1985.
11. American Academy of Periodontology News 20, No. **2:**1, 1985.
12. Yamane, T., et al.: Fundamental and clinical studies on endosseous implant of new sapphire material, J. Oral. Implantol. **8:**232, 1979.
13. McKinney, R.V., Jr., Steflik, D.E., and Koth, D.L.: Ultrastructural surface topography of the single crystal sapphire endosseous dental implant, J. Oral Implantol. **11:**327, 1983-84.
14. Mishima, A., Yamane, T., and Yamanovchi, H.: Alpha alumina sapphire implant: clinical development and its historical background, J. Oral Implantol. **11:**516, 1983.
15. Akagawa, Y., et al.: Tissue reaction to implanted biomaterials, J. Prosthet. Dent. **53:**681, 1985.
16. Schulte, W.: The intraosseous $Al_2O_3$ (Frialit) Tuebingen implant: developmental status af-

ter eight years (I), Quintessence Inter. **12:**1, 1984, Report 2267.
17. Helmeke, G., et al.: Generalization of biomechanical rules for the fixation of bone, joint, and tooth replacements, J. Biomed. Mat. Res. **14:**537, 1980.
18. Tracy, B.M., and Doremues, R.H.: Direct electron microscopy studies of the bone-hydroxlapatite interface, J. Biomed. Mat. Res. **18:**719, 1984.
19. Denissen, H., et al.: Dense apatite implants: the bonding to alveolar bone, Implantologist **2:**56, 1981.
20. Denissen, H., et al.: The interface of permucosal dense apatite ceramic implants in humans, J. Biomed. Mat. Res. **18:**147, 1984.
21. Ducheyne, P., et al.: Effect of hydroxylapatite impregnation on skeletal bonding of porous coated implants, J. Biomed. Mat. Res. **14:**225, 1980.
22. Hahn, J.: Clinical experience with the Titanodont subcortical implant system, J. Oral Implantol. **11:**72, 1983-84.
23. Kirsch, A.: The two-phase implantation method using IMZ intramobile cylinder implants, J. Oral Implantol. **11:**197, 1983.
24. Sutter, F., Schroeder, A., and Straumann, P.: ITI hollow cylinder system principles and methodology, J. Oral Implantol. **11:**166, 1983.
25. Babbush, C.A.: Titanium plasma spray screw implant system for reconstruction of the edentulous mandible, Dent. Clin. North Am. 117, 1986.
26. Schroeder, A., et al.: The reactions of bone, connective tissue, and epithelium to endosteal implants with titanium sprayed surfaces, J. Max. Surg. **9:**15, 1981.
27. Ledermann, P.: Titanium-coated screw implants as alloplastic endosteal retention elements in the edentulous problematic mandible, (I) & (II), Quintessence Inter. **12:**895, 1981.
28. Kopp, C.D.: Stent-assisted CT in three phases of osseointegration, Acad. Osseointegration Vols. 1, 2, Winter, 1985.

## ADDITIONAL SUGGESTED READINGS

Adell, R., et al.: A 15-year study of osseointegrated implants in the treatment of the edentulous jaw, Int. J. Oral Surg. **10:**387, 1981.

Albrektsson, T., et al.: The long-term efficacy of currently used dental materials: a review and proposed criteria of success, Int. J. Oral Max. Implants **1:**11, 1986.

Ericcson, I., et al.: A clinical evaluation of fixed-bridge restorations supported by a combination of teeth and osseo-integrated titanium implants, J. Clin. Periodontol. **13:**307, 1986.

Ingber, A.: The osseointegration implant system and its influence upon occlusal design, Alpha Omegan **78:**73, 1985.

Koth, D., McKinney, R., and Steflik, D.E.: The single crystal sapphire endosseous dental implant. III. Preliminary human clinical trials, J. Oral Implantol. **11:**10, 1983-84.

Laney, W.R., et al.: Dental implants: tissue-integrated prosthesis utilizing the osseointegration concept, Mayo Clinic Proc. **61:**91, 1986.

McKinney, R., Jr., and Koth, D.: The single crystal sapphire endosteal dental implant: material characteristic and 18-month experimental animal trials, J. Prosthet. Dent. **47:**69, 1982.

Piecuch, J., et al.: Experimental ridge augmentation with porous replamineform hydroxylapatite, J. Biomed. Mat. Res. **18:**39, 1984.

Steenberghe, D. van, editor: Tissue integration in oral and maxillo-facial reconstruction, Amsterdam, 1986, Elsevier Science Publication.

Sullivan, D.Y.: Prosthetic considerations for the utilization of osseointegrated fixtures in the partially edentulous arch, Internat. J. Oral Max. Implants **1:**39, 1986.

Symington, J.M., et al.: Applications of osseointegrated implants: a preliminary report on 35 cases, J. Can. Dent. Assoc. **52:**139, 1986.

Verbist, D., Steenberghe, D. van, and Coppes, L.: The applicability of the osseointegration principle in edentulous people, J. Head Neck Path. **1:**128, 1982.

# PART EIGHT

## Maintenance

# CHAPTER 49

# The treated patient: maintenance and expectations; clinical trials; retrospective studies

**Reevaluation**
Pocket depths
Mobility
Restorative procedures
Tissue color, texture, and form
Oral hygiene
Roentgenograms and pulp testing
Conclusion

**Maintenance phase**
Extended transitional treatment
Use of auxiliaries
Recall examination
Treatment by a periodontist
Retreatment
Degree of success

**Concept of cure**
Illustrative cases
Comparative studies of surgical and nonsurgical treatment

**Retrospective studies**
Loss of questionable teeth
Loss of teeth with furcation involvement
Loss of nonfurcated questionable teeth
Findings
Conclusion

**Reliability of diagnostic methods**

**Summary**

---

Treatment of most periodontal diseases, particularly periodontitis, can be divided into two main phases. The first phase, which may last from a few weeks to several months, is the *corrective phase* of therapy. Its aim is to restore the periodontal status to one that is relatively free of inflammation and readily maintainable in a healthy state by the combined care of the patient and the therapist. The second phase is the *maintenance phase*, intended to prevent or minimize the recurrence of periodontal disease by controlling factors known to contribute to the disease process.

## Reevaluation

On completion of the active phase of periodontal treatment, the patient should be reexamined and reevaluated to make sure that optimal health has been established before proceeding with sequential dental treatment or discharge. The reexamination should include recharting for probing (pocket) depths, attachment levels, and tooth mobility; notation of tissue color, texture, form, and tooth hypersensitivity; occlusal stability; and evaluation of the patient's ability to perform oral hygiene adequately. Roentgenograms and pulp testing may also be included. Record the findings on the initial examination chart in a different-colored ink or on a separate chart. A comparison of pretreatment and posttreatment chartings will permit you to evaluate the effectiveness of treatment. The patient's periodontal health would include firm teeth, shallow sulci free of bleeding or exudate, with tooth and occlusal stability. An impression of the posttreatment prognosis for both the short and long term can be gained from the patient's response to treatment and past history. The restorative treatment plan can be finalized and the posttreatment maintenance schedule established.

## POCKET DEPTHS

Posttreatment sulcular probing depths should be minimal, perhaps not to exceed 3 mm.[1,2] If residual pocket depth exists, the involved areas should be retreated. Exceptions to this rule may be made in patients in whom physical or emotional status, advanced age, or extrinsic anatomic considerations make complete pocket elimination unfeasible. In some advanced cases of periodontal disease, total elimination of probing depth may not be possible. In these instances, however, other criteria for gingival health should be met and the objective of treatment might be to prolong the life of the dentition.

In some patients deep pockets may be maintainable, and in other patients deep pockets are indicative of recurrent disease. Although the establishment of ideal periodontal health is the therapeutic goal, even a reduction in inflammation in some cases may have the potential to prolong tooth longevity though residual pockets may persist.[3,4]

## MOBILITY

Tooth mobility is often, but not always, reduced by treatment. Sometimes moderate or advanced looseness may remain unchanged.[5,6] Note the extent of mobility with due regard for the transient mobility that sometimes follows surgery. Continuing mobility of class 2 or more or progressive mobility may be an indication for splinting.

## RESTORATIVE PROCEDURES

The patient should be reevaluated for restorative procedures such as permanent splinting, replacement of missing teeth, or individual restorations. In some patients it is imperative that restorative dentistry be done as soon as possible after completion of periodontal therapy to reestablish the form and function of the masticatory system. In others it is wise to defer operative dentistry, so that a longer evaluation of response to treatment can be made. This is especially true when teeth with questionable prognoses must be incorporated as abutment teeth in a prosthesis.

The patient should be advised of the possible need for splinting or extensive restorative programs at the time of the original treatment plan consultation. There is rarely justification for such a need to come as a surprise to the patient at the end of treatment. The indications for splinting are usually evident at the time of the initial examination. Moreover, the patient has a right to understand the total extent of expenses before treatment. On the other hand, if the properly informed patient procrastinates when the time for splinting arrives, you may be required to assume a firm role so that the results of treatment are not forfeited. Nevertheless, the final decision is the patient's.

## TISSUE COLOR, TEXTURE, AND FORM

After the completion of periodontal therapy, the gingiva should be pink, firm, and securely attached to the teeth. Stippling, which varies between individuals and in its distribution in the gingiva, may be lost after surgery and then gradually reappear over a period of several months. The gingival margins should be thin and should taper to the teeth. The interdental papillae should be cone shaped and the gingiva festooned when viewed from the facial or buccal aspect of the teeth. Thick and irregular margins and poor papillary contour tend to favor plaque retention and recurrent pocket formation. Gingival grafts should be smooth and blend imperceptibly with the host gingiva.

Examine the proximity of the frenum, muscle attachments, vestibular fornix, and sublingual space to the gingival margin, because marginal surgery may inadvertently create positional relationships that are potentially harmful. A wide zone of gingiva in all areas is no longer considered mandatory to maintain gingival health,[7] but there are situations when firm "attached" gingiva appears to be necessary for adequate plaque control without tissue abrasion, and possibly to prevent gingival recession from continuing. The presence of gingiva seems to be particularly important when restorations extend into the gingival sulcus.[8]

### ORAL HYGIENE

Determine the effectiveness of the patient's oral hygiene by examining the teeth and tissues for debris, inflammation, and exudate. Take a plaque score and observe the patient's routine in plaque control. Some patients lack dexterity; others lack motivation.[9,10] In addition, gingival margins may have been positioned apically, and embrasure spaces opened. Splints or other forms of prostheses may be present. These factors all tend to make oral hygiene more difficult to perform as the need for it is increased. If any part of the oral hygiene procedure is not performed well, further instruction or a change in the prescribed procedures may be advisable. A patient who is not proficient in oral hygiene should not be dismissed from treatment because studies have indicated that gingival attachment levels can be maintained with regular professional care (scaling and plaque control) at very frequent intervals.[4,11-14]

### ROENTGENOGRAMS AND PULP TESTING

When periodontal treatment is to be followed by other forms of dentistry or the treatment period has been unusually long, retake roentgenograms. Observation of caries status and bone levels is then possible. In addition, test the vitality of pulps. The findings of these procedures can be compared with earlier findings to determine the prosthetic prognosis and to finalize the restorative treatment plan. The findings also serve as a record against which future changes can be measured.

If, on the other hand, the patient is to be discharged without further treatment, roentgenograms need not be taken for at least 2 years. Thereafter, full-mouth periodontal roentgenograms may be taken at regular intervals, between 3 and 5 years. Bite wings may be taken at more frequent intervals.

### CONCLUSION

The posttreatment examination will usually indicate that the treatment has been carried to a successful completion. Explain to the patient the gains of treatment and the importance of maintaining these gains.[15] Then place the patient on a maintenance schedule, and enter the record in the recall system.

When the examination reveals areas that have not been resolved to your complete satisfaction, these areas should be retreated if further treatment can remedy the situation. If, because of local anatomic factors or the physical or mental status of the patient, retreatment would be fruitless or damaging, you may have to regard the case as complete. Treatment is complete when a result that is optimal for the patient has been reached.

If transitional maintenance procedures, periodontal retreatment, or other dentistry are undertaken, reevaluation should be performed after their completion.

## Maintenance phase

Where destruction from disease has been extensive or when results of treatment are less than optimal, transitional procedures are indicated following active treatment. The treated patient is recalled at 2-week intervals for a "professional cleaning,"[4,16]

**Transitional maintenance**

which includes staining the mouth for plaque, showing the patient the areas neglected, and having the patient remove the plaque with an appropriate implement. The dentist or hygienist then carefully polishes the teeth with fine Silex. After several such visits, the time between appointments is extended. Two objectives are gained by transitional treatment: (1) the patient's oral hygiene technique is perfected and its importance is reemphasized, and (2) newly healed tissues are kept plaque free for several weeks, which improves the clinical response.[4,16-20]

## EXTENDED TRANSITIONAL TREATMENT

Certain situations call for an extended transitional phase. The patient who is to undergo orthodontic therapy after periodontal treatment should be seen frequently for polishing and scaling. Bone grafts or reattachment sites should be seen every other month or more frequently so that the involved area can be planed and curetted (Fig. 49-1). Patients undergoing involved restorative programs should be seen frequently

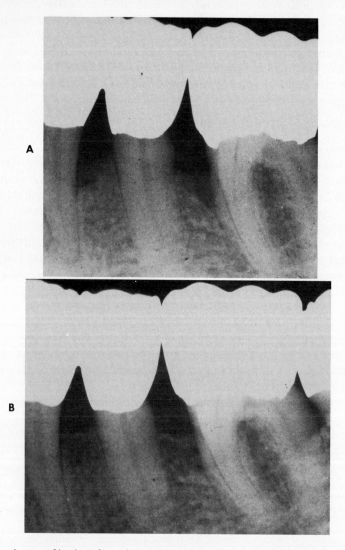

**Fig. 49-1.** When bone grafting is performed, the patient is placed in a transitional maintenance category initially. Débridement may be performed at 2-week intervals for 2 months, then monthly for 2 months. The patient is then placed on a 3-month maintenance schedule. **A,** Preoperative roentgenogram. **B,** Roentgenogram taken 1 year later. (Courtesy R. Chace, Winter Park, Florida.)

for polishing, scaling, and light curettage. A postrestorative appointment is necessary to check the periodontal status.

With the completion of all dental treatment, the state of dental health should be optimal. The expectation that the patient will continue at this level however, may not be completely realistic.[20,21] Germ-induced periodontal disease has a tendency to recur. The state of health can be modified with the passage of time by the various extrinsic and intrinsic changes that occur during the stages of a lifetime.

It is generally recognized that, in spite of the refinement of techniques of pocket elimination, some patients who have been treated for moderate or advanced periodontal disease may develop recurrences typically characterized by increased probing depth about individual teeth and at localized sites.[20] Often teeth with questionable long-term prognoses are provisionally retained. Occasionally entire dentitions with extremely advanced periodontal disease are treated when no possibility exists of completely eliminating pockets. Such compromise cases make the maintenance of periodontal health more difficult than the moderately involved case (Fig. 49-2). You and the patient should, by continued cooperative effort, seek to minimize detrimental changes to provide the patient with a healthy, functional dentition for life. The importance of excellent oral hygiene cannot be overemphasized. By diligent and successful plaque control, patients may retain in good health teeth that once had a doubtful prognosis. This requires proper and diligent habits on the part of the patient, as well as seeking out and obtaining proper and adequate dental care that is periodontally oriented.[15,21-25] To maintain periodontal health, *maintenance,* therapy must be continued indefinitely.[26-28]

**Teeth with questionable prognosis**

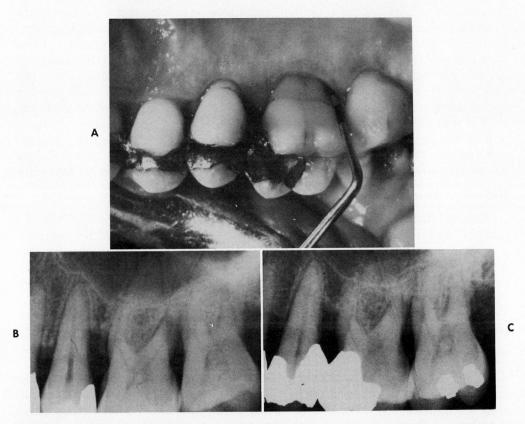

**Fig. 49-2.** Teeth with questionable prognoses are sometimes retained for many years. **A,** Maxillary molars with pocket depths of 6 mm and furcation invasion. **B,** Roentgenogram, 1963, **C,** Roentgenogram, 1977. (Courtesy R. Chace, Winter Park, Florida.)

Such care, consisting of periodic reexamination, preventive maintenance, and treatment, is successful in providing long-term periodontal health.[26-28] The arrangement that provides for notification and appointment of the patient for such purposes is known as the *recall system.*

**Recall system**

Each practice must have an effective recall system. When a patient misses a recall appointment, the receptionist must make every effort to reappoint as soon as possible. It is easy for any patient to delay a recall visit. The attitude of the receptionist is an important factor in stressing the necessity for maintenance. If every member of the office staff is imbued with the concept of preventive oral health care, the patient cannot fail to be impressed and motivated.

Treatment therefore consists of two phases: active treatment for the interception and cure of the disease process and periodic observation, supervision, and treatment calculated to prevent recurrence. The latter phase, often called *preventive maintenance,* will now be discussed.[11,24,29,30]

**Preventive maintenance**

The first year after treatment is a critical period, because the patient has already demonstrated susceptibility to periodontal disease, the causes of which tend to be persistent and recurrent. Moreover, oral hygiene habits are difficult to learn and unlearn. After periodontal treatment the first recall visit should be scheduled at 3 months. Longitudinal studies indicate that this is the desirable period for individuals susceptible to periodontal disease.[27,29,31-33] With excellent plaque control and maintenance of periodontal health, the interval may be occasionally lengthened to 4 or 6 months or longer. The frequency of visits should depend on the patient's ability and performance in home dental care, the clinical condition of the tissues, the rate of calculus deposition, and the presence of bleeding, inflammation, and increased probing depth.[33] Examine the patient frequently enough to prevent or intercept disease processes before they cause irreversible damage. In time, changes in the dental, psychologic, or intrinsic status of the patient may occur and completely alter the established equilibrium. In this regard, old causative factors may recur, or new ones may develop. Caries, particularly root caries, can be a vexing problem. Alterations may occur in bone level, tooth mobility, pocket depth, or number of teeth remaining in the mouth. Finally, acute conditions such as necrotizing ulcerative gingivitis, pericoronitis, periodontal abscess, pulpitis, or traumatic injury can occur with rapidity. The patient, of course, should return for treatment if any sign of disease becomes apparent. However, since signs of disease are not obvious to the patient, your careful observation and supervision are necessary.

## USE OF AUXILIARIES

Specially trained hygienists may be employed in maintenance of treated periodontal patients. Such hygienists must receive special training in periodontal screening examination, in instrumentation, and in knowledge of periodontics so that they can assume the role of preventive therapists. Even veteran hygienists need considerable extra training unless their experience has been with treatment and maintenance care of periodontal patients.

Periodontal assistants can also be trained to be preventive dental assistants, competent in plaque control instruction and x-ray technique.

## RECALL EXAMINATION

A typical appointment would begin with a short interview with the patient. Make inquiries as to any discomfort or dental treatment received since the patient was last seen and any changes in the patient's health or medications. A patient might forget to inform the dentist of serious health problems that have arisen since the last appointment unless questioned. Also record any important event in the patient's personal life. Patients appreciate such interest. An oral examination should follow.

Reexamine the patient at every recall. Note changes in probing depth on a recall chart at every recall visit. Routine complete chartings may be done every 12 to 24 months or more frequently if necessary. Make dated notations with a different-colored ink on the same chart or make a new chart. You will then be able to compare chartings with ease. Changes in numbers of pockets and probing depths should be noted. These and other tallies of mobility, caries, and extractions can be compared on an Examination Synopsis Sheet (see Fig. 28-22).

The recall examination should include the following:

1. Inspection of the oral cavity for neoplasms
2. Examination for caries
3. Reappraisal of tooth mobility
4. Examination of probing depths, attachment levels, and bleeding points
5. Checking of tissue color, consistency, and architecture
6. Evaluation of oral hygiene procedures
7. Examination of the occlusion
8. Testing of pulp vitality where indicated
9. Noting bone levels in sequential radiographs

You may need roentgenograms to properly perform the examination. Take a full-mouth series every third to fifth year. In addition, remember to remove all temporary splints (i.e., wire splints) and all temporarily cemented permanent splints to fully examine the covered teeth.

Every recall examination results in a diagnosis and reappraisal of the patient's condition, from which you may draw conclusions concerning the prognosis of the patient's dental health, the need for retreatment, and the choice of the time interval between maintenance appointments.

A dental hygienist may chart or make a periodontal screening examination, instruct in oral hygiene, perform root planing, and treat root sensitivity. However, the dentist must make the definitive examination, reexamine for deposits, and perform corrective occlusal adjustment or surgical retreatment where indicated.

**Recall treatment**

Unless the patient has an acute problem, attend first to the status of oral hygiene. If needed, give new instruction in plaque control. Using the chart, perform a light scaling, root planing, and gingival curettage wherever these are indicated. During the instrumentation, note the tone of the marginal gingiva if bleeding was encountered on probing and scaling. Note areas requiring extra attention. It is important that a record be made at each recall appointment so that changes from the baseline record are documented. An increase in sulcus depth or mobility is an alert to the dentist.

Scale the rest of the mouth and plane subgingival areas with fine, sharp curettes. When any roughness is encountered, plane it to an acceptable smoothness. At present, glasslike smoothness of the root surface is the only way the clinician can know that the surface has been cleansed. Smoothness of the root is important because it is the main indication that plaque and calculus have been removed. Polish the teeth with a fine, nonabrasive paste, and treat any area of sensitivity. Give the caries-susceptible patient a fluoride treatment or prescribe fluoride gel.

**Well-maintained periodontal health**

When the patient's periodontal condition has been maintained satisfactorily, all that is required is to remove deposits, smooth root surfaces, and polish the clinical crowns of the teeth. Cleanse and reinsert, as indicated, splints that have been removed. On occasion, minor occlusal alterations may be required.

**Evaluation of status of periodontal health**

A decision can now be made on the prognosis of the case. Does the patient need additional plaque control instruction? Is additional root planing or other treatment necessary? Should recall intervals be maintained at current intervals or be extended or shortened?

When recall procedures have been accomplished,[11,16,23,30,31] inform the patient of his/her current dental health status. This reappraisal, which concludes the appointment, serves to remind the patient of the necessity of continued supervision, and it stimulates dental cooperation in plaque control in the interim until the next recall. The patient should then be dismissed and the record reentered in the recall system.

## TREATMENT BY A PERIODONTIST

The general dentist may have referred the patient to a periodontist for treatment. On occasion after such treatment the periodontist may suggest maintaining the patient because of the severity of destruction or because of special problems that may exist, such as poor compliance with plaque control measures. On other occasions the periodontist may suggest sharing in the recall program with the general dentist. Patients who have had a mild involvement should be returned to the general dentist for maintenance.

**Transfer patients**

In our mobile society, patients treated elsewhere are seen frequently. Unless acute problems exist, initial treatment should be conservative. The patient's mouth should be charted, appropriate roentgenograms obtained, and a recall prophylaxis done. The patient's history and treatment records should be obtained from the referring dentist, and appropriate care given, consistent with the patient's current and past periodontal status, posttreatment responses, and current needs. The dentist should not hasten to intervene surgically without thorough evaluation.

## RETREATMENT

From time to time, findings of special significance will be made during the recall examination. These may indicate the presence of new lesions or extensions of the original disease. For example, bone may not regenerate in an intra-alveolar defect after grafting or reattachment procedures or there may be new areas of pocket formation and bone resorption. Mobility may be increased. Tissue changes may have been induced by the presence of fixed or removable prostheses. Caries or pulpal disease may occur. Changes in the patient's systemic status may alter capacity to withstand insults to the periodontium that were previously well tolerated. In these instances, develop a treatment plan based on the findings, and render treatment to extend the useful life of the dentition.

A patient may be considered cured if the disease has been arrested, bone loss is nonprogressive, and the patient functions in comfort.

**Immediate poor results**

At times the results of treatment may fall short of the projected goals. The failure to obtain optimal treatment effects or to maintain optimal periodontal health after successful treatment may be due to treatment or to events that follow. Some causes of an immediate poor result[16,22,25] are (1) misdiagnosis, incomplete examination, or inadequate record[34]; (2) inappropriate or incomplete treatment[34-37]; and (3) deficient oral hygiene by the patient.

**Recurrence**

The recurrence of periodontal disease after apparently successful treatment may be caused by any of the following:

1. Inadequate oral hygiene by the patient
2. Incomplete scaling and root planing in the maintenance program
3. Incomplete treatment or misdiagnosis
4. Inappropriate or improper dental restorations or prostheses
5. Failure to carry out associated prosthetic or restorative procedures
6. Intrinsic or other factors beyond your or the patient's control (e.g., diabetes or compromised immune responses, polymorphonuclear dysfunctions)
7. Persistence or reintroduction of certain microbial pathogens

Recurrent periodontal disease is characterized by one or all of the following symptoms:

1. Bleeding on probing
2. Increased probing depth
3. Continued attachment loss
4. Increased mobility
5. Purulent discharge from pockets

The cultural or microscopic examination of sulcular and pocket microbiota is being explored as a method of assessing periodontal health or disease.

According to the nonspecific plaque hypothesis,[38] any amount of dental plaque may be considered harmful. Consequently plaque control becomes synonymous with complete removal of plaque deposits. Recent research has shown that composition of the periodontal microbiota is variable, and that although certain bacterial forms are associated with disease, others tend to be more prevalent in health.[39-42] According to the specific plaque hypothesis,[38] plaque control may begin to take on a different meaning, namely the control of periodontal pathogens, rather than of all bacteria.[43]

Cultural, microscopic, or immunocytochemical monitoring of the periodontal microbiota can lead to the determination of whether potentially harmful bacteria have been successfully eliminated and whether the residual microbiota is compatible with health.

Phase contrast or dark-field microscopy of wet mount preparations of plaque samples have been used to detect disease activity.[44,45] It has been assumed that increased proportions of spirochetes or motile rods indicated active periodontal breakdown at a site. However, dark-field examination of plaque samples taken from sites of active periodontal breakdown (as determined by changes in the attachment level measurement) when compared with samples from inactive sites in the same individuals do not support this assumption. There is evidence, following the corrective phase of treatment, that patients with elevated proportions of spirochetes or motile rods are more susceptible to recurrences of periodontitis.[46] This information has been used to tailor recall intervals to periods short enough to keep these microbial morphotypes below critical levels.[47] Preliminary results from a study comparing the experimental schedule with fixed trimonthly recalls support the notion that optimal recall intervals average around 3 months.[47] However, the range varied widely from 1 month to more than 1 year. Before microscopic monitoring[44,45] can be recommended as a safe and effective method to schedule recall intervals,[48,49] additional clinical trials must be carried out.[47,50,51]

Similar results with cultural studies suggest that *Bacteroides gingivalis, Bacteroides intermedius,* and *Actinobacillus actinomycetemcomitans* can serve as indicator organisms for periodontitis. Research results[52-54] suggest these organisms can account for better than 90% of the cases of periodontitis. Furthermore, the degree of new attachment following corrective treatment of periodontal lesions seemed to be inversely correlated with the number of bacteria recoverable from the treated sites. Further clinical trials are needed to validate the safety and efficacy of this approach to scheduling maintenance visits compared to standard trimonthly visits. Future research tools may provide more accurate means of monitoring pathogen presence than do cultural analyses and dark-field examination (e.g., monoclonal antibodies, DNA probes).

## DEGREE OF SUCCESS

In periodontics, as in all healing arts, the degree of success is variable. It depends on the diagnostic and manipulative ability of the therapist,[36] the severity of the disease, the cooperation of the patient, the objectives of treatment, the intrinsic status of the patient, and the advancing state of the basic biologic principles and operative procedures on which all therapy rests.[30] If the useful life of the dentition has been prolonged significantly and no signs of pathologic conditions are present, treatment is successful. Even teeth with poor, guarded, or hopeless prognoses can sometimes be maintained for years. The superlative therapist is one who salvages a compromised tooth where others could not.

**Failure**

Failure occurs only when teeth can no longer function and must be extracted. Unsuccessful results may occur even in the most properly managed cases. Continued inflammation and loss of attachment apparatus or increased mobility in one or more areas are indicative of an unsuccessful result.

**Poor home dental care**

Although some unsuccessful results might have been avoided, others could not. Failures are sometimes caused by a lack of cooperation by the patient.[23,55] There is a recurrence of localized breakdown because of poor oral hygiene and undiagnosed diabetes (Fig. 49-3).

**Questionable teeth**

The therapist may not always be able to be completely accurate in making a diagnosis, and treatment plans may not provide for all eventualities. Attempts to treat teeth with a questionable prognosis cannot be successful in every case. The distinction between a questionable and a hopeless tooth may not be apparent.[56] Moreover, the treatment of questionable teeth is a high-risk situation; the patient should be apprised of this at the start of therapy.

**Therapeutic judgment**

Therapeutic judgment rests on clinical experience and a knowledge of biologic principles. In some instances the objectives of treatment for a specific patient are not achievable. In other instances the therapist lacks an understanding of the total situation and of the patient. In still other situations procedural tactics are secondary to insight and empathy. If these are not brought into play, expertise in technique is unavailing, and somehow each operation is performed at a maladroit time in a maladroit manner. The results in such cases can be quite devastating.

**Intrinsic factors**

Periodontal treatment frequently does not take intrinsic host factors sufficiently into account. Knowledge concerning these factors in the cause of periodontal disease is vague and even where it is being developed it is not yet readily transferable to the clinical situation.

Proper evaluation of the intrinsic factors is not yet available. Deficiencies in host defense such as neutrophil dysfunctions that are not readily identified may account for an increased frequency of recurrences in some patients. Pocket elimination and the creation of ideal anatomic contours even in the presence of good oral hygiene may not be sufficient to maintain the health of an immunologically deficient patient.

## Concept of cure

**Cure**

When is periodontal disease cured, and what constitutes a cure? When the signs and symptoms of periodontal disease have been removed and have been replaced by the signs of periodontal health and causative factors are controlled, a cure can be considered to have been achieved. Although the integrity of the tissues may be completely restored without any evidence of recession of bone and gingiva beyond the normal levels, more often the margins of these tissues will be found positioned somewhat apically. Although this may constitute a deformity in the architectural sense, it does not represent a manifestation of disease. Cure, then, is the attainment of a functional and healthy periodontal and dental status, with or without some loss of structural support, and the control of the factors responsible for the disease. It should be understood, however, that a cure is not always synonymous with permanent arrest of the disease. In fact, even well-maintained patients may on occasion develop an isolated lesion about a single tooth.[20,28] Variations in disease susceptibility occurs among patients, the causes of which may not be apparent or controllable.

We still do not know enough about the causative factors in juvenile periodontitis and desquamative gingivitis. In fact, on rare occasions, gingivitis or adult periodontitis may not respond to standard therapy. However, when further knowledge is developed, a greater degree of success may be expected.

## ILLUSTRATIVE CASES

Periodontal disease can be cured, and periodontal health can be maintained. However, every dentist experiences failure or partial failure on occasion. At other times the destructive lesions of periodontal disease may be so severe or so irregular in distribution that an ideal result cannot be achieved. This section shows some results that may be less than ideal so that you can gain a realistic and balanced view of the results of therapy.

The appearance of a patient's mouth before treatment is shown in Fig. 49-3, *A*. **Failure** After the completion of treatment, the criteria for periodontal health were met, and the patient was placed on a maintenance program. Over a 5-year period the patient suffered repeated relapses. A few were acute in nature (periodontal abscesses); most could be attributed to errors or omissions in oral hygiene: others could be explained

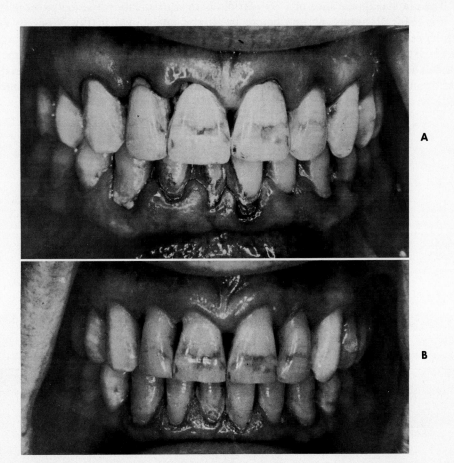

**Fig. 49-3. A,** Case of moderate periodontitis at the time of examination. **B,** Same case 2 years after treatment. Localized marginal inflammation is present. The patient practiced irregular and incomplete plaque removal and was later found to have diabetes.

only by the possible presence of intrinsic contributing factors. The severity of the inflammation and the extent of bone loss far outdistanced the amount of plaque. Finally, the patient was discovered to have diabetes.

Probably the diabetes predisposed this patient to exaggerated tissue responses to bacteria because of lessened resistance. The appearance of the patient's mouth 2 years after treatment (at the time of a recall appointment) can be seen in Fig. 49-3, *B*. Marginal inflammation and some fibrosis are evident. Maintenance of periodontal health in such a patient requires regular monitoring, frequent retreatment in localized areas, and control of the diabetes.

The dentition of a 26-year-old woman is shown in Fig. 49-4, *A*. The roentgenograms are shown in Fig. 49-4, *B*. The patient had been twice divorced and supported four children by working as a waitress. She appeared for treatment with a recurrent necrotizing ulcerative gingivitis. She had a history of dental neglect and had lost all but eight mandibular teeth. Initial treatment to reduce the acute phase of the disease had been performed and was followed by treatment to eradicate tissue deformities. The course of treatment was marked by broken appointments and irregular, inadequate oral hygiene. The patient changed jobs several times and finally left the city. Prognosis for this patient was poor. The possible role of emotional and stress factors in this patient's disease remained. The poor oral hygiene and an indifferent attitude might well have predisposed the patient to eventual loss of the remaining teeth.

**Success**

The clinical appearance of a 36-year-old man with advanced periodontitis is shown in Fig. 49-5. Roentgenograms before treatment are shown in Fig. 49-5, *B*. Pocket depths ranged up to 10 mm, and significant mobility patterns were present in many teeth. Extraction was advised for the mandibular right first premolar and the mandibular left second premolar because of tortuous pocket formation, up to 10 mm in depth, and because of the class 3 mobility of these teeth. The mandibular right second pre-

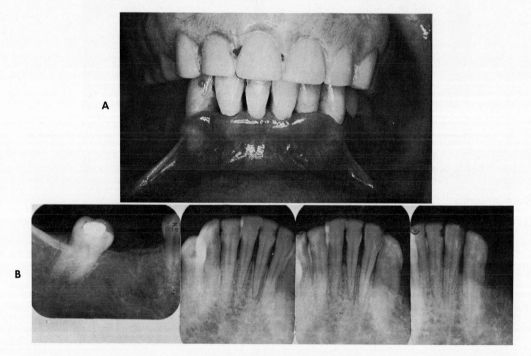

**Fig. 49-4.** **A,** Recurrent necrotizing ulcerative gingivitis in a 26-year-old woman. **B,** Roentgenograms showing loss of all but seven teeth because of neglect and lack of dental awareness. Alveolar bone destruction was horizontal and of moderate degree (35% to 40% about the incisors).

molar and the maxillary right first molar were given a poor prognosis. A guarded prognosis was projected for the rest of the dentition because of the severity of the disease, the complexity of the pocket formation and the extent of bone destruction (Fig. 49-5, *B*), and the variety of etiologic factors present. The patient had received dental treatment but was unaware of the presence of periodontal disease. He was informed of his condition and of the prognosis. His desire to keep his teeth was so great that he requested treatment despite the guarded prognosis. Extensive treatment consisting of repeated root planing, intensive oral hygiene coaching, provisional splinting, occlusal adjustment, and surgery was performed. Exacting attention was given to training in home dental care and to the reduction of tooth mobility. Two cast removable splints were constructed to control tooth mobility.

Nine years later the periodontal tissues were in good condition (Fig. 49-5, *C* and *D*). The gingivae were generally found to be pink, firm, and stippled. The patient was conscientious in home dental care and regularly followed a maintenance program. The initial guarded prognosis was changed to a more favorable prognosis, despite the considerable loss of tooth support. Gingival health (Fig. 49-5, *C* and *D*) was present 16 years later; roentgenograms indicate that bone levels were unaltered (Fig. 49-5, *E*). The patient continues to do well (23 years later).

## COMPARATIVE STUDIES OF SURGICAL AND NONSURGICAL TREATMENT

Studies conducted at the Universities of Michigan and Minnesota have compared the effectiveness of scaling and root planing, curettage, modified Widman flap, and pocket elimination surgery (gingivectomy and osseous surgery with and without apically positioned flaps) *on different tooth types and different probing depths.*

An 8-year posttreatment study of the modified Widman flap procedure (MWFP) indicated that all teeth did relatively well. The incisors did slightly better and the maxillary premolars did slightly worse.[32,57] Does this indicate a difference in response according to tooth type?

Treatment by scaling/root planing alone or followed by the MWFP (6½ years posttreatment)[58] yielded results of pocket deepening and more recession on molars with 4 to 6 mm pockets than on other teeth. Nonmolar teeth with pockets of 7 mm or greater had a larger reduction in pocket depth with the MWFP but there was no difference between tooth types with scaling alone. Both methods maintained pretreatment attachment levels.[58]

In a 2-year posttreatment study there was a minor reduction in pocket depth regardless of method used (surgical pocket elimination, MWFP, subgingival curettage, scaling and root planing) and an increased loss of attachment. Pockets of 4 to 6 mm had the greatest reduction in depth during the hygiene phase but depth was also reduced with either pocket elimination surgery or MWFP. Pockets of 7 mm or greater had the greatest reduction with pocket elimination surgery but attachment levels remained the same with all four methods. Scaling and root planing imposed the least discomfort and produced the least change in appearance. All four methods consumed the same treatment time. This study suggests that the most important factor in the maintenance of periodontal support is thorough mechanical cleaning of the root surfaces rather than surgery per se.[59]

In a 4-year study by the same group, shallow pockets (1 to 3 mm) tended to increase slightly in depth with either scaling or the MWFP and to experience a slight increase in the loss of attachment. Moderately deep pockets (4 to 6 mm) were reduced by either method and demonstrated a gain or maintenance of probing attachment levels. Deep pockets (≧7 mm) exhibited the greatest reduction in probing depth and greatest gain in attachment levels. Both procedures were effective in treating moderate and advanced periodontitis. The MWFP resulted in a greater pocket reduction and attachment gain

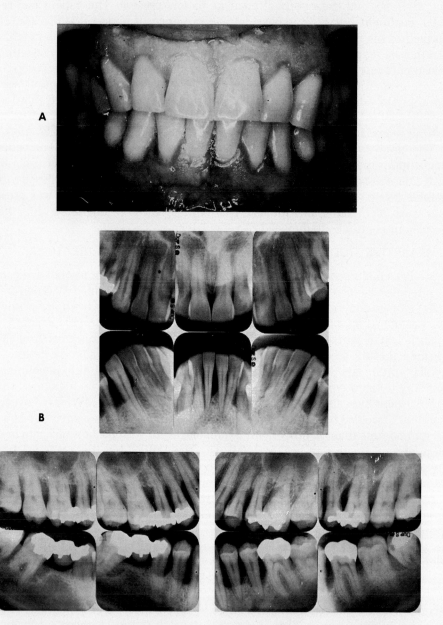

**Fig. 49-5.** **A,** Advanced bone destruction caused by periodontitis in a 36-year-old man. Despite regular visits to the dentist, the patient was unaware that he had periodontal disease. **B,** Roentgenograms at the time of examination show severe generalized bone destruction that is irregular in form and distribution. There are both horizontal and vertical patterns. Significant tooth mobility was also present.

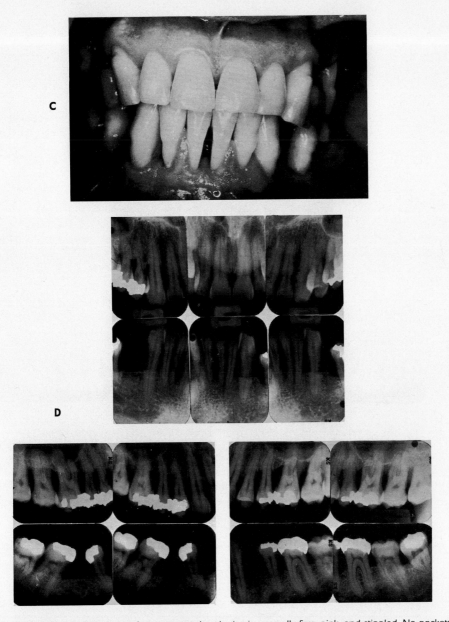

**Fig. 49-5, cont'd.    C,** Nine years after treatment the gingiva is generally firm, pink, and stippled. No pockets are present, but there are localized areas of inflammation of the marginal gingiva. Tooth mobility is controlled by two cast-removable splints. **D,** Roentgenograms 9 years after treatment showing a more regular bony profile. The bone levels have been maintained or have been improved.                                                *Continued.*

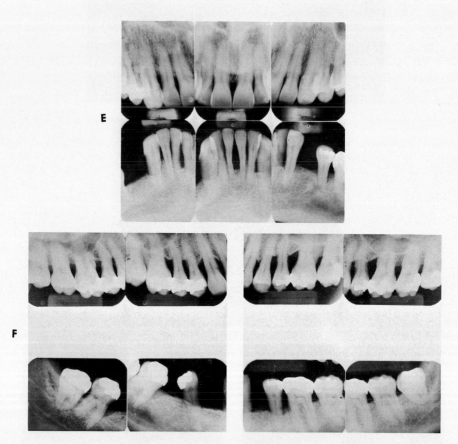

**Fig. 49-5, cont'd.** **E,** Roentgenograms 16 years after treatment with continued maintenance. Note that the bone levels have been maintained. The patient still wears cast-removable splints on the maxillary and mandibular teeth.

for the deeper pockets and a loss of clinical attachment for shallow pockets.[59,60]

In another 8-year study, probing depth reduction 1 year after treatment was sustained regardless of initial probing depth. The reduction in probing depth was greater for deep than for shallow pockets. A slight gain in attachment level occurred for moderate and deep pockets (more for the deep than for the moderate pockets). The MWFP tended to be most effective both for probing depth reduction and for preservation of attachment level for moderate pockets (4 to 6 mm) over the 8 years. For deep pockets (7 to 12 mm) both MWFP and pocket elimination surgery were equally effective in reducing probing depth and curettage only slightly less effective.[61] For 4- to 6-mm pockets, scaling and root planing alone or followed by MWFP were equally effective. Deep pockets were initially best reduced by flap. After 2 years there was no consistent difference in pocket reduction by either method. However, pocket reduction was sustained for 6½ years with MWFP and for 3 years with scaling/planing. Pockets of 1 to 3 mm had sustained attachment loss with the MWFP, while scaling/planing did not produce sustained attachment loss. In pockets of 4 to 6 mm attachment levels were sustained by both procedures but scaling/planing resulted in greater gain in attachment. Treatment of pockets $\geq 7$ mm by both procedures resulted in a gain of attachment with no difference between procedures.

Other studies[62,63] compared results after subgingival curettage, MWFP, and pocket elimination surgery (PES). For pockets 4 mm or deeper a reduction in pocket depth and a gain in clinical attachment was obtained following all three methods and was sustained for 8 years. No one method was consistently superior to the other two. PES did not enhance the prognosis for moderate and advanced pockets when compared with the more conservative measures.[62,63]

Experimental studies in monkeys indicated that placing Millipore filters to prevent the migration of the junctional epithelium was followed by new attachment of collagen fibers in cementum.[64] The regenerated periodontium formed in the apical portion of the wound in continuity with the original cementum layer. The cementum was thicker apically and thinner coronally. This new attachment was formed by the coronal migration of cells originating in the periodontal ligament.[65,66]

The gain in attachment may occur equally for many treatment methods (scaling and planing, scaling and planing with gingivectomy or with apically positioned flap with or without bone surgery, scaling and planing with MWFP with or without bone surgery).[67] The perceived gain in attachment level may be a false gain that simply reflects reduced penetrability of the probe following resolution of inflammation rather than the formation of a new connective tissue attachment.[65] The conclusion is that most patients maintained on an optimal level of oral hygiene can be cured of periodontal disease and its progression can be terminated irrespective of surgical technique used.[62] Patients schooled in proper plaque control measures and able to carry them out seem to do well on limited recall visits (every 4 to 6 months).[68]

Periodontal disease activity was monitored bimonthly to detect new bursts of destructive activity in sites with prior evidence of destructive periodontal disease. When bursts of activity were noted, treatment with systemic tetracycline and MWFP was instituted. Following such treatment the sites were again monitored bimonthly. This permitted classification of the sites into sites with good, intermediate, and poor response to treatment. Sites that responded poorly had elevated local humoral antibody to three or more of the gram-negative organisms tested (*Fusobacterium nucleatum, Eikenella corrodens, Bacteroides intermedius, Capnocytophaga sputigena*). Sites with good responses had greater proportions of *Actinobacillus actinomycetemcomitans, C. ochracea,* and *B. intermedius* before therapy while sites with poor responses had significantly elevated proportions of *F. nucleatum, Peptostreptococcus micros,* and *Streptococcus intermedius.* These findings must be treated with caution because of the small number of individuals studied, but they provide hints of tests that might be applied in the future that would detect poor responders in advance of therapy.[69]

While some studies report that new attachment occurs, others do not. One study compared the MWFP alone or combined with either frozen autogenous red marrow and cancellous bone or beta tricalcium phosphate implants with root planing and soft tissue curettage. It reported the formation of a long junctional epithelium with no new connective tissue attachment.[70] Such a long junctional epithelium does not seem to be more susceptible to breakdown caused by plaque accumulation than does a normal (short) junctional epithelium.[71] Following root planing and mucoperiosteal flaps, a long junctional epithelium may reform to the level of or beyond preexisting calculus but the connective tissue attachment does not reform coronal to that level.[72]

Scaling and root planing were almost equally effective alone as when combined with the MWFP in establishing a clinically healthy gingiva and preventing further loss of attachment. Pockets of less than 4 mm were frequently produced postoperatively. Probing depth reduction was more pronounced in deep than in shallow pockets. Deep pockets became more shallow following surgery than they did following scaling and root planing. Deep pockets exhibited a greater gain in attachment level than did shallow pockets. In pockets of 4 mm or less scaling and planing did not produce loss of attachment while such loss did occur with the MWFP.[73]

Data of this type is extremely interesting and is bound to be altered as advances are made in plaque chemotherapy and in bone-grafting and bone regenerative techniques.

Results of these studies should not be confused with absolute comparisons of the effectiveness of techniques. Further studies conducted by varying groups of differing therapeutic schools evaluated by "double-blind" examination techniques are needed to make valid comparisons. The studies cited tend to establish differences in the response of mild, moderate, and deep pockets to therapy and differences in the effect of therapy on different tooth types (e.g., molars vs. incisors). In addition they appear to indicate that pocket elimination surgery reduces pockets most effectively and maintains attachment levels least effectively. The more conservative measures maintain attachment levels more effectively and eliminate pockets less effectively.

## Retrospective studies

Clinical experience is of great value because it provides a background and comparison of relatively similar cases over a period of many years. Such studies demonstrate pathways that the majority of patients can be expected to follow.[74]

Hirschfeld and Wasserman have reported two retrospective studies of patients treated for periodontal disease. The second study reported in the fifth edition of this text[74] surveyed 565 patients who were treated initially more than 20 years before the study was initiated. There were 371 females and 194 males. The periods of maintenance ranged from 20 to 58 years, with an average of 27.2 years and a median of 25 years. Observations of 158 patients were made for more than 30 years; 30 patients were observed for more than 40 years; and 7 were first treated more than 50 years before the study.

The age of patients initially ranged from 12 to 70, with an average of 40.3 years and a median age of 41. At that time 345 patients (61%) were between 35 and 50.

At the time of the final survey the average age was 67.5 years. It is interesting that 238 patients (42%) were over 70, and 46 (8%) were over 80 years old. This indicates that the patients were maintained for the greater part of their adult lives.

The dentitions of most of the 565 patients were nearly complete at initial treatment: 174 patients had more than 28 teeth, and 427 (75%) had more than 24 teeth. The average number of teeth present was 26.3.

The severity of periodontal disease at the time of initial examination was divided into categories:

1. *Early:* pockets of 4 mm or less, generally with gingival inflammation and subgingival calculus
2. *Intermediate:* pockets of 4 to 7 mm about a number of teeth
3. *Advanced:* pockets deeper than 7 mm and furcation involvement of at least one tooth

Of the 565 patients, 438 (77.7%) had advanced periodontal disease; only 8.3% had early disease.

On the basis of response the study population was distributed as follows:

|  | Number of patients | Percent |
|---|---|---|
| WM (well maintained) | 414 | 73.2 |
| D (downhill) | 115 | 20.4 |
| ED (extreme downhill) | 36 | 6.4 |

No relationship of sex distribution, age, or period of maintenance to the posttreatment trend could be determined.

The teeth lost, based on a response group, showed marked differences. In the WM group (almost three fourths of the patients) only 0.7 teeth per person were lost (Chart 2, p. 1114). Of the entire study population, 242 patients (42.6%) lost no teeth over the average period of 27 years. On the other hand, 36 patients in the ED group averaged 12.9 teeth lost per person. In the total study population of 565 patients, 8.1% of the teeth were lost (2.5 per person).

The loss of teeth from periodontal causes during the period was determined by comparison chartings and from the treatment history. Teeth lost during the initial treatment were not counted. If no specific information was found in the records, it was assumed the tooth was lost for periodontal reasons.

Initially, 14,866 teeth were present. Overall, 1397 teeth were lost (2.5 per patient).

**Table 49-1** Percentage of each tooth type lost during maintenance period

|  | Present after initial treatment | Number lost during maintenance period | Percent lost |
|---|---|---|---|
| 8 \| 8* | 404 | 68 | 16.8 |
| 7 \| 7 | 952 | 184 | 19.3 |
| 6 \| 6 | 861 | 140 | 16.3 |
| 5 \| 5 | 1018 | 61 | 6.0 |
| 4 \| 4 | 1045 | 66 | 6.3 |
| 3 \| 3 | 1153 | 42 | 3.6 |
| 2 \| 2 | 1110 | 61 | 5.5 |
| 1 \| 1† | 1127 | 60 | 5.3 |
| 1 \| 1‡ | 1162 | 73 | 6.3 |
| 2 \| 2 | 1182 | 39 | 3.4 |
| 3 \| 3 | 1192 | 9 | 0.8 |
| 4 \| 4 | 1142 | 18 | 1.6 |
| 5 \| 5 | 1065 | 30 | 2.8 |
| 6 \| 6 | 764 | 77 | 10.1 |
| 7 \| 7 | 958 | 107 | 11.2 |
| 8 \| 8§ | 532 | 75 | 14.1 |

From Hirschfeld, L., and Wasserman, B.: A long term survey of tooth losses in 600 treated periodontal patients, J. Periodontol. **49:**226, 1978.
*Maxillary third molars.
†Maxillary central incisors.
‡Mandibular central incisors.
§Mandibular third molars.

| Tooth type | Initially present | Lost | Percent lost | Tooth type | Initially present | Lost | Percent lost |
|---|---|---|---|---|---|---|---|
| 8⌋ | 164 | 10 | 6.1 | ⌊8 | 174 | 15 | 8.6 |
| 7⌋ | 409 | 40 | 9.8 | ⌊7 | 402 | 51 | 14.9 |
| 6⌋ | 364 | 25 | 6.9 | ⌊6 | 373 | 29 | 7.7 |
| 5⌋ | 431 | 7 | 1.6 | ⌊5 | 439 | 10 | 2.3 |
| 4⌋ | 442 | 8 | 1.8 | ⌊4 | 443 | 4 | 0.9 |
| 3⌋ | 481 | 0 | 0 | ⌊3 | 482 | 0 | 0 |
| 2⌋ | 467 | 1 | 0.2 | ⌊2 | 465 | 6 | 1.3 |
| 1⌋ | 474 | 2 | 0.4 | ⌊1 | 471 | 6 | 1.3 |
| 1⌉ | 482 | 7 | 1.5 | ⌈1 | 485 | 5 | 1.0 |
| 2⌉ | 498 | 4 | 0.8 | ⌈2 | 490 | 2 | 0.4 |
| 3⌉ | 497 | 0 | 0.0 | ⌈3 | 495 | 0 | 0 |
| 4⌉ | 472 | 5 | 1.0 | ⌈4 | 482 | 1 | 0.2 |
| 5⌉ | 439 | 5 | 1.1 | ⌈5 | 450 | 4 | 0.9 |
| 6⌉ | 327 | 18 | 5.5 | ⌈6 | 318 | 13 | 4.1 |
| 7⌉ | 402 | 17 | 4.2 | ⌈7 | 406 | 22 | 5.4 |
| 8⌉ | 225 | 8 | 3.5 | ⌈8 | 215 | 17 | 7.9 |

A

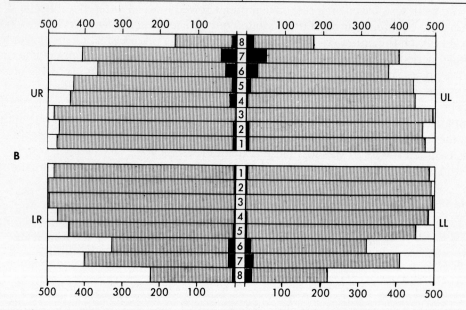

B

**Chart 2.** **A,** Well-maintained group (499 patients). Tooth loss from periodontal disease, by tooth type. **B,** Teeth in the WM group that were present initially *(gray areas)* but were lost during the study period *(black areas).* (From Hirschfeld, L., and Wasserman, B.: J. Periodontol. **49:**226, 1978.)

Of the teeth lost, 771 had questionable prognoses at initial examination.

The data was in accord with that reported in an earlier study of 600 patients who had been treated for an average of 22 years and a minimum of 15 years.[75] The types and locations of teeth lost are shown in Table 49-1. There is remarkable bilateral symmetry of periodontal disease and tooth loss. A considerable difference clearly exists in tooth loss according to position in the arch. Upper molars have the highest loss rates, lower molars somewhat less, and lower cuspids and first bicuspids far less, approximately one twelfth of the upper molars.

As the initial survey, reported in 1978, progressed, it became clear that the post-treatment course of patients differed markedly. Thus the totals provided only limited and somewhat misleading information. The sample was then divided on the basis of response to therapy into the following groupings:

| Tooth type | Initially present | Lost | Percent lost | Tooth type | Initially present | Lost | Percent lost |
|---|---|---|---|---|---|---|---|
| 8⌐ | 26 | 14 | 53.8 | ⌐8 | 29 | 20 | 68.9 |
| 7 | 54 | 31 | 57.4 | 7 | 54 | 31 | 57.4 |
| 6 | 51 | 29 | 56.8 | 6 | 47 | 31 | 65.9 |
| 5 | 61 | 11 | 18.0 | 5 | 53 | 8 | 15.0 |
| 4 | 62 | 15 | 24.2 | 4 | 60 | 14 | 23.3 |
| 3 | 71 | 10 | 14.1 | 3 | 71 | 7 | 9.8 |
| 2 | 66 | 11 | 16.6 | 2 | 68 | 13 | 19.1 |
| 1 | 66 | 10 | 15.1 | 1 | 68 | 12 | 17.6 |
| 1 | 75 | 16 | 21.3 | 1 | 75 | 15 | 20.0 |
| 2 | 73 | 8 | 10.9 | 2 | 75 | 8 | 10.6 |
| 3 | 75 | 2 | 2.6 | 3 | 76 | 2 | 2.6 |
| 4 | 73 | 3 | 4.1 | 4 | 69 | 0 | 0 |
| 5 | 66 | 6 | 9.0 | 5 | 65 | 5 | 7.6 |
| 6 | 47 | 15 | 31.9 | 6 | 45 | 9 | 20.0 |
| 7 | 58 | 20 | 34.5 | 7 | 55 | 24 | 43.6 |
| 8⌐ | 36 | 18 | 50.0 | ⌐8 | 36 | 17 | 47.3 |

**A**

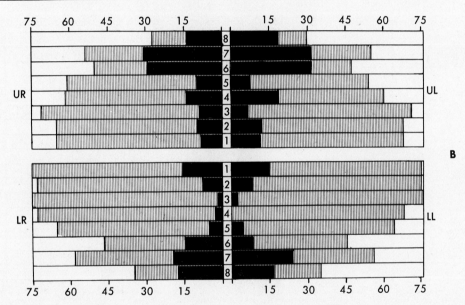

**B**

**Chart 3.** **A,** Downhill group (76 patients). Tooth loss from periodontal disease, by tooth type. **B,** Teeth in the D group that were present initially *(gray areas)* but were lost during the study period *(black areas).* (From Hirschfeld, L., and Wasserman, B.: J. Periodontol. **49:**226, 1978.)

1. Well-maintained (WM) group, 0 to 3 teeth lost (Chart 2, p. 1114)
2. Downhill (D) group, 4 to 9 teeth lost (Chart 3, above)
3. Extreme downhill (ED) group, 10 to 23 teeth lost (Chart 4, p. 1116)

The pattern of tooth loss is interesting. There is great variation in mortality of the teeth in different positions in the arch and remarkable symmetry of loss. The numbers of teeth originally present in each position in the arches of the WM group, as well as the numbers of teeth lost, are listed in Chart 2, p. 1114. The data demonstrate the loss according to tooth type. The dentitions of the WM group were relatively intact at the beginning of the study, with sizable numbers of only first and third molars missing. Over the average span of 27 years, no cuspids were lost in this group of 414 patients. Relatively few incisors and bicuspids were lost.

When compared to the WM group, the D group (Chart 3, above) of 115 patients showed essentially the same pattern of tooth loss, but relatively more incisors, upper

| Tooth type | Initially present | Lost | Percent lost | Tooth type | Initially present | Lost | Percent lost |
|---|---|---|---|---|---|---|---|
| 8⌐ | 5 | 4 | 80.0 | ⌐8 | 6 | 5 | 83.3 |
| 7⌐ | 16 | 16 | 100.0 | ⌐7 | 17 | 15 | 88.2 |
| 6⌐ | 13 | 13 | 100.0 | ⌐6 | 13 | 13 | 100.0 |
| 5⌐ | 20 | 15 | 75.0 | ⌐5 | 19 | 10 | 52.6 |
| 4⌐ | 20 | 14 | 70.0 | ⌐4 | 18 | 11 | 61.1 |
| 3⌐ | 24 | 13 | 54.1 | ⌐3 | 24 | 12 | 50.0 |
| 2⌐ | 23 | 16 | 69.6 | ⌐2 | 21 | 14 | 66.6 |
| 1⌐ | 24 | 16 | 66.6 | ⌐1 | 24 | 14 | 58.4 |
| 1⌐ | 23 | 14 | 60.9 | ⌐1 | 22 | 16 | 72.7 |
| 2⌐ | 23 | 8 | 34.8 | ⌐2 | 23 | 9 | 39.1 |
| 3⌐ | 23 | 2 | 8.7 | ⌐3 | 25 | 3 | 12.0 |
| 4⌐ | 23 | 5 | 21.7 | ⌐4 | 23 | 4 | 17.4 |
| 5⌐ | 22 | 7 | 31.8 | ⌐5 | 23 | 3 | 13.0 |
| 6⌐ | 13 | 10 | 76.9 | ⌐6 | 14 | 12 | 85.7 |
| 7⌐ | 18 | 11 | 61.1 | ⌐7 | 19 | 13 | 68.4 |
| 8⌐ | 8 | 6 | 75.0 | ⌐8 | 12 | 9 | 75.0 |

**A**

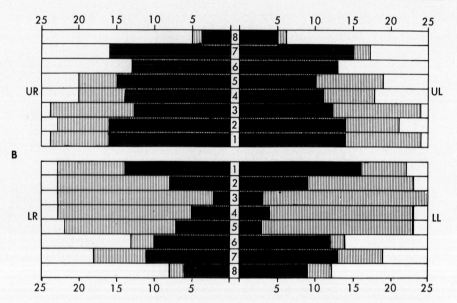

**B**

**Chart 4. A,** Extreme downhill group (25 patients). Tooth loss from periodontal disease, by tooth type. **B,** Teeth in the ED group that were present initially *(gray areas)* but were lost during the study period *(black areas)*. (From Hirschfeld, L., and Wasserman, B.: J. Periodontol. **49:**226, 1978.)

cuspids, and bicuspids were lost. The teeth most resistant to loss were the mandibular cuspids and the first bicuspids.

In the ED group (Chart 4, above) of 36 cases, tooth loss was less selective. Most maxillary teeth had similar frequency of loss. Although most of the lower molars and incisors were lost, the relative resistance of the mandibular cuspids and first bicuspids was apparent.

## LOSS OF QUESTIONABLE TEETH

In the well-maintained group of 414 patients, 279 teeth were lost (0.7 per patient). Of the teeth lost, 80% (225 teeth) had been diagnosed originally as having a questionable prognosis because of furcation involvement, severe mobility, or pocket depth of 7 to 9 mm (with poor root length). Only 54 (20%) of the teeth lost had been considered to have a favorable prognosis.

In the downhill group, in which an average of 5.7 teeth per patient had been lost, 55% (351 teeth) were considered questionable originally. In the extreme downhill group, in which 12.9 teeth per patient were lost, only 42.2% of the teeth lost had been considered questionable originally.

## LOSS OF TEETH WITH FURCATION INVOLVEMENT

There were 810 maxillary and 548 mandibular teeth with furcation involvement initially. Of these, 360 maxillary and 196 mandibular teeth were lost.

In the WM group it can be seen that 20% of the maxillary first and mandibular first and second molars with furcation involvements were lost. However, 25% of the maxillary second molars were lost. It is apparent that, although most of the molars lost in the WM group had furcation involvements originally, only 23% of such molars were lost. Proportionately more third molars were lost, since there were many possibilities for their extraction (e.g., prosthetic reasons or extrusion), which might have been associated with periodontal disease but were not primarily periodontal. The proportion of furcated teeth lost was much greater in both the D and the ED groups.

## LOSS OF NONFURCATED QUESTIONABLE TEETH

Of 767 single-rooted teeth and molars without furcations that were originally classified as having questionable prognoses, 216 (27.3%) were lost. In examining individual tooth loss in each response group, it is interesting that, although 23 cuspids in the WM group originally had so much destruction that they were marked questionable, not one was lost. In fact, only 12.9% of the questionable nonfurcated teeth were lost in this group, whereas 60% were lost in the D group, and 85.4% in the ED group. Questionable maxillary incisors were more resistant to loss in the WM group than were mandibular incisors.

From the initial and final chartings for noting tooth loss, it was not discernible whether the loss had occurred early in the long maintenance period or at intervals. To see what had happened to the patients, 352 patients from the first survey were surveyed again. Notations then could be made of teeth lost since the charting in the first survey.[74]

The 352 patients were divided approximately in the same way as were the 565 patients of the total group regarding sex, age, initial dentition, and initial severity of disease. The posttreatment response groups had almost the same percentages as the total group. It is apparent that in all the response groups, approximately half as many teeth were lost in the 6-year period between surveys.

## FINDINGS

Following are conclusions that have been drawn from several retrospective[74,75] surveys:

1. There is a remarkable bilateral symmetry of tooth loss.[75] This is not unexpected since many studies of the incidence and severity of periodontal disease have also demonstrated bilateral symmetry.[28,76,77]
2. A great variation exists in the loss of the individual teeth in different positions in the arch.
3. Patients with periodontal breakdown have gingival inflammation more often than patients without breakdown. However, the teeth with the most inflammation and the teeth with most breakdown were not necessarily the same.
4. The posttreatment course of patients with the same initial status could be markedly different. The figures presented indicate that 5 out of 6 patients can be expected to do

well with treatment, but it is not possible to predict accurately which patient will deteriorate.

5. Periodontal disease is often cyclic. Several patients with severe destruction at age 40 responded well to the initial treatment, had no further breakdown for more than 20 years, but then suddenly had a period of periodontal destruction and tooth loss. Other patients responded well for 5 years and then had exacerbations of the disease alternating with periods of remission. The patients in Hirschfeld and Wasserman's study had their initial treatment before 1956,[74] when periodontal surgery was not routine and the surgery that was done consisted principally of gingivectomy. There was no grafting of bone and very little mucogingival surgery. The benefits of antibiotic therapy were not available during the treatment of many of these patients (Chart 5, opposite).

6. Contrary to the most widely accepted opinion, no relation exists between periodontal destruction and deep overbite, crossbite, or any type of generalized malocclusion.[28] Of course, severe trauma of a particular tooth in any of these relationships can occur.

The question, "What is a questionable tooth?" is interesting. In Hirschfeld and Wasserman's long-term survey,[74] teeth that originally had pocket depth of over 7 mm, furcation involvements, or 2 degrees of mobility were considered questionable.

Of these nonfurcated questionable teeth, few were lost in well-maintained patients, whereas almost all were lost in downhill cases. Thus factors differentiating downhill from other cases must be investigated.

Obviously patients with aggressive periodontal disease (extremely downhill case histories) constitute a special population when compared with either normal or well-maintained populations.

## CONCLUSION

The long maintenance span of these[74] patients clearly indicates that most treated periodontal patients can expect to go through life with functioning dentitions. Other studies support the conclusions of Hirschfeld and Wasserman.[26,78-80,81] In general, the rate of tooth loss in untreated patients and in treated patients who receive no maintenance care is greater than that in treated patients and maintained patients.[78,79,82] The practice of treatment without maintenance is of questionable value.[79] Treatment leads to a slower rate of bone loss.[80] Pockets tend to recur more frequently in the maxilla than in the mandible and more frequently in molars than the other teeth in the dentition. Pockets redevelop more frequently in teeth with initial pockets of 6 mm or greater. Older patients appear to be more vulnerable to pocket recurrence than do patients under 40 years of age.[83]

## Reliability of diagnostic methods

**Sensitivity**

**Specificity**

The value of a diagnostic test (e.g., probing, mobility, monitoring of microbiota) depends on its sensitivity and specificity. *Sensitivity* is defined as the ability of a test to detect patients with the disease. The ability to exclude patients without the disease is defined as *specificity*. All tests have a number of false positive and false negative outcomes. Critical evaluation considers the ability of a diagnostic procedure to detect patients with diseases while simultaneously excluding patients without disease. As can be seen this is of major importance in the diagnosis of periodontal disease where the testing methods are relatively crude and when a number of mistaken diagnoses are likely to occur. Critical evaluation depends on the *decision matrix,* the *receiver operating characteristic curve* (ROC) and *information theory.*

**Decision matrix**

The *decision matrix* logically relates the diagnostic test to the clinical outcome. It plots true positives (TP) and true negatives (TN) against false positives (FP) and false negatives (FN). A good diagnostic test has a high TP and a low FP ratio and correctly

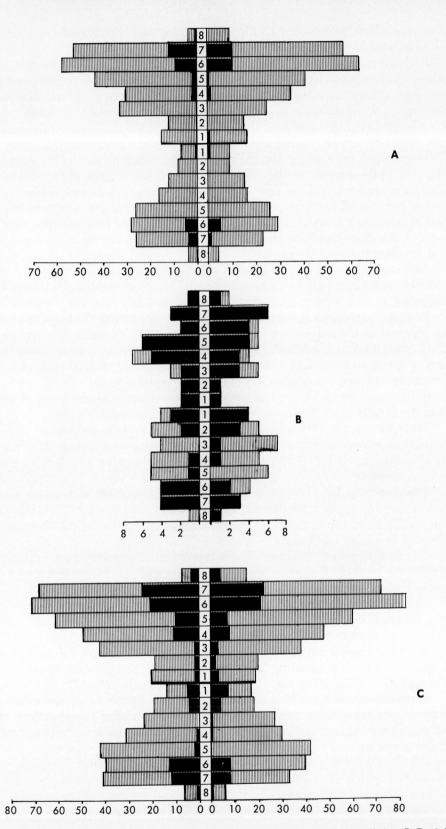

**Chart 5.   A,** Teeth in the well-maintained group that were treated surgically and subsequently lost. **B,** Teeth in the extreme downhill group that were treated surgically and subsequently were lost. **C,** Teeth in all three groups that were treated surgically and subsequently were lost. (From Hirschfeld, L., and Wasserman, B.: J. Periodontol. **49:**226, 1978.)

identifies a large portion of patients with the disease without including among them patients who do not have the disease.[84]

Because most tests yield a continium of findings and because any one of several points can be chosen to classify and differentiate diseased from nondiseased patients, the point chosen depends on how dangerous the disease is. If the disease is very dangerous we would want to include as many true positives as possible even at the expense of including some patients who are false positives. To chose the cut-off point one plots TP/FP, which is the *ROC curve*. The higher the ratio is, the better the test. The expense of the therapy and the possible discomfort as well as the impact on the longevity of the patient (or the dentition) are deciding factors. If the cost of missing a diagnosis is high and the cost of mistakenly treating a patient is low, one would choose one cut-off point, whereas if the value of treating the patient is low and the cost of treatment is high, one would not want to include false positives and another point on the curve would be chosen.[84] A good diagnostic test should have a specificity and sensitivity greater than 0.9.

*Information theory* may be used to select a cut-off point on the ROC curve. This includes additional tests or even preliminary therapy to reduce the uncertainty of a diagnosis.[84]

**Receiver operating characteristic curve**

Disagreements among diagnosticians occur in every field and these disagreements are reduced as the reliability of the diagnostic method increases.[85-87] The measure of reliability of diagnostic methods in periodontics has not yet been ascertained. Reliability and accuracy indicate that inflammation or plaque are present without accurately indicating whether or not bacterially induced progressive periodontal disease is present. Until such tests are developed one will not be able to fully evaluate the need for therapy or of the relative effectiveness of varying forms of treatment.

The true positive (TP) ratio is the proportion of positive tests in all patients who actually have the disease; the probability that patients with disease will be identified by a positive test is $P(T+/D+)$.* The true positive ratio expresses the sensitivity of the examination.

The true negative (TN) ratio $T-/D-$ is the proportion of negative tests in all patients who do not have the disease. The probability is $P(T-/D-)$* and this measures the specificity of the examination. It measures the fraction of patients correctly diagnosed as having no disease.

The false-negative (FN) ratio is the proportion of negative tests in patients with the disease $T-/D+$. The probability that patients with the disease will have a negative test is $P(T-/D+)$.*

The false-positive ratio (FP) $T+/D-$ is the proportion of positive tests in patients who do not have the disease. The probability that a patient without disease will incorrectly be identified as being ill is $P(T+/D-)$.*

A good diagnostic examination has a high TP ratio and a low FP ratio. It identifies a large number of diseased patients without incorrectly including healthy ones. TP/FP = likelihood ratio. The higher the ratio the better the test.

In periodontics it is possible for a patient to have plaque accumulation and inflammation without periodontal disease pathogens being present. Therefore tests that simply measure inflammation or quantity of plaque may have low likelihood ratios and thus be poor tests.

Few tests have simple binary outcomes; most yield a continuous scale of values, of which any one of several points can be selected as a cut-off point to distinguish patients with and without disease. This depends on the costs of classifying a diseased person as normal vs. classifying a normal person as being diseased.

---

*D+ = disease present          T+ = tests positive (abnormal)
 D- = disease absent           T- = tests negative (healthy)

If we select a cut-off point that makes the test very sensitive, to detect as many people with the disease as possible, the number of false positives unavoidably increases. For example, if increasing probing depths of 1 to 6 mm are used as cut-off points to classify periodontally diseased from nondiseased patients, the higher the cut-off point the greater will be the percentages of true positives and false negatives. But because the number of false negatives is increased as higher probing depths are chosen as cut-off points, the likelihood ratio diminishes. If decreasing probing depths are used as cut-off points, the same problem is encountered as when 4 mm is defined as healthy and 5 mm as diseased. As the number of false positives increases, the test becomes less specific (e.g., it does not correctly identify a healthy patient) (Fig. 49-6).

To help choose the most advantageous cut-off point we must plot the TP/FP or TN/FN that produces the ROC curve (Fig. 49-7).

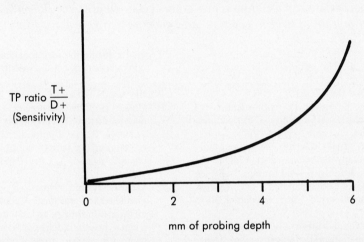

**Fig. 49-6.**  When diagnosis of periodontal disease is made on the basis of pocket depth, as the cut-off point in millimeters is increased, the percentage of true positives increases but the number of false negatives increases also.

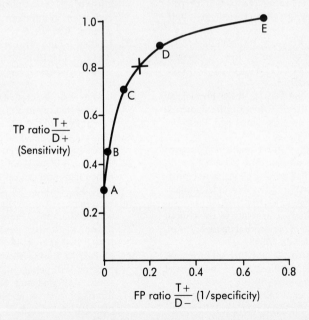

**Fig. 49-7.**  Hypothetical receiver operating characteristic (ROC) curve. At one point, A, the test has poor sensitivity but good specificity. At point E, the test has high sensitivity but poor specificity. Optimal cut-off point is shown by x. (Reprinted, by permission from McNeil, B.J., Keeler, E., and Adelstein, S.J.: N. Engl. J. Med. **293:**211, 1975.)

For a test to be diagnostically useful, it should have a specificity and sensitivity greater than 0.9. Consequently probing depths, bleeding points, and radiographic evidence of bone loss remain as *indications* of periodontal disease. *Conclusive tests have yet to be developed* and then their correlation with pocket depths and other clinical indicators has to be established. Then and only then can we develop standards for the evaluation of therapy.

## Summary

Notwithstanding occasional negative results, periodontal treatment usually meets with predictable success. The period of preventive maintenance, including occasional instances of retreatment, extends the success of treatment and the useful life of the natural dentition.[3,74] Moreover, the recall examination and reevaluation serve to unify all dental therapy around a common preventive goal—*to preserve the patient's natural dentition in a state of health, comfort, and good appearance for a lifetime.*

### REFERENCES

1. Waerhaug, J.: The interdental brush and its place in operative and crown and bridge dentistry, J. Oral Rehab. **3:**107, 1976.
2. Waerhaug, J.: Effect of toothbrushing on subgingival plaque formation, J. Periodontol. **52:**30, 1981.
3. Oliver, R.C.: Tooth loss with and without periodontal therapy, Periodont. Abstr. **17:**8, 1969.
4. Nyman, S., Rosling, B., and Lindhe, J.: Effect of professional tooth cleaning on healing after periodontal surgery, J. Clin. Periodontol. **2:**80, 1975.
5. Everett, F.G., and Stern, I.B.: When is tooth mobility an indication for extraction? Dent. Clin. North Am. **13:**791, 1969.
6. Nyman, S., and Lindhe, J.: Persistent tooth hypermobility following completion of periodontal therapy, J. Clin. Periodontol. **3:**81, 1976.
7. Dorfman, H.S., Kennedy, J.E., and Bird, W.C.: Longitudinal evaluation of free autogenous gingival grafts: a four year report, J. Periodontol. **53:**349, 1982.
8. Maynard, J.G, and Wilson, R.D.: Physiologic dimensions of the periodontium fundamental to successful restorative dentistry, J. Periodontol. **50:**170, 1979.
9. Derbyshire, J.C.: Patient motivation in periodontics, J. Periodontol. **41:**630, 1970.
10. Awwa, I., and Stallard, R.E.: Periodontal prognosis, educational and psychological implications, J. Periodontol. **41:**183, 1970.
11. Parks, S.R.: The responsibility of the patient in the treatment of periodontal disease, J. Am. Dent. Assoc. **85:**230, 1957.
12. Ramfjord, S.P., et al.: Subgingival curettage versus surgical elimination of periodontal pockets, J. Periodontol. **39:**167, 1968.
13. Ramfjord, S.P., et al.: Results following three modalities of periodontal therapy, J. Periodontol. **46:**522, 1975.
14. Morrison, E.C., et al.: The significance of gingivitis during the maintenance phase of periodontal treatment, J. Periodontol. **53:**31, 1982.
15. Sorrin, S.: Success or failure in periodontal therapy, N.Y. Dent. J. **29:**271, 1959.
16. Chace, R.: The maintenance phase of periodontal therapy, J. Periodontol. **22:**234, 1951.
17. Axelsson, P., and Lindhe, J.: The significance of maintenance care in the treatment of periodontal disease, J. Clin. Periodontol. **8:**281, 1981.
18. Lindhe, J., and Nyman, S.: The effect of plaque control and surgical pocket elimination on the establishment and maintenance of periodontal health: a longitudinal study of periodontal therapy in cases of advanced disease, J. Clin. Periodontol. **2:**67, 1975.
19. Rosling, B., Nyman, S., and Lindhe, J.: The effect of systematic plaque control on bone regeneration in infrabony pockets, J. Clin. Periodontol. **3:**38, 1976.
20. Lindhe, J., and Nyman, S.: Long-term maintenance of patients treated for advanced periodontal disease, J. Clin. Periodontol. **11:**504, 1984.
21. Wilson, T.G., Jr., et al.: Compliance with maintenance therapy in a private periodontal practice, J. Periodontol. **55:**468, 1984.
22. Ogilvie, A.L.: Recall and maintenance of the periodontal patient, Periodontics **3:**198, 1967.
23. Thomas, B.O.A.: What is periodontal maintenance care and whose responsibility is it? J. West Soc. Periodontol. **11:**8, 1963.
24. Sternlicht, H.C.: Evaluating long-term periodontal therapy, J. Prev. Dent. **2:**4, 1975.
25. Chace, R.: Retreatment in periodontal practice, J. Periodontol. **48:**7, 410, 1977.
26. McFall, W.T., Jr.: Tooth loss in 100 treated patients with periodontal disease: a long-term study, M. Periodontol. **53:**539, 1982.
27. Ramfjord, S.P., et al.: Longitudinal study of periodontal therapy, J. Periodontol. **44:**66, 1973.
28. Wasserman, B.H., et al.: Relationship of oc-

clusion to periodontal disease: II. periodontal status of the study population, J. Periodontol. **42:**371, 1971.

29. Gottsegen, R.: A fresh look at the maintenance phase of periodontal therapy, Alpha Omegan **76:**85, 1983.

30. Cross, W.G.: Some causes of failure in periodontal treatment, Parodontopathies **18:**127, 1966.

31. Ramfjord, S.P., et al.: Oral hygiene and maintenance of periodontal support, J. Periodontol. **53:**26, 1982.

32. Pihlstrom, B.L., Oliphant, T.H., and McHugh, R.B.: Molar and non-molar teeth compared over 6½ years following two methods of periodontal therapy, J. Periodontol. **55:**499, 1984.

33. Schick, R.A.: Maintenance phase of periodontal therapy, J. Periodontol. **52:**576, 1981.

34. Bradley, R.E.: Periodontal failures related to improper prognosis and treatment planning, Dent. Clin. North Am. **16:**33, 1972.

35. Kramer, G.M.: Dental failures associated with periodontal surgery, Dent. Clin. North Am. **16:**13, 1972.

36. Ward, H.L., and Kirsch, S.: Factors influencing negative tissue response after periodontal therapy, J. Periodontal. **33:**379, 1962.

37. Rateitschak, K.H.: Misserfolge bei der Parodontaltherapie und ihre Ursachen, Parodontopathies **18:**149, 1966.

38. Loesche, W.J.: The bacterial etiology of dental decay and periodontal disease: the specific plaque hypothesis. In Clark, J.W., editor, Clinical dentistry. Vol. 2, Philadelphia, 1982, Harper & Row.

39. Listgarten, M.A.: Structure of the microbial flora associated with periodontal health and disease in man, J. Periodontol. **47:**1, 1976.

40. van Palenstein-Heldermann, W.H.: Microbial etiology of periodontal disease, J. Clin. Periodontol. **8:**261, 1981.

41. Savitt, E.D., and Socransky, S.S.: Distribution of certain subgingival microbial species in selected periodontal conditions, J. Periodont. Res. **19:**111, 1984.

42. Listgarten, M.A., and Helldén, L.: Relative distribution of bacteria at clinically healthy and periodontally diseased sites in humans, J. Clin. Periodontol. **5:**115, 1978.

43. Loesche, W.J.: Clinical and microbiological aspects of chemotherapeutic agents used according to the specific plaque hypothesis, J. Dent. Res. **58:**2404, 1979.

44. Rams, E., et al.: Long-term effects of microbiologically modulated periodontal therapy on advanced adult periodontitis, J. Am. Dent. Assoc. **111:**429, 1985.

45. Keyes, P.H.: Microbiologically monitored and modulated periodontal therapy, Gen. Dent. **33:**105, 1985.

46. Listgarten, M.A., and Levin, S.L.: Positive correlation between the proportions of subgingival spirochetes and motile bacteria and susceptibility of human subjects to periodontal breakdown, J. Clin. Periodontol. **8:**122, 1981.

47. Listgarten, M.A., et al.: Comparative longitudinal study of two methods of scheduling maintenance visits: two-year data. J. Clin. Periodontol. **13:**692, 1986.

48. Keyes, P.H., and Rams, T.E.: A rationale for management of periodontal diseases: rapid identification of microbial "therapeutic targets" with phase-contrast microscopy, J. Am. Dent. Assoc. **106:**803, 1983.

49. Rams, T.E., and Keyes, P.H.: A rationale for the management of periodontal diseases: effects of tetracycline on subgingival bacteria, J. Am. Dent. Assoc. **107:**37, 1983.

50. Listgarten, M.A.: A perspective on periodontal diagnosis, J. Clin. Periodontol. **13:**175, 1986.

51. Listgarten, M.A., Schifter, C.C., and Laster, L.: 3-year longitudinal study of the periodontal status of an adult population with gingivitis, J. Clin. Periodontol. **12:**225, 1985.

52. Slots, J., and Genco, R.J.: Black-pigmented *Bacteroides* species, *Capnocytophaga* species, and *Actinobacillus actinomycetemcomitans* in human periodontal disease: virulence factors in colonization, survival and tissue destruction, J. Dent. Res. **63:**412, 1984.

53. Slots, J.: *Actinobacillus actinomycetemcomitans* and *Bacteroides gingivalis* in advanced periodontitis in man, Dtsch. Zahnärztel. Z. **39:**615, 1984.

54. Slots, J., et al.: The occurrence of *Actinobacillus actinomycetemcomitans, Bacteroides gingivalis* and *Bacteroides intermedius* in destructive periodontal disease in adults, J. Clin. Periodontol. **13:**570, 1986.

55. Trott, J.R.: Biological approach to dental practice: Periodontics, J. Can. Dent. Assoc. **28:**687, 1962.

56. Everett, F.G., and Hall, W.B.: Grenzen der Behandlung parodontotischer Zahne, Deutscher Zahnärztekalender, Munich, 1973, Urban & Schwarzenberg.

57. Ramfjord, S.P., et al.: Results of periodontal therapy related to tooth type, J. Periodontol. **51:**270, 1980.

58. Pihlstrom, B.L., et al.: Comparison of surgical and nonsurgical treatment of periodontal disease: a review of current studies and additional results after 6½ years, J. Clin. Periodontol. **10:**524, 1983.

59. Hill, R.W., et al.: Four types of periodontal treatment compared over two years, J. Periodontol. **52:**655, 1981.

60. Pihlstrom, B.L., Ortiz-Campos, C., and McHugh, R.B.: A randomized four-year study of periodontal therapy, J. Periodontol. **52:**227, 1981.

61. Knowles, J.W., et al.: Results of periodontal treatment related to pocket depth and attachment level: eight years, J. Periodontol. **50:**225, 1979.

62. Rosling, B., et al.: The healing potential of periodontal tissues following different techniques of periodontal surgery in plaque-free dentitions: a 2-year clinical study, J. Clin. Periodontol. **3**:233, 1976.

63. Knowles, J.: Comparison of results following three modalities of periodontal therapy related to tooth type and initial pocket depth, J. Clin. Periodontol. **7**:32, 1980.

64. Magnusson, I., et al.: Connective tissue attachment formation following exclusion of gingival connective tissue and epithelium during healing, J. Periodontol. Res. **20**:201, 1985.

65. Karring, T., et al.: New attachment formation on teeth with a reduced but healthy periodontal ligament, J. Clin. Periodontol. **12**:51, 1985.

66. Gottlow, J., et al.: New attachment formation as the result of controlled tissue regeneration, J. Clin. Periodontol. **11**:494, 1984.

67. Westfelt, S, et al.: Improved periodontal conditions following therapy, J. Clin. Periodontol. **12**:283, 1985.

68. Raeste, A.-M., and Kilpenen, E.: Clinical and radiographic long-term study of teeth with periodontal destruction treated by a modified flap operation, J. Clin. Periodontol. **8**:415, 1981.

69. Haffajee, A.D., Socransky, S.S., and Ebersole, J.L.: Survival analysis on periodontal sites before and after periodontal therapy, J. Clin. Periodontol. **12**:553, 1985.

70. Caton, J., Nyman, S., and Zander, H.: Histometric evaluation of periodontal surgery. II. Connective tissue attachment levels after four regenerative procedures, J. Clin. Periodontol. **7**:224, 1980.

71. Magnusson, I., et al.: A long junctional epithelium—a locus minoris resistentiae in plaque infection, J. Clin. Periodontol. **10**:333, 1983.

72. Steiner, S.S., Crigger, M., and Egelberg, J.: Connective tissue regenertion to periodontally diseased teeth. II. Histologic observations of cases following replaced flap surgery, J. Periodontol. **16**:109, 1981.

73. Lindhe, J., et al.: Healing following surgical/non-surgical treatment of periodontal disease: a clinical study, J. Clin. Periodontol. **9**:115, 1982.

74. Hirschfeld, L., and Wasserman, B.: Long-term survey of tooth loss in 565 treated periodontal patients. In Grant, D., Stern, I., and Everett, F.: Periodontics, ed. 5, St. Louis, 1979, The C.V. Mosby Co., p. 931.

75. Hirschfeld, L., and Wasserman, B.: A long term survey of tooth loss in 600 treated periodontal patients, J. Periodontol. **49**:226, 1978.

76. Wade, A.B.: Validity of anterior segment scores in epidemiologic studies, J. Periodontol. **37**:55, 1966.

77. Bossert, W.A., and Marks, H.H.: Prevalence and characteristics of periodontal disease in 12,800 persons under periodic dental observation, J. Am. Dent. Assoc. **52**:429, 1956.

78. Buckley, L.A., and Crowley, M.J.: A longitudinal study of untreated periodontal disease, J. Clin. Periodont. **11**:523, 1984.

79. Becker, W., Becker, B.E., and Berg, L.E.: Periodontal treatment without maintenance: a reconstructive study in 44 patients, J. Periodontol. **55**:505, 1984.

80. Becker, W., Berg, L.E., and Becker, B.E.: The long-term evaluation of periodontal treatment and maintenance in 95 patients, Int. J. Perint. Restor. Dent. **4**:54, 1984.

81. Goldman, M.J., Ross, E.F., and Goteiner, D.: Effect of periodontal therapy on patients maintained for 15 years or longer: a retrospective study, J. Periodontol. **57**:347, 1986.

82. DeVore, C.H., et al.: Bone loss following periodontal therapy in subjects without frequent periodontal maintenance, J. Periodontol. **57**:354, 1986.

83. Halazonetis, T.D., et al.: Pocket formation 3 years after comprehensive periodontal therapy: a retrospective study, J. Periodontol. **56**:515, 1985.

84. McNeil, B.J. Keeler, E., and Adelstein, S.J.: Primer on certain elements of medical decision making, N. Engl. J. Med. **293**:211, 1975.

85. Koran, L.M.: Increasing the reliability of clinical data and judgements, Ann. Clin. Res. **8**:69, 1976.

86. Koran, L.M.: The reliability of clinical methods, data and judgements. I, N. Engl. J. Med. **293**:642, 1975.

87. Koran, L.M.: The reliability of clinical methods, data and judgements. II, N. Engl. J. Med. **293**:695, 1975.

## ADDITIONAL SUGGESTED READINGS

Bailit, H. et al.: Is periodontal disease the primary cause of tooth extraction in adults? J. Am. Dent. Assoc. **114**:40, 1987.

Goodson, J.M.: Clinical measurements of periodontitis, J. Clin. Periodontol. **13**:446, 1986.

Haffajee, A.F., and Socransky, S.S.: Frequency distributions of periodontal attachment loss: clinical and microbiological features, J. Clin. Periodontol. **13**:625, 1986.

Isador, F., and Karring, T.: Long-term effect of surgical and non-surgical periodontal treatment: a 5-year clinical study, J. Periodont. Res. **21**:462, 1986.

Ralls, S.A., and Cohen, M.E.: Problems in identifying "bursts" of periodontal attachment loss, J. Periodontol. **57**:746, 1986.

Ramfjord, S.P.: Surgical pocket elimination: still a justifiable objective? J. Am. Dent. Assoc. **114**:37, 1987.

van der Velden, U., Abbas, F., and Winkel, E.G.: Probing considerations in relation to susceptibility to periodontal breakdown, J. Clin. Periodontol. **13**:894, 1986.

# INDEX

---

Page numbers in *italics* indicate boxes and illustrations.
Page numbers followed by *t* indicate tables.

## O

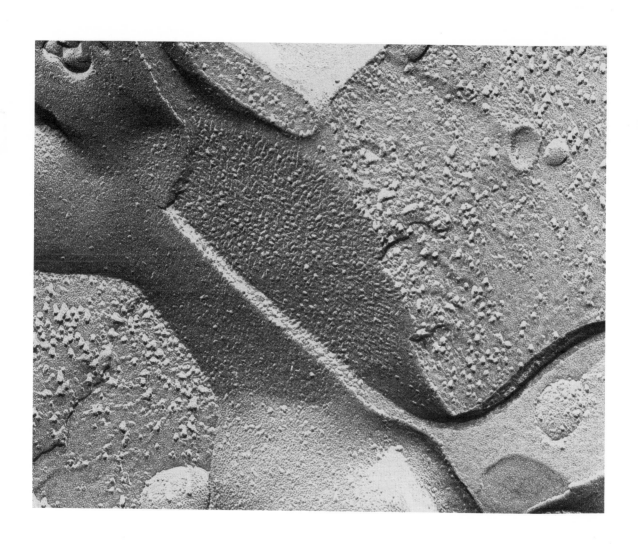